Orthotics and Prosthetics
in Rehabilitation

Orthotics and Prosthetics in Rehabilitation

MICHELLE M. LUSARDI, Ph.D., P.T.

Associate Professor of Physical Therapy, Department of Physical Therapy and Human Movement Sciences, College of Education and Health Professions, Sacred Heart University, Fairfield, Connecticut

CAROLINE C. NIELSEN, Ph.D.

Health Care, Education, and Research Consultant, Bonita Springs, Florida; Former Associate Professor and Director, Graduate Program in Allied Health, University of Connecticut, Storrs

Foreword by
JOAN E. EDELSTEIN, M.A., P.T.

Associate Professor of Clinical Physical Therapy and Director, Program in Physical Therapy, College of Physicians and Surgeons, Columbia University, New York

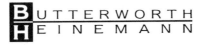

Boston • Oxford • Auckland • Johannesburg • Melbourne • New Delhi

Butterworth–Heinemann supports the efforts of American Forests and the Global ReLeaf program in its campaign for the betterment of trees, forests, and our environment.

Library of Congress Cataloging-in-Publication Data

Lusardi, Michelle M.
   Orthotics and prosthetics in rehabilitation / Michelle M. Lusardi, Caroline C. Nielsen ; foreword by Joan E. Edelstein.
     p. ; cm.
   Includes bibliographical references and index.
   ISBN 0-7506-9807-1
    1. Orthopedic apparatus. 2. Prosthesis. 3. Orthopedic implants. 4. Physically handicapped--Rehabilitation. I. Nielsen, Caroline C. II. Title.
   [DNLM: 1. Orthotic Devices. 2. Prostheses and Implants. 3. Rehabilitation. WE 172 L968o 2000]
   RD755 .L87 2000
   617'.9--dc21

                                      00-024895

British Library Cataloguing-in-Publication Data
A catalogue record for this book is available from the British Library.

The publisher offers special discounts on bulk orders of this book.
For information, please contact:
Manager of Special Sales
Butterworth-Heinemann
225 Wildwood Avenue
Woburn, MA 01801-2041
Tel: 781-904-2500
Fax: 781-904-2620

For information on all Butterworth–Heinemann publications available, contact our World Wide Web home page at: http://www.bh.com

10 9 8 7 6 5 4 3 2

Printed in the United States of America

To celebrate the life of my father, Philip Andrew Ouellette
January 3, 1926–January 16, 1999

"When a man walks in integrity and justice,
happy are the children who follow him!"
(Proverbs 20:7)

M.M.L.

To Svend Woge Nielsen
A true partner who nourishes my spirit and achievements
with his constant understanding and belief in me

C.C.N.

Contents

SECTION III
Prosthetics in Rehabilitation

Contributing Authors

Edmond Ayyappa, M.S., C.P.O.
Assistant Clinical Professor of Physical Medicine and Rehabilitation, University of California, Irvine, College of Medicine, Irvine; Director, Prosthetic and Orthotic Clinical Services, Desert Pacific Health Care System, VA Medical Center, Norwalk, California

William J. Barringer, M.S., C.O.
Associate Professor of Orthopedic Surgery and Rehabilitation and Chief of Orthotics, University of Oklahoma Health Sciences Center, Oklahoma City

Gary M. Berke, M.S., C.P.
Assistant Professor of Orthopaedic Surgery and Rehabilitation and Chief of Prosthetics, University of Oklahoma Health Sciences Center, Oklahoma City

Jennifer M. Bottomley, Ph.D., M.S., P.T.
Core Faculty, Division on Aging, Harvard Medical School, Boston; Geriatric Rehabilitation Program Consultant, Geriatric Wellness and Rehabilitation, Wayland, Massachusetts

Karen M. Brewer, P.T.
Former Senior Physical Therapist, National Rehabilitation Hospital, Washington, D.C.

James H. Campbell, Ph.D., C.O.
Director of Product Development, Engineering, and Technical Services, Becker Orthopedic, Troy, Michigan

Kevin Christensen, M.D.
Assistant Professor of Orthopaedic Surgery, University of Texas Southwestern Medical Center, Parkland Hospital, and Children's Medical Center, Dallas

Thomas V. DiBello, B.S., C.O.
President, Dynamic Orthotics and Prosthetics LLC, Houston

Joan E. Edelstein, M.A., P.T.
Associate Professor of Clinical Physical Therapy and Director, Program in Physical Therapy, College of Physicians and Surgeons, Columbia University, New York

John Fergason, C.P.O.
Director, Division of Prosthetics-Orthotics, Department of Rehabilitation Medicine, University of Washington School of Medicine, Seattle

Patrick Flanagan, C.O.
Orthotic Prosthetic Centers, BioConcepts, Inc., Burr Ridge, Illinois

Juan C. Garbalosa, Ph.D., P.T.
Assistant Professor of Physical Therapy, University of Hartford, West Hartford, Connecticut; Research Consultant, New Britain General Hospital, New Britain, Connecticut; Director, Gait Laboratory, Center for Reconstructive Foot Surgery, Plainville, Connecticut

Donna Q. Gavin, C.O.
Certified Orthotist, BioConcepts, Inc., Burr Ridge, Illinois

Thomas M. Gavin, C.O.
Teaching Associate, Department of Orthopaedic Surgery, Loyola University Chicago Stritch School of Medicine, Maywood, Illinois; Research Orthotist, Orthopaedic Biomechanics Laboratory, Veterans Administration Hospital, Hines, Illinois

Thomas M. Harrigan, P.T., C.P.O.
Seacoast Rehabilitation Services, Orthotic and Prosthetic Center, York, Maine

Carolyn B. Kelly, P.T.
Coordinator, Neuropathic Foot Program, Hartford Hospital, Hartford, Connecticut

John F. Knecht, M.A., P.T., A.T.C.
Clinical Specialist, Health South–Physical Therapy and Sports Medicine Associates, Manchester, Connecticut

Géza F. Kogler, Ph.D., C.O.
Assistant Professor of Clinical Surgery and Director, Orthopaedic Bioengineering Research Laboratory, Southern Illinois University School of Medicine, Springfield

Frances J. Lagana, D.P.M.
Active Medical Staff, Department of Surgery, Winchester Hospital, Winchester, Massachusetts; Chief of Service, Podiatric Medicine and Surgery, Massachusetts Hospital School, Canton

Robert S. Lin, C.P.O.
Clinical Associate Professor, School of Allied Health Professions, University of Connecticut, Storrs; Director of Pediatric Clinical Services and Academic Programs, Department of Orthotics and Prosthetics, Connecticut Children's Medical Center, Hartford

Robert D. Lipschutz, B.S.M.E., C.P.
Curriculum Coordinator and Prosthetic and Biomechanics Instructor, Newington Certificate Program in Orthotics and Prosthetics, Newington Orthotics and Prosthetics Systems, Newington, Connecticut; Senior Staff Prosthetist and Myoelectric Specialist, Limb Enhancement Clinic, Connecticut Children's Medical Center, Hartford

Michelle M. Lusardi, Ph.D., P.T.
Associate Professor of Physical Therapy, Department of Physical Therapy and Human Movement Sciences, College of Education and Health Professions, Sacred Heart University, Fairfield, Connecticut

Sheila A. MacGregor, O.T.R., L.M.S.
Occupational Therapist, Hebrew Home and Hospital, West Hartford, Connecticut

John W. Michael, M.Ed., C.P.O.
Instructor, Allied Health Program, Century College, White Bear Lake, Minnesota; President, CPO Services, Inc., Chanhassen, Minnesota

Olfat Mohamed, Ph.D., P.T.
Associate Professor of Physical Therapy, California State University, Long Beach

Caroline C. Nielsen, Ph.D.
Health Care, Education, and Research Consultant, Bonita Springs, Florida; Former Associate Professor and Director, Graduate Program in Allied Health, University of Connecticut, Storrs

Roberta Nole, M.A., P.T., C.Ped.
Stride Physical Therapy and Pedorthic Center, Middlebury, Connecticut

Laura L. F. Owens, B.S., M.S.
Physical Therapist, Genesis ElderCare Rehabilitation Services, Windsor, Connecticut

Avinash G. Patwardhan, Ph.D.
Professor of Orthopaedic Surgery and Rehabilitation and Director, Musculoskeletal Biomechanics Laboratory, Loyola University Chicago Stritch School of Medicine, Maywood, Illinois

Richard Psonak, M.S., C.P.O.
Director of Orthotics and Prosthetics, Mississippi Methodist Rehabilitation Center, Jackson

Julie D. Ries, M.A., P.T., G.C.S.
Assistant Professor of Physical Therapy, Marymount University, Arlington, Virginia; Physical Therapist, INOVA-VNA Home Health, Sterling, Virginia

Melvin L. Stills, C.O.
Assistant Professor (Retired) of Orthopaedic Surgery, University of Texas Southwestern Medical Center, Dallas; Orthotist, Parkland Memorial Hospital, Zale Lipshy University Hospital, and Children's Medical Center, Dallas

David M. Thompson, M.S., P.T.
Assistant Professor of Physical Therapy, University of Oklahoma Health Science Center, Oklahoma City

Jessie M. VanSwearingen, Ph.D., P.T.
Associate Professor of Physical Therapy, University of Pittsburgh School of Medicine, Pittsburgh

R. Scott Ward, Ph.D., P.T.
Associate Professor and Director, Division of Physical Therapy, University of Utah School of Medicine, Salt Lake City; Physical Therapist, Intermountain Burn Center, University of Utah Health Sciences Center, Salt Lake City

Richard I. Weiner, M.D.
Chairman of Surgery, Winchester Hospital, Winchester, Massachusetts; Clinical Associate Professor of Surgery, Tufts University School of Medicine, Boston

Foreword

Contemporary rehabilitation encompasses an ever-widening spectrum of clinical responsibilities, particularly to patients who are candidates for orthoses or prostheses. Excellent patient care requires that clinicians be familiar with new methods of assessing the patient's needs, advanced technology, and progressive means of treating patients. The newest device, however, may not be the most suitable choice for a given patient. Consequently, the clinician needs to evaluate the appropriateness of a range of devices or procedures in light of established therapeutic practice. The fundamental aim of this book is to enable aspiring and practicing clinicians to determine and implement the approach that is most appropriate for each patient who might require an orthosis or prosthesis.

Rehabilitation is not a solo specialty. Collaboration of many health professionals is especially important for rational prescription and application of prostheses and orthoses. Because devices can be made of many different materials, it is important that the clinician understand the principal attributes of various plastics and metals, particularly how the choice of material affects the fit, function, and ease of altering devices. Other basic considerations pertain to clinical gait assessment, which is the foundation for prescription and utilization of lower-limb orthoses and prosthesis. Teaching a child or adult to use a device is more effective if one understands how people learn a motor skill. Fostering efficient use of a device involves assessing and improving the patient's endurance.

Although orthoses are prescribed to serve many therapeutic purposes, the essential function of all such appliances is the application of force to the body. The amount of force, the sites of application, and the means of controlling force application all contribute to the impact of the orthosis on the wearer's mobility, function, and acceptance of the device. Rational prescription should be based on a thorough evaluation of the patient, including physical and psychosocial attributes. The patient who returns to the rehabilitation department carrying the unworn orthosis is a mute testimony to the importance of gathering critical data before ordering a device.

The editors have recruited a talented group of experts who explore orthotic considerations that apply to disorders of the lower and upper limbs and the trunk. A multitude of orthoses are described, together with the clinical factors that will guide clinicians in making a wise selection.

Prostheses also apply force to the body. They serve to replace missing limb segments. The first duty of the rehabilitation team, whenever possible, is to prevent amputation, and thus the need for a prosthesis. In the United States, the majority of prostheses are worn by adults with lower-limb amputation resulting from peripheral vascular disease. By identifying patients at risk for amputation, clinicians can do much to prevent or forestall limb loss. Rational care before, during, and after amputation surgery has a lifelong effect on the patient's function. Prosthetic options for the various levels of lower-limb amputation make evident that the clinician and patient face many decisions. Clinicians are guided to weigh options when selecting componentry, and are encouraged to treat the patient in a holistic manner. Clinicians who treat children or adults with upper-limb amputations for limb anomalies will also gain a detailed perspective.

For students and experienced clinicians alike, *Orthotics and Prosthetics in Rehabilitation* opens the door to optimum clinical care, whether the setting is the hospital, rehabilitation center, long-term care facility, or the home. The challenge of harmonizing the patient's needs with an ever-changing armamentarium is rewarded when the youngster with transradial amputation rides a tricycle, or a middle-aged salesperson returns to work with improved foot comfort, or a 70-year-old man with transtibial amputation walks to the corner store.

Joan E. Edelstein, M.A., P.T.

Preface

One of the challenges and joys for professionals in the field of rehabilitation is the ability to see possibility for patients who are faced with significant neuromuscular and musculoskeletal pathology or impairment. An appropriately designed and carefully fit orthosis or prosthesis can be an important component of our intervention to minimize the impact of a functional limitation or disability on the quality of life of the patients for whom we care.

Advances in technology, materials, design, and fabrication processes for orthoses and prostheses, along with the demand for greater efficiency in provision of health care services, create an imperative for health professionals to update their knowledge about orthotic and prosthetic options. These changes illustrate the importance of interdisciplinary care, in which special knowledge and skills of a variety of health professionals can be brought together to best serve the needs of patients and their families, as a vehicle for the most effective patient care.

This volume has its roots in more than 10 years of laboratory manuals and course syllabi prepared for clinical science courses at the University of Connecticut and our frustration, as instructors, with the text resources available during that time. Our goal in preparing the manuscript for this book has been to provide a detailed resource for students in rehabilitation fields, as well as a comprehensive reference for clinicians. We have attempted to organize the information presented from a functional, rather than a technical, perspective so that new designs and materials can be fit easily into the scheme as development occurs.

The first section of the book provides a foundational understanding of the field of orthotics and prosthetics and of the materials used and of the fabrication process. Readers will recognize the importance of effective assessment of gait dysfunction as the foundation for orthotic and prosthetic prescription, intervention, and outcomes assessment. They will also appreciate the significance that energy expenditure plays in the selection of an orthosis or prosthesis, especially for patients who are elderly or have cardiopulmonary/cardiovascular impairment.

In the second section, the indications for orthoses and the underlying biomechanical principles of orthotic design are explored. The importance of appropriate footwear as the foundation for most lower extemity orthoses is considered, and a functional scheme for prescription of and training for the various lower extremity and spinal orthoses is developed. Finally, the reader is introduced to the use of orthoses in fracture management, in the care of patients with burns, and in the management of patients with impairments of the wrist and hand.

The third section of the book focuses on rehabilitation of patients with amputation. Initially, the etiology of amputation, the management of patients at risk of amputation, and strategies for immediate postoperative care and early prosthetic fitting for patients who have had amputation are explored. Then readers are introduced to prosthetic options for patients with amputation. Chapters are organized to assist the reader in developing an organizational schema for understanding design, alignment, and selection of appropriate components from among many available options. Readers are also introduced to strategies for functional prosthetic training for patients with amputation, including gait assessment strategies to identify patient or prosthetic "cause" of gait dysfunction. Readers first learn about distal amputations of the lower limb and move proximally through transtibial and transfemoral levels, considering the impact of joint loss on prosthetic control, stance phase stability, and energy expenditure during ambulation. The book concludes with several chapters focusing on the needs of patients with high-level and bilateral lower extremity amputation, children with limb deficiency, and prosthetic options for patients with upper extremity amputation.

One of the strengths of this work is its true interdisciplinary perspective. The contributors are professionals from the fields of orthotics and prosthetics, physical and occupational therapy, and medicine and surgery. We hope that readers will gain an appreciation of the unique knowledge and skills of our colleagues across these disciplines and that this will serve as a foundation for effective collaborative practice and interdisciplinary patient care. Interdisciplinary teaming has enriched our clinical practice and teaching, for us as individuals, for our students, and for the patients we care for. Our wish is that this work will encourage our readers to embrace interdisciplinary and collaborative practice in their own practice settings.

Michelle M. Lusardi
Caroline C. Nielsen

Acknowledgments

The work of creating *Orthotics and Prosthetics in Rehabilitation* began as a simple two-page outline more than 4 years ago. Given the professional paths we have taken since its conception, the writing and editing of this book have been, at times, a Herculean task. In all projects of this size and scope, successful completion is founded on the support and assistance provided by many individuals along the way. We gratefully, if inadequately, acknowledge the following:

- Colleagues from the Physical Therapy Program, the Graduate Program in Allied Health, and the Orthotics and Prosthetics certificate program at the University of Connecticut. Special thanks go to Pam Roberts, Rita Wong, Polly Fitz, and Priscilla Douglas for their belief in possibilities as we began this project.
- Colleagues from the Physical Therapy and Nursing programs at Sacred Heart University, who provided unwavering encouragement, valuable advice, and forgiveness for missed deadlines and short tempers during the lengthy manuscript preparation process. Special thanks to Michael Emery, Pam Levangie, Donna Bowers, Beverly Fein, Salome Brooks, Gary Austin, David Cameron, Linda Strong, and Julie Pavia.
- Robin C. Seabrook, Executive Director of the National Commission on Orthotic/Prosthetic Education, for her insight and vision of the future of orthotic/prosthetic education and her constant support of this project, and William Barringer, for his efforts in developing and implementing this vision among the community of practitioners, and Ronald Altman for his initial creative thoughts on interdisciplinary education.
- Clinical colleagues who have helped us learn about orthotic and prosthetic care and who have willingly shared their expertise and energy with our students. Special thanks to Carolyn Kelly, Robert Lin, Richard Psonak, Robert Lipschutz, John Zenie, Ian Engelmann, and David Rooney for their commitment to clinical education and interdisciplinary patient care.
- The students from the University of Connecticut and Sacred Heart University who have explored the field of orthotics and prosthetics in our classrooms; their thirst for knowledge and desire for excellence in patient care have been the true catalyst for this project.
- Each of our contributors, for their willingness to take the time to share their knowledge and clinical expertise in their chapters, for their enthusiasm for the project, and for their patience and perseverance over the many, many months of manuscript preparation, editing, and production.
- J.C. Bender, physical therapist and illustrator extraordinaire, who created the original illustrations for this work. His ability to turn our preliminary ideas and very rough sketches into an ideal illustration is miraculous.
- The medical editors at Butterworth–Heinemann, Mary Drabot and Leslie Kramer, for their patience and expectancy, words of encouragement, technical assistance, and gentle reminders as this project moved from concept to reality. Thanks also to Barbara Murphy, who helped us to believe we could and should attempt this project in the first place.
- And most important, to the members of our families who have steadfastly encouraged, graciously suffered, and joyfully celebrated with us during the writing and editing process:

  My mother, Elizabeth Ouellette, who, by her loving example, has taught me how much caring for others can be joyful work. My daughter, Karen Elizabeth, whose love of learning and celebration of difference enliven my spirit. And my husband, Lawrence, whose belief in me makes anything possible. —M.M.L.

  My husband, Svend, for his endless support, and for contributing his expertise in pathology. And my children, Frederick, Elizabeth, and Caroline, who have not only endured but enthusiastically supported my endeavors. —C.C.N.

*Orthotics and Prosthetics
in Rehabilitation*

I

Building Baseline Knowledge

1

Orthotics and Prosthetics in Rehabilitation: The Multidisciplinary Approach

CAROLINE C. NIELSEN

Today's health care environment emphasizes maximizing patient outcomes while containing costs. In this complex environment, current and evolving patterns of health care delivery focus on a team approach to the total care of the patient. Downsizing in health care, reorganization from traditional functional structures to patient-focused structures, and use of total quality management approaches that reward group participation over individual efforts contribute to the increased emphasis on interdisciplinary team care.[1] Today, practicing allied health professionals are expected to collaborate in diverse health care settings.

For a health care team to function effectively, each member must develop positive attitudes toward interdisciplinary collaboration. Key attitudes for the collaborating health professional include (1) understanding the functional roles of each health care discipline within the team and (2) establishing respect and value for each discipline's input in the decision-making process of the health team.[2] Rehabilitation, particularly related to orthotics and prosthetics, lends itself well to interdisciplinary teaming because the total care of patients with complex disorders requires a wide range of knowledge and skills. The prosthetist, the orthotist, and the physical therapist are important participants in the rehabilitation team. Understanding the roles and professional responsibilities of each of these disciplines maximizes the ability of the team to function effectively to provide comprehensive care for the patient. In this chapter, the professions of orthotics and prosthetics are defined, the history and development of the profession and the parallel development of physical therapy are described, and professional roles and attitudes in the team approach to rehabilitation are discussed.

ORTHOTISTS AND PROSTHETISTS

Every year more than 125,000 people lose a limb to an accident or disease. Currently, more than 1.5 million peo-

ple in the United States have had an amputation.[3] In addition, many other people require special devices to help them walk, regain active lives, or participate effectively in athletic activities.

Prosthetists and orthotists are allied health professionals who custom make and fit prostheses (artificial limbs) and orthoses (braces). Along with physical therapists, occupational therapists, and other health care professionals, they are integral members of the rehabilitation team who are responsible for returning the patient to a productive and meaningful life.

Definition

Prosthetists are allied health professionals who provide care to patients with partial or total absence of a limb by designing, fabricating, and fitting the patient with a prosthesis, or artificial limb. The prosthetist creates the design to fit the individual's particular functional and cosmetic needs; selects the appropriate materials and components; makes all necessary casts, measurements, and modifications (including static and dynamic alignment); evaluates the fit and function of the prosthesis on the patient; and teaches the patient how to care for it (Figure 1-1).

Orthotists are allied health professionals who provide care to patients with neuromuscular and musculoskeletal impairments that contribute to functional limitation and disability by designing, fabricating, and fitting the patient with an orthosis, a custom-made brace. The orthotist is responsible for evaluating the patient's functional and cosmetic needs, designing the orthosis, and selecting appropriate components; fabricating, fitting, and aligning the orthosis; and educating the patient on appropriate use (Figure 1-2).

In 1999, more than 3,362 certified prosthetists and orthotists were practicing in the United States (American Orthotic and Prosthetic Association, National Office, Alexandria, VA; personal communication, December

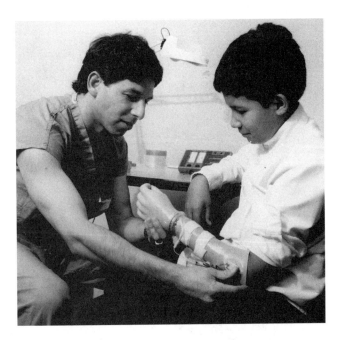

FIGURE 1-1

The prosthetist evaluates, designs, fabricates, and fits a pros-thesis specific to a patient's functional needs. Here the pros-thetist double-checks electrode placement sites for a myoelectric upper extremity prosthesis in a child with amputation of the left forearm.

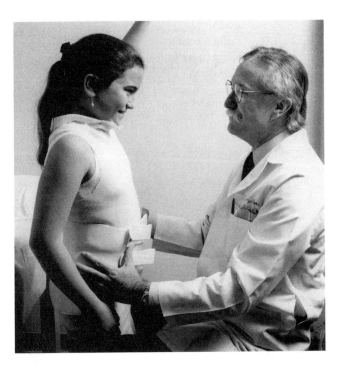

FIGURE 1-2

Once an orthosis has been fabricated, the orthotist evaluates its fit on the patient to determine if it meets prescriptive goals and can be worn comfortably during functional activities or if additional modifications are necessary. Here the orthotist is fit-ting a spinal orthosis and teaching his young patient about proper donning and wearing schedules for her new orthosis.

1999; Table 1-1). At present, approximately 10% of the current practitioners are women, although the number of women entering the field is increasing. An individual who enters the fields of prosthetics and orthotics today must complete advanced education and residency programs before becoming eligible for certification. Registered assis-tants and technicians in orthotics and/or prosthetics assist the certified practitioner with patient care and fabrication of orthotic and prosthetic devices.

History

The emergence of orthotics and prosthetics as a health pro-fession has followed a course similar to that of the profes-sion of physical therapy. Development of both professions is closely related to three significant events in world his-tory: World War I, World War II, and the development and spread of polio in the 1950s. Unfortunately, it has taken war and disease to provide the major impetus for research and development in these key areas of rehabilitation: phys-ical and occupational therapy, orthotics, and prosthetics.

The roots of prosthetics can be traced to early black-smiths, armor makers, and other skilled artisans or to the individuals with amputations themselves, who fashioned

some sort of replacement limb from materials at hand. During the Civil War, more than 30,000 amputations were performed on Union soldiers injured in battle; at least as many occurred among injured Confederate troops. At that time, most prostheses consisted of a carved or milled wooden socket and foot. Many were procured by mail order from companies in New York or other manufac-turing centers at a cost of $75–100 each.[4] Before World War II, prosthetic practice required much hands-on work and craftsman's skill. D. A. McKeever, a prosthetist who practiced in the 1930s, described the process: "You went to [an amputee's] house, took measurements and then carved a block of wood, covered it with rawhide and glue, and sanded it." During his training, McKeever spent 3 years in a shop carving wood: "You pulled out the inside, shaped the outside, and sanded it with a sandbelt."[5] Until World War II, the practice of prosthetics was dependent on the skills of individual craftsmen.

Although the profession of physical therapy has its roots in the early history of medicine, World War I was a major impetus to its development. During the war, female "physical educators" volunteered in physicians' offices and army hospitals instructing patients in corrective exercises. After the war ended, a group of these Reconstruction Aides, as they were called, joined together to form the American Women's Physical Therapy Association. In 1922, the association changed its name to the American Physiotherapy Association, opened membership to men, and aligned itself closely with the medical profession.[6]

World War II, and the period following, was a time of significant growth for the professions of physical therapy, prosthetics, and orthotics. During the war, many more physical therapists were needed to treat the wounded and rehabilitate those who were left with functional impairments and disabilities. The Army became the major resource for physical therapy training programs, and the number of physical therapists serving in the armed services increased more than sixfold.[7] The sheer numbers of soldiers who required braces or artificial limbs during and after the war increased the demand for prosthetists and orthotists as well.

After World War II, a coordinated program for persons with amputations was developed. In 1945, a conference of surgeons, prosthetists, and scientists organized by the National Academy of Sciences revealed that little scientific effort had been devoted to the development of artificial limbs. A "crash" research program was initiated, funded by the Office of Scientific Research and Development and continued by the Veterans Administration. A direct result of this effort was the development of the patellar tendon-bearing prosthesis for individuals with transtibial (below knee) amputation and the quadrilateral socket design for those with transfemoral (above knee) amputation. This program also included education of prosthetists, physicians, and physical therapists to develop skills in fitting and training of patients using these new prosthetic designs.[8] The needs of soldiers injured in the wars in Korea and Vietnam ensured continuing research, further refinements, and development of new materials. The development of myoelectrically controlled upper extremity prostheses and the advent of modular endoskeletal lower extremity prostheses occurred in the post–Vietnam War era.

The development of the profession of orthotics mirrors the field of prosthetics. Early "bracemakers" were also artisans, such as blacksmiths, armor makers, and patients, who used much the same materials as the prosthetist: metal, leather, and wood. By the eighteenth and nineteenth centuries, splints and braces were also mass produced and sold through catalogues. Frequently, these bracemakers were also known as *bonesetters* until surgery replaced manipulation and bracing in the practice of orthopedics. "Bracemaker" then became a profession with a particular role distinct from that of the physician.[4]

TABLE 1-1

Orthotists and Prosthetists Certified by the American Board for Certification Practicing in the United States in 1991 and 1999

	1991		1999	
	Number	*Percent*	*Number*	*Percent*
CP	864	32.4	1,093	32.5
CO	1,009	37.8	1,164	34.6
CPO	795	29.8	1,105	32.9
Total	2,668	100.0	3,362	100.0

CP = certified prosthetist; CO = certified orthotist; CPO = certified prosthetist/orthotist.
Source: From American Orthotic and Prosthetic Association, National Office, Alexandria, VA. Personal communication, December 1999.

The current term *orthotics* emerged in the late 1940s and was officially adopted by American orthotists and prosthetists when the American Orthotic and Prosthetic Association was formed to replace its professional predecessor, the Artificial Limb Manufacturers' Association. *Orthosis* is a more inclusive term than *brace*, and its use reflects the development of devices and materials for dynamic control in addition to stabilization of the body. In 1948, the American Board for Certification in Orthotics and Prosthetics was formed to establish and promote high professional standards.

The polio epidemics of the 1950s played a role in the further development of the physical therapy profession, but the effects of these epidemics were perhaps the strongest motivating factor in the development of orthotics. By 1970, many new techniques and materials, some adapted from industrial techniques, were being used to assist patients in coping with the effects of polio. The scope of practice in the field of orthotics is extensive, including working with children with muscular dystrophy, cerebral palsy, and spina bifida; patients of all ages recovering from severe burns or fractures; adolescents with scoliosis; athletes recovering from surgery or injury; and older adults with diabetes, cerebrovascular accidents, severe arthritis, and other disabling conditions.

Like physical therapists, orthotists and prosthetists practice in a variety of settings. The most common setting is the private office, where the professional offers services to patients in conformity with the attending physician's referral or prescription. Many large institutions, such as hospitals, rehabilitation centers, and research institutes, have a department of orthotics and prosthetics with onsite staff to provide services to patients. The prosthetist or orthotist might also be a supplier or fabrication manager in a central production laboratory. In addition, some orthotists and prosthetists serve as full-time faculty in one of the eight programs that are available for orthotic/prosthetic entry level training or in one of the programs available at the Master of Science degree level. Others also serve as clinical educators in a variety of facilities for the year-long residency program that is required before the certification examination.

Prosthetic and Orthotic Education

With rapid advances in technology and in health care, the role of the prosthetist and orthotist has grown from a focus on the technological aspects to a more inclusive role as a member of the rehabilitation team. Patient evaluation, education, and treatment now play a significant role in the responsibilities of practitioners. Most technical tasks are completed by technicians who work in the office laboratory or at an increasing number of central fabrication facilities. The advent and availability of prefabrication systems also reduce the amount of time that the practitioner expends in crafting new prostheses and orthoses.[4]

Current educational requirements reflect these changes in orthotic and prosthetic practice. Entry into professional training programs requires completion of a baccalaureate degree from an accredited college or university, with a strong emphasis on prerequisite courses in the sciences. Professional education in orthotics or prosthetics requires an additional academic year for each discipline. Along with the necessary technical courses, students study research methodology, kinesiology and biomechanics, musculoskeletal and neuromuscular pathology, communication and education, and current health care issues. Orthotics and prosthetics programs are most often based within academic health centers or in colleges or universities with hospital affiliations. After completion of the academic program, a year-long residency begins during which new clinicians gain expertise in pediatrics and adult care, in the acute, rehabilitative, and chronic phases of care. On completion of the educational and experiential requirements, the student is eligible to sit for the certification examinations. Today, the physical therapist and the orthotist or prosthetist must understand the language, roles, and concerns of all the potential members of the rehabilitation team, including the orthopedic surgeon or neurologist, occupational therapist, social worker, nurse, and dietitian, as well as the patient and family.

CHARACTERISTICS OF THE HEALTH CARE TEAM

The enormous explosion of knowledge in health care, particularly in rehabilitation, has led to increasing specialization in many fields. The interdisciplinary health care team concept has evolved, in part, because no single individual or discipline can have all of the necessary expertise and specialty knowledge that are required for high-quality care,

especially the care of patients with complex disorders. Effective team functioning begins during the education of each individual health professional. The rapid change that is occurring in health care practice reinforces the need for interdisciplinary education; in addition to discipline-specific skills and knowledge, the student must be aware of the interrelationships among health professionals. Students must develop an understanding of and appreciation for the contributions of the other rehabilitation disciplines in the assessment and treatment of the patient and management of patient problems. One of the major barriers to effective team functioning is a lack of understanding or misconception of the roles of different disciplines in the care of the whole patient.[9] A clear understanding of the totality of the health care delivery system and the role of each professional within the system increases the potential effectiveness of the health care team. A group of informed, dedicated health professionals working together to set appropriate goals and initiate patient care to meet these goals uses a model that exceeds the sum of its individual components.[10]

Almost all health care today is provided in a team setting. This integrated approach facilitates appreciation of the patient as a person with individual strengths and needs rather than as a dehumanized diagnosis or problem. The diverse perspectives and knowledge that are brought to the rehabilitation process by the members of the interdisciplinary team provide insight into all aspects of the patient's concerns. Conceptually, all members of the health care team contribute equally to patient care: The contribution of each is important and valuable; otherwise quality of patient care and efficacy of intervention would be diminished. Although one member of the team may take an organizing or managing role, decision making occurs by consensus building and critical discussion.[11] Professionals with different skills function together with mutual support, sharing the task and responsibility of patient care.

Effective use of team-based health care assumes that groups of health care providers, representing multiple disciplines, can work together to develop and implement a treatment plan for the patient that is comprehensive and integrated. This requires professionals, who traditionally have worked independently and autonomously, to function effectively in an interdependent relationship with members of other disciplines.[12] This may not be an easy task to accomplish because of the considerable potential for dysfunction.

One definition of *team*, found in the *Oxford English Dictionary*, describes "beasts of burden yoked together." Pearson and Jones[13] define a team in more positive terms as "a small group of people who relate to each other to contribute to a common goal." A number of factors are important influences on a health professional's perception of team membership as being beasts of burden or members who contribute toward a common goal. Much of our understanding of team

TABLE 1-2

Formal and Informal Factors That Influence Dynamics of the Multidisciplinary Work Group

Formal (Visible) Influences	Informal (Submerged) Influences
Policies of the group or institution	Informal relationships among team members
Objectives of the group	Communication styles of team members
Formal systems of communication	Power networks within the group
Job descriptions of group members	Individual values and beliefs
	Goals/norms of individuals in the group

Source: Adapted from P Pearson, K Jones. The primary health care non-team? Dynamics of multidisciplinary provider groups. BMJ 1994;309:1387.

function is drawn from organization and management research literature, the theories of which provide insight and information on how interdisciplinary teams operate and the factors that facilitate or inhibit their effectiveness.

The factors that tend to limit the effectiveness of a work group include large group size, poor decision-making practices, lack of fit between group members' skills and task demands, and poor leadership.[14,15] Other formal and informal factors influence team dynamics as well. Formal factors, those that are tangible or visible, include the policies and objectives of the group or its parent organization, the systems of communication available to the group, and the job descriptions of its members. Informal (submerged) factors, although often less obvious, are equally as influential on group process. These factors include the informal relationships among team members, power networks within and external to the group, and the values, beliefs, and goals of individuals within the group[13] (Table 1-2). Team-building initiatives are often focused on the formal or visible areas, but informal communication, values, and norms play key roles in the functioning of the health care team.

A variety of characteristics and considerations also enhance the effectiveness of the interdisciplinary health care team. In addition to having strong professional backgrounds and appropriate skills, team members must appreciate the diversity within the group, taking into account age and status differences and the dynamics of individual professional subgroups.[16] The size of the team is also important: The most capable and effective teams tend to have no more than 12 members. Team members who know each other and are aware of and value each other's skills and interests are often better able to share in setting and achieving goals. Clearly defined goals and objectives about the group's purpose and primary task, combined with a shared understanding of each member's roles and skills, increase the likelihood of effective communication.

One of the most important characteristics of an effective health care team is the ability to accommodate personal and professional differences among members and to use these differences as a source of strength.[11] The well-functioning team often becomes a means of support,

growth, and increased effectiveness for the physical therapist and other health professionals who wish to maximize their strengths as individuals while participating in professional responsibilities.

Rehabilitation Team

The interdisciplinary health care team has become essential in the rehabilitation of patients whose function would be enhanced by an orthosis or prosthesis. The complexity of the rehabilitation process and the multidimensional needs of patients frequently demand the expertise of many different professional disciplines. The rehabilitation team is often shaped by the typical needs and characteristics of the patient population that it is designed to serve. The health disciplines most often represented in the team include an orthopedic or vascular surgeon; neurologist; the patient's primary physician; a prosthetist and/or orthotist; nurses; a physical and/or occupational therapist; a dietitian; a social worker; a vocational counselor; and, most important, the patient (Figure 1-3). Each of the professionals has an important role to play in the rehabilitation of the patient. Patient education is often one of the primary concerns of the team: Understanding their condition's process and prognosis and the treatment options that are available to them helps patients to be active partners in the rehabilitation process rather than passive recipients of care. Patients and their families are best able to define their needs and concerns and to communicate them to the other team members. Each member of the team has the responsibility to contribute to this education so that the patient has the information needed for an effective partnership and positive outcome of rehabilitation efforts.

Evidence that those patients who feel prepared and informed are most likely to comply with treatment interventions, and often have the most positive health outcome, is found in research studies across a wide variety of medical conditions and health disciplines. Ideally, patient education about amputation and prosthetics begins in advance of, or at least immediately after, the amputation surgery.[17] A national survey of people with amputations (n = 109)

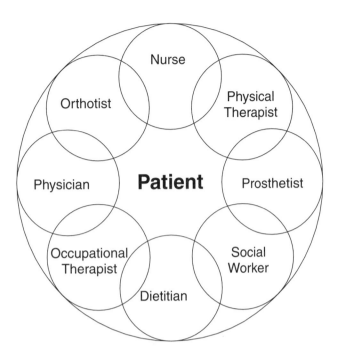

FIGURE 1-3

A clear understanding of the role responsibilities and unique skills and knowledge of each member of the rehabilitation team, combined with open and effective communication, are key characteristics of the successful health care team.

revealed that information is often scarce at this crucial time.[18] Individuals with recent amputations are often caught in an information gap in the days between surgery and the initial process of prosthetic prescription and fitting. Only approximately 50% of patients with a new amputation received information about the timing and process of rehabilitation or about prosthetic options before or immediately after amputation.[18] Interestingly, the health professional most frequently cited as a provider of information at the time of amputation was the physical therapist (25%), followed by the physician (23%). The health professionals cited as most helpful after amputation were the prosthetist (65%) and the

physical therapist (23%; Table 1-3). Clearly, one of the most valued contributions of the physical therapist, in addition to the traditional roles in facilitating a patient's mobility and independence, is as a provider of early information about the timing and process of prosthetic fit and training.

The respondents in this study desired to be active participants in treatment planning and rehabilitation decision making, in partnership with the health care team. The keys to the patient's successful participation in the rehabilitation team are efforts to provide more information and opportunity for open communication; both are likely to enhance patient satisfaction and compliance and the achievement of a positive clinical outcome.

Coordinated care by a multidisciplinary team is just as essential for effective rehabilitation of children as it is for adults. For children with myelomeningocele or cerebral palsy, the broad knowledge base available through team interaction provides a stronger foundation for tailoring interventions to the changing yet ongoing developmental needs of the child and family.[19] The optimum delivery of care to these children is best provided in the multidisciplinary setting in which the various specialists can provide a truly collaborative approach. Orthopedic surgeons, neurologists, orthotists, prosthetists, physical therapists, occupational therapists, nurses, dietitians, social workers, psychologists, and special education professionals may all be involved in setting goals and in formulating and carrying out the treatment plan.

The concept of a multidisciplinary pediatric clinic team was formulated as World War II came to an end.[20] This structure has evolved further over the years and is particularly effective for the more complex orthotic and prosthetic challenges. A "mini-team" consisting of the patient's physician, a physical therapist, and a prosthetist/orthotist can usually be assembled even in a small town with few facilities. Regardless of its size, an effective team views the child from a holistic perspective, with the input from each subspecialty being of equal value. Under these circumstances, the setting of treatment priorities, such as whether prosthetic fitting or training in single-handed

TABLE 1-3

Health Professionals Cited as Sources of Information to Persons with Amputations (n = 109)

Health Discipline	Provided Information at Time of Amputation		Most Helpful after Amputation	
	Number	*Percent*	*Number*	*Percent*
Physical therapist	24	25	22	23
Prosthetist	18	19	63	65
Surgeon/family physician	22	23	28	29
Others with amputation	21	22	7	7

Source: Adapted from CC Nielsen. A survey of amputees: functional level and life satisfaction, information needs, and the prosthetist's role. J Prosthet Orthot 1991;3:125.

tasks is most appropriate at a child's current age or developmental level, is based on the particular needs of the individual rather than on local custom.[21]

Clearly, the team is a diverse group of health care professionals, each bringing his or her particular skills to bear on the needs of the patient. Each member of the team must understand the role and responsibilities of the other members. Clear and frequent communication is essential for this team to function effectively.

CONCLUSION

The development of interdisciplinary teams in health care practice today is prevalent and often required. The use of teams has evolved in part because no one person or discipline can have expertise in all the areas of specialty knowledge that are required for high-quality care. This is particularly true in orthotic/prosthetic rehabilitation, in which complex issues require the resources of a variety of specialists. For health professionals to work together in a collaborative and cooperative manner, particular attitudes and attributes are essential.[22] These attitudes include (1) openness and receptivity to the ideas of others; (2) an understanding of the roles and expertise of other professionals in the team, as well as value and respect for them; (3) interdependence and acceptance of a common commitment to comprehensive patient care; and (4) willingness to share ideas openly and to take responsibility.

In this chapter, we have explored the influence of these attitudes on the team approach to rehabilitation. The contributions of a physical therapist, as an integral member of the rehabilitation team, to the holistic care of the patient can be enhanced by an understanding of orthotics and prosthetics. Collaboration, mutual respect, and an understanding of the roles and responsibilities of colleagues engender productive teamwork and improved outcomes for the rehabilitation patient.

REFERENCES

1. Fitz PA, Smey JW, Douglas PD, Gillespie PW. A Case Study in Core Curriculum: Twenty Years and Counting. In Core Curricula in Allied Health. Washington, DC: Pew Health Professions Commission, 1995;139–164.
2. Stubblefield C, Houston C, Haire-Joshu D. Interactive use of models of health-related behavior to promote interdisciplinary collaboration. J Allied Health 1994;23:237–243.
3. American Orthotic and Prosthetic Association. You Can Make a Difference in People's Lives: Become an Orthotist or Prosthetist. Alexandria, VA: Orthotics and Prosthetics National Office, 1995.
4. Shurr DG, Cook TM. Prosthetics and Orthotics. Norwalk, CT: Appleton & Lange, 1990;1–5.
5. Retzlaff K. AOPA celebrates 75 years of service to O&P. Orthotics and Prosthetics Almanac 1992;Nov:45.
6. Myers RS. Historical Perspective, Assumptions, and Ethical Considerations for Physical Therapy Practice. In RS Myers (ed), Saunders Manual of Physical Therapy Practice. Philadelphia: Saunders, 1995;3–7.
7. Hazenhyer IM. A history of the American Physiotherapy Association. Part IV: Maturity, 1939–1946. Phys Ther Rev 1946;26:174–184.
8. Wilson BA. History of Amputation Surgery and Prosthetics. In JH Bowker, JW Michael (eds), Atlas of Limb Prosthetics: Surgical, Prosthetic and Rehabilitation Principles. St. Louis: Mosby–Year Book, 1992;3–15.
9. McFadden FO, Skoloda, TE, Schubel C. Educational Programming in Geriatrics to Enhance Interdisciplinary Team Functioning. In The Seventh Annual Conference on Interdisciplinary Health Team Care: Conference Proceedings. Chicago: University of Illinois at Chicago, 1985.
10. Douglas PD. The Core Concept. In NE Farber, EJ McTernan, RO Hawkins (eds), Allied Health Education. Springfield, IL: Thomas, 1989;87–97.
11. Purtillo R. Health Professional and Patient Interaction. Philadelphia: Saunders, 1990;27–29.
12. Alexander JA, Lichtenstein R, Jinnet K, D'Aunno TA. The effects of treatment team diversity and size on assessment of team functioning. Hospital and Health Services Administration 1996;41(1):37.
13. Pearson P, Jones K. The primary health care non-team? Dynamics of multidisciplinary provider groups. BMJ 1994;309:1387.
14. Hackman JR. Groups That Work (& Those That Don't): Creating Conditions for Effective Team Work. San Francisco: Jossey-Bass, 1990.
15. Goodman PS, Devadas RA, Hughson TLG. Groups and Productivity: Analyzing the Effectiveness of Self-Managing Teams. In JP Campbell, JR Campbell (eds), Productivity in Organizations. San Francisco: Jossey-Bass, 1988;295–327.
16. Fried B, Rundall T. Group and Teams in Health Services Organizations. In SM Shortell, AD Kaluzny (eds), Health Care Management, Organization, Design and Behavior (3rd ed). Albany: Delmar, 1994.
17. Nielsen CC. Factors affecting the use of prosthetic services. J Prosthet Orthot 1989;1(4):242–249.
18. Nielsen CC. A survey of amputees: functional level and life satisfaction, information needs, and the prosthetist's role. J Prosthet Orthot 1991;3(3):125–129.
19. Banta JV, Lin RS, Peterson M, Dagenais T. The team approach in the child with myelomeningocele. J Prosthet Orthot 1990;2(4):365–375.
20. American Academy of Orthopedic Surgeons. Atlas of Limb Prosthetics. St. Louis: Mosby, 1981;493.
21. Michael J. Pediatric prosthetics and orthotics. Phys Occup Ther Pediatr 1990;10(2):123–146.
22. Bassoff BZ. Interdisciplinary education as a facet of health care policy: the impact of attitudinal research. J Allied Health 1983;12(4):280–286.

2

Materials and Technology

Géza F. Kogler

A fundamental concept that is common to orthotics, prosthetics, and rehabilitation is the restoration of normal form and function after injury or disease. To accept this philosophic challenge, the field of orthotics and prosthetics has evolved into a uniquely specialized profession. In addition to training in the basic biologic and medical sciences, an orthotist/prosthetist has an understanding of biomechanics, kinesiology, and the material sciences complemented by highly developed technical skills. Knowledge of the physical properties of materials and the techniques to manipulate and use them is essential to the design and fabrication of orthoses and prostheses. Within the profession, the subject of material science and technologies as it relates to orthotics and prosthetics is exhaustive and could not possibly be given justice within the scope of this text. Instead, the topic is presented as a general overview so that the rehabilitation clinician can develop a basic understanding of current design and fabrication processes used by orthotists and prosthetists in their work.

ORTHOTICS AND PROSTHETICS IN THE TWENTIETH CENTURY

Orthotics and prosthetics have a rich history of research and development; many innovative devices have been designed to restore function and provide relief from various medical ailments. Although progress can be documented throughout human history, the most significant contributions to orthotic/prosthetic sciences were made in the twentieth century, stimulated by the aftermath of the world wars. Injured veterans who returned home from battle with musculoskeletal and neuromuscular impairments or traumatic amputation dramatically increased the demand for orthotic prosthetic services. Although World War I stimulated some clinical progress in the two disciplines, notable scientific advancements did not occur until the second World War. To improve the quality and performance of assistive devices at the end of World War II, particularly for veterans with amputation, the United States government sponsored a series of research and development projects under the auspices of the National Academy of Sciences (NAS) that would forever change the manner in which orthotics and prosthetics would be practiced.[1]

An extensive research effort was initiated by the NAS in late 1945, when a consensus conference revealed that few modern scientific principles or developments had been introduced in prosthetics.[2] Research and educational committees were formed to advise and work with the research groups between 1945 and 1976. Universities, the Veterans Administration, private industry, and other military research units were subcontracted to conduct various prosthetic research projects. In summarizing the most notable achievements in prosthetics during this period, Wilson[3] cited the development of the total contact transfemoral socket, the quadrilateral socket design and hydraulic swing phase knee-control units for transfemoral prosthesis; the patellar tendon-bearing (PTB) transtibial prosthesis, the solid-ankle cushioned-heel (SACH) prosthetic foot, several new designs for Syme's prosthesis, and the Canadian hip-disarticulation prosthesis. He also notes the implementation of immediate postsurgical and early fitting as having a significant impact on the rehabilitation process for persons with lower extremity amputation. The most notable improvements in upper extremity prosthetics were the lyre-shaped three-jaw chuck terminal device and more efficient harnessing systems. Modular components and advances in bioengineering have permitted increased use and availability of the myoelectric prosthesis since it was first proposed in 1950.[4]

Of the wealth of scientific advances made during this intensive research period, the most important is related to greater attention to the biomechanics of prosthetic alignment and socket design.[5] According to Wilson,[2] "The introduction of socket designs based on sound biomechanical analyses to take full advantage of the functions and properties of the stump in conjunction with the rationale for alignment undoubtedly represents the greatest achievement in prosthetics since World War II."

Although the focus of the NAS Artificial Limb Program was in prosthetics, it was anticipated that these efforts would also benefit orthotics. A formal research directive in orthotics did not begin until 1960. Biomechanical principles developed for the PTB prosthesis were immediately introduced in orthotics at the Veterans Administration Prosthetic Center with the PTB orthosis to unload the foot-ankle complex axially.[6] The concept of fracture bracing or cast bracing began at approximately the same time and is now common practice for orthopedic management of fractures.[7,8] Clinical aspects of orthotic practice were also considered as a systematic approach to prescription formulation was established with the development of the technical analysis forms. Nomenclature to describe an orthosis and its function was standardized to identify the body segments it encompassed with the desired biomechanical control mechanisms.[9]

The introduction of new materials led to further advances in the field shortly after World War II. The use of thermosetting plastics in prosthetics permitted the development of the suction socket suspension system.[10] Transparent plastics offered a new approach to diagnostic and fitting evaluation techniques such as the transparent prosthetic socket (test socket) and the transparent face mask for patients with thermal injuries. In orthotics, the addition of thermoplastics led to numerous innovative designs of ankle-foot orthoses (AFOs) in the 1960s and 1970s. The custom plastic AFO was an important technological advance in lower extremity orthotics. The physical characteristics of thermoformable plastics allowed biomechanical controls to match the prescription for improved function. The mechanical properties of an orthosis could be controlled by the layout of the trimlines of a device or structural reinforcements through specially placed corrugations that could be incorporated into its surface geometry. Advances have been steady in the area of material engineering and continue to have an impact on orthotics and prosthetics. Numerous prosthetic feet have been introduced as elite athletes demand increased performance capabilities from their prosthetic components. Innovative designs for some prosthetic feet have been possible, in part due to the diversity of carbon composite technology complemented by sound engineering design.

The development of CAD/CAM (computer-aided design–computer-aided manufacture) systems for orthotics and prosthetics, which began in the 1970s, was another major technological advance when one considers the long tradition of custom hand-crafted devices in the profession. In the late 1980s and early 1990s, as the availability of computers became more economical, facilities began to integrate CAD/CAM systems into their practices. CAD/CAM systems have now been designed for most orthotic and prosthetic applications, often with specialized digitizers, scanners, and milling equipment to accommodate the unique needs of a particular device. The current trend within the profession is that orthotic prosthetic practices use the CAD portion to digitize and manipulate the data, then subcontract the production of a device from a central fabrication company for its computer-aided manufacture. The art and workmanship that have distinguished the orthotist/prosthetist from other health professionals for most of the twentieth century continue to evolve as CAD/CAM technologies improve the design, manufacture, and diagnostic aspects of the field.

Orthotics and prosthetics have played an important historical role in the development of orthopedics and rehabilitation. Fundamental concepts that evolved from orthotic and prosthetic advancements are now basic principles in rehabilitation. Orthotics and prosthetics have evolved as sister professions because the technical skills and knowledge base to prescribe, fabricate, and fit the respective mechanical devices are similar. Because of this, it is not surprising that material and technological advancements have been transferred between these two rehabilitation specialties.

MATERIALS

In the first part of the twentieth century, orthoses were constructed primarily of metal, leather, and fabric, and prostheses were manufactured from wood and leather. In the last 50 years, tremendous technological advancements have been made in the material sciences. The demand for strong and lightweight components in the aerospace and marine industries has produced a variety of new materials that possess mechanical properties suitable for use in the construction of orthoses and prostheses. New plastics have led to revolutionary advancements in the profession, permitting increased durability and strength and significant cosmetic improvements. Although a multitude of materials are now available, traditional ones are still in wide use; material selection is dependent in part on the individual needs of each clinical situation. In a rehabilitation team setting, the orthotist and prosthetist are responsible for choosing the appropriate materials and components for fabrication because their experience and training are quite specialized in this area.

In this chapter, we present an overview of the general types of materials used in orthotics and prosthetics for rehabilitation professionals. For specific technical information, the reader is referred to publications of the American Society for Testing and Materials (ASTM).[11] To understand the strength requirements for orthotic and prosthetic components, the International Organization for Standardization (ISO) has established industry standards for consumer and patient protection.[12]

The types of materials that are used most commonly in current orthotic and prosthetic practice include leathers, metals, woods, thermoplastic and thermosetting materials, foamed plastics, and viscoelastic polymers. In deciding which of the available materials are most appropriate for a given patient's circumstances or needs, the orthotist or prosthetist considers the following characteristics of materials:[13]

Strength: the maximum external load that the material can support or sustain. Strength is especially important in lower limb devices, in which loading forces associated with gait can be very high, or when heavy use of the orthotic or prosthetic device is anticipated.

Stiffness: the amount of bending or compression that occurs on loading (stress/strain or force to displacement ratio). The stiffer a material, the less flexible or less likely it is that deformation will occur during wear. When provision of significant external stability is desirable (for example, in a fracture brace or a rigid prosthetic frame), a stiff material is often chosen. When conformation to body segments is necessary (for example, in a posterior leaf-spring AFO or a flexible transfemoral prosthetic socket), a more flexible material is used.

Durability (fatigue resistance): the ability of a material to withstand repeated cycles of loading or unloading during functional activities. Repeated loading compromises the material's strength and increases risk of failure or fracture of the material. Fatigue resistance is especially problematic in the presence of interface of materials with different characteristics.

Density: a material's weight per unit volume. This is one of the prime determinants of energy cost during functional activities while wearing a prosthetic or orthotic device. Although the goal is to provide as lightweight a device as possible, the need for strength, durability, and/or fatigue resistance may require that a denser material be chosen.

Corrosion resistance: the degree to which the material is susceptible to chemical degradation. Many of the materials used for orthoses or prostheses retain heat, so that perspiration becomes a problem. For some patients who require lower extremity devices, incontinence may also be a concern. Materials that are impervious to moisture are easier to clean than those that are porous.

The ease of fabrication of materials is also an important consideration. Certain materials can be easily molded or adjusted for a custom fit; others require special equipment or techniques to shape the material as desired.

Leather

Leather is manufactured from the skin and hides of various animals. Tanning methods and the type of hide determine the final characteristics of the leather. As an interface material for an orthosis or a prosthesis, vegetable-tanned leather is used to protect the skin from irritation. Chrome-tanned leather is implemented for supportive purposes when strength and resiliency are needed. Additional chemical processes can be incorporated during manufacturing to produce leathers that are waterproof or porous and flexible or stiff. Qualities that have made leather favorable for use in orthoses and prostheses are its dimensional stability, porosity, and water vapor permeability.[14] These desirable features have made leather a frequently used material within orthopedics, and it continues to be a material of choice in many current devices. Today, leather is used for supportive components, such as suspension straps, belts, and limb cuffs. Leather is also used to cover metallic structures such as pelvic, thigh, and calf bands. For foot orthoses and shoe modifications, leather is often preferred over synthetic substitutes because of its superior "breathe-ability" characteristics.

Another important attribute of leather is its moldability. Although numerous techniques are available to mold leather, the most common one used in orthotics and prosthetics is to stretch it over a plaster cast after it has been mulled (dampened or soaked) in water. When the water evaporates from the molded leather, its dried shape is maintained, and the leather can be trimmed to the desired dimensions. To increase strength and durability, leather can be reinforced by lamination with plastics or other leathers. Similarly, if padding is desired over bony regions of the body, foamed plastics or felt can be sandwiched between layers of leather for comfort or to distribute applied forces over a larger surface area. Three basic skills are required for crafting orthotic or prosthetic components of leather: cutting, sewing, and molding. A technique specific to leather work is that of skiving or thinning the edge on the flesh side of the hide. Finishing methods such as these contribute to the final appearance of the leather work and the device.

Metals

The types of metal used in the fabrication of orthoses and prostheses can be categorized into three groups: steel and its alloys, aluminum, and titanium or magnesium alloys. These metals may or may not share similar characteristics. If metals are incorporated into an orthosis or prosthesis, the choice of metal is determined by the needs and preferences of the particular patient.

Steel

The general term *steel* refers to any iron-based alloy material. Carbon alloys have carbon added to the composition of steel. The term *alloy steel* is used when other materials are included in the material manufacture. Alloy steels are further defined as low-alloy or high-alloy steels. Steels have properties of strength, rigidity, ductility, and durability. Their high density (weight) and susceptibility to corrosion are the major disadvantages. Many different types of steel are available to meet various engineering needs. To assist in identifying the composition and type of material, the American Iron Steel Institute–Society of Automotive Engineers has established a four-digit numbering system. The first two digits in the number indicate the type of steel, and the last two digits identify the carbon content. For alloy steels, the first digit identifies the major alloy and the second digit indicates the percentage of the major alloying element.

The carbon content of steel is the major determinant of its ductile and yield strength characteristics. Yield strength is an offset measure in a stress-strain curve where strain occurs without an increase in stress. Ductility is the property of a material to deform in the inelastic or plastic range. Low carbon content (0.05–0.10%) produces high ductility and a low yield strength.[15] As the carbon concentration increases, yield strength increases and ductility is reduced. Heat treatments can alter the properties of carbon steel by increasing yield strength and reducing ductility. The mechanical properties of low-alloy steels fall between those of carbon steels and high-alloy steels. High strength-weight ratios are possible with the high-alloy steels, an important characteristic for repetitive loading situations. These types of steels are used for some orthotic and prosthetic joint components. High-alloy steels are not very resistant to corrosion and are often more difficult to fabricate.

Stainless steel is a steel alloy that contains 12% or more of chromium, a material that increases resistance to corrosion and oxidation. Chromium produces a light oxide film on the surface that deters deterioration of the base metal. Because durability and protection from corrosion are highly desirable, stainless steels are used extensively within orthotics and prosthetics to enhance longevity of devices. Two types of stainless steel, martensitic steel and ferretic steel, have chromium as the predominate alloying element. Because martensitic steel can be hardened by heat treatment, this type of stainless steel is the only one used in orthotics and prosthetics. Stainless steels are used for orthotic and prosthetic joints, support uprights, and band material.

Aluminum

Aluminum alloys are well suited for orthotics and prosthetics due to their high strength-weight ratio and resistance to corrosion. As with steels, the properties of aluminum are dependent on alloying compositions, heat treatments, and cold working. *Wrought* and *cast* are terms used to describe the two major types of aluminum alloys. Alloys are further subdivided into those that are heat treatable and those that are non–heat treatable. The low-ductility and low strength of cast aluminum are ideal for prefabricated prosthetic components and in some assemblies for moving parts. Wrought aluminum alloys are used in orthotics and prosthetics for structural purposes such as prosthetic pylons, orthotic uprights, and upper extremity devices. The high-compression bending stresses of lower extremity prosthetics are well suited to the use of wrought aluminum alloys.

Although aluminum alloys are very resistant to atmospheric and some chemical corrosion, urine, perspiration, and other bodily fluids are corrosive. Acids and alkalis in these body fluids deteriorate the natural protective oxides on the material's surface, making the aluminum susceptible to corrosion. To deter corrosion in aluminum and to resist abrasive wear, various hard coatings, such as anodic or oxide finishes, can be applied. Mechanical finishes, such as polishing, buffing, and sandblasting, offer attractive cosmetic appearances for devices.

Titanium and Magnesium

Components made of titanium alloys have become more prevalent in prosthetics but are rarely used in orthotics. Although titanium alloys are stronger than those of aluminum and have comparable strength to some steels, their density is 60% that of steel.[16] Titanium alloys are also more resistant to corrosion than are aluminum and steel. It is important to note, however, that titanium alloys are often more difficult to machine and fabricate. Because of this, titanium is most often used in prefabricated prosthetic components, when strength and light weight are of concern. Titanium is also more expensive than aluminum and steel, which has been a limiting factor for its use.

Magnesium alloys are lighter than those of aluminum and titanium, are corrosion resistant, and have a lower modulus of elasticity than does aluminum. The modulus of elasticity (Young's modulus) is defined as the ratio of unit stress to unit strain in a stress-strain curve's elastic range; materials with low modulus values are associated with lower rates of fatigue under conditions of repeated stress. Although some of these features are promising, magnesium alloys have not yet been widely used in orthoses and prostheses.

Wood

Wood possesses many desirable characteristics for use in prosthetics. Its wide availability, strength, light weight, and ability to be shaped easily have continued to be of benefit in prosthetics socket and component construction, even with the introduction of thermoplastics. The wood used in prosthetics must be properly cured, free of knots, and relatively strong. Yellow poplar, willow, basswood (linden), and balsa are most commonly used. Hardwoods have been reserved for prosthetic applications in which structural strength is essential, most often in certain types of prosthetic feet or as reinforcement for knee units. The keel prosthetic feet are fabricated of maple and hickory. The SACH foot has a hardwood keel that is bolted to the prosthetic shank, creating a solid structural unit for standing and ambulation.

Plastics

One of the most important production-related characteristics of an orthotic or prosthetic material is its ability to be molded over a positive model. Because plastics can be readily formed, they are a very popular, widely used material for orthoses and prostheses. Plastics are grouped into two categories: thermoplastics or thermosetting materials.[17–19]

Thermoplastics

Thermoplastic materials are formable when they are heated but become rigid after they have cooled. Thermoplastics are classified as either low-temperature or high-temperature materials, depending on the temperature range at which they become malleable. Low-temperature thermoplastics become moldable at temperatures less than 149°C and often can be molded directly on the patient's limb, whereas high-temperature materials require heating to much higher temperatures and must be molded over a positive model of the patient's limb.[18] One advantage of thermoplastic materials is that they can be reheated and shaped multiple times, making it possible to make minor adjustments of an orthosis or prosthesis during fittings. Thermoplastics are the material of choice for "shell" designs, in which structural strength is required. Some of the more popular materials used are acrylic, copolymer, polyethylene, polypropylene, polystyrene, and a variety of vinyls.

Certain low-temperature thermoplastics, those moldable at temperatures less than 80°C, can be applied and shaped directly to the body. Some of the most commonly available materials include Kydex (Rohm & Haas, Philadelphia, PA), Orthoplast (Johnson & Johnson, Raynham, MA), and Polysar (Bayer, Pittsburgh, PA). These materials are most often reserved for orthotic devices that are designed to provide temporary support and protection. Their susceptibility to repetitive stress, high loads, and temperature changes usually limit their use to spinal and upper extremity orthoses. Because these devices are molded directly on the patient, no casting is necessary, and the time required from measurement to finished product is greatly reduced. Another important convenience afforded by low-temperature thermoplastic materials is that no special equipment is required: Hot water heated in an electric frying pan, a heat gun, and sharp scissors are all that are necessary to produce a functional splint or orthosis.

High-temperature plastics are frequently used in the production of orthotics and prosthetics. The most commonly used materials include polyethylene, polypropylene (homopolymer, copolymer), polycarbonate, acrylic, acrylonitrile-butadiene-styrene, acrylics, polyvinyl acetate, polyvinyl chloride, and polyvinyl alcohol.

Polypropylene is a rigid plastic material that is relatively inexpensive, lightweight, and easy to thermoform. Polypropylenes are further characterized as homopolymers or copolymers. They are one of the most widely used plastics in orthotics. The material has a white opaque color and is available in sheets of various thicknesses, from 1 mm to 1 cm. Polypropylene is impact resistant and can endure several million cycles of repetitive flexes. This attribute has been extremely useful in orthotics for hinge joints and spring assists in AFOs. The material is, however, susceptible to ultraviolet light and extreme cold and is sensitive to scratches and nicks. In prosthetics, the light weight of polypropylene makes it ideal for components such as sockets, pelvic bands, hip joints, or knee joints. Polypropylene is commonly used for prefabricated AFOs and preformed modular orthotic systems.

The long fatigue life of polyethylene during repeated loading situations makes this material suitable for a number of orthotic and prosthetic applications. Prosthetic sockets, orthotic hinge joint components, and compression shells for clamshell design orthoses are common uses of the polyethylene plastics. Several densities of polyethylene are available from various manufacturers. Low-density polyethylene is used for upper extremity and spinal orthoses under the trade names Vitrathene (Stanley Smith & Co, Ltd, Isleworth, UK) and Streiflen (FG Striefeneder KG, Munich, Germany). High-density polyethylene, Subortholen (Wilh. Jul. Teufel GmbH, Stuttgart, Germany), is used for spinal and lower extremity orthoses. The ultra high-density poly-ethylenes such as Ortholen (Wilh. Jul. Teufel GmbH) is used principally for lower extremity orthoses.

Thermosetting Materials

Thermosets are plastics that are applied over a positive model in liquid form and then chemically "cured" to solidify and maintain the desired shape. To enhance their structural properties, thermosets are often impregnated into various fabrics using a process of lamination. Although this group of plastics has inherent structural stability, their rigidity precludes modification by heat molding; their shape can only be changed by grinding. Thermosetting plastics cannot be reheated without destroying their physical properties. Some of the most common thermoset resins used to produce rigid orthoses are acrylic, polyester, and epoxy. Because acrylic resins are strong, lightweight, and somewhat pliable, they offer a different set of characteristics than those of polyester resins. Using lamination, acrylic resin can create a thin but strong structural wall for a prosthetic socket or component of an orthotic. If frequent adjustments are anticipated, however, thermoforming plastics are chosen instead. Fiberglass, nylon, aramid fiber (Kevlar; DuPont, Wilmington, DE), and carbon graphite are the materials used in conjunction with the thermoset plastic to give it added strength. Collectively, they are often referred to as *composites* or *laminates*. Thermosets are used more frequently in prosthetics than are orthotics, for which the advantages of thermoforming plastics have significantly decreased the use of thermosets.

Foamed Plastics

Foamed plastics can be used as a protective interface between the orthotic or prosthetic and the skin, especially over areas that are vulnerable to pressure, such as bony prominences. Foamed plastics are grouped into two classes: open and closed cell. Cells are created in rubber or polymers in a high-pressure gassing process.[18] The microcell structure allows the foamed plastic material to be displaced in several planes, which is an ideal physical property for the reduction of shear forces. In an open-cell foam, the cells are interrelated (as in a kitchen sponge), whereas in a closed-cell foam the cells are independent or separate from each other. Because closed-cell foams are impervious to liquids, they are less likely to absorb body fluids such as perspiration or urine; however, they do act as insulators and can be hot when worn for extended periods.

An orthopedic grade of polyethylene foam was introduced in the 1960s by a British subsidiary of the Union Carbide Company.[20] These closed-cell foams are available in a wide array of durometer hardnesses (durometer refers to a spring indenture post instrument that is used to measure the resistance to the compression/hardness of a material). Polyeth-

ylene foams are commercially available under trade names such as Plastazote (Hacketstown, NJ), Pe-Lite, Evazote (Bakelite Xylonite Ltd., Croydon, UK), or Aliplast (Alimed Inc., Dedham, MA), as well as others. The various polyethylene foams are used in the manufacture of soft and rigid orthoses, depending on the density of the material. Plastazote is a low-temperature heat-formable foam that has been used successfully in the treatment and prevention of neuropathic foot lesions.[21-24] Its light weight and forgiving quality to bony prominences make it a desirable interface for the insensate foot. For a complete review of the use of Plastazote in lower limb orthotics and prosthetics, the reader is referred to Hertzman.[21]

Closed-cell foams are also made with synthetic rubbers or polychloroprenes. Neoprene is available in various densities, making the low-durometer versions suitable as liners for orthoses, whereas the firmer materials are used for posts or soling for shoes. Spenco (Spenco Medical Corp., Waco, TX) is a microcellular neoprene foam that reduces shear forces to the foot's plantar surface and the occurrence of foot blisters in athletes.[25] The nylon (polyamide)-covered neoprene acts as a shock absorber while also reducing friction on the foot's plantar surface.[20] Although few of these materials are heat moldable, most can be conformed without difficulty to the shallow contours of foot orthoses.

Lynco (Apex Foot Products Corp., South Hackensack, NJ) is an open-cell neoprene foam that dissipates heat more efficiently than its closed-cell cousin; however, it does not attenuate shock as well as Spenco.[20] Polyurethane open-cell foams are alternatives for topcovers for foot orthoses. They provide good shock absorption and dissipate heat well. Some of the commercially available open-cell polyurethane foams include Poron (The Rogers Co., Rogers, CT), PPT (Professional Protective Technologies, Deer Park, NY), and Vylite (Steins Foot Specialties, Newark, NJ).

Several studies that compare materials used to fabricate orthoses have been conducted.[26-30] In 1982, Campbell et al.[26] conducted compression tests on 31 materials to determine their suitability for insoles in shoes. Materials were classified according to stiffness under the categories "very stiff," "moderately deformable," and "highly deformable." The moderately deformable group of plastics was deemed the most beneficial as an insole material, which included 19 of the tested foamed plastics. Campbell et al. concluded that these materials could relieve stress from bony prominences and transfer the loads to the adjacent soft tissues more effectively than could the very stiff or highly deformable materials.

Viscoelastic Polymers

A viscoelastic solid is a material that possesses the characteristics of stress relaxation and creep. Stress relaxation occurs when a material that is subjected to a constant deformation requires a decreasing load with time to maintain a steady state.[31] Creep refers to the increase in deformation with time to a steady state as a constant load is applied.[31] Sorbathane (Triad Research Inc., Strasburg, PA), widely used as an insole material, is made of a noncellular polyurethane derivative that possesses good shock-attenuating characteristics.[31] Viscolas (Chattanooga Corp., Chattanooga, TN), another type of viscoelastic solid, has been found to attenuate skeletal shock at heel strike in the tibia to half the normal load.[15,32] Two other viscoelastic polymers that are used to fabricate orthotic prosthetic components are Viscolite (Polymer Dynamics, Inc., Lehigh Valley, PA) and PQ (Riecken's Orthotic Laboratories, Evansville, IN).

PRESCRIPTION GUIDELINES

The formulation of a prescription for an orthosis or prosthesis greatly influences the potential functional outcome for the patient: It is critical that rehabilitation objectives and design criteria are considered carefully. Physicians, therapists, orthotists, and prosthetists who are involved in developing a prescription for an orthotic or prosthetic device must have a sound understanding of orthotics and prosthetics to treat patients effectively with these devices. Assessment of the patient's functional deficit includes a thorough evaluation of his or her present physical status, including muscle strength testing, range of motion measures, and documentation of other physical impairments that would affect the fit or performance of the device. Equally important to the physical examination is the consideration of any individual needs of the patient and an understanding of how the treatment will affect daily activities. To increase the success of treatment, the patient and other rehabilitation team members must reach a consensus on the type of device and the associated training and education required for optimal functional outcome.

Orthotic Prescription

The Committee on Prosthetics and Orthotics of the American Academy of Orthopaedic Surgeons developed a technical analysis form to standardize the process of patient evaluation. This evaluation protocol documents the biomechanical deficits of the patient and provides the basic information needed for orthotic prescription formulation. This systematic approach has two major objectives: (1) to define the anatomic segments that the orthosis will encompass and (2) to describe accurately the biomechanical controls that are needed for treatment. The underlying principle of this assessment is that

orthoses should be designed to control only those movements that are considered abnormal while permitting free motion in anatomic segments that are not impaired.

Technical analysis forms have been developed for three general regions of the body: upper limb, lower limb, and spine. The forms are four pages long with the same basic approach for formulating an orthotic prescription (Figure 2-1). The first page has sections for recording general patient information and noting major physical impairments. The major impairment section characterizes any functional limitations such as skeletal structure, sensation, or joint contracture. This information provides an overview of the patient's clinical presentation. Pages two and three contain diagrams of the respective anatomic segments for which an orthotic prescription is being considered. Each skeletal region is represented in three planes of motion: coronal, sagittal, and transverse. On either side of the figures, square boxes at the level of the joints are used to note volitional force (V), hypertonicity (H), proprioception (P), and range of motion. Page four consists of a summary of the functional disability, treatment objectives, orthotic recommendation, and a key for the biomechanical controls of function.

Voluntary movements of muscles are assessed using conventional muscle testing techniques. Muscle strength can be recorded using either the standard descriptive or numeric muscle grading systems, depending on regional preferences. Two types of motion are recorded on the forms: rotary and translatory. According to McCollough,[33] all points of the distal segment move in the same direction, following the same path shape and distance during translatory motion. During rotary motion, one point of the distal segment (or its imaginary extension) remains fixed while other points move in an arc around it. Translatory motion is recorded with linear arrows in the direction of the distal segment's movement relative to its proximal counterpart. The linear arrows are placed below the circle (representing the joint axis) for translatory motion. If translatory force acts in the vertical axis, the linear arrow is placed to the side of the circle. Rotary motion and the related degree of range of motion are documented via an arrow within a "protractor"-type arrangement for each joint. The established normal range of motion for each joint is shaded on the form for comparative reference. If a fixed contracture or fusion of the joint is present, a double linear arrow is used.

Hypertonicity of muscle groups in each of the body segments is described using a functionally based letter scale.[33] A designation of mild tonicity (M) is given when any hypertonus that is present is thought to be functionally insignificant. Moderate tonicity (Mo) indicates that tone might have some functional value, assisting the patient in holding an item during minor tasks. A designation of severe tone (S) indicates that normal function is not at all possible. The patient's proprioceptive ability is described in a similar way, as absent (A), impaired (I), or normal (N) for each of the body segments of interest.

The final page of the technical analysis form contains space for an overview of functional impairments, a checklist of the orthotic treatment objectives, and a chart that details the orthotic recommendation. The desired orthotic control for each body segment is indicated by a specific letter; as many as seven types of orthotic controls can be incorporated into the design of an orthosis. The terms and descriptions of these controls are indicated in the key. If the orthotic recommendation section is completed correctly, the chart will indicate the body segments that the device will encompass and the desired biomechanical control of function needed. Any comments on the specific design requirements or materials, or both, can be detailed in the remarks section of the form.

For the orthotist, the prescription is the blueprint from which the design of a device is based. It specifies the force system requirements needed to achieve the treatment objectives independent of material selection or production processes. Although an in-depth biomechanical assessment may not always be necessary, a system based on these principles is a logical and objective method for formulating an orthotic prescription.

Prosthetic Prescription

The formulation of a prosthetic prescription requires a different evaluative process. Prosthetic prescription is dependent on an in-depth understanding of components and materials, as well as their indications and contraindications for use. Ideally, prosthetic prescription begins before amputation surgery, so that the residual limb is of appropriate length and healing is adequate for optimal prosthetic use. Factors such as vascular supply, anticipated activity level, intelligence, vocation, and age are also important to consider. Range of motion, flexible and fixed contracture, functional strength, skin condition, girth measurements, pain, and sensation of the residual limb and the intact limb are evaluated.

An important part of prosthetic prescription is component selection. The diversity of prosthetic foot-ankle units and knee mechanisms for lower extremity prosthetics, and the variety of terminal devices for the upper extremity, can present difficult decisions for those who are unfamiliar with their intended application. Therefore, the prosthetist is often relied on for recommendations on components, because he or she is usually most familiar with their specifications and limitations. Many prosthetic teams have developed data collection forms to standardize the prosthetic prescription process. Redhead[34] suggests that the prescription for a prosthesis consider each of the major "prescription options." Examples of the specifications delineated by Redhead for a transfemoral prosthesis are type of limb, socket material and design, suspension, knee joints, knee controls, ankle joints, feet, and cosmesis.

For new prosthetic wearers, the interdisciplinary team is essential for rehabilitation, training, and education. For individuals who are successful prosthetic users in need of a new prosthesis, fewer members of the team may be involved.

FABRICATION PROCESS

Once a prescription for a custom orthosis or prosthesis has been determined, the fabrication process begins. The traditional fabrication process is composed of a series

FIGURE 2-1 ➤

The technical analysis form provides a systematic method of data collection for the development of prescriptions for lower extremity orthoses. The form is used to identify existing musculoskeletal and neuromuscular impairments, including deformity, restriction of joint rotary and translatory range of motion in all three planes of movement, volitional strength, and the level of hypertonicity. The specific functional limitations to be addressed by the recommended orthosis are also identified. Once the prescription is developed, the form serves as a guideline for fabrication and fitting of the orthosis. (AC = anterior cruciate ligament; AFO = ankle-foot orthosis; A.S.S. = anterior superior iliac spine; FO = foot orthosis; H = hypertonicity; HKAO = hip-knee-ankle orthosis; LC = lateral collateral ligament; MC = medial collateral ligament; MTP = medial tibial plateau; P = proprioception; PC = posterior cruciate ligament; V = volitional force.) (Reprinted with permission from Committee on Prosthetics Research and Development. Report of the Seventh Workshop Panel on Lower Extremity Orthoses of the Subcommittee on Design and Development, National Research Council–National Academy of Sciences, 1970; and McCollough NC III. Biomechanical Analysis Systems for Orthotic Prescription. In American Academy of Orthopaedic Surgeons, Atlas of Orthotics: Biomechanical Principles and Application [2nd ed]. St. Louis: Mosby, 1985;35–75.)

TECHNICAL ANALYSIS FORM　　　　**LOWER LIMB**　　　　**Revised March 1973**

Name_____ No._____ Age _____ Sex_____

Date of Onset_____ Cause_____

Occupation _____ Present Lower-Limb Equipment_____

Diagnosis _____

_____

_____

Ambulatory ☐　　　　Non-Ambulatory ☐

MAJOR IMPAIRMENTS:

A.　Skeletal
　　1.　Bone and Joints:　　Normal ☐　　Abnormal_____
　　2.　Ligaments:　　Normal ☐　　Abnormal ☐　　Knee: AC ☐　　PC ☐　　MC ☐　　LC ☐
　　　　　　　　　　　　　　　　　　　　　　　　　Ankle: MC ☐　　LC ☐

　　3.　Extremity Shortening:　None ☐　　Left ☐　　Right ☐
　　　　Amount of Discrepancy:　A.S.S.-Heel_____　A.S.S.-MTP_____　MTP-Heel_____

B.　Sensation:　Normal ☐　　Abnormal ☐
　　1.　Anesthesia ☐　　Hypesthesia ☐　　Location:_____
　　　　Protective Sensation:　　Retained ☐　　Lost ☐
　　2.　Pain ☐　　Location:_____

C.　Skin:　Normal ☐　　Abnormal: _____

D.　Vascular:　　Normal ☐　　Abnormal ☐　　Right ☐　　Left ☐

E.　Balance:　　Normal ☐　　Impaired ☐　　Support:_____

F.　Gait Deviations: _____

_____

G.　Other Impairments: _____

─────────────────── **LEGEND** ───────────────────

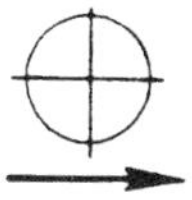

= Direction of Translatory Motion

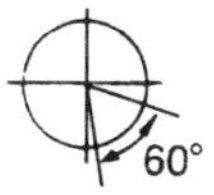

= Abnormal Degree of Rotary Motion

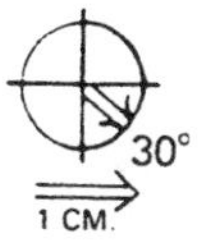

= Fixed Position

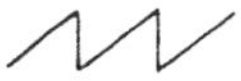

= Fracture

Volitional Force (V)
N　= Normal
G　= Good
F　= Fair
P　= Poor
T　= Trace
Z　= Zero

Hypertonic Muscle (H)
N　= Normal
M　= Mild
Mo = Moderate
S　= Severe

Proprioception (P)
N　= Normal
I　= Impaired
A　= Absent

D　= Local Distension or Enlargement

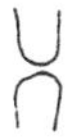

= Pseudarthrosis

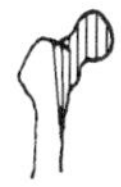

= Absence of Segment

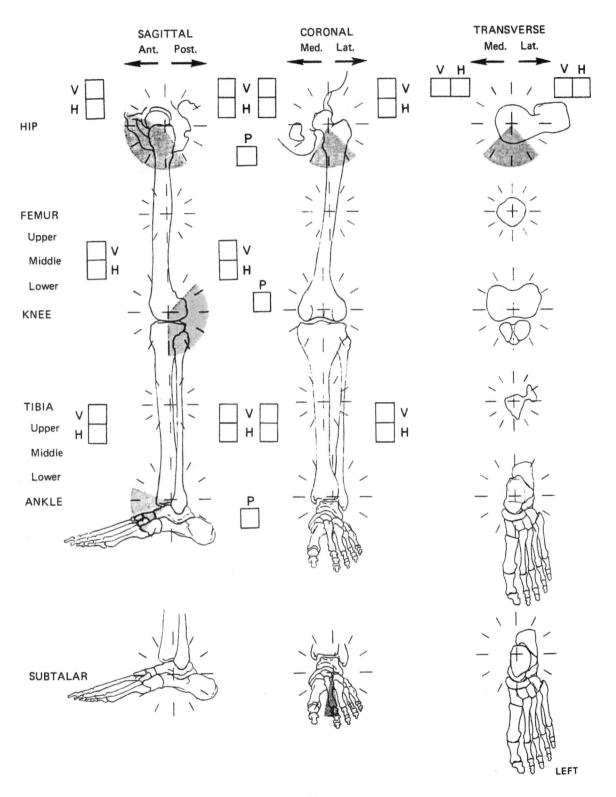

FIGURE 2-1 *(Continued)*

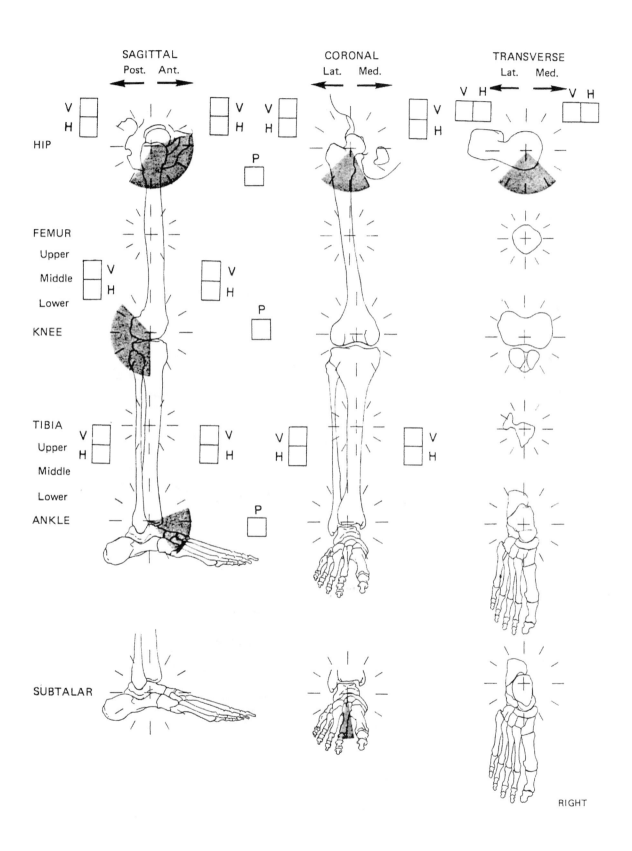

Summary of Functional Disability _____

_____

_____

_____

_____

_____

Treatment Objectives:

Prevent/Correct Deformity ☐   Improve Ambulation ☐

Reduce Axial Load   ☐   Fracture Treatment ☐

Protect Joint   ☐   Other _____

ORTHOTIC RECOMMENDATION

LOWER LIMB			FLEX	EXT	ABD	ADD	ROTATION Int.	ROTATION Ext.	AXIAL LOAD
HKAO	Hip								
KAO	Thigh								
	Knee								
AFO	Leg								
	Ankle		(Dorsi)	(Plantar)					
		Subtalar					(Inver.)	(Ever.)	
FO Foot		Midtarsal							
		Met.-phal.							

REMARKS:

_____   _____
Signature   Date

KEY: Use the following symbols to indicate desired control of designated function:

F = FREE   — *Free* motion.

A = ASSIST   — Application of an external force for the purpose of increasing the range, velocity, or force of a motion.

R = RESIST   — Application of an external force for the purpose of decreasing the velocity or force of a motion.

S = STOP   — Inclusion of a static unit to deter an undesired motion in one direction.

v = Variable   — A unit that can be adjusted without making a structural change.

H = HOLD   — Elimination of all motion in prescribed plane (verify position).

L = LOCK   — Device includes an optional lock.

FIGURE 2-1 *(Continued)*

of six steps. The process begins with making accurate measurements of the limb, followed by taking a negative impression (cast). Next, a three-dimensional positive model of the limb or body segment is created, and then it is modified to incorporate the desired controls. The orthosis or prosthetic socket is then created around the positive. The final step is the fitting of the device to the patient. In some instances, further modification or adjustment is necessary to achieve optimal fit and function of the device.

Measurement

Measurements are most often referenced from readily palpable bony landmarks. Important measurements include the length, successive circumferences, and mediolateral as well as anteroposterior dimensions of the body segment for which the orthotic or prosthetic device is being created. Although many measurements can be obtained with simple tools, such as a tape measure, specialized measurement devices, such as electronic scanning devices, have been developed to enhance accuracy and reproducibility. Measurements are recorded on forms that are specific to the body segment being treated, such as the technical analysis form described previously. These measurements are used in two ways: as a reference when modifications to the positive cast are needed and to determine the placement of the perimeter trimlines of the device.

Negative Mold

A negative impression is a mold taken of an actual body part that is used to create the three-dimensional positive cast or model necessary for fabrication of the orthosis or prosthesis. This negative impression is most often taken using plaster of Paris bandage or a fiber resin tape, although in some instances direct impressions are used as an alternative. Creation of a negative impression has four steps. First, a layer of tubular stockinet or a stocking is placed over the skin, as both a protective interface and to control the position of soft tissue structures within the cast. Tubular stockinets are available in sizes that range from small diameter for the pediatric limb to large diameter for the adult torso. When a direct impression technique is being performed, a topical separator such as petroleum jelly can be used as an interface to minimize the risk of capturing cuticle hair in the impression. Second, bony prominences or other important guiding landmarks are marked on the body segment with indelible ink.

These marks transfer to the inside of the negative mold and from there to the surface of the positive model (Figure 2-2A).

Once the limb or body segment has been prepared, a thin layer of plaster of Paris or fiber resin tape is applied (Figure 2-2B). This procedure differs from that of fracture casts in one important way: The goal is to achieve an "intimate" fit that captures the actual contours of the limb or body segment, so that no protective padding is required. Rolls of elasticized plaster can be wrapped circumferentially in no more than two or three layers. Alternatively, strips of the material can be laid along the length of the limb or body segment. Most impression casting materials are readily available in roll form, although special versions have been produced for specific types of impression procedures such as the fiber resin sock for an AFO. As the molding material is applied, the clinician smoothes the surface, following the normal shape of the limb. While the mold hardens, the clinician supports the limb or segment in the desired position, sometimes applying a light corrective force. As an example, the desired limb position of an orthosis incorporating the ankle joint might be in subtalar and talocrural neutral. If a patellar tendon-bearing socket design is desired for a transtibial prosthesis, an extra force applied just distal to the patella marks its desired location on the resulting positive mold. Once the cast is hardened sufficiently, it is removed carefully from the limb segment, preserving its shape and contours and checked for alignment (Figures 2-2C and 2-2D).

It is essential that the clinician who takes the negative impression has a thorough understanding of the forces that will be applied to the anatomic segments involved, to ensure optimal fit and function of the orthosis or prosthesis. Estimates of soft tissue compression and skeletal alignment changes need to be considered carefully during the negative impression procedure. A skilled and experienced professional uses clinical judgment to create a negative impression, not only to capture the shape of the anatomic segment but also to apply an efficient force system to improve or maximize function. Basic design decisions must be made before the impression procedures so that any special accommodations required for the desired functional outcome can be incorporated.

Special negative impression techniques have been developed for specific purposes. Polystyrene foam impression blocks are one of the common methods of acquiring an impression of the plantar surface of the foot.[35] For patients who are recovering from facial burns, fabrication of a facial orthotic designed to deliver even steady pressure during

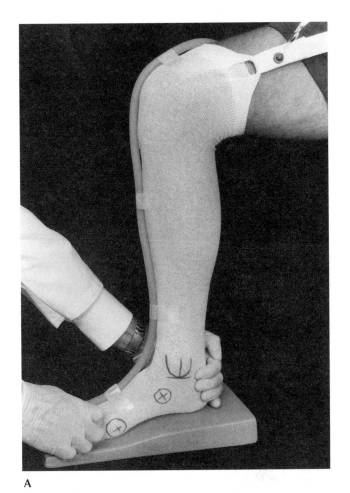
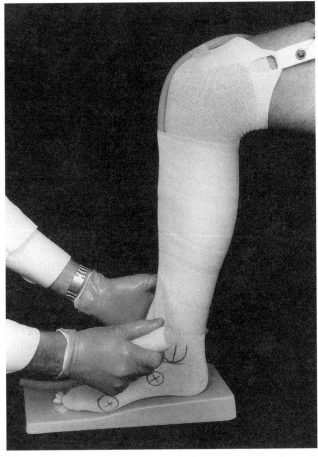

A   B

FIGURE 2-2

The procedure for taking a conventional negative impression begins with placing a layer of cotton stockinette over the limb and marking bony prominences with an indelible water-soluble transfer pencil (A). Surgical tubing is positioned on the anterior aspect of the limb to serve as a guideline for cast removal and to protect the shin, and the limb is positioned on a shoe "last" impression in preparation for circumferential application of a plaster of Paris bandage or fiber resin casting tape (B). The impression board allows the foot to assume the contours of a shoe during molding, for an optimal foot/shoe/ankle-foot orthotic interface.

the period of scar maturation requires a highly detailed mold of the face. Alginate impressions, also referred to as *moulage techniques*, similar to those used in dentistry, are often used.

Fabricating and Modifying the Positive Model

Conventional methods for creating a positive cast are well established. The negative impression is prepared by sealing the mold so that it can accept liquid plaster of Paris. A separator material (i.e., silicone, soap) is added to the inner walls of the mold before the plaster of Paris is poured so that it can be removed more easily once the positive

model has set. Once the cast has solidified, the negative impression is stripped away and discarded. The anatomic landmarks and reference points marked on the limb or body segment with indelible pencil and transferred from the patient to the negative impression are again transferred to the positive model. A mandrel (post) is embedded into the setting plaster of the positive model. This mandrel is used to hold the model for cast rectification and the rest of the production processes.

Model rectifications remove artifacts produced during the molding or impression process and bring the cast to specification of the measured values taken from the patient. Once the positive model has been rectified, fur-

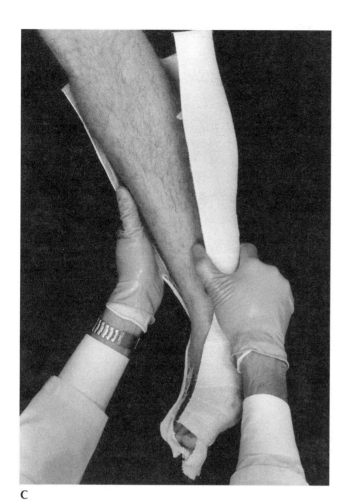

C

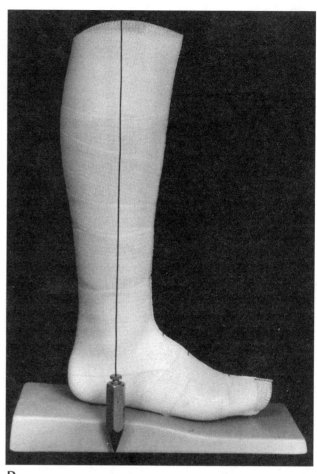

D

FIGURE 2-2 (Continued)
*Once the cast is "set," a cast saw is used to open the front of the cast (**C**), and the negative impression is removed carefully from the limb. The anterior edges are closed, and the ankle-foot alignment of the negative impression is verified with a plumb line (**D**).*

ther modifications can be made based on the design of the orthosis or prosthesis that is being fabricated. During the negative impression procedure, soft tissue may have been manipulated for specific applications of force or pressure to be incorporated into the final orthosis or prosthesis. Although the positive model represents a three-dimensional shape of a respective body segment, it cannot relay information about the density of the tissue that it will interface. In general, additional plaster is added where relief of pressure is desired (for example, over bony prominences) (Figure 2-3A) or is removed where additional forces are to be applied (Figure 2-3B). When the orthosis or prosthesis is formed over the model,

an area of relief for a more intimate fit is achieved. Although some guidelines have been established with regard to the amount of material to be removed or added to the positive model, the clinical experience of the prosthetist or orthotist is relied on for this stage of the process. The positive model can also be modified to reconfigure surface geometry to improve the strength of the finished product. Once design changes have been incorporated into the model, its surface is prepared for component production. This involves removing any surface imperfections with abrasive tools and abrasive sanding screen to ensure that the surface that will contact patient skin will be smooth. The positive cast is then ready to be used

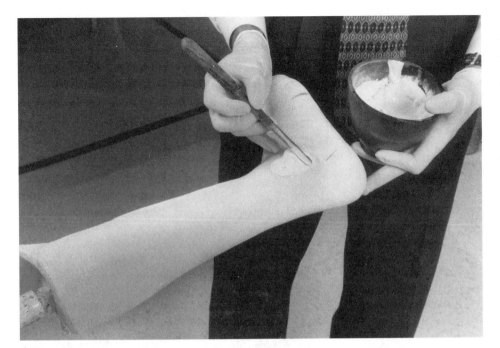

A

FIGURE 2-3
In the rectification of a positive model, plaster of Paris added over pressure-sensitive areas, such as the lateral malleolus (A), results in a "relief" in the finished orthosis. Modification of the positive model by removal of material with a plaster rasp over pressure-tolerant areas (B) increases intimacy of fit for better loading or stabilizing of the limb.

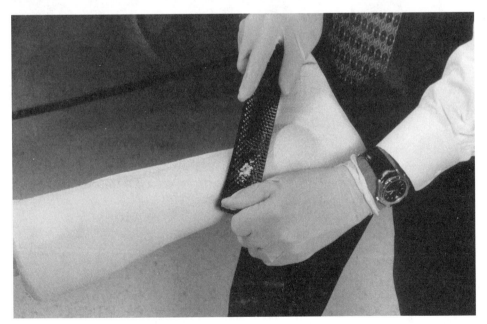

B

as a form from which different materials can be shaped to produce an interface component.

Fabrication

The fabrication process used with the positive model is dependent on the material selected for the device.

Thermoforming is a common production method used in orthotics and prosthetics. Thermoplastic sheet material is heated in an oven until it has reached its "plastic" state, then shaped over a positive model by changing the air pressure difference across its surface (vacuum forming; Figure 2-4A). Once the plastic has cooled and returned to its solid state, trimlines are delineated on

FIGURE 2-4
*Once a sheet of thermoplastic material has been heated, it is dropped over the rectified positive model (**A**) and the edges of the thermoplastic are sealed. Negative pressure created by a vacuum pump removes any trapped air and draws the polypropylene to the surface of the positive model. When the material has cooled, trimlines are drawn on the formed plastic (**B**), using measurements taken during the initial evaluation as well as bony landmarks as a guide. Note the corrugations incorporated to strengthen the orthosis at the ankle.*

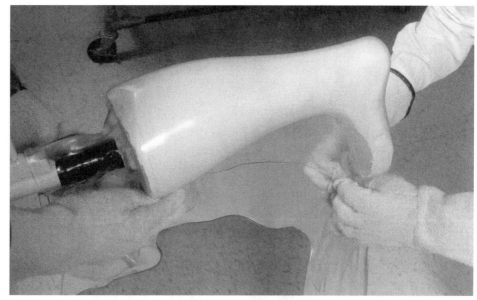

A

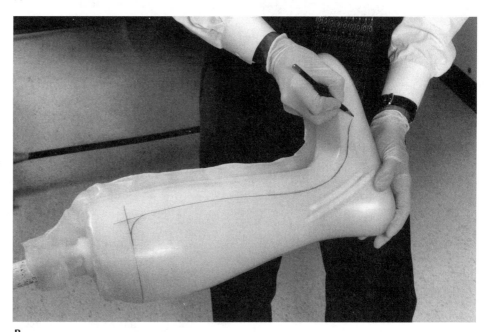

B

the formed plastic before the edges are finished and smoothed (Figure 2-4B).

CAD/CAM

In the 1960s, an alternative method of prosthetic fabrication, using computers, was first introduced. Early CAD/CAM methods used stereophotography and digitization to create a numerical model, which guided a milling machine in the creation of a positive model of the residual limb.[2] A more complete concept of fabrication and manufacture of a prosthesis were developed at the University College London in the late 1970s and early 1980s.[36] After establishing a system for automated production of a prosthesis called *Rapidform*, the London

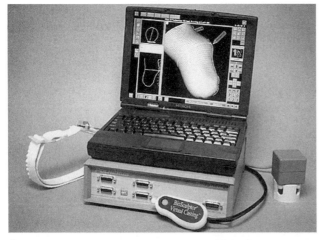

A

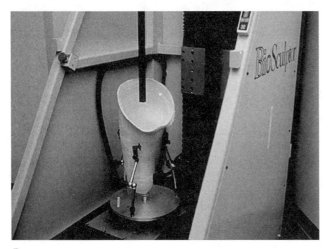

B

FIGURE 2-5

Examples of the use of CAD/CAM (computer-aided design–computer-aided manufacture) data acquisition systems. A digital model of the residual limb (A) can be captured using a laptop computer, appropriate signal processor components, and a hand-held digitizer. Laser digitization (B) can be used to capture accurately the contours of a conventional negative impression of a residual limb. (Photographs courtesy of BioSculptor Corporation, Coral Gables, FL.)

research group conceived a completely automated fabrication process using appropriate prosthetic alignment data.[37] In the United States, the Veterans Administration began funding research projects in the 1980s to investigate further the potential of CAD/CAM in orthotics and prosthetics. Advances were also made in private industry as the availability of personal computers became widespread. Since the late 1980s and through the 1990s,

manufacturers have designed a multitude of CAD/CAM systems for various applications in orthotics and prosthetics. Advances in computer hardware, processors, and software have made CAD/CAM systems fast and efficient as well as an economical alternative for fabrication of devices for many orthotic and prosthetic practices.

Today, most CAD systems use a scanning device to record digital information of a body segment for CAM. The primary components of a CAD/CAM system consist of a digitizing device, computer, and milling machine. Surface contours of the anatomic segment are recorded with various digitization devices: optical laser scanners, surface-contacting stylus, and pneumatically operated mechanical posts. Digital information acquired from a scan of a body segment is processed by the computer and translated into a triordinate data point file. This file is used by the computer to create a graphic image in the form of a surface contour plot.[38] The data are then relayed to a milling unit to carve an orthosis/prosthesis for a positive model.

Data Acquisition

Each of the many digitizers used for data acquisition are designed for a specific task or to handle certain anatomic regions. Noncontact laser digitizers that are capable of circumferential scanning are well suited for measurement of cylindrical shapes such as those found in limb prosthetics or spinal orthotics. An optical-laser camera mechanism images the surface topography of the body segment and records the measured data points in a computer. Special holding fixtures and bars to aid in patient comfort and safety are part of each system. An apparatus that is designed to scan the torso for a spinal orthosis usually requires a different setup than that of a limb prosthesis. Some scanners are capable of digitizing directly from the patient's body segment, whereas other systems take measurements from a negative impression or mold of the segment (Figure 2-5). Compact, hand-held contact digitizers have been introduced by several CAD/CAM manufacturers. These units allow the clinician to digitize a body segment by direct contact with the skin. Hand-held contact digitizers are described as a wand, pen, stylus, and/or pointer. Contact digitizers often have special attachments to scan certain shapes or measurement tools, such as calipers, for acquiring anteroposterior or mediolateral dimensions. Their versatility permits data acquisition of complex shapes. In some systems, hand-held digitizers can be used in conjunction with a laser scan.

The use of digitizers in the production of foot orthoses is also becoming more common. Several systems have been developed for data acquisition for the foot, based on differences in technique and philosophy in foot orthosis design. For full weight-bearing or partial weight-bearing techniques, pneumatically operated mechanical posts are used to digitize the foot's plantar surface (Amfit Corp, San Jose, CA). Orthotic contoured shapes such as metatarsal domes can be evaluated during the digitization procedure to determine optimal position and comfort before fabrication. An optical-laser scanner situated under a Plexiglas platform has also been used for scanning the foot when a weight-bearing technique is desired (Bergmann Orthotic Laboratories, Northfield, IL). Because this system is also capable of scanning the foot with non–weight-bearing methods without the platform, it is quite versatile in clinical practice.

In many instances, the orthotist/prosthetist is restricted to surface geometry and palpation of underlying anatomic structure to interpret the position of skeletal and soft tissue structures of the body segment. Magnetic resonance imaging (MRI) and computed tomography (CT) have been used to create a three-dimensional computer model and assist in making design decisions of a mechanical device (Figure 2-6). Data files from these scans are converted to a working format for specific graphic and modeling programs. Although this capability may not be practical for all applications, it may offer insight into areas of further research and development in the field.

Shape-Manipulation Software

The ability to modify the three-dimensional model of a patient's body segment permits the clinician to incorporate the desired biomechanical controls into an orthosis or prosthesis. The amount of force applied to a specific area is dependent in part on manipulation of the digital three-dimensional model. A variety of software packages are now available to assist orthotists and prosthetists in designing the most appropriate modifications for a given patient. Generic modification templates or custom-designed templates can be used to make a wide range of revisions to the data. The clinician can incorporate reliefs for bony prominences of the limb or trunk or can change the geometry of the shape to enhance structural strength characteristics in final orthosis or prosthesis. Trimlines can be delineated so that technicians who are involved in assembly of components can complete a device without further instruction.

Milling and Production

Once the digital model is in place, the milling apparatus creates the actual orthotic or prosthetic device. Because

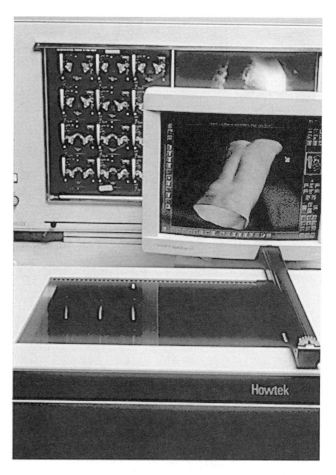

FIGURE 2-6
Computed tomographic (CT) or magnetic resonance imaging (MRI) images can be used to create a digitized computer model of a body segment for various orthotic or prosthetic CAD/CAM (computer-aided design–computer-aided manufacture) applications. The components of this type of system include an image scanner (foreground), *a computer monitor for display of digitized images (e.g., the torso;* center right), *and the CT or MRI images being used* (background). *(Photograph courtesy of BioSculptor Corporation, Coral Gables, FL.)*

each type of orthosis or prosthesis usually has specific milling parameters, a different setup may be required for each. For instance, the long rounded shape of a transtibial or transfemoral socket is often manufactured using a lathe-type milling machine (Figure 2-7). In contrast, foot orthoses are manufactured by an end mill setup because their plate-like structure and production processes create different finishing needs. The production laboratory needs to be large enough to have separate milling stations for each type of orthosis or prosthesis. This manufacturing limitation has led to the establishment of lab-

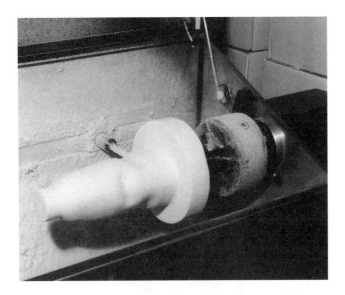

FIGURE 2-7
A positive model for a transtibial prosthetic socket being carved on a computer-controlled milling/lathe machine. (Photograph courtesy of Prosthetic Designs, Inc., Clayton, OH.)

oratory production companies that mill the positive model and manufacture the orthoses or prostheses from computer data files transmitted by modem. Computer production networks can often offer reduced fabrication time and decreased production times, making the use of CAD/CAM economically feasible even for small orthotic/prosthetic facilities. Special production equipment is available that partially automates the thermoforming processes of some components. In the thermoforming machine for prosthetic sockets, a preformed polypropylene shell travels upward on a mechanical platform to an oven that heats the plastic to its formable temperature. The heated shell is then lowered over the positive model of the residual limb and vacuum formed for an intimate fit.

CAD/CAM in orthotics and prosthetics will play an important role in clinical and research settings. Although the development of CAD/CAM in orthotics and prosthetics has a history that spans more than two decades, only since the 1990s has it become an integral part of some clinical practices. Systems that have been designed for virtually all prosthetic and orthotic applications can be integrated with CT, MRI, and other medical imaging technologies. The technological advancements of CAD/CAM offer the orthotist/prosthetist an additional clinical fabrication and research tool. Although this sophisticated equipment can contribute greatly to certain clinical and manufacturing tasks, successful fitting of a device is dependent on proper data input and prescription formulation.

MAINTENANCE OF ORTHOSES AND PROSTHESES

Routine care and maintenance of orthoses and prostheses are important for proper function and long-term use of a device. An orthotic/prosthetic maintenance program usually includes servicing by the orthotist/prosthetist and the patient. The service schedule is dependent on the specific orthosis or prosthesis, the materials from which it is made, the durability of the components incorporated (such as a prosthetic knee unit), and the knowledge and ability of the patient and caregivers. Patient instructions on the daily care of their devices should include cleaning and inspection. Proper patient education of basic fitting criteria and instructions on donning and doffing a device allow the patient to evaluate the fit of a device during routine use. Orthoses and prostheses need to be inspected weekly for any defects, stress risers (nicks, scratches), loose screws, or weakened rivets. Any device that has mechanical components and moving parts and is subjected to repetitive loading requires periodic servicing; it is less expensive to recognize and fix early signs of a problem than it is to replace a device that has failed because of a lack of proper maintenance. Informing patients of potential problems that are associated with the use of their orthosis or prosthesis and how to resolve minor problems can prevent serious problems from arising.

Most plastic components should be cleaned with a mild antibacterial soap and rinsed thoroughly with cold water. Extra moisture is dried with a towel, and the orthosis or prosthesis is then air dried. Heat can distort some plastics: Patients should be warned not to use electric hairdryers to dry their device. Similarly, devices should not be left near direct heat sources, such as radiators, wood stoves, or any appliance that generates heat when running. They must also be protected from intense direct sunlight.

Leather liners and covers are cleaned weekly with a leather "saddle" soap. One should not use leather softeners unless thus instructed by the orthotist because they can compromise function of some straps and cuffs. Water-repellent treatments and protectants for leather often contain skin irritants and should not be used on leather components that directly contact the body.

Most orthoses and prostheses are designed to apply a corrective or stabilizing force to a body segment during wear. For some patients, especially those with fragile skin or scarring, this pressure may increase the risk of skin irritation or damage. The risk of skin problems differs from device to device and on the general health and skin condition of the individual who is wearing the orthosis or prosthesis. To minimize problems with skin intolerance of these extra forces, most new orthotic or prosthetic users begin with an intermittent wearing schedule. A treatment plan that incorporates a gradual buildup of orthotic or prosthetic use can avert complications such as excessive redness, chafing, and blisters. For patients with high risk or a history of skin problems, a variety of preventative measures (for example, foam or silicone interface liners) can be incorporated into the orthotic or prosthetic system.

Most custom orthoses or prostheses are designed to achieve a very intimate fit with the body segment that they encompass. Changes in the physical condition of a patient can significantly alter the fit and function of a device. Compromised fit occurs most often when the patient has had significant growth, weight gain or loss, muscle atrophy, edema, structural degeneration, or trauma. Periodic evaluations are necessary to ensure that fit and function are maintained in the months and years after the initial fitting. Semiannual or annual checkups should be part of a treatment plan for definitive orthotic and prosthetic devices.

To maintain proper function of a lower extremity prosthesis, special attention is needed in several areas. The alignment of a prosthesis is usually based on a specific heel height: Variations from the prescribed heel height (when footwear is changed) often lead to functional problems during gait. In the same way, moderate to excessive wear of the shoe at the heel also compromises performance. The condition of footwear must be monitored carefully and frequently. The prosthesis should be free of dirt, sand, and other debris to ensure that joint mechanisms and their movements are not inhibited. Socket attachment and suspension systems need daily attention because they are usually prone to accumulation of lint, dirt, and other debris. If the prosthesis or any of its components are subjected to water, the device should be dried thoroughly to prevent permanent damage. Rubber bumpers in prosthetic feet deteriorate over time and use and must be replaced regularly. The prosthetist can advise patients on specific parts that require regular maintenance.

The care of the socket portion of a prosthesis should be done faithfully to avoid potential skin problems, especially infection, on the residual limb. When special liners are used with a prosthesis, specific instructions for cleaning are necessary, as materials used vary greatly. For patients who are fitted with suction sockets or special socket attachment mechanisms, the joining components or threads should be cleaned with a soft brush or rag to remove debris.

SUMMARY

In this chapter, we have explored the materials and methods that are most commonly used in the prescription, measurement, and production of orthoses and prostheses. The type of design, materials, and components is selected to facilitate best the functional goals of the patient who is to wear the device. The foundation for effectiveness of the orthosis or prosthesis is careful measurement of the body segment (by casting or by CAD/CAM) and careful modification of the resulting model for optimal fit. For an individual who is being fit for his or her initial orthosis or prosthesis, the shared decision making of the rehabilitation team, including the patient and caregivers, is essential. An orthosis or prosthesis that is difficult to don or is quite uncomfortable to wear is more likely to be found standing in a closet or pushed under a bed than on the patient for daily use.

REFERENCES

1. Committee on Artificial Limbs. National Research Council: Terminal Research Reports on Artificial Limbs (Covering the Period from April 1, 1945 through June 30, 1947). Washington, DC: National Research Council, 1947.
2. Wilson AB. History of Amputation Surgery and Prosthetics. In JH Bowker, JW Michael (eds), Atlas of Limb Prosthetics. Surgical, Prosthetic, and Rehabilitation Principles (2nd ed). St. Louis: Mosby, 1992;3–15.
3. Wilson AB. Prosthetics and Orthotics Research in the U.S.A. In International Conference on Prosthetics and Orthotics. Cairo: S.O.P. Press, 1972;268–273.
4. Rang M, Thompson GH. History of Amputations and Prostheses. In JP Kostuik, R Gillespie (eds), Amputation Surgery and Rehabilitation. The Toronto Experience. New York: Churchill Livingstone, 1981;1–12.
5. Eberhart HD, Inman VT, Dec JB, et al. Fundamental Studies of Human Locomotion and Other Information Relating to the Design of Artificial Limbs. A Report to the National Research Council. Berkeley, CA: Committee on Artificial Limbs, University of California, 1947.
6. Kay HW. Clinical applications of the Veterans Administration Prosthetic Center patellar tendon-bearing brace. Artif Limbs 1971;15(1):46–67.
7. Mooney V, Nickel VL, Harvey JP, Snelson R. Cast-brace treatment for fractures of the distal part of the femur. J Bone Joint Surg 1970;52A(8):1563–1578.
8. Sarmiento A, Sinclair WF. Tibial and Femoral Fractures–Bracing Management. Miami: University of Miami School of Medicine, 1972.
9. Committee on Prosthetics Research and Development. Report of the Seventh Workshop Panel on Lower Extremity Orthoses of the Subcommittee on Design and Development, National Research Council–National Academy of Sciences, 1970.
10. Eberhart HD, McKennon JC. Suction-Socket Suspension of the Above-Knee Prosthesis. In PE Klopsteg, PD Wilson (eds), Human Limbs and Their Substitutes. New York: McGraw-Hill International, 1954.
11. American Society of Testing and Materials (ASTM) Standards, Philadelphia, PA.

12. International Organization for Standardization (ISO). Prosthetics-Orthotics. ILI Infodisk, Paramus, NJ.

13. Shurr DG, Cook TM. Methods, Materials, and Mechanics. In Prosthetics and Orthotics. Norwalk CT: Appleton & Lange, 1990;17–29.

14. O'Flaherty F. Leather. In American Academy of Orthopaedic Surgeons, Orthopaedic Appliances Atlas. Ann Arbor, MI: JW Edwards, 1952;17–28.

15. Redford JB II. Orthotics Etcetera (3rd ed). Baltimore: Williams & Wilkins, 1986.

16. Murphy EF, Burnstein AH. Physical Properties of Materials including Solid Mechanics. In American Academy of Orthopaedic Surgeons, Atlas of Orthotics: Biomechanical Principles and Application (2nd ed). St. Louis: Mosby, 1985;6–33.

17. Compton J, Edelstein JE. New plastics for forming directly on the patient. Prosthet Orthot Int 1978;2(1):43–47.

18. Lockard MA. Foot orthoses. Phys Ther 1988;68(12): 1866–1873.

19. Peppard A, O'Donnell M. A review of orthotic plastics. Athletic Training 1983;18:77–80.

20. Levitz SJ, Whiteside LS, Fitzgerald TA. Biomechanical foot therapy. Clin Podiatr Med Surg 1988;5(3):721–736.

21. Hertzman CA. Use of Plastizote in foot disabilities. Am J Phys Med 1973;52(6):289–303.

22. Jopling UH. Observation on the use of Plastizote insoles in England. Lepr Rev 1969;40:175–176.

23. Mondl AM, Gardiner J, Bisset J. The use of Plastizote in footwear for leprosy patients. A preliminary report. Lepr Rev 1969;40(3):177–181.

24. Tuck UH. The use of Plastizote to accommodate foot deformities in Hansen's disease. Lepr Rev 1969;40(3):171–173.

25. Spence WR, Shields MN. Insole to reduce shearing forces on the soles of the feet. Arch Phys Med Rehab 1968;49(8); 476–479.

26. Campbell G, Newell E, McLure M. Compression testing of foamed plastics and rubbers for use as orthotic shoe insoles. Prosthet Orthot Int 1982;6(1):48–52.

27. Campbell G, McLure M, Newell EN. Compressive behavior after simulated service conditions of some foamed materials intended as orthotic shoe insoles. J Rehab Res 1984; 21(2):57–65.

28. Leber C, Evanski PM. A comparison of shoe insole material in pressure relief. Prosthet Orthot Int 1986;10(3):135.

29. Pratt DJ, Rees PH, Rodgers C. Assessment of some shock absorbing insoles. Prosthet Orthot Int 1986;10(1):43.

30. Rome K. Behavior of orthotic materials in chiropody. J Am Podiatry Assoc 1990;80(9):471–478.

31. Cinats J, Reid DC, Haddow JB. A biomechanical evaluation of sorbathane. Clin Orthop Rel Res 1987;Sept.(222): 281–288.

32. MacLellan GE, Bybyan B. Management of pain beneath the heel and Achilles tendonitis with visco-elastic heel insert. Br J Sports Med 1981;15(2):117.

33. McCollough NC III. Biomechanical Analysis Systems for Orthotic Prescription. In American Academy of Orthopaedic Surgeons, Atlas of Orthotics: Biomechanical Principles and Application (2nd ed). St. Louis: Mosby, 1985;35–75.

34. Redhead RG. Prescription Criteria, Fitting, Check-Out Procedures and Walking Training for the Above-Knee Amputee. In G Murdoch, RG Donovan (eds), Amputation Surgery and Lower Limb Prosthetics. Oxford: Blackwell Scientific, 1988.

35. Schuster RO. Neutral plantar impression cast: methods and rationale. J Am Podiatry Assoc 1976;6(66):422–426.

36. Davies RM, Lawrence RB, Routledge PE, Knox W. The Rapidform process for automated thermoplastic production. Prosthet Orthot Int 1985;9(1):27–30.

37. Davies RM. Computer aided socket design: the UCL system. In RM Davies (ed), Annual Report of the Bioengineering Centre, Roehampton, England, 1986;9–12.

38. Davis FM. In-office computerized fabrication of custom foot supports. The AMFIT system. Clin Podiatr Med Surg 1993;10(3):393–401.

3

Clinical Assessment of Pathologic Gait

EDMOND AYYAPPA AND OLFAT MOHAMED

The first attempts to analyze gait, recorded in the *Rig Veda* more than 3,500 years ago, most likely reflect attempts to enhance mobility through early orthotic or prosthetic intervention. This classic prose chronicles the story of Vispala, a fierce female warrior whose leg, lost in battle, was replaced by an iron prosthesis that enabled her return to the front to fight again.[1]

Gait assessment is used to describe the patterns of movement that control progression of the body in walking. Bipedal gait requires a combination of automatic and volitional postural components. This can result in either asymmetric reciprocal movements of the lower limbs (seen in walking or running) or symmetric, simultaneous two-legged hopping. Kangaroos are bipeds that are successful two-legged hoppers.[2] Homo sapiens have reached the zenith of movement efficiency in bipedal walking and running using reciprocal patterns of motion. The integration of numerous physiologic systems is needed for successful locomotion. Normal walking requires stability to provide antigravity support of body weight in stance, mobility of body segments, and motor control to sequence multiple segments while transferring body weight from one limb to another. Gait characteristics are influenced by the shape, position, and function of neuromuscular and musculoskeletal structures and by the ligamentous and capsular constraints of the joints. The primary goal in gait is energy efficiency in forward progression, using a stable kinetic chain of joints and limb segments working congruently to transport its passenger unit (the head, arms, and trunk).

Understanding the process of walking can help us improve the performance efficiency of persons with musculoskeletal and neuromuscular impairments. Gait assessment in orthotic and prosthetic treatment provides an accurate description of walking patterns for a given patient. Assessment also identifies primary or pathologic gait problems and helps to differentiate them from compensatory strategies. Skilled gait assessment is necessary for selection of appropriate orthotic or prosthetic components, alignment parameters, and identification of other variants that might enhance an individual's ability to walk. Clinical gait assessment contributes to the development of a comprehensive treatment plan, with the ultimate goal of optimal energy efficiency and appropriate pathomechanical controls during walking, balancing cosmesis with overall function.

TERMINOLOGY OF HUMAN WALKING

Step length, stride length, cadence, and velocity are important, interrelated, quantitative kinematic measures of gait. Step length and stride length are not synonymous. *Step length* is the distance from the floor-contact point of one (ipsilateral, originating) foot in early stance to the floor-contact point of the opposite (contralateral) foot: the distance from right heel contact to left heel contact. *Stride length* is the distance from floor contact on one side to the next floor contact on that same side: the distance from right heel contact to the next right heel contact. Stride length contains a left and a right step length. A reduction in functional joint motion or the presence of pain or muscle weakness can result in reduction in stride or step length, or both. Pathologic gait commonly produces asymmetries in step length between the two lower limbs.

Cadence is defined as the number of steps taken in a given unit of time, most often expressed in steps per minute. *Velocity* is defined as the distance traveled in a given unit of time, the rate of forward progression, and is usually expressed in centimeters per second or meters per minute. Velocity is the best single index of walking ability. Reductions in velocity correlate with joint impairments and with many acute pathologies. Velocity can also be qualitatively described as free, slow, or fast. An individual's free walking speed is his

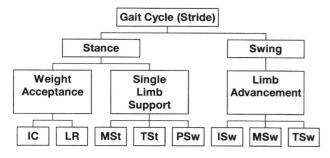

FIGURE 3-1

A complete gait cycle can be viewed in terms of the three functional tasks of weight acceptance, single limb support, and limb advancement. The gait cycle can also be described in phasic terms of initial contact (IC), loading response (LR), midstance (MSt), terminal stance (TSt), preswing (PSw), initial swing (ISw), midswing (MSw), and terminal swing (TSw). The PSw phase is a transitional phase between single limb support and limb advancement.

or her normal self-selected (comfortable) walking velocity. Fast walking speed describes the maximum velocity possible for a given individual. Slow walking speed describes a velocity below the normal self-selected walking speed. For healthy individuals, fast walk velocity may be as much as 44% faster than free walking speed.[3] In people with musculoskeletal and neuromuscular impairment that affects gait, often much less of a difference is found between free and fast gait velocity.

Double limb support is the period of time when both feet are in contact with the ground. It occurs twice during the gait cycle, at the beginning and the end of each stance phase. As velocity increases, double limb support time decreases: When running the individual has rapid forward movement with little or no period of double limb support. Individuals with slow walking speeds spend more of the gait cycle in double support. *Step width*, or width of the walking base, typically measures between 5 and 10 cm from the heel center of one foot to the heel center of the other foot. A wide walking base may increase stability but also reduces energy efficiency of gait. The *ground reaction force (GRF) vector* is the mean load-bearing line, which takes into account both gravity and momentum. It has magnitude as well as directional qualities. The spatial relationship between this line and a given joint center influences the direction in which the joint tends to rotate. The rotational potential of the forces that act on a joint is called a *torque* or *moment*.

GAIT CYCLE

A variety of conceptual approaches have been used to understand the walking process. Saunders et al.[4] and Inman et al.[5] define the functional task of walking as translation of the center of gravity through space in a manner that requires the least energy expenditure. They identify six determinants or variables that affect energy expenditure: pelvic rotation, pelvic tilt, knee flexion in stance phase, foot and ankle interaction with the knee, and lateral pelvic displacement. Individually and collectively, these determinants have an impact on energy expenditure and the mechanics of walking. Although they help us to understand the process of walking, the determinants do not by themselves offer a practical clinical solution to address the problems of assessment of pathologic gait.

A comprehensive system that is useful in describing normal and abnormal gait was developed by the pathokinesiology and physical therapy departments at Rancho Los Amigos Medical Center over the last several decades.[6-8] The Rancho system serves as the descriptive medium for this chapter (Figure 3-1). Because velocity affects many parameters of walking, the description of normal gait assumes a comfortable self-selected velocity. At free walking velocity, the individual naturally enlists the mannerisms and the speed that provide maximum energy efficiency.

The gait cycle is considered to be the period of time between any two identical events in the walking cycle. Initial contact is traditionally selected as the starting and completing event. Each gait cycle is divided into two periods, stance and swing. Stance is the time when the foot is in contact with the ground and constitutes approximately 60% of the gait cycle. Swing denotes the time when the foot is in the air, and it constitutes the remaining 40% of the gait cycle. Five subphases occur within the stance period: initial contact (IC), loading response (LR), midstance (MSt), terminal stance (TSt), and preswing (PSw). Swing phase is divided into three subphases: initial swing (ISw), midswing (MSw), and terminal swing (TSw). PSw, however, prepares the limb for swing advancement and in that sense could be considered a preparatory component of swing phase. Three functional tasks are achieved during these eight gait phases: weight acceptance in early stance, single limb support in mid- to late stance, and limb advancement during swing.

Functional Task 1: Weight Acceptance

IC and LR are the subphases of stance involved in the task of weight acceptance. Effective transfer of body weight onto the limb as soon as it contacts the ground requires initial limb stability and shock absorption and the preservation of forward momentum.

Initial Contact

IC is a single point in time, the instant that the foot of the leading lower limb touches the ground. Most motor function during IC is preparation for LR. At IC, the ankle is in neutral position, the knee is close to full extension, and the hip is flexed thirty degrees. The sagittal plane GRF vector lies posterior to the ankle joint, creating a plantar flexion moment (Figure 3-2). Eccentric contraction of the pretibial muscles (tibialis anterior and long toe extensors) holds the ankle and subtalar joint in neutral position. At the knee, the GRF vector is anterior to the joint axis, which creates a passive extensor torque. Muscle contraction activity of the quadriceps and hamstring muscle groups continues from the previous TSw to preserve the neutral position of the knee joint. A flexion moment is present around the hip joint, because the GRF vector falls anterior to the joint axis. Gluteus maximus and hamstring muscles are activated to restrain the resultant flexion torque.

Loading Response

LR occupies approximately 10% of the gait cycle and constitutes the period of initial double limb support. Two functional tasks occur during LR: (1) controlled descent of the foot toward the ground and (2) shock absorption as weight is transferred onto the stance limb (Figure 3-3). The momentum generated by the fall of body weight onto the stance limb is preserved by the *heel rocker* (first rocker) of the stance phase. Normal IC at the calcaneal tuberosity creates a fulcrum about which the foot and tibia move. The bony segment between this fulcrum and the center of the ankle rolls toward the ground as body weight is dropped onto the stance foot, preserving the momentum that is necessary for forward progression. Eccentric action of the pretibial muscles regulates the rate of ankle plantar flexion, and the quadriceps contract to limit knee flexion. The action of these two muscle groups provides controlled forward advancement of the lower extremity unit (foot, tibia, and femur). During the peak of LR, the magnitude of the vertical GRF exceeds body weight. To absorb the impact force of body weight and to preserve forward momentum, the knee flexes 15–18 degrees and the ankle plantar flexes to 10 degrees. The hip maintains its position of 30 degrees of flexion. Contraction of the gluteus maximus, hamstrings, and adductor magnus prevents further flexion of the hip joint.

Functional Task 2: Single Limb Support

Two phases are associated with single limb support: MSt and TSt. During this period the contralateral foot is in swing phase, and body weight is entirely supported on the stance limb. Forward progression of body weight over the stationary foot while maintaining stability must be accomplished during these two subphases of stance.

Midstance

MSt begins when the contralateral foot leaves the ground and continues as body weight travels along the length of the stance foot until it is aligned over the forefoot, approximately 20% of the gait cycle (Figure 3-4). This pivotal action of the *ankle rocker* (second rocker) advances the tibia over the stationary foot. Forward movement of the tibia over the foot is controlled by the eccentric contraction of the soleus, assisted by the gastrocnemius. During this phase, the ankle moves from its LR position of 10 degrees of plantar flexion to approximately 7 degrees of dorsiflexion. The knee extends from 15 degrees of flexion to a neutral position. The hip joint moves toward extension, from 30 to 10 degrees of flexion. With continued forward progression, the body weight vector moves anterior to the ankle, creating a dorsiflexion moment. Eccentric action of the plantar flexors is crucial in providing limb

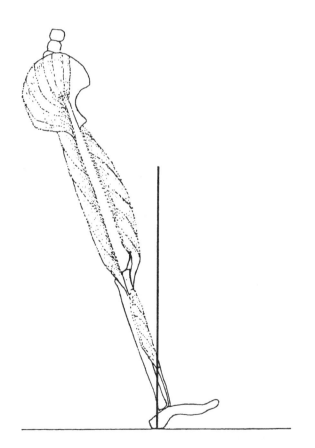

FIGURE 3-2

At initial contact, the ground reaction force (GRF) line is posterior to the ankle and anterior to the knee and hip with activation of pretibial, quadriceps, hamstring, and gluteal muscles. Note that the length of the GRF line represents its magnitude.

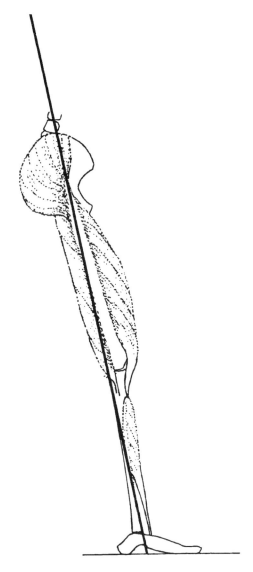

FIGURE 3-3

Loading response phase results in an increased magnitude of the vertical force, which ultimately exceeds body weight. Activity of the same muscle groups elicited at initial contact increases steadily as the vertical force increases.

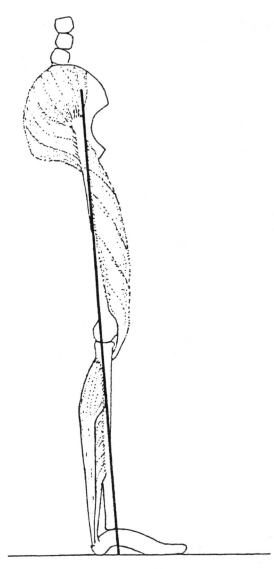

FIGURE 3-4

In early midstance, the vertical force begins to decrease and the triceps surae, quadriceps, and gluteus medius and maximus are active.

stability as the contralateral toe-off transfers body weight onto the stance foot. By the end of MSt, the vector moves anterior to the knee (creating passive stability of the limb) and posterior to the hip (reducing the demand on the hip extensors). The gluteus maximus, active in early MSt, yields to this passive hip extension as the hip nears vertical alignment over the femur. Vertical GRF is reduced in magnitude at MSt because of the upward momentum of the contralateral swing limb. In the coronal plane, activity of hip

abductors during MSt is essential to provide lateral hip stability and a level pelvis.

Terminal Stance

TSt, the second half of single limb support, begins with heel rise and ends when the contralateral foot contacts the ground. As the body vector approaches the metatarsophalangeal joint, the heel rises and the phalanx dorsiflexes (extends). The metatarsal heads serve as an axis of

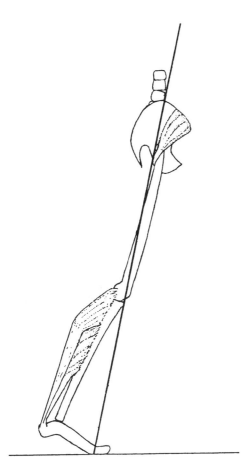

FIGURE 3-5
Terminal stance produces a second peak in vertical force, exceeding body weight, with high activity of the triceps surae, which maintain the third rocker. The tensor fascia lata restrains the increasing posterior hip vector.

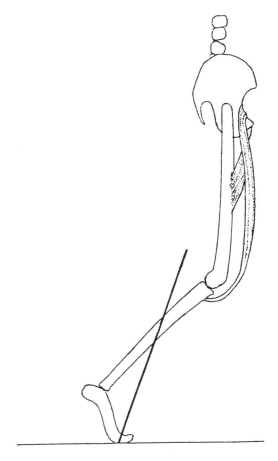

FIGURE 3-6
Contralateral loading results in limited muscle activity during preswing. The rectus femoris and adductor longus initiate hip flexion. Knee flexion is passive, resulting from the planted forefoot and mobile proximal segments.

rotation for body weight advancement (Figure 3-5). This is referred to as the *forefoot* or *toe rocker* (third rocker of gait). The forefoot rocker serves as an axis around which progression of the body vector advances beyond the area of foot support, creating the highest demand on calf muscles (gastrocnemius and soleus) of the entire gait cycle. During TSt, the ankle continues to dorsiflex until it reaches 10 degrees of dorsiflexion. The knee is fully extended, and the hip moves into slight hyperextension. Forward fall of the body moves the vector further anterior to the ankle, creating a large dorsiflexion moment. Stability of the tibia on the ankle is provided by the eccentric action of calf muscles. The trailing posture of the limb and the presence of the vector anterior to the knee and posterior to the hip provide passive stability at hip and knee joints. The tensor fascia lata serves to restrain the posterior vector at the hip. At the end of TSt, the vertical GRF reaches a sec-

ond peak greater than body weight, similar to that which occurred at the end of LR.

Functional Task 3: Limb Advancement

Four phases contribute to limb advancement: PSw, ISw, MSw, and TSw. During these phases the stance limb leaves the ground, advances forward, and prepares for the next IC.

Preswing

PSw, the second period of double limb support in gait, occupies the last 10% of the stance phase. It begins when the contralateral foot contacts the ground and ends with ipsilateral toe-off. During this period the stance limb is unloaded and body weight is transferred onto the contralateral limb (Figure 3-6). The ankle moves rapidly from its TSt position of dorsiflexion into 20 degrees of plantar

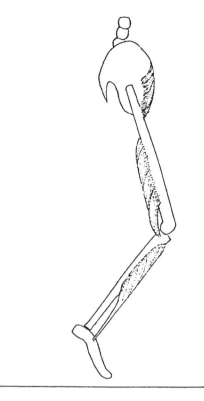

FIGURE 3-7
During initial swing, the pretibial muscles, short head of the biceps femoris, and iliacus are active in initiating limb advancement and providing swing clearance.

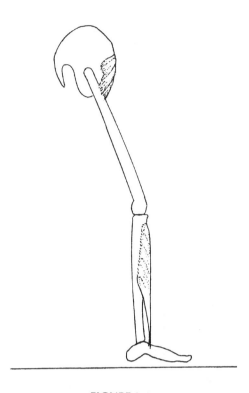

FIGURE 3-8
A vertical tibia signals the end of the period of midswing. Here contraction of the iliacus preserves hip flexion while pretibial muscle activity maintains foot clearance.

flexion. During this subphase, plantar flexor muscle activity decreases as the limb is unloaded. Toward the end of PSw, the vertical force is diminished such that plantar flexors are quiescent. There is no "push-off" in normal reciprocal free walk bipedal gait.[6] The knee also flexes rapidly to achieve 40 degrees of flexion by the end of PSw. The GRF vector is at the metatarsophalangeal joints and posterior to the knee, and the resultant knee flexion is mainly passive. Knee flexion during this phase prepares the limb for toe clearance in the swing phase. PSw hip flexion is initiated by the rectus femoris and the adductor longus, which also decelerates the passive abduction created by contralateral body weight transfer. The sagittal vector extends through the hip as the hip returns to a neutral posture.

Initial Swing
Approximately one-third of the swing period is spent in ISw. It begins the moment the foot leaves the ground and continues until maximum knee flexion occurs, when the swinging extremity is directly under the body (Figure 3-7). Concentric contraction of pretibial muscles begins to lift the foot toward dorsiflexion from its initial 20 degrees to 5 degrees of plantar flexion. This is necessary for foot clearance as the

swing phase begins. Knee flexion, resulting from action of the short head of the biceps femoris, also assists in toe clearance. The knee continues to flex until it reaches a position of 60 degrees of flexion. Contraction of the iliacus brings the hip into 20 degrees of flexion. Contraction of the gracilis and sartorius during this phase assists hip and knee flexion.

Midswing
During MSw, limb advancement and foot clearance continue. MSw begins at maximum knee flexion and ends when the tibia is vertical. Knee extension, coupled with ankle dorsiflexion, contributes to foot clearance while advancing the tibia (Figure 3-8). Continued concentric activity of pretibial muscles ensures foot clearance and moves the foot toward the neutral position. Momentum creates an extension moment, advancing the lower leg toward extension from 60 degrees to 30 degrees of flexion, with the quadriceps quiescent. Mild contraction of hip flexors continues to preserve the hip flexion position.

Terminal Swing
In the final phase, TSw, the knee extends fully in preparation for heel contact (Figure 3-9). Eccentric contraction of the hamstrings and gluteus maximus decelerates the

thigh and restrains further hip flexion. Activity of the pretibial muscles maintains the ankle at neutral to prepare for heel contact. In the second half of TSw, the quadriceps become active to facilitate full knee extension. Hip flexion remains at 30 degrees.

PATHOLOGIC GAIT DEVIATIONS

Clinicians often use qualitative descriptive terms to characterize the gait deviations and compensations of pathologic gait. Some of these terms help to identify specific primary problems. Others describe compensatory strategies used by patients to solve gait difficulties created by a variety of primary problems.

Trendelenburg's gait occurs in the stance phase, when the trunk leans to the same side as the hip pathology (ipsilateral lean). This is a compensatory strategy used when the gluteus medius and its synergists (gluteus minimus and tensor fascia lata) cannot stabilize the pelvis adequately during stance.[9] Normally, the drop of the contralateral pelvis is limited to 5 degrees by the strong response of the hip abductor musculature. To support the pelvis, the hip abductor muscles must generate a force that is 1.5 times the body weight.[10] A weak or absent gluteus medius leads to postural substitution of trunk lean over the weight-bearing hip joint. This reduces the external varus moment created by a GRF line that falls medial to the joint center. Without this postural compensation, clearance becomes a problem for the swinging contralateral limb. Rarely, Trendelenburg's gait is caused by overactive hip adductors (adductors longus, magnus, brevis, and gracilis).

The *circumduction gait* is a swing phase deviation in which hip abduction is combined with a wide arc of pelvic rotation. It occurs when there is a "relative" long swing limb and is often associated with inadequate knee flexion or poor hip flexion motor control. A plantar flexion contracture at the foot or a stiff knee or hip joint can contribute to circumduction. This combination of abduction and pelvic rotation can provide a compensatory method of the usual limb advancement process. The motion can be observed as a lateral arc of the foot in the transverse plane, which begins at the end of PSw and ends at IC on the same limb. The arc reaches the apex of its lateral movement at MSw. The typical pattern is a mixture of a wide base of support with the foot abnormally outset and may include an ipsilateral pelvic drop. It is possible for a contracture of the contralateral adductors to create this deviation by pulling the pelvis toward the contralateral femur and demanding a compensatory ipsilateral abducted position relative to the pelvis. A severe leg length discrepancy can result in an exaggerated pelvic tilt from the contralateral stance leg, which obligates the swing limb to an

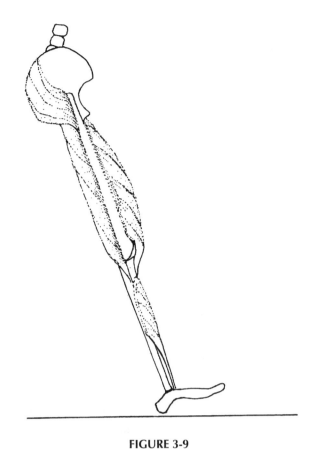

FIGURE 3-9
At terminal swing, the gluteus maximus, hamstrings, quadriceps, and pretibial muscles are active to prepare for limb placement and the ensuing loading response.

increased abduction position. Circumduction and abduction create a significant energy cost penalty, increasing lateral displacement of the center of gravity.

Vaulting is exaggerated heel elevation of the stance foot, sometimes in combination with increases in stance limb hip and knee extension, with the goal of raising the pelvis to clear the contralateral swing limb. It occurs when the functional length of the swing limb is relatively longer than that of the stance limb. It also occurs when swing limb advancement is impaired or delayed by inadequate motor control of hip or knee flexion, or both, or in the presence of a plantar flexion contracture of the swing leg. It may compensate for pelvic obliquity or leg length discrepancy.

Antalgic gait is a strategy used to avoid pain during walking. It is frequently seen at LR when the patient reduces single limb support time on the affected limb. If the pain occurs during a particular period in stance, that specific time period is diminished. Antalgic gait caused by pain that originates around the hip might translate into a lateral lean to permit the patient to get the center of gravity over the support point, the head of the femur. If the pain occurs during the extreme end range of a particular joint motion, that motion is diminished. For example, if full extension produces pain, the knee would be maintained in slight flexion throughout the gait cycle.

A variety of abnormal gait patterns are associated with abnormal muscle tone (spasticity, rigidity, hypotonicity) or muscle weakness. *Scissors gait* describes a pattern of poor control in limb advancement or tracking of the swing leg characterized by the crossing, or scissoring, of the lower limbs. It is common in spastic/paretic pathologies. *Steppage gait* occurs when weakness or paralysis of the dorsiflexor musculature demands exaggerated hip and knee flexion of the proximal joints to accomplish swing clearance. It is most easily observed in late MSt. In *crouch gait* exaggerated knee and hip flexion is exaggerated throughout the gait cycle. Crouch gait is often seen in combination with a toe-walking stance in spastic diplegic cerebral palsy. It has been attributed to a combination of overactivity of the hamstrings and weakness of calf muscles. Although use of an orthosis can successfully control abnormal motion in the sagittal plane (for example, in steppage gait), orthoses are less effective in controlling the abnormal transverse, rotational, and/or coronal limb placement problems observed in scissors or crouch gait. In *ataxic gait* there is a failure of coordination or irregularity of muscular action of the limb segments. It may be secondary to cerebellar dysfunction or loss of joint proprioception. Ataxia often becomes accentuated when the eyes are closed or vision is otherwise impaired.

METHODS OF QUANTITATIVE GAIT ANALYSIS

Quantitative analysis seeks to understand the process of walking with measurable parameters collected through instrumentation. Perhaps the potential to assess gait through quantified measurement emerged prehistorically with the sunrise to sunset movement of a lone traveler on foot or with the hailing chant of each advancing step of a marching army. Such basic techniques would have enabled measurement of walking velocity (distance traversed per unit of time) and cadence (steps per unit of time). Marks,[11] a New York City prosthetist, offered a more precise qualitative description of pathologic gait in 1905, when he described the gait process in eight organized phases and discussed the implications of prosthetic component design on the function of walking. Marks praised "kinetoscopic" photography as a potential diagnostic tool for optimizing pathologic gait. Today we record gait parameters with instruments as common as a stopwatch or as complex as

the simultaneous integration of three-dimensional kinematics, kinetics, and electromyographic (EMG) methods. The primary emphasis of clinical assessment has been on the use of accessible techniques and inexpensive technologies. A simple, inexpensive footprint mat has been used for decades to record barefoot plantar pressures. Individual or multiple mats can record step and stride length as well as walking base width for clinical use. A qualitative contribution has been made by video technology, particularly with slow-motion capabilities. Recent development of inexpensive video gait assessment software has clinical quantitative applications as well. The system measures joint angles in two dimensions. Because walking is a three-dimensional function, however, it may have limited value for comprehensive assessments and as a research tool.

Perhaps the best-kept secret in the energy cost arsenal is the physiologic cost index (PCI). It is easily calculated as follows:

$$PCI = \frac{(walking\ pulse - resting\ pulse)}{gait\ speed}$$

It is one of the most sensitive indicators of energy cost of gait. Winchester et al.,[12] who compared two different orthotic designs by measuring a wide variety of metabolic parameters, used the PCI to identify a statistically significant difference of the two devices when all other measured parameters failed to produce such differences. Pulse and respiratory rate taken at rest and after timed intervals during normal comfortable gait can also help assess exertion levels.

Technology in Gait Assessment

Perhaps the most user-friendly and economically accessible family of measurement tools with broad clinical application are the emerging pressure technologies. A thin plastic array can slip nearly unnoticed between the plantar surface of the foot and an orthosis or the insole of the shoe (Figure 3-10). This array, connected to a computer via a lead wire, can measure dynamic pressure patterns and record critical events throughout the walking cycle. A prosthetic version can provide pressure measurements at 60 individual sites within a socket and record those measurements during multiple events of the gait cycle. The clinical relevance lies in identifying critical gait events, temporal measurements, and skin-loading pressure patterns. Because of the ease in collection of temporal and plantar pressure readings and relatively modest cost, this approach may well replace microswitch technologies in the future and be increasingly accessible to therapists, prosthetists, and orthotists for clinical use.

The "high-tech" side of quantitative gait analysis has traversed a surprisingly long road. The birth of instrumented kinematic, EMG, and temporal performance analysis began in the 1870s with E. J. Marey, who first performed movement analysis of pathologic gait using photography.[13] He also developed the first myograph for measuring muscle activity and the first foot-switch collection system for measuring temporal (time-distance)-related gait events. The foot-switch system was an experimental shoe that measured the length and rapidity of the step and the pressure of the foot on the ground. Eadweard Muybridge,[14] working at Stanford University in the 1880s, used synchronized multiple camera photography with a scaled backdrop to capture on film and assess the motion of subjects walking. Other major advances into instrumented gait analysis were made by Scherb, who performed hand muscle palpation using a treadmill in 1920, and Adrian, who in 1925 advocated the use of EMG to study the dynamic action of muscles.[15] Modern gait technology began in 1945, when Inman and colleagues initiated the systematic collection of normal and amputee data in the outdoor gait laboratory at the University of California at Berkeley. Since then, researchers and clinicians have increasingly used the growing array of gait technologies to measure the parameters of human performance in normal and pathologic gait. A full-service gait laboratory gathers information on six performance parameters in walking: (1) temporal, (2) metabolic, (3) kinematic, (4) kinetic, (5) EMG, and (6) pressure.[16]

Temporal Data Collection

Temporal (time-distance) parameters enable the clinician to summarize the overall quality of a patient's gait. In the gait laboratory, temporal data can be collected with microswitch embedded pads taped to the bottom of a patient's shoes or feet that record the amount of time that the patient spends on various points of the sole over a measured distance. Stride length, velocity, cadence, percentage of the gait cycle spent in single and double limb support, and general stance progression patterns can be measured and assessed. Tendencies toward excessive inversion, eversion, or prolonged heel-only time can be noted and may suggest modifications to alignment or components of prostheses or orthoses to normalize such gait patterns. A temporal data collection system is particularly cost efficient, clinically meaningful, and affordable. Temporal data can be, and often are, part of another system such as EMG or motion analysis.

Metabolic Data Collection

Metabolic data reflect the physiologic "energy cost" of walking. The traditional measures of energy cost are oxygen consumption, total carbon dioxide generated, and

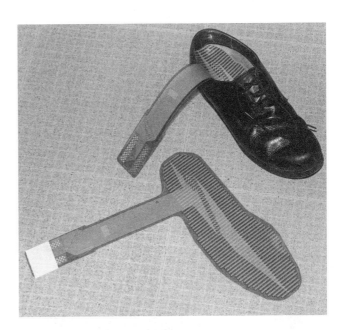

FIGURE 3-10

An in-shoe pressure-sensing array can help to identify areas of high pressure concentration. This information assists the design of an orthosis to modify pressure dynamics during the stance phase of gait.

heart rate. Other relevant factors include volume of air breathed and respiration rate. All of these parameters are viewed in terms of velocity and distance walked over the collection period. Historically, metabolic data were collected while the patient walked on a treadmill, wearing umbilical devices. In recent years, due to the known influence of treadmill collection in altering gait velocity from that of normal, energy cost data are more likely to be obtained on an open track of a measured distance with the patient ambulating in a free walk or natural cadence (Figure 3-11). The primary limitation of energy cost as an assessment tool is that, although it can inform the investigator about body metabolism relative to the patient's gait, it cannot explain why or how an advantage or disadvantage was obtained. Waters[17] demonstrated that an individual with Syme's level amputation uses less oxygen to traverse a given distance than someone with a transtibial amputation but could not explain why. For that explanation, other gait parameters must be examined. Energy cost measures cannot easily identify widely variant prosthetic foot designs worn by the same patient, whereas kinematic, kinetic, and EMG data typically can.[18]

Kinematic and Kinetic Systems

Most kinematic systems provide joint and body segment motion in graphic form. This information includes sagit-

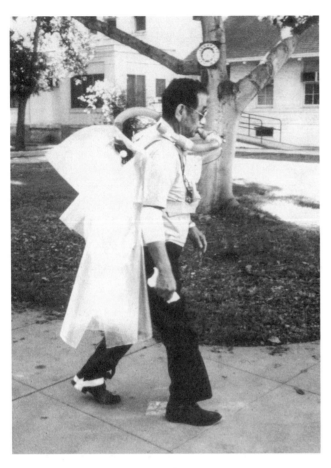

FIGURE 3-11

The Douglas bag method collects exhaled gases for later analysis as the patient walks in a circular walkway. Heart rate and other metabolic variables are monitored by radio telemetry.

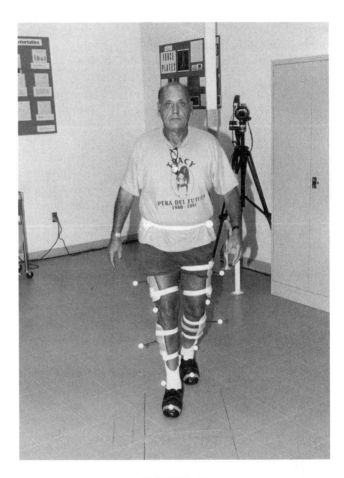

FIGURE 3-12

This patient is instrumented with reflective spheres. An infrared camera system can track limb segment motion as the patient walks across the field of view.

tal, coronal, and transverse motions that occur at the ankle, knee, hip, and pelvis. The patient is instrumented with reflective spheres that are placed on well-recognized anatomic landmarks (Figure 3-12). Typically, an infrared light source is positioned around each of several television cameras. This light is directed to the reflective spheres on the patient, which in turn are reflected into the cameras. Each field of video data is digitized, the markers are identified manually by an operator, and the coordinates of the geometric center of each marker are calculated. Resultant data are displayed as animated stick figures that represent the actual motions produced by the patient. The operator can freeze any frame and enlarge the image at any joint to examine gait patterns in greater depth. The operator can extract raw numbers that represent joint placement and motion in space or produce a printout showing joint motion in all planes plotted against the per-

centage of the gait cycle. Angular velocities, accelerations, and joint and segment linear displacements can be calculated. Data from other systems (force platforms and EMG) collected during the same time sequence as the motion data are often integrated with the kinematics.

Kinetic information is obtained from one or more force platforms, which collect data on vertical force, fore-aft shear, and mediolateral shear. The contribution of kinetic data can be profound. Fore-aft shear is very useful in establishing appropriate transtibial prosthetic alignment in the sagittal plane. For this purpose the analyst would anticipate a balanced magnitude and timing of the braking and propulsive patterns. Collection of data from two consecutive steps requires dual force plates. The typical force platform system can obtain power calculations or center of pressure graphs or can be combined with kinematic data to show joint moments. This is useful in measuring the dynamic joint control of an individual throughout stance. Some kinetic software offers specialized programs for specific purposes such as stability analysis, which provides information about center of gravity shift relative to time.

Electromyography

EMG data may be the single most important technology in terms of understanding the direct physiologic effect of gait variants. Patterns of muscle activity in patients with abnormal gait are compared to well-established norms. Knowledge of the timing and intensity of the muscle activity throughout the gait cycle may guide gait training, orthotic or prosthetic prescription, and dynamic orthotic or prosthetic alignment aimed at reduction of excessive, ill-timed, or prolonged muscle activity. EMG data are also helpful in guiding decisions about surgical intervention (dorsal rhizotomy, tendon lengthening, or osteotomy) in children with cerebral palsy.

Pressure Sensing Technology

Pressure sensing technologies offer the clinician tremendous insights into the treatment of patients at risk for amputation because of vascular disease and diabetic neuropathy and can assist vascular surgeons and orthopedic foot fellows in limb salvage through more appropriate custom-designed prophylactic orthoses. This area is one of the more recent and clinically promising technologies for the assessment team.

Over the last several decades, technologies have significantly improved understanding of pathologic gait, offered strong evidence for the efficacy of various treatment approaches, and enhanced patient care. Advocates of a more universal application of the high-end technologies in the clinical setting have yet to make a compelling case, particularly in the current climate of cost containment. Perhaps the strongest argument for gait technology in our present era lies in its use for outcome measurement in the justification of legitimate therapeutic treatment approaches as well as orthotic and prosthetic applications.

QUALITATIVE GAIT-BASED ASSESSMENT

Qualitative methods for identification and recording of gait deviation have played a role in patient care for decades. In 1925, Robinson[19] described 11 pathologic gait patterns and attempted to correlate them with specific disease processes. In 1937, Boorstein[20] identified 14 disease processes that could be diagnosed with the help of gait assessment. He described seven major gait deficit groups, attributing the term *steppage gait* to the French

physician Charcot and the identification of *waddling gait* in hip dysplasia to Hippocrates.[20] In the late 1950s, Blair Hangar, the founder of Northwestern University's School of Prosthetics and Orthotics, and Hildegard Myers, a physical therapist at Rehabilitation Institute of Chicago, collaborated to develop the first comprehensive system of clinical gait analysis for persons with transfemoral amputation. They identified 16 gait deviations and suggested numerous patient and prosthetic causes for each. Their work, developed into an educational film and handbook in 1960, has been a model for subsequent instructional videos and assessment systems in prosthetics (Hangar HB. Personal conversation, July 1996).[21] Brunnstrom's[22] comprehensive gait analysis form for hemiplegic gait, published in 1970, is a checklist of 28 deviations seen at the ankle, knee, and hip that are common after stroke.

Early work in observational gait analysis received a significant impetus from Dr. Jacquelin Perry[23] as an outgrowth of basic research data published in 1967. In the late 1960s, Dr. Perry and a group of physical therapists from the Rancho Los Amigos Medical Center Physical Therapy Department developed an organized format for systematically applied observational gait analysis. Initially, their work focused on the development of an in-house training program for students and personnel who were new to the rehabilitation hospital. The first Normal and Pathological Gait Syllabus was published by the Professional Staff Association of Rancho Los Amigos Hospital in 1977.[7] Subsequent revisions have included additional basic gait data and gait interpretation. This syllabus uses parameters of normal gait as a comparative standard for abnormal or pathologic gait. It focuses on identifying gait deviations that affect the three functional tasks of walking: (1) weight acceptance, (2) single limb support, and (3) swing limb advancement. A form listing the most commonly occurring gait deviations in each subphase of gait is used to record any observed gait deviations that interfere with these functional tasks (Figure 3-13). Problems in each of the six major body segments are noted with a check in one of the boxes, beginning with the toes, then the ankle, knee, hip, pelvis, and trunk. This format allows the clinician to consider systematically the following questions:

- Are the toes up, inadequately extended, or clawed?
- Is there forefoot-only contact (toe walking), foot-flat contact, foot slap, excess plantar flexion, or dorsiflexion? Is heel off, foot drag, or contralateral vaulting present?
- Is knee flexion adequate, absent, limited, or excessive? Is extension inadequate? Does the knee wobble, hyper-

Gait Analysis: Full Body

Rancho Los Amigos Medical Center
Physical Therapy Department

Reference Limb:
L ☐   R ☐

☐ Major Deviation
▓ Minor Deviation

		Weight Accept		Single Limb Support		Swing Limb Advancement			
		IC	LR	MSt	TSt	PSw	ISw	MSw	TSw
Trunk	Lean: B/F								
	Lateral Lean: R/L								
	Rotates: B/F								
Pelvis	Hikes								
	Tilt: P/A								
	Lacks Forward Rotation								
	Lacks Backward Rotation								
	Excess Forward Rotation								
	Excess Backward Rotation								
	Ipsilateral Drop								
	Contralateral Drop								
Hip	Flexion: Limited								
	Excess								
	Inadequate Extension								
	Past Retract								
	Rotation: IR/ER								
	Ad/Abduction: Ad/Ab								
Knee	Flexion: Limited								
	Excess								
	Inadequate Extension								
	Wobbles								
	Hyperextends								
	Extension Thrust								
	Varus/Valgus: Vr/Vl								
	Excess Contralateral Flex								
Ankle	Forefoot Contact								
	Foot-Flat Contact								
	Foot Slap								
	Excess Plantar Flexion								
	Excess Dorsiflexion								
	Inversion/Eversion: Iv/Ev								
	Heel Off								
	No Heel Off								
	Drag								
	Contralateral Vaulting								
Toes	Up								
	Inadequate Extension								
	Clawed								

MAJOR PROBLEMS:

Weight Acceptance

Single Limb Support

Swing Limb Advancement

Excessive UE Weight Bearing ☐

Name _____

Diagnosis _____

© 1996 LAREI, Rancho Los Amigos Medical Center, Downey, CA 90242 extend, or produce an extension thrust (recurvatam)? Is varum or valgum present, or is excessive contralateral flexion seen?

- Is hip flexion adequate, absent, limited, or excessive? Is adequate extension seen? Is retraction of the thigh during TSw from a previously attained degree of flexion seen? Can internal or external rotation, abduction, or adduction be observed?
- Does the pelvis hike? Does it tilt anteriorly or posteriorly? Is forward or backward rotation seen? Does it drop to the ipsilateral or contralateral side?
- Does the trunk lean or rotate backward or forward? Does it lean laterally to the right or left?

Qualitative gait assessment is an important component of preorthotic assessment, because it assists the clinician in identifying the functional task and the subphase of gait that is problematic and can be addressed with orthotic intervention. Similarly, findings of observational gait analysis can identify the need for adjustment of prosthetic alignment.

FUNCTION-BASED ASSESSMENT

Holden et al.[24] suggest that gait performance goals for patients with neurologic impairments are best measured against values from impaired rather than healthy subjects. Treatment goals are adjusted for the individual patient's diagnosis, etiologic factor, ambulation aid, and functional category. In separate studies, Brandstater et al.[25] and Holden et al.[24] found that patients with the greatest number of gait deviations did not have the lowest temporal gait values. A great deal of energy is often expended by physical therapists, prosthetists, and orthotists in an attempt to achieve gait patterns of "optimal quality." Holden suggests that hard-won qualitative gait improvements may bring with them secondary losses in time-distance parameters, such as slower velocity and reduced step length. The fundamental issue is whether temporal gait efficiency or cosmesis should be the preferred goal. Certainly, in cases in which patients are nominal walkers and in which therapy, surgery, and orthotics or prosthetics have been maximized, general gait efficiency is far more important than reduction in compensatory gait deficits.

In the past, symmetry and reciprocity have been significant treatment goals. Wall and Ashburn[26] maintain that "an ideal objective in the functional rehabilitation of hemiplegia is the reduction of the asymmetrical nature of movement patterns." Measuring pathologic gait against normal gait values is a useful means of providing an overall clinical picture. In setting treatment goals, however, measuring a patient's performance against that patient's own best possible outcome is more reasonable. How does one anticipate a given patient's best possible outcome? This requires collection of accurate data to establish pre- and post-treatment profiles for a wide variety of involvement levels within each pathology. Olney and Richards[27] suggest that large groups of instrumented studies be undertaken to identify clusters of biomechanical features associated with functional performance during walking.

Time-distance parameters have enormous potential for setting outcome goals. Variations in time-distance values are often pathology specific. Asymmetries in hemiplegia, for example, are obviously greater than in most other types of pathologies. Variables that are reported to affect temporal measurements in normal healthy subjects include age, sex, height, orthotic use, or type of assistive device. Brandstater et al.[25] and Holden et al.,[24] in separate studies of pathologic patients, found no significant difference in temporal performance based on sex or age.

Corcoran et al.[28] measured temporal parameters of subjects with hemiplegia under two gait conditions: with and without their ankle-foot orthosis (AFO). Patients with hemiplegia had significantly faster gait velocity when wearing their orthosis than when walking without it.[28] A similar study of healthy unimpaired subjects wearing an AFO found reduced step length. Apparently subjects without central nervous system pathology altered their movement strategy to decrease movements at the knee in an effort to minimize shearing forces in the AFO.[29] Reduced step length can minimize force exerted by the brace along the posterior aspect of the calf band.[30]

Holden et al.[24] suggest that grouping subjects by motor ability or functional category is more important than grouping by other means. They have developed the Massachusetts General Hospital (MGH) functional ambulation classification system.[24] Six functional categories are defined in their system: A score of (1) indicates nonfunc-

◄ **FIGURE 3-13**

The Rancho gait analysis system seeks to identify and record any observable activity that interferes with the three functional tasks of walking: weight acceptance, single limb support, and swing limb advancement. (Reprinted with permission from Los Amigos Research and Education Institute, Rancho Los Amigos Medical Center. Observational Gait Analysis Handbook. Downey, CA: Los Amigos Research and Education Institute, Rancho Los Amigos Medical Center, 1989;55.)

tional ambulation. Patients who require the assistance of another for support and balance are scored with a (2). A score of (3) indicates that light touch assistance is required, and (4) means that the patient needs verbal cueing or occasional safety assistance. To be scored as a (5), the patient must be independent in ambulation on level surfaces, and (6) means that the patient is independent in ambulation on all surfaces, including stairs and inclines. This is a function-based assessment index that does not rely on instrumentation or specialized training for categorization.

It is important to recognize similarities and differences in purpose and design of the various gait assessment methods. The gait-based methods, such as the Rancho observational gait assessment, seek to identify and differentiate pathologic versus compensatory mechanisms and, therefore, guide the specific surgical, therapeutic, orthotic, or prosthetic interventions for a particular patient. Functional indices, such as the MGH functional ambulation classification system, may be a means of evaluating treatment efficacy. The cost of gait assessment through comprehensive instrumented procedures often precludes its general use in the clinical arena. Observational analysis through gait-based assessment will remain a viable and important contribution to clinical care for many years to come.

CLINICAL EXAMPLES OF GAIT DEFICIENCIES: IMPACT OF FUNCTIONAL TASKS DURING GAIT

Several clinical examples of gait deficiencies have been selected to illustrate some of the more common pathology-based variants in gait performance: (1) pretibial flaccid paralysis, (2) hemiplegia, (3) cerebral palsy, and (4) spina bifida. As might be expected, each example demonstrates common gait characteristics specific to its particular pathology while at the same time presenting variants from that profile. The discussion is based on information gathered by foot-switch stride, kinematic, and observational gait analysis.

Case Study: A Patient with Flaccid Paralysis of Pretibial Muscles

A patient with a diagnosis of inherited sensorimotor neuropathy is evaluated. Examination of muscle function and strength reveals relatively symmetric distal impairment. Manual muscle test scores include "trace" activity of dorsiflexion muscles bilaterally, "poor" plantar flexion on the left, and "fair+" plantar flexion on the right. Knee and hip strength is "normal." For foot-switch stride analysis, the patient walks without his usual orthoses. In the trailing

left limb, the posterior compartment fails to support the forefoot lever arm so that the tibia progresses forward with limited heel off in late stance. This creates excessive knee flexion and limits the step length of the contralateral limb. The net effect of this inadequate forefoot rocker is a reduction in velocity. Lack of support of the trailing forefoot allows depression of the center of gravity. At the same time, dorsiflexion weakness on the right creates early, abrupt plantar flexion (foot slap) with premature contact of the first metatarsal. The variance between plantar flexor strength of the left and right limbs is demonstrated by difference in single limb support times. The stronger right calf participated in 39.8% (0.416 seconds) of the gait cycle, whereas the weaker left calf committed itself to only 31.4% (0.328 seconds). This subtle timing discrepancy in gait was not readily identifiable in observational analysis. In right MSw, while the left foot is in supporting posture, the classic steppage gait characteristics of a flail forefoot are seen. Compensatory swing clearance is accomplished through excessive hip and knee flexion. When the patient wears his orthosis (a dorsiflexion assist thermoplastic AFO on the right and a dorsiflexion stop–plantar flexion resist thermoplastic AFO on the left) results of foot-switch temporal analysis are quite different. Velocity, cadence, and stride length increase slightly. The asymmetry between right and left single limb support times decreases because the AFO provides external support of the trailing left limb. The energy-inefficient steppage gait and unsightly foot slap are diminished as well.

Clinical Characteristics of Gait in Hemiplegia

For most patients who are recovering from stroke (cerebrovascular accident [CVA]), improvement in the quality of gait is related to the natural history of the pathologic process and the impact of gait retraining in rehabilitation. In the week immediately after CVA, only 24–38% of patients are able to ambulate independently.[31] After weeks of rehabilitation, more than 50% are able to walk without assistance, especially if using an appropriate AFO and assistive device.[32] At the 6-month mark, more than 80% of patients with CVA are functionally independent in ambulation.[33]

The many variations of limb control observed during the gait of patients who are recovering from a CVA can be explained by one or more of the following factors: primitive locomotor patterns, impaired postural responses, abnormal postural tone with various degrees of spasticity and rigidity, inappropriately timed muscle contractions, and diminished muscle strength. One of the primary determinants of gait dysfunction in post-CVA hemiplegia is whether the patient has some degree of selective control of specific muscles rather than activation of abnormal synergy patterns (mass flexion or extension). Patients with hemiplegia often have difficulty grading the magnitude of a particular muscle contraction with respect to other muscle contractions. Because of hyperactivity of muscle spindle/stretch reflex in the presence of spasticity, the ability to move toward dorsiflexion with forward progression of the tibia during stance may be counteracted by contraction of plantar flexors into a position of equinus. Spasticity, although difficult to measure, can be described for clinical purposes using the Ashworth Spasticity Scale.[34] The baseline level 0 indicates no measurable tone. A designation of level 1, mild tone, is given when a muscle "catches" with an abrupt passive movement into flexion or extension. A level 2 designation indicates marked abnormal tone but flexible range of motion, and level 3 is characterized by pronounced tone and difficult passive movement. Level 4 denotes a limb that is held rigidly in either flexion or extension.

The orthotic goal for patients with hypertonicity of the lower extremity after a CVA is to control ankle motion and preposition for tibial advancement. Two orthotic strategies are commonly used: (1) provision of an AFO with a locked ankle component set in slight dorsiflexion or (2) use of an articulated AFO that allows slight ankle motion around the neutral position. When ankle joint motion is limited or blocked by an orthosis, stability in stance improves; however, forward progression of the tibia is compromised, and step length is reduced. Modifications to the shoe, such as application of a rocker bottom sole or elevation of the heel, can compensate by mimicking the second rocker of gait.

Over the course of rehabilitation, the patient with hemiplegia often experiences changes in tone, joint flexibility, pain or discomfort, fear or confidence, motor strength or weakness, and quality of proprioception. Six stages of motor recovery in hemiplegia have been identified by Brunnstrom.[35] In the first stage, no voluntary movement of limbs is present. In the second, movement reappears but is limited by pronounced muscle weakness or spasticity, or both. The patient is usually not yet ready for functional ambulation. In the third stage, spasticity coexists with limb synergy motion. Typically a mass extensor pattern is seen in the lower limb. As the patient continues to improve in the fourth stage, spasticity may be reduced as the patient begins to be able to move out of stereotypical synergy patterns. In stage 5, selective control outside mass synergy patterns becomes more consistent and more functional. With recovery complete, in stage 6, the patient may achieve coordinated controlled movement. Because of the dynamic nature of the recovery process, the ability to adjust or alter orthotic alignment or characteristics is very desirable. It is not unusual that an orthosis prescribed early in rehabilitation becomes inappropriate or creates further gait dysfunction at a later stage. Once rehabilitation is complete and the patient has achieved stability in walking patterns, definitive biomechanical needs are identified, and the adjustability of the orthosis is less important.

The extension synergy pattern places the lower extremity in excessive extension at the hip and knee and the foot in equinovarus. This reduces the amount of knee flexion and dorsiflexion during swing, necessitating a compensatory strategy, such as circumduction, to provide swing phase clearance.[36] The rigidity of the ankle leaves the patient with inadequate dorsiflexion mobility as well as vastly reduced plantar flexion excursion during PSw and early swing. Stance time is considerably reduced on the hemiplegic/paretic side, and the quadriceps, gastrocnemius, gluteus maximus, and semitendinous muscles are inappropriately active throughout stance.[37] The activity of most lower limb muscle groups on the hemiplegic/paretic side is increased compared to normal patterns of muscle activation. Excessive hip flexion at MSt on the hemiplegic/paretic side shifts the GRF line anteriorly, producing a knee extension moment that interferes with forward progression. The hemiplegic/paretic side also displays less hip adduction in single limb support, which compromises lateral shift toward the affected side.[37] Brandstater et al.[25] describe reduced velocity, cadence, stride length, and single limb support time on the affected side, with consequent increased single limb support and reduced step length on the sound side. Hirschberg and Nathanson[37] demonstrated that an appropriate AFO improves the quality of gait by increasing step length and stance time as well as reducing swing time of the affected side. Velocity of gait improves when the AFO is placed in slight dorsiflexion. When spasticity is not problematic, an AFO that permits some plantar flexion normalizes IC to LR timing and prevents an unstable knee flexion moment in early stance. Because knee extensor strength often equals or exceeds hip extensor strength after CVA, most patients with hemiplegia can be managed effectively with an AFO rather than a knee-anklefoot orthosis.[38] Muscle strengthening is less important in achieving improved walking characteristics in hemiplegia than is the retraining of normal movement patterns in gait.[39]

Case Study: A Patient with Hemiplegia

A patient is referred to the gait laboratory for evaluation 13 months after a CVA damaged the sensorimotor cortex of the left hemisphere. Currently, he is a community ambulator (MGH functional ambulation classification level 6) who walks with the aid of an AFO and quad cane. In the clinical examination, his spasticity becomes apparent when his ankle moves toward a neutral position (Ashworth spasticity scale level 3). The orthosis he received early in rehabilitation, and continues to use, is locked in slight plantar flexion. Although this ankle angle delays tibial advancement and forward progression in stance, the patient has come to rely on its contribution to stability at proximal joints.

The patient's gait with the AFO is evaluated by foot-switch testing. Extensor synergy patterns contribute to function by providing a degree of stability in stance but also reduce efficiency of gait by limiting normal stance progression beginning with the first rocker period (Figure 3-14A). Duration heel-only time of the first rocker (IC to the foot-flat position at the end of LR) is approximately one-sixth of a second on the hemiplegic side, significantly less than normal heel-only time. Heel-only time on the intact side is roughly three times greater than that on the hemiplegic side. Forward progression during MSt is halted at the second rocker when spasticity prevents the necessary dorsiflexion of the ankle (Figure 3-14B). As the patient moves into TSt, when metatarsophalangeal break (concurrent with heel off) should allow progression onto the forefoot, the third rocker is also relatively blocked. This lack of mobility of the metatarsophalangeal joints and inadequate third rocker results in a loss of knee flexion, necessary for an effective PSw, for which the patient is unable to compensate. Of the 60 degrees of knee flexion that is necessary for the swing phase clearance, 35 degrees should be achieved passively during PSw. For patients with hemiplegia, the loss of this positional flexion is an additional challenge to clearance, beyond that produced by the equinus position of the ankle. Any attempts to compensate by "hip hiking" are likely to be inefficient and unsuccessful. These rocker limitations reduce step length of the sound side, leading to premature double limb support. The corresponding MSw knee flexion on the hemiplegic side is also reduced. The patient demonstrates a much reduced stance time on the affected side (62% gait cycle) versus the sound side (71% gait cycle) and a reduced single limb support time on the affected side (28% gait cycle) versus the sound side (38% gait cycle).

Clinical Characteristics of Gait in Patients with Spastic Diplegic Cerebral Palsy

Children with spastic diplegic cerebral palsy often have significant spasticity as well as marked weakness of the antigravity muscles in both lower extremities. This combination is a precursor of joint contracture. The clinical term often used to describe the typical gait of a patient with diplegia is *crouch gait*: Marked internal rotation of the femur and tibia occurs throughout the gait cycle, the knees remain in flexion throughout stance, and the ankles remain in plantar flexion during stance (toe walking) and

swing. Gage[40] clearly documented the high energy cost of flexed knee gait. The pathologic combination of an equinus ankle, positive Trendelenburg's hip, and stiff knee gait often produces various combinations of compensatory hiking of the pelvis, external rotation of the foot, and circumduction of the swing limb. This pattern has been attributed to tightness and overactivity of the distal hamstrings, alone or in combination with the hip flexors.[41] Some patients with diplegia ambulate using a "jump gait" pattern, using somewhat less hip and knee flexion than do patients with crouch gait but with prolonged ankle dorsiflexion rather than plantar flexion. Jump gait is often a postoperative manifestation of bilateral tendo Achillis lengthening without concurrent release of hip and knee contractures. Common compensatory strategies in jump gait include vaulting and circumduction. In crouch and jump gait, the GRF line falls progressively behind the knee joint center during single limb support of the stance phase. This creates an excessive demand on the quadriceps for stance phase stability. One surgical strategy that is used to correct jump gait combines hip flexion releases, hip flexion release lengthening of the distal hamstrings, and correction of external rotation. Postoperatively, the patient is fitted for floor reaction AFOs.[42] Ideally, the Achilles tendon is lengthened to neutral dorsiflexion position and the patient protected in AFOs for 1 year postoperatively. The scissoring pattern, which is also a common gait deviation in children with diplegia, is aggravated by spastic hip flexors and adductors, as the widened base of support reduces the efficiency of their line of pull. Orthotic solutions provide limited assistance in limb tracking and rotational control. Those that attempt to control rotation must cross the hip joint, adding significant weight and bulk, as well as increasing difficulty in donning and doffing.

Case Study: A Patient with Spastic Diplegic Cerebral Palsy

A 10-year-old with spastic diplegic cerebral palsy is referred to the gait laboratory for evaluation to assist his orthopedist in deciding whether corrective surgery is indicated. The boy currently ambulates independently, without assistive devices, wearing bilateral AFOs. A typical crouch gait pattern is observed during observational gait analysis. Foot-switch analysis confirms diminished heel contact with no heel-only time on the left and no heel contact at all on the right. Clinical examination reveals a combination of overactive hamstrings and weak gastrocnemius and soleus (Figure 3-15A). The flexion of hips and knees increases the need for proximal stabilization, resulting in compensatory hyperextension of the trunk and posterior arm placement

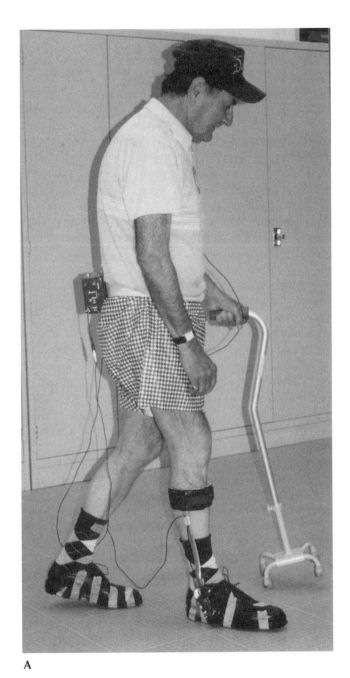
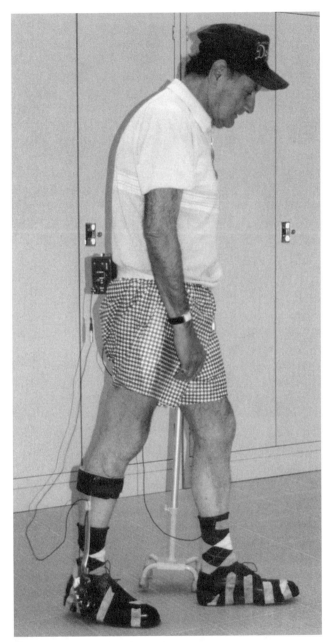

A   B

FIGURE 3-14

*In this patient with hemiplegia after CVA, the first rocker from initial contact to foot flat (**A**) is abrupt as a result of extensor patterns and limb rigidity. Extensor pattern at the ankle (**B**) translates into a failure to yield into dorsiflexion toward the end of the second rocker. Third rocker heel elevation will also be reduced, and lack of mobility reduces the step length of the contralateral limb.*

(Figure 3-15B). Because the ankles are held in equinus, the final rocker propels tibial advancement, despite limitation in ankle mobility. The patient spends most of the stance phase in TSt and PSw; consequently, double limb support time is vastly increased. This patient has not had surgical release of gastrocnemius. Even with surgery, impairment of motor control may continue to be problematic, so that dorsiflexion may not work in concert with the knee flex-

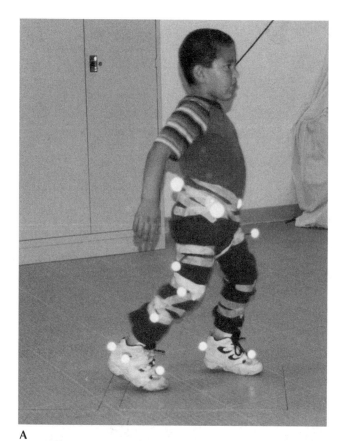 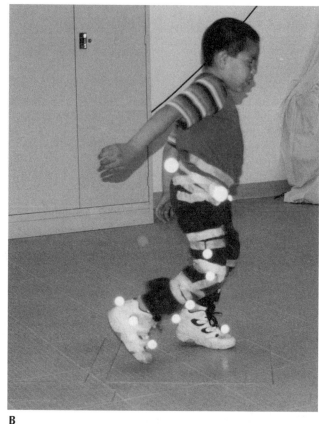

A   B

FIGURE 3-15

*In children with spastic diplegia, classic crouch gait (**A**) is characterized by increased hip and knee flexion in combination with toe walking. Postural substitutions in crouch gait (**B**) may include increased lumbar lordosis, trunk extension, and posterior arm placement.*

ion to provide a heel-toe gait pattern. Gastrocnemius release without concurrent releases of the hip and knee contractures usually leads to short step lengths with a compensatory increase in cadence. Spastic hip flexors, also serving as adductors, create a mild scissors effect during each swing limb advancement. Ambulation with bilateral AFOs, which the patient prefers, increases step length and reduces knee flexion compared to ambulation with no orthosis.

Clinical Characteristics of Gait in Children with Spina Bifida

Spina bifida (myelomeningocele) occurs when vertebral arches fail to unite early in gestation. Clinically, this leads to partial or complete paralysis at or below the level involved. The most common impairment is a flaccid paralysis, with loss of proprioception and exteroception (pain, temperature sensation, light touch, and pressure

sensation). Many children with spina bifida have significant ambulatory deficiencies; more than 50% require an orthosis of some kind to ambulate.[43] Assessment for orthotic support begins as soon as the child attempts to gain an erect posture. Severity of gait dysfunction is dependent on the level of involvement of the spinal cord. When the L-5 and S-1 nerve roots are affected, the gluteus maximus, hip abductors, and triceps surae are lost, the hamstrings are present but weak, and sensory loss is limited to the plantar surface of the feet. The plantar flexor deficit requires setting limits to dorsiflexion range of motion through orthotic joint control. This limitation of dorsiflexion allows the patient to establish hip stability through extension accomplished with trunk lordosis. Without it, the patient would fall forward unopposed. Lateral stability is achieved through crutches and a wide walking base. When the L-3 and L-4 root nerves are affected, hamstring function, hip extension, knee flexion, plantar flexion, and dorsiflexion are completely lost.

The resulting footdrop cannot be adequately compensated for in swing by knee flexion. Hip flexion, adduction, and knee extension are intact but may be weak. At the L-3 level weak knee flexion from the gracilis may also be present. These children benefit early from standing frames; later, they often are able to ambulate with orthotic assistance. Adequate stabilization of the foot and ankle is achieved through orthotic application of a locked ankle in neutral or slight dorsiflexion. Trunk lordosis is a compensatory strategy that is used to stabilize the hip during stance. The muscular imbalance at the hip increases the likelihood of flexion contracture, which, in turn, amplifies the need for even more compensatory lordosis. Extreme hip flexion contracture may ultimately preclude ambulation. If contractures at the hip, knee, and ankle are minimal and the child gains trunk control, he or she will be able to stand erect but will rely on trunk alignment for static balance and forearm crutches for further stability. A child with lesions that involve L-1 and L-2 levels has little lower limb function other than weak hip flexors. These children often begin upright function with a parapodium or swivel walker and can later progress to a reciprocal gait orthosis. The swing-through gait with bilateral hip-knee-ankle-foot orthoses has been shown to be less efficient than a reciprocal gait orthosis for thoracic level spina bifida.[44]

Case Study: A Child with Spina Bifida

An active 9-year-old with myelomeningocele at L-5 returns to the gait laboratory as part of an ongoing research study to document changes in gait characteristics over time. He currently ambulates wearing bilateral AFOs set in a neutral ankle position, using Loftstrand crutches in a four-point reciprocal gait pattern. Comparative foot-switch testing reveals that, without crutches, stride length and velocity are reduced. External rotation of both limbs is present throughout the gait cycle. With or without crutches, he has no measurable fifth metatarsal or toe contact on either limb in his typical stance phase weight-bearing patterns. Passive external rotation is present at the hip as well as abducted limb placement as he advances over the forefoot. His abducted limb placement and wide-based gait provide increased stability at a cost of excessive loading on the posteromedial aspect of the feet. Like many children with spina bifida, he spends excessive time in heel contact, largely to the exclusion of lateral forefoot weight bearing. This loading and shear pattern often leads to callusing and eventual neuropathic breakdown in adult life. His fastest gait velocity (55 m/min) is approximately 60% of normal free gait velocity. During swing phase, external rota-

tion of the limb is marked. The flail foot is held in slight dorsiflexion during TSw through the support of the AFO.

CONCLUSION

These clinical examples of gait deficiencies have demonstrated some of the complexity and variety that challenge the clinician daily. Each patient presents unique combinations of pathologic and compensatory deficits. A combination of simple quantitative measure (cadence and velocity, step length, stride length and width, and double support time), systematic qualitative gait analysis (Rancho Los Amigos observational gait assessment protocol), functional measures of energy cost (PCI), and level of assistance (MGH functional ambulation profile) are essential clinical tools. They help the clinician to differentiate primary pathologies from secondary compensations, guide orthotic prescription and therapeutic intervention, and assess efficacy of treatment. Instrumented gait assessment is an important part of preoperative assessment and research in orthotic and prosthetic design. In addition, the data collected in gait laboratories are building a database that can provide information necessary to build accurate outcome estimations for many groups of patients. The current challenge is for the clinic team to gain the broadest possible knowledge base in analytical gait assessment and to serve the patient as a team, considering each patient as an individual.

Acknowledgments
The authors express grateful appreciation to Sue Rouleau, P.T., and the Physical Therapy Department of Rancho Los Amigos Medical Center for assistance in identifying patient models and to Jacquelin Perry, M.D., and Los Amigos Research and Education Institute for permission to duplicate the Rancho full-body gait analysis form.

REFERENCES

1. Shastri JL (ed). Hymns of the Rig Veda. Griffith RTH (trans). Varanasi, India: Motilal Banarsidas, 1976;72–80.
2. McMahon TA. Muscles, Reflexes, and Locomotion. Princeton, NJ: Princeton University Press, 1984;168–171.
3. Finley FR, Cody K, Finizie R. Locomotive patterns in elderly women. Arch Phys Med Rehabil 1969;50(3):140–146.
4. Saunders JB, Inman VT, Eberhart HD. The major determinants in normal and pathological gait. J Bone Joint Surg 1953;35A:543–558.
5. Inman V, Ralston HJ, Todd F. Human Walking. Baltimore: Williams & Wilkins, 1981;1–128.
6. Perry J. Gait Analysis; Normal and Pathological Function. Thorofare, NJ: Slack, 1992;2–128.

7. Los Amigos Research and Education Institute. Observational Gait Analysis Handbook. Downey, CA: Professional Staff Association, Rancho Los Amigos Medical Center, 1989;1–55.

8. Perry J. Integrated Function of the Lower Extremity including Gait Analysis. In RL Cruess, WA Rennie (eds), Adult Orthopedics. New York: Churchill Livingstone, 1984;1161–1207.

9. Winter DA. Energy generation and absorption at the ankle and knee during fast, natural, and slow cadences. Clin Orthoped 1983;May(174);147–154.

10. Merchant AC. Hip abductor muscle force. An experimental study of the influence of hip position with particular reference to rotation. J Bone Joint Surg 1965;47A;462–476.

11. Marks AA. Manual of Artificial Limbs. New York: AA Marks, 1905;17–20.

12. Winchester PK, Carollo JJ, Parekh RN, et al. A comparison of paraplegic gait performance using two types of reciprocating gait orthoses. Prosthet Orthot Int 1993;17(2):101–106.

13. Braun M. Picturing Time, Work of Etienne-Jules Marey, 1830–1904. Chicago: University of Chicago Press, 1995;24–84.

14. Muybridge E. Muybridge's Complete Human and Animal Locomotion. New York: Dover, 1887;20–78.

15. Sutherland DH. Historical perspective of gait analysis (lecture handouts). Interpretation of Gait Analysis Data, Oct 17, 1994;1–2.

16. Ayyappa E. Gait lab technology: measuring the steps of progress. Orthot Prosthet Almanac 1996;45(2);28–56.

17. Waters RL. Energy Expenditure. In J Perry (ed), Gait Analysis. Thorofare, NJ: Slack, 1992;443–489.

18. Torburn L, Perry J, Ayyappa E, Shanfield S. Below-knee amputee gait with dynamic elastic response prosthetic feet: a pilot study. J Rehab Res Dev 1990;27(4):369–384.

19. Robinson GW. A study of gaits. J Kans Med Soc 1925; 25(12);402–406.

20. Boorstein SW. Abnormal gaits as a guide in diagnosis. Hebrew Physician 1937;1:221–227.

21. Northwestern University Prosthetic Orthotic Center. Gait Analysis Instructional Film. Chicago: Northwestern University Prosthetic Orthotic Center, 1960. (Handbook published by Ideal Picture Co, Chicago.)

22. Brunnstrom S. Movement Therapy in Hemiplegia; Neurophysiological Approach. New York: Harper & Row, 1970;103.

23. Perry J. The mechanics of walking: a clinical interpretation. Phys Ther 1967;47(9):777–801.

24. Holden MK, Maureen K, Gill KM, Magliozzi MR. Gait assessment for neurologically impaired patients; standards for outcome assessment. Phys Ther 1986;66(10):1530–1539.

25. Brandstater M, deBruin H, Gowland C. Hemiplegic gait: analysis of temporal values. Arch Phys Med Rehabil 1983; 64(12):583–587.

26. Wall JC, Ashburn A. Assessment of gait disabilities in hemiplegics: hemiplegic gait. Scand J Rehabil Med 1979;11(3): 95–103.

27. Olney SJ, Richards C. Hemiparetic gait following stroke. Part 1: Characteristics. Gait & Posture 1996;4:136–148.

28. Corcoran PJ, Jebsen RH, Brengelmann GL. Effects of plastic and metal leg braces on the speed and energy cost of hemiparetic ambulation. Arch Phys Med Rehabil 1970;51(2): 69–77.

29. Lehmann JF, Condon SM, Price R, deLateur BJ. Gait abnormalities in hemiplegia: their correction by ankle-foot orthoses. Arch Phys Med Rehabil 1987;68(11):763–771.

30. Lee K, Johnston R. Effect of below-knee bracing on knee movement: biomechanical analysis. Arch Phys Med Rehabil 1974;55(4):179–182.

31. von Schroeder HP, Coutts RD, Lyden PD, Billings E Jr. Gait parameters following stroke: a practical assessment. J Rehabil Res Dev 1995;32(1):25–31.

32. Burdett RG, Borello, France D, et al. Gait comparison of subjects with hemiplegia walking unbraced, with ankle foot orthosis, and with air-stirrup brace. Phys Ther 1988;68(8): 1197–1203.

33. Wade DT, Wood VA, Helleer A, et al. Walking after stroke: measurement and recovery over the first 3 months. Scand J Rehabil Med 1987;19(1):25–30.

34. Ashworth B. Preliminary trial of carisoprodol in multiple sclerosis. Practitioner 1964;192(4):540–542.

35. Brunnstrom S. Movement Therapy in Hemiplegia; Neurophysiological Approach. New York: Harper & Row, 1970;34–55.

36. Lehmann JF, Warren CG, Hertling D, McGee M. Craig-Scott orthosis: a biomechanical and functional evaluation. Arch Phys Med Rehabil 1976;57(9):438–442.

37. Hirschberg GG, Nathanson K. Electromyographic recording of muscular activity in normal and spastic gaits. Arch Phys Med Rehabil 1952;33:217.

38. Perry J. Lower extremity bracing in hemiplegia. Clin Orthop 1969;63(4):32–38.

39. Bobath K. The facilitation of normal postural reactions and movements in the treatment of cerebral palsy. Physiotherapy 1964;50:246.

40. Gage JR. Gait Analysis in Cerebral Palsy. New York: Cambridge University Press, 1991.

41. Ounpuu S, Muik E, Davis RB, et al. Rectus femoris surgery in children with cerebral palsy. Part 1: The effect of rectus femoris transfer location on knee motion. J Pediatr Orthop 1993;13(3):325–330.

42. Sutherland DH. Common gait abnormalities of the knee in cerebral palsy. Clin Orthop 1993;March(288):139–147.

43. Knutsson E, Richards C. Different types of disturbed motor control in gait of hemiparetic patients. Brain 1979;102(2):405–430.

44. Mazur JM, Sienko-Thomas S, Wright N, Cummings RJ. Swing-through versus reciprocating gait patterns in patients with thoracic-level spina bifida. Zeitschrift fur Kinderchirurgie 1990;1(12):23–25.

4

Exercise, Energy Cost, and Aging in Orthotic and Prosthetic Rehabilitation

Jessie M. VanSwearingen and Michelle M. Lusardi

Most individuals who use orthotic or prosthetic devices have impairments of the musculoskeletal or neuromuscular systems that limit the efficiency of their movement and increase the energy cost of their daily and leisure activities. The separate and interactive effects of aging, inactivity, and/or cardiac or pulmonary disease can further compromise the capacity for muscular "work," tolerance of activity, and ability to function. Consider the case of a 79-year-old woman with insulin-controlled type II diabetes referred for physical therapy evaluation after transfemoral amputation following a failed femoropopliteal bypass who has been on bed rest for several weeks because of her multiple surgeries. The physical effort required by rehabilitation and prosthetic training may initially feel overwhelming to this patient. Preprosthetic ambulation with a walker is likely to increase heart rate (HR) quickly to or above the upper limits of a safe target HR for aerobic training in patients who have become deconditioned by prolonged inactivity. It is important for the physical therapist, orthotist, and prosthetist to recognize factors that can be successfully modified to enhance performance and activity tolerance when making decisions about prescription and intervention strategies. It is also important that aerobic fitness be a key component of the rehabilitation program of patients who are using a prosthesis or orthosis for the first time. Finally, it is important that rehabilitation professionals recognize and respond to the warning signs of significant cardiopulmonary dysfunction during treatment and training sessions.

This chapter has four objectives:

1. To provide a functional view of the cardiopulmonary system and define the key components of cardiopulmonary function and energy expenditure
2. To review the age-related changes in cardiopulmonary function in the older adult and their functional consequences

3. To provide an overview of cardiopulmonary conditioning principles that are useful in treatment planning for older and/or deconditioned patients
4. To explore the energy costs of orthotic and prosthetic use, as they are related to cardiopulmonary function and its impact on rehabilitation outcome

Although the anatomic and physiologic changes in the aging cardiopulmonary system are important to our discussion, our focus is on the contribution of cellular and tissue-level changes to performance of the cardiopulmonary system. This functional view provides a conceptual framework for answering four essential questions: Can the patient do physical work? If so, what is the energy cost of doing this work? Is it possible to become more efficient or more able to do physical work? What impact does the use of an orthosis or prosthesis have on energy use and cost during functional activities?

OXYGEN TRANSPORT SYSTEM

The foundation for the functional view of the cardiopulmonary system is the equation for the oxygen transport system (Figure 4-1). Aerobic capacity (Vo_2max) is the body's ability to deliver and use oxygen (maximum rate of oxygen consumption) to support the energy needs of demanding physical activity. Vo_2max is influenced by three factors: the efficiency of ventilation and oxygenation in the lungs, how much oxygen-rich blood can be delivered from the heart (cardiac output, or CO) to active peripheral tissues, and how well oxygen is extracted from the blood to support muscle contraction and other peripheral tissues during activity (arterial-venous oxygen difference, or AVo_2diff).[1,2] Aerobic capacity can be represented by the formula:

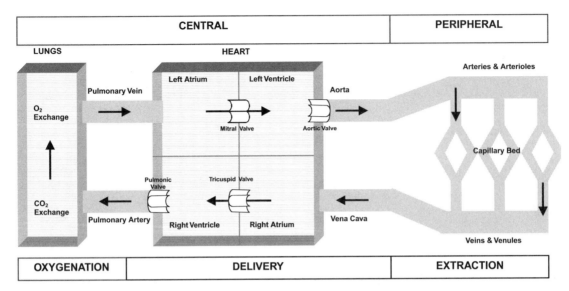

$$\text{Work capacity: } \text{V}_{\text{O}_2}\text{max} = \text{CO} \times \text{AV}_{\text{O}_2}\text{diff}$$
$$(\text{HR} \times \text{SV}) \times (\text{C}_\text{a}\text{O}_2 - \text{C}_\text{v}\text{O}_2)$$

FIGURE 4-1

Functional anatomy and physiology of the cardiorespiratory system. After blood is oxygenated in the lungs, the left side of the heart contracts to deliver blood, through the aorta and its branches, to active tissues in the periphery. Oxygen must be effectively extracted from blood by peripheral tissues to support their activity. Deoxygenated blood, high in carbon dioxide, returns through the vena cava to the right side of the heart, which pumps it to the lungs for reoxygenation. Aerobic capacity (V$_{O_2}$max) is the product of how well oxygen is delivered to cardiac output (CO) and extracted by arterial-venous oxygen difference (AV$_{O_2}$diff) active tissues. (HR = heart rate; SV = stroke volume.)

$$\text{V}_{\text{O}_2}\text{max} = \text{CO} \times \text{AV}_{\text{O}_2}\text{diff}$$

The energy cost of doing work is based on the amount of oxygen consumed for the activity, regardless of whether the activity is supported by aerobic (with oxygen) or anaerobic (without oxygen) metabolic mechanisms for producing energy. V$_{O_2}$max provides an indication of the maximum amount of work that can be supported.[1,2]

CO is the product of two elements: the HR; the number of times that the heart contracts, or beats per minute (bpm); and the stroke volume (SV), the amount of blood pumped from the left ventricle with each beat (measured in milliliters or liters).[1,3] Cardiac output is expressed by the formula:

$$\text{CO} = \text{HR} \times \text{SV}$$

As a product of HR and SV, CO is influenced by four factors: the amount of blood returned from the periphery through the vena cava, the ability of the heart to match its rate of contraction to physiologic demand, the efficiency or forcefulness of the heart's contraction, and the ability of the aorta to deliver blood to peripheral vessels. The delivery of oxygen to the body tissues to be used to produce energy for work is, ultimately, a function of the central components of the cardiopulmonary system.[1]

The second determinant of aerobic capacity, the AV$_{O_2}$diff, reflects the extraction of oxygen from the capillary by the surrounding tissues. The AV$_{O_2}$diff is determined by subtracting the oxygen concentration on the venous (postextraction) side of the capillary bed (C$_v$O$_2$) from that of the arteriole (pre-extraction) side of the capillary bed (C$_a$O$_2$), according to the formula

$$\text{AV}_{\text{O}_2}\text{diff} = \text{C}_\text{a}\text{O}_2 - \text{C}_\text{v}\text{O}_2$$

The smaller vessels and capillaries of the cardiovascular system are involved in the process of the extraction of oxygen from the blood by the active tissues. The extraction of oxygen from the blood to be used to produce energy for the work of the active tissues is a function of the peripheral components of the cardiopulmonary system.[1]

During exercise or a physically demanding activity, CO must increase to meet the need for additional oxygen in the more active peripheral tissues. This increased CO is a result of a more rapid HR and a greater SV: As the return of blood to the heart increases, the heart contracts more forcefully, and a larger volume of blood is pumped into the aorta by the left ventricle. Chemical and hormonal changes that accompany exercise enhance peripheral shunting of blood to the active muscles, and oxygen depletion in muscle facilitates transfer of oxygen from the capillary blood to the tissue at work.[1,3,4]

The efficiency of central components, primarily of CO, accounts for as much as 75% of VO_2max. Peripheral oxygen extraction (AVO_2diff) contributes the remaining 25% to the process of making oxygen available to support tissue work.[5] In healthy adults, under most bodily conditions, more oxygen is delivered to active tissues (muscle mass) than is needed.[1,5] For patients who are significantly deconditioned or who have cardiopulmonary or cardiovascular disease, the ability to deliver oxygen efficiently to the periphery as physical activity increases may be compromised. With normal aging, there are age-related physiologic changes in the heart itself that limit maximum attainable HR. Because of these changes, it is important to assess whether and to what degree SV can be increased effectively if rehabilitation interventions are to be successful.

AGE-RELATED CHANGES IN HEART STRUCTURE

With advanced age, some cellular and tissue changes and some physiologic changes in the cardiovascular system become apparent. However, clearly identifying how many of the changes are due to aging, are related to cardiovascular disease, or are due to the influence of a habitually sedentary lifestyle is difficult, especially with a high incidence of cardiovascular disease among older adults. Review of the research literature suggests that age-related structural changes in the cardiovascular system occur in five areas: the myocardium, the cardiac valves, the coronary arteries, the conduction system, and the coronary vasculature (i.e., arteries).[6-9]

Cells of the myocardium of advanced age show microscopic signs of degeneration, including the accumulation of lipid deposits and lipofuscin.[9,10] Unless excessive, such deposits have not been associated with abnormalities of heart function.[8,10] Minimal atrophy of cardiac muscle cells has been observed. In contrast, the left ventricular myocardium frequently hypertrophies, increasing the diameter of the left atrium. These changes are associated with an increase in the weight and size of the heart.[11-13] Thickening of the left ventricle and widening of the left atrium have been attributed to cardiac tissue responses to an increased systolic blood pressure (SBP) and to reduced compliance of the left ventricle.[14,15]

The four valves of the aged heart often become fibrous and thickened at their margins, as well as somewhat calcified. Calcification of the aorta at the base of the cusps of the aortic valve (aortic stenosis) is clinically associated with the slowed exit of blood from the left ventricle into the aorta.[6-8,16] Such aortic stenosis contributes to a functional reduction in CO. A baroreflex mediated increase in SBP attempts to compensate for this reduced CO.[8] Over time, the larger residual of blood in the left ventricle after each beat (increased end systolic volume, ESV) eventually weakens the left ventricular muscle.[17] The weakened left ventricular muscle must work harder to pump the blood out of the ventricle into a more resistant peripheral vascular system.[6,8,9]

Calcification of the annulus of the mitral valve can restrict blood flow from the left atrium into the left ventricle during diastole.[6] As a result, end diastolic volume (EDV) of blood in the left ventricle is decreased because the left atrium does not completely empty. Over time, this residual blood in the left atrium elongates the muscle of the atrial walls and increases the diameter of the atrium of the aged heart.[6,8,14]

Age-related changes of the coronary arteries are similar to those in any aged arterial vessel: an increase in thickness of vessel walls and tortuosity in its path.[8,9] These changes tend to occur earlier in the left coronary artery than in the right.[6,7] When coupled with atherosclerosis, these changes may compromise the muscular contraction and pumping efficiency and effectiveness of the left ventricle during exercise or activity of high physiologic demand.

Age-related changes in the conduction system of the heart also have substantial impact on cardiac function.[6,8] The typical 75-year-old has less than 10% of the original number of pacemaker cells of the sinoatrial node.[6,18] Fibrous tissue builds within the internodal tracts as well as the atrioventricular node, including the bundle of His and its main bundle branches. As a consequence, the exquisite ability of the heart to coordinate the actions of all four chambers of the heart may be compromised.[6,8,9]

Age-related changes in the arterial vascular tree, demonstrated most notably by the thoracic aorta and eventually the more distal vessels, disrupt the smooth flow of blood from the heart toward the periphery. Arterial vessels become less effective in transporting blood to the periphery.[8,9] As the endothelial cells of the intima (inner layer, vessel lining) become less parallel to the longitudinal axis of the vessel, blood flow becomes turbulent. Deposits of collagen and lipid, as well as fragmentation of elastic fibers in the intima and media (middle layer) of larger arterioles and arteries, further compromise the functionally important "rebound" characteristic of arterial vessels.[9] Rebound normally facilitates directional blood flow through the system, preventing the backward reflection of fluid pressure waves of blood.[8] A critical outcome of this loss of elasticity is an increased vulnerability of the aorta, which, distended and stiffened, cannot effectively resist the tensile force of left ventricular ejection.[8,9] Not surprisingly, the incidence of abdominal aortic aneurysms rises sharply among older adults.

AGE-RELATED CHANGES IN THE PHYSIOLOGY OF THE HEART

Compared to the structural changes, the physiologic changes in the cardiovascular system are few; however, their impact on performance of the older adult can be substantial. The nondiseased aging heart continues to be a good pump, maintaining its ability to develop effective tension (myocardial contractility). The response of cardiac muscle to calcium (Ca^{++}) is preserved and its force-generating capacity maintained.[8,9] Two aspects of myocardial contractility do, however, change with aging: the rate of tension development in the myocardium slows, and the duration of contraction and relaxation is prolonged.[6,8,9]

One of the most marked aging changes in cardiovascular function is the reduced sensitivity of the heart to sympathetic stimulation, specifically to the stimulation of beta-adrenergic receptors.[8,9,19] Age-related reduction in beta-adrenergic sensitivity includes a decreased response to norepinephrine and epinephrine released from sympathetic nerve endings in the heart, as well as a decreased sensitivity to any of these catecholamines circulating in the blood.[19,20] Normally, norepinephrine and epinephrine are potent stimulators of ventricular contraction. An important functional consequence of the change in receptor sensitivity is less efficient cardioacceleratory response, which leads to a lower HR at submaximal and maximal levels of exercise or activity.[6,8,9] The time for HR rise to the peak rate is prolonged, so that more time is needed to reach the appropriate HR level for physically demanding activities. A further consequence of this reduced beta-adrenergic sensitivity is less than optimal vasodilation of the coronary arteries with increasing activity.[19,21] In peripheral arterial vessels, beta-adrenergic receptors do not appear to play a primary role in mediating peripheral vasodilation in the working muscles.[22]

Age-related change in the cardiovascular baroreceptor reflex also contributes to prolongation of cardiovascular response time in the face of an increase in activity (physiologic demand).[9,21] The baroreceptors in the proximal aorta appear to become less sensitive to changes in blood volume (pressure) within the vessel. Normally, any drop in proximal aortic pressure triggers the hypothalamus to begin a sequence of events that leads to increased sympathetic stimulation of the heart. Decreased baroreceptor responsiveness may increase an elderly patient's suscep-

tibility to orthostatic (postural) and postprandial (after eating) hypotension or compromise their tolerance of the physiologic stress of a Valsalva maneuver associated with breath holding during strenuous activity.[9,19,21] Clinically, this is evidenced by lightheadedness when rising from lying or sitting, especially after a meal, or if one has a tendency to hold one's breath during effortful activity.

The consequences of age-related physiologic changes on the cardiovascular system can often be managed effectively by routinely using simple lower extremity warm-up exercises before position changes. Several repetitions of ankle and knee exercises before standing up, especially after a prolonged time sitting (including for meals) or lying down (after a night's rest), help to maximize blood return to the heart, facilitating cardiovascular function for the impending demand. In addition, taking a bit more time in initiating and progressing difficulty of activities may help the slowed cardiovascular response time to reach an effective level of performance. Scheduling physical therapy or physical activity for times more remote from mealtimes might also be beneficial for patients who are particularly vulnerable to postprandial hypotension.

FUNCTIONAL CONSEQUENCES OF CARDIOVASCULAR AGING

What are the functional consequences of cardiovascular aging for older adults participating in exercise or rehabilitation activities? This question can best be answered by focusing on what happens to the CO. The age-related structural and physiologic changes in the cardiovascular system give rise to two loading conditions that influence CO: cardiac filling (preload) and vascular impedance (afterload).[9]

Cardiac filling/preload determines the volume of blood in the left ventricle at the end of diastole. The most effective ventricular filling occurs when pressure is low within the heart and relaxation of the muscular walls of the ventricle is maximal.[9] Mitral valve calcification, decreased compliance of the left ventricle, and the prolonged relaxation of myocardial contraction can contribute to a less effective filling of the left ventricle in early diastole. Doppler studies of the flow of blood into the left ventricle in aging adults demonstrate decreased rates of early filling, an increased rate of late atrial filling, and an overall decrease in the peak filling rate.[6,23] When compared to healthy 45- to 50-year-old adults, the early diastolic filling of a healthy 65- to 80-year-old is 50% less.[6,23] This reduced volume of blood in the ventricle at the end of diastole does not effectively stretch the ventricular muscle of the heart, compromising the Frank-Starling mechanism and the myocontractility of the left ventricle.[24] The functional outcome of decreased early diastolic filling and the reduced EDV is a comparative decrease in SV, one of the determinants of CO and, subsequently, work capacity (VO_2max).[6,8,17]

High vascular impedance and increased afterload can disrupt the flow of blood as it leaves the heart toward the peripheral vasculature. Increased afterload is, in part, a function of age-related stiffness of the proximal aorta, an increase in systemic vascular resistance (elevation of SBP, hypertension), or a combination of both of these factors.[8,9] Ventricular contraction that forces blood flow into a resistant peripheral vascular system produces pressure waves in the blood. These pressure waves reflect back toward the heart, unrestricted by the stiffened walls of the proximal aorta.[8] The reflected pressure waves, aortic stiffness, and increased systemic vascular resistance collectively contribute to an increased afterload in the aging heart.[6] Increased afterload is thought to be a major factor in the age-associated decrease in maximum SV, hypertrophy of the left ventricle, and prolongation of myocardial relaxation (e.g., slowed relaxation in the presence of a persisting load on the heart).[6,9]

An unfortunate long-term consequence of increased afterload is weakening of the heart muscle itself, particularly of the left ventricle. Restricted blood flow out of the heart results in a large residual volume (RV) of blood in the heart at the end of systole when ventricular contraction is complete. Large ESVs gradually increase the resting length of the ventricular cardiac muscle, effectively weakening the force of contraction.[8,9,19,25]

Left ventricular ejection fraction (LVEF) is the proportion of the blood pumped out of the heart with each contraction of the left ventricle, which is expressed by the equation

$$LVEF = \frac{EDV - ESV}{EDV}$$

At rest, the LVEF does not appear to be reduced in older adults. Under conditions of maximum exercise, however, the rise in LVEF is much less than in younger adults.[17,26] This reduced rise in the LVEF with maximal exercise clearly illustrates the impact that preload and afterload functional cardiovascular age-related changes have on performance. A substantial reduction in EDV, an expansion of ESV, or a more modest change in both components could account for the decreased LVEF of the exercising older adult as follows:

$$\downarrow EDV = \downarrow LVEF$$

$$\uparrow ESV = \downarrow LVEF$$

When going from resting to maximal exercise conditions, the amount of blood pumped with each beat for young healthy adults increases to 20–30% from a resting LVEF of 55% to an exercise LVEF of 80%. For a healthy older adult, in contrast, LVEF typically increases less than 5% from rest to maximal exercise.[17,26] The LVEF may actually decrease in the majority of adults who are older than 60 years of age.[26] As LVEF and CO decrease with aging, so does the ability to work over prolonged periods (functional cardiopulmonary reserve capacity) because the volume of blood delivered to active tissue decreases (Figure 4-2). Functional reserve capacity is further compromised by the long-term effects of inactivity and by cardiopulmonary pathology. The contribution of habitual exercise to achieving effective maximum exercise LVEF is not well understood but may be important: Rodeheffer et al.[17] report that the decline in maximum exercise LVEF may not be as substantial for highly fit older adults.

PULMONARY FUNCTION IN LATER LIFE

Several important age-related structural changes of the lungs have a significant impact on pulmonary function.[27] The production of elastin, which is the major protein component of the structure of the lungs, decreases markedly in late life. The elastic fibers of the lung become fragmented, and functionally, the passive elastic recoil or rebound, which is so important for expiration, becomes much less efficient. The elastic fibers that maintain the structure of the walls of the alveoli also decrease in number. This loss of elastin means loss of alveoli and consequently less surface area for the exchange of oxygen. The deficits in elastic recoil and alveolar surface area for oxygen exchange may be further compounded by increased stiffness (loss of flexibility) of the thoracic rib cage, which houses the lungs. Although the stiffened rib cage may be as much a consequence of a sedentary lifestyle as age alone, lack of flexibility compromises inspiration and offers no assistance or compensation for the decrease in the elastic recoil of the expiratory phase.[27] With less recoil for expiration, and reduced flexibility for inspiration, the ability to work is compromised in two ways (Figure 4-3). First, vital capacity (VC), the maximum amount of air that can be voluntarily moved in and out of the lungs with a breath, is decreased by 40–50%. Second, RV, the air remaining in the lungs after a forced expiration, is increased by 30–50%. This combination of reduced movement of air with each breath and increased air remaining in the lung between breaths leads to higher lung-air carbon dioxide content and, eventually, lower oxygen saturation of the blood after air exchange. The increase in RV also has an impact on the muscles of inspiration: The dome of the diaphragm flattens, and the accessory respiratory mus-

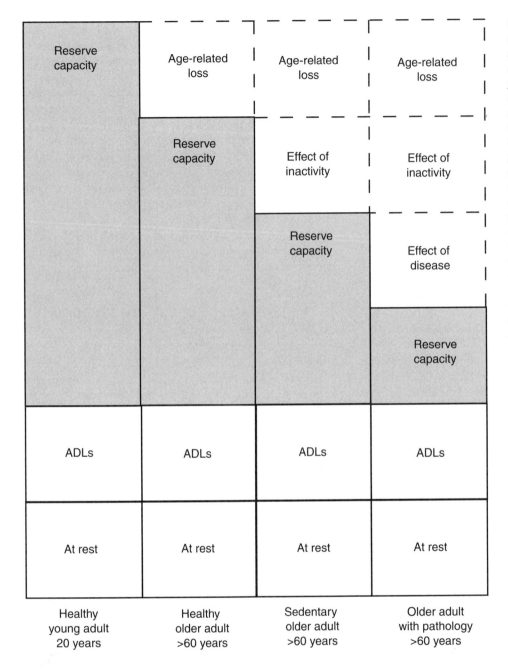

FIGURE 4-2
Comparison of the effects of aging, inactivity, and cardiopulmonary disease on functional reserve capacity, expressed as cardiac output (CO; liters per minute). At rest, the heart delivers between 4 and 6 liters of blood per minute to peripheral tissues. This may double during many activities of daily living (ADLs). In a healthy young person, the CO may increase to as much as 24 liters per minute to meet metabolic demands of sustained exercise. This reserve capacity decreases to approximately 18 liters per minute in healthy fit elders after the age of 60. A sedentary lifestyle decreases functional reserve capacity further. Superimposed cardiopulmonary disease further limits the ability to do physical work, in some cases approaching or exceeding cardiopulmonary reserve capacity. (Adapted from SC Irwin, CC Zadai. Cardiopulmonary Rehabilitation of the Geriatric Patient. In CB Lewis [ed], Aging the Health Care Challenge. Philadelphia: Davis, 1990;190.)

cles are elongated. As a result of these length changes, the respiratory muscles work in a mechanically disadvantageous range of the length-tension curve, and the energy cost of the muscular work of breathing rises.[27]

Functionally, the amount of air inhaled per minute (minute ventilation) is a product of the frequency of breathing times the tidal volume (volume of air moving into and out of the lungs with each, usual breath). In healthy individuals, the increased ventilatory needs of low-intensity activities are usually met by an increased depth of breathing (i.e., increased tidal volume).[1,27] Frequency of breathing increases when increased depth alone cannot meet the demands of activity, typically when tidal volume reaches 50–60% of the VC.[28] For the older adult with reduced VC who is involved in physical activity, tidal volume quickly exceeds this level so that frequency of breathing increases much earlier than would be demonstrated by a young adult at the same intensity of exercise.[27] Because the energy cost of breathing rises sharply with the greater respiratory muscle work associated with an increased respira-

A: Lung Volumes in Young Adults

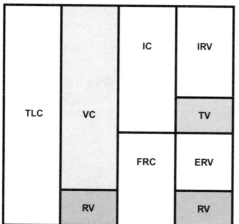

B. Lung Volumes in Older Adults

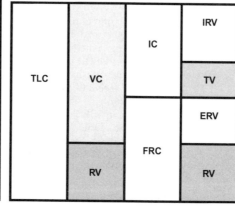

FIGURE 4-3

Changes in the distribution of air within the lungs (volume) have an impact on an older adult's efficiency of physical work. Loss of alveoli and increasing stiffness of the rib cage result in a 30–50% increase in residual volume (RV) and a 40–50% decrease in vital capacity (VC). VC includes three components: Inspiratory reserve volume (IRV) and expiratory reserve volume (ERV) tend to decrease with aging, whereas resting tidal volume (TV), the amount of air in a normal resting breath, tends to be stable over time. Total lung capacity (TLC) and inspiratory capacity (IC) tend also to decrease, whereas functional residual capacity (FRC) increases. Over time, the physiologic consequences of these changes make the older adult more vulnerable to dyspnea (shortness of breath) during exercise and physically demanding activity.

tory rate, an important consequence of increased frequency of breathing is fatigue.[29] This early reliance on an increased frequency of breathing, combined with a large RV and its higher carbon dioxide concentration in lung air, results in a physiologic cycle that further drives the need to breathe more often. Overworked respiratory muscles are forced to rely on anaerobic metabolism to supply their energy need, resulting in a buildup of lactic acid. Because lactic acid lowers the pH of the tissues (acidosis), it is also a potent physiologic stimulus for increased frequency of breathing.[29-31] The older person can be easily forced into a condition of rapid, shallow breathing (shortness of breath) to meet the ventilatory requirements of seemingly moderate-intensity exercise.

IMPLICATIONS FOR INTERVENTION

Two questions come to mind in considering implications of changes in the aged cardiopulmonary system and an older person's ability to do physical work. First, what precautions should be observed to avoid cardiopulmonary complications? Second, what can be done to optimize cardiopulmonary function for maximal physical performance?

Precautions

Because of the combined effects of the age-related changes in the cardiovascular and cardiopulmonary systems, the high incidence of cardiac and pulmonary pathologies in later life, and the deconditioning impact of bed rest and inactivity, older patients who require orthotic or prosthetic intervention may be vulnerable if exercise or activity is too physiologically demanding. Although most older adults are able to tolerate and respond positively to exercise, exercise is not appropriate in a number of circumstances (Table 4-1).

Estimating Workload: Heart Rate and Rate Pressure Product

One of the readily measurable consequences of the reduced response of the heart to sympathetic stimulation in later life is a reduction in the maximal attainable HR.[6,8,32] This reduction in maximal HR also signals that an older person's HR reserve, the difference between the rate for any given level of activity and the maximal attainable HR, is limited as well. This means that, for older patients involved in rehabilitation programs, the distance between resting and maximal HR is narrowed. One method of estimating maximal (max) attainable HR is

TABLE 4-1
Signs and Symptoms of Exercise Intolerance

Category	Cautionary Signs/Symptoms	Contraindications to Exercise
Heart rate	< 40 bpm at rest	Prolonged at maximum in activity
	> 130 bpm at rest	
	Little HR increase with activity	
	Excessive HR increase with activity	
	Frequent arrhythmia	Prolonged arrhythmia or tachycardia
ECG	Any recent ECG abnormalities	Exercise-induced ECG abnormalities
		Third-degree heart block
Blood pressure	Resting SBP > 180 mm Hg	Resting SBP > 200 mm Hg
	Resting DBP > 100 mm Hg	Resting DBP > 110 mm Hg
	Lack of SBP response to activity	Drop in SBP > 20 mm Hg in exercise
	Excessive BP response to activity	Drop in DBP during exercise
Angina	Low threshold for angina	Prolonged/intense angina in activity
		New jaw, shoulder, or left arm pain
Respiratory rate	Dyspnea > 35 breaths/min	Dyspnea > 45 breaths/min
Blood gas values	O_2 saturation < 90%	O_2 saturation < 86%
Other symptoms	Mild to moderate claudication	Severe, persistent claudication
	Onset of pallor	Cyanosis, severe pallor, or cold sweat
	Facial expression of distress	Facial expression of severe distress
	Lightheadedness or mild dizziness	Moderate to severe dizziness, syncope
	Postactivity fatigue > 1 hr	Nausea, vomiting
	Slow recovery from activity	Onset of ataxia, incoordination
		Increasing mental confusion
Acute illness	Fever > 100°F	< 2 days after myocardial infarction
		< 2 days after pulmonary embolism
	Recent mental confusion	Acute thrombophlebitis
	Abnormal electrolytes (potassium)	Acute hypoglycemia
		Digoxin toxicity

bpm = beats per minute; DBP = diastolic blood pressure; ECG = electrocardiogram; HR = heart rate; SBP = systolic blood pressure.
Source: Adapted from EA Hillegass, HS Sadowsky. Essentials of Cardiopulmonary Physical Therapy. Philadelphia: Saunders, 1994;166; and J Watchie. Cardiopulmonary Physical Therapy: A Clinical Manual. Philadelphia: Saunders, 1995;16.

$$Max\ HR = 220 - age$$

For healthy individuals, the recommended target HR for aerobic conditioning exercise is between 60% and 80% of maximal attainable HR. For many older adults, especially those who are habitually inactive, resting HR may be very close to the recommended range for exercise exertion.[1] Consider an 80-year-old individual with a resting HR of 72 bpm. His maximal attainable HR is approximately 140 bpm (220 – 80 years). A target HR for an aerobic training level of exertion of 60% of maximal HR would be 84 bpm. His resting HR is within 12 beats of the HR for aerobic training. Functionally, this means that an activity as routine as rising from a chair or walking a short distance on a level surface may represent physical work of a level of exertion equated with moderate- to high-intensity exercise. Because of the reduction in maximal attainable HR with age, older adults may be working close to their VO_2max range even in usual activities of daily living.[17]

Because HR essentially signals the work of the heart, with each beat representing ventricular contraction, increased HR relates closely to increased heart work and increased oxygen consumption by the myocardium.[1,32] Given that afterload on the heart increases with age, the overall work of the heart for each beat is likely greater as well.[6,8,9,17] A more representative way to estimate the work of the heart during activity for older adults is the rate pressure product (RPP),[33–36] using HR and SBP as follows:

$$RPP = HR \times SBP$$

The linear relationship between VO_2max and HR for younger adults actually levels off for older adults.[37] Because of this, HR alone cannot accurately reflect the physiologic work that the older patient experiences; the RPP provides a clearer impression of relative work.[36] For older individuals with HR reserve limited by age, adjusting activity to keep the rise in HR within the lower end of the HR reserve is wise, especially for those with known coronary artery compromise.

Blood Pressure as a Warning Sign

An older person's blood pressure (BP) must also be considered. Hypertension, particularly increased SBP, is common in older adults. SBP also provides a relative indication of the level of afterload on the heart.[8,38,39] Resting blood pressure can be used to indicate whether an older person can safely tolerate increased physiologic work. Patients with a resting BP of more than 180/95 mm Hg may have difficulty with increased activity. A conservative estimate of the safe range of exercise suggests that exercise should be stopped if and when BP exceeds 220/110 mm Hg, although some consider 220 mm Hg too conservative a limit for older adults.[32] SBP should rise with increasing activity or exercise.[33] The older adult with limited HR reserve must increase SV to achieve the required CO.[3,4,6,17,26] SBP rises as SV increases and blood volume in the peripheral vasculature rises.[8] If SBP fails to rise or actually decreases during activity, this is a significant concern.[32] The drop or lack of change in SBP indicates that the heart is an ineffective pump, unable to contract and force a reasonable volume of blood out of the left ventricle. Continuing exercise or activity in the presence of a dropping SBP returns more blood to a heart that is incapable of pumping it back out to the body. Elevated diastolic blood pressure suggests that the left ventricle is maintaining a higher pressure during the filling period.[6,8] Early diastolic filling during preload will be compromised,[8,9,23] and the heart will be unable to capitalize on the Frank-Starling mechanism to enhance the force of ventricular contraction.[17,26]

Respiratory Warning Signs

Dyspnea, or shortness of breath, is an important warning sign as well. Age-related changes in the pulmonary system increase the work of breathing, and breathing becomes less efficient as work increases.[29] Because an older patient is prone to shortness of breath, recovering from shortness of breath during exercise may be very difficult. Breathing more deeply requires a disproportionately greater amount of respiratory muscle work, which further increases the cost of ventilation.[27,30,31] The use of supplemental oxygen by nasal cannula for the postoperative or medically ill patient who is beginning rehabilitation may be quite beneficial. Oxygen supplementation may prevent or minimize shortness of breath, enabling the older patient to tolerate increased activity better and to participate in rehabilitation more fully. During this oxygen-assisted time, any conditioning exercise to improve muscular performance (especially if combined with nutritional support) delivers blood to the working tissues and improves tissue oxygenation, ultimately aiding pulmonary function. Improved muscular conditioning and cardio-

vascular function may prevent or delay onset of lactic acidemia and the resultant increased desire to breathe that would trigger shortness of breath.[29]

Optimizing Cardiopulmonary Performance of the Older Patient

For most older adults, conditioning or training is an effective way to improve function, although some may need a longer training period to accomplish their desired level of physical performance as compared to younger adults.[40-43] Physical conditioning, in situations of acute and chronic illness, enables the older person to do more work and better accomplish desired tasks or activities.

Older patients, including those who are quite debilitated, experience improvement in physical performance as a result of conditioning exercise.[41] For some, significant gains are made as work capacity increases from an initial state below the threshold needed for function, such that an older person appears to make greater gains than a younger individual in similar circumstances.[44] In many cases, the cardiopulmonary system efficiency gained through conditioning means the difference between independence and dependency, functional recovery and minimal improvement, life without extraordinary means and life support, and, for some older patients, life and death.

The physiologic mechanisms for achieving the conditioned responses of the old may vary slightly from those of the young. With increasing activity or exercise in the submaximal range, older adults demonstrate greater increases in SV and less rise in HR than do young adults.[8,17,23,26,32] This increase in SV is accomplished with an increased EDV, usually without change in the ESV.[8,17,23] Increasing the EDV enhances the force of ventricular contraction by the Frank-Starling mechanism, which, in turn, increases CO despite the age-related impairment of the cardioaccelatory responses, which limits the rise in HR.[6,8,17,23,26] An increased preload, which improves CO, is the usual outcome of training at any age because improved conditioning of the peripheral musculature prevents distal pooling of blood, and increased resting tension of the muscles facilitates blood return.[1,3,4,32]

Preparation for Activity and Exercise

Simple lower extremity exercise as a warm-up before any functional activity or training session enhances the preload of the heart in a similar way. Any gentle, repetitive, lower extremity motions (e.g., ankle "pumps" in dorsiflexion/plantar flexion, knee flexion/extension, or cycling movements of the legs) before transfer or ambulation activities, before upper trunk and upper extremity activities, or as part of

TABLE 4-2
Borg Scales: Ratings of Perceived Exertion

Linear Scale		Ratio Scale	
Value	Description	Value	Description
6	No exertion	0	No effort at all
7–8	Extremely light effort	1	Very little (very weak) effort
9–10	Very light effort	2	Light (weak) effort
11–12	Light effort	3	Moderate effort
13–14	Somewhat hard effort	4	Somewhat strong effort
15–16	Heavy or hard	5–6	Strong effort
17–18	Very hard effort	7–8	Very strong effort
19	Extremely hard effort	9	Extremely strong effort
20	Maximum exertion	10	Maximal exertion

Source: Adapted from G Borg, D Ottoson. The Perception of Exertion in Physical Work. London: McMillan, 1986.

the warm-up portion of an aerobic or strength training exercise effectively improve the EDV. This increased EDV compensates in part for age-related preload problems, which might otherwise compromise work capacity.

Additionally, the muscular work of preliminary lower extremity exercise initiates the electrolyte and hormonal changes that promote the metabolic changes and vasodilation in peripheral tissues necessary to support aerobic metabolism for meeting energy demands of the task.[1,32,41] Peripheral oxygen exchange improves as much as 16% with regular exercise training.[17] The peripheral vasodilation associated with exercise helps to check the rise in afterload on the heart and also minimizes the development of lactic acidemia and the resulting drive to breathe more rapidly.[30,31]

As submaximal levels of exercise increase toward maximal exercise, SV continues to increase, maintaining CO.[3,4,17,23,26] When cardiopulmonary disease is present in addition to aging, however, this continued increase in SV is likely to be blunted.[1,6,32] Under these circumstances, the reduced sensitivity of the heart to sympathetic stimulation limits the force of contraction of the ventricle, so that the ejection fraction decreases and the ESV rises slightly.[8,26]

MONITORING THE CARDIORESPIRATORY RESPONSE TO EXERCISE

Consistent monitoring of the cardiopulmonary response is an essential component of rehabilitation interventions aimed at optimizing endurance or fitness of older frail or deconditioned patients. The positive effects of training only occur when the older person is appropriately chal-

lenged by the exercise or activity. According to the principle of overload, functional improvements occur only when the body is asked to do more than the customary workload for that individual.[1,5] For a patient who has been on prolonged bed rest and is quite deconditioned, simple lower extremity exercises while sitting upright may be as challenging as training for a marathon in a healthy young adult. The level of physiologic exertion is relative to the individual's customary work. Providing the physiologic overload necessary to produce improvements in performance, while avoiding a decline in performance because of exercise-induced fatigue or exhaustion, means recognizing the individual level of exertion.

Heart Rate and Blood Pressure

Maximum oxygen consumption (VO_2max) is the most accurate and sensitive measure of the individual workload, but the special equipment and technology needed to determine VO_2max are not typically available in routine clinical practice.[1,5,32] Although the linear relationship between HR and VO_2max plateaus so that HR becomes an inaccurate reflection of the workload for older adults, HR does partially indicate the work of the heart.[32,36,37] For a rapid clinical impression of the physiologic burden of an activity or exercise, HR is helpful as long as the clinician recognizes its limitations when using the measure with elders. Pre-exercise or activity BP provides some indication of likely afterload against which the heart will be working.[8,9,32,33] Continuing to monitor BP during the activity helps the clinician to recognize if the exercising cardiovascular system can meet the requirements of an increasing workload.[32] Calculation of the RPP may be a more accurate estimate of workload.[33–36]

Perceived Exertion

Ratings of perceived exertion are also effective indicators of the level of physiologic exertion experienced by patients who are exercising or involved in a strenuous physical activity[32,45,46] (Table 4-2). These scales ask individuals to assess subjectively how much effort they are expending during an exercise session or activity, with higher ratings indicating greater effort. Similar scales have been developed to assess breathlessness, fatigue, and discomfort or pain during exercise (Table 4-3). In the clinical use of these ratings of perceived exertion, many older persons using ratings of perceived exertion tend to overestimate their true physiologic stress, as indicated by their HR during exercise sessions.[32,45] Clinicians who appropriately, but bravely, recommend exercise for older adults relying on perceived exertion to limit the activity safely may find this phenomenon comforting.

TABLE 4-3
Ratio Scales of Perceived Breathlessness, Fatigue, or Discomfort during Exercise

Value	Breathlessness/Dyspnea	Fatigue	Discomfort or Pain
0	No breathlessness at all	No fatigue at all	No pain or discomfort
1	Very light breathlessness	Very light fatigue	Very little (weak) pain
2	Light breathlessness	Light fatigue	Little (weak) discomfort
3	Moderate breathlessness	Moderate fatigue	Moderate discomfort
4	Somewhat hard to breathe	Somewhat hard	Somewhat strong discomfort
5–6	Heavy breathing	Heavy work/fatigue	Strong discomfort or pain
7–8	Very heavy breathing	Very heavy fatigue	Very heavy discomfort
9	Very, very breathless	Very, very fatigued	Very, very hard discomfort
10	Maximum breathlessness	Maximally fatigued	Maximal discomfort or pain

Source: Adapted from E Dean. Mobilization and Exercise. In D Frownfelter, E Dean (eds), *Principles and Practice of Cardiopulmonary Physical Therapy* (3rd ed). St. Louis: Mosby, 1996;282.

Exercise Testing Protocols

Standard exercise testing protocols are appropriate for assessment of the status of conditioning of the cardiovascular system and exercise tolerance of older adults.[32,47] A treadmill test, cycle ergometer, or step test can be used or adapted for use in assessing cardiovascular performance of the older patient, unless the specific clinical setting or associated musculoskeletal dysfunction (e.g., balance problems, arthritic joints, or lower extremity muscle weakness) precludes this type of testing. A brief, sitting step test has been successfully used as an alternative to standard stress testing because it better accommodates the physical performance of more older patients and is practical to perform in any clinical setting.[32,48]

Careful monitoring of HR and BP before the sitting step test, at predetermined points during testing, at the completion of a brief bout of exercise, and a short while into recovery from the exercise bout, provides a comprehensive picture of cardiovascular function of any given older patient. This information often proves important in clinical decision making and program planning. Similarly, careful monitoring of HR and BP before, during, and after a bout of exercise during rehabilitation allows the clinician to compare the pattern of responses to the expected pattern for conditioned adults.[49] Normal exercise-induced cardiovascular responses include a slow rate of rise of HR, a rise in SBP, and minimal (if any) rise in diastolic BP during the exercise bout. For the conditioned older adult, HR and SBP should return toward pre-exercise values during the immediate postexercise recovery period on the order of 50% of the changes during exercise. The pattern of change in the RPP for the exercise bout and recovery period may be an even more descriptive measure of the cardiovascular response.

It is unreasonable to expect patients who are significantly deconditioned, can barely tolerate sitting for 30 minutes, are short of breath after 10 repetitions of simple lower extremity exercises while sitting, or are fatigued after 5 minutes of a sitting step test to be fully able to participate in gait and balance training. How can older individuals who are working at 90% or more of their maximum target HR be truly concerned with much more than delivering oxygen to the working tissues? Deconditioned individuals who are working at a high intensity in simple, well-known tasks have seriously restricted energy reserves; they are likely to have difficulty with focus and attention, processing, of the therapist's directions and supporting muscle activity, all necessary components for motor learning in performing a new skill such as gait training with a prosthetic device. Under these circumstances, emphasis must first be placed on improving cardiovascular conditioning, to improve energy reserves so that subsequent functional training with an orthosis or prosthesis has greater likelihood of a successful outcome.

PHYSICAL PERFORMANCE TRAINING FOR OPTIMAL RECOVERY OF FUNCTION

The same principles of training that are used with young adult athletes can be adapted and applied to frail or deconditioned older patients who are recovering from amputation or a neuromuscular event necessitating a prosthesis or orthosis. The two goals are to develop enough aerobic capacity to do work and to ensure efficient muscle function to produce work.[1,32] These concepts can guide any single rehabilitation session as well as the progression of the rehabilitation program over time. An understanding of exercise for improving fitness and of the few physiologic age-related changes in cardiopulmonary function provide a foundation for exercise prescription, which then is individualized based on current exercise tolerance of a specific older patient. This strategy can likely optimize the performance and the recovery of older adults in rehabilitation.

An effective strategy to improve cardiopulmonary response to exercise and activity for older patients who are deconditioned by bed rest, acute illness, or sedentary lifestyle begins with a warm-up of continuous alternating movements using large muscle groups, particularly of the lower extremities. The goal of such activity is facilitation of the preload and SV; any increase in SV realized through this training regimen helps an older patient to maximize cardiovascular function despite age-associated limitations in HR, cardioacceleratory responses, and baroreceptor sensitivity.

For healthy young adults the recommended regimen for aerobic conditioning and endurance training involves at least three sessions per week of 30–60 minutes' duration in activities that use large muscles (running, cycling, swimming, brisk walking) and keep HR in a target range between 60% and 80% of the individual's maximal attainable HR.[50] This may be unreasonable for an older adult who is recovering from an acute illness, is habitually sedentary, or is coping with age- or pathology-related impairments of cardiac or pulmonary function. Evidence suggests that, for older adults who are deconditioned, slower but significant improvement in work capacity can occur at exercise intensities as low as 30–45% of maximal HR.[40,51–53] The work of Sidney and Shephard[54] suggests that, although high-frequency high-intensity exercise can maximize increase in work capacity (VO_2max), high-intensity exercise performed less frequently and low-intensity exercise performed more frequently can yield positive endurance training effects. Evidence is also growing of improvement in oxygen extraction and muscle function when elders are involved in regular endurance training.[43]

In addition to aerobic conditioning, the rehabilitation program might include exercises that focus on flexibility. One of the goals of stretching and flexibility exercise for older adults is to preserve or restore any limited joint mobility that would otherwise limit essential functions. This is especially important for energy-efficient gait with lower limb orthoses or prostheses: Contracture of the hip, knee, or ankle has an impact on the alignment of orthotic and prosthetic components and often leads to greater sway and smaller stride length during gait, significantly increasing the energy cost or workload of walking. As flexibility of the trunk and thorax improves, a more effective alignment of the diaphragm and improved elastic recoil of the chest wall will have a positive impact on VC and inspiratory reserve volume and minimize RV, reducing the work of breathing and improving ventilation.

Muscle strengthening can begin as soon as the aerobic conditioning appears adequate to oxygenate the peripheral muscular tissue sufficiently. Assessment of the adequacy of peripheral oxygenation might include monitoring the coloring of the distal extremities before and during exercise and noting whether cramping or claudication occurs during exercise. One of the most sensitive indicators of appropriate intensity and duration of exercise is whether the activity can be increased without a marked rise in respiratory rate or onset of shortness of breath; a potent stimulus for frequency of breathing is the pH of the exercising tissues, with decreases as lactic acid builds up during anaerobic exercise.[30,31]

Two factors should be considered when including strengthening exercises in a rehabilitation program. First, is there adequate muscle strength for consistent and safe performance of the motor tasks needed for functional independence (including the use of assistive devices)? Second, is the muscle mass large enough to support a VO_2max that allows activities of daily living to represent a light to modest work intensity level? For many older people who have lost muscle mass (whether as a result of disuse and sedentary lifestyle or because of recent health problems that limit activity), development of more muscle mass increases lean body mass and improves the basal metabolic rate, improving overall health, fitness, and functional status.[28,32]

ENERGY COST OF GAIT

The human body is designed to be energy efficient during upright bipedal gait. Muscles of the trunk and extremities are activated by the central nervous system in a precise rhythmic cycle to move the body forward while maintaining dynamic stability, adapting stride length and gait speed to the constraints and demands of the task, the force of gravity, and the environment.[55,56] The advancing foot is lifted just enough to clear the surface in swing, and muscle activity at the stance-side hip and lower torso keeps the pelvis fairly level and the trunk erect, minimizing vertical displacement of the body's center of mass.[57] Normal arthro- and osteokinematic relationships between body segments ensure a narrow base of support in quiet stance and relaxed walking, and reciprocal arm swing counterbalances the dynamic pendular motion of the lower extremities, ensuring that the center of mass progresses forward with minimal mediolateral sway.[57–60] Much of the energy cost of walking is related to the muscular work performed to keep the center of mass moving forward with a minimum of vertical and mediolateral displacement.[57,61] Any musculoskeletal or neuromuscular pathology that interferes with alignment of body segments, the carefully controlled sequential activation of muscles, or the effectiveness of muscle contraction increases the energy cost of walking. As vertical displacement and mediolateral sway increase and gait deviations occur, muscles must work harder to keep the center of mass moving forward despite displacing moments. As muscle work increases, the cardiopulmonary system responds to this physiologic demand with increased HR, SV, and respiratory rate. Any orthosis or prosthesis that adds mass to or alters movement of the lower extremity potentially increases the work of walking. It is important to note, however, that for individuals with neuromuscular dysfunction, walking with an appropriate orthosis may actually require less energy than walking without it.[61]

Measuring Energy Costs of Walking

Measurement of physiologic energy expenditure by direct calorimetry is not realistic in all but the most sophisticated research laboratory settings. Instead, several indirect indicators have been found to be reliable estimates of the energy cost and the efficiency of gait in research and clinical applications. These include calculation of oxygen consumption (VO_2max) and oxygen cost while walking, monitoring blood lactate levels, calculating the physiologic cost index (PCI) of walking, and monitoring heart and respiratory rates during activity.

Oxygen Rate and Oxygen Cost

The most precise indirect measurements of energy and gait efficiency use special equipment (e.g., a portable spirometer or a Douglas bag) to monitor ventilatory volumes and to measure how much oxygen is taken in and carbon dioxide exhaled during physical activity. This type of testing is usually done while the subject or patient walks or runs on a treadmill or track or cycles on a stationary bicycle. The rate of oxygen consumption (O_2 rate), measured as volume of oxygen consumed per unit of body weight in 1 minute (ml/kg/min), provides an index of intensity of physical work at any given time.[61] VO_2max is the highest rate of oxygen uptake possible and is determined by progressing the exercise test to the point of voluntary exhaustion, when the age-adjusted maximum attainable HR is approached or reached.[62,63] If oxygen consumption during gait is low, an individual is likely to be able to walk long distances. If it is high, however, the distance of functional gait is likely to be limited. The oxygen cost of walking is determined by dividing the rate of oxygen consumption by the speed of walking. Oxygen cost reflects efficiency of gait, the amount of energy expended to walk over a standard distance (ml/kg/m).[61] Most of what we currently understand about energy expenditure when using a prosthesis or orthosis is based on studies that have measured oxygen rate and oxygen cost of walking.

Serum Lactate

The energy efficiency of walking is also assessed by evaluation of serum carbon dioxide and lactate levels as indicators of anaerobic energy production. The energy (adenosine triphosphate [ATP]) required for muscle contraction during gait can be derived from a combination of aerobic oxidative and anaerobic glycolytic pathways. The aerobic oxidative pathway, which depends on oxygen delivery to active muscle cells, is the most efficient source of energy, producing almost 19 times as much ATP as the anaerobic pathway.[61] In healthy fit individuals, this aerobic pathway is more than able to meet energy requirements of relaxed walking. If energy demands of an exercise or activity are met by aerobic oxidation, the activity can be sustained for long periods with relatively low levels of fatigue. As activity becomes strenuous (i.e., as gait speed or surface incline increases) and the need for energy begins to exceed the availability of oxygen for aerobic oxidation, additional energy is accessed through anaerobic metabolism. This transition to anaerobic metabolism is reported to begin at work levels of 55% of VO_2max in healthy, untrained individuals but may begin at 80% of VO_2max in highly trained athletes.[64] When the ability to deliver oxygen is compromised by the physical deconditioning of a sedentary lifestyle or by cardiac, pulmonary, or musculoskeletal pathology, anaerobic glycolysis becomes a primary source of energy at lower levels of work.[65] Whenever the anaerobic pathway is the major source of energy, blood levels of lactate and carbon dioxide rise, lowering blood pH and increasing the respiratory exchange ratio (CO_2 production/O_2 consumption).[66] Under these conditions, the ability to sustain activity is limited, with an earlier onset of fatigue as workload increases. Serum lactate levels are most often used in studies of assisted ambulation using hybrid orthotic/functional electrical stimulation systems for those with spinal cord injury.

Physiologic Cost Index and Heart Rate

Another clinical indicator of the energy cost of walking is the PCI, which is calculated as follows:[67]

$$PCI = \frac{(HR\ walking - HR\ resting)}{gait\ speed}$$

Measured in beats per meter, the PCI reflects the effort of walking; low values suggest energy-efficient gait. For children between 3 and 12 years of age, the mean PCI at self-selected or preferred gait speed has been reported to be between 0.38 and 0.40 beats per meter.[68,69] High correlation between the PCI, percent maximum HR, and oxygen rate ($r = 0.91$, $p > .005$) in able-bodied children and children with transtibial amputation supports its validity as an indicator of energy cost for children.[70] Comparison of preoperative and postoperative PCI values has been used to assess the long-term outcome of orthopedic surgery for children with cerebral palsy.[71] The PCI was originally used to assess gait restrictions in adults with rheumatoid arthritis and similar inflammatory joint disease.[67] The PCI has also been used to assess the effect of different assistive devices on the effort of walking[72] and to evaluate the short- and long-term impact on neuromuscular stimulation on the ability to walk and run in children and in older adults with hemiplegia.[73-75] Most recently, the PCI is being used in the research and development of reciprocal gait orthosis/functional electrical stimulation systems for individuals with spinal cord injury.[76-78]

High correlations between HR and oxygen consumption during gait have been reported for children and for healthy young adults at a variety of gait speeds.[79,80] Although this suggests that HR monitoring may be a reliable substitute for oxygen rate determination, it should be used with caution in older adults because of the age-related changes in cardiopulmonary function discussed earlier in this chapter. This is especially true for older adults with heart disease who are being managed with medications that further blunt HR response. The rate-pressure product or the physiologic cost index may be more appropriate indicators of the energy cost of walking in these circumstances.

Energy Expenditure in Normal Gait

The energy requirements of walking vary with age and with gait speed (Figure 4-4). Oxygen consumption is highest in childhood but decreases to approximately 12 ml/kg/min in healthy adults and elders.[81] When oxygen consumption during walking is expressed as a percent of Vo_2max, a slightly different picture emerges. For a healthy, untrained young adult, oxygen consumption at a comfortable walking speed may be 32% of Vo_2max, whereas for an older adult walking at a similar speed, oxygen consumption may be as much as 48% of Vo_2max.[57,82] For functional gait, if walking is to cover large distances or is to be sustained over long periods of time, oxygen consumption must be less than 50% of that individual's Vo_2max so that aerobic oxidation will be used as the primary source of energy.[5] At comfortable gait speeds, older adults are working nearer the threshold for transition to anaerobic metabolism than are younger adults. If some form of gait dysfunction is superimposed, increasing the energy cost of gait, the work of walking will transition to anaerobic glycolysis unless a cardiovascular conditioning program is included in the rehabilitation program.

For individuals without neuromuscular or musculoskeletal impairment, the relationship between the energy

cost of walking and gait speed is nearly linear[81,83] (Figure 4-5). Gait is most efficient, as indicated by oxygen cost (O_2 rate/velocity), at an individual's self-selected or customary walking speed; energy requirements increase whenever gait speed is much slower or much faster.[84,85] The customary walking speed of most individuals with neuromuscular or musculoskeletal impairments is often much slower, a strategy that minimizes the rate of energy used during walking. As a result of slower speed, however, it takes longer to cover any given distance. Any impairment that reduces gait speed leads to increased oxygen cost, even if oxygen rate remains close to normal[86-89] (Table 4-4).

The weight and design of the prosthesis or orthosis are also determinants of energy cost of gait. The impact of added mass on the energy cost of gait is dependent on where the load is placed: Extra weight loaded on the trunk (such as a heavy backpack) changes oxygen rate during walking less than would a smaller load placed around the ankle.[90] This highlights the importance of minimizing weight of lower extremity orthoses and prostheses to keep the energy cost of walking within an individual's aerobic capacity.[91]

Work of Walking with an Orthosis

When discussing the energy cost of walking with an orthosis, it is important to remember that, for those with significant neuromuscular or musculoskeletal impairment, the energy cost of walking without the orthosis is typically higher than walking with an appropriate orthosis.[92,93] One of the determinants of energy cost when walking with a cast or an orthosis is the degree of immobility that the orthosis imposes on the ankle, knee, and hip and the associated change in gait speed.[89] For individuals with restriction of knee motion because of a cast or orthosis, the energy cost of gait can be reduced by placing a shoe lift on the contralateral limb.[94]

For individuals with spinal cord injury, the potential for functional ambulation appears to be determined by four conditions: the ability to use a reciprocal gait pattern, the adequacy of trunk stability, at least fair hip flexor strength bilaterally, and fair quadriceps strength of at least one limb. This corresponds to an ambulatory motor index (AMI) score of 18 of 30 possible points, or 60% of "good" lower extremity strength.[95] In this instance, gait may be possible with bilateral ankle-foot orthoses (AFOs) or an AFO and knee-ankle-foot orthosis combination. Those with spinal cord injury at mid to low thoracic levels with AMI scores of less than 60% often require bilateral knee-ankle-foot orthoses, with Loftstrand or axillary crutches in a swing-through gait pattern to ambulate. Waters[61]

FIGURE 4-4

*Comparison of comfortable gait speed (**A**, upper bar) and fast gait speed (**A**, lower bar) and associated oxygen consumption (**B**) and oxygen cost (**C**) for four age groups: children (6–12 years), adolescents (13–19 years), adults (20–59 years), and older adults (60–80 years). (Based on data reported by RL Waters, BR Lunsford, J Perry, R Byrd. Energy-speed relationships of walking: standard tables. J Orthop Res 1988;6:215–222.)*

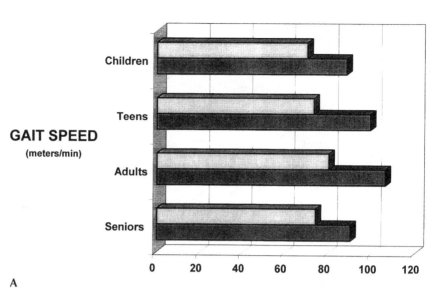

A

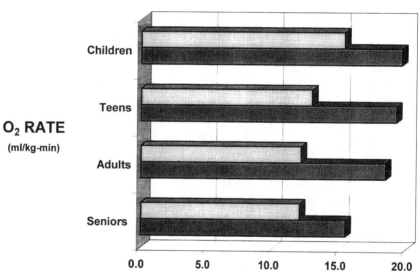

B

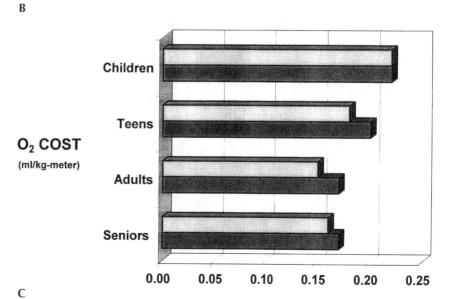

C

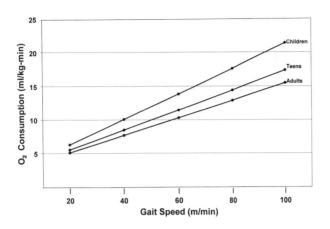

FIGURE 4-5

Relationship between gait speed and oxygen consumption (O_2 rate). The differences in O_2 rate between children and adults (20–80 years) are attributed, in part, to differences in body composition. (Derived from gait-velocity regression formulas reported by RL Waters. Energy Expenditure. In J Perry [ed], Gait Analysis: Normal and Pathological Function. Thorofare, NJ: Slack, 1992;443–489.)

reports a near linear positive relationship between AMI scores and gait velocity, as well as a somewhat curvilinear inverse relationship between AMI score and oxygen rate (% above normal), and oxygen cost. For persons with spinal cord injury who have the potential for functional ambulation, continued cardiovascular conditioning after discharge from rehabilitation improves the efficiency of walking, as reflected in lower oxygen cost and improvement in gait speed.[96,97] The development of reciprocal gait orthoses and "parawalkers," at times augmented by functional electrical stimulation, has also made modified ambulation possible for those with injury at mid- and upper thoracic levels.[98–102] The high energy cost of the intense upper extremity work using crutches to propel the body forward during swing and maintain upright position in

stance, however, restricts functional ambulation as a primary means of mobility.

Gait pattern appears to be one of the determinants of functional ambulation in children with myelodysplasia: Swing-through gait with crutches is 33% more energy efficient (O_2 rate) than four-point reciprocal gait; however, the speed and energy cost of wheelchair propulsion are most similar to that of able-bodied walking.[103] The type of orthosis also has an impact on the energy cost of walking for children with myelodysplasia: Oxygen rate during walking with a conventional hip-knee-ankle-foot orthosis is as much as six times that of normal, whereas the oxygen rate of walking with a reciprocal gait orthosis is twice that of normal.[104] The high energy cost of ambulation in children with myelomeningocele may have an impact on more than mobility: In a study that compared the impact of functional ambulation with orthotics and assistive devices or wheelchair mobility in the school environment, performance on visuomotor tasks was less accurate when ambulation was the primary means of mobility.[105]

The movement dysfunction associated with stroke, cerebral palsy, and other neuromuscular impairments tends to reduce gait speed, with the degree of slowing determined by the severity of neuromuscular impairment.[106,107] As abnormal movement patterns and impaired postural responses compromise the cyclic and dynamic flow of walking, the higher levels of muscle activity that are required to remain upright and to move forward increase the energy cost of gait. Reduction of gait speed is a functional strategy to keep energy expenditure within physiologic limits. In the research literature, the oxygen rate (consumption) of persons with stroke who walk at a reduced gait speed is reported to be close to that of elders who walk at their customary gait speed.[61,106] Oxygen cost, however, is significantly higher: 54 ml/kg/m after stroke, as compared to 0.16 ml/kg/m for elders without impairment.[61,106] When compared to unimpaired individuals who walk at similar speeds, persons with hemiplegia wearing an AFO use 52% more energy; when they walk with-

TABLE 4-4

Gait Speed, Oxygen Rate, Oxygen Cost, and Efficiency of Gait Associated with Restriction in Range of Motion

Condition	"Normal" Range of Motion	Ankle Arthrodesis	Knee Immobilization	Hip Arthrodesis
Gait speed (m/min)	80	67	64	67
O_2 rate (ml/kg/min)	12.1	12.0	12.7	14.7
O_2 cost (ml/kg/m)	0.151	0.166	0.200	0.223
Gait efficiency	100	91.0	75.5	76.7

Source: Adapted from FR Waters. Energy expenditure. In J Perry (ed), Gait Analysis: Normal and Pathological Function. Thorofare, NJ: Slack, 1992;462.

TABLE 4-5
Gait Speed, Oxygen Consumption, and Oxygen Cost in Prosthetic Gait: Comparison of Etiology and Level of Unilateral Amputation

Etiology and Level: Parameter	Traumatic Transtibial	Traumatic Transfemoral	Dysvascular Transtibial	Dysvascular Transfemoral
Waters et al., 1976[112]				
Gait speed (m/min)	71	52	45	36
O_2 rate (ml/kg/min)	12.4	10.3	9.4	10.8
O_2 cost (ml/kg/m)	0.16	0.20	0.20	0.28
Torburn et al., 1995[113]				
Gait speed (m/min)	82.3	—	61.7	—
O_2 rate (ml/kg/min)	17.7	—	13.2	—
O_2 cost (ml/kg/m)	0.22	—	0.21	—

out an orthosis, their energy cost can increase to as much as 65% more than unimpaired gait.[108]

Individuals with spastic diplegic cerebral palsy often walk in a "crouch gait" pattern, maintaining abnormal knee and hip flexion throughout the gait cycle. In stance, as a result of this flexed posture, a large flexion moment occurs as the weight line passes anterior to the hip and posterior to the knee joint. The muscular work that is necessary to remain upright during stance, counteracting the effects of gravity at the hip and knee, significantly increases the energy cost of walking.[61,109] As in adults with stroke, gait speed and stride length are markedly reduced. Bilateral thermoplastic AFOs, designed to stabilize the knee in stance, appear to improve the energy efficiency of gait in children with spastic diplegia (as determined by the PCI); however, energy cost remains much higher than that of children without impairment.[93] For some children, quality of gait can be further enhanced when hinged AFOs are worn instead of solid ankle AFOs: Forward progression of the tibia from mid to terminal stance increases stride length and gait speed, enhancing the energy efficiency of gait.[110]

Work of Walking with a Prosthesis

The characteristics of gait and the energy cost of walking with a prosthesis are related to the etiology and the level of amputation. The gait speed, stride length, and cadence of persons with lower extremity amputation who walk with a prosthesis are typically lower than those of individuals without impairment, regardless of the cause of amputation.[111] In most instances, individuals with traumatic amputation demonstrate a more energy-efficient gait than those with amputation as a result of vascular or neuropathic disease.[112,113] Additionally, biomechanical and energy efficiency of prosthetic gait decreases as amputa-

tion level increases: Preservation of the anatomic knee joint appears to be especially important.[61,111,114,115] A classic study by Waters et al.[112] (Table 4-5) demonstrated that, for young adults with traumatic transtibial amputation, gait speed, oxygen rate, and oxygen cost were quite close to normal values reported by Perry.[57] For those with traumatic transfemoral or dysvascular amputation, diminishing gait speeds kept oxygen consumption close to that of normal adult gait; however, oxygen cost increased well beyond the normal value of 0.15 mg/kg/m.[112] Although gait speeds reported in a more recent study by Torburn et al.[113] are much higher, the difference in performance between traumatic and dysvascular groups was consistent. Other studies report oxygen costs of prosthetic gait at between 28% and 33% above normal for individuals with transtibial amputation[116,117] and between 60% and 110% above normal for individuals with transfemoral amputation.[118–120] Although the relationship between gait speed and oxygen rate (consumption) in prosthetic gait is linear, just as it is in unimpaired gait, the slope is significantly steeper.[121] The clinical implication of this relationship is that the rate of energy consumption and of cardiac work, at any gait speed, is higher for those with amputation and that the threshold for transition from aerobic to anaerobic metabolism is reached at lower gait speeds.[122]

Several explanations are possible for the differences in prosthetic gait performance after traumatic versus dysvascular amputation. Because those with dysvascular amputation are typically older than those with traumatic amputation, differences in performance may be the result of age-related changes and concurrent cardiovascular disease in the dysvascular group.[116,123,124] For many older patients with dysvascular amputation, the energy source for walking with a prosthesis may be anaerobic rather than the more efficient aerobic metabolic pathways.[113] A larger cardiac and respiratory functional reserve capacity in younger persons with traumatic transtibial amputation may permit them to meet the increased metabolic demands of prosthetic use, as proximal muscle groups work for longer periods at higher intensities to compensate for the loss of those at the ankle.[113,121,125]

It is important to recognize that for most individuals with unilateral transtibial and transfemoral amputation, regardless of age or etiology of amputation, the energy cost of walking with a prosthesis is less than that expended when walking without it using crutches or a walker.[112] For most patients with a new transtibial amputation, the ability to ambulate before amputation is the best predictor of tolerance of the increased energy cost of walking with a prosthesis after surgery.[123] For some older individuals with transfemoral amputation and concurrent cardiovascular or respiratory disease, and for those with bilateral amputation at transfemoral/transtibial or bilateral transfemoral levels, wheelchair mobility may be preferred.[126–128]

During the 1990s, significant efforts have been made to reduce the energy cost of prosthetic gait by developing dynamic response (energy storing) prosthetic feet and cadence-responsive prosthetic knee units, using lightweight but durable materials in prosthetic sockets and components and improving the fit and alignment of the prosthesis. The flexible keels of most dynamic response prosthetic feet are designed to mimic those of normal ankle mobility, such that mechanical energy stored by compression during stance is released to enhance "push-off" in the terminal stance.[129] The impact of different prosthetic foot designs on the energy cost is not clear, however. Comparison of gait characteristics of the solid-ankle cushioned-heel (SACH) foot (Kingsley Manufacturing Co, Costa Mesa, CA) and the Flex-Foot (Aliso, Viejo, CA) in children with unilateral transtibial amputation walking at preferred (0.9 m/sec) and fast (1.3 m/sec) gait speed suggests that dynamic response feet should reduce the energy cost of gait.[130] In a study that compared the Seattle (Seattle Limb Systems, Poulsba, WA) and SACH foot in children, however, no differences in the work of walking were found.[131] Similarly, for adults with transtibial amputation, the FlexFoot functioned more like an anatomic ankle than did four other dynamic response feet and the SACH foot, but little difference in stride, velocity, or energy cost was noted.[113,125,132,133] It is important to note, however, that the materials and design of most dynamic response feet may enable transtibial prosthetic users to jump, run, and use a step-over step pattern in stair climbing; these activities are difficult or not possible with a traditional SACH foot.[134–137] Additionally, many individuals with transtibial amputation wear their prosthesis for longer periods during the day and report less fatigue in prolonged walking when using a prosthesis with a dynamic response foot.[123]

Evidence that the new ischial containment transfemoral socket designs improve the quality and efficiency of prosthetic gait, as compared to the traditional quadrilateral socket, is accumulating. Most ischial containment sockets attempt to stabilize the femur in a position close to the normal adduction angle during stance, enhancing the ability of hip abductors to stabilize the pelvis and reducing lateral sway during stance.[138] These two factors appear to reduce the energy cost of prosthetic gait as compared to the traditional quadrilateral socket.[114,139]

SUMMARY

An understanding of normal cardiopulmonary function and how it changes in aging, as a result of sedentary lifestyle or pathologic conditions, provides a necessary foundation for rehabilitation professionals working with patients who require an orthosis or prosthesis to walk. In this chapter we have reviewed the anatomy and physiology of the cardiopulmonary system, with attention to age-related changes, energy expenditure, and principles of aerobic conditioning for older adults.

Optimal performance of the cardiopulmonary system is influenced by three interrelated factors. First, the patient must have sufficient flexibility and mobility of the trunk for efficient and uncompromised ventilation. Second, adequate mobility of the extremities and excursion of the joints must be present for efficient performance of functional tasks. Third, the patient must have enough muscle mass, strength, and endurance to support the performance of the activity and function of the heart. Immediate and ongoing interventions that functionally enhance preload by returning blood to the older heart and avoidance of conditions (isometric muscle contraction and Valsalva maneuvers, for example) that unnecessarily increase afterload can result in marked improvement in physical performance of the older person. With these conditions, as well as compensation for the beta-adrenergic receptor–reduced sensitivity with a prolonged period of warm-up exercises, an older person is capable of physical performance that is quite similar to that of younger counterparts and essential for the process of recovery of function for the optimal outcome of rehabilitation.

The energy cost and efficiency of gait are affected by aging, by deconditioning of a sedentary lifestyle, and by neuromuscular and musculoskeletal impairments that alter motor control or the biomechanics of walking. Although an orthosis that restricts joint motion increases the energy cost in unimpaired individuals, the same orthosis leads to more efficient gait in those with neuromuscular impairment. Determinants of efficiency of prosthetic gait include the level and etiology of the amputation. Reduction of gait speed when using an orthosis or prosthesis helps to maintain oxygen consumption at close to normal levels; however, this tends to compromise overall efficiency of gait, as indicated by oxygen cost. Attention to the principles of cardiovascular conditioning, including monitoring the response to exercise so that patients are challenged appropriately, optimizes the outcomes of rehabilitation programs.

REFERENCES

1. Fox EL, Mathews DK. The Physiological Basis of Physical Education and Athletics (3rd ed). Philadelphia: Saunders, 1981.
2. Astrand P, Cuddy T, Saltin B, Stenberg J. Cardiac output during submaximal and maximal work. J Appl Physiol 1964;19:268–274.
3. Ekblom B, Hermansen L. Cardiac output in athletes. J Appl Physiol 1968;25(5):619–625.
4. Ekblom B, Astrand P, Saltin B, et al. Effect of training on circulatory response to exercise. J Appl Physiol 1968; 24(4):518–528.
5. Astrand P, Rodahl K. Textbook of Work Physiology: The Physiological Bases of Exercise (3rd ed). New York: McGraw-Hill, 1986.
6. Kitzman DW. Aging and the heart. Dev Cardiol 1994;1(1):1–15.
7. Kitzman DW, Edwards WD. Age related changes in the anatomy of the normal human heart. J Gerontol 1990;45(1):M33–39.
8. Lakatta EB, Mitchell JH, Pomerance A, Rowe GG. Human aging: changes in structure and function. III. Characteristics of specific cardiovascular diseases in the elderly. J Am Coll Cardiol 1987;10(2supplA):42–47.
9. Wei JY. Cardiovascular anatomic and physiologic changes with age. Top Geriatr Rehab 1986;2(1):10–16.
10. Anversa P, Miller B, Ricci R, et al. Myocyte cell loss and myocyte hypertrophy in the aging rat heart. J Am Coll Cardiol 1986;8(6):1441–1446.
11. Kitzman DW, Scholz DG, Hagen PT, et al. Age-related changes in normal human hearts during the first ten decades. Part II (Maturity): a quantitative anatomic study of 765 specimens from subjects 70–99 years old. Mayo Clin Proc 1988;63(2):137–146.
12. Labovitz AJ, Pearson AC. Evaluation of left ventricular diastolic function: clinical relevance and recent Doppler echocardiographic insights. Am Heart J 1987;114(4):836–851.
13. Nixon JV, Hallmark H, Page K, et al. Ventricular performance in human hearts aged 61–73 years. Am J Cardiol 1985;56(15):932–937.
14. Gardin JM, Henry WL, Savage DD, et al. Echocardiographic measurements in normal subjects: evaluation of an adult population without clinically apparent heart disease. J Clin Ultrasound 1979;7(6):439–447.
15. Lakatta EG. Do hypertension and aging have similar effect on the myocardium? Circulation 1987;75(suppl 1):69–77.
16. Selzer A. Changing aspects of the natural history of valvular aortic stenosis. N Engl J Med 1987;317(2):91–98.
17. Rodeheffer RJ, Gerstenblith G, Becker LC, et al. Exercise cardiac output is maintained with advancing age in healthy human subjects: cardiac dilation and increased stroke volume compensate for a diminished heart rate. Circulation 1984;69(2):203–213.
18. Shiaishi I, Takamatsu T, Minamikawa T, et al. Quantitative histological analysis of the human sinoatrial node during growth and aging. Circulation 1992;85(6):2176–2184.
19. Lakatta EG. Altered autonomic modulation of cardiovascular function with adult aging; perspectives from studies ranging from man to cells. In HL Stone, WB Weglicki (eds), Pathobiology of Cardiovascular Injury. Boston: Martinus Nijhoff, 1985;441–460.
20. Tsunoda K, Abe K, Golto T. Effect of age on the renin-angiotensin-aldosterone system in normal subjects; simultaneous measurement of active and inactive renin, renin substrate, and aldosterone in plasma. J Clin Endocrinol Metab 1986;62(2):384–389.
21. Shimada K, Kitazumi T, Ogura H. Differences in age-dependent effects of blood pressure on baroreflex sensitivity between normal and hypertensive subjects. Clin Sci 1986;70(5):763–766.
22. Guyton AC. Textbook of Medical Physiology. Philadelphia: Saunders, 1986.
23. Kitzman DW, Higginbotham MB, Sullivan MJ. Aging and the cardiovascular response to exercise. Cardiol Elderly 1993;1:543–550.
24. Petersdorf RG, Adams RD, Braunwald E, et al. Harrison's Principles of Internal Medicine (10th ed). New York: McGraw-Hill, 1983.
25. Nichols WW, O'Rourke MF, Avolio AP. Effects of age on ventricular-vascular coupling. Am J. Cardiol 1985; 55(9):1179–1184.
26. Port S, Cobb FR, Coleman E, Jones RH. Effect of age on the response of the left ventricular ejection fraction to exercise. N Engl J Med 1980;303(20):1133–1137.
27. Zadia CC. Pulmonary physiology of aging: the role of rehabilitation. Top Geriatr Rehab 1985;1(1):49–57.
28. Shepherd RJ. The cardiovascular benefits of exercise in the elderly. Top Geriatr Rehab 1985;1(1):1–10.
29. Stulberg M, Carrieri-Kohlman V. Conceptual approach to the treatment of dyspnea: focus on the role of exercise. Cardiopulmonary Phys Ther 1992;3(1):9–12.
30. Wasserman K, Casaburi R. Dyspnea: physiological and pathophysiologic mechanisms. Ann Rev Med 1988;39:503–515.
31. Casaburi R, Patessio A, Ioli F. Reductions in exercise lactic acidosis and ventilation as a result of exercise training in patients with obstructive lung disease. Am Rev Respir Dis 1991;143(1):9–18.
32. Pollock ML, Wilmore JH (eds). Exercise in Health and Disease. Philadelphia: Saunders, 1990.
33. Naughton J. Exercise Testing: Physiological, Biomedical, and Clinical Principles. Mount Kisco, NY: Futura, 1988.

34. Kitamura K, Jorgensen CR, Gobel FL, et al. Hemodynamic correlates of myocardial oxygen consumption during upright exercise. J Appl Physiol 1972;32(4):516–522.

35. Ellestad MH. Stress Testing: Principles and Practice (3rd ed). Philadelphia: Davis, 1986.

36. DeVries HA. Phyiology of Exercise (4th ed). Dubuque, IA: WMC Brown, 1986.

37. Tonino RP, Driscoll PA. Reliability of maximal and submaximal parameters of treadmill testing for the measurement of physical training in older persons. J Gerontol 1988;42(2):M101–104.

38. Materson BJ. Isolated systolic blood pressure: new answers, more questions. J Am Geriatr Soc 1991;39(12):1237–1238.

39. Applegate WB, Davis BR, Black HR. Prevalence of postural hypotension at baseline in the systolic hypertension in the elderly program (SHEP) cohort. J Am Geriatr Soc 1991; 39(11):1057–1064.

40. Badenhop DT, Cleary PA, Schaal SF, et al. Physiological adjustments to higher- or lower-intensity exercise in elders. Med Sci Sports Exerc 1983;15(6):496–502.

41. Hagberg JM, Allen WK, Seals DR. A hemodynamic comparison of young and older endurance athletes during exercise. J Appl Physiol 1985;58(6):2041–2046.

42. Julius S, Amery A, Whitlock LS, Conway J. Influence of age on the hemodynamic response to exercise. Circulation 1967;36(2):222–230.

43. Seals DR, Hagberg JM, Hurley BF, et al. Endurance training in older men and women. 1: Cardiovascular responses to exercise. J Appl Physiol 1984;57(4):1024–1029.

44. Higginbotham MB, Morris KG, Williams RS. Physiologic basis for the age related decline in aerobic work capacity. Am J Cardiol 1986;57(4):1374–1379.

45. Borg G. Perceived exertion as an indicator of somatic stress. Scand J Rehabil Med 1970;2(3):92–97.

46. Borg G, Ottoson D. The perception of exertion in physical work. London: McMillan, 1986.

47. Fleg JL. Diagnostic and prognostic value of stress testing in older persons. J Am Geriatr Soc 1995;43(2):190–194.

48. Smith EL, Gilligan C. Physical activity perception for the older adult. Physician Sports Med 1993;11:91–101.

49. Arnheim DD. Modern Principles of Athletic Training (6th ed). St. Louis: Mosby, 1985.

50. Karvonen M, Kentala E, Mustala O. The effects of training on heart rate: a longitudinal study. Ann Med Exp Fenn 1957;35:307.

51. Yerg JE, Seals DR, Hagberg JM, et al. Effects of endurance exercise training on ventilatory function in the older individual. J Appl Physiol 1985;58(3):791–794.

52. Frontera WR, Evans WJ. Exercise performance and endurance training in the elderly. Top Geriatr Rehab 1986;2(1):17–32.

53. Seals DR, Hagberg JM, Hurley BF, et al. Effects of endurance training on glucose tolerance and plasma lipid levels in older men and women. JAMA 1984;252(5):645–649.

54. Sidney KH, Shephard RJ. Frequency and intensity of exercise training for elderly subjects. Med Sci Sports 1978; 10(2):125–131.

55. Palta AF. Neurobiomechanical Bases for the Control of Human Movement. In A Bronstein, T Brandt, M Woollacott (eds), Clinical Disorders of Balance, Posture, and Gait. London: Arnold, 1996;19–40.

56. Bianchi L, Angelini D, Orani GP, Lacquaniti F. Kinematic coordination in human gait: relation to mechanical energy cost. J Neurophysiol 1998;79(4):2155–2170.

57. Perry J. Basic Functions. In J Perry (ed), Gait Analysis: Normal and Pathological Function. Thorofare, NJ: Slack, 1992;19–48.

58. Norkin CC, Levangie PK. Gait. In Joint Structure and Function: A Comprehensive Analysis (2nd ed). Philadelphia: Davis, 1992;448–495.

59. Winter DA, Quanbury AO, Reimer GD. Analysis of instantaneous energy of normal gait. J Biomech 1976;9(4): 252–257.

60. Rose J, Gamble JG. Human Walking (2nd ed). Baltimore: Williams & Wilkins, 1994.

61. Waters RL. Energy Expenditure. In J Perry (ed), Gait Analysis: Normal and Pathological Function. Thorofare, NJ: Slack, 1992;443–489.

62. Sidney KH, Shepherd RJ. Maximum and submaximum exercise tests in men and women in the seventh, eighth and ninth decades of life. J Appl Physiol 1977;43(2):280.

63. Thomas SG, Cunningham DA, Rechnitzer PA, et al. Protocols and reliability of maximal oxygen uptake in the elderly. Can J Sport Sci 1987;12:144.

64. Saltin B, Blomquist G, Mitchell JH, et al. Response to submaximal and maximal exercise after bedrest and training. Circulation 1968;38(suppl 7):1–78.

65. Davis JA. Anaerobic threshold: review of the concept and directions for future research. Med Sci Sports Exerc 1985;17(1):6–8.

66. McArdle WD, Datch FI, Katch VL. Exercise Physiology. Philadelphia: Lea & Febiger, 1986.

67. Steven MM, Capell HA, Sturrock RD, MacGregor J. The physiological cost of gait (PCG): a new technique for evaluating non-steroidal anti-inflammatory drugs in rheumatoid arthritis. Br J Rheumatol 1983;22(3):141–145.

68. Butler P, Engelbrecht M, Major RE, et al. Physiological cost index of walking for normal children and its use as an indicator of physical handicap. Dev Med Child Neurol 1984;26(5):607–612.

69. Jeng SF, Liao HF, Lai JS, Hou JW. Optimization of walking in children. Med Sci Sports Exerc 1997;29(3): 370–376.

70. Engsberg JR, Herbert LM, Grimston SK, et al. Relation among indices of effort and oxygen uptake in below knee and able-bodied children. Arch Phys Med Rehabil 1994;75(12):1335–1341.

71. Nene AV, Evans GA, Patrick JH. Simultaneous multiple operations for spastic diplegia. Outcome and functional assessment of walking in 18 patients. J Bone Joint Surg Br 1993;75(3):488–494.

72. Hamzeh MA, Bowker P, Sayeqh A, et al. The energy cost of ambulation using 2 types of walking frames. Clin Rehabil 1988;2:119–123.

73. Carmick J. Clinical use of neuromuscular electrical stimulation for children with cerebral palsy: lower extremity. Phys Ther 1993;73(8):505–513.

74. Burridge JH, Taylor PN, Hagan SA, et al. The effects of common peroneal nerve stimulation on the effort and speed of walking: a randomized controlled clinical trial with chronic hemiplegic patients. Clin Rehabil 1997;11(3):201–210.

75. Burridge J, Taylor P, Hagan S, Swain I. Experience of clinical use of the Odstock dropped foot stimulator. Artif Organs 1997;21(3):254–260.

76. Yang L, Condie DN, Granat MP, et al. Effects of joint motion constraints on normal subjects and their implications on the further development of hybrid FES orthosis for paraplegic persons. J Biomech 1996;29(2):217–226.

77. Nene AV, Jennings SJ. Physiological cost index of paraplegic locomotion using the ORLAU ParaWalker. Paraplegia 1992;30(4):246–252.

78. Stallard J, Major RE. The influence of stiffness on paraplegic ambulation and its implications for functional electrical stimulation walking systems. Prosthet Orthot Int 1995;19(2):108–114.

79. Rose J, Gamble JG, Medeiros J, et al. Energy cost of walking in normal children and in those with cerebral palsy: comparison of heart rate and oxygen uptake. J Pediatr Orthop 1989;9(3):276–279.

80. Rose GK. Clinical gait assessment. J Med Eng Technol 1983;7(6):273–279.

81. Waters RL, Lunsford BR, Perry J, Byrd R. Energy-speed relationships of walking: standard tables. J Orthop Res 1988;6(2):215–222.

82. Astrand A, Astrand I, Hallback I, Kilbon A. Reduction in maximal oxygen uptake with age. J Appl Physiol 1973;35(5):649–654.

83. Corcoran PJ, Gelmanan B. Oxygen reuptake in normal and handicapped subjects in relation to the speed of walking beside a velocity controlled cart. Arch Phys Med Rehabil 1970;51(2):78–87.

84. Holt KG, Hamill J, Andres RO. Predicting the minimal energy cost of human walking. Med Sci Sports Exerc 1991;23(4):491–498.

85. Duff Raffaele M, Kerrigan DC, Corcoran PJ, Saini M. The proportional work of lifting the center of mass during walking. Am J Phys Med 1996;75(5):375–379.

86. Waters RL, Perry J, Conaty P, et al. The energy cost of walking with arthritis of the hip and knee. Clin Orthop 1987;2(14):278–284.

87. Gussoni M, Margonato V, Ventura R, Veicsteinas A. Energy cost of walking with hip joint impairment. Phys Ther 1990;70(5):295–301.

88. Waters RL, Barnes G, Husserl T, et al. Comparable energy expenditure following arthrodesis of the hip and ankle. J Bone Joint Surg 1988;70(7):1032–1037.

89. Waters RL, Campbell J, Thomas L, et al. Energy cost in walking in lower extremity plaster casts. J Bone Joint Surg 1982;64(6):896–899.

90. Inman VT, Ralston HJ, Todd F. Human Walking. Baltimore: Waverly, 1981.

91. Waters RL, Lunsford BR. Energy Expenditure of Normal and Pathological Gait: Application to Orthotic Prescription. In JH Bowker, JW Michael (eds), Atlas of Orthotics. St. Louis: Mosby, 1985.

92. Luna-Reyes OB, Reyes TM, So FY, et al. Energy cost of ambulation in healthy and disabled Filipino children. Arch Phys Med Rehabil 1988;69(11);946–949.

93. Mossberg KA, Linton KA, Friske K. Ankle foot orthoses: effect of energy expenditure of gait in spastic diplegic children. Arch Phys Med Rehabil 1990;71(7):490–494.

94. Abudulhadi HM, Kerrigan DC, LaRaia PJ. Contralateral shoe-lift: effect on oxygen cost of walking with an immobilized knee. Arch Phys Med Rehabil 1996;77(7):760–762.

95. Hussey RW, Stauffer ES. Spinal cord injury: requirements for ambulation. Arch Phys Med Rehabil 1973;54(12):544–547.

96. Yakura JS, Waters RL, Adkins RH. Changes in ambulation parameters in spinal cord injury individuals following rehabilitation. Paraplegia 1990;28(6):364–370.

97. Waters RL, Yakura JS, Adkins RH. Gait performance after spinal cord injury. Clin Orthop 1993;March(228):87–96.

98. Nene AV, Patrick JH. Energy cost of locomotion using the ParaWalker—electrical stimulation "hybrid" orthosis. Arch Phys Med Rehabil 1990;71(2):116–120.

99. Banta JV, Bell KJ, Muik EA, Fezio J. Parawalker: energy cost of walking. Eur J Pediatr Surg 1991;1(suppl 1):7–10.

100. Hirokawa S, Grimm M, Le T, et al. Energy consumption in paraplegic ambulation using the reciprocal gait orthosis and electrical stimulation of the thigh muscles. Arch Phys Med Rehabil 1990;71(9):687–694.

101. Winchester P, Caroolo JJ, Habasevich R. Physiological costs of reciprocal gait in FES assisted walking. Paraplegia 1994;32(10):680–686.

102. Yang L, Granat MH, Paul JP, Condie DN, Rowley DI. Further development of hybrid functional electrical stimulation orthoses. Artif Organs 1997;21(3):183–187.

103. Williams LO, Anderson AD, Campbell J, et al. Energy cost of walking and wheelchair propulsion by children with myelodysplasia: comparison to normal children. Dev Med Child Neurol 1983;25(5):617–624.

104. Katz DE, Haideri N, Song K, Wyrick P. Comparative study of conventional HKAFO versus RGO for children with high level paraparesis. J Pediatr Orthop 1997;17(3):377–386.

105. Franks CA, Palisano RJ, Darbee JC. The effect of walking with an assistive device and using a wheelchair on school performance in students with myelomenigocele. Phys Ther 1991;71(1):570–579.

106. Hash D. Energetics of wheelchair propulsion and walking in stroke patients. Orthop Clin North Am 1978;9(2):372–374.

107. Ryerson SD. Hemiplegia. In DA Umphred (ed), Neurological Rehabilitation (3rd ed). St. Louis: Mosby, 1995;681–721.

108. Mauritz KH, Hesse S. Neurological Rehabilitation of Gait and Balance Disorders. In AM Bronstein, T Brandt, MH Woollacott (eds), Clinical Disorders of Balance, Posture and Gait. London: Arnold, 1996;236–250.

109. Campbell J, Ball J. Energetics of walking in cerebral palsy. Orthop Clin North Am 1978;9(2):374–377.

110. Knutson LM. The effects of fixed and hinged ankle foot orthoses on gait myoelectric activity and standing joint alignment in children with cerebral palsy. Doctoral dissertation, University of Iowa, Iowa City, IA, 1993.

111. Winter DA, Sienko SE. Biomechanics of below-knee amputee gait. J Biomech 1988;21(5):361–367.

112. Waters RL, Perry J, Antonelli D, Hislop H. The energy cost of walking of amputees: influence of level of amputation. J Bone Joint Surg 1976;58(1):42–46.

113. Torburn L, Powers CM, Guiterrez R, Perry J. Energy expenditure during ambulation in dysvascular and traumatic below-knee amputees: a comparison of five prosthetic feet. J Rehabil Res Dev 1995;32(2):111–119.

114. Ward KH, Meyers MC. Exercise performance in lower extremity amputees. Sports Med 1995;20(4):207–214.

115. Esqienazi A. Geriatric amputee rehabilitation. Clin Geriatr Med 1993;9(5):731–743.

116. Ganguli S, Datta SR, Chatterjee B. Performance evaluation of amputee-prosthesis system in below knee amputees. Ergonomics 1973;16(6):797–810.

117. Shurr DG, Cook TM. Below Knee Amputation and Prosthetics. In Prosthetics and Orthotics. Norwalk, CT: Appleton & Lange, 1990;53–82.

118. Otis JC, Lane JM, Kroll MA. Energy cost during gait in osteosarcoma patients after resection and knee replacement and after above the knee amputation. J Bone Joint Surg 1985;67A(4):606–611.

119. Fisher SV, Gullickson G. Energy cost of ambulation in health and disability: a literature review. Arch Phys Med Rehabil 1978;59(3):124–133.

120. Jaeger SM, Vos LD, Rispens P, Hof AL. The relationship between comfortable and most metabolically efficient walking speed in persons with unilateral above knee amputations. Arch Phys Med Rehabil 1993;74(5):521–525.

121. Molen NH. Energy/speed relation of below knee amputees walking on a motor driven treadmill. Int Z Angewandte Physiol 1973;31(3):173–185.

122. Czerniecki JM. Rehabilitation of limb deficiency. 1: Gait and motion analysis. Arch Phys Med Rehabil 1996; 77(35suppl):S29–37, S81–82.

123. May BJ. Lower Extremity Prosthetic Management. In Amputation and Prosthetics: A Case Study Approach. Philadelphia: Davis, 1996;139–185.

124. Andrews KL. Rehabilitation in limb deficiency. 3: The geriatric amputee. Arch Phys Med Rehabil 1996;77(3):S14–17.

125. Torburn L, Perry J, Ayyappa E, Shanfield SL. Below knee amputee gait with dynamic elastic response feet: a pilot study. J Rehabil Res Dev 1990;27(4):369–384.

126. Dubow LL, Witt PL, Kadaba MP, et al. Oxygen consumption of elderly persons with bilateral below knee amputation: ambulation vs. wheelchair propulsion. Arch Phys Med Rehabil 1983;64(6):255–259.

127. Nissen SJ, Newman WP. Factors influencing reintegration to normal living after amputation. Arch Phys Med Rehabil 1992;73(6):548–551.

128. Nitz JC. Rehabilitation outcomes after bilateral lower limb amputation for vascular disease. Physiotherapy Theory & Practice 1993;9(3):165–170.

129. Gitter A, Czerniecki JM, DeGroot DM. Biomechanical analysis of the influence of prosthetic feet on below knee amputee walking. Am J Phys Med Rehabil 1991;70(3):142–148.

130. Schneider K, Zernicke RF, Setoguchi Y, Oppenheim W. Dynamics of below-knee child amputee gait: SACH foot versus Flex foot. J Biomech 1993;26(10):1191–1204.

131. Colborne GR, Naumann S, Longmuir PE, Berbrayer D. Analysis of mechanical and metabolic factors in the gait of congenital below knee amputees: a comparison of SACH and Seattle feet. Am J Phys Med Rehabil 1992; 71(5):272–278.

132. Barth DG, Shumacher L, Sienko-Thomas S. Gait analysis and energy cost of below-knee amputees wearing six different prosthetic feet. J Prosthet Orthot 1992;4(2):63–75.

133. McFarlane PA, Nielsen DH, Shurr DG, Meier K. Gait comparisons for below-knee amputees using a FlexFoot versus a conventional prosthetic foot. J Prosthet Orthot 1991; 3(4):150–161.

134. Wirta RW, Mason R, Calvo K, Goldbranson FL. Effect on gait using various prosthetic ankle foot devices. J Rehabil Res Dev 1991;28(2):13–24.

135. Czerniecki JM, Gitter A. The impact of energy storing prosthetic feet on below knee amputation gait. Arch Phys Med Rehabil 1989;70(13):918.

136. Czerniecki JM, Gitter A, Murno C. Joint moment and muscle power output characteristics of below knee amputees during running: the influence of energy storing prosthetic feet. J Biomech 1991;24(1):63–75.

137. Torburn L, Schweiger GP, Perry J, Powers CM. Below knee amputee gait in stair climbing: a comparison of stride characteristics using five different prosthetic feet. Clin Orthop 1994;June(303):185–192.

138. Flandry F, Beskin J, Chambers RB, et al. The effect of the CAT-CAM above knee prosthetic on functional rehabilitation. Clin Orthop 1989;Feb(239):249–262.

139. Gailey RS, Lawrence D, Burditt C, et al. The CAT-CAM socket and quadrilateral socket: a comparison of energy cost during ambulation. Prosthet Orthot Int 1993;17(2):95–100.

II

Orthotics in Rehabilitation

5

Principles of Orthotic Design

Michelle M. Lusardi

An orthosis, an external device used in rehabilitation of patients with neuromuscular and musculoskeletal disorders, can be prescribed for a variety of reasons. For patients with rheumatoid arthritis or an acute injury, an orthosis can be used to "rest" an inflamed joint and its surrounding tissues. It is often prescribed in the postoperative management of patients with surgical fusion or reconstructive surgery to immobilize the affected body part. An orthosis can be used to project a joint made vulnerable by ligamentous instability or to control joint motion in the presence of weakness or abnormal tone. Orthoses can serve as stabilizing substitutes for muscles that are weakened by a disease process or provide the foundation for use of an assistive device. Some orthoses provide additional kinesthetic feedback to remind the patient to move (or not to move) in certain ways or postures. An orthosis that applies strategically placed forces to a limb or body segment can also be used to correct alignment or to prevent further deformity.

To make informed decisions about whether a particular orthosis would be appropriate for a patient with gait dysfunction or other functional limitation, rehabilitation professionals must understand two things: (1) the basic biomechanical principles of joint motion and (2) the underlying design of the orthosis and its impact on the joint. Orthotists, therapists, physicians, and patients and their caregivers must discuss and come to agreement on which design and component options would best meet the patient's functional needs. A number of important questions must be raised and answered: How and where does the orthosis apply force to provide stability or to control movement at a particular joint? In what planes of movement does the orthosis have an effect? Will it be most important for the orthosis to restrict movement completely or to allow movement in a limited range, or will movement be supported or unrestricted? How does application of an orthosis to control motion at one joint or limb segment impact on

those that are proximal or distal to it? What impact does the orthosis have on each of the subphases of gait? Are the biomechanical "tradeoffs" or consequences imposed by the device outweighed by the benefits of its use? Given the patient's physical condition and potential for growth, as well as the likelihood of change in status or progression of his or her condition, what types of orthotic materials would be most appropriate?

The goal of this chapter is to help the reader identify the characteristics of an effective orthosis and to understand how an orthosis is biomechanically designed so that it can effectively meet the patient's functional needs. To do this, we begin with a review of some basic kinesiologic principles as they apply to the function of joints during movement and to the design of the orthosis. The chapter concludes with a discussion of factors that influence the fit and function of orthoses.

WHAT MAKES AN "IDEAL" ORTHOSIS

Although no orthotic design can restore "normal" function in the presence of neuromuscular or musculoskeletal impairment, an effective and well-designed orthosis enhances mobility and, it is hoped, improves quality of life. From a patient's perspective, there are two important determinants of success: whether the orthosis is comfortable during use and how well it meets his or her needs and goals. Does the orthosis enable the patient to accomplish the tasks and be involved in activities that are important to him or her, without undue discomfort, skin irritation, or fatigue or other orthosis-induced concerns?[1] Even the most technically advanced orthosis will remain in the patient's closet or under the bed if it is too hot to wear for long periods of time, too heavy on the limb, too cumbersome to use for more than a short period, or if wearing the orthosis causes discomfort or pain. Patients are most likely to use an orthosis that fits well, is dependable during function, is easy to don and doff, and is simple to clean and maintain. Many patients also appreciate orthoses that are "cosmetic" and can be worn without being too obvious to others.

From the perspective of the rehabilitation team, an important determinant of success is how well the orthosis does what it has been designed to do. Does the orthosis support or protect a joint or limb during movement as intended? How effective is it in controlling movement in the presence of spasticity or weakness? How well does the orthosis maintain or correct alignment and reduce the risk of deformity? Does the patient's functional status improve when it is worn? Can the orthosis accomplish its intended goals without causing secondary problems, such as skin irritation, breakdown, or discomfort at other joints? The rehabilitation team is also interested in the ease of fabrication and adjustment. How quickly and efficiently can the orthosis be fabricated and delivered to the patient for use? How economical is the orthosis in terms of materials, cost, and the time and skill requirements for fabrication? Can the orthosis be adjusted as the patient grows or as functional status changes? How durable are the materials and components used in orthosis? What are the anticipated maintenance requirements of the device?

The answers to these questions are founded on understanding of normal joint structure and function, the kinematics of gait, the pathomechanics that result from the patient's pathology or collection of impairments, and the biomechanics of orthotic design.

DESCRIBING MOTION

Human movement can be categorized as being rotatory, translatory, curvilinear, or as a general plane motion. Joint motion is rotatory or angular when it takes place around an axis in a curved path. In true rotatory movement, all points on the distal limb segment move around the joint axis in concert, at the same time and at a constant distance from the axis of rotation. An example of true rotary motion is a door that is being opened or closed; all parts of the door move concurrently, inscribing an arc, in a fixed path, at a constant distance from the hinge. Few joints in the human body, however, move in purely rotatory motion.[2]

Translatory or linear motion occurs when the moving object, like a joint surface, moves in a straight line. An object that is being pushed or pulled across a level surface is moving in a linear or translatory path. Although few human motions are entirely translatory, the line of pull of most muscles create a sizable translatory component to voluntarily controlled joint motion.

When rotatory and translatory motion are combined in a single joint, such that the axis of motion changes, the motion that occurs is described as curvilinear. An example of curvilinear motion is the gliding that occurs as the tibial plateau moves around the larger femoral condyles during flexion and extension of the knee.

General plane motion occurs when a limb segment rotates around an axis at the same time that it is translating (moving) through space. An example of general plane motion of the lower extremity is the motion used to kick a soccer ball: Rapid knee extension (a rotatory motion) occurs as the entire limb is moving forward (a translatory motion) toward the ball.

To understand joint movement, kinesiologists often diagram each of the forces that act on a limb segment at a particular time. Each of these forces can be resolved into its rotatory and translatory components. Rotatory force vectors are drawn perpendicular to the bony lever, whereas translatory force vectors are typically drawn parallel to the bony lever. These force vectors are discussed in more detail shortly.

Planes, Direction, and Magnitude of Motion

Traditionally, human movement is described as occurring in one or more of the three cardinal planes of motion, referenced to anatomic position of the body (Figure 5-1). The *sagittal plane* divides the body into fairly symmetric left and right sides. On a three-dimensional graph, sagittal plane movement would occur in the "z" plane around an axis of rotation in the frontal plane. Elbow and knee flexion and extension are examples of motions that, for the most part, occur in the sagittal plane. The *frontal* or *coronal plane* divides the body into front (ventral) and back (dorsal) halves. On a three-dimensional graph, frontal plane motion occurs in the "y" plane around an antero-posterior axis of motion. Lateral bending (side bending) and abduction/adduction of the extremities are examples of motion in the frontal plane. The third plane of motion is *transverse plane motion*, which occurs in the "x" plane on a three-dimensional graph, around a longitudinal axis of rotation. Trunk rotation and internal or external rotation of the hip are examples of motions that occur primarily in the transverse plane.

Given the shape of articular surfaces and the line of pull of most muscles, rarely does functional movement occur purely in one plane: Most human movement is multidimensional, blending motion in all three planes to meet a particular movement goal. Theoretically, each joint has six potential degrees of freedom: two directions of motion in each plane. The shape and structure of each joint vary so that movement does not happen equally in all planes.

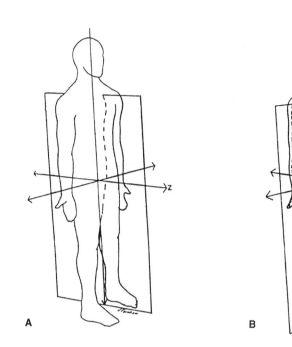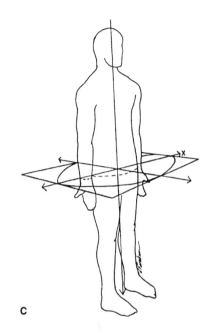

FIGURE 5-1

(A) Sagittal plane motions, such as knee extension, occur around an axis of rotation in the frontal plane. (B) Frontal plane motion, such as lateral bending of the trunk or abduction of the hip, occurs around an anteroposterior axis of rotation. (C) Transverse plane motion, such as trunk rotation or internal rotation of the hip, occurs around a longitudinal axis of motion. (Adapted with permission from CC Norkin, PK Levangie. Joint Structure and Function: A Comprehensive Analysis [2nd ed]. Philadelphia: Davis, 1992;6.)

Additionally, during closed chain activities such as gait, motion at one joint is often "coupled" (has an influence on) motion at the joints that are proximal and distal to that joint. An example of this is the relationship between pronation of the foot and internal (medial) rotation of the tibia in standing and gait.[3,4]

Joint motion can be assessed in a variety of ways. Observation of active movement provides evidence of muscle strength and control, as well as the constraints imposed by soft tissue structures around the joint. Passive movement of the limb segment or single joint provides further evidence of the influence of muscle tone, biomechanical stability of the joint, or restriction of motion resulting from contracture or deformity. The total active and passive excursion of the joint can be measured using a goniometer as number of degrees of range of motion. Norms for expected range of motion of each joint of the body have been established and are used as a reference in clinical decision making.[5] For some conditions, such as idiopathic scoliosis, range of motion can be measured most accurately using x-ray films rather than during active or passive movement. Angular speed (the number of degrees of joint movement that occur per second) is often used as an indicator of joint function in motion analysis and may be especially important for gait analysis. Joint

play motions, performed either at the end of range or at the point in the range at which ligaments and joint capsule become taut, are additional indicators of joint function and are used to evaluate ligamentous stability or soft tissue dysfunction that has an impact on joint motion.[6] All of these methods of assessing magnitude of joint motion provide important information for the orthotic prescription and fabrication process.

UNDERSTANDING MOVEMENT: MOBILITY AND STABILITY

One way to describe human movement is to think of the skeleton, the body's framework, as a system of many levers.[2] Movement can occur at a single joint in the articulation of two bony levers (e.g., isolated knee flexion) or across an entire limb, involving multiple joints with overlapping or shared bony levers (e.g., the combination of dorsiflexion, knee flexion, and hip flexion that is necessary when ascending a set of stairs). During most functional activities, some joints or segments must be constrained for stability, whereas others must be moved to accomplish the intended task or goal. A joint or limb

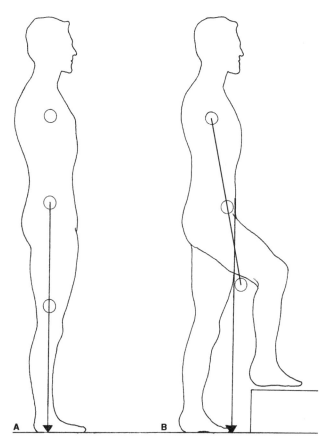

FIGURE 5-2

(A) The body's center of mass in quiet standing is just anterior to the S2 level of the sacrum. (B) As the leg is lifted toward a stair, the COM of the body shifts forward. If an orthosis adds mass to the limb, the limb's COM will shift further distally within the segment, and the body's COM will shift to a slightly more anterior position as a result.

is at rest or is stable when the forces that act on the limb are in equilibrium, when the forces acting on that limb sum to zero. Movement occurs when unequal or unopposed forces act on the limb or body segment.

If we define a "force" as a push or pull applied by one object on another, we can identify a number of forces or structures that act on the body simultaneously: gravity, muscle contraction, ligamentous tension, and the external forces imposed by orthoses or by contact with other still or moving objects. Each force can be described as a vector, in terms of its point of application, direction (line of action), and magnitude.[2] The force's moment arm is the perpendicular distance from a joint's center (axis) of motion to the force vector (i.e., the shortest distance). The larger this moment arm, the more powerful the influence that a

force will have on a limb segment. To understand how a force influences a particular joint, the force must be resolved into its rotatory and translatory components.

Gravity and Center of Mass

One of the most important forces that acts on the body is gravity, the attraction of the earth's mass for the mass of objects on or near the earth. Gravity acts continuously on the body at an acceleration magnitude of 32 ft/sec^2. Body weight (w = mass $\times$ 32 ft/sec^2) is, in effect, the vector that results from the force of gravity. Gravity's vector is often referred to as the *line of gravity*. Traditionally, kinesiologists and physicists describe a single point of application for gravity, which occurs at an object's center of gravity (COG) or center of mass (COM). When considering the influence of gravity on the body, we can identify the COM for an individual segment, for the whole limb, or for the entire body.[7] For adults who are standing quietly, the approximate position of the body's COM is just anterior to the S2 level of the sacrum.

It is important to understand that the location of the COM is determined by the body's position in space and contact with the supporting surface: The position of the COM changes as body position or type of activity changes. In a forward reach, for example, the COM moves forward as the arms are lifted and even farther forward if mass (such as a full bag of groceries) is added to the arms. When a lower extremity is lifted to ascend stairs, the COM moves slightly upward and forward from its "at rest" position anterior to S2 (Figure 5-2). An orthosis worn on the ascending limb increases the mass of the limb, shifting its COM to a more distal position and the body's COM slightly toward that limb. The COM of patients who are immobilized in a "halo" cervical thoracic orthosis shifts upward from the S2 level because of the added mass of the orthosis' framework around the patient's head.

Earlier, we learned that a force can be divided into a rotatory and a translatory component. Consider an individual sitting on a dock, gently swinging her legs over the water. At the most anterior point of the arc, at 45 degrees of knee flexion, gravity's rotatory component acts to swing the lower leg backward (into more knee flexion), while the translatory component will distract or separate the femoral and tibial articular surfaces. At the bottom of the arc, in approximately 90 degrees of knee flexion, the force of gravity is almost entirely translatory, separating joint surfaces at the knee. As the swing reaches its posterior maximum, the rotatory component of gravity causes the lower leg to swing forward (toward knee extension), and the translatory motion separates joint surfaces once again. In this situation, the impact of the translatory component of gravity is counteracted by tension in the ligaments that stabilize the knee and the soft tissue of the joint capsule.

When the line of gravity (also known as the *weight line*, a downward vector from the COM) falls within an individual's base of support, the body is in a state of relative stability. When activity moves the line of gravity beyond the edges of the base of support, action of some type must occur to restore stability. One strategy used to restore the COM within the confines of the base of support during movement is the activation of postural muscles. Postural muscle contraction applies counteractive forces to limb segments that oppose gravity or act to realign body segments. Another strategy would be to use assistive devices to enlarge the base of support, so that the COM is once again within the larger base of support.

Muscles, Tendons, and Ligaments

The point of application of forces created by muscle contraction is the muscle's tendinous attachment to the bone of a limb or body segment. The muscle's line of pull is determined by the arrangement of muscle fibers within the muscle belly: In muscles with multiple bellies, the muscle's force vector is a composite of the vectors of each individual belly. In the quadriceps femoris, for example, the line of pull for the rectus femoris and vastus intermedius is generally parallel with the femur, whereas the vastus lateralis and vastus intermedius exert an oblique pull on the quadriceps tendon (Figure 5-3). The resultant quadriceps vector positions the patella to be an efficient pulley for knee extension and provides the power to accomplish that extension.

During an open chain concentric contraction, most muscles of the human body act as third-class lever systems: The distance between their point of attachment and the joint center (effort arm) is significantly shorter than the distance between the segment's COG and the joint center (resistance arm)[2] (Figure 5-4). Although the mechanical inefficiency of a third-class lever system means that the muscle must generate a great deal of force to move the limb, it also ensures that the distal limb moves quickly through a large arc of movement. Most functional tasks require just this type of movement through space. In an eccentric contraction, a controlled "letting go" of limb position, the force of gravity acting at the COG of the segment is the end point of the effort arm, whereas the muscle's attachment is the end point of the resistance arm, forming a second-class lever. For muscles, the distance between the joint axis and the muscle's point of attachment changes as the limb moves through its range of motion. This means that the length of the moment arm of the muscle varies as well: The muscle is not equally efficient or powerful at all points in the range of motion. A muscle is able to develop maximum torque when its moment

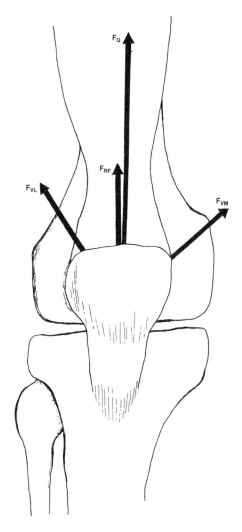

FIGURE 5-3

Schematic diagram of the force vectors created by contraction of the rectus femoris (F_{RF}), vastus lateralis (F_{VL}), and vastus medialis (F_{VM}), along with the composite force vector for the entire quadriceps femoris (F_Q). The line of pull is determined by the arrangement of fibers within the muscle and by their attachment to the quadriceps tendon.

arm is at maximum value, the point at which its line of pull is perpendicular to the bony lever it is moving.

In the human body, most muscles generate a line of pull that is closer to being parallel than perpendicular to the limb segment (lever) to which the muscle is attached. We can resolve the force of muscle contraction into its rotatory component (which acts perpendicular to the lever) and its translatory component (which acts parallel to the lever). For most muscles, the translatory force is greater than the rotatory force, contributing to joint compression and stability during functional activity.

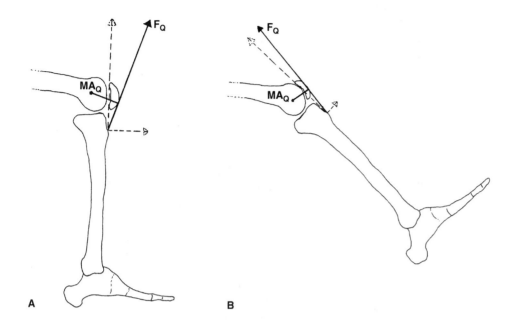

A

B

FIGURE 5-4

*Even though the patella acts as an anatomic pulley, increasing the overall distance from the center of the knee joint axis to the line of pull of the patellar tendon, the relative length of the quadriceps moment arm decreases as the knee extends from (**A**) 90 degrees of flexion toward (**B**) 45 degrees of flexion. MA_Q = moment arm of the quadriceps; F_Q = force vector of the quadriceps.*

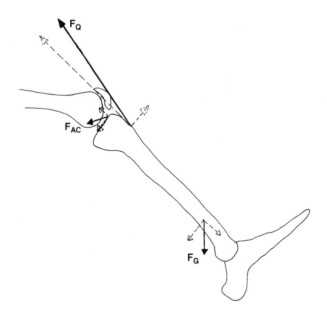

FIGURE 5-5

In this diagram, three of the forces that act on the knee during active knee extension are diagrammed. Gravity (F_G) acts at the lower limb's center of mass. The quadriceps femoris (F_Q) acts at the attachment of the patellar tendon. The anterior cruciate ligament (F_{AC}) acts at its point of attachment to the tibia. Each force has been resolved into its rotatory and translatory components. For effective knee extension, the posterior translatory forces must balance the anterior translatory force, and the upward acting rotary force of the quadriceps must be more than the downward rotary force of gravity. (Adapted with permission from CC Norkin, PK Levangie. Joint Structure and Function: A Comprehensive Analysis [2nd ed]. Philadelphia: Davis, 1992;53.)

The passive tension exerted on a joint by its capsule and supporting ligaments can also be diagrammed as a force with rotatory and translatory components (Figure 5-5). One of the important functions of ligaments is to provide dynamic stability during movement, protecting the joint from excessive movement when forces such as muscle contraction or gravity are acting on the levers on either side of the joint. As fibroelastic connective tissue, ligaments are susceptible to failure under conditions of prolonged elongation or when a sudden or excessive loading force exceeds their elastic limits.[8] Orthoses are often used to protect a joint for excessive translatory movement when ligamentous laxity or damage is present. Functional knee orthosis used for patients with anterior cruciate ligament deficiency is an example of such use.

Use of Forces in Orthotic Design

Most orthotic designs use a balanced parallel force system to control joint motion. These force systems operate, in effect, as a first-class lever system. In a three-point loading or control system, a proximal and a distal force applied in the same direction are countered by (or balanced against) a third force applied in the opposite direction at a point somewhere in between them.[9,10] Each plane and direction of motion that the orthosis attempts to control has a three-point loading system (Figure 5-6). Some orthotic designs use an additional force, acting as a balanced four-point system, to allow better control of rotatory and translatory motion of the joint or to provide effective control of motion in multiple planes (Figure 5-7).

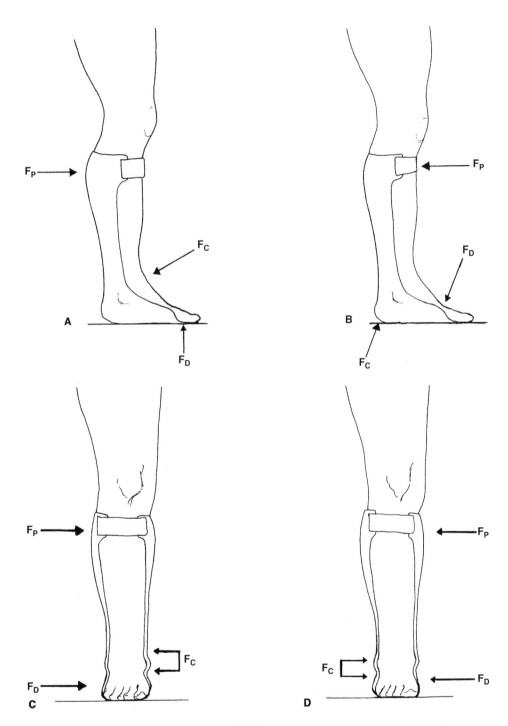

FIGURE 5-6

*Force system in a molded thermoplastic solid-ankle AFO design. (**A**) Plantar flexion is controlled during swing phase by a proximal force (F_P) at the posterior calf band and a distal force at the metatarsal heads (F_D) that counter a centrally located stabilizing force (F_C) applied at the anterior ankle by shoe closure. (**B**) For control of dorsiflexion during stance phase (i.e., forward progression of tibia over the foot), F_P is applied at the proximal tibia by the anterior closure, F_D at the ventral metatarsal heads by the toe box of the shoe, and counterforce F_C at the heel, snugly fit in the orthosis. (**C**) The force system for eversion (valgus) locates F_D along the fifth metatarsal, F_P at the proximal lateral calf band, and F_C on either side of the medial malleolus. (**D**) To control inversion (varus) of the foot and ankle, F_D is applied by the distal medial wall of the orthosis against the first metatarsal, F_P at the proximal medial calf band, and F_C at the distal lateral tibia and calcaneus/talus, on either side of the lateral malleolus.*

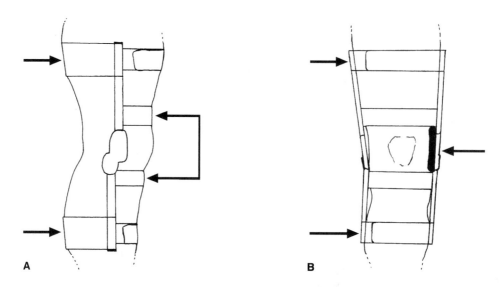

FIGURE 5-7
(A) For a patient with instability of the knee, this four-point control system is designed to control sagittal plane translatory motion between the tibia and femur. Distributing the counterforce on either side of the knee joint axis reduces shearing forces at the knee joint while simultaneously controlling knee flexion. (B) The same orthosis controls valgus at the knee in the frontal plane using a three-point control system. Note the enlarged medial pad that is used to distribute F_C comfortably over a large area. Rotation of the tibia in the transverse plane cannot be controlled effectively by this design. To provide complete control of tibial rotation, the orthosis would have to incorporate the foot and ankle as well.

Each orthosis is designed to apply force of a particular magnitude at a specific point or place on the limb or body segment. These forces impact on the joint indirectly, through the contact between orthosis (via straps, pads, bands, or total contact fit) and the soft tissue structures of the limb (skin, muscle, fat, fascia, tendons, and bone). Many molded ankle-foot orthoses (AFOs) are designed to use the shoe as a means of closure to apply the desired force to the foot. The loading forces of a three- or four-point control system on a limb segment or joint may be substantial; even low pressure sustained over long periods of time can lead to tissue deformation and breakdown.[8] For this reason, orthotic forces are often distributed over as much surface area of the limb as possible, to keep pressures applied by the orthosis within levels that are tolerable to soft tissue and comfortable for the patient during wear. This is especially important for patients with sensory loss, cognitive impairment, or compromised circulation, who may have increased vulnerability to skin breakdown. Most orthotic designs incorporate "reliefs" for areas of bony prominence or use padding to cushion or distribute forces that would otherwise be excessive.

As a first-class lever system, the magnitude of each of the forces in the control system is inversely related to the distance between its point of application and the axis of movement. To be in equilibrium, the forces in the system must sum to zero. Consider, as an example, a knee orthosis designed to control genu recurvatum (Figure 5-8). The central force in the system is an anteriorly directed force applied at the posterior knee. The opposing paired posteriorly directed forces are applied at the anterior femur and the anterior tibia. Although these forces can be applied anywhere along the shaft of the femur and tibia, the magnitude of the required force decreases as the point of application is moved upward on the femur and downward on the tibia. If the forces are in equilibrium, the central force applied at the posterior knee will be twice the magnitude of either of the other forces. The potentially negative impact of this force on soft tissues of the knee is minimized by distributing the force over a large surface area via padding. Orthoses with long levers tend to be more comfortable for the patient during wear, although the length of the orthosis is also related to ease of donning and doffing and to cosmesis.

Because most human movement is multiplanar, with an axis of joint motion offset from any single plane, no orthosis can perfectly match or mimic the biomechanical motion of the anatomical joint. As a result, the forces applied by the orthosis and the reactive forces that originate from the limb segment will be mismatched.[11,12] Because these applied and reactive forces are, to some extent, noncollinear, any three- or four-point force sys-

FIGURE 5-8

Magnitude of forces necessary to control recurvatum decreases as the point of application is moved from (A) close to the central force at the knee axis to (B) a position more proximal on the femur and distal on the tibia. Because the system is in equilibrium, moving the forces away from the joint axis also reduces the magnitude of the central force in this three-point force system.

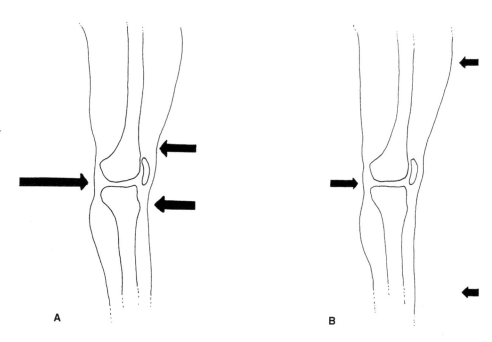

A   B

tems applied by an orthosis to a limb in an effort to control joint motion will have a desired (corrective, controlling) and undesired (deforming) impact. These effects are best understood in terms of bending moments and shearing forces.

The bending moment, which is greatest at the point of application of the center force in a three-point system, represents the location of maximum orthotic control or correction. A separate bending moment is present in each plane of motion that the orthosis attempts to control. The efficiency of an orthosis in controlling or correcting motion is influenced by the distance between the joint axis and the point of application of each of the forces. We have already discovered the magnitude of the force needed if the orthosis is to achieve the desired level of correction or control decreases as the lever arm (distance from the joint axis to the point of force application) increases. The location of the point of application of the central force, where the bending moment is maximal, is also important to consider: The controlling or corrective forces are most effective (and least deforming) if the central force and the maximum bending moment coincide (are congruent with) with the actual joint axis. When a discrepancy occurs, the resulting shear forces and torques will have an impact on the joint and its support structures that must be taken into account, to maximize patient comfort and compliance and to minimize the long-term consequences of these shearing forces on joint and soft tissue integrity. This is most often accomplished by careful placement of the straps

or bands used to apply the force system, attention to their widths and depths, the "initimacy" of fit of the orthosis, and the degree of tightness that is necessary to secure the orthosis and apply the desired forces.

When the goal of an orthosis is to support motion, rather than to immobilize a joint, the relationship between the anatomic and orthotic joint is an important consideration in orthotic design as well. Because most anatomic joints have a triplanar or polycentric axis and most orthotic joints are single axis designs, incongruence necessarily occurs between the axes of the joint and the orthosis at some point in the range of motion, even in the most carefully designed orthosis. The torque that results from this mismatch can, over time, have significant impact on the integrity of soft tissue and articular surfaces of the joint that the orthosis is trying to control. Because of this, an important component of long-term follow-up for patients who depend on orthoses for function is careful periodic reassessment of joint condition and function.

LOWER EXTREMITY ORTHOSES AND GAIT

Any time that a lower extremity orthosis changes joint motion, it is also likely to, in some way, change progression through the gait cycle. A solid-ankle AFO, which holds the ankle in a neutral position, facilitates toe clearance during swing and optimally positions the limb for heel strike at initial contact. In loading response, however, the fixed ankle cannot move into plantar flexion to reach foot flat, hampering the first rocker of gait. Instead, the rigid orthosis causes the tibia to accelerate forward quickly so that the forefoot contacts the ground. As a consequence, disruption of the normal shock absorption mechanism occurs with a potential disruption of postural stability in early stance. With the progression from midstance to terminal stance, the fixed angle of the ankle prevents forward progression of the tibia over the foot. Disruption of this second rocker of gait hampers forward progression of the COM and ultimately reduces step length of the opposite swinging limb. If the orthosis has a relatively stiff extended toe plate, the extension (dorsiflexion) of the toes that is necessary for continued forward progression and heel rise may be blocked as well. The stance phase "tradeoffs" of a solid-ankle AFO can be addressed by footwear: Shoes with a compressible heel and rocker sole are effective substitutes when the rockers of gait are constrained by an orthosis.

Ambulation with a knee-ankle-foot orthosis with a locked knee has an impact on stance and on swing phase of gait. With a knee that is prevented from flexing during loading response, the "shock absorption" eccentric function of the quadriceps is compromised, and impact forces are transmitted upward to the hip and low back. Stance phase stability during midstance and terminal stance is ensured by the locked knee, but the relative shortening of the limb that usually occurs as a result of knee flexion in preswing is prevented. Similarly, swing limb clearance becomes problematic in initial swing and midswing because the knee remains in extension, and the patient must use a compensatory strategy, such as circumduction or vaulting, to advance the limb successfully.

Most patients who are fitted with lower extremity orthoses, such as a solid-ankle AFO or a knee-ankle-foot orthosis with a locked knee, have musculoskeletal-based biomechanical dysfunction or neuromuscular impairments of motor control that themselves compromise functional ambulation. Whenever an orthosis is prescribed, the relative merits of an orthotic design are weighed carefully against the constraints imposed by the device. For this reason, orthotists and therapists strive to determine which orthosis can maximally enhance the patient's function with the minimal possible external support or control. An orthosis that does too much is as problematic as an orthosis that does too little to assist or improve function and is likely to end up in the closet or under the bed rather than being worn.

Other Important Considerations

The energy cost associated with the use of an orthosis is related to its weight as well as to the impact of the ortho-

sis on joint motion and gait. Weight of the orthosis is determined by the materials used in its fabrication and by how much of the limb is encompassed by the device. The high-temperature thermoplastic and lightweight composites and metal alloys that have replaced traditional metal and leather lower extremity orthoses have had an extremely positive impact on energy expenditure during gait, making ambulation a feasible goal for patients with a wider variety of diagnoses.

It is also important to realize that, in many instances, control of a proximal joint is possible without having to bring the orthosis above the level of that joint, which adds more mass (and weight) to the limb as it moves through space. Consider, for example, a patient with a complete spinal cord injury at T10 who has no volitional muscle function at the hips, knees, or ankles. This patient is able to stand and ambulate (with crutches) when fitted with a pair of knee-ankle-foot orthoses set to stabilize the ankles in 10–15 degrees of dorsiflexion and the knees in extension. The combination of the ankle fixed in dorsiflexion and a locked knee creates a forward inclination of the entire lower extremity. When this resting posture is coupled with an exaggerated lumbar lordosis and forward pelvis, the axis of hip motion is well anterior to the line of gravity. The resultant extensor moment at the hip is enough to stabilize the hip in stance. Because of this alignment stability, it is not necessary to add a hip joint and pelvic band to the orthosis.

For patients with hip control who have difficulty in maintaining knee extension in stance because of impairment of motor control or muscle function, a similar "less is more" principle is used. A solid-ankle AFO or an anterior floor reaction AFO that fixes the ankle in slight plantar flexion may functionally eliminate the need to bring the orthosis above the knee and up the thigh for stability in stance. If the ankle is fixed in slight plantar flexion, the forward progression of the tibia over the foot during stance is blocked. Because stance is a closed chain activity, this translates into an extensor moment at the knee. This slight plantar flexion often provides just enough extensor stability during early stance, when the weight line falls behind the axis of the knee joint, to allow the patient to swing through with the opposite limb. Without this plantar flexion, early stance phase stability may be sacrificed and the opposite swing phase shortened in an effort to remain upright on an unstable limb.

SUMMARY

An orthosis can be prescribed for patients with many different impairments and functional limitations of the neuromuscular or musculoskeletal system. In deciding among possible orthotic designs and components, the first step is to define clearly the goal of the orthosis. Whether the orthosis is used to protect an unstable or healing joint, to immobilize or unload a limb segment, to allow motion within a restricted range of motion, or to substitute for inadequate muscle strength or motor control, the impact of the orthosis' force system on the limb must be considered. Ideally, the force system used in the orthotic design is able to apply judiciously only that amount of force necessary to accomplish its goal, and the forces are applied in such a way that bending moments are effective and shearing or torque forces that act on the joint are minimal. To evaluate whether an orthosis is effective, the orthotist and therapist must be aware of normal function of the joints involved, as well as any existing deformities that might have an impact on orthotic design. As an external device, orthoses often increase the physiologic "work" of walking and can constrain movement in advantageous and in unwanted ways. The "costs" of orthotic wear must be outweighed by the perceived benefits (from a patient's point of view) if the orthosis is going to be used, as intended, for improving function.

REFERENCES

1. Shurr DG, Cook TM. Methods, Materials, and Mechanics. In Prosthetics and Orthotics. Norwalk, CT: Appleton & Lange, 1990;17–30.

2. Norkin CC, Levangie PK. Basic Concepts in Biomechanics. In Joint Structure and Function: A Comprehensive Analysis. Philadelphia: Davis, 1992;1–56.

3. Oatis CA. Biomechanics of the foot and ankle under static conditions. Phys Ther 1988;68(12):1815–1821.

4. Rodgers MM. Dynamic foot biomechanics. J Orthop Sports Phys Ther 1995;21(6):306–316.

5. Norkin CC, White DJ. Measurement of Joint Motion: A Guide to Goniometry (2nd ed). Philadelphia: Davis, 1995.

6. Hall RC, Nitz AJ. Basic Concepts of Orthopedic Manual Therapy. In TR Malone, T McPoil, AJ Nitz (eds), Orthopedic and Sports Physical Therapy (3rd ed). St. Louis: Mosby, 1997;191–210.

7. Soderberg GL. Kinesiology Application to Pathological Motion. Baltimore: Williams & Wilkins, 1986.

8. Norkin CC, Levangie PK. Joint Structure and Function. In Joint Structure and Function: A Comprehensive Analysis. Philadelphia: Davis, 1992;57–91.

9. Trautman P. Lower Limb Orthoses. In JB Redford, JV Basmajian, P Trautman (eds), Orthotics: Clinical Practice and Rehabilitation Technology. New York: Churchill Livingstone, 1995;13–39.

10. Nawoczenski DA. Introduction to Orthotics: Rationale for Treatment. In DA Nawoczenski, ME Epler (eds), Orthotics in Functional Rehabilitation of the Lower Limb. Philadelphia: Saunders, 1997;1–14.

11. Byars EF, Snyder RD, Plants HL. Engineering Mechanics for Deformable Bodies (4th ed). New York: Harper & Row, 1983;224–237.

12. Smith EM, Juvinall RC. Mechanics of Orthotics. In JB Redford (ed), Orthotics Etcetera (3rd ed). Baltimore: Williams & Wilkins, 1986;26–32.

6

Assessment Strategies for Lower Extremity Orthoses

MICHELLE M. LUSARDI

Lower extremity orthoses are prescribed for patients with diverse diagnoses and functional limitations, of many ages and abilities and with diverse physical characteristics. The purpose of an orthotic prescription varies as well (Table 6-1). For a certain patient, the primary goal of the orthosis might be to protect a joint that is biomechanically unstable and vulnerable to injury or a limb segment that is healing after injury. For another, the goal might be to use the orthosis to apply corrective forces when the patient has a risk of developing a deformity or to halt the progression of an existing deformity. For a third, an orthosis might be a substitute when weakness or paralysis prevents a muscle from functioning as it should. In another situation, an orthosis can enhance function by controlling limb position in the presence of spasticity, positioning the limb for a more efficient swing phase and preparing it for a more "normal" initial contact at the heel. Finally, an orthosis might be used to provide stability for patients who would otherwise be unable to function in an upright posture, to immobilize a limb segment after orthopedic surgery following fracture, or to correct a musculoskeletal deformity.

Given the diverse characteristics and functional needs of the many patients who might benefit from the use of an orthosis, individualized prescription ensures that an orthosis will meet the expectations of the patient and health care team. The foundation for this individualized prescription is a careful evaluation of the patient's musculoskeletal and neuromuscular status, as well as an assessment of current functional status and estimation of future potential. This information helps the orthotist, therapist, physician, patient, and family to define the goals of orthotic intervention clearly for each patient and then to make informed choices about design and components. This evaluation and discussion of options also help to ensure that the orthosis created for the patient will meet expectations and that all members of the team understand the ways that the orthosis will, or will not, have an impact on function.

The therapist and orthotist often have complementary roles in preorthotic assessment. Having worked with the patient in inpatient or outpatient rehabilitation settings, the therapist develops an in-depth understanding of the patient's motor control and functional status. The therapist begins to define the goals of orthotic intervention and may have initial impressions about the design or components that might be appropriate. The orthotist, in addition to assessing joint and limb function and taking specific measurements necessary for fabrication of a custom orthosis, asks questions that help to clarify the goals of orthotic intervention. The orthotist also has the most up-to-date information and a wealth of clinical experience about design and components to best address the patient's needs and functional goals. Patients and their family members or caregivers bring practicality into the decision-making process in their concern about how difficult the orthosis might be to don and doff, and to maintain and care for.

In this chapter, we present an overview of data collection and evaluation in preparation for orthotic prescription. The information presented reflects the roles of the orthotist and the therapist in preorthotic assessment so that the reader can develop an appreciation of the entire evaluative process. We begin with assessment of musculoskeletal and neuromuscular impairment, continue with strategies for functional assessment, and conclude with a discussion of other factors that are important in decision making and orthotic prescription.

STRATEGIES FOR ASSESSMENT OF IMPAIRMENTS

To design the most effective orthosis, the orthotist needs specific information about limb segment alignment, joint range of motion, limb length and girth, ligamentous

TABLE 6-1
Goals of Orthotic Management

To protect a joint or limb segment
To correct alignment in flexible deformity
To substitute for functional losses
To enhance function in the presence of impairment
To stabilize or immobilize a limb segment or the trunk

stability, and muscle function. Because orthoses apply external forces to the limb, the orthotist must also evaluate sensory function and skin integrity. If either (or both) sensation or skin condition is compromised, precautions must be built in to the orthosis to minimize risk of skin breakdown and vascular compromise. To provide the least necessary orthotic support, the orthotist must have a clear understanding of muscle strength and tone, both when the patient is at rest and when the patient is active and moving. Most of the examination methods used in the preorthotic assessment are standard or routinely used orthopedic or neuromuscular assessment strategies. Occasionally, additional information, such as x-ray or electromyographic findings, are also important in the prescription process.

JOINT FUNCTION AND INTEGRITY

For patients who require an orthosis because of musculoskeletal or neuromuscular dysfunction, assessment begins with careful evaluation of joint function, including range of motion and the factors that can contribute to limitation of motion or joint instability. Information about the spatial relationship of articular surfaces, the axis of motion of the joints, the alignment of limb seg-

ments, and any discrepancies in limb or segmental length and girth is important in the development of an individualized orthotic prescription.

Range of Motion

Therapists and orthotists use similar strategies to assess joint range of motion. Observation of the patient's active movement begins to identify where limitations may occur that require further assessment. Passive movement of the patient's limb through its gross arcs of motion further identifies potential problem areas. Special attention is given to excursions of the hip, knee, and ankle that are necessary for "normal" progression through stance and swing[1] (Table 6-2).

In most instances, the orthotist or therapist chooses to take definitive *goniometric measurements* of the joints that will be controlled or directly influenced by the orthosis.[2] Normal range of motion of the hip, knee, and ankle joints is summarized in Table 6-3. In addition to measuring total excursion of the joint, goniometric assessment identifies where a limitation begins or whether the joint is hypermobile. With application of a slight gentle overpressure as a limb segment reaches the end of passive range of motion, the examiner compares the *end feel* of the patient's joint to the end feel (bone to bone, soft tissue approximation, or tissue stretch) that is typical for that joint.[3] Assessment of *joint play*, the accessory movements necessary for normal volitional joint motion, provides additional information about possible factors that contribute to limitation of joint motion.[3] Special tests can also be used to assess joint function and contracture, as well as the impact of passive insufficiency of two-joint muscles on the function of the lower extremity.

TABLE 6-2
Critical Lower Extremity Joint Range of Motion during the Gait Cycle

Phase and Subphase	Hip	Knee	Ankle	MTP
Stance				
Initial contact	25–30 degrees flexion	Full extension	Neutral	Neutral
Loading response	25–30 degrees flexion	15 degrees flexion	10 degrees plantar flexion	Neutral
Midstance	Neutral	Full extension	5 degrees dorsiflexion	Neutral
Terminal stance	15–20 degrees extension	Full extension	10 degrees dorsiflexion	30 degrees extension
Preswing	Neutral	30–40 degrees flexion	20 degrees plantar flexion	60 degrees extension
Swing				
Initial swing	15 degrees flexion	60 degrees flexion	10 degrees plantar flexion	Neutral
Midswing	25–30 degrees flexion	25 degrees flexion	Neutral	Neutral
Terminal swing	25–30 degrees flexion	Full extension	Neutral	Neutral
Maximum excursion	30 degrees flexion	60 degrees flexion	10 degrees dorsiflexion	60 degrees extension
	20 degrees extension	Full extension	20 degrees plantar flexion	Neutral

MTP = metatarsal-phalangeal.
Source: Adapted from VT Inman, HJ Ralston, F Todd. Human Walking. Baltimore: Williams & Wilkins, 1981; and Pathokinesiology Department and Physical Therapy Department of Rancho Los Amigos Medical Center. Observational Gait Analysis. Downey, CA: Los Amigos Research and Education Institute, 1993.

TABLE 6-3
Normal Range of Motion of Lower Extremity Joints

Joint	Motion	Magee[6–8] (active; degrees)	Hoppenfeld[9–11] (passive; degrees)	AAOS[12] (degrees)	Norkin et al.[2,13] (passive; degrees)
Hip	Flexion	110–120	120	120	120–135
	Extension	10–15	30	30	10–30
	Abduction	30–50	45–50	45	30–50
	Adduction	30	20–30	30	10–30
	External rotation	40–60	45	45	45–60
	Internal rotation	30–40	35	45	30–45
Knee	Flexion	135	135	135	130–140
	Extension	0	0–5	0	5–10
	Ext. rotation	10	10	—	40*
	Int. rotation	10	10	—	30*
Ankle	Dorsiflexion	20	20	20	20
	Plantar flexion	50	50	50	30–50
	Supination	45–60	—	—	—
	Pronation	15–30	—	—	—
	Inversion	—	—	35	—
	Eversion	—	—	15	—
	Subtalar inversion	5	5	5	—
	Subtalar eversion	5	5	5	—
Foot	Forefoot adduction	20	20	—	—
	Forefoot abduction	10	10	—	—
	Hallux MTP extension	70	70–90	70	—
	Hallux MTP flexion	45	45	45	—
	MTP extension[2–5]	—	—	40	—
	MTP flexion[2–5]	—	—	40	—

AAOS = American Academy of Orthopedic Surgeons; MTP = metatarsal-phalangeal.
*Passive external (lateral) and internal (medial) rotation of the tibia on the femur measured at 90 degrees of knee flexion.

The *Thomas test* is used to detect flexion contracture at the hip. The patient is positioned supine on the examination table, lying close to the edge on the "test" limb side. Both knees are drawn upward to the chest to stabilize the lumbar spine in neutral or slight posterior tilt. The examiner monitors pelvic motion as one limb is passively extended. Movement of the pelvis toward anterior tilt indicates contracture of the iliopsoas muscle. Extension of the knee as the limb is lowered suggests tightness of the rectus femoris.[14] The angle between the thigh and table surface (at the point that the pelvis begins to move) is an estimate of the contracture.[6,9]

The *Ober test* is used to detect contracture of the iliotibial band and tightness of the tensor fascia lata. The patient is positioned in side-lying position with the limb to be examined uppermost. The examiner flexes the knee to 90 degrees and, keeping the hip in a neutral position, passively abducts the limb. Normally, when the limb is released, it falls into an adducted position. If the limb does not drop completely, contracture of the iliotibial band or tensor fascia lata is likely.[2,5,14]

Soft tissue contracture or tightness in muscles that cross two joints limits range of motion when the muscle is elongated by simultaneous motion of both joints. Passive insufficiency of a tight or shortened rectus femoris muscle limits knee flexion when the hip is in an extended position.[13] Rectus femoris tightness may be observed during the Thomas test (described previously) or during passive knee flexion while the patient is in a prone position. Passive insufficiency of the hamstring muscle groups (semimembranosus, semitendinosis, and biceps femoris) limits excursion of straight leg raise.[14]

In evaluating the need for (and the consequences of) application of a lower extremity orthosis, it is important to keep in mind the minimum necessary range of motion during key functional activities. Efficient gait requires 60 degrees of knee flexion during the transition from stance into swing for adequate swing clearance.[4,5] Climbing stairs in a step-over-step pattern requires an 80-degree excursion between knee flexion and extension.[5] Comfortable sitting in and rising from a standard desk or office chair requires at least 90 degrees of knee flexion.[13,15] Rising from the floor may require more than 100 degrees of knee flexion.[16,17]

The passive tension of the gastrocnemius and soleus muscles and their Achilles tendon at the posterior ankle has an impact on knee motion during stance and other functional activities. When plantar flexion tightness or contracture limits dorsiflexion, forward progression of the tibia over the foot in a closed chain motion during the transition from midstance to terminal stance is compromised. The resulting extensor moment at the knee prevents the knee flexion that is required to prepare for relative limb shortening during swing. For patients who have a limitation of plantar flexion motion (usually a result of trauma, arthritis, or other joint deformity), the ability to attain full knee extension, which is required for stability during midstance, is compromised.[13] It is important to measure dorsiflexion range of motion in an extended knee and a flexed knee position: Tightness of the gastrocnemius muscle results in a decrease in available range of motion when the knee is extended.[14]

Any orthosis that crosses or controls the ankle joint (foot orthosis, AFO, or knee-ankle-foot orthosis [KAFO]) must take into account the range of motion and alignment of the patient's foot. The orthotist assesses the patient's ability to achieve a subtalar neutral position, the relative position of the calcaneus to the tibia in quiet standing (calcaneovarus or calcaneovalgus), and the relationship between the rear foot and the forefoot. He or she is also concerned with the height and flexibility of the longitudinal arch (pes planus, pes cavus, or pes equinus) and the integrity of the transverse arch at the anterior tarsals as well as at the midshaft of the metatarsals. Assessment of forefoot function determines whether a hallux valgus, hallux limitus, or hallux rigidus will require accommodation in the design or structure of the orthosis. Patients with weakness of the intrinsic muscles or long-standing biomechanical abnormalities of the foot may have hammer and claw toe deformities that must be accounted for in orthotic fitting and in footwear.

It is also important to compare the range of motion measured passively to joint excursion performed by active contraction of muscles. Many musculoskeletal or neuromuscular conditions impact on strength or control of motion during volitional movement of the limb. The desire for optimal biomechanical alignment in an orthosis must, at times, be tempered by the patient's ability to use or control the limb during functional activities.

Ligamentous Stability

The integrity of supportive ligaments is an important determinant of the design and the trimlines of a lower extremity orthosis. If a patient has demonstrable mediolateral instability at the ankle, for example, the orthotist would likely choose to fabricate a thermoplastic ankle-foot orthosis (AFO) with a trimline at or slightly anterior to the malleoli, or a traditional metal double-upright AFO,

to protect and support the talocrural joint effectively. Mediolateral instability at the knee is best controlled if the proximal trimline of the orthosis is midthigh or higher and the distal trimline extends at least to midcalf level. The strategies used to assess ligamentous stability of patients who require a lower extremity orthosis are the same as those used to assess joint stability when musculoskeletal impairments occur as a result of injury.

Hip Joint Stability

The hip joint supports the mass of the upper body during standing, walking, and other functional activities and transmits forces between the pelvis and the bones of the lower extremity during closed chain activities while the head is maintained upright at the midline.[13] The stability of the hip joint (coxofemoral joint) is determined, to a large extent, by its ball-and-socket structure: The head of the femur moves within the deep acetabulum with its horseshoe-shaped labrum. The actual articulation is between the superior surface of the femoral head and the superior concavity of the slightly anteverted acetabulum. The stability of the joint is enhanced by its particularly dense, strong articular capsule, which is reinforced by the iliofemoral, pubofemoral, and ischiofemoral ligaments.

Instability of the hip joint is most often a result, not of ligamentous laxity, but of the excessively shallow and malaligned acetabulum associated with congenital dislocation of the hip. In nonreduced congenital hip dislocation, the head of the femur is positioned above and behind the acetabulum. Patients with bilateral, nonreduced, congenital hip dislocation may assume increased lumbar lordosis as a compensatory strategy to achieve stability in stance.[6]

In newborns, the assessment for congenital hip dislocation begins with a passive movement of the hips into a flexed, abducted, and internally rotated position. The examiner then applies an upward pressure into the greater trochanter. A "click" or jerky motion as this force is applied, accompanied by additional movement into abduction (Ortolani's sign), suggests that reduction in a lax or congenitally dislocated hip has been accomplished[6,9,18] (Figure 6-1). For children up to 6 months old, the test position is modified to assess each hip individually (Barlow's test). The test begins with the hip flexed to 90 degrees and the knee fully flexed. The examiner passively moves the limb into abduction and applies pressure inward at the greater trochanter; a click or jerky motion suggests reduction of a dislocated femoral head. The severity of hip instability is assessed by then applying a backward/outward pressure against the inner thigh to determine if the femoral head will dislocate. Asymmetry or apparent length differences in a toddler positioned in the supine position with the hips flexed to 90 degrees and the knees fully flexed

(Galeazzi's or Allis's test) suggest possible unrecognized congenital hip dislocation. Noticeable differences in passive abduction range of motion when the hip is flexed at 90 degrees (Hart's sign/abduction test) also suggest hip dislocation, especially if asymmetry of the gluteal folds and upper thigh is also present.

In older children, adolescents, and adults, hip instability and potential dislocation are assessed in two ways. The patient is positioned supine with the hip and knee flexed to 90 degrees. The examiner gently pushes downward through the knee. Normally, very little motion occurs; if telescoping or pistoning is seen as the downward pressure is applied and released (Dupuytren's test), hip instability or dislocation is suspected. Another assessment strategy visualizes a line between the ischial tuberosity and the anterosuperior iliac spine (ASIS) of the pelvis (Nélaton's line). If the greater trochanter is palpated above this line, either congenital dislocation or coxa vara is suspected.

Knee Joint Stability

The somewhat asymmetric size and incongruent shape of the articular surfaces and menisci of the knee joint render it much less inherently stable than the hip joint.[13] Stability of the knee is a function of a strong joint capsule, two pairs of ligaments, and the muscles and tendons that act on the knee joint. The medial collateral ligament (MCL; stretched between the medial femoral condyle and the proximal medial tibia) stabilizes the slightly flexed and extended knee against valgus forces during function. The MCL also protects the knee from becoming excessively extended, limits external (lateral) rotation and anterior displacement of the tibia, and anchors the medial meniscus within the knee joint. The lateral collateral ligament (LCL; between the lateral femoral condyle and the proximal lateral tibia) stabilizes the slightly flexed or extended knee against varus stresses during function and helps to limit lateral rotation and posterior displacement of the tibia. The anterior cruciate ligament (ACL; from the anterior tibia to the posterior inner surface of the lateral femoral condyle) restrains forward displacement of the tibia on the condyles and controls rotation of the tibia. The posterior cruciate ligament (PCL; from the posterior tibia to the inner surface of the medial femoral condyle) restrains posterior displacement of the tibia on the condyles, especially if the knee is in an extended position. Like the ACL, the PCL appears to contribute to control of tibial rotation on the condyles, playing a role in the "screw home" mechanism in full knee extension.[13]

Integrity of the collateral ligaments is assessed by applying an external valgus (MCL) or varus (LCL) force to the knee joint (Figure 6-2). The patient's limb is supported in slight flexion with the foot stabilized between the exam-

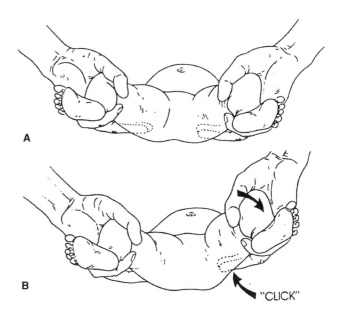

FIGURE 6-1

Test position for congenital hip dislocation in the newborn. (A) The hip is moved into flexion, abduction, and internal rotation. (B) A "click" when upward pressure is applied at the greater trochanter suggests that the dislocation has been reduced. (Reprinted with permission from DJ Magee. Orthopedic Physical Assessment [3rd ed]. Philadelphia: Saunders, 1997;477.)

iner's arm and trunk. Application of a valgus (inwardly directed) force on the lateral knee produces a palpable medial gap in the MCL-deficient knee joint. Application of a varus (outwardly directed) force at the medial knee produces a palpable lateral gap in an LCL-deficient knee joint. Laxity or injury of the MCL results in greater joint instability than does a deficient LCL.[10]

The anterior drawer test is used to evaluate the integrity of the ACL and accessory structures of the knee. The patient is placed in the supine position with the hip flexed to 45 degrees, knees flexed to 90 degrees, and feet flat on the surface of the examination table or mat. The examiner stabilizes the foot and then gently pulls the proximal tibia forward at the posterior knee. Excessive forward motion (more than 6 mm) suggests insufficiency of the anterior cruciate along with the posterior joint capsule, MCL, and other supporting structures.[7,10] Repeating the test with the lower leg externally rotated assesses the integrity of the posteromedial joint capsule. Repeating the test with the lower leg internally rotated assesses integrity of the posterolateral joint capsule.[7,10] An alternative test position is supine, with the hip and knee flexed to 90 degrees and the lower leg snugly supported between the examiner's arm and trunk.[19] The examiner slowly applies an upward force, as if to lift the buttocks from the

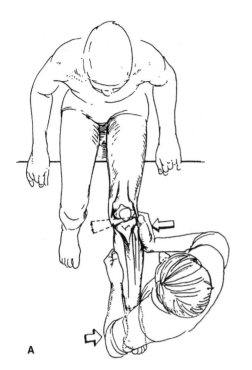

A

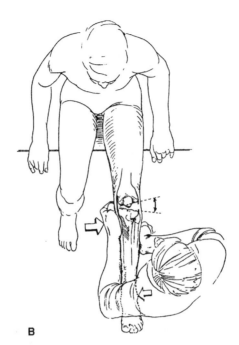

B

FIGURE 6-2
*(A) A palpable medial gap on application of a valgus force indicates insufficiency of the medial collateral ligament.
(B) Increased lateral gaping on application of a varus force indicates insufficiency of the lateral collateral ligament. (Reprinted with permission from S Hoppenfeld. Physical Examination of the Spine and Extremities. Norwalk, CT: Appleton-Century-Crofts, 1976;185.)*

supporting surface. When an audible snap or jerking feeling (Finochetti's jumping sign) accompanies excessive anterior motion of the tibia, a damaged meniscus is suspected.[20]

The posterior drawer test is used to evaluate the integrity of the PCL of the knee. The test position is the same as that of the anterior drawer test. Instead of pulling forward from behind the knee, the examiner pushes backward on the anterior surface of the proximal tibia. Excessive motion suggests deficiency of the PCL and similar stabilizing structures.[10] The reverse Lachman's test position, performed with the patient lying prone, is an alternative for assessment of PCL integrity.[21] The examiner passively flexes the knee to 30 degrees, stabilizes the femur against the support surface, and then applies an upward force at the proximal tibia while watching and feeling for posterior displacement. For an in-depth discussion of assessment of ligamentous and capsular integrity of the knee, the reader is referred to Magee,[7] Strobel and Stedtfeld,[20] or Greenfield.[21]

Ankle Joint Stability

The stability of the ankle (talocrural) joint is a product of three components: (1) the structure of the talocrural joint itself (the medial and lateral condyles and the size and shape of the articular surfaces); (2) several strong, strategically placed ligaments; and (3) the tendons that cross the ankle joint. Medially, the stabilizing structures include the MCL (deltoid) ligament, tibialis posterior tendon, flexor digitorum longus tendon, and flexor hallucis longus tendon. Laterally, the examiner will find the LCL liga-

ments (anterior talofibular, calcaneofibular, and posterior talofibular ligaments) and the peroneus longus and brevis tendons. The Achilles tendon and its bursa are the posterior components of the ankle. Structures of the anterior ankle include the tendons of the tibialis anterior, extensor hallucis longus, and extensor digitorum longus muscles. Structures on the sole or plantar surface that have an impact on ankle and foot function during gait include the plantar calcaneonavicular ligament (spring ligament) and the plantar aponeurosis

The ankle anterior drawer test evaluates the integrity of the anterior talofibular ligament. The patient is positioned in supine with the heel of the foot off of the supporting surface. The examiner stabilizes the distal tibia/fibula against the support surface, supports the foot in 20 degrees of plantar flexion, and then lifts the forefoot upward to move the talus forward in the mortise.[21] An alternative strategy positions the patient as in the drawer test for the knee, stabilizing the foot against the support surface and then applying a backward force just proximal to the ankle to elicit posterior movement of the mortise on the talus.[11] The integrity of this ligament can also be tested while the patient is in the prone position with the feet over the edge of the support surface.[22]

Gross lateral instability of the ankle is a result of insufficiency of the anterior talofibular and the calcaneofibular ligaments. To assess the integrity of these ligaments, the examiner passively inverts the calcaneus while stabilizing the distal tibia and fibula. Medial gapping or rocking of the talus in the ankle mortise suggests deficiency of these two medial ligaments. It is important to note that the third medial ligament, the posterior talofibular ligament, is rarely insufficient unless significant trauma or dislocation of the ankle joint has occurred.[11] Integrity of the MCL (deltoid) ligament is assessed by passive eversion performed while the lower leg is stabilized. Excessive lateral gapping suggests insufficiency or damage of one or more components of the deltoid ligament.

Pain on palpation of specific ligaments usually suggests inflammation due to recent injury. Hypermobility of the joints of the ankle and foot may be apparent when passive range of motion and accessory motions are assessed.[23] These may be the long-term results of abnormalities of structural alignment from musculoskeletal or neuromuscular impairment. For a more complete discussion of ankle and foot structure and function, the reader is referred to Magee,[8] or McPoil.[24]

ALIGNMENT OF LIMB SEGMENTS

In patients with long-standing muscular imbalances or abnormal tone, malalignments or deformities of the joints

or excessive torsion of the femur or of the tibia and fibula are likely to have developed. Effective and comfortable lower extremity orthoses are designed to accommodate existing fixed alignment or rotational deformities, while supporting the joints and limb segments enough to minimize progression of deformity over time.

Alignment of the Hip

The alignment relationship between the proximal femur (femoral head and neck) and the distal femur is described in two ways: as the angle of inclination and as the angle of torsion. It is important to recognize that although these angles are characteristics of the femur, an abnormal angle of inclination or torsion will likely have a functional impact on the hip, knee, talocrural, and subtalar joints (Table 6-4).

The angle of inclination is measured in the frontal plane as the angle formed between the long axis of the femoral neck and the long axis of the femoral shaft. At birth, the normal angle of inclination is approximately 150 degrees. This angle decreases to approximately 125 degrees in early and mid-adulthood and 120 degrees in later life.[13] In coxa valga, the angle of inclination is greater than expected,

TABLE 6-4
Functional Consequences of Femoral Malalignment

Abnormality	Resultant Postures	Potential Compensatory Strategy
Angle of inclination		
Coxa vara	Anterior pelvic rotation	Pelvic posterior rotation (ipsilateral)
	Shorter limb length (ipsilateral)	Lumbar rotation (ipsilateral)
	Medial (internal) femoral torsion	Hip and knee flexion (contralateral)
	Subtalar joint pronation	Genu recurvatum (contralateral)
		Plantar flexion (ipsilateral)
		Subtalar supination (ipsilateral)
		Subtalar pronation (contralateral)
Coxa valga	Posterior pelvic tilt	Anterior pelvic rotation (ipsilateral)
	Long limb length (ipsilateral)	Lumbar rotation (contralateral)
	Lateral (external) femoral torsion	Hip and knee flexion (ipsilateral)
	Subtalar joint supination	Genu recurvatum (ipsilateral)
		Plantar flexion (contralateral)
		Subtalar supination (contralateral)
		Subtalar pronation (ipsilateral)
Angle of torsion		
Anteversion	Medial (internal) femoral torsion	Lumbar rotation (ipsilateral)
	Medial (internal) tibial torsion	External rotation of femur or pelvis
	Lateral patellar subluxation	External rotation of tibia
	Subtalar joint pronation	External rotation at the knee
	In toeing in stance and gait	Lateral (external) tibial torsion
Retroversion	Lateral (external) femoral torsion	Lumbar rotation (contralateral)
	Lateral (external) tibial torsion	Internal rotation of femur or pelvis
	Subtalar joint supination	Internal rotation of tibia
	Out toeing in stance and gait	Internal rotation at the knee

Source: Adapted from DJ Magee. Orthopedic Physical Assessment (3rd ed). Philadelphia: Saunders, 1997;476; and C Riegger-Kruch, JJ Keysor. Skeletal malalignments of the lower quarter: correlated and compensatory motions and postures. J Orthop Sports Phys Ther 1996;23:166–167.

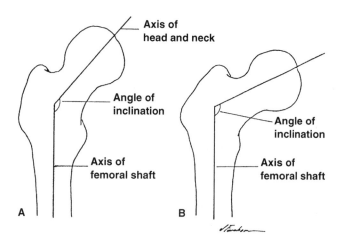

FIGURE 6-3

(A) Normal angle of inclination between the neck and shaft of the femur is 125 degrees in adults. (B) A pathologic increase in the angle of inclination is called coxa valga, *and a pathologic decrease in the angle of inclination is called* coxa vara. *(Reprinted with permission from CC Norkin, PK Levangie. The Hip Complex. In CC Norkin, PK Levangie (eds), Joint Structure and Function: A Comprehensive Analysis [2nd ed]. Philadelphia: Davis, 1992;305.)*

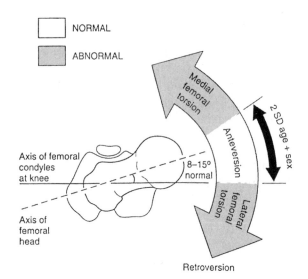

FIGURE 6-4

Normal relationship between the axis of the femoral neck and the axis of the femoral condyles (viewed as if looking down the center of the femoral shaft) is between 8 and 15 degrees of anteversion. Excessive anteversion leads to medial (internal) femoral torsion. Insufficient angulation, retroversion, is associated with lateral (external) femoral torsion. (Reprinted with permission from LT Staheli. Medial femoral torsion. Orthop Clin North Am 1980;11:40.)

whereas in coxa vara the angle is more acute (less) than expected (Figure 6-3).

In adults with a normal angle of torsion, the neck of the femur is positioned in approximately 8–15 degrees of anteversion (measured as the angle between the axis of the femoral head and the axis of the femoral condyles; Figure 6-4). When a patient is placed in the supine position, the patella is relatively parallel to the supporting surface, and the foot and toes are upright, perpendicular to the supporting surface. In standing, the patient's patella is forward facing and centered, and the foot and toes are aligned. It is important to note that the relationship between the femoral neck and long axis of the femur changes over time from approximately 30 degrees of anteversion in infancy and toddlerhood to the "normal" 8- to 15-degree position of adulthood.[6,13]

When excessive femoral anteversion is present, however, the angulation of the femoral neck is greater than 15 degrees. The limb appears to fall into internal rotation when the patient lays in the supine position, and the patella and foot "point" toward the midline (Figure 6-5). Passive movement of the hip finds limited external rotation range of motion, with excessive internal rotation range of motion (total excursion may be within expected limits). Femoral anteversion is manifested in the distal femur as internal or medial femoral torsion. Retroversion occurs when the angle between the axis of the femoral neck and the

axis of the femoral condyles is less than the normal 8–15 degrees. In the supine position, the patient's limbs appear to fall into excessive external rotation, with the patella and foot incline away from the midline. Passive motion of the hip reveals excessive external rotation with limited internal rotation. Femoral retroversion is manifested distally in the femur as external or lateral femoral torsion.

One method that can be used to assess whether anteversion of the femoral neck is present is the *Craig test*, also known as the *Ryder test*. The patient is placed in the prone position, with the knee supported in 90 degrees of flexion so that the lower limb is vertical. While palpating the posterior edge of the greater trochanter, the examiner gently rotates the limb until the trochanter reaches its most lateral position or is parallel to the support surface. The number of degrees that the lower limb has moved from the vertical position provides an estimate of hip anteversion.[6]

Alignment of the Knee

Malalignment of the knee can occur in all three planes of motion. Genu recurvatum occurs when knee extension exceeds normal limits, hyperextending beyond 5–10 degrees in the sagittal plane.[13] Genu valgus and genu varus

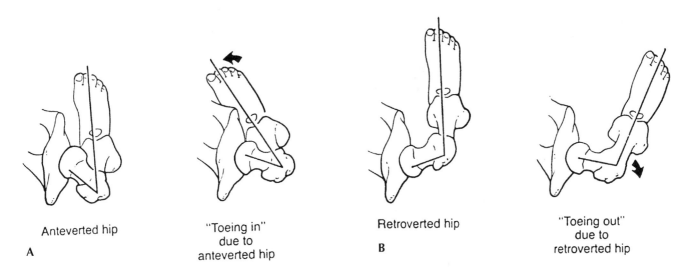

Anteverted hip

A

"Toeing in"
due to
anteverted hip

Retroverted hip

B

"Toeing out"
due to
retroverted hip

FIGURE 6-5

(A) When excessive anteversion is present, the patient's limb appears to be internally rotated or in toeing when the head of the femur is well seated in the acetabulum. (B) With retroversion, the patient's limb appears to fall into external rotation. (Reprinted with permission from DJ Magee. Orthopedic Physical Assessment [3rd ed]. Philadelphia: Saunders, 1997;475.)

are angulational abnormalities that are described by the relationship between the long axis of the femur and the tibia in the frontal plane. Abnormal tibial torsion occurs in the transverse plane around the long axis of the bone. The altered postures or joint motions associated with malalignments are summarized in Table 6-5. Alignment has an important developmental component: Angular relationships of limb segments change significantly from birth to adulthood.[25] Age and motor development must be taken into account in using alignment information to develop an orthotic prescription or design.

Genu recurvatum is observed in the lateral view of the patient's lower extremity in quiet standing. Although slight hyperextension of both knees (up to 10 degrees) is a normal finding, excessive hyperextension appears as "backward bow" of the femur/tibia articulation.[10] The severity of genu recurvatum is measured with a goniometer. Genu recurvatum is more common in female than in male patients, especially in those with relative laxity of the knee ligaments. An apparent recurvatum may be a postural compensation for excessive lumbar lordosis.

From infancy until functional walking has begun, the normal alignment of the lower limb is in slight genu varum with an associated in toeing. Once a child (without neuromuscular impairment) begins to cruise and walk, the amount of genu varum gradually decreases. By the age of 18 months, the axes of the femur and tibia coincide, and the child stands in a wide base with straight limbs. By the age of 30 months, a physiologic genu valgum has developed, often accompanied by a protective in toeing. By the age of 4–6 years, the

physiologic genu valgum has been reduced, and the child stands with a narrow base and a straight limb.[25]

In adults, the anatomic or longitudinal axis of the femur is tilted slightly into an adducted position, creating a physiologic genu valgus (measured as the angle of intersection of the longitudinal axis of the femur and of the tibia at the medial knee) of 185–190 degrees (Figure 6-6). On x-ray, normal alignment measured as the tibiofemoral shaft angle is between 6 and 10 degrees (Figure 6-7). The fact that the mechanical axis of the lower extremity passes through the centers of the hip, knee, and ankle joints ensures equal weight distribution between the medial and lateral condyles in the normally aligned knee joint.[13] When the medial valgus angle increases into abnormal genu valgus, compression of the lateral joint surfaces and distraction of medial joint and soft tissue structures occur. Conversely, when the medial valgus angle is reduced into abnormal genu varum, compression of the medial joint surfaces and distraction of lateral joint and soft tissue structures occur.

Frontal plane alignment of the knee can be clinically evaluated by placing the patient in the standing position, so that the patellae are facing directly forward and the medial aspects of the knees and the medial malleoli are as close together as possible. Genu valgus is likely if the knees touch and the ankles do not, especially if the distance between the ankles is more than 3.5 in. If genu varum is present, the knees will be separated when the ankles are together.

Normal tibial torsion (measured as the difference in positions of the knee and ankle axes) is between 12 and 15 degrees, which means that the ankle mortise is approxi-

TABLE 6-5

Functional Consequences of Malalignment of the Knee

Abnormality	Resulting Postures	Potential Compensatory Strategies
Genu recurvatum	Increased anterior pelvic tilt Posterior inclination of tibia Plantar flexion	Thoracic kyphosis Trunk flexion in standing Posterior pelvic tilt
Genu varum	Lateral angulation of tibia Medial (internal) tibial torsion External rotation of hip (ipsilateral) Abduction of hip (ipsilateral)	Medial rotation of pelvis (ipsilateral) Subtalar supination for heel contact Forefoot valgus
Genu valgus	Lateral (external) tibial torsion Lateral patellar subluxation Subtalar pronation, pes planus Adduction of hip (ipsilateral) Internal rotation of hip (ipsilateral) Rotation of lumbar spine (contralateral)	Lateral rotation of pelvis (ipsilateral) In toeing in gait (to limit medial-lateral sway) Subtalar supination for heel contact Forefoot varus
Medial tibial torsion (internal)	Subtalar pronation with related lower quarter rotation In toeing Metatarsus adductus	Functional forefoot valgus Subtalar supination with relaxation of lower quarter rotation
Lateral tibial torsion (external)	Subtalar supination with related lower quarter rotation Out toeing	Functional forefoot varus Subtalar pronation with relaxation of lower quarter rotation

Source: Adapted from DJ Magee. Orthopedic Physical Assessment (3rd ed). Philadelphia: Saunders, 1997;476; and C Riegger-Kruch, JJ Keysor. Skeletal malalignments of the lower quarter: correlated and compensatory motions and postures. J Orthop Sports Phys Ther 1996;23:166–167.

mately 15 degrees externally rotated relative to the axis of knee motion.[7,10] When excessive internal rotation of the tibial shaft is present, the mortise may face forward or slightly inward, and in toeing during stance and in gait is likely. With excessive external tibial torsion, the mortise is more than 15 degrees externally rotated, and out toeing is likely.

One clinical indicator of excessive external tibial torsion is the "too many toes sign": If more than the fourth and fifth toe can be visualized on a posterior view of the patient's foot position while in quiet stance, excessive external tibial torsion should be suspected. Tibial torsion can also be assessed with the patient placed in the sitting position with the feet dangling; the examiner looks downward, visualizing the positions of the knee axis between condyles and the ankle axis between malleoli. Normally, the forefoot is pointing forward or just slightly laterally. If medial tibial torsion is present, the forefoot points inward. Conversely, in lateral tibial torsion, the forefoot is turned outward. To assess tibial torsion while the patient is lying supine, the examiner visualizes the relative positions of the axes of the knee joint (the femoral condyles in frontal plane/patella upward) and the ankle joint (the angle of intersection of the line between the malleoli and the line parallel to the floor). Visualization of tibial torsion in small children may be enhanced if a child is positioned in the prone position, with the knee flexed and the ankle in the subtalar neutral position.[7,10]

Torsional deformities of the femur and tibia are likely to develop in children with neuromuscular diagnoses such as cerebral palsy or myelomenigocele because of habitual abnormal postures and movement patterns. Children with cerebral palsy who have impaired postural control often prefer a "W" sitting position because this provides a stable base of support for play and other functional activities. In this position, the hips are flexed and maximally internally rotated and the knees are maximally flexed. As a result, compression of the lateral knee joint and distraction of the medial knee joint and soft tissue structures occur, increasing the likelihood of genu valgus. If the child's feet are turned outward, away from midline, excessive lateral (external) tibial torsion is likely to develop. If the child tucks the feet under the pelvis, there is a risk of excessive medial (internal) tibial torsion.

Ankle and Forefoot Alignment

Alignment abnormalities and torsional deformities of the hip and knee have a significant impact on the alignment and function of the talocrural, subtalar, and transverse tarsal joints of the foot. Most lower extremity orthoses that cross the ankle joint are designed with a neutral position of the talocrural and subtalar joints. During the preorthotic assessment, the orthotist evaluates alignment and relationships of the ankle, rear foot, and forefoot to differentiate functional and fixed deformities. Weight-bearing and non–weight-bearing assessment strategies are used to determine the patient's ability to achieve a subtalar neutral position and to identify uncompensated or compensated malalignment of the rear foot (calcaneovarus, calcaneovalgus, rear foot varus, rear foot valgus) and

FIGURE 6-6
(A) Normal alignment of the adult knee is in slight physiologic genu valgus. (B) In an abnormal genu valgus alignment, the medial angle measurement is greater than 190 degrees. (C) In genu varum, the medial angle is less than 180 degrees.

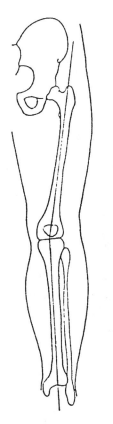 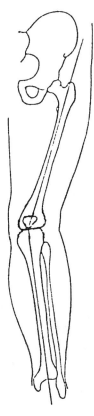 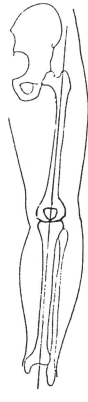

A Normal Knee
185°-190°

B Genu Valgus
> 190°

C Genu Varum
< 180°

forefoot (varus, valgus, or adductus). The orthotist also looks for potential abnormalities that affect the longitudinal arch (pes planus, pes cavus, or pes equinus) and the tranvserse arch and notes forefoot deformities (hallux valgus, hallux limitus, or hallux rigidus; claw toes; hammertoes) that may require accommodation. For a detailed discussion of ankle and foot kinematics and assessment, the reader is referred to Chapter 8 or to Magee.[8]

Age and motor development must be considered when assessing ankle and foot alignment during preorthotic evaluation. During infancy, the foot is normally pronated, with minimal out toeing (Ficke angle of 5 degrees) and a relatively straight or slightly adducted forefoot footprint.[27] With the development of the longitudinal arch comes a shift toward supination, an increase in out toeing (Ficke angle of 12–18 degrees), and a more neutral footprint pattern.

LEG LENGTH

In standing, the optimal functional position of the lower trunk and lower extremity begins with a level pelvis and equal leg lengths. It is common, however, to find evidence

of a pelvic obliquity and leg length discrepancy in children and adults with neuromuscular impairment. During the preorthotic assessment, the orthotist differentiates an apparent obliquity or leg length discrepancy (associated with malalignment, deformity, or contracture) from an actual leg length discrepancy as a contributor to pelvic obliquity. To do this, the orthotist or therapist assesses segmental and total leg length, first with the patient standing and then with the patient in the supine position.

In standing, the examiner palpates bony landmarks on the left and right sides of the pelvis (iliac crests, anterior supererior iliac spine [ASIS], posterosuperior iliac spines [PSIS]) to identify whether a pelvic obliquity related to leg length discrepancy may be present. Comparison of the standing heights of the greater trochanter of the femur, the popliteal crease of the posterior knee, the head of the fibula, and the malleoli of the ankle helps to identify possible length discrepancies within the limb segments. When the patient is in the supine position, overall leg length is measured between the ASIS and medial malleolus of the ankle. Segmental length is measured between two neighboring bony landmarks. Femoral length is measured from the ASIS or greater trochanter to the fibular head, tibial tubercle, or

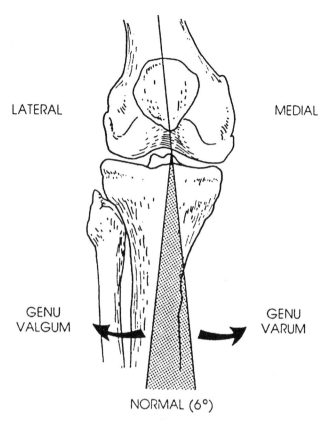

FIGURE 6-7
Severity of frontal plane malalignment at the knee is measured by the tibiofemoral angle. (Reprinted with permission from DJ Magee. Orthopedic Physical Assessment [3rd ed]. Philadelphia: Saunders, 1997;512.)

medial knee joint line. Tibial length is measured from the head of the fibula or tibial tubercle to a malleolus. Segmental length discrepancies become more apparent when the patient's limbs are positioned in "hooklying" with the knees flexed to 90 degrees while the feet remain flat against the examining table.

SENSORY ASSESSMENT

Assessment of sensory function is performed to ascertain whether the patient will be able to monitor accurately the impact of forces being applied to the lower extremity by the orthosis. Patients who are unable to detect areas of high pressure or skin irritation when they are wearing an orthosis are at risk of developing blisters, abrasions, bruises, or neuropathic ulcerations that compromise skin integrity and increase the risk of infection. Sensory function is diminished in areas of skin graft, scar tissue, or callus. Patients with paresthesia or hyperesthesia may not

easily tolerate the contact between the orthosis and the skin surface. The patient's current and past medical history determines whether a screening of sensory function or definitive sensory testing should be performed.[27,28]

Examples of diagnoses that compromise sensation or perception include diabetic polyneuropathy and other peripheral neuropathies, nerve root impingement, spinal cord injury and myelomeningocele, multiple sclerosis involving sensory tracts, or head injury and hemiplegia that damage the sensory or perceptual cortices, thalamus, or associated pathways. Acuity of sensation and perception tends to diminish with aging, perhaps as a result of loss or damage of peripheral receptors or slower conduction velocity and information processing within the central nervous system (CNS).[29] Older patients with concurrent impairments of somatosensation, proprioception, and vision often have compromised dynamic anticipatory and reactionary postural control even if the individual impairments are mild.[30]

The reliability of sensory testing is influenced by the patient's vision and hearing, language comprehension, level of consciousness and ability to concentrate, cognitive function and ability to understand the testing procedure, motivation, and level of anxiety during testing.[27,28] Sensory testing is best performed in a quiet environment in which the patient is relaxed and comfortable, can concentrate, and will not be unduly distracted. The patient must understand the testing procedure and how he or she should respond; demonstration on an area of intact sensation is often quite helpful. During the sensory examination, the orthotist or therapist determines which of the sensory modalities are impaired, the areas of the body that are affected and boundaries of the sensory impairment, the severity of sensory loss, and the patient's awareness or understanding of the sensory impairment. The extent of sensory impairment is often recorded on a body chart that may include dermatome or peripheral nerve maps (Figure 6-8). Descriptive terminology used to rate severity of sensory loss is defined in Table 6-6.

The examiner attempts to apply the stimulus for the sensation being tested in a random, slightly unpredictable manner, altering timing to avoid rhythmic patterns that might help the patient to predict stimulus application. In most instances (except for kinesthetic or perceptual tests based on mimicry) the patient's vision is obscured during testing. The boundaries of sensory dysfunction are most accurately determined if testing begins in areas of impaired or absent sensation and moves into areas where sensation is intact.[27] In many cases, this means that testing begins distally and moves proximally on the limb.[28]

Typically, "primitive" exteroceptive sensation carried out in the anterolateral/spinothalamic system (pain, sharp/dull discrimination, light touch, and temperature) is tested first. An open safety pin or wooden cotton-tipped

FIGURE 6-8

Comparison of the sensory dermatome map (left) and sensory peripheral nerve map (right) of the anterior and posterior body surfaces. (Reprinted with permission from NB Reese. Muscle and Sensory Testing. Philadelphia: Saunders, 1999;424–425).

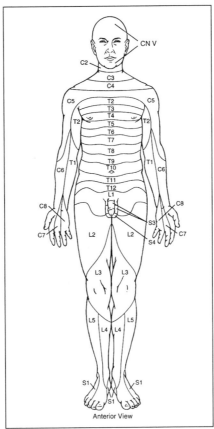

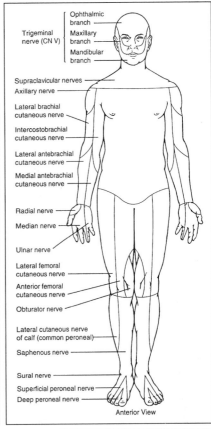

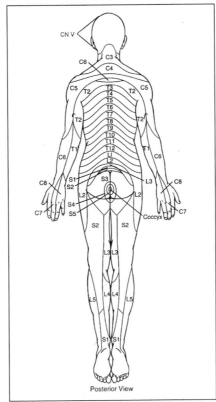

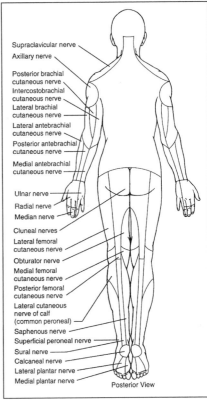

TABLE 6-6
Definition of Terms Used to Describe Sensory Impairment

Term	Definition
Analgesia	Loss of ability to perceive pain
Anesthesia	Loss of tactile and pain sensation
Astereognosis	Inability to recognize an object using touch
Causalgia	Painful burning sensation in the distribution of a peripheral nerve
Hypalgesia/hyperalgesia	Reduced/heightened sensitivity to painful stimuli
Hypesthesia/hyperesthesia	Reduced/heightened sensitivity to tactile or other sensory stimuli
Paresthesia	Abnormal sensation (numbness, tingling) without obvious cause

Source: Adapted from TJ Schmitz. Sensory Assessment. In SB O'Sullivan, TJ Schmitz (eds), Physical Rehabilitation: Assessment and Treatment (3rd ed). Philadelphia: Davis, 1994;90.

swab is used to test "pain" sensation and ability to discriminate sharp or dull sensation. The patient is instructed to say "yes" each time a sharp stimulus is perceived. Alternately, the patient may be asked to say "sharp" or "dull" to identify which type of stimulus has been applied. A cotton ball is gently touched to the skin surface to assess light touch, and the patient responds "yes" each time a stimulus is perceived. Testing of thermal sensation requires a "hot" (hot water filled) and "cold" (ice filled) test tube. The patient says "hot" or "cold" whenever the stimulus is perceived.

Proprioception and kinesthesia (including vibration) carried in the dorsal column/medial lemniscus system are assessed next. A vibrating 128-Hz tuning fork gently held against a bony prominence provides evidence of the integrity of the peripheral and central components of the dorsal column system. Patients are instructed to indicate when they are no longer able to perceive vibration. Impaired vibratory sensation has been associated with increased risk of neuropathic ulcer formation.[31] To test proprioception, the examiner passively changes the patient's limb position and then asks the patient to describe the end position or to mimic the position with the other extremity. Care must be taken to minimize additional tactile clues by using circumscribed manual contacts. Limb position varies over multiple repetitions to ensure that initial, mid-, and terminal ranges of motion are tested at proximal, intermediate, and distal joints of the limb.[28] Kinesthesia, the ability to detect direction of movement, is tested by asking the patient to describe what is happening as the limb is being passively repositioned. Eval-

uation of "cortical" sensation, such as two-point discrimination, tactile location (where the stimulus is being applied), and stereognosis (recognition of an object by its form and function using tactile senses) may not be as important in orthotic prescription as in other rehabilitation interventions. The use of Semmes-Weinstein filaments helps to determine whether the patient has sufficient "protective sensation" or is at risk of developing neuropathic ulcers on the soles of the foot because of repetitive low-pressure application by the orthosis or shoe.[32]

Defining the severity and scope of lower extremity sensory impairment guides the orthotist's selection of materials and plan for modification and rectification of the positive model on which the orthosis is to be molded. An intimate fit between the orthosis and limb reduces the risk of skin irritation and breakdown during orthotic wear. Achieving a truly intimate fit is especially important for patients with neuropathy and vascular compromise. Any patient who is referred for assessment and fitting of a lower extremity orthosis must also be screened for visual and upper extremity sensory and motor function. Patients with visual impairment may require contrasting, colored Velcro strapping or large D-rings to don and doff the orthosis independently. Similarly, adaptive strategies for donning and doffing may have to be developed for those who have difficulty using their hands because of sensory impairment, weakness, pain, or deformity resulting from stroke, arthritis, or other neuromuscular or musculoskeletal pathologies.

SKIN CONDITION AND VASCULAR SUPPLY

During the preorthotic assessment, the orthotist carefully notes the overall condition of the patient's skin and supportive soft tissue. Special attention is given to open or healing traumatic, neuropathic, or surgical wounds and to healed areas that may be pressure intolerant due to scarring. Significant bony prominences are also noted so that adequate relief areas can be incorporated into the orthosis. The overall health and viability of the skin are assessed by skin color, temperature, hydration, and turgor (resiliency) and by the pattern of hair distribution or loss and the condition of the nails.

The patient's past and present medical history may suggest arterial, venous, or lymphatic disease that requires more detailed evaluation. Adequacy of arterial vascular supply is initially screened by assessment of skin temperature, capillary refill time, and palpation of lower extremity arterial pulses (dorsalis pedis, posterior tibial, popliteal, and femoral).[33] If there are significant differences or asymmetry in distal to proximal skin temperatures of the limbs, poor or nonpalpable distal pulses, prolonged capillary refill time, and skin signs that suggest arterial insufficiency, the patient may need to be referred for further vascular evaluation. The reader is referred to Chapter 20 or to Wong[34] for further information on evaluation of vascular status and skin and wound care. For patients with fragile or pressure intolerant skin or impaired vascular supply, the orthotist might incorporate strategies to distribute forces over larger surface areas into the orthotic design or use pressure distributing materials to protect the skin and reduce the impact of shearing or torque forces during orthotic wear.

MOTOR FUNCTION

To gain an understanding of the patient's motor function, the therapist and orthotist evaluate muscle tone of the limbs and trunk when the patient is at rest and during functional activities, test deep tendon reflex (DTR) responses, assess the influence of abnormal CNS reflexes on posture and movement, and evaluate muscle strength and muscle endurance.

Muscle Tone and Reflexes

Muscle tone is traditionally tested as the muscle's resistance to passive movement. For patients with upper motor neuron lesions, such as stroke or cerebral palsy, muscle tone (spasticity) is velocity dependent: Little resistance may be seen if the passive movement is slow and gentle, but significant cogwheel "giving and catching" occur if the passive movement is quick and forceful.[35] When a lower motor neuron lesion (as in peripheral nerve damage, cauda equina level spinal cord injury, or myelomeningocele/spina bifida) is present, muscle tone is described as "flaccid" (no tone). Immediately after an acute spinal cord injury or stroke, muscle tone may be reduced significantly and can be described as flaccid or (more accurately) hypotonic. Lesions or damage to the brain stem or cerebellum can result in consistent hypotonicity (low tone). During rehabilitation after an upper motor neuron lesion, tone may become abnormally high, which is described as hypertonicity or spasticity. The baseline muscle tone of patients with cerebellar dysfunction is typically hypotonic, especially in the muscles around proximal joints (limb girdle) and trunk.[36] The muscle tone of patients with extrapyramidal disorders ranges from unpredictably fluctuating (athetosis or choreoathetosis) for patients with diseases of the basal ganglia to consistent rigidity and cocontraction for patients with Parkinson's disease.[37] It is also important to note the occurrence of involuntary movements, such as

resting or intention tremor or choreoathetosis, and of dystonic postures of the distal limb that might have an impact on the fit and function of a lower extremity orthosis.[38]

In addition to assessment of resting muscle tone, the orthotist and therapist are interested in understanding how tone changes or fluctuates over time or with functional activity.[39] The functional consequences of hypertonicity and the severity of abnormal tone can be quantified using the modified Ashworth scale.[40] Asking the patient to perform simple motor tasks, such as reaching for or pointing to an object with the involved limb or stepping over an obstacle on the floor illustrates whether normal or abnormal patterns of motion (synergies) are used to accomplish goal-directed movement.[41] Abnormal tone, muscle weakness, and decreased sensory input contribute to the malalignment of limb segments: Many patients with upper motor neuron lesions stand on a lower limb dominated by extensor synergy, which alters calcaneal position and subtalar joint alignment. The orthotist and therapist must consider the ways in which baseline muscle tone and dynamic muscle function are likely to change if the patient's foot and ankle are supported in a more optimally aligned position.[39]

One of the clinical assessment strategies for evaluation of muscle spindle function and resting muscle tone is DTR testing (Table 6-7). The patient's limb is positioned, in a relaxed state, so that the muscle of interest is moderately elongated, in or near its midrange. The examiner applies a quick and forceful tap to the muscle's tendon with a reflex hammer. The amplitude and quality of motor response are graded using an ordinal descriptive scale (Table 6-8). Consistent DTR responses of 4 + or more suggest an upper motor neuron lesion involving the pyramidal (voluntary) motor system. The use of a Jendrassik's maneuver (isometric contraction of upper extremity muscles or clenching of the teeth) can enhance DTR responses that are diminished or otherwise difficult to elicit.[3,27] Flaccidity and absence of DTR response are suggestive of a lower motor neuron problem involving the nerve root, spinal nerve, peripheral nerve, neuromuscular junction and, in some cases, the muscle itself. DTRs have been described as "pendular" (having larger than expected arcs of motion) in patients with cerebellar dysfunction.[36] In other CNS pathologies, such as Parkinson's disease, DTR responses may be normal despite significant movement dysfunction.[37]

In patients with intact neuromuscular function, DTRs are expected to be symmetric and similar in magnitude from distal to proximal joints.[42] An asymmetric DTR pattern between the left and right extremities or a significant difference (more than one grade) between distal and proximal reflex responses is an indicator of underlying neuromuscular dysfunction.[42] It is important to recognize that,

TABLE 6-7
Deep Tendon Reflexes of the Lower Extremity

Muscle	Location of Tendon Tap	Expected Response	Level
Quadriceps femoris	Patellar tendon	Knee extension	L3-L4
Hamstrings (medial)	Semimembranosus tendon	Knee flexion	L5-S1
Hamstrings (lateral)	Biceps femoris tendon	Knee flexion	S1-S2
Posterior tibialis	Posterior tibialis tendon behind medial malleolus	Plantar flexion/inversion	L4-L5
Gastrocnemius/soleus	Achilles tendon	Plantar flexion	S1-S2

in certain muscles, DTRs may be difficult to elicit, even for the skilled examiner. Responses to DTR testing often vary within the same individual, depending on level of arousal at the time of testing. Muscle tone increases in times of stress or anxiety and tends to decrease with relaxation or during sleep.[43] Because the evaluation process can be anxiety producing for many patients (especially children), it is important to ask patients and family members about muscle function during routine daily activities to achieve an accurate impression of usual muscle function.

For patients with CNS dysfunction, such as cerebral palsy or stroke, it is also important to assess the presence and influence of pathologic developmental reflexes on muscle function and movement[44] (Table 6-9). Certain pathologic reflexes, such as a positive Babinski's response, indicate an impairment in the pyramidal motor system. A positive Babinski's

TABLE 6-8
Grading Scale for Deep Tendon Reflex Responses

Grade	Descriptive Criteria
0	No response; no visible or palpable muscle contraction, even with reinforcement (e.g., Jendrassik's maneuver)
1+	Minimal response, muscle contraction without joint movement; reinforcement often required to strengthen evidence of muscle contraction
2+	Normal response; muscle contraction results in slight joint movement
3+	Brisk response; easily elicited, moderate to strong muscle contraction leads to noticeable movement of the distal limb segment
4+	Hyperactive response; very strong and brisk muscle contraction with large joint excursion, often with one or more beats of clonus of the distal limb segment
5+	Sustained clonus

Source: Adapted from NB Reese (ed). Techniques of the Sensory Exam. In Muscle and Sensory Testing. Philadelphia: Saunders, 1999;421–445; and RT Ross, How to Examine the Nervous System (3rd ed). Stamford, CT: Appleton & Lange, 1999.

response is normal in newborns and may persist in children who are nonambulatory.[45] Patients with CNS dysfunction may learn to rely on other pathologic reflexes, such as the tonic neck reflexes, to establish and maintain enough muscle tone and power (abnormal though it may be) to accomplish a functional goal.[39] The use of an orthosis may initially limit function for patients who have learned to use their abnormal developmental reflexes for function. One of the goals of orthotic intervention may be to facilitate development of effective "normal" motor strategies in place of reliance on abnormal or dysfunctional motor strategies.[39]

Muscle Strength and Endurance

During the preorthotic assessment, the orthotist and therapist also evaluate functional muscle strength and muscular endurance. Traditional "make or break" manual muscle tests or hand-held dynamometry may be useful for patients with lower motor neuron pathology (such as post polio syndrome, muscular dystrophy, or Guillain-Barré syndrome) when muscle function is likely to change over time.[14,46] In patients with CNS dysfunction, results of manual muscle testing may be influenced by abnormal reflex activity, spasticity of antagonistic or agonistic muscles, stereotypical movement patterns, or postural dyscontrol.[47] The validity and reliability of standard manual muscle testing in patients with abnormal tone are controversial.[48,49] In this population it may be more appropriate to evaluate several other aspects of muscle function and motor control. These include the patient's ability to perform concentric, holding, and eccentric muscle contractions; how smoothly the patient is able to reverse direction of movement by activating antagonistic muscle groups; and whether the patient is able to use and control cocontraction of agonistic and antagonistic muscle groups when a task requires stability. Functional assessment helps to identify how strength changes throughout an active range of motion, as well as how dynamic strength varies with position and type of activity and whether muscular fatigue is likely to compromise function.

TABLE 6-9
Pathologic Reflexes Seen in Patients with Central Nervous System Dysfunction

Reflex	*Stimulus*	*Positive Response*
Babinski's	Stroking lateral border of the sole	Extension of hallux Fanning of second to fifth toes
Startle	Sudden loud or harsh noise	Mass extension response of extremities and trunk
Flexor withdrawal	Noxious stimulus on sole of foot	Mass flexion pattern of ipsilateral extremity
Crossed extension	Noxious stimulus on sole of foot	Opposite extremity flexes as ipsilateral limb extends
Positive supporting reaction	Repeated loading of ball of the foot	↑ Extensor synergy
Asymmetric tonic neck reflex	Rotation of the head and neck	↑ Extensor tone of "face" limbs ↑ Flexor tone of "skull" limbs
Symmetric tonic neck reflex	Flexion/extension of head and neck	↑ UE flexion and LE extension ↑ UE extension and LE flexion
Tonic labyrinthine supine reflex	Prolonged supine position	Gradual ↑ extension tone of trunk/limbs
Tonic labyrinthine prone reflex	Prolonged prone position	Gradual ↑ flexion tone of trunk/limbs

↑ = increased; UE = upper extremity; LE = lower extremity.

The impact of paralysis or paresis of each involved muscle or muscle group on lower limb alignment in standing and during each subphase of gait must be assessed carefully.[50] Imbalances in strength or muscle tone in antagonistic muscles increase the risk of malalignment of limb segments, including development of angular and torsional deformities, soft tissue contracture, and differences in leg length during growth periods. Orthoses for patients with lower motor neuron lesions must be lightweight, supportive or assistive of existing muscle function, carefully aligned for congruence with anatomic joint axis, and designed for optimal alignment of limb segments and prevention of deformity. For growing children with neuromuscular dysfunction, the risk of developing soft tissue contracture or angular or torsional deformity of the lower extremity is powerfully influenced by imbalances of strength and abnormal tone. Orthoses for children and adults with neuromuscular dysfunction must also be designed with optimal alignment, facilitation of efficient motor function, and energy cost in mind.[39,51]

Functional Assessment

Although much of the information collected in the pre-orthotic assessment focuses on impairments that might be addressed by orthotic information, an understanding of a patient's functional status and functional limitation is just as important in developing the appropriate orthotic prescription. An orthosis that corrects malalignments or protects unstable or vulnerable joints well but in doing so prevents the patient from accomplishing the important tasks and activities will end up in the closet or under the bed instead of on the limb. The orthotist and therapist must develop an understanding of how the patient currently

functions, as well as the types of activities that the patient is required or would like to perform, to make appropriate choices among orthotic component and design options.

Functional assessment of children and adults with neuromuscular disorders who may benefit from a lower extremity orthosis begins with observation and assessment of postural control under static and dynamic (anticipatory and reactionary) conditions.[52] It is important to understand the patient's ability to achieve and maintain antigravity postures and the efficacy of righting and equilibrium responses during a variety of functional activities.[41,51,53] How does the patient create or achieve postural stability? Are "abnormal" reflexes or postures used to "fix" a limb or trunk segment, or has the patient developed compensatory strategies to create stiffness when postural control mechanisms are inefficient?[51] What is likely to happen if an orthosis changes alignment of limb segments or alters access to compensatory movement patterns? Efficacy of postural control may be different when sitting and standing are compared. It is also important to gain a sense of how large the patient's functional "sway envelope" might be: How far and in which directions can the patient consistently and functionally shift the center of mass before activating an equilibrium response to "recenter" within the base of support.[54,55]

The next considerations are how the patient changes position and what impact the addition of an orthosis might have on movement strategy and functional ability during transitional activities. Children often move from sitting or standing to the floor and back during play or school activities. It may be that an orthosis designed to facilitate a more functional gait pattern will restrict range of motion at the ankle, knee, or hip, limiting the joint excursion typically used to move to or from the floor. Patients of all ages must be able to move safely and efficiently from sitting to standing. One of the musculoskeletal determinants of this functional task is adequate knee flexion and ankle dorsiflexion, which allow the foot to be positioned far under the seated pelvis for smooth transfer of body weight onto the foot.[15] The patient who requires an orthosis that restricts ankle or knee range of motion may benefit from functional retraining to adapt motor strategies for these important functional tasks.

The most important functional component of the pre-orthotic evaluation is a comprehensive gait analysis. Observational gait analysis provides information about difficulties that the patient may be having with the three major functional tasks of gait: weight acceptance in early stance, stability during single limb support, and swing limb advancement.[5] Observation of gait also identifies problems with critical events in each of the subphases of gait (see Table 6-2). Therapists and orthotists must distinguish between primary gait problems that might be effectively addressed by an orthosis and abnormal gait patterns that may be a compensatory strategy. In making a choice among the many designs and components for lower extremity orthoses, the orthotist and therapist select those that effectively address the primary gait dysfunction with minimal compromise of progression through the entire gait cycle.

It is also helpful to record typical quantitative kinematic characteristics of the patient's gait (stride length, step length, step width, foot angle, step or stride time, double support time, velocity, and cadence) as a baseline for later assessment of the impact of the orthosis on gait. If the patient has been evaluated in a formal gait laboratory, kinetic information (ground reaction forces, joint torques/moments, center of pressure excursion, and work) and electromyography-collected patterns of muscle activity are also valuable in the decision-making process for orthotic prescription.

Functional assessment of gait continues with an exploration of how often and how far the patient walks during a typical day and whether the patient is able to vary speed, change direction, and manage nonlevel surfaces, including stairs, grass/sidewalks, and ramps. If a patient uses an ambulatory aid (a cane, crutches, or walker), the device and pattern of walking used are documented as well.

Finally, the orthotist and therapist must consider the patient's ability to don and doff and to care for the orthosis. Information about sensory function of the upper extremities, vision and perception, and fine motor control guides the selection of closure strategies for the orthosis. Questions about who is likely to apply the device must be posed. Ideally, the orthosis will be designed so that it can be applied with relatively minimum effort, keeping the patient's tone, flexibility, postural control, and fine motor function in mind. How likely is the orthosis to be worn, for example, if a caregiver must struggle to move the patient's hypertonic limb into significant hip and knee flexion to position the ankle in "neutral" to don the orthosis? What will happen if the patient lives alone and assistance with dressing is not routinely available?

The adequacy of fit of the orthosis over time is also an important consideration, especially if the patient is a growing child or adolescent. Many thermoplastic AFO and KAFO designs require intimate fit of the foot in the orthosis and are carefully aligned to ensure congruence between anatomic and orthotic joint axes. As a child grows, the fit of the orthosis changes, evidenced by difficulty in donning, discomfort during gait when bony prominences are no longer protected within relief areas, and compromised orthotic control of motion. Patients and caregivers must understand the importance of skin inspection and be encouraged to contact the orthotist or therapist when concerns about fit arise. Routine follow-up appointments in an orthotic clinic identify when a new orthosis is indicated for a growing child.

SUMMARY

We have identified the many components of a comprehensive preorthotic assessment. In developing an appropriate orthotic prescription, the orthotist and therapist must have a thorough understanding of the patient's diagnosis and prognosis. Systematic examination of the musculoskeletal system identifies pertinent biomechanical or anatomic impairments, constraints, or concerns (joint contracture or deformity, ligamentous instability, compromised muscle function, and limitations for weight bearing) that have an impact on choice of orthotic design or components. Examination of the neuromuscular system provides information about abnormalities of tone, sensory impairment, compromised postural control, and difficulties with motor control. Because orthoses apply forces to control limb alignment and motion, skin condition and integrity are also assessed. Observational and quantitative gait analysis helps the orthotist and therapist to understand the ways in which musculoskeletal and neuromuscular impairments compromise the patient's mobility and functional status. A clear understanding of the patient's or caregiver's functional goals for the orthosis is essential. Discussion about how an orthosis may or may not address these functional goals helps to assure satisfaction with the orthosis to be fabricated. With the information collected in the preorthotic assessment, the orthotist develops a specific orthotic prescription for the patient.

The next step in the process is the application of a cast to create a negative mold of the limb and the creation of a plaster of Paris positive model. The positive model is modified and rectified based on the findings and goals developed during the preorthotic assessment, and the orthosis is fabricated. At the initial fitting, observational and quantitative gait assessment help the orthotist and therapist to begin to assess the efficacy of the orthosis in meeting the goals developed during preorthotic assessment. An initial wearing schedule is developed, gradually increasing the time "in brace." The therapist incorporates functional and gait training with the new orthosis into the patient's plan of care to ensure that the orthosis is meeting the patient's goals. Finally, follow-up visits with the orthotist for re-evaluation and orthotic maintenance are scheduled.

REFERENCES

1. Perry J. Total Limb Function. In Gait Analysis: Normal and Pathological Function. Thorofare, NJ: Slack, 1992;149–168.
2. Norkin CC, White DJ. Measurement of Joint Motion: A Guide to Goniometry (2nd ed). Philadelphia: Davis, 1995.
3. Magee DJ. Principles and Concepts. In Orthopedic Physical Assessment (3rd ed). Philadelphia: Saunders, 1997;1–52.
4. Inman VT, Ralston HJ, Todd F. Human Walking. Baltimore: Williams & Wilkins, 1981.
5. Pathokinesiology Department and Physical Therapy Department of Rancho Los Amigos Medical Center. Observational Gait Analysis. Downey, CA: Los Amigos Research and Education Institute, 1993.
6. Magee DJ. Hip. In Orthopedic Physical Assessment (3rd ed). Philadelphia: Saunders, 1997;460–505.
7. Magee DJ. Knee. In Orthopedic Physical Assessment (3rd ed). Philadelphia: Saunders, 1997;506–598.
8. Magee DJ. Lower Leg, Ankle and Foot. In Orthopedic Physical Assessment (3rd ed). Philadelphia: Saunders, 1997; 599–672.
9. Hoppenfeld S. Physical Examination of the Hip and Pelvis. In Physical Examination of the Spine and Extremities. Norwalk, CT: Appleton-Century-Crofts, 1976;143–170.
10. Hoppenfeld S. Physical Examination of the Knee. In Physical Examination of the Spine and Extremities. Norwalk, CT: Appleton-Century-Crofts, 1976;171–196.
11. Hoppenfeld S. Physical Examination of the Foot and Ankle. In Physical Examination of the Spine and Extremities. Norwalk, CT: Appleton-Century-Crofts, 1976;197–236.
12. American Academy of Orthopedic Surgeons. Joint Motion: Method of Measuring and Recording. Chicago: American Academy of Orthopedic Surgeons, 1965.
13. Norkin CC, Levangie PK. Joint Structure and Function: A Comprehensive Analysis (2nd ed). Philadelphia: Davis, 1992.
14. Kendall FP, McCreary EK, Provance PG. Muscles Testing and Function (4th ed). Baltimore: Williams & Wilkins, 1993.
15. Hughes MA, Schenkman ML. Chair rise strategies in the functionally impaired elderly. J Rehabil Res Dev 1996;33(4):409–412.
16. VanSant AF. Rising from a supine position to erect stance: description of adult movement and a developmental hypothesis. Phys Ther 1988;68(2):185–192.
17. VanSant AF. Age differences in movement patterns used by children to rise from a supine position to erect stance. Phys Ther 1988;68(9):1330–1339.
18. LeVeau B. Hip. In JK Richardson, ZA Iglarish (eds), Clinical Orthopedic Physical Therapy. Philadelphia: Saunders, 1994;333–398.
19. Weatherwax RJ. Anterior drawer sign. Clin Orthop 1981;154:318–319.
20. Strobel M, Stedtfeld HW. Diagnostic Evaluation of the Knee. Berlin: Springer-Verlag, 1990.
21. Greenfield BH. Sequential Evaluation of the Knee. In BH Greenfield (ed), Rehabilitation of the Knee: A Problem Solving Approach. Philadelphia: Davis, 1993;44–65.
22. Gungor T. A test for ankle instability: brief report. J Bone Joint Surg 1988;70B(3):487.
23. Frost HM, Hanson CA. Technique for testing the drawer sign in the ankle. Clin Orthop 1977;March/April(123):49–51.
24. McPoil TG. The Foot and Ankle. In TR Malone, T McPoil, AJ Nitz (eds), Orthopedic and Sports Physical Therapy (3rd ed). St. Louis: Mosby, 1997;259–294.
25. Tachdjian MO. Pediatric Orthopedics. Philadelphia: Saunders, 1972.
26. Tachdjian MO. Clinical Pediatric Orthopedics: The Art of Diagnosis and Principles of Management. Stamford, CT: McGraw-Hill, 1997;1–86.
27. Berryman Reese N. Techniques of the Sensory Exam. In Muscle and Sensory Testing. Philadelphia: Saunders, 1999;421–445.
28. Schmitz TJ. Sensory Assessment. In SB O'Sullivan, TJ Schmitz (eds), Physical Rehabilitation: Assessment and Treatment (3rd ed). Philadelphia: Davis, 1994;83–96.
29. Jackson-Wyatt O. Brain Function, Aging, and Dementia. In DA Umphred (ed), Neurological Rehabilitation (3rd ed). St. Louis: Mosby, 1995;722–746.
30. Shumway-Cook A, Woollacott M. Aging and Postural Control. In Motor Control: Theory and Practical Applications. Baltimore: Williams & Wilkins, 1995;169–184.
31. Young MJ, Breddy JL, Veves A, Boulton AJ. The prediction of diabetic foot ulceration using vibration perception threshold. Diabetes Care 1994;17(6):557–560.
32. Mueller MJ. Identifying patients with diabetes mellitus who are at risk for lower extremity complications: use of Semmes-Weinstein monofilaments. Phys Ther 1996;76(1):68–71.
33. McCullough J. Peripheral Vascular Disease. In SB O'Sullivan, TJ Schmitz (eds), Physical Rehabilitation: Assessment and Treatment (3rd ed). Philadelphia: Davis, 1994;361–373.
34. Wong RA. Chronic Dermal Wounds in Older Adults. In AA Guccione (ed), Geriatric Physical Therapy. St. Louis: Mosby, 1993;307–330.
35. Katz R, Rymer Z. Spastic hypertonia; mechanisms and measurement. Arch Phys Med Rehabil 1989;70(2):144–155.
36. Urbscheit NL, Oremland BS. Cerebellar Dysfunction. In DA Umphred (ed), Neurological Rehabilitation (3rd ed). St. Louis: Mosby, 1995;657–680.
37. Adams RD, Victor M, Ropper AH. Abnormalities of Movement and Posture Due to Disease of the Basal Ganglia. In

Principles of Neurology (6th ed). New York: McGraw-Hill, 1997;64–83.

38. Lusardi MM. Tremors, Chorea, and Other Involuntary Movements. In TL Kauffman (ed), Geriatric Rehabilitation Manual. New York: Churchill Livingstone, 1999;155–164.

39. Huber SR. Therapeutic Application of Orthotics. In DA Umphred (ed), Neurological Rehabilitation (3rd ed). St. Louis: Mosby, 1995;893–910.

40. Bohannon RW, Smith M. Interrater reliability of a modified Ashworth scale of muscle spasticity. Phys Ther 1987; 67(2):206–207.

41. Ryerson SD. Hemiplegia. In DA Umphred (ed), Neurological Rehabilitation (3rd ed). St. Louis: Mosby, 1995;681–721.

42. Ross RT. How to Examine the Nervous System (3rd ed). Stamford, CT: Appleton & Lange, 1999.

43. Umphred DA. The Limbic Complex: Influence over Motor Control and Learning. In Neurological Rehabilitation (3rd ed). St. Louis: Mosby, 1995;92–117.

44. Byarm LE. Developmental Therapy Approaches: Neurodevelopmental Therapy. In LA Kurtz, PW Dowrick, SE Levy, ML Batshaw (eds), Handbook of Developmental Disabilities. Gaithersburg, MD: Aspen, 1996;249–259.

45. Adams RD, Victor M, Ropper AH. Normal Development and Deviations in Development of the Nervous System. In Principles of Neurology (6th ed). New York: McGraw-Hill, 1997;573–607.

46. Daniels L, Worthingham C. Muscle Testing: Techniques of Manual Examination (4th ed). Philadelphia: Saunders, 1980.

47. O'Sullivan SB. Motor Control Assessment. In SB O'Sullivan, TJ Schmitz (eds), Physical Rehabilitation: Assesment and Treatment (3rd ed). Philadelphia: Davis, 1994;111–132.

48. Rothstein J, Riddle D, Finucane S. Commentary: is the measurement of muscle strength appropriate in patients with brain lesions? Phys Ther 1989;69(3):230–231.

49. Bohannon RW. Is the measurement of muscle strength appropriate in patients with brain lesions? Phys Ther 1989; 69(3):225–229.

50. Prosthetics and Orthotics staff. Lower Limb Orthotics. New York: Post-graduate Medical School, New York University, 1986.

51. Styer-Acevedo J. Physical Therapy for the Child with Cerebral Palsy. In JS Techlin (ed), Pediatric Physical Therapy (3rd ed). Philadelphia: Lippincott, 1999;107–162.

52. Woollacott MH. Postural Control Mechanisms in the Young and Old. In PW Duncan (ed), Balance: Proceedings of the APTA Forum. Alexandria, VA: American Physical Therapy Association, 1990;23–28.

53. Winker PA. Head Injury. In DA Umphred (ed), Neurological Rehabilitation (3rd ed). St. Louis: Mosby, 1995;421–453.

54. Allison L. Balance Disorders. In DA Umphred (ed), Neurological Rehabilitation (3rd ed). St. Louis: Mosby, 1995;802–837.

55. Maki BE, McIllroy WE. The Role of Limb Movements in Maintaining Upright Stance: The Change in Support Strategy. In Balance: An American Physical Therapy Association Mongraph. Alexandria, VA: American Physical Therapy Association, 1997;58–77.

7

Footwear: Foundation for Lower Extremity Orthotics

Jennifer M. Bottomley

The most essential element of clothing in any person's wardrobe is shoes. No other article of clothing is designed to fit so precisely. Continuous pressure from tight shoes can produce ulceration and deformities. Ill-fitting shoes can create shear forces that lead to skin breakdown, can create and facilitate toe and foot deformities, and can lead to falls.[1] Shoes perform the vital functions of transferring body weight to the floor during walking and of protecting the wearer from any hazards in the environment. A well-designed shoe is the necessary foundation for many lower extremity orthotics and for prosthetic alignment and energy-efficient gait. This chapter discusses the components and characteristics of shoes, how to ensure proper fit, and how to choose appropriate footwear for patients with foot dysfunction and deformity.

COMPONENTS OF A GOOD SHOE

A suitable pair of shoes minimizes stress on all portions of the feet, provides support, and acts as a shock absorber of ground reaction forces.[2] The basic parts of a shoe are the sole, upper, heel, and last. Each of these parts is further divided into component parts or areas that are required for proper shoe design (Figure 7-1). Each component is crucial to the prescription of appropriate shoes for the person's individual needs.

Sole

The sole protects the plantar surface of the foot. The traditional sole consists of two pieces of leather sewn together with compressible cork between. An additional layer, the insole, is situated next to the foot in most shoes. A heavy thick sole protects the foot against walking surface irregularities. The rigidity or stiffness of the sole is also important: Although it needs to be durable, it should not be so rigid as to interfere with the toe rocker of the metatarsophalangeal (MTP) hyperextension during terminal stance and preswing phases of gait. Various areas of the sole are identified by location. The *welt* is the inside piece of the external sole; the *outsole* is the portion that is most external. The area that lies between the heel and the ball of the shoe is known as the *shank*. The shank of the sole is commonly fabricated to provide reinforcement and shape using such materials as spring steel, steel and leatherboard, or wood strips between the welt and the outsole. The purpose of the shank is to prevent collapse of the material between the heel and the ball of the foot and the provision of extra support. In most athletic shoes the sole is rubber to provide maximal traction. Rubber soles absorb shock, thereby minimizing heel impact forces.

Upper

The upper, which is divided into the *vamp, tongue,* and *rear quarters,* covers the dorsum of the foot. The vamp extends from the insole forward. The tongue is an extension of the vamp in a blucher-style closure, but in the bal-type oxford, the tongue is separate (Figure 7-2). The blucher-style closure can be opened slightly more than the bal oxford closure to allow the foot into the shoe. The toe of the vamp is often covered with a separate piece of leather called the *tip.* The rearward line of the tip may be straight or winged. The vamp is joined to the quarters, which make up the sides and back of the upper. The two quarters are joined at a back seam. The design of the shoe dictates the shape and size of the quarters. For the oxford shoe, the outside quarter is cut lower than the inside to avoid contact with the malleoli. In the bal oxford, the back edges of the vamp cover the forward edges of the quarter. The forward edges of the quarters are on the top of the vamp in the blucher style of shoe. The blucher

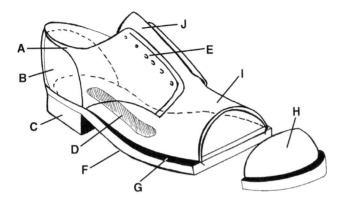

FIGURE 7-1

Basic parts of a shoe. The upper is made up of the quarter (A) and its reinforcing counter (B), which stabilize the rear foot within the shoe; the closure (E) and tongue (J) across the mid-foot; and the shaft (vamp; I) and toe box (H), which enclose the forefoot. The exterior outsole (F) is often reinforced with a steel shank (D) and is attached to the upper at the welt (G). The standard heel (C) is ¾ in. high.

closure is preferable. This design has a separation between the distal margins of the lace stays, thus offering a wide inlet, making the shoes easier to don and doff and readily adjustable in circumference. High shoes are required when mediolateral stability is needed.

Heel

The heel is located beneath the outer sole under the anatomic heel. The heel base is usually rigid rubber, plastic, or wood with a resilient plantar surface. The individual with limited ankle motion may benefit from a compressible heel base to absorb shock and achieve plantar flexion during the early stance phase. A broad low heel maximizes stability and minimizes stress on the metatarsal heads. Most lower extremity orthotics and prosthetic feet are designed

for a specific heel height; efficacy of the orthotic or quality of the prosthetic gait can be significantly compromised if used with shoes that have higher or lower heels.

Reinforcements

Strategic shoe reinforcements contribute to foot protection. Toe boxing at the distal vamp shields the toes and prevents the anterior portion of the vamp from losing its shape. The toe box can also be increased in depth to protect and accommodate any toe deformities. The heel counter reinforces the quarters to help secure the shoe to the anatomic heel. The medial counter helps support the medial arch of the shoe, and the heel counter aids in controlling the rear foot. The convex shank piece stiffens the sole between the distal border of the shoe heel and the MTP joints and aids in supporting the longitudinal arch.

Lasts

Shoes are constructed over a model of the foot stylized from wood, plaster, or plastic that is called a *last*. Manufacturers are now converting to computer-aided last designs. Regardless of the origin of the last, it determines the fit, walking ease, and appearance of the shoe. Commercial shoes are made over many different lasts in thousands of size combinations. Most shoes are made with a medial last, which means that the toe box is directed inward from the heel (Figure 7-3). Shoes can also be obtained that have a conventional last, straight last, inflared or medial last, or outflared or lateral last.

FASHION VERSUS FUNCTION

A revolution to create comfortable and "healthy" shoes has occurred within the shoe industry.[3] The epidemic of footwear-related health problems, a result of long-term wearing of

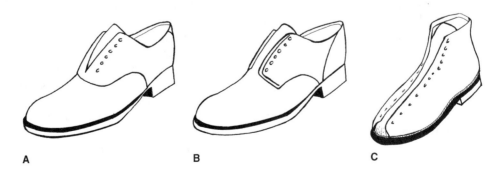

FIGURE 7-2

Three types of shoe closures. (A) In the bal oxford style, the tongue is a separate piece sewn to the vamp and anterior edges of the quarters. (B) In the blucher style, the tongue is an extension of the vamp and can be opened slightly wider. (C) For patients with rigid ankle orthotics, fixed deformity, or fragile neuropathic feet, the lace to toe (surgical) style may be necessary.

FIGURE 7-3
The last determines the shape of the shoe. (A) In a conventional last, the forefoot is directly slightly lateral (L) to the midline. (B) A straight last is symmetric around the midline. (C) An inflared last directs the forefoot medially, and (D) an outflared last directs it more laterally than a conventional last. (M = medial.)

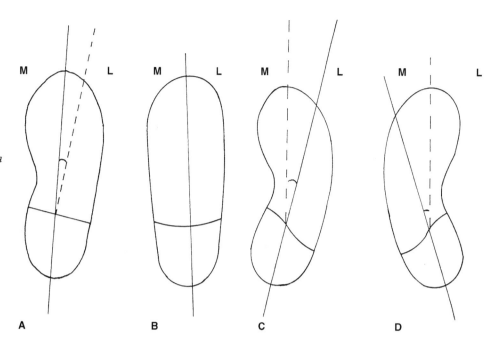

improperly fitting shoes, costs more than $3 billion annually in surgery. Even the most savvy, health-conscious women sometimes buy shoes for looks, not fit. A survey of 356 women concluded that nearly 90% of women wore shoes that were one to two sizes too small. This trend contributes significantly to the development of bunions, hammertoes, claw toes, mallet deformities, corns and calluses, and other disabling foot problems in mid- and later life.[4,5]

Enhancing Function

Foot stability is critical to minimizing ankle injury, excessive pronation, and slipping of the heel during the gait cycle. A well-designed shoe provides a broad heel base, ankle collar, and close-fitting heel counter. A keystone of a good shoe is its ability to absorb shock. The construction of and materials used for the insole, midsole, and outer sole determine the amount of shock absorption that the shoe will provide.

A good shoe must be flexible and be able to provide stability with every step. Flexible construction is especially important in the sole, to enhance the toe rocker in late stance phase. The sole should also provide adequate traction as it contacts the ground, especially in early stance as body weight is transferred onto the foot. A coefficient of friction that is sufficient to minimize slips and near slips is vital. Heel height can create stress on the forefoot during gait: Heels of more than 1.5 in. exponentially increase weight-bearing forces on the metatarsal heads.[6]

The ability of a shoe to handle moisture is also an important consideration: For optimal foot health and com-

fort, perspiration must be wicked away and, at the same time, external moisture must be kept out. The upper should be soft and pliable. Modern tanning techniques can create strong but supple uppers that surround the feet supportively and protectively without rubbing and chafing, while allowing the foot to breathe.

Orthotic-Related Function

A molded insole contributes to foot stability, shock absorption, and a transfer of shear forces away from problem areas. Orthotics can enhance the function of the shoes. The principles and practices of orthotic prescription in commonly occurring conditions of the foot are presented in Chapter 8.

PROPER FITTING OF A SHOE: "IF THE SHOE FITS"

The two primary determinants of proper shoe fit are shoe shape and shoe size. Shoe shape refers to the shape of the sole and the upper. Proper fit is achieved when shoe shape is matched to foot shape. Shoe size is determined by arch length, not by overall foot length.[7] The proper shoe size is the one that accommodates the first metatarsal joint in the widest part of the shoe. Properly fitting shoes are important in avoiding foot discomfort and deformity and are absolutely essential in individuals with arthritis, diabetes, and other foot disorders.

Great variability is found in human foot size and shape. Mass-produced shoes, however, are formed over fairly standard lasts that give a shoe its special size and shape. In the well-fit shoe, the shape determined by the last approximates the human foot. The design and construction of the shoe should allow for a roomy toe box; it should be wide enough for normal toe alignment and ½ in. longer than the longest toe. Proper fit of the forefoot in the shoe can be a critical factor in reducing the incidence of bunions, hammertoes, and other forefoot deformities. In general, the shoe should be wide enough to accommodate the widest part of the forefoot. A tracing of the foot (standing) should fit within an outline of the shoe bottom.

Proper fit presupposes proper design, shape, and construction and is fundamentally wedded to availability in widths as well as lengths. It is important that the clinician cultivate a consumer mindset that realizes the medical importance of modifying the old cliché, "if the shoe fits, wear it," to "if the shoe fits, wear it, and if it doesn't, order it in the correct size."

Determining Measurements

The average shoe salesperson does not offer to measure the foot, instead relying on the consumer to know his or her foot size. Because foot size changes over time, it is important to measure both feet for length and width periodically. Many shoe styles that are available in retail shoe stores do not appropriately match the shape of an individual's foot. As a result, comfort and protection are compromised in the name of "style." This is especially problematic in the presence of foot deformity. Hallux valgus is a foot deformity that is aggravated by wearing shoes that are too narrow across the metatarsal heads and triangularly shaped in the toe box. Shoes should be wide enough to allow the material of the upper that surrounds the widest region of the forefoot (i.e., the metatarsal heads) to be compressed at least one-sixteenth of an inch before bony contact is made. Likewise, at least a ½-in. space should be present between the tip of the longest toe and the front of the toe box in weight bearing (generally the width of the thumb).

In the United States, 12 standard shoe widths are manufactured, ranging from the very narrow AAAAA to the very wide EEEE—that is, AAAAA, AAAA, AAA, AA, A, B, C, D, E, EE, EEE, EEEE. Most retail stores stock shoes of midrange widths (A–E). Patients with narrow or wide feet often have difficulty finding shoes of the optimal width. Standard shoe sizes are available in half-size increments, from an infant's size 0 to men's size 16 in U.S. sizes. The difference in length between half sizes is ⅟₁₆ in., with adjustments made in girth measurements accordingly. Standard shoe-sizing classifications are made by groups and lasts: infants' sizes 0–2; boys' sizes 2½–6; girls' sizes 2½–9; women's

sizes 3–10; and men's sizes 6–12. Sizes larger than women's size 10 and men's size 12 can be special ordered. A U.S. women's shoe size is usually three half sizes smaller than the corresponding men's size (e.g., women's size 9 is the same as a men's size 7 ½). European and U.K. manufacturers use a different numbering system. The comparison of European and U.K. women's to men's sizes is based on centimeters (e.g., women's size 38 EUR/5.0 UK is the same as men's size 40 EUR/5.0 UK). Table 7-1 compares the standard sizes for U.S., European, and U.K. shoe manufacturers, in addition to the measures for each size.

Foot Contour

Foot contour changes throughout the life cycle. Aging, pregnancy, obesity, and everyday stresses on the foot cause it to get wider. Deformities such as bunions increase the width and shape of the foot, and splaying of the metatarsal heads create a collapse of the transverse arch, further increasing the width of the forefoot.[8] Forefoot height may increase in the presence of toe deformities. Deformities such as pes planus (foot flattening) or pes cavus (high arches) change the contour of the midfoot. The shape of the foot needs to be considered and accommodated when an individual is measured for shoes. Often a "combined last," in which the last in the toe box is different from the rear foot counter, is required to accommodate the contour of the foot. The relationship of the forefoot to the rear foot is an important consideration in determining if the shoe shape, provided by the last, corresponds to the shape of the foot. Shoes with medial, straight, or lateral lasts can be ordered to best meet patient needs.

Obesity and Edema

The additional mechanical stress of carrying excess weight takes its toll on the feet, often resulting in problems such as plantar fasciitis, arthritis and bursitis, heel pain, neuroma, and gait changes.[5] Frey et al.[5] found that a weight gain of as little as 9 pounds over a 5-year period increased foot size by one full size. Obesity has been shown to increase the length and the width of the foot. The Frey study also revealed that although women tended to adjust for length increases by purchasing a longer shoe, they rarely increased shoe width. The net result over the 5-year study period included increased incidence of calluses, corns, bunions, hammertoes, ingrown toenails, and neuromas.

Obesity also has an impact on gait patterns. Persons with obesity demonstrate increased step width, increased ankle dorsiflexion with reduced plantar flexion, increased Q angles at the knee, increased hip abduction angles, increased abducted foot angles, greater out toeing, a tendency for

TABLE 7-1

Comparison of Standardized Shoe Sizes

United States	Europe	United Kingdom	Centimeters
Women's sizes			
3	34.0	1.0	20.0
3½	34.5	1.5	20.5
4	35.0	2.0	21.0
4½	35.5	2.5	21.5
5	36.0	3.0	22.0
5½	36.5	3.5	22.5
6	37.0	4.0	23.0
6½	37.5	4.5	23.5
7	38.0	5.0	24.0
7½	38.5	5.5	24.5
8	39.0	6.0	25.0
8½	39.5	6.5	25.5
9	40.0	7.0	26.0
9½	40.5	7.5	26.5
10	41.0	8.0	27.0
Men's sizes			
6	40.0	5.0	24.0
6½	40.5	5.5	24.5
7	41.0	6.0	25.0
7½	41.5	6.5	25.5
8	42.0	7.0	26.0
8½	42.5	7.5	26.5
9	43.0	8.0	27.0
9½	43.5	8.5	27.5
10	44.0	9.0	28.0
10½	44.5	9.5	28.5
11	45.0	10.0	29.0
11½	45.5	10.5	29.5
12	46.0	11.0	30.0

flat-footed weight acceptance early in the gait cycle, increased touchdown angles, more eversion at the subtalar joint, and a faster maximum eversion velocity. These gait changes may be an attempt to increase stability during gait. The net effect, however, is an increased incidence of overuse injuries as a result of everyday activities.[9]

Proper shoe fitting is essential for preventing secondary foot problems that stem from ill-fitting shoes. Overweight individuals should be encouraged to have their feet measured regularly, particularly if they have had a significant weight gain. It is often helpful to shop for shoes at the end of the day when feet are at their largest, to fit standing to the largest foot, and to make sure that a ½-in. space is present between the end of the longest toe and the edge of the toe box. The shoes should be comfortable the moment they are put on.

Fluctuation in foot size in individuals with edema (e.g., those with kidney dysfunction or congestive heart failure or any patient who is taking diuretic medication) creates a challenge when fitting shoes. The contour of the foot is constantly changing. For someone with severe edema, a

Thermold (P. W. Minor Shoes, Batavia, NY) Velcro closure shoe/sandal (Figure 7-4) is recommended to accommodate and support the foot and prevent the undue pressures that are imposed by a shoe that becomes too small over the course of the day.

CONSEQUENCES OF THE ILL-FITTING SHOE

The national obsession with beauty has created some not-so-beautiful sites on feet, such as bunions, hammertoes, and neuromas. This is particularly the case for women who often select poorly fitting shoes in an attempt to have the foot appear to be smaller, daintier, and narrower than it actually is. In Frey et al.'s study,[5] 90% of women surveyed wore shoes that were too small by one or two width and length sizes; 80% of these women had foot problems. Snow et al.[10] report that 90% of 795,000 surgeries for bunions, hammertoes/claw toes/mallet toes, neuromas, and Taylor bunions were directly attributed to wearing

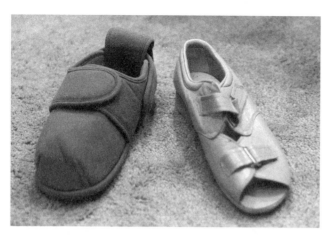

FIGURE 7-4
Thermold (P. W. Minor Shoes, Batavia, NY) Velcro closure shoe/sandal. Adjustable Velcro closures are recommended to accommodate edematous feet and prevent tissue damage due to high pressure.

ill-fitting shoes. Foot problems, including bunions, lesser toe deformities, and neuromas, are the primary consequences of wearing shoes that are not a proper fit. Clearly, many of these problems would be prevented by habitual use of properly fitting shoes.

SPECIAL CONSIDERATIONS

Feet come in many shapes, sizes, and conditions of health. The biomechanical and functional characteristics of feet change over an individual's lifetime and must also be reflected in shoe choice. The foot of an infant must adapt to weight bearing, especially as walking becomes functional. The foot of a child continues to adapt as normal growth changes alignment of pelvis, femur, and tibia. The influence of hormones during pregnancy also has an impact on structure and function of the foot. Finally, the combined influence of the aging process and of diseases that are common in later life can create special footwear needs for the elderly.

Pediatric Foot

Many pediatric and lower extremity foot disorders are minimally symptomatic and do not require treatment, whereas others require more aggressive management. An understanding of the natural history of many of these disorders is important in establishing the appropriate footwear for toddlers and children as they begin to walk and run.

In toeing is a problem caused by positional factors in utero and during sleep, muscle imbalances due to paralytic disorders, and decreased range of motion in the lower kinetic chain. It may also be due to metatarsus adductus, internal tibia torsion, or internal femoral torsion.

Metatarsus adductus is characterized by a bean-shaped foot that results from adduction of the forefoot. In most children (approximately 85%), this disorder resolves itself spontaneously.[11] If it does not improve over the first 6–12 weeks of life, the treatment of choice is an outflared shoe. The bones of the foot are soft and can be corrected with positioning in the outflared shoe (reverse last) or Bebax shoe (Camp Healthcare, Jackson, MI).

Internal tibial torsion is a twist between the knee and the ankle. Generally, this torsion disappears by the age of 5 years. Torsion can be exacerbated by abnormal sitting and sleep postures with the foot turned inward. (Note: Some of the best athletes are in toers.) The Dennis Browne bars or the counter rotation splint is used in combination with a reverse last shoe to remodel the bones during growth. Persistent severe toeing created by internal tibial torsion requires a derotational osteotomy of the tibia/fibula in the supramalleolar region.

Internal femoral torsion can also be the cause of in toeing with a twist between the knee and hip. Neither splints nor shoes are effective in treatment of torsion. Habitual sitting in the "W" position (for example, when a child is watching television or playing games on the floor) can aggravate the problem. Children with internal femoral torsion should be encouraged to sit "X" legged as an alternative.

Out toeing occurs in children who sleep in the frog position and have soft tissue contractures around the hip. This is usually a hip or a long bone torsion problem and is not impacted by footwear.

Toe walking can be the result of an in utero shortening or a congenital shortening of the Achilles tendon but can also be an early sign of cerebral palsy, muscular dystrophy, or Charcot-Marie-Tooth disease.[11] Up until the age of 4 years, the ability to stretch the tendon is well preserved, and conservative treatment includes stretching, casting, ankle-foot orthoses, and/or a night splint. Z-plasty lengthening is performed if conservative interventions fail. Shoe prescription objectives follow the same principles as those in the older adult with Achilles tendonitis (see Achilles Tendonitis, Bursitis, and Haglund's Deformity).

Flexible flatfoot appears to reflect generalized, hereditary ligamentous laxity.[12] Treatment for flatfootedness in children has changed over time. Currently, the shoe used to treat flatfoot is designed to correct heel valgus, support the arch, and pronate the forefoot in relation to the rear foot. Forefoot pronation is achieved by using a lateral shoe wedge combined with a medial heel wedge. A scaphoid pad supports the arch, and a strong medial counter prevents medial rollover. A Thomas heel is often used to provide additional support for the arch.

Calcaneovalgus is a congenital positional deformity. The heel is in severe valgus, and the foot is dorsiflexed so much that it rests against the anterolateral aspect of the tibia. Calcaneovalgus is usually secondary to intrauterine position. Most cases correct spontaneously. Treatment of the severe cases includes stretching and serial casting. A few severe cases, if left untreated, persist into adolescence as a flat foot (pes planus).

An *accessory navicular bone* is a small ossicle at the medial tuberosity of the navicular. Individuals with an accessory navicular bone often complain of pressure and discomfort when wearing shoes. Often, placement of a prefabricated arch support in the shoe lifts the arch just enough to minimize rubbing on the shoe.

Hallux valgus (bunions) is most often the consequence of rear foot valgus, leading to varus of the first metatarsal. The conservative approaches to treating this condition in children are orthotics and a comfortable shoe, with a good heel counter to maintain the heel in subtalar neutral.

Curly toes involve the congenital shortening of the flexor tendons. Treated conservatively, flexors are stretched, and a rocker-like insole is used in the shoe to support the toes in extension. Shoes need to have extra depth with plenty of room in the toe box.

Shoe prescription for these biomechanical problems of the foot and lower extremity in childhood is as valuable as a conservative corrective intervention. Overall, if a child's foot is developing normally and does not exhibit any signs of an abnormality, a soft-soled shoe is appropriate.[13,14] If some degree of abnormality exists, a more supportive, rigid shoe is indicated for toddlers. In general, the stiffer the heel counter, the more effective the intervention.

The most common prescription shoe for young children is a straight last shoe. This type of shoe is roomy enough to accommodate pads or wedges. In addition, a straight last shoe does not generate any abnormal forces against the child's foot.

Foot during Pregnancy

During pregnancy, women may experience problems in the lower extremity, including edema, leg cramps, restless legs syndrome, joint laxity, and low back pain. As a result, foot pain is a common problem in the pregnant woman.[15] One of the most important considerations for shoes for the pregnant individual is provision of maximum shock absorption. Gel-cushioned running shoes are recommended, especially if the woman continues to jog or walk for exercise. Expectant mothers are also advised to exercise on soft surfaces to prevent problems caused by repetitive pounding on unforgiving surfaces.

High-heeled shoes exaggerate the lordotic curve and are inadvisable during pregnancy. Many women possess an intuitive level of common sense when it comes to wearing comfortable shoes during pregnancy. As weight distribution shifts with advancing pregnancy, especially if edema occurs, many women choose to wear shoes with laces or a Velcro closure. Athletic and walking shoes provide good support, excellent cushioning, and a solid heel counter. If a heel is desired for special occasions, a 1-in. or lower heeled shoe should be recommended. Many comfortable and attractive low-heeled dress shoes are now manufactured so that the expectant mother need not sacrifice fashion for function. Even a low, but tiny, tapered heel can cause a women to wobble as she walks.

Many women find that their foot has "grown" during pregnancy: After having returned to prepregnancy weight and clothing, their shoes no longer fit. Measurements often reflect an increase in shoe length of one-half to a full size. The stress of extra body weight coupled with ligamentous laxity can reduce arch height, adding length to the foot. This process is a normal age-related change in foot structure, associated with wear and tear of the body over time, which is hastened during pregnancy. The hormonally induced tissue laxity of pregnancy leads to a broader forefoot as the metatarsal heads separate and the distal transverse arch flattens and to a longer foot as the longitudinal arch is less efficiently supported by soft tissue structures. For this reason, pregnant women are advised to wear a larger shoe size, with a square or deeper toe box, or both, especially if edema is also a problem.

Garbalosa and McClure[16] found that almost 80% of the general population has a forefoot varum deformity. This foot deformity displaces the center of gravity forward, which can increase stress on the back during pregnancy. Forefoot varum deformity produces instability whenever the center of gravity is moved anteriorly over the forefoot in weight bearing, forcing the foot into exaggerated pronation.[17] The net effect of the hormonal changes, pregnancy-induced forward displacement of the center of gravity, and the presence of forefoot varum is increased strain on the axial skeleton and reduced efficiency of gait. An orthotic to support the metatarsal heads and medial longitudinal arch, placed in shoes with good shock absorption ability, can help to decrease foot discomfort and prevent injury to the low back during pregnancy.

Foot in Later Life

Foot problems are one of the most common complaints of the elderly. The foot is also the most frequently neglected area of evaluation by most health care practitioners. In a study of patients who resided in a long-term care facility,

40% did not own properly fitting shoes. A subsequent survey indicated that the majority of community elders preferred to wear slippers and did not own adequate footwear.[18]

Gait disorders are a major cause of morbidity and mortality in the elderly, significantly contributing to the risk of disabling injury.[19] Gait changes, poor health, and impaired vision are the major predictors for falls.[20] Many older persons attribute their problems with walking to pain or to a sense of unsteadiness, stiffness, dizziness, numbness, weakness, or impaired proprioception.[20]

Physical therapists work with patients to maximize their functional abilities and mobility. Treating foot pain and dysfunction can be a fundamental contributor to becoming functional in ambulation. As Helfand[21] so eloquently stated, "Ambulation is many times the key or the catalyst between an individual retaining dignity and remaining in a normal living environment or being institutionalized."

Gait and foot problems in the elderly are associated with diseases that are common in later life and with the aging process itself. Examples of conditions that can compromise gait and foot function include the residuals of congenital deformities, ventricular enlargement, spinal cord diseases, joint deformities, muscle contractures, peripheral nerve injuries, peripheral vascular disease, cerebrovascular accidents, trauma, ulcers, arthritis, diabetes, inactivity, and degenerative and chronic diseases.[19] The anatomic and biomechanical considerations of podogeriatrics focus on the interrelationships of the rear foot, midfoot, and forefoot, established by osseous, muscle, and connective tissue structures. Movement of one joint influences movement of other joints in the foot and ankle. Soft tissue structures establish an interdependency of the foot and ankle to the entire lower limb. As tissues age, they become stiffer, less compliant, weaker, and more vulnerable to breakdown.

Foot contour alters with aging: The foot gets wider, and bunions and splaying occur from collapse of the transverse arch.[22] Forefoot height increases in the presence of toe deformities. Fat pads under the metatarsal joints atrophy and shift position distally, whereas the calcaneal fat pad atrophies and shifts laterally. These changes leave bony prominences that are vulnerable to breakdown. In the diabetic patient, development of Charcot's joint (neuropathic arthropathy) is a relatively painless, progressive, and degenerative destruction of the tarsometatarsal or MTP joints.[23,24] With the sensory losses that are common in diabetes, these joints are subjected to extreme stresses without the benefits of normal protective mechanisms. Capsular and ligamentous stretching, joint laxity, distention, subluxation, dislocation, cartilage fibrillation, osteochondral fragmentation, and fracture occur.[25] Hyperemia increases the blood supply, which promotes resorp-

tion of bone debris with resorption of normal bone as well. The foot often fuses in a deformed rocker bottom shape, vulnerable to pseudoarthrosis, instability, abnormal weight bearing surfaces, ulcerations, and infections.[26]

The majority of foot problems in geriatric patients can be managed with proper shoe fitting and minimal shoe modifications. The most inexpensive footwear for this patient population is running or walking shoes. These are less expensive and fit within a fixed income budget.[27] They provide good foot support and can be purchased with Velcro straps for closure if hand function or foot edema is a problem. The Thermold shoe is also a blessing for all the pathologic and structural deformities with which the elderly patient must deal.

CHOOSING APPROPRIATE FOOTWEAR AND SOCKS

A vast, and somewhat bewildering, variety of "off the shelf" footwear is available from which consumers can choose. Many shoes are designed with certain types of activities in mind. Understanding the design and construction, as well as ensuring proper fit, enhances foot health and minimizes the risk of foot dysfunction, injury, and pain.

Athletic Shoe Gear

Many people jump into fitness activities "feet first" and develop blisters, calluses, and other foot injuries because of inappropriate footwear. A well-fit, activity-appropriate athletic shoe enhances enjoyment of the activity by protecting and supporting the foot and minimizing injury. Athletic shoes are designed for specific activities. A running shoe is designed with a high-force heel impact and forward foot movement in mind; the various shoe models have specific features that are designed for different surface conditions and distances in running. Basketball shoes do not provide as much cushioning as do running shoes but instead focus on foot support during quick lateral movement. Aerobic shoes are also designed for lateral movement but provide more cushioning for the impact anticipated on the ball of the foot. Shoe soles are also designed for the surface on which the activity is performed. Some shoes are manufactured as cross-training shoes so that they can go from the workout in the gym to jogging but are not designed for high-mileage runners.

Determining the foot type is important in prescribing the best shoe. For individuals with a flat low-arched foot, a shoe that provides maximum stability to prevent the foot from rolling in with each step is required. High-arched feet demand a shoe that is more flexible. "Normal" feet do best in a shoe that combines the last to accommodate the heel and the forefoot and that has forefoot flexibility. The size and shape of the toe box must also be considered: Enough room should be available in the toe box to prevent blisters, ulcers, and chafing of the toes. Shoes made from materials that "breathe" so that perspiration can escape are desirable. Athletic shoes are best used only for their intended activity and should be replaced at regular intervals to maximize their effectiveness.

Most athletic footwear is available in medium widths. A few manufacturers provide shoes in several widths. Children's athletic footwear is available in narrow, medium, and wide widths. Women's athletic footwear is available in AA, B, and D widths. Men's athletic footwear is available in B, D, EE, and EEE widths. The key element in proper fit of athletic shoes is comfort from the moment the shoe is put on, with no break-in period needed. The shoe should also provide adequate support and shock absorption for the sport or activity that is being pursued.

Walking Shoes

A well-designed walking shoe provides stable hind foot control, ample forefoot room, and a shock absorption heel and sole. This type of footwear may be specifically designed by an athletic footwear manufacturer or even by an orthopedic footwear manufacturer. Walking shoes are available in a variety of widths and in several different lasts. Long medial counters, Thomas heels, and crepe soles can be used to modify this type of shoe gear to meet specific patient needs.

Dress Shoes

Despite the fashionable preference for shoes with narrow or pointed toes and slim high heels, the most foot-friendly dress shoe for women is a rounded-toe Mary Jane style with boxy heels. A good dress shoe approximates the shape of the individual's foot and provides flexibility and sufficient shock absorption. Prerequisites of a good dress shoe include a roomy toe box, low stable heel, proper width in the ball of the foot area, flexible outsole with skid-proof bottoms, and arch support.[28]

Triangular toe boxes and high heels, no matter how dainty, are best avoided because they can and do cause deformity. For a high-heeled shoe to stay on the foot, it must fit closely around the toes, resulting in no room for anything but the foot. The foot is virtually unsupported at the distal end of the shank, and extreme high pressure is present under the metatarsal heads. Heels higher than 2 in. make any kind of orthosis ineffectual.[29] Because the angle of the foot causes the heel of the orthosis to lift up, high heels transform an orthotic into a catapult.

Although orthoses can help to relieve metatarsal and heel pain and provide arch support, they do not offer any corrective features in a shoe that is designed so unnaturally for the human foot.[10]

Socks

The sock is often overlooked when shoes of any kind are prescribed. Socks can aid in shock absorption, shield the skin from abrasion by the shoe stitching and lining, and prevent skin irritation from shoe dyes and synthetic leather materials. Additionally, clean, freshly laundered socks are integral to a sanitary foot environment. Unbleached, white cotton socks are ideal because they lack dyes, are hypoallergenic, and absorb perspiration readily. Cotton socks also provide ample toe room, unlike socks that are made from stretchable fabric, which often crowds the toes.

The size and style of socks also influence foot health. Socks that are too short crowd the toes; those that are too long wrinkle within the shoe, creating potential shear pressure points. If knee-high socks are worn, the proximal band must not be unduly restrictive; similarly, the use of circumferential garters to hold socks can impede circulation to the foot. Any holes worn into the sock also potentially create shear pressures and should be discarded. Mended holes in socks, because of the difference in thickness and materials, can irritate delicate skin. An open hole at the toes pinches and constricts the digits, with excessive friction at the edges of the hole.

The Thor-lo (Thor-lo Inc., Statesville, NC) sock is specially designed to support and cushion the insensitive foot or athletic/military foot that is exposed to repetitive frictional forces. Use of these specially designed socks not only reduces the frictional shearing forces but also significantly decreases vertical ground reaction pressure forces, preventing blistering and ulceration.[30–35] Extra high-density padding functions as a natural fat pad, reducing the deteriorating effects of shearing forces and the pressure and friction in the toe area. The Thor-lo concept of stockings is beneficial for patients with insensitive feet. It has also been used for individuals involved in aerobic exercise, baseball, basketball, cycling, golf, hiking, trekking and climbing, skiing, tennis, walking, and running.

PRESCRIPTION FOOTWEAR, CUSTOM-MOLDED SHOES, AND SHOE MODIFICATIONS

Alteration of foot function and alignment can be accomplished with foot orthoses of the appropriate materials, prescription shoes, and/or shoe modifications. These modalities are used to relieve pain and improve balance and function during standing and locomotion. These alternatives are indicated when a transfer of forces from sensitive to tolerant areas is needed to reduce friction, shock, and shear forces; to modify weight transfer patterns; to correct flexible foot deformities; to accommodate for fixed foot deformities; and to limit motion in painful, inflamed, or unstable joints.

When special protective or prescription footwear is being considered, the functional objectives must be clearly stated so that the appropriate specific prescription can be developed. Careful examination of the foot helps the clinician to identify pathology or mechanical factors, or both, that need to be addressed and to choose the appropriate materials and footwear styles to meet the patient's specific needs.

Moldable Leathers

Thermold is an example of prescription footwear that can be used to protect feet that are vulnerable due to vascular insufficiency, neuropathy, or deformity (Figure 7-5). It is a cross-linked, closed cell polyethylene foam laminated to the leather upper of the footwear that can be heat molded directly to the foot. This makes modification for foot deformity easily managed and far less expensive than custom molding. Thermold shoes are also available in extra depth styles, with a removable ¼-in. insole. Extra depth shoes enable adequate room for custom-made insoles or orthoses to become an intricate adjunct to the footwear. In some instances, the Thermolds can be used as an alternative to the custom-molded footwear.

Custom-Molded Shoes

Some foot problems cannot be accommodated in conventional footwear, and the best solution is custom-molded footwear. This footwear is molded directly over a plaster reproduction of the foot rather than over a standard last. Special modifications, such as toe fillers, Plastazote (Zoteforms, Inc., Hacketstown, NJ), rocker bars, and elevations, can be added during manufacturing to meet the specific requirements of each foot. Because of this process, custom-molded shoes are made to conform to the foot shape in all respects (Figure 7-6). Custom orthopedic shoes represent the ultimate combination of function and aesthetics. Incorporating biomechanics and craftsmanship, shoes can redistribute weight, restrict joint motion, facilitate ambulation, and decrease the probability of neuropathic ulceration.[36]

Plastazote Shoe or Sandal

For patients with insensitive or ulcerated feet, or both, a "healing sandal" or Plastazote shoe is often prescribed. This custom shoe is fabricated using a plaster cast of the individual's foot for construction.[37] Temporary protective footwear, such as a Plastazote boot or shoe or a healing sandal, is often used during neuropathic ulcer wound healing to allow for ambulation without pressure on the healing area, especially for patients who are unable to walk or noncompliant with non–weight-bearing ambulation.

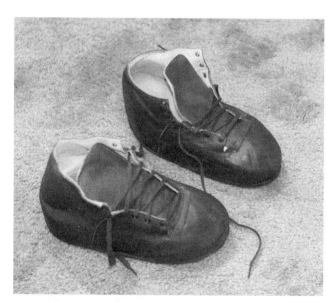

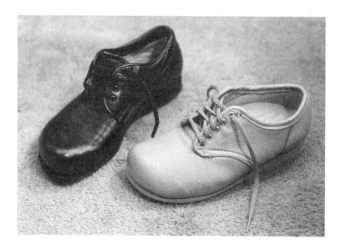

FIGURE 7-5
Thermold shoes (P. W. Minor Shoes, Batavia, NY). These shoes allow for easy modification to accommodate foot deformities.

FIGURE 7-6
Examples of custom-molded shoes. These shoes are prescribed when foot deformities are too severe for accommodation in a conventional shoe.

Shoe Modifications

A variety of shoe modifications can be used to address functional and anatomic deformities of the foot and leg. Clearly stated objectives, based on careful evaluation, ensure that the appropriate shoe modifications are chosen.

Lifts for Leg Length Discrepancy

For patients with leg length discrepancy of ⅜ in. or more, a full-length external lift can be mounted to the sole of the shoe on the shorter limb to equalize leg length and reduce proximal stresses at the hips and spine. If the length difference is less than ⅜ in., the discrepancy can usually be accommodated with an orthotic heel wedge worn inside the shoe. If the discrepancy is a result of a unilateral equinus deformity, a heel wedge can be attached to the external surface of the shoe. Leg length discrepancy is a common result of a hip fracture, congenital anomaly, or biomechanical imbalance such as pelvic rotation, hip anteversion or retroversion, or unilateral foot pronation. The level of the pelvis and absolute and relative measures of leg length should be part of a a comprehensive gait evaluation.

Heel Wedging

Wedging is used to alter lines of stress to facilitate a more normal gait pattern. The most effective wedges range from ⅛ in. to ¼ in. in thickness at their apex. Larger wedges tend to cause the foot to slide away from the wedge toward the opposite side of the shoe, drastically reducing the effectiveness of the modification. Wedging is useful for children with a rotational problem, such as tibial torsion. In adults, wedges are used for accommodation in conditions such as a fixed valgus deformity of the calcaneus (Figure 7-7).

A medial heel wedge is used when flexible valgus of the calcaneus is present (Figure 7-8A). As the wedge elevates the medial heel, a resultant varus tilt acts on the calcaneus, preventing excessive pronation of the foot. A lateral heel wedge is used when flexible varus of the calcaneus is present (Figure 7-8B). Elevation of the lateral heel

decreases the medial drive on floor contact at heel strike, tipping the calcaneus into valgus. A full heel wedge is sometimes used in the presence of fixed or functional equinus deformity. The goal of wedging is to obtain a subtalar neutral position during the stance phase of gait.

Sole Wedging

Wedging can also be used to modify midfoot and forefoot position. A medial sole wedge produces an inversion effect on the forefoot. This wedge is positioned along the medial aspect of the footwear, from a point just proximal of the first metatarsal head to the midline of the footwear (Figure 7-8C). Conversely, a lateral sole wedge creates an eversion effect at the forefoot. This wedge is placed proximal to the fifth metatarsal head to the midline of the footwear. The apex of this wedge is the fifth metatarsal head (Figure 7-8D).

A Barton wedge (Figure 7-8E) is used in the presence of severe, flexible pronation deformities, such as those seen in pes planus, when control of the midfoot is the goal. The Barton wedge, usually made with ³⁄₁₆-in. leather, extends along the medial side of the foot to the midtarsal joint and tapers laterally just anterior to the cuboid bone. It provides support to the navicular and helps to invert the calcaneus. It is used when it is necessary to shift body weight laterally. When a Barton wedge is used, the shoe must have a firm medial counter. The Barton wedge can be incorporated in an internally placed lateral heel wedge for patients with fixed calcaneal varus or clubfoot deformity. Because an internal wedge is closer to the target deformity, it creates a positive force of greater magnitude than is possible with the external Barton wedge: Instead of tilting the footgear, the wedge tilts the calcaneus into the desired position.

Steel Spring

The steel spring, an external shoe modification, is a piece of flexible metal that is ¹⁄₁₆ in. in depth and 1 in. in width, extending along the length of the footwear. It is usually placed between the insole and outsole of the shoe to restrict flexion of the sole. The need to enhance the strength of the shoe shank is often required to control the foot when lower extremity bracing is necessary. A steel spring is frequently helpful in assisting an individual who has hemiplegia with forward propulsion during the vertical pathway of the foot, from initial contact through midstance and into push off/terminal stance.

Metatarsal Bars and Rocker Bottoms

A metatarsal bar is a block of material (usually stacked pieces of leather or rubber) that is attached to the sole of the shoe. Its placement proximal to the metatarsal heads

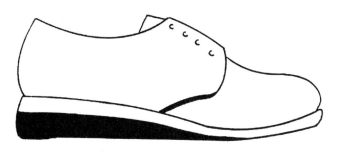

FIGURE 7-7
A heel wedge provides elevation of the heel for equinus deformity.

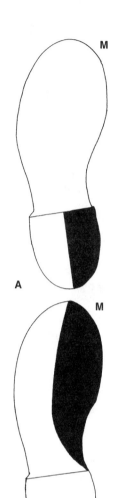

A

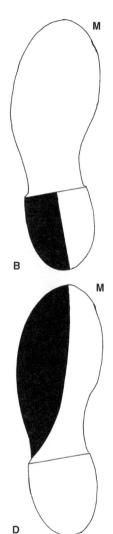

B

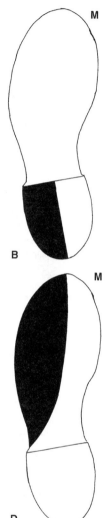

C

D

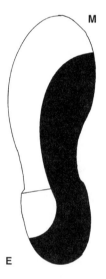

E

FIGURE 7-8

*Examples of heel and sole wedge modifications. A medial (M) heel wedge (**A**) is used when flexible valgus of the calcaneus is present; a lateral heel wedge (**B**) is used for flexible varus of the calcaneus. Medial sole wedges (**C**) create an inversion effect of the forefoot, whereas lateral sole wedges (**D**) create an eversion effect. A Barton wedge (**E**) supports the navicular bone and helps invert the calcaneus, shifting the body weight laterally.*

significantly reduces pressure at the metatarsal heads during the push-off phase of the gait cycle. The curved distal edge of the metatarsal bar is designed to follow the curve of the metatarsal heads. It is commonly used to adapt shoes worn by patients with transmetatarsal amputations, fixed arthritic deformities, diabetes, forefoot deformities such as hallux rigidus, and neuromas. The placement of a metatarsal bar or rocker facilitates push-off by simulating forward propulsion in the absence of metatarsal flexibility.

Rocker bottoms are made of either lightweight crepe or leather (Figure 7-9). These modifications are flush with the heel and toe, in an arch with an apex of ½–⅝ in. The rocker bar redistributes body forces over the entire plantar surface of the foot while in weight bearing. It facilitates a smooth roll during the stance phase of gait, while reducing sheer stress and trauma to the mid- and forefoot. It is often used to modify shoes worn by patients with par-

tial foot amputations, arthritis, and diabetes. It is also used for patients who have any lower extremity orthotic that limits forward progression of the tibia over the foot and toes during mid- and late stance phase. For patients with diabetes, a rigid rocker sole (a steel spring heel to toe with the toes extended and a rocking axis near the center of the foot) can be used to help distribute body weight and compel knee flexion at toe-off, reducing the length of stride and sheer stress on the metatarsal heads.

Thomas Heels

The Thomas heel is designed to improve foot balance and to relieve excessive pressure on the shank portion of the footwear. Applied as either a lateral or a medial flare of the heel, its goal is to increase stability during gait by assimilating subtalar neutral. A laterally flared heel is used with a rear foot varus to decrease the incidence of inversion injuries.

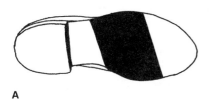
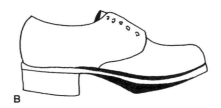
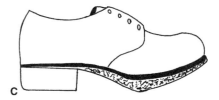

FIGURE 7-9

*Examples of rocker bottom soles. A metatarsal bar (**A**) prevents undue pressure at the metatarsal heads during push-off in late stance. A rigid leather rocker sole (**B**) or an extended crepe rocker bar (**C**) redistributes body weight over the entire plantar surface, facilitating a smoother and more normal gait pattern while reducing stress and trauma in the forefoot.*

A medially flared heel is used with a rear foot valgus to decrease the incidence of eversion injuries (Figure 7-10). For instance, a medial flare from the heel to the sustentaculum tali prevents excessive pronation of the foot during gait.

Offset Heels and Shoe Counters

The offset heel is a modification used to help correct valgus or varus deformities. It offers a broad support base, especially at the superior surface of the heel, where the broad buildup against the shoe's counter provides reinforcement either medially or laterally. A heel counter is an extension along the medial or lateral borders of the shoe from the heel to the proximal border of the fifth or the first metatarsal head. This shoe modification strengthens the shank portion of the footwear for better control of the hind foot. The heel counter is often used in combination with the appropriate Thomas heel. A counter can also be placed medially or laterally in the midfoot region. A patient whose gait exhibits excessive pronation, such as is common in rheumatoid arthritis, may require a firm medial counter to prevent the shoe from collapsing medially and to assist in realigning the foot into a neutral position.

Brace Attachments

For some patients with neuromuscular dysfunction (e.g., hemiplegia, paraplegia, or multiple sclerosis), a traditional, metal, double-upright lower extremity brace can be prescribed. If it is, the shoe must be modified: A U-shaped brace bracket (stirrup) is attached to the shoe by means of three copper rivets, one on the heel and two in the shank. The metal is riveted through the outsole to the insole. To accomplish this, the heel is removed and the plate of the brace is attached. The groove is then cut through the heel, and the heel is reattached. The appropriate orthotic ankle joint is then attached to uprights of the stirrup.

Shoe Stretching

Shoes with leather uppers can be stretched almost one full width. Although a shoe cannot be truly lengthened, it can be made to feel longer with a toe box stretcher device that

looks like the shape of the foot and is inserted into the shoe to expand it (Figure 7-11). After the leather is moistened or softened, this device effectively raises and slightly rounds the toe box. Frequently, the pressure of a flat toe box on the toes is more problematic than the length of the shoe. Specific points in the shoe can be softened and expanded by placing an "expansion knob" on the toe-box stretcher or using a ball-and-socket device. Site-specific stretching is particularly helpful for patients with toe deformities such as hallux valgus, hammertoe, mallet toe, claw toe, overlapping toes, and Taylor bunion deformity.

Blowout Patches and Gussets

Patients with foot deformities who prefer conventional shoes to Thermold shoes may find temporary pain relief if a blowout patch or gusset is applied to their shoe. The shoe leather around the area of deformity is cut away and replaced with a softer blowout patch or gusset of moleskin, soft leather, or suede.

FOOTWEAR IN THE CONSERVATIVE MANAGEMENT OF COMMON FOOT DEFORMITIES AND PROBLEMS

Conservative management of common forefoot, midfoot, and rear foot deformities often involves modification of shoes or prescription footwear, or both. Specific footwear strategies that are useful for several common foot problems are described in the following section.

Problems in the Forefoot

The most common footwear variation used for abnormalities in the forefoot is a high toe box. High toe boxes are available in a variety of footgear, including athletic sneakers, comfort shoes, Thermolds, and prescription footwear. To accommodate forefoot deformity optimally, the maximum height of the abnormal toes must be measured in a weight-bearing position. Tables of manufac-

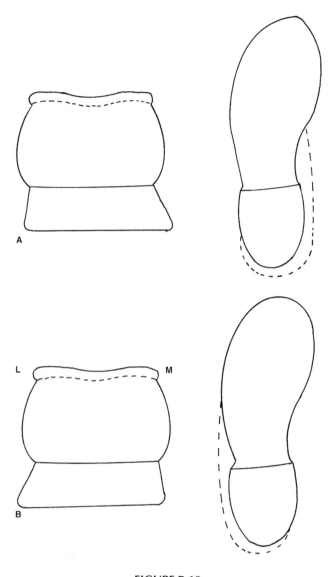

FIGURE 7-10
Examples of Thomas heels. (A) A medial (M) flared heel pro-vides a broader base of support and prevents eversion of the ankle. (B) A lateral (L) flared heel prevents inversion of the ankle.

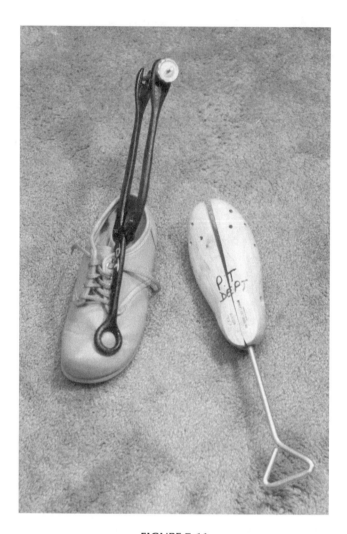

FIGURE 7-11
Tools that are used to stretch leather shoes. Stretching often pro-vides adequate accommodation for deformities in conventional shoes. The toe box stretcher (right) can increase width by one size. The ball-and-socket device (left) is used to stretch specific points that correspond to the forefoot and toe deformity.

tured shoes by toe box space are available that can guide the clinician in recommending shoes that most closely match patient needs.[38]

Metatarsalgia

Metatarsalgia is pain around the metatarsal heads that results from compression of the plantar digital nerve as it courses between the metatarsal heads. Excessive weight bearing with atrophy of the metatarsal fat pad can result in irritation of the nerves and potentially lead to devel-opment of a neuroma. The three major objectives in shoe prescription for patients with metatarsalgia are (1) to trans-fer pressure from painful sensitive areas to more pressure-tolerant areas, (2) to reduce friction by stabilizing the MTP joint, and (3) to stabilize the rear foot and midfoot to reduce pressure on the metatarsal heads. Characteristics of the shoe of choice include wide width to reduce pres-sure on the transverse metatarsal arch, long fitting to elim-inate plantar flexed MTP joints, cushion soles to enhance shock absorption, and a high toe box to allow forefoot flexion and extension. Additionally, the shoe should include a long medial counter to stabilize the rear foot, a lower heel to minimize pressure at the metatarsal heads, and preferably thermoldable leather to accommodate deformities. Shoe modifications often include a transverse metatarsal bar to redistribute pressure from metatarsal heads to metatarsal shafts and shorten stride and a rocker sole to reduce motion of painful joints.

Sesamoiditis

Sesamoiditis is an inflammation around the sesamoid bones under the first metatarsal head. It often results from a loss of soft tissue padding under the first metatarsal head and from toe deformities such as hallux valgus and hallux rigidus. The objective of shoe prescription for patients with sesamoiditis is to redistribute weight-bearing forces from the first MTP joint and its sesamoids to the long medial arch and shafts of the lesser metatarsals. A transverse metatarsal bar is used to redistribute pressure from metatarsal heads to metatarsal shafts and to shorten stride. A rocker sole can be used to reduce motion of the painful hallux joint.

Morton's Syndrome

With repetitive irritation of the plantar digital nerve between the first and second metatarsal heads, a neuroma is likely to develop. This condition is known as *Morton's syndrome*. The three major objectives in shoe prescription for patients with Morton's syndrome are (1) to redistribute weight from the lesser metatarsals (especially the second and third) to the proximal phalanx of the hallux, (2) to stabilize the rear foot by maintaining subtalar joint neutral, and (3) to accommodate forefoot varus or a dorsiflexed first metatarsal, or both. Shoe prescription includes a long medial counter for rear foot support and stability; a straight or flared last to accommodate foot shape; a high, wide toe box to reduce compression across the transverse metatarsal arch; a large enough shoe size to accommodate the long second toe; and a Thomas heel or wedge sole to support the medial longitudinal arch. A medial heel and medial sole wedge may be necessary when symptoms are severe.

Morton's (Interdigital) Neuroma

Overstretching of the digital nerves in extreme toe extension at the proximal phalanx can also result in the development of a neuroma. Two objectives should be considered for patients with Morton's neuroma. First, the patient must obtain relief from the pain and burning, especially in the third interspace of the MTP joint. Second, compression of the digital nerve as it passes between the heads of the third and fourth metatarsals needs to be reduced. To achieve these goals, the shoe should be wide enough to eliminate transverse compression and have enough length to reduce plantar flexion of the MTP joints. A long medial counter can help to reduce pronation; a cushioned sole increases shock absorption, and a low heel unloads pressure on the metatarsals. Elastic laces may be helpful in allowing expansion of the forefoot. Shoe modifications for Morton's neuroma might include a metatarsal bar to elevate the metatarsals and redistribute weight or a metatarsal rocker bar to immobilize the metatarsals, or both.

Metatarsalgia of the Fifth Metatarsophalangeal Joint

Like the metatarsalgia described previously, metatarsalgia of the fifth MTP joint results in plantar digital nerve irritation at the interdigital space of the fourth and fifth metatarsal heads. When metatarsalgia of the fifth MTP joint is present, the goals of intervention are to redistribute weight forces to the fifth metatarsal shaft and to provide a broad base of support along the lateral border of the foot. The optimal shoe has a last with enough lateral flare to accommodate the lateral aspect of the foot and fifth metatarsal shaft, a firm lateral counter, and a firm leather or rubber sole. Possible shoe modifications include a lateral heel and sole flare ending proximal to the fifth metatarsal head to provide a broader base of support. Lateral heel and sole wedges may be useful for patients with a flexible foot.

Hallux Rigidus (Limitus)

Degenerative joint disease of the first MTP joint causes pain, loss of mobility, and eventually fusion of the joint. Osteophyte formation on the dorsal aspects of the metatarsal head and base of the proximal phalanx can be quite painful and result in a loss of extension. For patients with hallux rigidus or limitus, the goals are to limit motion of the hallux and first MTP joint and to reduce pressure on the dorsal and plantar aspects of the hallux and first MTP joint. To accomplish this, the shoe should have a high and wide toe box and Thermold or soft leather uppers. When significant deformity is present, a steel shank from heel to phalanx of the hallux and a rigid rocker sole with compensating heel elevation may be necessary.

Hallux Valgus (Bunions)

A prominent bony formation on the medial aspect of the first MTP joint can result from lateral deviation of the hallux and from foot pronation. This deformity is often associated with long-term wearing of shoes with a triangular toe box. Five objectives should be considered in the prescription of shoes for patients with hallux valgus:

(1) to reduce friction and pressure to the first MTP joint, (2) to eliminate abnormal pressure from narrow-fitting shoes, (3) to reduce pronation of the foot from heel strike to midstance, (4) to correct eversion, and (5) to relieve posterior tibial tendon and ligamentous strain. Patients with hallux valgus benefit from shoes with high, wide toe boxes and Thermold or soft leather uppers. A combined last with increased last width in the toe box and a smaller heel for better control of the subtalar joint may also be indicated. Additionally, the choice of a shoe that is longer and wider helps to accommodate deformity; a lower heel to reduce forefoot pressure and a reinforced medial counter help to prevent pronation.

Hammertoes, Claw Toes, and Mallet Toes

Hammertoe deformity is characterized by hyperextension of the MTP joint, flexion of the proximal interphalangeal (PIP) joint, and extension of the distal interphalangeal (DIP) joint. This results in high load during weight bearing at the plantar metatarsal heads and at the plantar surface of the distal phalanx. Claw toe deformity features hyperflexion of the PIP and DIP joints, although the MTP joint can be hyperextended or hyperflexed. Mallet toe deformity results from hyperextension of the MTP joint, flexion of the PIP, and a neutral position of the DIP, so that weight bearing is on the tip of the distal phalanx. Deformities of the lesser toes can be problematic, especially for patients with compromised circulation and neuropathy. For these individuals, there are two major goals: (1) to transfer pressure away from the metatarsal heads, the PIP joints, and the distal phalanx joints, and (2) to encourage flexion of the MTP joints and extension of the PIP joints. Patients with lesser toe deformities should wear shoes with a high, wide toe box made of Thermold or soft leather to reduce the likelihood of microtrauma over the bony prominences. The shoe should also be long enough to allow flexion of MTP joints and extension of PIP joints rather than cramping the toes. Finally, a soft cushion outsole and low heel further reduce pressure on the metatarsal heads. Commonly used shoe modifications for lesser toe deformities include metatarsal bars to reduce pressure to metatarsal heads and shift weight bearing to metatarsal shafts and a rocker bar or rocker sole to accommodate rollover on fixed deformity.

Problems in the Midfoot

Shoe prescription or modifications, or both, are also helpful in management of midfoot dysfunction and deformity. The most commonly encountered problems include pes planus (flatfoot), pes equinus, pes cavus, and plantar fascitis.

Pes Planus

Pes planus is pronation of the midfoot that results in a failure of the foot to supinate during midstance. The longitudinal arch flattens, causing a splaying of the forefoot and lateral deviation of the metatarsals. This deformity can be either flexible or fixed (rigid).

For patients with a flexible pes planus, the goals of intervention are to reduce pronation from heel strike to midstance, to correct eversion, to relieve tension on the posterior tibial tendonitis, and to relieve ligamentous strain. To do these things, the shoe should offer a long medial heel counter, a Thomas heel (medial extension) or a firm wedge sole, and a straight last. A custom shoe is recommended for severe cases. Shoe modifications may include a medial heel wedge to correct eversion and reduce pronation or a medial heel and sole flare in extreme cases.

Because of the fixed nature of a rigid pes planus, the goals are somewhat different: to relieve ligamentous strain, to relieve arch pain, and to correct eversion of the foot. The optimal shoe should offer a broad shank (extra wide midfoot), a straight last, and a long medial counter. Additionally, a wedge sole is applied to reduce the load on the metatarsal heads, to stabilize the intertarsal joint, and to provide a dorsiflexion assist.

Pes Equinus

In pes equinus, the plantar flexor muscles and Achilles tendon are tightened, which limits dorsiflexion of the ankle and results in a plantar flexion deformity. For patients with a flexible pes equinus, the footwear prescribed attempts to reduce ankle plantar flexion, reduce the load on the metatarsal heads, and stabilize the subtalar joint. This can be accomplished in a shoe with a low heel. A rocker bottom can be applied to the sole to provide a dorsiflexion assist and further reduce load on the metatarsal heads.

When the pes equinus deformity is rigid or fixed, the goals of footwear intervention change. Instead of trying to reduce plantar flexion, a posterior platform supports the rear foot from heel strike to midstance and mimics the dorsiflexion needed at toe-off. It is important to contain the entire foot in the shoe, reducing the load on the metatarsal heads. For patients with unilateral deformity, it is also important to equalize the relative leg length difference between the normal and the equinus foot through all phases of gait. Shoe prescription for patients with a fixed equinus deformity includes a Cuban (elevated) heel to provide a platform and deep quarter or high-top shoes. If modifications are necessary, they might include posterior heel elevation on the equinus side, as well as on the contralateral limb, to facilitate swing of the involved limb and reduce pelvic obliquity.

Pes Cavus

Pes cavus is an exaggerated longitudinal arch. It can lead to a plantar flexed forefoot with retraction of the toes and severe weight-bearing stresses on the metatarsal heads and heel. Patients with pes cavus benefit from shoes that provide a broad platform for stability; reduce loading at the heels, lateral borders, and metatarsal heads; and accommodate the deformed foot within the shoe. The shoe should also have a firm heel counter to maintain rear foot stability and a modified curved last to accommodate foot shape. Custom-molded shoes are recommended in severe cases. Possible shoe modifications for patients with pes cavus include a lateral flare to provide a platform for greater stability, a cushion sole to absorb shock on the heel and metatarsal heads, and a metatarsal bar to shift weight from the metatarsal heads.

Plantar Fascitis

Plantar fascitis is inflammation of the plantar fascia at its insertion to the medial aspect of the calcaneus. This inflammatory process can lead to the development of calcification at that insertion, commonly referred to as a *heel spur*. Plantar fascitis is often a consequence of loss of the longitudinal arch in conditions such as pes planus or of undo stresses created in the forefoot with tightness of the gastrocnemius and soleus muscles or an elevated longitudinal arch. To reduce the painful signs and symptoms of plantar fascitis, the goals of intervention are to transfer weight-bearing pressure from painful to more tolerant areas, to reduce tension on the plantar fascia and Achilles tendon, to control pronation from heel strike to midstance, and to maintain the subtalar joint in a neutral position. The shoe prescribed for plantar fascitis has a long medial heel counter to limit heel valgus, a high heel to reduce tension on the plantar fascia and Achilles tendon, and adequate length to minimize compression and promote supination from midstance to toe-off. The type of shoe modifications that may be useful include a posterior heel elevation to reduce tension on the plantar fascia and Achilles tendon.

Problems in the Rear Foot

The most common dysfunctions and deformities of the rear foot that can be addressed by footwear prescription or modification include arthrodesis, Achilles tendonitis or bursitis, and Haglund's deformity (pump bump).

Arthrodesis

Arthrodesis is a loss of mobility at the ankle mortise, the junction of the talus with the tibia and fibula. This deformity prevents motion at the ankle in all planes. When arthrodesis of the ankle is present, the major objectives are to provide effective shock absorption at heel strike, to improve comfort and efficiency of push-off, and to accommodate any shortening or residual equinus. Shoes that address the problems of arthrodesis have a reinforced counter and may have a medial or a lateral flared heel, or both, to provide greater stability. Some patients benefit from a high-top shoe as well. Modifications that protect the foot and facilitate a more normal gait pattern include application of a cushioned heel to absorb shock and simulate plantar flexion after heel strike and a rocker sole to mimic the dorsiflexion needed in late stance phase.

Achilles Tendonitis, Bursitis, and Haglund's Deformity

Undo stresses of the Achilles tendon, direct pressure of a too-short shoe, and/or tightness of the gastrocnemius and soleus muscles can result in tendonitis or bursitis. Haglund's deformity is an osseous formation at the insertion of the Achilles tendon at the calcaneus. The goals of shoe prescription for patients with Achilles tendonitis, bursitis, and/or Haglund's deformity (pump bump) are similar: to reduce tension on the Achilles tendon, to provide dorsiflexion assist at heel strike and at toe-off, to reduce abnormal pronation, and to reduce pressure and friction (shear) at the insertion of the calcaneus. Patients with these problems require a slightly higher heel to reduce dorsiflexion; a long medial counter to limit subtalar motion, a longer shoe size to reduce compression pressure, and a backless shoe to prevent irritation of the pump bump. The types of shoe modifications that may be helpful include a posterior heel elevation to reduce tension on the Achilles tendon or a foam-filled posterior heel counter.

IMPORTANT DIAGNOSIS-RELATED CONSIDERATIONS IN SHOE PRESCRIPTION

Prescription footwear and shoe modifications are also extremely useful tools to protect joints, prevent skin problems, and enhance normal function of patients who are coping with arthritis and gout or diabetes and peripheral vascular disease. Adaptations to footwear may also be helpful for patients with hemiplegia, partial foot amputations, or congenital deformities.

Arthritis

Arthritis, whether degenerative, rheumatoid, or traumatic, leads to destruction of joints. In working with patients with arthritis of the foot, the goals of intervention are to prevent or limit abnormal motion, to accommodate for arthritic deformities, and to cushion impact loading and reduce microtrauma within the joint.[39] A reinforced counter can help to limit subtalar motion; a high-top design shoe can also help to limit ankle motion. Extra depth shoes may be needed to accommodate deformities of the midfoot and forefoot. Thermoldable leather is preferable if deformities need further accommodation. The application of a rocker bottom helps to improve push-off by shortening the distance between the heel and the MTP joint. It also reduces the total ankle motion required for push-off. Shock-absorbing accommodative orthotics can be placed inside the shoe, and a cushion heel can be added to absorb even more force at heel strike, as well as to limit ankle and subtalar motion. A flared heel can reduce medial/lateral movement at the subtalar joint.

Gout

For patients with gout, the treatment objectives are similar to those for patients with arthritis: preventing or limiting motion of painful or inflamed joints, accommodating foot deformities, and cushioning the impact of loading on the involved joints. A reinforced counter to limit subtalar motion or a high-top design to limit overall ankle motion should be considered. An extra depth shoe of thermoldable leather is best able to accommodate deformities without creating pain and discomfort over sensitive joints. A rocker bottom can be applied to assist push-off, prevent pedal joint movement, and reduce ankle motion required for push-off. Shock-absorbing accommodative orthotics and a cushion heel provide even more comfort and protection of inflamed joints during gait.

Diabetes

The loss of protective sensation in patients with diabetic neuropathy creates significant vulnerability to injury from repetitive microtrauma. Protection of the plantar surface of the diabetic foot from microtrauma is of paramount importance. Patients with diabetic neuropathy often have significant weakness of intrinsic muscles, and forefoot deformities such as claw toes develop, which are susceptible to breakdown in areas of excessive shoe pressures. The risk of nonhealing, infection, and subsequent amputation is quite high; prevention is the most effective treatment strategy. Total-contact full-foot orthotics using soft, shock-absorbing materials helps to distribute weight-bearing pressures over the entire plantar surface of the foot

away from the vulnerable bony prominences. A Thermold leather shoe is recommended for the insensitive diabetic foot. (See Chapter 20 for comprehensive management of vulnerable feet.)

Peripheral Vascular Disease

Because the ability to heal is compromised in patients with peripheral vascular disease, any irritation or ulceration exponentially increases the risk of infection and subsequent amputation. Here, too, prevention of skin breakdown and protection of the vulnerable foot are the primary goals. The ability to fit and protect the foot effectively is further challenged by fluctuating edema. A Thermold sandal with Velcro closure is often recommended for patients with peripheral vascular disease–related edema as a safe and effective alternative to standard shoes. If edema is not a problem, a soft Thermold shoe protects the plantar surface of the foot from repetitive pressures and accommodates deformities that are at risk for shoe pressure–related trauma. Because hypersensitivity is often a problem with circulatory pathologies in the lower extremities, a shoe that cushions the foot may be helpful. Elastic shoelaces allow expansion of the shoe for patients with minimal edema-related fluctuations in foot size.

Hemiplegia

The patient with hemiplegia after a cerebrovascular accident (stroke) may have inadequate or excessive tone of the lower extremity. Many need orthotic intervention to control the foot and ankle in some or all phases of gait, to accommodate for any fixed deformities and to cushion impact loading at initial contact. Footwear is selected to enhance orthotic function or, in some instances, to have a direct impact on mild dysfunction. A reinforced heel counter helps to limit subtalar motion and stabilize the foot on heel strike. A flared heel or high-top shoe may be recommended to enhance foot placement and stance stability. A rigid shoe shank may be required for some types of lower extremity orthoses. In the presence of an equinus deformity, a heel lift on the shoe provides total contact during weight bearing and facilitates stability. In severe deformities of the ankle, a custom-molded shoe may be the only alternative. The most common ankle-foot orthoses used in hemiplegia tend to increase shoe length, width, and depth by a half to a whole size. Often the insole can be replaced with an insert foundation, to garner a little more room for the orthosis within the shoe. Extra depth shoes are particularly helpful for patients who are faced with difficulty in donning their orthosis and shoe because of upper extremity dysfunction in hemiplegia.

Amputation and Congenital Deformity

The foot that is shortened surgically or is congenitally deformed is a management challenge because the weight-bearing surface is reduced or altered, increasing the likelihood of tissue breakdown with repeated loading in gait. The type of protective footwear used can range from an over-the-counter extra depth shoe for a mild deformity to a custom-molded shoe for a severe deformity. When the feet are of unequal size, it is more difficult to fit them without buying two pairs of shoes or having custom footwear made. If the difference between the feet is no more than one size in length, the larger size can be used with toe padding for the shorter deformed or amputated foot or with an orthosis to accommodate the deformity (Figure 7-12). Frequently, the shorter foot is also wider and would need to be accommodated by the appropriate orthosis custom molded to the shoe. A toe filler prevents the shortened foot from sliding within the shoe during gait but also increases the risk of skin breakdown. It is crucial that the first MTP joint be aligned with the "toe break" point in the shoe. If the foot falls posterior to the toe break, stress is concentrated at the distal end of the foot, increasing the chance of pressure imposition by the "filler."

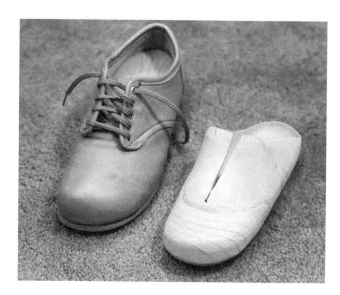

FIGURE 7-12
A toe filler can be used on a foot that has been shortened by amputation or congenital deformity.

READING THE WEAR ON SHOES

For the clinician who is faced with decisions about modifying, repairing, or replacing footwear, examination of patterns of wear and erosion provides important information. Deterioration of the shoe itself impairs tactile sensibility and position sense judgment.[40] Shoes that have outlasted their purpose often create abnormal forces and shearing that increase the risk of repetitive microtrauma to the skin and joints of the foot and ankle. Analysis of the wear and erosion of the shoe is a prescriptive tool in advising, prescribing, and modifying a shoe to fit the needs of the individual.

SUMMARY

The shoe is an essential interface between the foot and the ground that protects the foot from trauma and supports the structures of the foot as an individual walks, runs, and changes direction. Fashionable footwear, especially for women, often compromises, rather than enhances, foot function. Foot function and footwear needs have a developmental aspect as well: An understanding of how the foot changes over the life span and of the special needs of children, pregnant women, and the elderly is essential. Knowledge about the components of the shoe and their variations, the criteria for proper fitting, and the relationship between shoe design and activity-related demands is an important tool for clinical practice. Physical therapists are often called on to recommend footwear for patients with special needs. A baseline knowledge of shoe characteristics and modifications for certain types of deformities or diagnoses enhances this ability.

REFERENCES

1. Finlay OE. Footwear management in the elderly care programme. Physiotherapy 1986;72(4):171–178.
2. Fuller EA. A review of the biomechanics of shoes. Clin Podiatry Med Surg 1994;11(2):241–258.
3. Black E, Black E. Comfort shoes: the long overdue revolution. Biomechanics 1995;2(10):27–33.
4. Frey C. If the shoe fits . . . . Biomechanics 1995;2(4):26–28.
5. Frey C, Thompson F, Smith J, et al. American Orthopaedic Foot and Ankle Society Women's Shoe Survey. Foot Ankle 1993;14(2):78–81.
6. Snow RE, Williams KR. High heeled shoes: their effect on center of mass, position, posture, three-dimensional kinematics, rearfoot motion, and ground reaction forces. Arch Phys Med Rehabil 1994;75(5):568–576.
7. Janisse DJ. The art and science of fitting shoes. Foot Ankle 1992;13(5):257–262.
8. Herman HH, Bottomley JB. Anatomical and biomechanical considerations of the elder foot. Top Geriatr Rehabil 1992;7(3):1–13.

9. Frey C, Chan C, Carrasco N. Obesity: do weight gains lead to lower extremity pain? Biomechanics 1996;3(1):30–35.

10. Snow RE, Williams KR, Holmes GB Jr. The effects of wearing high heeled shoes on pedal pressure in women. Foot Ankle 1992;13(2):85–92.

11. Shapiro S. Pediatrics: a reasoned approach to common lower limb disorders. Biomechanics 1995;2(5):18–21.

12. Rao UB, Joseph B. The influence of footwear on the prevalence of flat foot: a survey of 2300 children. J Bone Joint Surg 1992;74(4):630–631.

13. Valmassy RL. Pediatric biomechanics. Podiatry Today 1989;May:86–92.

14. Valmassy RL. The use of gait plates for in-toed and out-toed deformities. Clin Podiatry Med Surg 1994;11(2):211–217.

15. Black E, Cooke Anastasi S. Pregnancy and the lower extremities. Biomechanics 1995;2(4):22–25, 68–69.

16. Garbalosa JC, McClure MH. The frontal plane relationship of the forefoot to the rearfoot in an asymptomatic population. J Sports Phys Ther 1994;20(4):200–206.

17. Rothbart BA, Hansen KH, Yerratt MK. Resolving chronic low back pain: the foot connection. Am J Podiatry Med 1995;5(3):84–90.

18. Karpman R. Geriatric prefab. Biomechanics 1995;2(5):53–58.

19. Sudarsky L, Ronthal M. Gait disorders among elderly patients. Arch Neurol 1993;40(2):740–743.

20. Hough JC, McHenry MP, Kammer LM. Gait disorders in the elderly. Assoc Prescription Footwear 1987;35(6):191–196.

21. Helfand AE. Common Foot Problems in the Aged and Rehabilitative Management. In TF Williams (ed), Rehabilitation in the Aging. New York: Raven, 1984;291–303.

22. Edelstein JE. Foot care for the aging. Phys Ther 1988;68(12):1882–1886.

23. Frykerg RG, Kozak GP. The Diabetic Charcot Foot. In Kozak GP, Hoar CS, Rowbotham JL, et al. (eds), Management of Diabetic Foot Problems. Philadelphia: Saunders, 1984;103–112.

24. Frykerg RG. Podiatric Problems in Diabetes. In Kozak GP, Hoar CS, Rowbotham JL, et al. (eds), Management of Diabetic Foot Problems. Philadelphia: Saunders, 1984;45–67.

25. Gramuglia VJ, Palmarozzo PM, Rzonca EC. Biomechanical concepts in the treatment of ulcers in the diabetic foot. Clin Podiatry Med Surg 1988;5(3):613–626.

26. Bailey TS, Yu HM, Rayfield EJ. Patterns of foot examination in a diabetes clinic. Am J Med 1985;78(3):371–374.

27. Bottomley JB, Herman H. Making simple, inexpensive changes for the management of foot problems in the aged. Top Geriatr Rehabil 1992;7(3):62–77.

28. Seale KS. Women and their shoes: unrealistic expectations? Instructional Course Lectures, American College of Podiatry, Oct 1995;44:379–384.

29. Corrigan JP, Moore DP, Stephens MM. Effect of heel height on forefoot loading. Foot Ankle 1993;14(3):148–152.

30. Herring KM, Richie DH. Friction blisters and sock fiber composition: a double-blind study. J Am Podiatry Med Assoc 1990;80(2):3–7.

31. Richie DH, Herring KM. Friction Blisters and Sock Construction. Presented at the annual meeting of the American Academy of Podiatric Sports Medicine, Miami, FL, May 29, 1990.

32. Herring KM, Richie DH. Friction Blisters and Sock Fiber Composition: A Single-Blind Study. Part 2. Presented at 75th annual meeting of the American Podiatric Medical Association, Las Vegas, NV, August 15, 1990.

33. Murray HJ, Veves A, Young MJ, et al. Role of experimental socks in the care of the high-risk diabetic foot. Diabetes Care 1993;16(8):1190–1192.

34. Veves A, Masson E, Fernando D, Boulton AJM. Use of experimental padded hosiery to reduce abnormal foot pressures in diabetic neuropathy. Diabetes Care 1989;12(9):16–19.

35. Veves A, Masson E, Fernando D, Boulton AJM. Studies of experimental hosiery in diabetic neuropathic patients with high foot pressures. Diabetic Med 1990;7(3):324–326.

36. White J. Custom shoe therapy. Current concepts, designs, and special considerations. Clin Podiatry Med Surg 1994;11(2):259–270.

37. Breuer U. Diabetic patient's compliance with bespoke footwear after healing of neuropathic foot ulcers. Diabete Metab 1994;20(4):415–419.

38. Kaye RA. The extra-depth toe box: a rational approach. Foot Ankle Int 1994;15(3):146–150.

39. Michelson J, Easley M, Wigley FM, Hellmann D. Foot and ankle problems in rheumatoid arthritis. Foot Ankle Int 1994;15(11):608–613.

40. Robbins S, Waked E, McClaran J. Proprioception and stability: foot position awareness as a function of age and footwear. Age Ageing 1995;24(1):67–72.

8

Functional Foot Orthoses

ROBERTA NOLE AND JUAN C. GARBALOSA

HISTORY OF THE FUNCTIONAL FOOT ORTHOSIS

The use of foot orthoses as an effective treatment tool for biomechanical dysfunction of the feet developed throughout the twentieth century. Early on, the goal of orthotic management was to redistribute plantar foot forces to alleviate discomfort in pressure-sensitive areas. Little consideration was given to the specific foot abnormality that led to the pathology.[1] Researchers in the early 1900s began fabricating metal foot braces in an attempt to control motion at specific joints of the foot and prevent pathology.[2] These devices, although functional, were often not well tolerated by the patient because of the rigidity of the materials and the lack of attention given to the brace design. In 1948, Schreber and Weineman first identified forefoot invertus (varus) and evertus (valgus) as primary foot deformities that required correction by an orthosis.[3] In the 1960s, Dr. Merton Root developed neutral impression casting techniques, positive cast modifications, and posting (mechanical correction) techniques. The standards that he established have enhanced orthotic comfort and function.[3] During the past few years, the use of functional foot orthoses has increased considerably, as theories linking the mechanics of the foot and ankle and the etiology of musculoskeletal disorders have evolved.[4]

This chapter has six learning objectives: (1) The major anatomic structures of the foot and the basic biomechanical principles associated with these structures are presented. (2) The effects of extrinsic and intrinsic deformities and of abnormal pronation on the function of the foot during the various phases of gait are compared and contrasted. (3) The essential components of a lower extremity evaluation of intrinsic foot deformities are described. (4) Abnormal pronation and the pathologic conditions that contribute to abnormal pronation in gait are defined. (5) The components of a foot orthosis are identified, and

the general goals of orthotic intervention and the specific purposes of several common orthotic interventions are discussed. (6) Current research literature related to the efficacy of functional foot orthoses is reviewed.

FOOT STRUCTURE

The foot is a complex of bones interconnected by a series of articulations and supported by soft tissue structures. The foot complex is structurally subdivided into three functional components: the rear foot, the midfoot, and the forefoot. Several important articulations of the foot (talocrural, subtalar, midtarsal, first and fifth rays) are triplanar. The axes of rotation in triplanar joints are not perpendicular to any of the cardinal planes of the human body. Because of their alignment, motion about triplanar joints leads to simultaneous movement in all three cardinal planes of the body.[5] The amount of motion that is evident in any single plane is related to the pitch (inclination) of the triplanar axis from the respective cardinal plane.[6] Triplanar motion occurs in three-dimensional space; the breakdown of triplanar motion into its three constituent cardinal plane movements is artificial.

Because motion about a triplanar axis is three dimensional, motion in the three cardinal planes occurs simultaneously. Blocking any one component of triplanar motion, in a single cardinal plane, prevents movement in the other two planes as well. This concept, the "all or nothing rule," is the premise for orthotic posting or wedging.[5] Theoretically, the addition of a post or wedge to an orthosis blocks the frontal plane component of triplanar motion, which in turn blocks or limits the triplanar motion of pronation. An understanding of the principles of foot orthotics is based on knowledge of the functional anatomy of the foot. This section reviews the pertinent anatomic

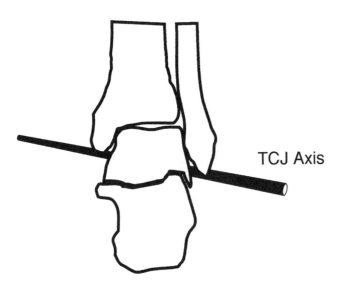

FIGURE 8-1

Posterior view of the osseous components and axis of the talocrural joint (TCJ). The osseous components of the TCJ are the tibia medially and superiorly, the fibula laterally, and the talus inferiorly. The axis of the joint passes in a posterolateral to anteromedial direction through the tips of the lateral and medial malleoli. (Used with permission from Juan C. Garbalosa, Ph.D., P.T., University of Hartford, West Hartford, CT.)

and biomechanical aspects of the components of the foot and their interconnections.

Talocrural Joint

The talocrural joint (TCJ) connects the foot to the lower leg: It is the articulation of the tibia, fibula, and talus. The TCJ has a triplanar axis of rotation. In neutral position, the TCJ axis passes through the tips of the medial and lateral malleoli, pitched 10 degrees from the transverse plane and 20–30 degrees from the frontal plane[7-10] (Figure 8-1). Although sagittal plane plantar flexion and dorsiflexion are the primary motions at this joint, the slight inclination of the TCJ axis of rotation results in concomitant transverse and frontal plane motion as well. During plantar flexion, the foot adducts and inverts; with dorsiflexion it abducts and everts.[11] Normal range of motion (ROM) of the TCJ is between 12 and 20 degrees of dorsiflexion and 50 and 56 degrees of plantar flexion.[12,13] The primary ligamentous structures stabilizing and limiting the motion that occurs at the TCJ are the medial (deltoid) and lateral collateral ligaments.[14] For a more in-depth discussion of the function of these ligaments, the reader is referred to the work of Rasmussen and Tovberg-Jevsen.[14]

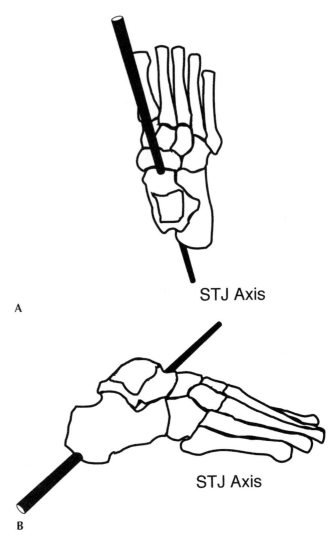

FIGURE 8-2

Superior (A) and lateral (B) views of the osseous structures in the rear foot: the superior talus and inferior calcaneus. Also pictured is the triplanar axis of the subtalar joint (STJ). Note the inclination of the axis from all three cardinal planes of the body. (Used with permission from Juan C. Garbalosa, Ph.D., P.T., University of Hartford, West Hartford, CT.)

Rear Foot

The two osseous structures of the rear foot are the calcaneus (inferior) and the talus (superior) (Figure 8-2). The articulation between the calcaneus and talus is the subtalar joint (STJ). Three joint surfaces are present in this articulation: posterior, anterior, and middle. The posterior joint surface has a concave talar and convex calcaneal portion, whereas the anterior and middle joint surfaces have convex talar and concave calcaneal arrangements. This structurally based articular geometry, along with the interosseous talocalcaneal ligament, limits the amount and type of motion at the STJ.[11,15] Other ligamentous structures that offer support to the STJ are the medial and lateral collateral and the posterior and lateral talocalcaneal ligaments.[16]

At the STJ, the triplanar axis of rotation is directed in an anterosuperior to posteroinferior direction, pitched 42 degrees from the transverse plane, 48 degrees from the frontal plane, and 16 degrees from the sagittal plane (see Figure 8-2). The location of the STJ axis in the human foot varies greatly. Manter[17] reports that the inclination from the transverse and sagittal planes varied from 29 degrees to 47 degrees and 8 degrees to 24 degrees, respectively.

The triplanar motions that occur at the STJ are supination and pronation. Supination of the weight-bearing foot leads to dorsiflexion and abduction of the talus with simultaneous inversion of the calcaneus. Pronation of the weight-bearing foot results in plantar flexion and adduction of the talus and eversion of the calcaneus.[5] Because of the variability in location of axis of rotation of the STJ, the component motions of supination and pronation vary as well. As the axis becomes more perpendicular to a particular cardinal plane, the motion occurring in that plane becomes more pronounced, whereas the other motions become less prominent.[18,19] If the axis of rotation inclined 29 degrees from the transverse plane and 8 degrees from the sagittal plane, the STJ axis would lie more perpendicular to the frontal plane. As a result, the amount of eversion and inversion seen would be greater than the amount of either abduction/adduction or plantar flexion/dorsiflexion. This variability often has an effect on coupled motion between the joints of the foot and the lower leg. During pronation and supination of the rear foot, the tibia and fibula rotate internally and externally in the transverse plane.[5,20,21] An increase in the frontal plane motion of the rear foot could cause a simultaneous increase in the transverse plane motion of the lower leg.

Midfoot

The two osseous structures of the midfoot are the cuboid and navicular bones. Two articulations between the midfoot and the rear foot (talonavicular and calcaneocuboid) form an important composite joint; the midtarsal joint (MTJ) or transverse tarsal joint (Figure 8-3). The articular surfaces of the talonavicular joint are convex-concave, whereas the surfaces of the calcaneocuboid joint are sellar shaped.[8,17] MTJ movement is supported and restricted by the bifurcate, short and long plantar, and plantar calcaneonavicular (spring) ligaments. The short and long plantar ligaments and the plantar calcaneonavicular ligaments also support the longitudinal and transverse plantar arches of the foot.[22]

Because the MTJ is a composite joint, motion occurs about two separate triplanar joint axes: a longitudinal and an oblique axis (see Figure 8-3). Functionally, movement of the forefoot about each joint axis can occur independently of the other. Manter[17] reports that the longitudinal axis was inclined superiorly 15 degrees from the transverse plane and medially 9 degrees from the sagittal plane, whereas the oblique axis was pitched superiorly 52 degrees from the transverse plane and medially 57 degrees from the sagittal plane. The predominant motion about the longitudinal axis is frontal plane inversion and eversion. Because of the slight deviation of the longitudinal axis from the three cardinal planes, insignificant amounts of adduction/abduction and of plantar flexion/dorsiflexion of the forefoot occur during inversion and eversion. Plantar flexion/dorsiflexion and abduction/adduction are the predominant movements around the oblique MTJ axis, with minimal concomitant inversion/eversion.[5,15]

These two joint axes produce the combined motion of supination and pronation of the MTJ. During supination and pronation, the forefoot inverts/everts about the longitudinal axis. The motion around the oblique axis is plantar flexion with adduction, and dorsiflexion with abduction. The amount of motion possible at the two MTJ axes depends on the position of the STJ. In STJ supination, the two joint axes are nearly perpendicular so that MTJ mobility is restricted. This mechanism helps to convert the forefoot into a rigid structure for propulsion during the push-off phase of gait.[17,23] When the STJ is pronated the joint axes are more parallel, allowing a greater degree of MTJ mobility.

Forefoot

The forefoot is comprised of all structures that are distal to the navicular and cuboid bones. It is subdivided into five rays and toes. The first through third rays consist of a cuneiform and its associated metatarsal bone. The fourth and fifth rays consist only of a metatarsal. The tarsometatarsal joints, the primary joints of the ray complexes, have two opposing planar surfaces.[5,22] The hallux, or first toe, has two bones (a proximal and distal phalanx) and two corresponding joints [metatarsophalangeal (MTP) and interphalangeal (IP)]. The lesser toes have three bones (proximal, middle, and distal phalanges) and three associated joints. The proximal articular surfaces of MTP and IP joints are convex, and the distal articular surface is concave.[5] Numerous soft tissue structures support these joints. Several excellent texts review the anatomy of the foot and ankle.[22,24,25]

Although each ray has its own axis of motion, the first and fifth rays are of particular interest. The triplanar axes of rotation of these two joints are almost perpendicular to each other. The axis of the first ray is pitched at a 45-degree angle from the sagittal and frontal planes; the primary motions possible are plantar flexion with eversion and dor-

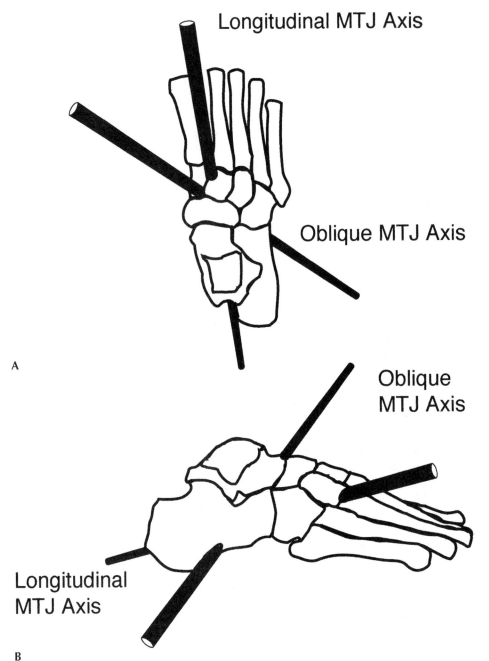

FIGURE 8-3
*A superior (**A**) and lateral (**B**)
view of the osseous components
of the midtarsal joint (MTJ).
The anterior portion of the MTJ
is comprised of the navicular
and cuboid bones, whereas the
posterior portion is comprised
of the calcaneus and talus. The
two axes of the MTJ, the
oblique and longitudinal axes,
are also depicted. Like the subtalar joint, both axes of the MTJ
are triplanar. (Used with permission from Juan C. Garbalosa,
Ph.D., P.T., University of Hartford, West Hartford, CT.)*

siflexion with inversion. Because the axis of the first ray is minimally pitched from the transverse plane, insignificant transverse motion occurs.[5] In contrast, the axis of rotation of the fifth ray is oriented at a 20-degree angle from the transverse plane and a 35-degree angle from the sagittal plane. The resulting motions combine inversion with plantar flexion and eversion with dorsiflexion. Less motion is present about the axis of rotation of the fifth ray than the first ray.[5]

The MTP joints have separate vertical and transverse axes of motion. Plantar flexion/dorsiflexion occurs at the transverse axis, whereas abduction and adduction take place around the vertical axis.[5,8,22] Normally, no frontal plane motion occurs at the MTP joints; any frontal plane motion leads to subluxation of the joints.[5]

Plantar Fascia and Arches of the Foot

The plantar aponeurosis is one of the most functionally important soft tissue structures of the foot. This sheath of fascia spans the foot along most of its plantar surface. Its proximal attachment is at the medial process of the cal-canean tuberosity. It passes distally along the plantar aspect of the foot, then divides into five slips for its distal attachment at the base of the proximal phalanges via the plantar pads.[26] This fascial sheath plays an extremely important role in providing the stability needed by the foot during the push-off phase of stance during gait and in supporting the longitudinal arch of the foot.

The medial longitudinal and transverse arches are formed by the ligamentous and osseous structures of a "normal" foot.[27] The medial longitudinal arch (MLA) extends from the calcaneus (posterior) to the first metatarsal head (anterior) and is supported by the plantar aponeurosis, short and long plantar ligaments, and the spring ligament. During weight bearing the height of the arch is reduced as the supporting ligamentous structures are elongated. The transverse arch reaches across the foot from medial to lateral borders. The height of the arch varies along the length of the foot: Its maximum height occurs at the cuboid-cuneiform bones of the midfoot, and its lowest point is at the metatarsal heads.

FUNCTION OF THE FOOT IN GAIT

The foot and ankle complex has three major functions in the gait cycle: attenuating the impact forces, maintaining equilibrium, and transmitting propulsive forces. For optimal biomechanical and energy-efficient performance, the joints of the foot and ankle must work in harmony. In early stance, the foot-ankle complex must decrease the shock that is transmitted to proximal structures, absorb the energy generated during initial contact (heel strike), and adapt to surface conditions encountered by the foot. In later stance, the foot and lower leg transmit propulsive forces generated by muscles of the lower extremity to the ground. The ability of the foot and lower leg to accomplish these functions depends, in part, on the integrity of the various structures of the foot. When the foot-ankle complex is unable to compensate for deficits in motion or structure, gait abnormalities result.

The kinematic, kinetic, and neuromuscular events of the normal human gait cycle have been described in many ways.[5,28,29] We focus on five distinct events: heel strike (initial contact), foot flat (loading response), midstance, heel-off (terminal stance), and toe-off (preswing). Heel strike occurs when the heel contacts the ground. Foot flat begins when the forefoot contacts the ground and ends at midstance, when the center of gravity is directly over the stance leg. Heel-off occurs when the heel first loses contact with the ground, and toe-off marks transition into swing phase.[5,29] During early swing phase, limb acceleration occurs until the malleoli are even with the stance leg. Subsequent deceleration slows the limb to prepare for the next heel strike.[28,29]

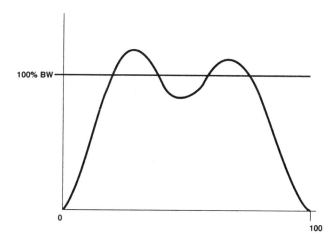

FIGURE 8-4

Typical vertical ground reaction pattern during walking. Note the bimodal shape of the ground reaction force. The first peak occurs at heel strike, and the second peak occurs during the push-off phase of gait. Note that the recorded ground reaction force represents the whole body center of mass acceleration. (BW = body weight.) (Reprinted with permission from GA Valiant. Transmission and Attenuation of Heelstrike Accelerations. In PR Cavanagh [ed], Biomechanics of Distance Running. Champaign, IL: Human Kinetics, 1990;225–249.)

Shock Absorption

The musculoskeletal structures of the lower extremity act from heel strike to midstance to attenuate impact forces.[5,28,30] Force plate recording of the ground reaction force (GRF) estimates the foot's ability to absorb energy and decelerate the lower leg. The push of the foot against the floor creates a GRF that has three components: vertical, medial/lateral, and fore/aft forces. The vertical component of a typical GRF record has a bimodal shape (Figure 8-4). The brief first peak results from the impact of the heel with the ground. Some of the vertical GRF is attributed to acceleration of the centers of mass of the foot and shank of the leg.

In early stance, from heel strike to foot flat, the STJ moves into pronation as the TCJ is plantar flexing.[5,28,31,32] The fibula and tibia internally rotate with respect to the foot.[20,21] Pronation of the STJ is controlled by eccentric contraction of the tibialis anterior, posterior tibialis, flexor hallucis longus, and flexor digitorum longus muscles.[5,28,33] Plantar flexion of the foot is controlled primarily by eccentric action of the tibialis anterior.[5,32] The combined muscle activity decelerates plantar flexion and pronation motion of the TCJ, STJ, and MTJ, slowing vertical and anterior movement of the center of mass of the foot and shank, decreasing impact forces encountered at heel strike.

The viscoelastic plantar fat pad absorbs some of the energy generated between heel strike and foot flat.[34] Pronation of the STJ flattens the arches of the foot, elongating plantar connective tissue structures. Because these tissues are viscoelastic, they also absorb some of the energy generated from heel strike to foot flat.

Adaptation to Surfaces

In everyday walking, the foot must be able to adapt quickly to many types of terrains and uneven surfaces. The key contributor to surface adaptation is STJ pronation, which unlocks the MTJ, permitting the joints of the foot to function in loose-packed positions and enabling the osseous elements to shift their relative positions.

At heel strike the forefoot is in a supinatory twist (inverted) about the longitudinal MTJ axis. Eccentric action of the anterior tibialis decelerates plantar flexion of the forefoot, lowering it to the ground. The MTJ becomes fully supinated at foot flat, as a result of eversion of the STJ and GRFs acting upward on the foot's medial border. Contraction of the extensor digitorum longus and peroneus tertius abduct and dorsiflex (pronates) the forefoot, locking it about the oblique MTJ axis and preparing the forefoot to receive the loading forces encountered at midstance.[5]

Propulsion

During midstance (foot flat to toe-off), the STJ is maximally pronated and begins to resupinate. At this time, the GRF maintains the MTJ in a pronated position about its oblique axis. At the same time, a pronatory twist is initiated at the longitudinal axis by concentric action of the peroneals. The MTJ locks in a fully pronated position around the longitudinal axis just before heel rise, as the STJ reaches its neutral position. The MTJ must remain locked in this position throughout propulsion, as the peroneals contract to lift the lateral side of the foot from the ground and transfer weight medially to the other foot. As the heel is raised from the ground, the rear foot continues to supinate (talus abducts and dorsiflexes) as the lower limb rotates externally. This coupled motion necessitates supination of the MTJ about the oblique axis to maximize joint stability and convert the foot into a rigid lever for propulsion.

Supination of the STJ occurs with concentric action of the tibialis posterior, flexor hallucis longus, and flexor digitorum longus and soleus, as well as the antagonistic functioning of the peroneus brevis.[5,28] The concentric activity of the gastrocnemius and soleus muscles causes the foot and lower leg to experience a vertical acceleration. Propulsive forces generated by the foot and lower leg are transmitted to the floor.[5,28,32] The second peak of a GRF curve (see Figure 8-4) corresponds to propulsion in late stance phase.

Supination of the STJ and locking of the MTJ about the longitudinal axis place the foot in a closed-packed posi-

tion, transforming the foot into a rigid lever.[5,10,20,28] This transformation is aided by the action of the plantar aponeurosis as it wraps around the metatarsal heads. During heel-off, the MTP joints extend (dorsiflex), creating a "windlass effect." This compresses joints of the mid- and forefoot, facilitating the transition from flexibility to rigidity, which is required for effective push-off.[10,15,20,26,27]

BIOMECHANICAL FOOT AND ANKLE EXAMINATION

Biomechanical examination of the foot and ankle has three components: a non–weight-bearing assessment, a static weight-bearing assessment, and a dynamic gait analysis. Five common intrinsic foot deformities can be identified by biomechanical examination: rear foot varus, forefoot varus, forefoot valgus, equinus deformity, and plantar flexed first ray.

The theoretical model that forms the basis of biomechanical foot and ankle examination emerged from the work of Merton Root et al.[5] The major assumption of Root's model is that proper foot function is contingent on a neutral STJ position, defined as the point of maximum congruence in the articulation of the talus and navicular.[8,26,5,35] This subtalar joint neutral (STN) position was thought to minimize stress to the surrounding joints, ligaments, and tendons and to be most efficient with regard to muscle function and attenuation of the impact forces at heel strike.[35,36] Neutral STJ position represents the point at which the foot converts from a mobile adapter to a rigid lever.[5,36] According to Root's traditional theory, ideal or normal foot alignment occurs just before heel-off during gait, when the STJ is in the neutral position and the MTJ is fully locked.[5] Root describes deviations from normal foot alignment as "intrinsic" foot deformities, which can lead to aberrant lower extremity function and musculoskeletal pathology.[5,36]

Currently, much debate is taking place regarding the validity of Root's criteria for normalcy and his supposition that the STJ is in the neutral position between the midstance and heel-off phases of the gait cycle. The reliability of the measurement techniques that are used to determine the neutral position has also been questioned.[37–39]

Before prescribing a biomechanical foot orthosis, the clinician must understand the source of the pathology or deformity. Toward that end, a full patient history is taken and a comprehensive biomechanical examination is performed.[40] After this, resultant pathomechanical abnormalities of the condition are identified and benefits of orthotic intervention are established.

A biomechanical examination consists of three basic components: (1) a static non–weight-bearing examination, (2) a static weight-bearing examination, and (3) a dynamic gait assessment (Figure 8-5). The non–weight-bearing examination involves visual inspection of the basic architecture of the foot and ankle. Any bony deformities or prominence of the joints, rays or toes, and callosities are noted. Through goniometric procedures the examiner locates the STN position and identifies which, if any, intrinsic foot deformities are present. In the static weight-bearing examination, compensatory mechanisms that result from intrinsic deformities are assessed as the foot is subjected to GRFs. During the dynamic gait assessment, extrinsic factors that affect foot function (e.g., muscle imbalances or weaknesses, proximal structural deformities, kinesthetic or proprioceptive losses, etc.) are observed.

NON–WEIGHT-BEARING EXAMINATION

The non–weight-bearing goniometric examination is performed with the subject prone. The lower extremity being assessed is positioned with the knee extended and the foot 6–8 in. off the treatment table. Placing the contralateral lower extremity in a figure-four position orients the ipsilateral lower extremity in the frontal plane, reducing the influence of proximal rotational limb disorders on measurement.[41]

Examination of the Rear Foot

The first goniometric measurements of the non–weight-bearing examination assess rear foot (STN) position and STJ mobility, based on calcaneal positioning in the frontal plane. Frontal plane motion of the calcaneus is used because it is one of the largest and easiest components of triplanar STJ motion to measure directly. The stationary arm of a goniometer is aligned with an imaginary bisection of the lower one-third of the tibiofibular complex, and the mobile arm is aligned with an imaginary bisection of the posterior surface of the calcaneus.[41] The axis of the goniometer is aligned at the STJ axis, just above the superior border of the calcaneus but beneath the level of the medial and lateral malleoli (Figure 8-6). Some evaluators use calipers and a pen to mark the skin of the patient over the midlines of girth of the lower leg and calcaneus.[42] The authors prefer to use visual bisections to reduce the potential for error due to skin distortion.

Subtalar Neutral Position
STJ neutral position can be determined either by the palpation method or by a mathematical model. Both methods use standard goniometric procedures. In the palpation

method, the examiner identifies the anteromedial and anterolateral aspects of the talar head using the thumb and index fingers of the hand closest to the patient's midline. The anteromedial aspect of the talar head is located by placing the thumb just proximal to the navicular tuberosity, approximately 1 in. below and 1 in. distal to the medial malleolus. In STJ pronation, the anteromedial talar head becomes prominent beneath the thumb, and an anterolateral sulcus, representing the sinus tarsi, is apparent. The index finger is placed in this sulcus, where the talar head is found to protrude when the foot is fully supinated. The thumb and index finger of the other hand grasp the fourth and fifth metatarsal heads, moving the foot in an arc of adduction and inversion (supination) and abduction and eversion (pronation). STN is the point where the talar head is equally prominent anteromedially and anterolaterally.[36,41,42] The examiner then "loads" the foot by applying a dorsally directed pressure against the fourth and fifth metatarsal heads until slight resistance is felt. The loading procedure locks the MTJ against the rear foot, mimicking GRFs of midstance.[5,43] The angular relationship between the bisection of the calcaneus and the bisection of the lower one-third of the leg is measured using a goniometer (see Figure 8-6) and is recorded on the evaluation form as rear foot "STN position."

Root described a mathematical model for determining STN position using a quantitative goniometric formula.[5,36] First, end-ROM calcaneal inversion and eversion are determined by goniometric measurement. Total calcaneal ROM is the sum of the inversion and eversion values. The STN position is determined as the calcaneus is moved into inversion at one-third of the total calcaneal ROM. For example, if end-range calcaneal inversion is 25 degrees and end-range calcaneal eversion is +5 degrees, total calcaneal ROM is then 30 degrees. STN position is calculated to be at 5 degrees calcaneal inversion (e.g., one-third the distance from its fully everted position).

The reliability and clinical validity of these models are debated.[36,39,41,44-47] The authors agree with Diamond et al.'s[47] findings that acceptable reliability is possible but requires practice and experience. Although the palpation method takes less time to perform, it requires more advanced manual skills and experience. The mathematical model may be more reliable for the entry-level practitioner.

Calcaneal Range of Motion
Calcaneal inversion and eversion ROM occur primarily at the STJ, with lesser contributions from the TCJ. Measurements are assessed in the prone position, using the same anatomic landmarks and lines of bisection as for STN assessment. The examiner grasps the calcaneus in one hand, fully inverting it in the frontal plane until end

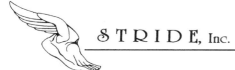

$\mathscr{S}\text{TRIDE}$, Inc.

Physical Therapy and Pedorthic Services
530 Middlebury Road • Suite 102 • Middlebury, CT 06762
TEL.: (203) 598-0070 • FAX: (203) 598-0075

BIOMECHANICAL FOOT EVALUATION

Patient: _____ Phone: _____

Address: _____

Age: _____ Height: _____ Weight: _____ Shoe size: _____ Shoe Style: _____

Occupation: _____ Activity level: _____ Sports: _____

Referring Practitioner: _____ Date of Evaluation: _____

Diagnosis: _____

I. NON-WEIGHTBEARING EVALUATION

	Left	**Right**

Rearfoot:

STN position	_____ varus	_____ varus
calcaneal inversion	_____ degrees	_____ degrees
calcaneal eversion	_____ degrees	_____ degrees
rearfoot dorsiflexion	_____ degrees	_____ degrees

Forefoot:

STN position   _____ varus/valgus   _____ varus/valgus

locking mechanism
⊢———+———+———⊣   ⊢———+———+———⊣
poor   fair   normal   rigid   poor   fair   normal   rigid

MTJ dorsiflexion   _____ degrees   _____ degrees

First Ray:

STN position and mobility   oooo(○)   (○)oooo

hallux dorsiflexion   _____ degrees   _____ degrees

Arch Position:

⊢———+———⊣   ⊢———+———⊣
low   med   high   low   med   high

Toe Position/Deformities: _____   _____

Lesions/Shoe Wear: **Calluses:**   L   R

R   L   L   R

A

FIGURE 8-5

Biomechanical examination form outlining components of the **(A)** *non–weight-bearing and* **(B)** *weight-bearing assessment. (Ante = femoral anteversion; ASIS = anterior superior iliac spine; DLS = double limb stance; Gastroc = gastrocnemius; G.T. = greater trochanter; ITB= iliotibial band; M.M. = medial malleolus; MTJ = midtarsal joint; PSIS = posterior inferior iliac spine; RCS = relaxed calcaneal stance; Retro = femoral retroversion; SLS = single limb stance; STN = subtalar neutral; T.T. = tibial tubercle; VAR = varus; VAL = valgus.) (Used with permission from Stride, Inc., Middlebury, CT.)*

II. WEIGHTBEARING EVALUATION

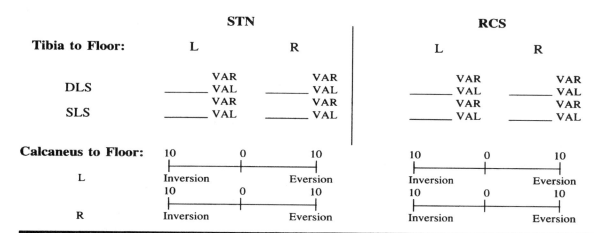

	STN		RCS	
Tibia to Floor:	L	R	L	R
DLS	____ VAR ____ VAL	____ VAR ____ VAL	____ VAR ____ VAL	____ VAR ____ VAL
SLS	____ VAR ____ VAL	____ VAR ____ VAL	____ VAR ____ VAL	____ VAR ____ VAL

Calcaneus to Floor:

L

10	0	10
Inversion		Eversion

10	0	10
Inversion		Eversion

R

10	0	10
Inversion		Eversion

10	0	10
Inversion		Eversion

III. SOFT TISSUE RESTRICTIONS

	L	R		L	R
Iliopsoas	____	____	**Hip Rotation (Hips 90°, Knees 90°)**		
Rectus Femoris	____	____	Internal	____	____
ITB	____	____	External	____	____
Hamstring	____	____	**Hip Rotation (Hips 0°, Knees 90°)**		
Gastroc	____	____	Internal	____	____
Soleus	____	____	External	____	____

IV. POSTURAL OBSERVATIONS

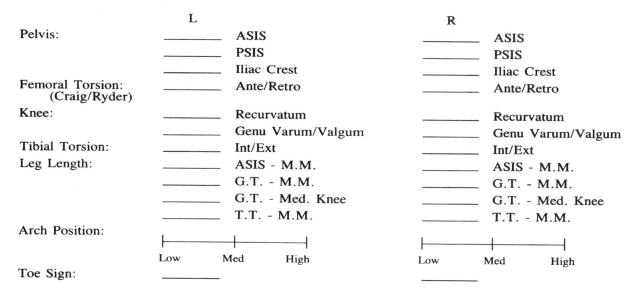

	L		R	
Pelvis:	____	ASIS	____	ASIS
	____	PSIS	____	PSIS
	____	Iliac Crest	____	Iliac Crest
Femoral Torsion: (Craig/Ryder)	____	Ante/Retro	____	Ante/Retro
Knee:	____	Recurvatum	____	Recurvatum
	____	Genu Varum/Valgum	____	Genu Varum/Valgum
Tibial Torsion:	____	Int/Ext	____	Int/Ext
Leg Length:	____	ASIS - M.M.	____	ASIS - M.M.
	____	G.T. - M.M.	____	G.T. - M.M.
	____	G.T. - Med. Knee	____	G.T. - Med. Knee
	____	T.T. - M.M.	____	T.T. - M.M.

Arch Position:

Low	Med	High

Low	Med	High

Toe Sign: ____   ____

B

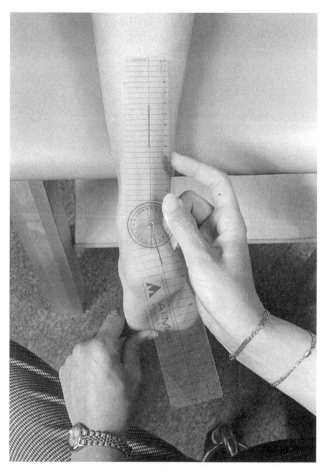

FIGURE 8-6

Non–weight-bearing goniometric technique. A loading force applied by the examiner over the fourth and fifth metatarsal heads locks the forefoot on the rear foot, while the examiner's opposite hand operates the goniometer to measure subtalar joint neutral position and calcaneal range of motion. The examiner is seated at the distal end of the treatment table, with chair height adjusted to position the subject's foot at chest level.

ROM is achieved and a goniometric measurement is taken.[46] The procedure is repeated for calcaneal eversion. The TCJ must be maintained in a 0-degree or mildly dorsiflexed position while measuring to lock it in a closed-packed position and better isolate STJ motion.[48] The normative values reported are 20 degrees for calcaneal inversion and 10 degrees beyond vertical for eversion.[5]

Values of calcaneal eversion are larger when assessed in a full weight-bearing position. Some researchers suggest that this position is more clinically valid.[37,46] Assessment of calcaneal eversion in the weight-bearing position, however, represents a total "functional" pronation/eversion that is the summation of motion occurring at the STJ and compensatory motion occurring extrinsic to the STJ (e.g., TCJ, MTJ, etc.). Passive assessment of calcaneal eversion in non–weight bearing remains the most accurate method to determine the degree of composite pronation acquired from the STJ itself.

Ankle: Talocrural Joint Range of Motion
In normal walking, the TCJ is maximally dorsiflexed just before heel rise when the knee is fully extended and the STJ is in a nearly neutral position.[5,49] When and whether an actual STN position ever occurs during gait is disputed.[37] The use of a standard position of knee extension and STN, however, offers a consistent point of reference when assessing TCJ dorsiflexion. According to most sources, a minimum of 10 degrees TCJ dorsiflexion is required for normal gait; anything less is classified as an equinus deformity.[5,49-52] A minimum of 20 degrees of plantar flexion is also required for normal gait.[5]

Ankle dorsiflexion is measured in a non–weight-bearing position with the STJ held in neutral and the knee extended. The examiner forcefully dorsiflexes the ankle with active assistance from the subject. Active assistance encourages reciprocal inhibition of the calf muscle group and is essential for accurate measurement.[49] Traditional goniometric techniques for measurement of dorsiflexion place the proximal arm of the goniometer along the lateral aspect of the fibula, the distal arm along the lateral border of the fifth metatarsal, and the axis distal to the lateral malleolus.[53] The authors suggest that an alternative placement of the distal arm of the goniometer along the inferolateral border of the calcaneus more effectively isolates true TCJ dorsiflexion. This value is recorded as "rear foot dorsiflexion." Forefoot dorsiflexion is measured by repositioning the distal arm along the lateral aspect of the fifth metatarsal. This method allows the examiner to identify contributions or restrictions in sagittal plane motion from the oblique axis of the MTJ.

If ankle dorsiflexion is less than 10 degrees when measured with the knee extended, remeasurement with the knee flexed may rule out soft tissue restriction of the gastrocnemius-soleus complex.[5,49] If dorsiflexion values are consistent in both positions, the limitation is likely a result of osseous equinus formation of the ankle.

During gait, ankle dorsiflexion occurs as a closed kinetic chain as the tibiofibular complex moves forward over a fixed foot. Some have suggested that it would be more accurate to assess ankle dorsiflexion in a weight-bearing position.[37,50] The weight-bearing technique measures the angle between the tibia and the floor as the subject leans forward with the foot flat on the floor. Baggett and Young[50] found poor correlation between non–weight-bearing and weight-bearing values of ankle dorsiflexion and concluded that the non–weight-bearing measurement had no clinical value. The authors suggest that both measures have clinical value, although the weight-bearing technique does have several limitations. In assessing weight-bearing dorsiflexion, unwanted compensations are often difficult to control and may mask true TCJ limitations. The non–weight-bearing technique allows the examiner to assess end feel and joint play, as well as mechanical blocks or joint laxity, providing additional information that is not accessible in the weight-bearing examination.

Rear Foot Deformities

Normal rear foot position is one in which STN is 1–4 degrees of varus.[38,39,45,46] Larger values are classified as "rear foot varus deformity." Root proposed that the etiology of a rear foot varus deformity was ontogenetic failure of the calcaneus to derotate sufficiently during early childhood development.[5,43,54] Because this deformity is a torsional structural malalignment of the calcaneus, not a joint-related problem, the TCJ and STJ lines remain congruent when observed in the non–weight-bearing STN position. Because this deformity is structural, it cannot be corrected or reduced by joint mobilization or a strengthening program. Instead, it can be managed with a functional foot orthosis that partially supports the calcaneus in its inverted alignment while preventing excessive STJ pronation.

Assessment of calcaneal ROM is fundamentally predicting the quality of motion and the integrity of the STJ. Moreover, measuring calcaneal motion into eversion allows the examiner to determine whether a rear foot deformity is compensated or uncompensated (Figure 8-7). In a compensated rear foot varus deformity, the calcaneus fully everts to vertical or beyond in weight bearing because the STJ possesses an adequate amount of pronatory motion to compensate for the deformity. A compensated rear foot varus deformity of 10 degrees (STN position) would require that the STJ pronate or evert at least 10 degrees to enable the medial condyle of the calcaneus to achieve ground contact in weight bearing. Such excessive pronatory motion causes medial gapping and lateral constriction at the STJ line and a medial bulge of the talus as it moves into adduction and plantar flexion.

In an uncompensated rear foot varus deformity, the calcaneus remains fixed in its inverted STN position with no eversion motion at the STJ. A partially compensated rear foot varus deformity allows for partial STJ eversion so that the medial condyle of the calcaneus does not completely contact the ground on weight bearing. Alternative compensatory motion, extrinsic to the STJ, is then necessary to achieve weight bearing on the medial aspect of the foot. One of the common compensations is an acquired soft tissue (valgus) deformity of the forefoot caused by a plantar flexed first ray. Other sources of compensatory motion can occur at the MTJ or proximally at the knee, hip, or sacroiliac joints.

An equinus deformity occurs when less than 10 degrees of ankle dorsiflexion is available as a result of osseous or muscular problems.[50,52,55,56] Clubfoot (talipes equinovarus) is a congenital osseous deformity that presents with varus deformities of the rear foot and forefoot, rear foot equinus, and an inverted and adducted forefoot.[57,58] The angular relationship between the body and the head and neck of the talus is decreased, and the navicular is shifted medially. Muscular forms of equinus include congenital or acquired soft tissue shortening or muscle spasm.[52,56] Tissue contracture or shortening occurs in contractile tissues (gastrocnemius, soleus, and plantaris) and noncontractile tissues (teno Achilles and plantar fascia).[50,52]

Compensation for an equinus deformity occurs at the foot through pronation, perpetuating soft tissue contractures. The STJ is forced to pronate maximally to gain as much sagittal plane dorsiflexion as possible. Although foot pronation improves acquisition of dorsiflexion from the STJ, the amount is often inadequate. Pronation of the STJ does, however, allow the MTJ to unlock, creating an unstable midfoot and allowing further acquisition of dorsiflexion and forefoot abduction from the oblique axis of the MTJ.[52] Other compensatory strategies for equinus deformity include knee flexion (especially in patients with cerebral palsy), early heel rise, toe walking, shortened stride length of the contralateral lower limb, and toe-out walking.[28,36,52] Clinical consequences of long-term ankle equinus include many conditions that are normally associated with the excessively pronated foot: plantar fasciitis, heel spurs, bunions, and capsulitis.[52]

Examination of the Forefoot

Forefoot position is assessed with the STJ held in neutral position. Because the first and fifth rays have independent axes of motion, forefoot orientation is defined by the planar relationship of the second, third, and fourth rays to the bisection line of the calcaneus.

Neutral Forefoot Position

If the forefoot is properly balanced, the plane of the three central metatarsals will be perpendicular to the bisection of the calcaneus when in STN (Figure 8-8). In a forefoot varus deformity, the forefoot is excessively supinated or inverted, whereas in a forefoot valgus the forefoot is excessively pronated or everted.

Mobility Testing: Locking Mechanism

As discussed previously, when isolating STN position, the examiner attempts to lock the MTJ by applying a dor-

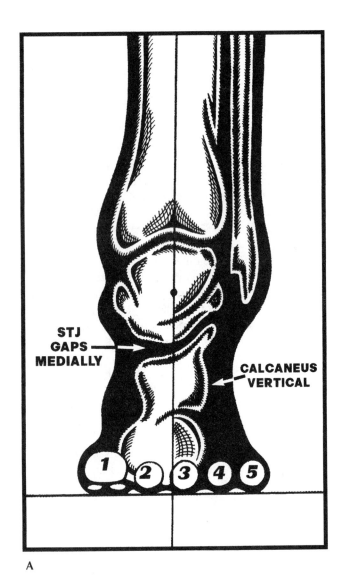

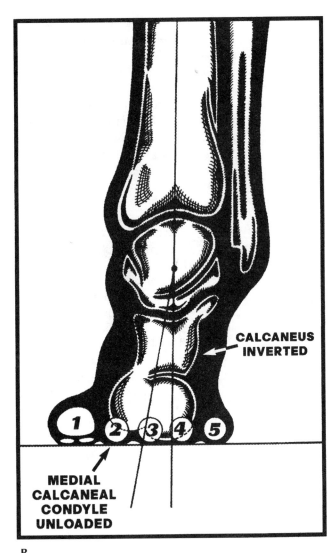

A   **B**

FIGURE 8-7

(A) In relaxed calcaneal stance, compensation for a rear foot varus is normally subtalar joint (STJ) pronation. (B) In an uncompensated rear foot varus, the STJ cannot pronate and instead may develop compensatory midtarsal joint pronation about the longitudinal joint axis. (Used with permission from Stride, Inc., Middlebury, CT.)

sally directed loading pressure with the thumb and index fingers over the fourth and fifth metatarsal heads of the subject's foot (see Figure 8-6). Applying force to only the fifth metatarsal head simply dorsiflexes the fifth ray about its independent axis, without achieving the proper locking mechanism.[5,35] The loading force is gently applied until tissue slack is taken up from the normally plantar flexed resting position of the ankle; overload of the forefoot with too much force results in excessive dorsiflex-

ion and abduction of the foot. This places the forefoot in an excessively pronated position and gives a false valgus orientation.

Although many forefoot measurement devices are commercially available, forefoot orientation can be accurately assessed with a standard goniometer.[45] To assess the forefoot to rear foot relationship, the proximal arm of the goniometer is aligned along the bisection of the calcaneus, with the axis just below its distal border. The distal arm

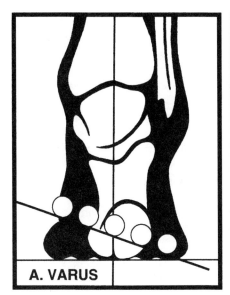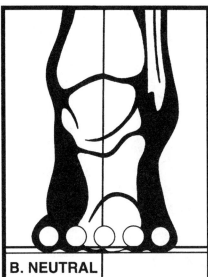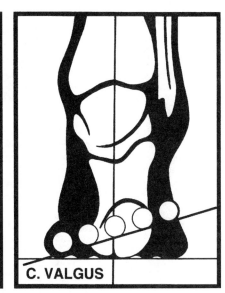

FIGURE 8-8

*In subtalar joint neutral, the normal orientation of the forefoot to the calcaneus (**B**) is perpendicular. Excessive supination/inversion of the forefoot, in subtalar joint neutral, would indicate a forefoot varus (**A**), whereas excessive pronation/eversion of the forefoot would indicate a forefoot valgus (**C**). (Used with permission from Stride, Inc., Middlebury, CT.)*

is positioned in the plane of the three central metatarsal heads (Figure 8-9). The angular displacement is recorded on the evaluation form under "STN position" for the forefoot assessment (see Figure 8-5).

Efficacy of foot function with a given forefoot orientation depends on the mobility of the MTJ and its ability to achieve a locking mechanism. In normal walking, the MTJ "locks" as heel rise begins so that the foot is converted into a rigid lever for propulsion. This lock requires that the STJ be in neutral position. Clinical assessment of MTJ mobility and locking mechanism is an advanced manual skill. Observations made during weight-bearing assessment (e.g., toe sign, navicular drop test, talar bulge) provide an elementary method to identify a loose MTJ that is unable to lock.

An ineffective locking mechanism at the MTJ can often be more clinically significant than the absolute degree of forefoot deformity. For example, a forefoot varus deformity of 3 degrees with a poor MTJ locking mechanism may be symptomatic, whereas an 8-degree forefoot varus deformity with a normal MTJ locking mechanism may not be.

Identifying Forefoot Deformities

The prevalence of forefoot deformity in subjects with and without symptoms is well established, although the distribution of deformities reported is not consistent.[45,59] It has also been observed that when forefoot deformities do occur bilaterally, they are not necessarily symmetric.

According to Root, MTJ deformities change the location of the lock of the forefoot against the rear foot. Although these osseous frontal plane deformities alter the direction of motion, they do not limit the total ROM of the MTJ.[5] In a forefoot varus deformity, the forefoot locks in a position that is inverted in relation to the rear foot.[5] It is the result of an ontogenetic failure of the normal valgus rotation of the head and neck of the talus in relation to its body during early childhood development.[5,43,54] Compensations for foot deformities are viewed in a relaxed weight-bearing position referred to as *relaxed calcaneal stance* (RCS). When excessive pronation of the STJ compensates for the deformity on weight bearing, the condition is called a *compensated forefoot varus* (Figure 8-10A). If the STJ cannot adequately pronate to accommodate the inverted position of the forefoot, the condition is called an *uncompensated forefoot varus*.[5] The medial forefoot does not contact the ground, and the lateral forefoot is subjected to excessive pressure. Thick callus develops beneath the head of the fifth metatarsal, and the risk of stress fracture is increased (Figure 8-10B). Plantar flexion of the first ray and pronation at the MTJ are common compensations that allow the medial forefoot to contact the ground. Ongoing repeated stress at the MTJ can lead to breakdown of the joint and excessive forefoot abduction and eversion.

Forefoot valgus is a frontal plane deformity that locks the forefoot in an everted position relative to the rear foot.[5]

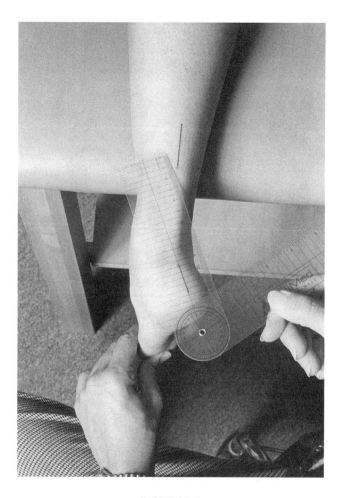

FIGURE 8-9

Measurement of forefoot orientation in subtalar joint neutral using a standard goniometer. The proximal arm of the goniometer is aligned with the bisection of the posterior surface of the calcaneus, and the distal arm parallels the plane of the metatarsal heads. The axis lies beneath the distal aspect of the calcaneus.

Root proposed that this deformity is a result of ontogenetic over-rotation of the talar head and neck in relation to its body during early childhood development.[5,43,54] Forefoot valgus can be a rigid or flexible deformity. In rigid forefoot valgus, the compensatory weight-bearing mechanism occurs at the STJ as excessive supination or calcaneal inversion. It is a result of excessive premature GRFs at the first metatarsal head, causing rapid STJ inversion and increasing loading forces beneath the fifth metatarsal head. Thick callosities are often present beneath the first and fifth metatarsal heads. In contrast, flexible forefoot valgus is usually an acquired soft tissue condition. It most often occurs as a consequence of uncompensated rear foot varus, as an attempt to increase weight bearing along the medial foot. Because this deformity is flexible, no compensatory

mechanism is necessary. Contact force beneath the first metatarsal head simply pushes it up out of the way, and the foot functions as if this condition were not present.

First Ray: Neutral Position and Mobility Testing

Assessment of first ray position is performed with the foot in STN position. Ideally, the first ray lies within the common transverse plane of the lesser metatarsal heads. To examine mobility of the first ray, the examiner holds the first metatarsal head between the thumb and index finger and performs a dorsal/plantar glide while stabilizing the lesser metatarsal heads with the other hand. Normally, first ray movement is at least one thumb width above and below the plane of the other metatarsal heads.[5]

Deformities of the First Ray

As stance phase is completed, activity of the peroneus longus creates a pronatory twist of the forefoot, stabilizing the medial column of the foot on the ground, locking the MTJ about its longitudinal axis, and converting the foot to a rigid lever for propulsion. Adequate plantar flexion of the first ray must be present for conversion to a rigid lever to occur. The amount of first ray plantar flexion needed is contingent on several factors. First, the more the foot inverts during propulsion, the further the first ray must plantar flex to make ground contact. Second, because elevation of the medial forefoot is related to foot width, wider feet require more first ray plantar flexion. Third, an excessively long second metatarsal also increases the distance that the first ray must plantar flex to make ground contact.[5]

In some instances, the first ray is inappropriately dorsiflexed above the plane of the other metatarsals, resulting in restriction of plantar flexion and impeding normal propulsion. The first ray may also be plantar flexed below the plane of the other metatarsals. In uncompensated rear foot varus, for example, the eversion motion of the calcaneus is insufficient, the medial condyle fails to contact the ground, and there is excessive weight bearing on the lateral border of the foot. The peroneus longus contracts to pull the first metatarsal head toward the ground in an attempt to load the medial side of the foot. This is possible because of the cuboid pulley system[5] (Figure 8-11). When the STJ remains abnormally pronated in late stance phase, orientation of the cuboid tunnel is altered, and the mechanical advantage of the peroneus longus is lost. The MTJ cannot lock up, and the foot remains unstable throughout propulsion.

The presence of a rigid plantar flexed first ray sometimes results in a functional forefoot valgus (Figure 8-12). The compensatory mechanism for this condition is similar to that for rigid forefoot valgus: STJ supination or calcaneal inversion on weight bearing to lower the lateral aspect of the foot to the ground.

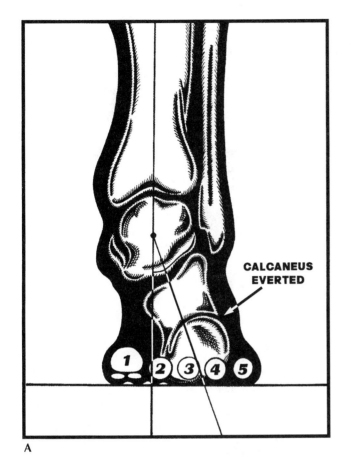 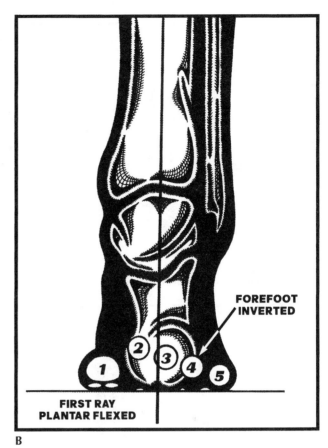

FIGURE 8-10

(A) In relaxed calcaneal stance, compensation for a forefoot varus deformity is normally subtalar joint pronation, resulting in an everted calcaneus. (B) In an uncompensated forefoot varus, the subtalar joint is unable to compensate. Instead, the first ray plantar flexes to achieve weight bearing medially on the foot. (Used with permission from Stride, Inc., Middlebury, CT.)

Assessment of the Hallux

In normal gait, dorsiflexion of the hallux occurs during the late propulsive phase as the body moves forward over the foot. Sagittal plane motion of the hallux is assessed as passive ROM. The stabile arm of the goniometer is positioned along the medial first metatarsal and the mobile arm along the medial proximal phalanx of the hallux. The axis is medial to the first MTP joint.[53] Sufficient force is applied to bring the hallux to its end ROM. Normal range of hallux dorsiflexion is between 70 and 90 degrees.[5,53]

Deformities of the Hallux

In hallux limitus deformity, pathomechanical functioning of the first MTP joint prevents the hallux from moving through its full range of dorsiflexion during propulsion. Repetitive trauma to the first MTP joint can lead to anky-losis, or hallux rigidus. Functional hallux limitus is a condition in which full first MTP ROM is present when non–weight bearing, but a functional restriction of hallux dorsiflexion occurs during gait. Functional hallux limitus disrupts the normal windlass mechanism described previously.[60,61]

Limitation of hallux dorsiflexion prohibits the normal progression of the foot and interferes with propulsion of the body over the hallux. Several gait compensations can overcome this limitation.[60,61] An abducted or toe-out gait pattern shifts propulsion to the medial border of the hallux. A pinched callus then develops from friction between the hallux and shoe during propulsion. Alternatively, the IP joint of the hallux may hyperextend, causing a callus in the sulcus of the IP joint.

Hallux abductovalgus (HAV) is a progressive acquired deformity of the first MTP joint that eventually results in

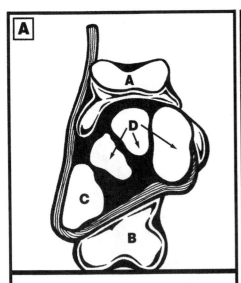

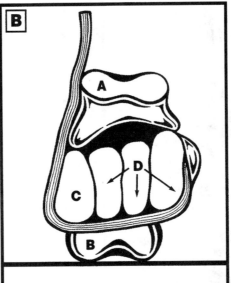

FIGURE 8-11
(A) Cuboid pulley mechanism in a normal foot. (B) In an abnormally pronated foot, the mechanical advantage of the peroneals is impaired. A = talus; B = calcaneus; C = cuboid; D = the cuneiforms. (Used with permission from Stride, Inc., Middlebury, CT.)

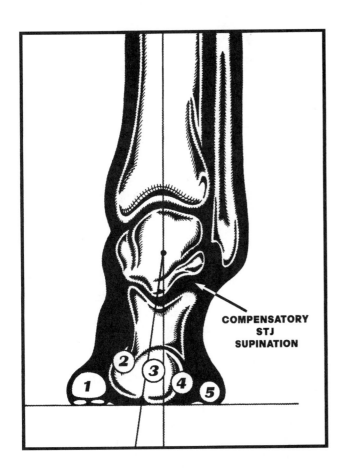

FIGURE 8-12
Plantar flexed first ray deformity in relaxed calcaneal stance. Compensation occurs at the subtalar joint (STJ), with lateral gapping and medial compression. (Used with permission from Stride, Inc., Middlebury, CT.)

a valgus subluxation of the hallux.[5,43] This deformity is caused by abnormal STJ pronation with hypermobility of the first ray.[5] There are several common misconceptions about HAV. One is that HAV is hereditary. In truth, the congenital osseous abnormalities that lead to aberrant STJ pronation are hereditary, but HAV itself occurs as a compensation to these other deformities. Another misconception is that HAV is caused by restrictive footwear. Although inappropriate or restrictive footwear can accentuate or speed the progression of HAV deformity when present, the deformity is frequently observed in populations in which shoes are not typically worn.[5,43]

Additional Observations in the Non–Weight-Bearing Examination

Several other important observations are made as the non–weight-bearing examination is completed. Non–weight-bearing arch height is observed for later comparison to weight-bearing arch height as a composite estimate of foot pronation. Toes are inspected for positional deformities such as hammertoes, claw toes, crossover deformity, and the presence of bunions or bunionettes. The plantar foot is checked for callus, plantar warts, or other signs of excessive pressure. The shoes are inspected for excessive or uneven wear patterns.

STATIC WEIGHT-BEARING EXAMINATION

The open chain kinetic motion evaluated in the non–weight-bearing examination is dramatically different from the functional sequence of events in the closed kinetic chain of standing and walking. Open kinetic chain pronation (calcaneal dorsiflexion, eversion, and abduction) and supination (calcaneal plantar flexion, inversion, and adduction) are triplanar motions around the STJ.[5,8,26] During closed kinetic chain pronation, internal rotation of the leg is coupled with talar adduction and calcaneal plantar flexion and eversion. Closed kinetic chain supination couples external rotation of the leg with talar abduction and calcaneal dorsiflexion and inversion. In the open kinetic chain, movement is initiated in the distal segment (the foot). In the closed kinetic chain, motion is initiated proximally (at the tibia and talus).[5]

Assessment of the lower extremity in a closed kinetic chain provides valuable insight as to how the body compensates for the intrinsic foot deformities or impairments of normal foot joint function identified in the non–weight-bearing examination. Improper foot functioning can lead to a complex series of compensations that influence not only the mobility patterns of the foot and lower leg but also the knee, hip, pelvis, and spine. A thorough closed kinetic chain examination includes static postural observations, dynamic motion testing, and gait assessment.

The individual being examined stands in a relaxed weight-bearing posture, referred to as *RCS*. The examiner observes the subject's preferred stance, noting postural alignment and foot placement angle. The subject then adjusts the stance position, if necessary, to assume equal weight-bearing double limb support, with feet 5–10 cm apart and oriented in neutral toe-in/toe-out foot placement angle. According to Gross,[36] this adjusted posture, with neutral foot placement angle, offers a better frame of reference for assessing planar alignment and enhances the reliability or consistency of the measurement. Postural alignment or body symmetry of the subject is evaluated in frontal, sagittal, and transverse planes.

Frontal Plane

The first part of the static weight-bearing examination considers alignment in the frontal plane: the angular relationship of the calcaneus and the tibia/fibula with respect to the floor and the relationship between the pelvis and the lower leg.

Calcaneal Alignment to the Floor

With the patient in double limb stance posture, a line bisecting the posterior surface of the calcaneus is visualized and the angular relationship between the line and the floor taken. Because the infracalcaneal fat pad often migrates (related to prolonged weight bearing), care must be taken to avoid errors in visual assessment (Figure 8-13). Palpation of the osseous medial, lateral, and inferior borders of the calcaneus helps to factor out skin stretching and fat pad

migration and improve measurement accuracy. Calcaneal alignment can also be quantified using a protractor to measure the degree of calcaneal tilt relative to vertical.[62]

The actual angular degree is not as important as the relative position or orientation of the calcaneus: The issue is whether the calcaneus is inverted, vertical, or everted relative to the floor during stance. The goal of this component of the examination is to assess the ability of the STJ to provide enough pronation to compensate for its neutral position. In the normal closed chain STN position, the calcaneus is in 1–4 degrees of varus (inversion). The STJ must have an equal amount of compensatory pronation to lower the medial condyle to the ground for a vertical calcaneus. If a patient has uncompensated rear foot varus of 10 degrees in STN as well as restricted calcaneal motion (–4 degrees) eversion, the STJ would not be able to achieve sufficient pronation or eversion in stance for normal calcaneal alignment. Instead the calcaneus would be in an inverted alignment relative to the floor. Inverted calcaneal position also occurs when a rigid forefoot valgus or rigid plantar flexed first ray deformity is present. STJ supination is a compensatory mechanism for both deformities. A forefoot varus deformity, however, requires excessive compensatory STJ pronation; calcaneal eversion occurs instead in weight bearing. The position of the calcaneus with respect to the floor provides insight into the type of STJ compensation present and can be correlated to the biomechanical findings of the non–weight-bearing examination. If the STJ is unable to pronate enough to compensate completely for a deformity, additional pronatory motion occurs at the MTJ[5,46] or by eversion tilting of the talus within the ankle mortise.[36] The functional rear foot unit (calcaneus and talus) may assume a valgus (everted) position relative to the floor, even if calcaneal eversion is restricted.

Tibiofibular Alignment

Structural malalignment proximal to the foot also contributes to abnormal foot pronation and overuse injuries. Tibial varum is a congenital osseous malalignment in which the distal third of the tibia is angled medially in the frontal plane. Tibial valgum occurs if the distal tibia inclines away from the midline.[36]

Alignment of the lower tibia can be measured with either a standard goniometer or a bubble inclinometer. The angular relationship between the visualized bisection of the distal one-third of the lower leg relative to the supporting surface is assessed[36,63] (Figure 8-14). Radiographic measurement of lower leg position is better correlated with clinically assessed tibiofibular position values than with isolated tibial position. McPoil et al.[64] conclude that radiographic measurement is the only accurate method to isolate true tibial varum and that clinical assessment more accurately reflects tibiofibular position.

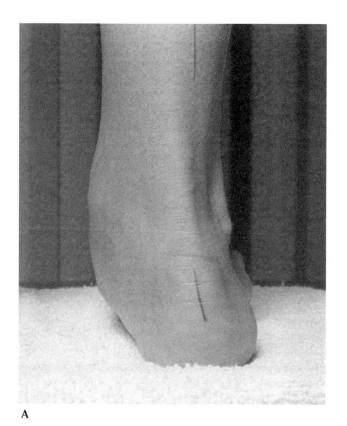

A

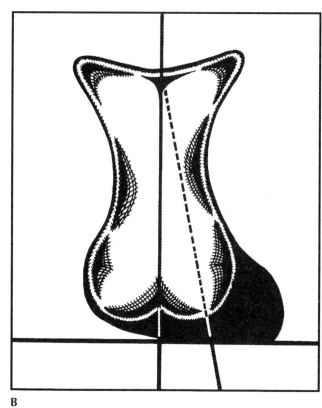

B

FIGURE 8-13

(A) Photograph of calcaneal alignment to floor. (B) Lateral migration of the infracalcaneal fat pad can give the illusion of an everted calcaneal to floor alignment. (Used with permission from Stride, Inc., Middlebury, CT.)

Test position is critical because variation in STJ alignment greatly influences tibiofibular varum measurement values. Tibiofibular varum values are larger in RCS (4.6–8.3 degrees) than in the STN (2.6–7.1 degrees) position,[63–65] possibly due to the combined effects of actual osseous malalignment and the varus leg alignment that is associated with compensatory STJ pronation in stance. The incidence of tibiofibular varum appears to be high, although no clear normative values have been established. Tomaro,[63] for example, found significant differences among bilateral values of tibiofibular varum that can lead to unilateral overuse syndromes.

The alignment of the distal third of the leg relative to the floor more accurately represents tibiofibular position than tibial position. Values assessed in STN reflect neutral tibiofibular alignment, whereas values assessed in RCS represent compensatory tibiofibular repositioning in response to STJ and MTJ pronation. High tibiofibular varum values measured in STN elevate the medial foot

from the supporting surface, requiring excessive compensatory foot pronation during gait. High tibiofibular varum values in RCS suggest excessive foot pronation, although the source of that pronation cannot be isolated.

Alignment of the Pelvis and Lower Leg

Evaluation of the symmetry of the anterior and superior iliac spines, iliac crests, greater trochanters, gluteal folds, popliteal creases, genu varum or valgum deformities, fibular heads, patellae, and malleolar levels is the final component of the frontal plane assessment. Asymmetric discrepancies often indicate sacroiliac joint dysfunction or leg length discrepancy, influencing foot position and function in the closed kinetic chain.

Sagittal Plane

The second component of the weight-bearing examination considers function in the sagittal plane. The exam-

FIGURE 8-14
Goniometric assessment of tibio-fibular varum. The proximal arm of the goniometer is aligned with the bisection of the distal one-third of the tibiofibular complex, and the distal arm is level with the floor. The axis of measurement shifts with the degree of varum or valgum deformity and may not always fall directly behind the calcaneus.

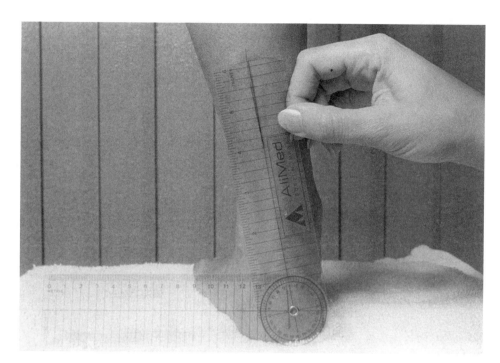

iner is looking for evidence of genu recurvatum or excessive knee flexion, navicular drop, talar bulge, and inadequate or excessive height of the longitudinal arch.

Genu Recurvatum or Flexion
Viewing stance from the side, the examiner observes the verticality of the tibia. In genu recurvatum the proximal tibia is aligned behind the axis of the TCJ.[36] This results in hyperextension of the knee and plantar flexion of the TCJ with relative shortening of the limb. Genu recurvatum also occurs as a compensation for equinus deformity at the ankle. When true leg length discrepancy is present, two types of compensation are possible. Genu recurvatum may adequately shorten the longer limb when the limb length difference is small. For larger limb length differences excessive knee flexion of the longer limb may be necessary.

Navicular Drop
The position of the navicular is ascertained using the navicular drop test as described by Brody.[66] It is a composite measure of foot pronation that focuses on the displacement of the navicular tuberosity as a subject moves from closed kinetic chain STN to RCS position. Excessive navicular displacement is associated with collapse of the MLA and may be correlated with midfoot pain or other

symptoms of excessive foot pronation.[36] The work of Subotnick[67] established an interdependency between MTJ and STJ function because of articulation of the navicular and cuboid with the talus and calcaneus. Brody[66] concluded that the navicular drop test was a valid assessment of STJ function in the closed kinetic chain. Although navicular drop occurs with STJ pronation that stems from intrinsic foot deformity, it can also be the result of muscle insufficiency or ligamentous laxity.[36]

To measure navicular drop, an index card is positioned perpendicular to the medial side of the foot, the level of the navicular tuberosity is marked in STJ neutral and in RCS, and the distance between the marks is calculated.[38] Normative studies by Mueller et al.[68] and Picciano et al.[38] report a mean navicular drop of between 7.3 and 9.0 mm. Mueller et al. suggest that a navicular drop of more than 10 mm should be considered abnormal.

Talar Bulge and Arch Height
When the STJ pronates excessively in stance, the talus moves into adduction and plantar flexion. Displacement of the talar head causes an observable medial bulge in the region of the talonavicular joint.[69] The height of the MLA normally decreases moderately in weight bearing as a result of normal STJ pronation. Pes planus deformity (flatfootedness) is a common condition characterized by exces-

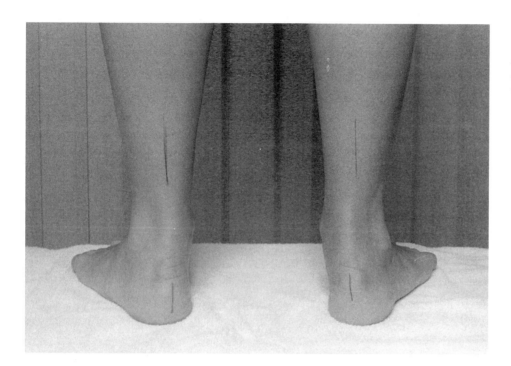

FIGURE 8-15

Toe sign, demonstrating excessive transverse plane motion as evidenced by the abducted position of the forefoot.

sive collapse of the MLA. A rigid flatfoot is a hereditary condition in which the MLA is low or absent in non–weight-bearing and weight-bearing positions. In a flexible flatfoot, the height of the MLA is normal in non–weight bearing but drops excessively in weight bearing because of abnormal STJ pronation. In normal foot alignment, the medial malleolus, navicular tuberosity, and first metatarsal head fall along the "Feiss line."[69] In a severely pronated foot, the navicular tuberosity lies below this Feiss line. In extreme cases the tuberosity may even rest on the floor.[69,70]

Transverse Plane

The final component of the static weight-bearing examination considers foot function in the transverse plane. The examiner looks for signs of excessive pronation or forefoot adduction and for torsional deformities of the lower extremities.

Toe Sign

The toe sign is a clinical indication of excessive pronation or abduction of the foot in the transverse plane. It is determined by the number of toes that can be seen, in a posterior view, when the patient is standing in RCS with a neutral foot placement angle.[58] Normally, no more than one and one-half toes are visible beyond the lateral border of the foot. If more toes can be seen, the foot may be

excessively pronated, causing excessive transverse plane motion or abduction of the foot (Figure 8-15). A false-positive toe sign can occur in the presence of a relative toe-out foot placement angle associated with lateral rotational deformities (e.g., femoral retroversion) or muscle imbalances that limit internal rotation of the hip (e.g., tight piriformis). Ensuring that the patient's patellae are oriented in the frontal plane before assessing toe sign reduces the risk of false-positive findings.

Torsional Deformities of the Lower Extremities

Transverse plane abnormalities of the femur and tibia also adversely affect normal foot functioning. The femoral shaft normally has 12 degrees of medial rotation relative to the femoral head and neck. Anteversion occurs when more than 12 degrees of rotation is present; retroversion occurs when there is less.[69] In normal transverse plane tibial alignment, the fibular malleolus is situated posterior to the tibial malleolus, for 20–30 degrees of lateral rotation.[69] Large amounts of internal tibial torsion or femoral anteversion increase medial rotational forces, causing abnormal foot pronation. Excessive external tibial rotation or femoral retroversion increases lateral rotational forces, causing abnormal foot supination.

To assess femoral torsion, the patient is positioned prone with the knee in 90 degrees flexion.[36] The examiner palpates the lateral border of the greater trochanter, then moves the patient's tibia inward (for hip external rotation) and outward (for hip internal rotation). At the point where the lateral aspect of the greater trochanter is most prominent, torsion is measured. The stationary arm of the goniometer is held parallel to the surface of the treatment table; the mobile arm bisects the proximal lower leg. The angular displacement represents femoral torsion. Normally, the femur is anteverted approximately 12 degrees, which results in a tibial alignment that appears to be internally rotated. If vertical alignment of the tibia is present, this indicates femoral retroversion.

To assess tibial torsion, the patient lies in the supine position with the ankle dorsiflexed to 90 degrees and the leg placed neutrally in the frontal plane. The examiner, at the end of the treatment table, holds the stationary arm of the goniometer parallel to the table surface. The mobile arm of the goniometer is aligned with the TCJ axis as it passes through the medial and lateral malleoli. This angular displacement represents tibial torsion. Normally, 20 degrees of external tibial torsion is present.

DYNAMIC GAIT ASSESSMENT

The final component of the clinical evaluation is observation of foot function during walking. Many clinicians videotape patients walking on a runway or treadmill to aid in accuracy of assessment. The function of the rear foot, midfoot, and forefoot is examined at each of the subphases of the gait cycle, with special attention to compensatory gait mechanisms.

FUNCTIONAL FOOT ORTHOSES

Although 4–6 degrees of triplanar STJ pronation is necessary to provide adequate shock absorption and accommodation to uneven ground terrain, persistent or recurrent abnormal pronation disrupts normal temporal sequencing of the gait cycle.[5,8,31,71] This disruption creates an unstable osseous and arthrokinematic situation that often leads to musculoskeletal pathology.[5,36] Compensatory motions occur in the primary plane of a given deformity. Frontal plane deformities (e.g., rear foot varus or forefoot varus) have a frontal plane compensatory motion, eversion at the STJ. Transverse plane deformities (e.g., torsional deformities of the hip, femur, or tibia) have transverse plane compensatory motion, adduction at the STJ. Sagittal plane deformities (e.g., ankle equinus) have sagittal plane compensatory motion, dorsiflexion at the STJ. Root's model suggests that single plane compensatory motion is beneficial, allowing adequate accommodation for a deformity.[5]

Because the STJ is a triplanar structure, however, movement in one plane leads to movement in the others as well. The associated motion of the other planes has the potential to become dysfunctional and destructive.[5]

A functional foot orthosis is an orthopedic device designed to promote structural integrity of the joints of the foot and lower limb by resisting the GRFs that cause abnormal skeletal motion during the stance phase of gait.[43] A foot orthosis attempts to control abnormal foot functioning during the stance phase by controlling excessive STJ and MTJ motion, decelerating pronation, and allowing the STJ to function closer to its neutral position at midstance.[72-74]

What Is Abnormal Pronation?

Five criteria are used to determine if pronation is abnormal. Pronation is considered to be an abnormal mechanical condition when

1. STJ pronation is more than the normal 4–6 degrees.[5,8,31,71]
2. The foot pronates at the wrong time, disrupting the normal sequencing of events during closed kinetic chain motion.
3. Pronation is recurrent, with each step contributing to repetitive microtrauma to musculoskeletal structures.
4. Pronation happens at a location other than the STJ (e.g., when MTJ pronation compensates for limited STJ motion).
5. Unnecessary destructive compensatory motion occurs in the other planes of motion of the STJ.[5]

Pathologic Conditions and Foot Function

Three pathologic situations lead to abnormal foot mechanics: (1) structural malalignment, (2) muscle weakness or imbalance, and/or (3) loss of structural integrity. Structural malalignment can be intrinsic or extrinsic to the foot or caused by abnormal mechanical forces.[5] Rear foot and forefoot varus and valgus, ankle equinus, and deformities of the rays are examples of intrinsic deformities. Congenital and developmental conditions, such as tibial varum or valgum, torsional deformities of the tibia or femur, or other conditions that occur above the foot and ankle, are extrinsic deformities. The types of abnormal mechanical forces that might contribute to pathomechanical foot function include obesity, leg length discrepancies, and genu valgum or varum. The goal of orthotic management when structural malalignment is present is preventative:

Control of aberrant or excessive STJ and MTJ motion forestalls the sequence of mechanical events associated with abnormal pronation or supination, minimizing the consequences of painful foot conditions.

A variety of upper and lower motor neuron diseases result in muscular weakness, abnormal muscle tone, or paralysis of the foot, with resultant instability of foot structure and reduced mechanical efficiency during gait.[40] In Charcot-Marie-Tooth disease (hereditary sensory motor neuropathy), for example, there is weakness of the foot intrinsics and peroneal and anterior tibial musculature.[75] As a result, patients with hereditary sensory motor neuropathy develop a "cavus" foot, with claw toes, metatarsus adductus, or other deformities of the rays.[40] When muscle weakness or imbalance is present, the examiner must identify its origin and extent, the specific soft tissue structures involved, the resultant mechanical foot deformities, and the potential to reduce them. An effective foot orthosis for a patient with muscular weakness deters the pathomechanical sequelae that result from such induced structural foot deformities.

Compromised joint integrity and mechanical instability can also be caused by musculoskeletal pathologies of the foot or ankle, including arthritis, acute trauma, or chronic repetitive injury. In rheumatoid arthritis, for example, joint deformity results from synovitis and pannus formation. Autodestruction of connective tissue weakens tendons, contributes to muscle spasm and shortening, and erodes cartilaginous surfaces. Eventually, joint dislocations will occur.[76]

The loss of protective sensation associated with peripheral neuropathy also contributes to compromised joint integrity. Patients with diabetes mellitus, chronic alcoholism, or Hansen's disease (leprosy) are particularly vulnerable. Inability to perceive microtrauma due to sensory compromise, weakness of instrinsic muscles of the foot, compromised autonomic control of the distal blood floor, and the poor nutritional and metabolic state of soft tissues combine to increase the risk of plantar foot ulceration. If neuropathic (Charcot's) osteoarthropathy occurs, significant bone and joint destruction, collapse of the midfoot, and a fixed rocker bottom deformity can result. Plantar ulceration at the apex of the collapsed cuneiforms or cuboid is common.[77]

Whenever mechanical instability is present, normal joint orientation is altered, and gait compensation shifts weight-bearing forces. A foot orthosis can be used to reduce pain, reduce weight-bearing stresses, control abnormal or excessive joint motion, or compensate for restricted motion.

GOALS OF ORTHOTIC INTERVENTION

The goals of orthotic intervention, regardless of the etiology of foot dysfunction, are to

1. Control the velocity of pronation
2. Redistribute plantar pressures
3. Support abnormal structural forefoot positions that lead to abnormal rear foot function in stance
4. Support abnormal rear foot deformities that cause excessive STJ pronation
5. Resist extrinsic forces of the leg that cause aberrant pronation and supination of the foot
6. Improve calcaneal positioning at heel strike
7. Reposition the STJ in neutral position just before heel rise
8. Fully pronate the MTJ, when the STJ is in neutral, to lock and stabilize the foot, converting it into a rigid lever for propulsion
9. Allow normal plantar flexion of the first ray, stabilizing the forefoot in response to the retrograde GRFs sustained during propulsion
10. Provide for a normal degree of contact phase shock absorption

The functional foot orthosis does not support the MLA of the foot; STJ pronation is controlled by the pressure of the rear foot post on the calcaneus at the sustentaculum tali. The ultimate goal is to stop, reduce, or slow down abnormal compensatory motion of the joints of the foot as the foot and leg interact with the GRFs.

MEASUREMENT AND FABRICATION PROCESS

The information gathered in the non–weight-bearing and static weight-bearing examinations and in gait analysis provides direction for orthotic prescription. To fabricate an orthosis, a simple plaster cast is used to make an accurate negative impression of the patient's foot in STN position. A positive model based on this impression is then prepared. Thermoplastic materials are heat molded over the model to form an orthotic shell. Accommodative padding, soft tissue supplements, and covering materials are added to address the patient's functional foot problem. The orthosis is fitted to the patient, and its effect on foot function during gait is evaluated. An early wearing schedule is devised, and an appointment for a recheck visit is scheduled.

Negative Impression

If a foot orthosis is to control abnormal pronation or supination effectively and minimize painful symptoms in gait, the negative foot impression must precisely duplicate the existing foot structure, including any intrinsic deformities. The goal of the foot impression is to capture the patient's STN position during the midstance phase of the gait cycle. Several methods are available for taking negative impressions: suspension technique, modified suspension technique, direct pressure technique, foam impression systems, semi–weight bearing, and in-shoe vacuum casts. Because maintenance of STN position and correct loading of the forefoot are difficult to control in weight-bearing impression techniques, suspension and direct pressure non–weight-bearing techniques appear to be the most reliable methods for making accurate negative impressions. The direct pressure technique, one of the easiest procedures to learn, captures STN position by loading the fourth and fifth metatarsal heads to mimic GRFs during midstance (Figure 8-16). For further information relating to alternative casting procedures the reader is referred to other resources.[78,79]

Direct Pressure Impression Technique

The patient is placed prone, in the figure-four position used for goniometric measurement. Two double-layer thickness wraps of 5-in. plaster of Paris bandage are used to make the negative cast. The first wrap is cut to surround the foot from just distal to the fifth metatarsal head, around the posterior heel, to just beyond the first metatarsal head. The second wrap is cut so that, when draped over the plantar surface of the forefoot, it overlaps the first wrap at the metatarsals.

The first wrap is thoroughly moistened with tepid water. Any wrinkles in the mesh are smoothed. The top edge of the plaster splint is folded ½ in., providing reinforcement to prevent distortion when the cast is later removed. The first wrap is draped over the heel, just below the malleoli, and along the borders of the foot to just beyond the first and fifth metatarsal heads. Because total contact with the sole of the foot is essential, the plaster is carefully smoothed along the sides of the foot, across its plantar surface, and around the curves of the malleoli.

The second wrap is moistened and draped around the forefoot, overlapping the distal edges of the first layer. Any excess bandage is folded into the sulcus of the toes. This layer should also have a wrinkle-free total contact with the foot and toes.

Once both wraps are in place, the foot is positioned in STN by maintaining appropriate forefoot loading pressure at the fourth and fifth metatarsal heads. The plaster splint is sufficiently hardened when an audible click is produced when it is tapped. The negative cast is then carefully removed. The skin is gently pulled around the reinforced top edge to loosen contact from the cast. A downward force over the superior border of the heel cup is exerted to free the heel from the cast. Then, a gentle forward force is provided to free the forefoot and remove the cast from the foot.

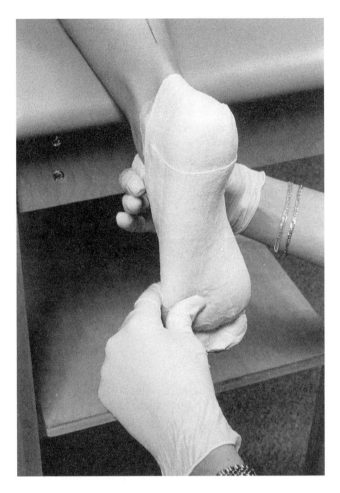

FIGURE 8-16

Negative cast impression via direct pressure technique. The foot is maintained in subtalar joint neutral position while the plaster hardens.

Errors to Avoid when Making a Negative Cast

Accuracy in the negative impression is the key to an effective orthotic. Although the casting procedure is a simple one, three common casting errors are made that compromise efficacy of orthotic design.

First, the foot may be inadvertently supinated at the longitudinal MTJ axis. This may be a result of contraction of the anterior tibialis, as the patient "helps" to hold the foot still. Alternatively, the loading force may be applied too far medially at the forefoot, creating a false forefoot varus. An orthosis manufactured from such a cast can cause excessive pressure plantar to the distal aspect of the first metatarsal shaft. It can also lead to lateral ankle instability or the development of a functional hallux limitus or HAV deformities.[80]

The second common casting error occurs when the foot is excessively supinated at the oblique MTJ axis. Improper

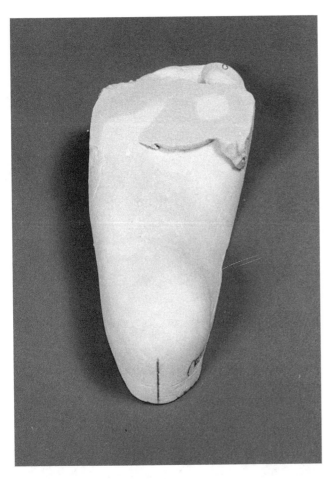

FIGURE 8-17
The modification process of forefront position on a positive cast.

peeled away, leaving a positive mold of the foot (Figure 8-17). Modifications to the positive cast assure an effective correction in foot alignment and function by redirecting forces through the foot. Those that are made to enhance comfort include plaster additions to relieve pressure-sensitive regions of the forefoot and MLA. Because the negative cast is taken in a non–weight-bearing position, it is also modified to allow for the elongation of the foot and expansion of the soft tissues in weight bearing. The cast is also modified to allow for normal plantar flexion of the first metatarsal during propulsion.[43,81] Intrinsic or extrinsic posts can be added for further correction of forefoot or rear foot deformity.

Forefoot Posting

Two techniques can be used to provide orthotic correction for forefoot deformity. Both are based on modification of the positive cast impression. The first, a traditional Root functional orthosis, uses an intrinsic correction. A plaster of Paris platform is applied to the positive cast at the level of the MTP joints to balance the abnormal forefoot to rear foot relationship (Figure 8-18). A lateral platform corrects forefoot valgus, and a medial platform corrects forefoot varus.[43] When the shell is pressed over the modified positive mold, it creates a convexity at the orthotic's distal anterior border. This posting technique achieves correction by effectively realigning the skeletal structure of the foot.[81] The intrinsic posting technique is often selected when shoe volume is limited, as with women's fashion footwear.

A second forefoot posting technique involves a variation of Root's original design, referred to as a *standard biomechanical orthosis*. In this technique a neutral platform is formed on the positive mold, but the existing valgus or varus position of the forefoot is maintained. An extrinsic forefoot post or wedge is attached to the bottom of the orthotic shell to support the forefoot in its position of deformity. In this manner unwanted compensatory motion is prevented by stabilizing the distal border of the orthosis (Figure 8-19A). Although an orthosis with an extrinsic correction takes up more space inside the shoe than does an intrinsically corrected orthosis, it affords the fabricator the advantage of ease in modification of the prescription if the patient has difficulty tolerating the original posting prescription.

Rear Foot Posting

As the foot contacts the ground and moves through stance during gait, GRFs act on the joints of the foot. An orthosis acts as an interface between the ground and the foot, creating its own orthosis reactive force. In a foot that pronates excessively, the foot orthosis is designed to decrease STJ pronation during weight bearing by creating a supina-

loading at the fourth and fifth metatarsal heads results in insufficient dorsiflexion of the forefoot. When this happens, transverse skin folds can be seen inside the negative cast at the MTJ. An orthosis manufactured from this cast creates an excessive sagittal plane angulation plantar to the calcaneocuboid joint (lateral longitudinal arch), with pain and irritation on weight bearing.[80]

The third error occurs when the STJ is excessively pronated during casting, placing the foot in a false forefoot valgus position. An orthosis manufactured from this cast does not capture neutral STJ position and is ineffective in controlling the symptoms of abnormal pronation.[80]

Positive Cast Modifications

Once a satisfactory negative impression of the patient's foot has been obtained, a positive cast is made and then modified. The hardened negative impression is filled with liquid plaster and allowed to dry. The negative cast is

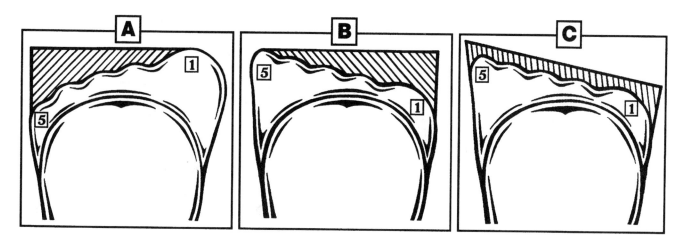

FIGURE 8-18

*Cross section at the level of the metatarsophalangeal joints, with first and fifth metatarsals labeled, demonstrating intrinsic modifications to the positive mold. (**A**) A lateral platform corrects forefoot valgus. (**B**) A medial platform corrects forefoot varus. (**C**) A neutral balancing platform maintains a forefoot alignment and serves as a base for extrinsic posts. (Used with permission from Stride, Inc., Middlebury, CT.)*

tion moment acting medial to the STJ axis.[2] This can be accomplished by adding an extrinsic rear foot post or wedge to the inferior surface of the heel cup or by modification of the plaster mold to incorporate an intrinsic rear foot post to the heel cup of the orthosis. A rear foot post effectively reduces rear foot pronation (eversion) during the contact phase of gait, as well as the angular velocity of eversion.[2,82,83]

Extrinsic rear foot posts are attached to the bottom of the orthosis shell beneath the heel (Figure 8-19B). A medial wedge or rear foot post increases orthosis reactive forces at the sustentaculum tali (medial to the STJ axis) to reduce abnormal STJ pronation. It also promotes stability of the heel by increasing the contact surface of the orthosis beneath the heel.[82,83] An intrinsic rear foot post can be made with a medial heel skive technique. A plaster modification is performed on the medial aspect of the heel of the positive mold to increase the amount of varus (medial) sloping within the heel cup of the orthosis in an effort to control pronation.[2] An intrinsic rear foot post reduces overall bulk of the orthosis for optimal fit within a shoe. A combination of intrinsic and extrinsic rear foot posting permits more correction than is possible with either method independently.

Orthotic Shell

To be effective, a functional orthosis must be made based on a neutral position model of the patient's foot. Prefabricated foot supports do not offer adequate control of foot motion or resistance to GRFs and therefore do not fulfill the criteria for a functional foot orthosis. A functional

custom orthosis, made of rigid or semirigid materials, can offer maximum resistance to weight-bearing forces and optimal realignment of foot structure. Accommodative orthoses, made of softer materials, support the arches of the foot and provide relief to pressure-sensitive areas, while offering minimal control of STJ motion.[84,85] A semifunctional orthosis is a hybrid of functional and accommodative orthotics that combines the motion effectiveness of a semirigid shell with soft posting and accommodative material to cushion the foot.

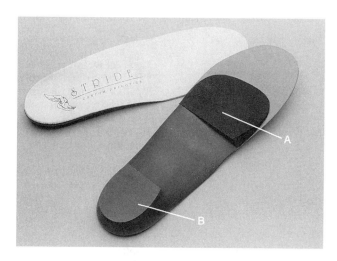

FIGURE 8-19

Standard biomechanical orthosis with an extrinsic forefoot post (A) and an extrinsic rear foot post (B).

Many studies have evaluated the effectiveness of the different types of orthotic materials in controlling rear foot mechanics and clinical symptoms.[84-88] Standards for the classification of materials (soft, semirigid, or rigid) have not yet been established. Olson[1] suggests that orthotic materials be classified by degree of rigidity.

A rigid orthosis achieves maximal motion control and biomechanical correction of a foot deformity, is lightweight, and takes up the least space within the shoe. Some clinicians are concerned that orthotics made of rigid materials are uncomfortable to the patient. Anthony[43] responds, "Practitioners who propose rigid devices to be patient intolerant are generally less acquainted with the theory of podiatric biomechanics and the correct diagnostics and prescription formularies that are critical for the provision of a truly functional foot orthosis."

Semirigid materials, such as polypropylene, TL-61, and TL-2100 (Medical Materials Corp., Camarillo, CA), are attractive alternatives to rigid orthotic shells. Polypropylene is a flexible olefin polymer that resists breakage. TL-2100 is a thermoplastic composite of resin and fiber that is harder and more rigid than polypropylene.[1]

Soft orthoses are often made of closed cell foams manufactured from heat-expanded polyethylene. Examples of such foams include Aliplast and Nickleplast (AliMed, Inc., Dedham, MA) and Plastazote (BXL Plastics Ltd, Croydon, UK), cross-linked polyethylene expanded foams that are available in many densities. Pelite (Durr-Fillover, Birmingham, AL) is an expanded, cross-linked, closed cell foam that can be heat molded in the fabrication of semi-flexible foot orthotics. Various rubberized or thermoplastic cork materials are also used.[1] Lightweight and available in different densities, these materials are effective in orthotics, in which accommodation and shock absorption are desirable. These same features limit the durability and the useful life of the orthotic, however, as these materials are prone to rapid and permanent shape deformation.[1]

Accommodative Padding and Soft Tissue Supplements

For some patients, extrinsic accommodative modifications are necessary to address a particular deformity. Examples of accommodative supplements are listed in Table 8-1.

Covering Materials

Once appropriate posts and supportive materials are attached to the shell of the orthosis, a covering material is applied to provide an interface with the skin of the foot. One commonly used orthosis-covering material is vinyl. Spenco (Spenco Medical Corp., Waco, TX) and various other fabric-covered neoprene materials are resistant to shearing and enhance shock absorption. They are often chosen as covering materials for certain sport orthoses when shear forces are expected to be high or for occupational situations that demand prolonged standing on hard surfaces.

TABLE 8-1

Accommodative Padding and Soft Tissue Supplements for Functional Foot Orthotics

Metatarsal mound	A dome-shaped addition in the form of a teardrop positioned with the apex just proximal to the metatarsal heads to support a collapsed transverse metatarsal arch. Often used to control symptoms of neuroma by reducing shearing of the metatarsals during contact phase. Reduction of the shearing eliminates irritation to the interdigital nerves of the forefoot.
2–5 Bar	A pad of uniform thickness placed beneath the second through the fifth metatarsal heads (MTHs) relieves pressure beneath the first MTH during propulsion. Used when there is a rigid plantar flexed first ray.
MTH cutout	A U-shaped pad positioned beneath a rigid plantar flexed MTH to relieve pressure from a painful callosity. Often used for hammertoe deformity.
Morton's extension	An extension of the plastic shell or the addition of an inlay made of dense material, beneath the shaft of the first metatarsal to the sulcus of the hallux. Often used for a dorsiflexed first ray or Morton's toe.
Heel cushion	Placed in the heel cup of the orthosis to enhance heel cushioning and shock absorption. Often made of the soft tissue–supplementing material Poron (Rodgers Co., Rogers, CT) or a viscoelastic polymer. Used when irritation or atrophy of the infracalcaneal fat pad is present or for calcaneal stress fracture.
Forefoot extension	A soft tissue–supplementing material such as Poron is added to the distal end of the orthosis shell to cushion the metatarsal heads or as a base for other forefoot inlays.
Scaphoid pad	A material of soft to medium density that is placed beneath the medial longitudinal arch to decelerate pronatory forces.

PRESCRIPTION PROCESS

During the stance phase of gait, 4–6 degrees of STJ pronation normally occurs. A fully compensated rear foot varus deformity of 10 degrees pronates at the STJ 10 degrees during gait to lower the medial condyle of the calcaneus to the ground, but only 6 degrees of this pronation is considered excessive. An appropriate orthotic design for varus deformities of the rear foot is a medial post or wedge. Because complete orthotic correction is not only difficult to achieve but often quite uncomfortable for the patient, the initial goal is often to create an orthosis that provides 50% correction of a rear foot deformity. To correct the excessive 6 degrees of pronation in this example, a medial rear foot post or wedge of 3 degrees would meet the goal of 50% correction.

If a patient with a rear foot varus deformity of 10 degrees is uncompensated to –5 degrees of calcaneal eversion, a medial or varus wedge of 3 degrees is not effective because the STJ would reach its end-range eversion motion (–5 degrees) before the orthotic provided support. To manage uncompensated rear foot deformity effectively, the varus wedge must be large enough to prevent the STJ from reaching its end ROM. In this example, a larger medial rear foot varus post or wedge of at least 5 degrees is necessary. When the rear foot is aggressively posted (more than 3 or 4 degrees of varus posting), the distal medial aspect of the orthosis shell loses contact with the ground, as if a forefoot varus deformity were present. In these circumstances, a medial forefoot post counteracts the induced apparent forefoot varus.

For forefoot varus deformities, a medial (varus) wedge or post is indicated. For forefoot valgus deformities, lateral (valgus) posts or wedges are used. Forefoot deformities can be corrected through intrinsic plaster modifications or extrinsic posting. For an orthosis to be accurately balanced so that it does not wobble, a forefoot deformity must be corrected to its fullest extent (e.g., an 8-degree forefoot varus deformity requires an 8-degree medial wedge or post). The addition of a large extrinsic post to the distal end of the orthotic shell often creates problems with shoe fit. One possible solution is to correct large forefoot deformities with a combination of intrinsic and extrinsic techniques. In this example, a 4-degree medial intrinsic plaster platform and a 4-degree extrinsic medial forefoot post or wedge would provide the desired correction without bulkiness. For patients with a forefoot varus deformity of 10 degrees or more, a semipronated or pronated negative cast can reduce the forefoot deformity to a more manageable degree.[78]

Plantar flexion of the first ray is managed according to the level of flexibility of the deformity. A fully flexible plantar flexed first ray deformity does not require orthotic intervention. A semirigid or rigid plantar flexed first ray deformity requires the addition of a metatarsal (second through fifth) bar inlay. The thickness of the inlay is determined by how far below the first metatarsal head lies relative to the plane of the remaining metatarsal heads. The orthotic intervention for patients with a rigid plantar flexed first ray and forefoot varus is an extended medial forefoot wedge. The forefoot post is modified with a cutout to accommodate the dropped first metatarsal head position. In some cases, a small forefoot varus deformity combined with a large, rigidly plantar flexed first ray deformity results in a functional forefoot valgus (see Figure 8-12).

Orthotic Checkout and Trouble Shooting

Delivery of an orthosis includes evaluation of its fit, comfort, and mechanical alignment. The shell of the orthosis should end just proximal to the metatarsal heads. The width is evaluated to ensure that normal first ray plantar flexion and propulsion are not compromised. The position of the orthosis within the shoe is also evaluated: Its volume, impact on heel height, points of excessive pressure, and tendency to cause pistoning during gait are considered. On initial fitting, many patients report that the orthosis feels slightly strange or unusual. The orthosis should not, however, cause undue discomfort. Fit and mechanical functioning of the orthosis are evaluated in standing and in walking. Patient education in appropriate break-in protocols and wearing schedules is also an important component of orthotic delivery. Usually, a new orthosis is worn for 2 hours on day one, 4 hours on day two, 6 hours on day three, and so forth, until the patient is able to wear the orthosis comfortably all day. A follow-up visit is scheduled after the patient has worn the orthosis for at least 2 weeks. By this time the patient should feel comfortable with use of the orthosis for normal activities of daily living. Thereafter, progressive increased use of the orthosis for all activities, including sport and occupational use, should be well tolerated. On occasion, adjustments are necessary to optimize patient comfort and mechanical alignment.

A FEW FINAL THOUGHTS

Recently, the efficacy of intervention through the use of foot orthoses has come into question. The effectiveness of a biomechanical foot orthosis is dependent on a sound understanding of the indications and contraindications of its use. Understanding the causes and effects of aberrant foot motion on pathologies of the foot is essential in determining the appropriate orthosis prescription and plan of care. Clinicians who do not carefully consider biomechanical principles and other factors that contribute to a patient's signs and symptoms may prescribe an ineffective or inappropriate orthosis. Information gathered from all three components of the biomechanical examination (non–weight bearing, static weight bearing, and dynamic gait assessment) is critical for orthotic design and prescription.

Historically, the principles and design of the Root functional orthosis and the biomechanical foot orthosis have had consistently effective clinical results. Root's model demands a keen understanding of foot biomechanics, careful prescription, and advanced fabrication skills. With this understanding and attention to detail, the end result is a lightweight, durable, cost-effective foot orthosis that substantially reduces the detrimental effects of aberrant foot motion.

REFERENCES

1. Olson WR. Orthotic Materials. In RL Valmassy (ed), Clinical Biomechanics of the Lower Extremities. St. Louis: Mosby–Year Book, 1996;307–326.
2. Kirby KA. The medial heel skive technique. Improving pronation control in foot orthoses. J Am Podiatry Med Assoc 1992;82(4):177–188.
3. Shuster RO. A history of orthopaedics in podiatry. J Am Podiatry Assoc 1974;64(5):322.
4. Rossi WA. Orthotics: the miracle cure-all? Footwear News 1995;22.
5. Root ML, Orien WP, Weed JH. Normal and Abnormal Function of the Foot (vol 2). Los Angeles: Clinical Biomechanics Corporation, 1977.
6. Burns ML. Biomechanics. In ED McGlamry (ed), Fundamentals of Foot Surgery. Baltimore: Williams & Wilkins, 1987;111–135.
7. Barnett CH, Napier JR. The axis of rotation at the ankle joint in man. Its influence upon the form of the talus and the mobility of the fibula. J Anat (Lond) 1952;86:1–9.
8. Hicks JH. The mechanics of the foot. Part I: The joints. J Anat 1953;87:345–347.
9. Isman RE, Inman VT. Anthropometric studies of the human foot and ankle. Bull Prosthet Res 1969;10–11:97–129.
10. Morris JM. Biomechanics of the foot and ankle. Clin Orthop 1977;122:10–17.
11. Norkin CC, Levangie PK. Joint Structure and Function. A Comprehensive Analysis (2nd ed). Philadelphia: Davis, 1992;379–419.
12. American Orthopedics Association. Manual of Orthopedic Surgery. Chicago: American Orthopedics Association, 1972; 69.
13. Boone DC, Azen SP. Normal range of motion of joints in male subjects. J Bone Joint Surg 1979;61A(5):756–759.
14. Rasmussen O, Tovberg-Jevsen I. Mobility of the ankle joint. Acta Orthop Scand 1982;53(1):155–160.
15. Lapidius PW. Kinesiology and mechanics of the tarsal joints. Clin Orthop 1963;30:20–35.
16. Kjaergaard-Andersen P, Wethelund J, Nielsen S. Lateral talocalcaneal instability following section of the calcaneofibular ligament: a kinesiologic study. Foot Ankle 1987;7(6):355–361.
17. Manter JT. Movements of the subtalar and transverse tarsal joints. Anat Rec 1941;80:397–410.
18. Phillips RD, Christeck R, Phillips RL. Clinical measurement of the axis of the subtalar joint. J Am Podiatry Assoc 1985;75(3):119–131.
19. Green DR, Carol A. Planal dominance. J Am Podiatry Med Assoc 1984;74(2):98–103.
20. Perry J. Anatomy and biomechanics of the hindfoot. Clin Orthop 1983;177:9–15.
21. Olerud C, Rosendahl Y. Torsion-transmitting properties of the hindfoot. Clin Orthop 1987;214:285–294.
22. Warwick R, Williams PL (eds). Gray's Anatomy (35th ed). Philadelphia: Saunders, 1973;373–385, 460–471, 571–585.
23. Elftman H. The transverse tarsal joint and its control. Clin Orthop 1960;16:41–45.
24. Sarafian SK. Anatomy of the Foot and Ankle: Descriptive, Topographic, Functional. Philadelphia: Lippincott, 1983.
25. Moore KL. Clinically Oriented Anatomy. Baltimore: Williams & Wilkins, 1980.
26. Hicks JH. The mechanics of the foot. Part II: The plantar aponeurosis and the arch. J Anat 1954;88:25–31.
27. Sarafian SK. Functional characteristics of the foot and plantar aponeurosis under tibiotalar loading. Foot Ankle 1987;8(1):1–4.
28. Perry J. Gait Analysis: Normal and Pathological Function. Thorofare, NJ: Slack, 1992;69–85.
29. Vaughn CL, Davis DL, O'Connor JC. Dynamics of Human Gait. Champaign, IL: Human Kinetics, 1992;7–14.
30. James SL, Jones DC. Biomechanical Aspects of Distance Running Injuries. In PR Cavanagh (ed), Biomechanics of Distance Running. Champaign, IL: Human Kinetics, 1990;249–271.
31. Wright DG, Desai M, Henderson WH. Action of the subtalar and ankle-joint complex during the stance phase of walking. J Bone Joint Surg 1964;46A(2):361–382.
32. Perry J, Hislop HJ. Principles of Lower Extremity Bracing. Washington, DC: American Physical Therapy Association, 1967;9–32.
33. Close JR, Todd FN. The phasic activity of the muscles of the lower extremity and the effect of tendon transfer. J Bone Joint Surg 1959;41A(2):189–208.
34. Valiant GA. Transmission and Attenuation of Heelstrike Accelerations. In PR Cavanagh (ed), Biomechanics of Distance Running. Champaign, IL: Human Kinetics Publishers, 1990;225–249.
35. D'Ambrosia RD. Orthotic devices in running injuries. Clin Sports Med 1985;4(4):611–619.
36. Gross MT. Lower quarter screening for skeletal malalignment. Suggestions for orthotics and shoewear. J Occup Sports Phys Ther 1995;21(6):389–405.
37. McPoil TG, Hunt GC. Evaluation and management of foot and ankle disorders. Present problems and future directions. J Occup Sports Phys Ther 1995;21(6):381–388.

38. Picciano AM, Rowlands MS, Worrell T. Reliability of open and closed kinetic chain subtalar joint neutral positions and navicular drop test. J Occup Sports Phys Ther 1993;18(4): 553–558.

39. Smith-Oricchio K, Harris BE. Interrater reliability of subtalar neutral, calcaneal inversion and eversion. J Occup Sports Phys Ther 1990;12(1):10–15.

40. Pratt D, Tollafield D, Johnson G, Peacock C. Foot Orthoses. In WA Wallace (ed), Biomechanical Basis of Orthotic Management. Oxford: Butterworth-Heinemann, 1993;70–98.

41. Wooded MJ. Biomechanical Evaluation for Functional Orthotics. In RA Donatelli (ed), The Biomechanics of the Foot and Ankle (2nd ed). Philadelphia: Davis, 1996; 168–183.

42. McPoil TG, Brocato RS. The Foot and Ankle. In JA Gould, GJ Davis (eds), Orthopaedics and Sports Physical Therapy. St. Louis: Mosby, 1985;322–325.

43. Anthony RJ. The Manufacture and Use of the Functional Foot Orthosis. Basel, Switzerland: Karger, 1991;1–178.

44. Elveru RA, Rothstein JM, Lamb RC. Goniometric reliability in a clinical setting. Subtalar and ankle joint measurements. Phys Ther 1988;68:672–677.

45. Garbalosa JC, McClure MH, Catlin PA, Wooden M. The frontal plane relationship of the forefoot to the rearfoot in an asymptomatic population. J Occup Sports Phys Ther 1994;20(4):200–206.

46. Lattanza L, Gray GW, Kantner RM. Closed versus open kinematic chain measurements of subtalar joint eversion. Implications for clinical practice. J Occup Sports Phys Ther 1988;9(9):310–314.

47. Diamond JE, Mueller MJ, Delitto A, Sinacore DR. Reliability of a diabetic foot evaluation. Phys Ther 1989;69:797–802.

48. Vitasalo JT, Kvist M. Some biomechanical aspects of the foot and ankle in athletes with and without shin splints. Am J Sports Med 1983;2(3):125–130.

49. Tiberio D. Evaluation of functional ankle dorsiflexion using subtalar neutral position. Phys Ther 1987;67(6):955–957.

50. Baggett BD, Young G. Ankle joint dorsiflexion. Establishment of a normal range. J Am Podiatry Med Assoc 1993;83(5): 251–254.

51. Hillstrom HJ, Perlberg G, Sieglers S, et al. Objective identification of ankle equinus deformity and resulting contracture. J Am Podiatry Med Assoc 1991;81:519.

52. Hill RS. Ankle equinus: prevalence and linkage to common foot pathology. J Am Podiatry Assoc 1995;85(6):295–300.

53. Hoppenfeld S. Physical Examination of the Spine and Extremities. Norwalk, CT: Appleton-Century-Crofts, 1976;197–235.

54. Tachdjian MO. The Child's Foot. Philadelphia: Saunders, 1985.

55. McGlamry ED, Kitting RW. Equinus foot. An analysis of the etiology, pathology, and treatment techniques. J Am Podiatry Assoc 1973;63:165.

56. Whitney AK, Green DR. Pseudo equinus. J Am Podiatry Assoc 1982;72:365.

57. Davidson RS. Deformities of the Child's Foot. In JG Sammarco (ed), Foot and Ankle Manual. Philadelphia: Lea & Febiger, 1991;296.

58. Donatelli RA. Abnormal Biomechanics. In RA Donatelli (ed), The Biomechanics of the Foot and Ankle. Philadelphia: Davis, 1990;32–65.

59. McPoil TG, Knecht HG, Schuit D. A survey of foot types in normal females between the ages of 18 and 30 years. J Occup Sports Phys Ther 1988;9(12):346–349.

60. Dananberg HJ. Gait style as an etiology to chronic postural pain. Part I: Functional hallux limitus. J Am Podiatry Med Assoc 1993;83(8):433–441.

61. Dananberg HJ. Gait style as an etiology to chronic postural pain. Part II: Postural compensatory process. J Am Podiatry Med Assoc 1993;83(11):615–624.

62. Gastwirth BW. Biomechanical Examination of the Foot and Lower Extremity. In RL Valmassy (ed), Clinical Biomechanics of the Lower Extremities. St. Louis: Mosby-Year Book, 1996;132–147.

63. Tomaro J. Measurement of tibiofibular varum in subjects with unilateral overuse symptoms. J Occup Sports Phys Ther 1995;21(2):86–89.

64. McPoil TG, Schuit D, Knecht HG. A comparison of three positions used to evaluate tibial varum. J Am Podiatry Med Assoc 1988;78:22–28.

65. Lohmann KN, Rayhel HE, Schneiderwind P, Danoff JV. Static measurement of tibial vara. Reliability and effect of lower extremity position. Phys Ther 1987;67:196–200.

66. Brody D. Techniques in evaluation and treatment of the injured runner. Orthop Clin North Am 1982;13(3): 541–558.

67. Subotnick SI. Biomechanics of the subtalar and midtarsal joints. J Am Podiatry Assoc 1975;65(8):756–764.

68. Mueller MJ, Host JV, Norton BJ. Navicular drop as a composite measure of excessive pronation. J Am Podiatry Med Assoc 1993;83(4):198–202.

69. Norkin C, Levangie P. Joint Structure and Function. A Comprehensive Analysis. Philadelphia: Davis, 1983;261–387.

70. Dahle LK, Mueller M, Delitto A, Diamond JE. Visual assessment of foot type and relationship of foot type to lower extremity injury. J Occup Sports Phys Ther 1991;14(2):70–74.

71. Close JR, Inman VT, Poor PM, Todd FN. The function of the subtalar joint. Clin Orthop 1967;50(1–2):159–179.

72. Donatelli R, Hurlbert C, Conaway D, Pierre R. Biomechanical foot orthotics. A retrospective study. J Occup Sports Phys Ther 1988;10(6):205–212.

73. Inman VT, Rolston HJ, Todd F. Human Walking. Baltimore: Williams & Wilkins, 1981.

74. Johnson MA, Donatelli R, Wooden M, et al. Effects of three different posting methods on controlling abnormal subtalar pronation. Phys Ther 1994;74(2):149–161.

75. Harper MC. Failed Treatment and Residual Deformity of the Midfoot and Hindfoot. In JG Sammarco (ed), Foot and Ankle Manual. Philadelphia: Lea & Febiger, 1991; 213–213.

76. Schumacher HR. Primer of the Rheumatoid Diseases (10th ed). Atlanta: The Arthritis Foundation, 1993;91.

77. Boulton A. Diabetic Neuropathy. In RG Frykberg (ed), The High Risk Foot in Diabetes Mellitus. New York: Churchill Livingstone, 1991;49–59.

78. Valmassy RL. Advantages and disadvantages of various casting techniques. J Am Podiatry Assoc 1979;69(12): 707–712.

79. McPoil TG, Schuit D, Knecht HG. Comparison of three methods used to obtain a neutral plaster foot impression. Phys Ther 1989;69(6):448–450.

80. Kirby KA. Troubleshooting Functional Foot Orthoses. In RL Valmassy (ed), Clinical Biomechanics of the Lower Extremities. St. Louis: Mosby–Year Book, 1996;327–348.

81. Philps JW. The Functional Foot Orthosis. Edinburgh: Churchill Livingstone, 1995;39–53.

82. Blake RL, Ferguson H. Extrinsic rearfoot posts. J Am Podiatry Med Assoc 1992;82(4):202–207.

83. Blake RL, Ferguson HJ. Effect of extrinsic rearfoot posts on rearfoot position. J Am Podiatry Med Assoc 1993;83(8):202.

84. Brown GP, Donatelli R, Catlin PA, Wooden MJ. The effects of two types of foot orthoses on rearfoot mechanics. J Occup Sports Phys Ther 1995;21(5):258–267.

85. Smith LS, Clarke TE, Hamill CL, Santopietro F. The effects of soft and semi-rigid orthoses upon movement in running. J Am Podiatry Med Assoc 1986;76(4):227–233.

86. Eng JJ, Pierrynowski MR. The effects of soft foot orthotics on three-dimensional lower-limb kinematics during walking and running. Phys Ther 1994;74(9):836–844.

87. Eng JJ, Pierrynowski MR. Evaluation of soft foot orthotics in the treatment of patellofemoral pain syndrome. Phys Ther 1993;73(2):62–70.

88. Rodgers MM, Leveau BF. Effectiveness of foot orthotic devices used to modify pronation in runners. J Occup Sports Phys Ther 1982;4(2):86–90.

9

Ankle-Foot Orthoses

ROBERT S. LIN

An ankle-foot orthosis (AFO) can be prescribed for patients with musculoskeletal or neuromuscular dysfunction to accomplish a variety of goals. For patients with an unstable ankle, whether from injury or muscular imbalance, an AFO can be used to support the foot and ankle, to maintain optimal functional alignment during activity, or to limit motion to protect healing structures. For patients with neuromotor dysfunction, the AFO can substitute for inadequate muscle function during key points in the gait cycle, can optimize alignment and help to manage abnormal tone, or can minimize the risk of deformity (e.g., equinovarus) associated with long-term hypertonicity. In this chapter, we focus on the AFO as a means to improve gait in children and adults with neuromuscular dysfunction, such as in cerebral palsy or after stroke. For a discussion of orthotic management of common musculoskeletal injuries of the ankle, the reader is referred to Epler.[1]

The development of a prescription for an AFO usually involves an interdisciplinary team (orthotist, therapist, physician, patient, and primary caregiver). The combined knowledge and skills of the team ensure that the prescription will best match orthotic design to the patient's functional needs. To create an optimal prescription, the team must consider a number of important issues. First, the biomechanical and neuromotor aspects of normal human locomotion must be thoroughly understood. With this foundation, team members are able to recognize primary gait pathologies and their most common compensations and to select appropriate components or design from among the many options. Second, an understanding of the specific disease or disorder is also essential; this includes the natural history and likely prognosis and the types of secondary musculoskeletal problems commonly encountered, as well as any cognitive or other multisystem involvement that may be associated with the disease. Practical issues, such as who will be responsible for applying (donning) or removing (doffing) the device and the ease with which this can be accomplished must also be considered if the optimal orthotic outcome is to be achieved.

PREREQUISITES OF FUNCTIONAL GAIT

Four fundamental prerequisites are necessary for safe, energy-efficient walking.[2] First, the lower limb must be stable enough to accept and support body weight during stance phase, especially in the period of single limb support. Second, clearance of the foot must be adequate during swing phase. Third, the foot must be properly pre-positioned in preparation for initial contact and loading response in early stance. Fourth, at the same time, precise control and adequate motion must be present at the foot, ankle, knee, and hip if step length is to be efficient and adequate. If any of these components is compromised, the energy cost of walking significantly increases, and safety during upright mobility becomes a concern. For some patients whose neuromuscular dysfunction substantially interferes with these prerequisites, functional ambulation may be an unrealistic goal unless an appropriate orthosis is provided.

Stability in Stance

When the support limb is in stance phase, it is called on to respond to the biomechanical forces that act on the body with substantial stability. In the presence of neuromotor or musculoskeletal dysfunction, an orthosis can effectively augment function by supporting anatomic structures that are prone to angulation or weakness, or both, during loading. The application of a three-point force mechanism of an AFO can moderate dynamic (nonfixed) functional defor-

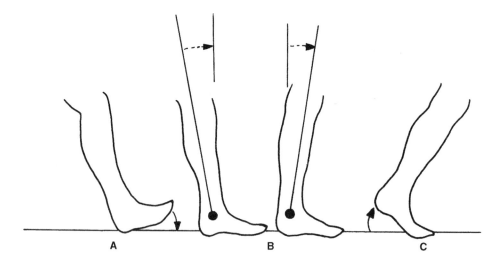

FIGURE 9-1
*Three transitional rocker periods occur as the body moves forward over the foot during stance. (**A**) During first rocker, the transition from swing into early stance, controlled lowering of the forefoot occurs, with a fulcrum at the heel. (**B**) During second rocker, controlled forward progression of the tibia over the foot occurs, with motion of the talocrural joint of the ankle. (**C**) In the third rocker, transition from stance toward swing occurs as the heel rises, with dorsiflexion of the metatarsophalangeal joints.*

mities, such as ankle varus, by optimally positioning the limb and providing an external support for effective single limb stance. A dynamic ankle varus deformity, which is commonly encountered in spastic cerebral palsy or after stroke, can be effectively controlled with the application of key forces with the orthosis. For example, the distal lateral force serves as a fulcrum for forces applied at the proximal-medial tibia and distal medial foot (see Figure 5-6). An additional force system controls dorsiflexion/plantar flexion position in the sagittal plane: The fulcrum is at the anterior ankle, and the counterforces are applied at the plantar surface of the foot and the posterior proximal calf.

Clearance in Swing

In normal gait, synergistic hip and knee flexion combined with dorsiflexion of the ankle (to a neutral position) during midswing provides just enough elevation for effective clearance of the foot. The ability to clear the foot without dragging or catching the toes is often compromised in patients with neuromuscular or musculoskeletal impairment. Weakness of dorsiflexor muscles, an abnormal extensor synergy pattern of the lower extremity, or both effectively "lengthen" the swing limb such that toe clearance cannot be achieved. An AFO of appropriate design and strength can position the foot and ankle to enhance clearance. An AFO cannot, however, compensate for inadequate knee or hip flexion.

Swing Phase Pre-Positioning

Preparation for initial contact, as swing phase ends, is similar in many ways to that of an airplane just before landing: The plane's nose is held slightly upward, its wings are level, and its tail is slightly down. At the end of swing

phase, while the extremity is "airborne," the ankle-foot complex is preparing to accept forces imposed during loading in early stance: The toes are up as a result of knee extension and ankle dorsiflexion to neutral, the foot is level without excessive inversion or eversion, and the heel is positioned to make first contact with the ground. Optimal alignment of the foot-ankle complex is essential for successful pre-positioning in preparation for stance.

Determinants of Step Length

Step length is determined by two things: appropriately timed activity of proximal musculature and the pendulum effect of the lower limb below the knee during swing. Sagittal plane stability at the talocrural joint in terminal stance and preswing also contributes to step length. As a first-class lever, a stable talocrural joint facilitates effective forward propulsion of the limb in swing. When this stability is compromised, propulsion is less effective and step length will be curtailed.

ROCKERS OF STANCE PHASE IN GAIT

Three transitional periods (rockers) occur during stance phase as the body progresses forward over the foot[2] (Figure 9-1). The first rocker (heel rocker) begins at initial contact and ends when the foot-flat position is achieved in loading response. During the first rocker, a controlled deceleration of the foot toward the floor occurs as well as an acceptance of body weight as the limb is loaded. In individuals with normal neuromotor function, eccentric contraction of the quadriceps and anterior tibialis prevents "foot slap" and protects the knee as ground reaction forces are translated upward toward the knee. During the second rocker (ankle rocker) the tibia advances over the ankle-foot complex, from approximately 10 degrees of plantar flexion at the end of loading response to 10 degrees of dorsiflexion at the end of midstance. The gastrocnemius-soleus complex contracts eccentrically to control the speed (deceleration) of forward tibial progression. The third and final rocker (toe rocker) begins as the heel rises off the ground surface, and body weight rolls over the first metatarsophalangeal joint through push-off in terminal stance. During fast walking, acceleration, rather than deceleration, actually occurs as active contraction of the gastrocnemius-soleus complex propels the foot and leg into swing phase.

Because most lower extremity orthoses provide external stability, they necessarily have an impact on the smooth transition through one or more of the stance phase rockers. Any disruption of forward progression compromises the mobility parameters of gait, such as step length, cadence, and single support time. An effective orthotic intervention attempts to balance the patient's need for external stability with the orthosis' potentially deleterious effects on mobility. The goal is to provide the minimal amount of stability necessary, so that the greatest amount of mobility is possible. For patients with dorsiflexion weakness, the primary gait problems are swing clearance, pre-positioning for initial contact, and controlled lowering of the foot in early stance. The optimal orthotic design would address these issues without restricting forward progression of the tibia in the second rocker or rolling over the forefoot in the third rocker. A patient with significant extensor hypertonicity and equinovarus, however, may have a greater need to control foot and ankle position throughout stance, such that all three rockers of gait may be compromised. Shoe modifications, such as a rocker bottom sole, can be used to compensate for some of this compromise in mobility. The rehabilitation team weighs the impact of stability provided by an orthosis on progression through stance with its impact on a patient's functional status: At times compromise is unavoidable if the patient's functional deficits are to be addressed effectively.

BIOMECHANICAL PRINCIPLES OF ANKLE-FOOT ORTHOSES

To understand the biomechanical principles of AFOs, one must understand the functional anatomy of the ankle-foot complex itself. Dorsiflexion and plantar flexion of the ankle occur as the talus rotates through the mortise of the ankle. The interior of the mortise is formed from the syndesmosis (fibrous articulation) between the distal tibia and the distal fibula. The medial malleolus is the downward extension of the tibia. The corresponding lateral

malleolus of the fibula is slightly longer and more posteriorly located. The shape of the articular surfaces of the talus and mortise, combined with spatial orientation of the malleoli, results in a joint axis that is slightly oblique. Because the axis of motion runs in an anteromedial to posterolateral direction, motion occurs in more than one plane. Dorsiflexion is associated with forefoot pronation with abduction and hind foot valgus, whereas plantar flexion is accompanied by forefoot supination with adduction and hind foot varus.

If a lower extremity orthotic includes mechanical ankle joints, it is essential that the axis of the mechanical joints be aligned, as closely as possible, to the obliquely oriented anatomic axis of motion (Figure 9-2). Although no mechanical ankle joints are able to model the multiplanar motion of the anatomic ankle exactly, approximating this axis reduces the likelihood of abnormal torque and shearing between the orthosis and limb during gait. Typically, a pair of mechanical joints is incorporated into the medial and lateral aspects of the orthosis. The distal border (tip)

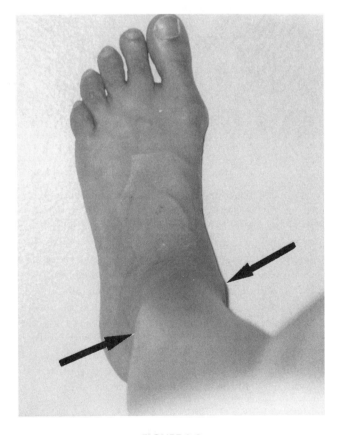

FIGURE 9-2
Alignment of the mechanical ankle joint axes must reflect the degree of external rotation/tibial torsion that is present in the transverse plane.

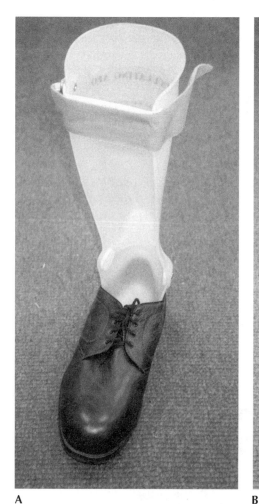

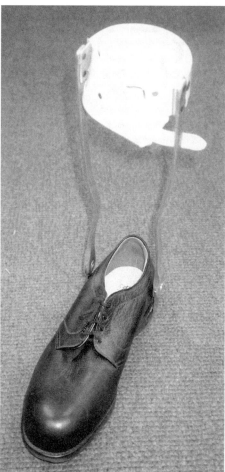

A   B

FIGURE 9-3
(A) A custom-molded, thermo-plastic, hinged-ankle ankle-foot orthosis closely follows the contours of the limb, with its intimate fit providing excellent motion control. (B) A conventional double upright hinged-ankle ankle-foot orthosis with shoe stirrup and calf band may be appropriate when limb volume fluctuates significantly.

of the medial malleolus is used as a reference point for placement of the mechanical joint in the coronal plane. A horizontal line that bisects the medial and lateral malleolus at the same height from the ground is used to position the lateral joint. In the transverse plane, the mechanical joint axes should be parallel to each other, to follow the line of progression and degree of external rotation dictated by the patient's tibial torsion. The specific mechanical joint heads are placed at approximately midline of the malleoli in the sagittal plane. If significant incongruency is present between the anatomic and mechanical axes, excessive motion of the extremity within the orthoses and a limitation of motion and efficiency of the mechanical joint often occur.

MATERIALS AND METHODOLOGIES

The development of thermoplastic materials has had a profound impact on the design and manufacture of lower extremity orthoses. Although AFOs can be constructed of a variety of materials, including metals, leathers, and thermosetting materials, the many advantages of thermoplastics have made them the material of choice for the majority of patients who require AFOs today. When compared to the metal double upright AFO designs of the polio era, today's themoplastic AFOs are significantly lighter weight, are much more cosmetic and comfortable to wear, and can be worn in more than one pair of shoes (Figure 9-3). A custom-molded AFO is heat formed over a positive model of the patient's own limb. The resulting intimate fit provides more effective control of the extremity than is possible with a traditional double upright AFO, with which control is limited by the structural integrity and fit of the patient's shoe. The closely fitting molded AFO effectively distributes forces exerted on the limb more broadly over the limb's surface area, reducing the potential of high pressure and skin breakdown. This is especially beneficial for patients with sensory impairment, who would not recognize discomfort and skin irritation from friction or high pressure within a shoe. The only true contraindication of a custom-molded thermoplastic design is significantly fluctuating limb size, associated with edema of the braced extremity. When the limb is at its lowest volume, the intimacy of fit can be lost so that excessive movement of the limb within the orthosis occurs. When the limb is significantly edematous, the intimate fit of the AFO may be too constricting, leading to pressure-related problems. In this instance, the total contact of a molded design may be inappropriate, and a conventional double upright system should be considered. Aside from this, continued development of new manufacturing techniques and the introduction of composite reinforcements clearly make thermoplastic the material of choice for construction of the majority of AFOs.

Thermosetting materials have also been used in the fabrication of AFOs (Figure 9-4). Manufacture of a thermoset AFO is a time- and labor-intensive process: Multiple layers of material must be laminated together; layers are often reinforced with glass or carbon fibers. Thermosetting materials are used when a high degree of stiffness is desired. It is important to note, however, that thermoset materials cannot be heat molded to adjust fit. These materials also tend to fail at points of high stress. In virtually all instances, a thermoplastic version can be fabricated in less time and for less cost than these other materials.

Custom-Molded Orthoses

AFOs can be prefabricated, custom fit, or custom molded. Custom-molded orthoses require casting of the affected body part to obtain a negative mold in the desired alignment. Once the cast is set and removed, it is filled with plaster of Paris to obtain a positive model of the patient's extremity. This positive model is rectified or modified to provide pressure relief in intolerant areas (e.g., around a bony prominence) or to apply corrective or stabilizing forces as dictated by the design of the orthotic. This modification sequence is the most critical design step in the determination of biomechanical forces and orthotic fit and function. The first step in the manufacture of a custom-molded AFO is casting for an accurate negative mold of the patient's limb. One or two rolls of plaster gauze wrap are smoothed over the limb, and then the limb is held in optimal alignment until the cast is set. The flexible tubing along the anterior leg is used as a guide for cast removal (see Figure 2-2).

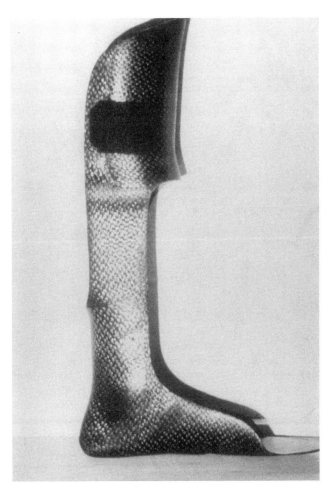

FIGURE 9-4

This floor reaction ankle-foot orthosis was fabricated using carbon graphite and fiberglass in a thermosetting process because of the desire to provide maximum stiffness. The combination of a solid-ankle design and an anterior wall produces a knee extension moment at midstance and enhances stance phase stability.

Prefabricated Orthoses

Prefabricated orthoses are mass produced in a variety of "typical" sizes and in a variety of materials. Most have generous contouring, although the degree to which they can be modified or adjusted to fit an individual patient varies. Although they are much less expensive than custom-molded AFOs, their ability to achieve desired control of motion as well as their durability can be compromised by the quality of material used and the lack of intimate fit. Prefabricated orthoses are often used by therapists as an evaluative tool to determine which orthotic design might best meet the patient's needs or as an interim device while a custom orthotic is being prepared.

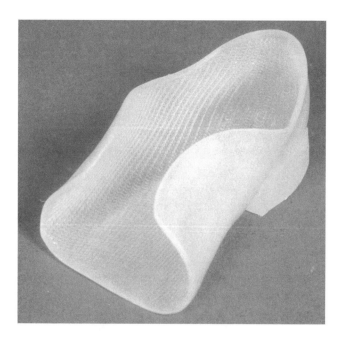

FIGURE 9-5

The University of California Biomechanics Laboratory orthosis is designed to position the calcaneus optimally for effective subtalar joint function. The deep heel cup, with its high medial and lateral trimlines, snugly holds the calcaneus. The orthosis also encompasses the joints of the midfoot, providing support for the longitudinal arch. In this example, a medial post (Gillette modification) has been added.

Custom-Fit Orthoses

Some manufacturers provide an orthotic "blank" that can be custom fit for a given patient using various heating or relieving techniques, or application of additional materials, to obtain as close a fit as possible. Although custom-fit devices provide better orthotic control than do most prefabricated versions, they often do not achieve the same accuracy of fit and degree of function that a custom-molded orthosis is able to provide.

Many factors influence the decision as to whether to choose a prefabricated, custom-fit, or custom-molded orthosis. The patient's functional needs are paramount but must be tempered by access to an orthotist for fit, education, and service; the rate of growth and need for ongoing adjustments; anticipated length of time that the orthosis will be required; likelihood of progression of dysfunction or evolution of deformity as it relates to preciseness of orthotic control; and, of course, cost of the orthosis. Many current health insurance plans have limitations in coverage for orthotic devices, leaving the patient with proportional out-of-pocket expense.

NAMING ANKLE-FOOT ORTHOSES

It is important to note that the acronyms used to name lower extremity orthotics describe joints that the orthotic encompasses, not necessarily all the joints in which functions are affected by the orthosis.[3] The foot orthosis category includes arch supports, biomechanical foot orthoses, University of California Biomechanics Laboratory (UCBL) orthoses, and heel cups. A supramalleolar orthosis (SMO) encompasses the ankle-foot complex but terminates just above the proximal border of the medial malleolus. An AFO may include a toe plate under the phalanges, a heel cup that holds the subtalar joint in neutral, a mechanical ankle joint with a plantar flexion stop, and a proximal trimline reaching a level just distal to the tibial tubercle on the anterior surface and an inch below the apex of the fibular head laterally. In addition to affecting function of the foot-ankle complex, this AFO also has a biomechanical impact at the knee and hip.

THE UCBL ORTHOSIS

Subtalar instability is a functional problem that can be effectively addressed by an orthotic intervention. In the 1970s, researchers at the University of California Biomechanics Laboratory developed a custom-molded shoe insert, now known as the *UCBL orthosis*[4] (Figure 9-5). The UCBL is very effective in controlling flexible calcaneal deformities (rear foot valgus or varus) as well as transverse plane deformities of the midtarsal joints (forefoot abduction or adduction).[5] The UCBL differs from the biomechanical foot orthosis described in the previous chapter in its intimate rear foot fit, which "grabs" the calcaneus, and its hold on the midfoot with high medial and lateral trimlines. The UCBL is based on the premise that the calcaneus is the key structure for subtalar joint orientation. The orthosis realigns the calcaneus, improving the angle of pull of the Achilles tendon, and proves a more stable foundation for the articular surfaces of the talus, navicular, and cuboids. The UCBL also is able to restore and support a supple longitudinal arch deformity. The Gillette modification, an external post positioned either on the medial or lateral border of the heel cup, can be used to apply additional rotatory moments to the calcaneus during weight bearing.

As with other custom orthoses, the UCBL begins with the patient's limb casted in a subtalar neutral position to provide a negative mold and create a positive model of the foot. Once the positive model is appropriately rectified and modified, thermoplastic material is heat molded, cooled, and trimmed to form the UCBL orthosis. The UCBL orthosis is most commonly used for dynamic control of coronal plane deformities at the subtalar joint. This type of orthosis is not effective for sagittal plane problems of the ankle and foot or when a patient has difficulty with swing phase clearance. In these instances, an orthosis with trimline above the ankle joint is necessary.

SUPRAMALLEOLAR ORTHOSES

The SMO is a relatively new orthotic design that has evolved from the UCBL in an effort to address sagittal plane problems and to facilitate foot clearance in swing. One design variant consists of a UCBL-like shoe insert modified with medial and lateral extensions. The medial and lateral extensions represent an attempt to improve control of subtalar valgus or varus by lengthening the proximal lever arm upward. A number of SMO designs are currently being used in clinical practice. Some versions include a mechanical ankle joint (Figure 9-6). One version, also called a *dynamic AFO* attempts to inhibit hypertonicity and dynamic equinovarus deformity by supporting normal triplanar motion of the ankle joint through stabilization of ankle position with nonjointed medial and lateral extensions.[6] Early evidence suggests that this version enhances biomechanical function of the foot during gait; however, its impact on abnormal tone is not as well supported.[7-9] The proximal trimlines of an SMO or dynamic AFO can be positioned anywhere between the superior aspects of the malleoli and just below the belly of the soleus.

The design of an SMO mimics the effect of a high-top sneaker or shoe but provides more intimate control of the ankle-foot complex because of its custom-molded fabrication. For children with mild to moderate neuromuscular impairment who are just beginning to ambulate, the SMO may provide enough control of coronal plane motion to enhance stability as the gait pattern matures, without the restrictions imposed by a full-height solid-ankle orthosis. Older children can be transitioned from an articulating AFO into an SMO if their gait pattern has matured and become stable. The SMO may be chosen for children with cerebral palsy who have had corrective orthopedic surgery and no longer require the external stability provided by their preoperative solid-ankle AFO. The SMO may also be indicated for patients with chronic inversion instability at the subtalar joint secondary to trauma, arthritic changes, peripheral neuropathy, or muscle disease.

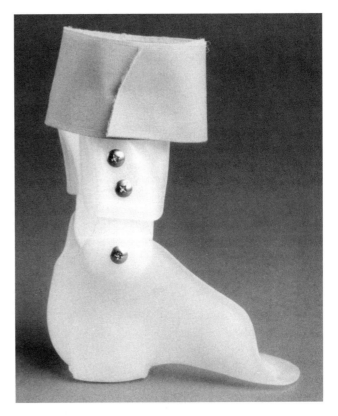

FIGURE 9-6

A low-profile supramalleolar orthosis with a mechanical ankle joint. Note the University of California Biomechanics Laboratory style foot orthosis with a medial post. Note also the relatively short lever arm of the proximal closure in controlling forward progression of the tibia through the period of midstance.

Controversy as to the effectiveness of the SMO centers on its impact on sagittal plane motion. The position of the ankle joint axis in an adult of average height is approximately 7 cm above the ground surface. If the SMO transverses this level with a definitive closure, it will limit sagittal plane motion of the ankle, and its impact on the rockers of gait may be profound. An additional concern is the patient's tolerance of forces applied at the proximal closure as the SMO controls forward progression of the tibia: The force on the anterior aspect of the tibia increases exponentially as the height of the proximal closure decreases (Figure 9-7). An SMO design that incorporates an elastic closure or a set of articulating mechanical ankle joints may enable tibial advancement over the foot. If control of tibial advancement in stance is a primary orthotic goal, a standard AFO, with a proximal trimline placed 1.0–1.5 in. below the apex of the fibular head, may be a more biomechanically effective and comfortable choice.

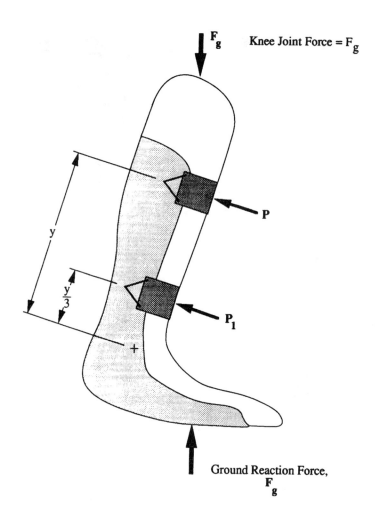

Knee Joint Force = F_g

Ground Reaction Force, F_g

FIGURE 9-7

Comparison of anterior forces at the proximal closure of a standard ankle-foot orthosis (P) and supramalleolar orthosis (P₁) in controlling forward advancement of the tibia during stance. The distance from the ankle axis (+) to the proximal closure of the supramalleolar orthosis (y/3) is one-third that of the standard ankle-foot orthosis (y). To counteract the collapsing moment that results from the force of gravity (F_g), the anterior force of the supramalleolar orthosis (P₁) must be nine times greater than the anterior force of the ankle-foot orthosis (P). The graph illustrates the exponential relationship between the anterior force (P) and lever arm (distance between the joint axis and the proximal closure, y).

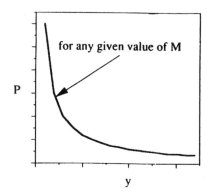

for any given value of M

$$\text{COLLAPSING MOMENT} = x \cdot F_g = M$$

$$\text{ORTHOTIC MOMENT} = y \cdot P = M$$

ANKLE-FOOT ORTHOSES

The orthosis most frequently fabricated for children and adults with neuromuscular disorders that have an impact on lower extremity function is the AFO. Although there are numerous variations in design details, most AFOs can be classified either as a static orthosis (prohibiting motion at the ankle) or a dynamic orthosis (permitting ankle motion, primarily in the sagittal plane). The solid-ankle AFO, the anterior floor reaction brace, and the patellar tendon-bearing (PTB) AFO are examples of static AFOs. Those in the dynamic group include posterior leaf spring and hinged-ankle (articulating) AFO designs.

STATIC ANKLE-FOOT ORTHOSES

The three orthoses in the static category hold the ankle in a fixed position, as close to neutral ankle, subtalar, and forefoot alignment as the patient is able to tolerate. These orthoses are able to assist swing clearance, effectively preposition the foot for initial contact and provide external stability for the ankle and knee during stance. The design of static orthoses, however, also compromises the first, second, and, to a lesser extent, third rocker of gait.

Solid-Ankle Ankle-Foot Orthoses

The solid-ankle AFO is designed to provide maximum immobilization of the ankle-foot complex in all three planes of motion. This AFO, usually fabricated from thermoplastic materials, encompasses as much of the lower leg and foot as possible, without making it too difficult to don the orthosis. The anteroposterior trimline of the solid-ankle AFO is usually placed at or near the midline of the medial and lateral malleolus (Figure 9-8). The proximal border is usually trimmed at 1.5 in. below the apex of the head of the fibula. For children with cerebral palsy, the foot plate can extend distally under the toes to reduce the likelihood of abnormal toe grasp reflex. For adults, the foot plate is usually trimmed just proximal to the metatarsal heads to facilitate the fit and donning of shoes. The ankle is held in a neutral 90-degree position, and the heel is well seated to control the position of the calcaneus and subtalar joint.

The solid-ankle AFO design incorporates four force systems to control the ankle (see Figure 5-6).[10] The force system that provides resistance to plantar flexion in swing has a fulcrum at the anterior ankle, with an upward counterforce on the plantar surface of the foot and anteriorly directed counterforce at the proximal posterior aspect of the orthosis. The foot section is designed to control excessive angular forces at the subtalar joints during stance.[11] The fulcrum of the varus/inversion control system is a medially directed force applied to the distal fibula and calcaneus across the lateral malleolus, with two laterally directed counterforces applied at the proximal medial tibia and the medial foot. The fulcrum of the valgus/eversion control system is a laterally directed force applied to the distal tibia and calcaneus just proximal to the medial malleolus, with two medially directed counterforces applied just below the fibular head proximally and at the lateral foot distally. Control in the transverse plane is also determined by the trimlines of the foot section. Midtarsal joint defor-

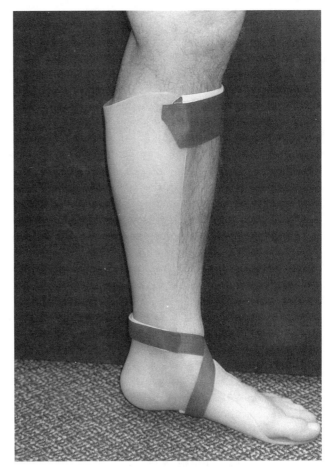

FIGURE 9-8

Custom-molded, solid-ankle ankle-foot orthosis holds the ankle in as close to optimal static alignment as possible for a given patient. Mediolateral ankle stability is a result of trimlines at the midline of the malleoli. Note the high medial border at the foot and the slight flaring just proximal to the medial malleolus. This strategy is used to counteract an abnormal, flexible subtalar valgus. The crossed Velcro strap anterior to the ankle helps to position the rear foot appropriately within the heel section of the orthosis.

mity and the resultant forefoot abduction or adduction can be effectively countered with trimlines that strategically encompass the shafts of the first and fifth metatarsals. If excessive subtalar valgus is present, the foot section incorporates a high medial wall and a flange just proximal to the medial malleolus. This strategy provides a greater surface area for distribution of the fulcrum of corrective forces applied by the orthosis, so that the patient is comfortable with the external stability provided by the orthosis. The fourth force system controls dorsiflexion during stance phase (and consequently facilitates knee extension in stance): There is a compressive force on the ankle section of the

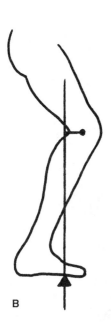
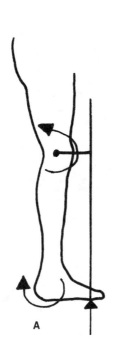
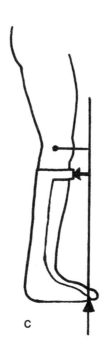

FIGURE 9-9

(A) In normal gait, knee stability at midstance is assisted by a ground reaction moment as the body moves over the foot, and the ground reaction force vector passes anterior to the knee. (B) When a patient walks in a "crouch gait" pattern, the ground reaction force vector passes behind the knee at midstance, creating a flexion moment at the knee, which must be counteracted to maintain upright position. The solid-ankle ankle-foot orthosis and the floor reaction orthotic designs (C) use a fixed ankle position to "harness" the ground reaction force, creating a large extension moment at the knee.

orthosis, an upward force of the sole of the foot, and a posteriorly directed force on the anterior proximal tibia.

A solid-ankle AFO is appropriate for patients who require total immobilization of the ankle-foot complex to be stable or functional in standing and during gait. The solid-ankle AFO effectively provides mediolateral stability at the ankle, prevents foot drop in swing by resisting plantar flexion, controls hyperextension of the knee (if set in a few degrees of dorsiflexion at the ankle), controls hyperflexion of the knee (if set in a few degrees of plantar flexion), and assists terminal stance by preventing a collapse into dorsiflexion at the end of stance. This orthosis is often prescribed for patients with neuromotor problems such as moderate to severe hypertonicity (spasticity), unpredictable fluctuating tone (athetosis), or postural instability and ataxia.[11,12] The solid-ankle AFO may also be appropriate for patients with very low tone or generalized weakness, who must rely on an external device to substitute for the stability that their own muscle activity cannot effectively provide. A solid-ankle AFO has also be used to protect the ankle and midfoot that are recovering from Charcot's arthropathy, for patients who need stabilization after foot or ankle surgery, or for those with ankle instability secondary to rheumatoid arthritis.[13] The calf component of the orthosis can be modified with a varus or valgus door or a padded tab for ambulatory patients with strong displacement of the subtalar joint on weight bearing. A Gillette modification can be added to the outer medial or lateral surface of the heel cup to influence valgus or varus attitude at the knee joint. A medial or lateral post (similar to those used in a biome-

chanical foot orthosis) can be incorporated into the foot section to equalize forefoot to rear foot relationships or to enhance biomechanical effects on the knee.

The solid-ankle AFO has a deleterious impact on all three rockers of gait. The ankle is held in a neutral position, at approximately 90 degrees, throughout all of the stance phase. This effectively prevents the controlled lowering of the foot toward the floor during loading response; instead, a rapid knee flexion may occur to achieve a foot-flat position quickly. If the orthosis is set in slight dorsiflexion in an effort to prevent recurvatum in early stance, the patient must have at least fair eccentric strength of the quadriceps to control the rapid knee flexion moment in loading response. The proximal closure, combined with the fixed ankle position, prevents forward progression of the tibia during midstance. If the distal trimlines extend to the metatarsal heads and the orthosis has a stiff toe plate, the third/toe rocker of the foot will also be limited. To counteract these limitations and improve the quality of gait, the patient's shoe can be modified with a cushion heel or a rocker bottom sole, or both.

Anterior Floor Reaction Ankle-Foot Orthoses

All AFO designs inherently use moments that result from the ground reaction force to provide some stability in stance. An anterior floor reaction AFO (also known as a *floor reaction orthosis, FRO*) is specifically designed to harness the ground (floor) reaction moment as a primary source of sagittal plane stability for the knee joint during stance.[14,15] The FRO relies on the plantar flexion–knee extension couple where a fixed, slightly plantar flexed ankle creates an extension moment at the knee (Figure 9-9; see Figure 9-4). The force systems that control foot and ankle position are the same as those described previously for a solid-ankle AFO.

The plantar flexion angle and the length and rigidity of the toe plate help to determine the magnitude of the resulting knee extension moment. When an FRO is set in neutral or a few degrees of plantar flexion, the tibia is restrained from advancing over the foot in the second rocker of gait, and the ground reaction force passes anterior to the knee earlier in stance phase. Additionally, as the length and stiffness of the toe plate increase, the third rocker of gait is also limited, and additional extension forces are brought to bear on the knee into extension in the latter half of stance phase. The anterior shell and mediolateral trimlines are padded at the proximal prepatellar areas, so that the extra extension force being transmitted to the knee in stance is more tolerable (Figure 9-10). The FRO can be fabricated as a single solid unit (which may be difficult to don) or as a solid-ankle AFO with an additional anterior shell that is snugly strapped in place. The latter variation may be appropriate if improvement is anticipated: The anterior shell can be removed and the orthosis used as a traditional solid-ankle orthosis.

For this orthotic design to be effective in stabilizing the knee, the vector of the ground reaction force must pass anterior to the knee axis: This may be problematic for patients with fixed flexion contracture of more than 10 degrees at the distal hamstring.[14] In this instance, the FRO resists dorsiflexion and knee flexion but does not create a true extension moment. The FRO is also inappropriate for patients who exhibit recurvatum or have structural instability of the knee joint. Because the FRO design limits ankle mobility and knee flexion, it may have a negative impact on balance reactions; if patients do not have effective postural control, an assistive ambulation device (such as a cane) may be required, especially if FROs are worn bilaterally.

As a result of the biomechanical advantages of the FRO design, a patient with little quadriceps function is able to be stable in stance, full weight bearing, without knee instability. This design has been successful in improving the quality and safety of gait for patients with poliomyelitis, peripheral neuropathy, and myopathy, as well as those with crouch gait from neuromuscular problems, as long as sufficient knee range of motion is possible.

Patellar Tendon-Bearing Ankle-Foot Orthoses

The PTB AFO is a modification of the solid-ankle design, with an additional anterior shell that incorporates the

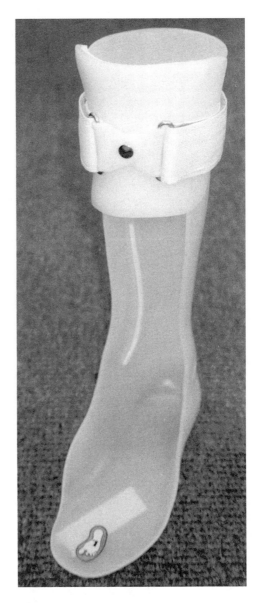

FIGURE 9-10

This floor reaction orthosis has a posterior shell similar to that of a solid-ankle ankle-foot orthosis. The combination of slight plantar flexion at the ankle and a stiff, long toe plate creates a plantar flexion–knee extension couple that acts in mid to late stance. The addition of a padded anterior shell more comfortably captures the resultant extension moment, stabilizing the knee. Note also the corrugation incorporated in the medial and lateral walls of the ankle-foot orthosis to provide additional rigidity to the orthosis.

weight-bearing principles of a PTB socket for a transtibial prosthesis.[16] The anterior shell of the PTB AFO is modified to include a "shelf" to support the medial tibial flare and a patellar tendon bar. The primary goal of the PTB AFO design is to reduce axial loading of the distal limb

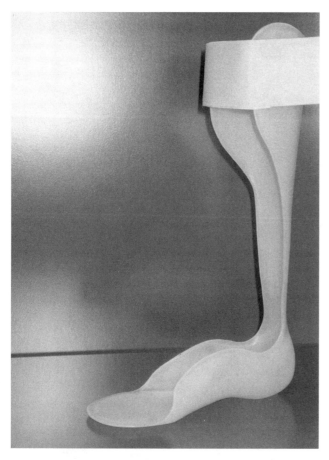

FIGURE 9-11
The posterior position and arc of the trimlines at the ankle, as well as the thickness of thermoplastic material used, determine the degree of flexibility of the posterior leaf spring ankle-foot orthosis. This design approximates the first and second rockers of stance phase and assists clearance and pre-positioning of the foot during swing.

during gait. The orthosis is oriented in approximately 10 degrees of knee flexion (with respect to vertical) so that a portion of body weight is loaded on the anterior shell of the AFO at the medial tibial flare and patellar tendon bar during stance. A portion of the axial loading forces is then transmitted down the metal uprights incorporated into the medial and lateral walls of the orthosis, reducing loading of the tibia, fibula, and bones of the foot.[17] This design has been used for patients with a Charcot's ankle, neuropathic ulcers on the plantar surface of the foot, slowly healing or nonunion fractures of the foot and ankle, ankle instability and pain associated with arthritis, and other conditions that require reduced weight bearing through

the foot-ankle complex. For this design to be effective, however, the anatomic knee must have structural and skin integrity to tolerate the extra loading forces applied by the PTB design. It is also important that the patient have adequate quadriceps strength for knee stability in early stance.

DYNAMIC ANKLE-FOOT ORTHOSES

The family of dynamic AFOs includes thermoplastic and conventional double upright orthotic designs. The feature that distinguishes dynamic from static AFOs is that they allow, or have the potential to allow, sagittal plane motion at the ankle. This is accomplished by incorporation of a mechanical ankle joint or, in the case of a posterior leaf spring orthosis (PLS), strategically minimized thermoplastic trimlines.

Posterior Leaf Spring Ankle-Foot Orthoses

The PLS is a thermoplastic AFO with medial and lateral trimlines placed well posterior to the midline of the malleoli (Figure 9-11). This design feature results in flexibility of the orthosis at the anatomic ankle joint. The degree of flexibility is determined by the thickness of the thermoplastic material used to construct the orthosis and the arc of the radius at the distal third of the AFO. During loading response, in the first rocker of early stance, the PLS substitutes for eccentric contraction of the muscles of the anterior compartment (primarily the tibialis anterior), providing a controlled lowering of the foot toward the ground. In the second rocker, the flexibility of the PLS allows the dorsiflexion necessary for tibial advancement over the foot during midstance. Once the limb is unweighted and the swing phase begins, the PLS holds the ankle at 90 degrees, assisting clearance and appropriately positioning the foot for the subsequent initial contact.[18,19]

Because of its posterior trimlines and flexibility at the ankle, the PLS cannot "contain" the calcaneus as well as a solid-ankle design. As a result, the PLS may not be as effective in controlling mediolateral foot position and may not be appropriate for patients with flexible deformity of the rear, mid-, or forefoot.[20]

If a patient requires some external mediolateral stability at the ankle, but not the rigid control of a solid-ankle AFO, the trimlines can be placed somewhere between those of a solid-ankle AFO and a PLS design. This design, known as a *semisolid AFO* or a *modified PLS orthosis*, has some of the functional characteristics of the solid-ankle and PLS AFOs. Although somewhat less flexible at the ankle than a PLS in loading response, this modified PLS design is able to provide some control of knee position during stance.

The conventional double upright counterpart to the PLS uses a spring mechanism incorporated into the mechanical ankle joint to assist dorsiflexion in swing, as well as to provide a smooth transition from heel strike/initial contact to foot flat at the end of loading response. The most commonly used conventional dorsiflexion assist joint is the Klenzak (Figure 9-12). The uprights are connected to the distal stirrup at the mechanical ankle joint. The stirrup is fixed between the heel and sole of the shoe. A coil spring and small ball bearing are placed in a channel in the distal uprights that runs toward the posterior edge of the stirrup. When the spring is compressed at initial contact and early loading response, it resists plantar flexion, allowing a controlled lowering of the foot to the floor. Recoil of the spring when the foot is unloaded in preswing and initial swing assists dorsiflexion for swing phase toe clearance.[20] The amount of dorsiflexion assist provided is determined by adjustment of a screw placed in the top of the channel to compress or decompress the spring further.

The PLS or dorsiflexion assist conventional AFO is chosen when the primary problem is weakness of dorsiflexion. Patients with peroneal nerve palsy, Charcot-Marie-Tooth disease, and various peripheral neuropathies are appropriate candidates for the PLS or dorsiflexion assist AFO. Patients with hypertonicity and neuromotor equinovarus, however, are better served by other orthotic designs: The flexible PLS is easily overpowered and rendered ineffective by abnormal tone. The PLS and dorsiflexion assist conventional AFO are equally effective substitutes for anterior compartment muscles. The choice of orthosis is determined by factors that include weight of the orthotic, functional strength of the proximal musculature, the need for total contact to protect the foot, the ability to interchange shoes, and the wearer's desire for cosmesis.

Articulating Ankle-Foot Prostheses

The articulating, or hinged-ankle, AFO is a thermoplastic orthotic design that incorporates a mechanical ankle joint placed between foot and calf sections of the orthosis. A variety of mechanical ankle joints are commercially available (Figure 9-13). Some require an overlap of the foot and calf, whereas others do not. Those with true articulations, such as the Oklahoma joint, have a single axis of motion that should be aligned as closely as

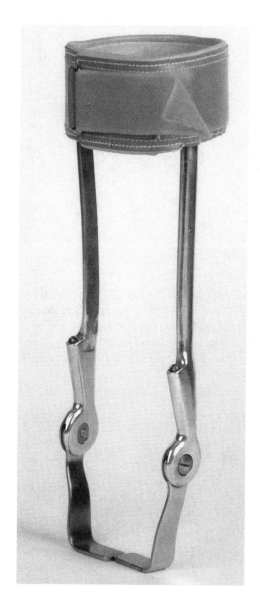

FIGURE 9-12
Conventional double upright dorsiflexion assist ankle-foot orthosis, with a single-channel Klenzak joint. Tightening the screw at the top of the channel compresses a spring to increase the amount of dorsiflexion assistance provided. This split stirrup would be fit into a shoe plate positioned between the sole and heel, making it possible for the patient to use the ankle-foot orthosis with more than one shoe.

possible to the anatomic ankle joint. Other orthotic joints, such as the Gillette joint, are flexible, nonarticulating, and axis-less.[10] The configurations of the foot and calf sections of an articulating AFO are essentially the same as those of the solid-ankle AFO. The width of the ortho-

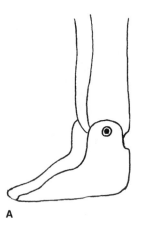 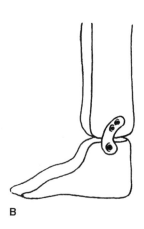 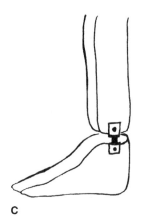

A   B   C

FIGURE 9-13

*Examples of mechanical ankle joints used in articulating ankle-foot orthoses. The overlap joint (**A**) and Oklahoma joint (**B**) are true single-axis joints, whereas the flexible Gillette mechanism (**C**) allows movement into dorsiflexion and plantar flexion without an actual articulation.*

sis at the ankle is usually marginally wider than a solid-ankle AFO because of the mechanical ankle joint. Most mechanical ankle joints allow dorsiflexion and plantar flexion (sagittal plane) motion. For this orthosis to function effectively, the patient must have at least 5 degrees of true ankle dorsiflexion, accomplished without compromise of subtalar or midtarsal joint position.[10] Because of the need for normal subtalar and midfoot arthrokinematics in the second rocker of gait, an articulating AFO is not usually appropriate in the presence of severe spasticity that limits ankle motion or if severe instability or if malalignment of the midfoot is present.[21] A 90-degree plantar flexion stop mechanism can be incorporated into the articulating AFO if prevention of plantar flexion is desired (for example, if spastic equinovarus is a concern). This is usually accomplished by an overlapping lip or pin stop mechanism (Figure 9-14).

Another version of the articulating AFO uses an adjustable posterior check strap to limit the excursion into dorsiflexion (Figure 9-15). If the check strap is maximally tightened, the orthosis functions much like a solid-ankle AFO. The check strap can be loosened, lengthened, or elasticized as neuromotor control improves, allowing only as much forward progression of the tibia in the second rocker as is safe and functional for the patient.[21] This adaptation makes the articulating AFO the most versatile of all thermoplastic designs. It is often prescribed for patients in the early stages of recovery from stroke, for children with cerebral palsy after orthopedic surgery to correct deformities, or for any other patient with a rapidly changing clinical picture in whom return of function is anticipated.

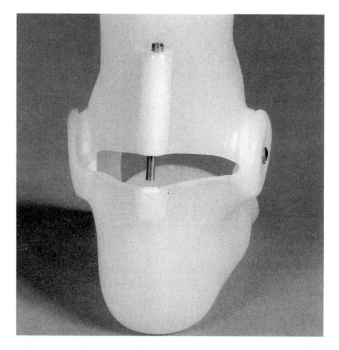

FIGURE 9-14

When control of plantar flexion is necessary, a posterior plantar flexion stop is incorporated into the articulating ankle-foot orthosis. In this example, a pin stop is used to limit plantar flexion, whereas the overlap mechanical ankle allows the dorsiflexion needed for an efficient second rocker of gait. The amount of plantar flexion motion is adjusted by how far the pin is screwed into the posterior channel.

Hybrid Plastic-Metal and Conventional Articulating Ankle-Foot Orthoses

The bichannel adjustable ankle locking joint (also referred to as a *double action ankle joint* or a *double Klenzak joint*) used in conventional double upright AFOs has also been adapted for use in thermoplastic designs[11,22] (Figure 9-16).

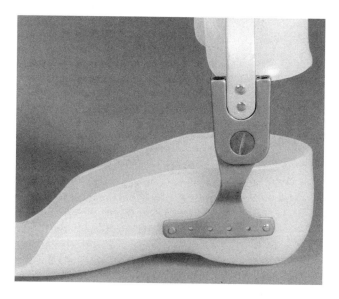

FIGURE 9-16
The double action joint can be used in a conventional, double upright, metal ankle-foot orthosis and a thermoplastic-metal, hybrid ankle-foot orthosis. Motion is assisted if a spring is compressed within the channel or can be blocked by placement of a steel pin within the channel.

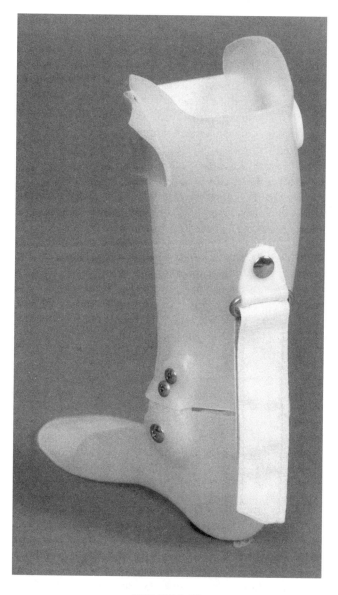

FIGURE 9-15
An articulating ankle-foot orthosis with Oklahoma joints and a Velcro closing posterior check strap. The mechanical ankle joint would permit free dorsiflexion and plantar flexion motion in the sagittal plane; however, plantar flexion is limited as the calf and foot components make contact. The amount of dorsiflexion possible can be adjusted as the patient progresses through gait training by loosening or elasticizing the check strap closure.

The double action mechanical joint has an anterior and a posterior channel. If motion assistance is desired, a wire spring is placed in the channel, and a screw is used to adjust compression until the desired level of assistance is achieved. If motion is to be blocked, a solid steel pin is inserted instead of the spring, to stop motion beyond a particular point in the range of motion. This mechanical ankle joint can be adjusted to meet individual patient needs, stopping plantar flexion and allowing or assisting dorsiflexion as neuromotor control dictates. The double action joint can also be set to block dorsiflexion (for example, to limit weight bearing on the anterior portion of the foot) or assist plantar flexion (for a patient with weakness of plantar flexors), should it be necessary. Because of its versatility and adjustability, the double action ankle joint is often chosen when change in a patient's functional status (improvement or deterioration) is anticipated.

A variety of other mechanical ankle joints are available for patients who require a conventional double upright AFO.[20] A simple single-axis joint can be used to provide mediolateral stability for the ankle while allowing free dorsiflexion and plantar flexion. Motion can be limited by adding a stop to the orthotic ankle joint to block either plantar flexion or dorsiflexion. Some orthotic ankle joints, such as the Friddle joint, can be adjusted to limit excursion between dorsiflexion and plantar flexion motion in increments of 7–9 degrees. A leather T-strap can be used in an attempt to position the rear foot more optimally within the shoe. Proximally, the conventional double upright AFO has a calf band and anterior closure, positioned approximately 1.5 in. from the apex of the fibular head.

SUMMARY: WHAT ARE THE CHARACTERISTICS OF AN EFFECTIVE ANKLE-FOOT ORTHOSIS?

Several characteristics are common to all effective AFOs, regardless of their specific design or the materials and methods used in their fabrication. First, the efficacy of the orthosis is directly related to the intimacy and consistency of its fit. For some patients, an additional figure-eight ankle strap or other form of augmented closure (in addition to an appropriately closed or tied shoe) may be necessary to keep the calcaneus well seated in the orthosis during all phases of gait. Even a minimal amount of pistoning or heel elevation within the orthosis during gait can lead to skin irritation, ulceration, or an increase of underlying extensor hypertonicity. Second, although thermoplastic AFOs are very effective in controlling a wide range of orthopedic deformities, this is dependent on a total contact intimate fit in all three planes of motion. Finally, the ability of an AFO to achieve maximum benefit is greatly influenced by the type and condition of the shoe. Many patients need to increase their shoe size one-half to a whole size to accommodate the orthosis. Although one of the benefits of thermoplastic AFOs is the ability to wear a variety of shoes, changing heel heights can dramatically alter the biomechanical function of the orthosis. A PLS, articulating, or solid-ankle AFO that is designed to be worn with an athletic or oxford type shoe that closes near the ankle is not as effective in a loafer or sandal with a more distal closure. Modification of the sole of a shoe can be used to counteract the limitations imposed by AFOs that restrict ankle motion. The addition of a cushion heel (similar to that used in prosthetic feet) can mimic the controlled lowering of the foot during first rocker. A rocker bar or rocker bottom placed at midfoot can simulate the second rocker, enhancing forward progression during the second half of stance phase. The orthotist and therapist share the responsibility for educating the patient and family about appropriate footwear, monitoring the condition of shoes, and evaluating the continuing efficacy of the orthosis in meeting the patient's functional needs over time.

The appropriately designed and fit AFO can have significant positive impact on the patient's mobility and functional status. Although thermoplastic designs are most often used, in some circumstances a conventional metal AFO may be more appropriate. The primary goal is to prescribe an orthosis that provides the appropriate external support for stability in stance and clearance in swing, with minimal compromise of the first (heel), second (ankle), and third (toe) rockers of gait. Factors that help to determine the appropriate design include the presence and degree of musculoskeletal impairment or deformity, the extent of impairment of motor control and hypertonicity, and the anticipated prognosis (growth, progression of the disease process, or likelihood of improvement). Thoughtful consideration of these factors results in a positive orthotic outcome for the patient and for members of the health care team.

REFERENCES

1. Epler ME. Orthoses for the Ankle. In DA Nawoczenksi, ME Epler (eds), Orthotics in Functional Rehabilitation of the Lower Limb. Philadelphia: Saunders, 1997;77–114.
2. Perry J. Gait Analysis: Normal and Pathological Function. Thorofare, NJ: Slack, 1992.
3. Bunch WH, Keagy RD, Kritter AE, et al. Atlas of Orthotics: Biomechanical Principles and Application (2nd ed). St. Louis: Mosby, 1985.
4. Carlson J, Berglund C. An effective orthotic design for controlling the unstable subtalar joint. Orthot Prosthet 1979;33(1):39–49.
5. Inman VT. Dual axis ankle control systems and the UCBL shoe insert: biomechanical considerations. Bull Prosthet Res 1969, Spring(10–11):130–146.
6. Knutson LM, Clark DE. Orthotic devices for ambulation in children with cerebral palsy and myelomeningocele. Phys Ther 1991;71(12):947–960.
7. Diamond MF, Ottenbacher KJ. Effect of a tone-inhibiting dynamic ankle-foot orthosis on stride characteristics of an adult with hemiparesis. Phys Ther 1990;70(7):423–430.
8. Hylton NM. Postural and functional impact of dynamic AFOs and FO in a pediatric population. J Prosthet Orthot 1989;2(1):40–53.
9. Mueller K, Cornwall M, McPoil T, et al. Effect of a tone-inhibiting dynamic ankle-foot orthosis on the foot loading pattern of a hemiplegic adult. J Prosthet Orthot 1992;4(2):86–92.
10. Trautman P. Lower Limb Orthotics. In JB Redford, JV Basmajian, P Trautman (eds), Orthotics: Clinical Practice and Rehabilitation Technology. New York: Churchill Livingstone, 1995;13–53.
11. Waters RL, Garland DE, Montgomery J. Orthotic Prescription for Stroke and Head Injury. In American Academy of Orthopedic Surgeons, Atlas of Orthotics, Biomechanical Principles and Application. St. Louis: Mosby, 1985;270–286.

12. Montgomery J. Orthotic management of the lower limb in head injured adults. J Head Trauma Rehabil 1987;2(2):57–61.
13. Carlson JM, Berglund C. An effective orthotic design for controlling the unstable subtalar joint. J Orthot Prosthet 1979;33(1):39–49.
14. Harrington E, Lin R, Gage J. Use of an anterior floor reaction orthosis in patients with cerebral palsy. Orthot Prosthet 1983;37(4):34–42.
15. Yang G, Chu D, Ahn J, et al. Floor reaction orthosis: clinical experience. Orthot Prosthet 1986;40(1):33–37.
16. McIlmurray WJ, Greenbaum W. A below knee weight bearing brace. Orthop Prosthet Appl J 1958;12(2):81–82.
17. Lehman JF. Lower Limb Orthotics. In JB Redford (ed), Orthotics Etcetera (3rd ed). Baltimore: Williams & Wilkins, 1975;317.
18. Waters RL, Garland DE, Montgomery J. Passive Drop Foot, Clinical Illustration: Trauma. In Rancho Los Amigos Medical Center Prosthetics and Orthotics Course Syllabus, Critical Decisions in Patient Management. Downey, CA: Professional Staff Association, 1985;6:10–12.
19. Lehman JF, Esselmen PC, Ko MJ. Plastic ankle foot orthosis: evaluation of function. Arch Phys Med Rehabil 1983;64(9):402–407.
20. Berger N, Edelstein JE, Fishman S, et al. Lower Limb Orthotics. Prosthetics and Orthotics. New York: NYU Postgraduate Medical School, 1986;129–163.
21. Weber D. Clinical Aspects of Lower Extremity Orthotics. Oakville, Ontario: Elgan, 1990.
22. Shurr DG, Cook TM. Lower Limb Orthotics. In Prosthetics and Orthotics. Norwalk, CT: Appleton & Lange, 1990;123–149.

10

Knee Orthoses

John F. Knecht

Although knee orthoses have long been used as a means of protection and stabilization of the knee joint, their effectiveness in preventing ligamentous injury or in stabilizing a knee with ligamentous insufficiency has not been well supported by research findings.[1,2] In 1984, the American Academy of Orthopaedic Surgeons developed a classification system that groups knee orthotics by their intended function.[3] *Prophylactic knee orthoses* are designed to reduce the risk of knee injury for those individuals who are engaged in "high-risk" activities, especially those individuals who have a history of previous knee dysfunction. *Rehabilitative knee orthoses* are used to protect a knee that has been injured or surgically repaired until adequate tissue healing has occurred. *Functional knee orthoses* attempt to provide biomechanical stability when ligaments are unable to do so during daily activities. This functional classification system continues to be helpful for physical therapists, orthotists, and athletic trainers who work with patients who have knee dysfunction.

The ability to select the most appropriate orthosis for a patient with knee dysfunction is founded on a clear understanding of normal knee structure and function. For this reason, we begin the chapter with a review of the anatomy and biomechanical stability of the knee and patellofemoral joints and the physiologic and accessory motions of the tibiofemoral and patellofemoral joints. We then examine the design and functional goals of prefabricated and custom-made knee orthoses and indications for knee orthoses in the management of common knee injuries and dysfunction. Finally, we explore strategies for clinical decision making in choosing an appropriate functional orthosis for active patients and athletes with ligamentous instability of the knee.

TIBIOFEMORAL JOINT

The knee joint is a hinge-like articulation between the medial and lateral condyles of the femur and the medial and lateral tibial plateau. Because of the shape and asymmetry of the condyles, the instantaneous axis of knee flexion/extension motion changes through the arc of motion. In open chain movements, the tibia rotates around the femoral condyles. In closed chain movements, an anatomic "locking" mechanism is present in the final degrees of extension, as the longer medial femoral condyle rotates medially on the articular surfaces of the tibia. The alignment between an adducted femur and relatively upright tibia creates a vulnerability to valgus stress in many weight-bearing activities. The capsule that encases the knee joint is reinforced by the collagen-rich medial and lateral retinaculum. The medial and lateral menisci are fibrocartilaginous, nearly ring-shaped disks that are flexibly attached around the edges of the tibial plateau (Figure 10-1). These menisci increase the concavity of the tibial articular surface, enhancing congruency of articulation with the femoral condyles to facilitate normal gliding and distribute weight-bearing forces within the knee during gait and other loading activities.[4] The menisci also play an important role in nutrition and lubrication of the articular surfaces of the knee joint.

Although contraction of the quadriceps and knee flexor muscle groups produces compressive forces that help to stabilize the knee, most of the stability of the knee is provided by two sets of ligaments. The collateral ligaments counter valgus and varus forces that act on the knee. The cruciate ligaments check translatory forces that displace the tibia on the femur. The location of attachments makes each of these ligaments most effective at particular places in the knee's normal arch of motion.[4]

Medial Collateral Ligament

The medial (tibial) collateral ligament (MCL) is a strong, flat membranous band that overlays the middle portion of the medial joint capsule (Figure 10-2A). It is most effective in counteracting valgus stressors when the knee is

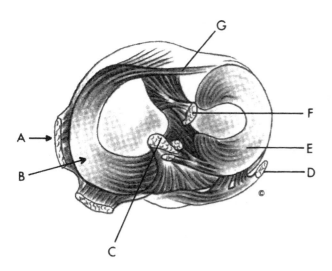

FIGURE 10-1

In this view of the surface of the tibia, we can identify (A) the medial collateral ligament, (B) the C-shaped medial meniscus on the large medial tibial plateau, (C) the posterior cruciate ligament with the accessory anterior and posterior meniscofemoral ligaments, (D) the tendon of the popliteus muscle, (E) the circular lateral meniscus on the smaller lateral tibial plateau, (F) the anterior cruciate ligament as it twists toward the inside of the lateral femoral condyle, and (G) the transverse ligament. (Reprinted with permission from BH Greenfield. Rehabilitation of the Knee: A Problem Solving Approach. Philadelphia: Davis, 1993;12.)

slightly flexed to fully extended. Approximately 8–10 cm in length, it originates at the medial epicondyle of the femur and attaches to the medial surface of the tibial plateau. The MCL can be subdivided into a set of oblique posterior fibers and anterior parallel fibers.

A bundle of meniscotibial fibers, also known as the *posterior oblique ligament*, runs deep to the MCL, from the femur to the midperipheral margin of the medial meniscus and toward the tibia. These fibers connect the medial meniscus to the tibia and help to form the semimembranosus corner of the medial knee.

Lateral Collateral Ligament and Iliotibial Band

The lateral (fibular) collateral ligament (LCL) resists varus stressors and lateral rotation of the tibia and is most effective when the knee is slightly flexed. The LCL runs from the lateral femoral condyle (the back part of the outer tuberosity of the femur) to the proximal lateral aspect of the fibular head (Figure 10-2B). The tendon of the popliteus muscle and the external articular vessels and nerves pass beneath this ligament.

The iliotibial band (ITB) is positioned slightly anterior to the LCL and is taut in all ranges of knee motion. Although the position of the ITB allows it to stabilize against varus forces as does the LCL, the ITB also appears to assist the anterior cruciate ligament (ACL), preventing posterior displacement of the tibia when the knee is extended.[5]

Anterior Cruciate Ligament

The ACL runs at an oblique angle between the articular surfaces of the knee joint and acts to prevent forward shift and excessive medial rotation of the tibia as the knee moves toward extension (Figure 10-3; see Figure 10-1). The ACL attaches to the tibia in a fossa just anterior and lateral to the anterior tibial spine and to the femur in a fossa on the posteromedial surface of the lateral femoral condyle. The ACL's tibial attachment is somewhat wider and stronger than its

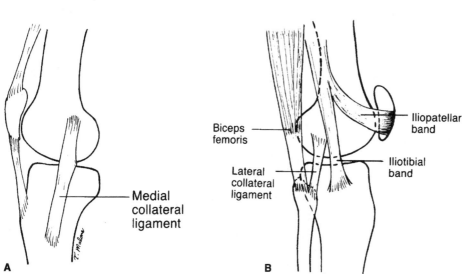

FIGURE 10-2

Positions of the (A) medial collateral ligament and (B) lateral collateral ligament and iliotibial band. (Reprinted with permission from CC Norkin, PK Levangie. Joint Structure and Function: A Comprehensive Analysis [2nd ed]. Philadelphia: Davis, 1992;347.)

femoral attachment. Some authors divide the fasciculi that make up the broad, somewhat flat ACL into two or three distinct bundles. The ligament's anteromedial band, with fibers running from the anteromedial tibia to the proximal femoral attachment, is most taut in flexion and relatively lax in extension. The posterolateral bulk (PLB), which begins at the posterolateral tibial attachment, is most taut in extension and relatively lax in flexion. An intermediate bundle of transitional fibers between the anteromedial band and PLB tends to tighten when the knee moves through the midranges of motion. This arrangement of fibers ensures tension in the ACL throughout the entire range of knee motion. The ACL is most vulnerable to injury when the femur rotates internally on the tibia when the knee is flexed and the foot is fixed on the ground during weight-bearing activities.[6]

Posterior Cruciate Ligament

The posterior cruciate ligament (PCL) restrains posterior displacement of the tibia in its articulation with the femur, especially as the knee moves toward full extension.[4] The PCL is shorter and less oblique in orientation than the ACL; it is the strongest and most resistant ligament of the knee. PCL fibers run from a slight depression between articular surfaces on the posterior tibia to the posterolateral surface of the medial femoral condyle (see Figures 10-1 and 10-3). Like the ACL, the PCL can be divided into anterior and posterior segments. The larger anterior medial band is most taut between 80 and 90 degrees of flexion and is relatively lax in extension. The smaller PLB travels somewhat obliquely across the joint, becoming taut as the knee moves into extension. The PCL plays a role in the locking mechanism of the knee, as tension in the ligament produces lateral (external) rotation of the tibia on the femur in the final degrees of knee extension. The PCL may also assist the collateral ligaments when varus or valgus stressors are applied to the knee.[4]

The meniscofemoral ligament, stretching between the posterior horn of the lateral meniscus and the lateral surface of the medial femoral condyle along with fibers of the PCL, has sometimes been described as a third cruciate ligament.[7] The anterior meniscofemoral band (ligament of Humphry) runs along the medial anterior surface of the PCL and may be up to one-third its diameter. The posterior meniscofemoral band (ligament of Wrisberg) lies posterior to the PCL and may be as much as one-half its diameter. The mensicofemoral ligaments act to pull the lateral meniscus forward during flexion of the weight-bearing knee, to maintain as much articular congruency as possible with the lateral femoral condyle.

Posterolateral Corner of the Knee

The lateral meniscus is somewhat more mobile than the medial meniscus because of the anatomy of the postero-

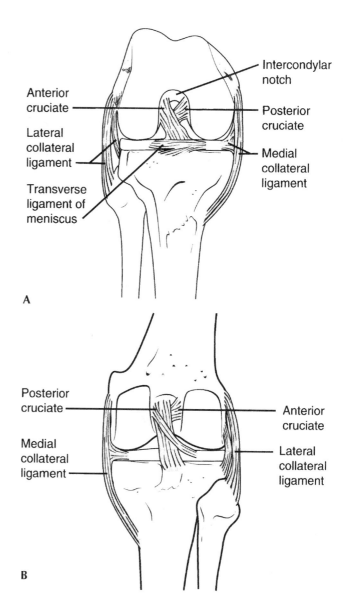

FIGURE 10-3
(A) Anterior view of the tibiofemoral joint in 90 degrees of knee flexion showing the menisci and the ligamentous structures that stabilize the knee. (B) Posterior view of the knee in extension. (Reprinted with permission from TJ Antich. Orthoses for the Knee; the Tibiofemoral Joint. In DA Nawoczenski, ME Epler [eds], Orthotics in Functional Rehabilitation of the Lower Limb. Philadelphia: Saunders, 1997;59.)

lateral corner of the knee. The arcuate complex and posterolateral corner run from the styloid process of the fibula, joining the posterior oblique ligament on the posterior aspect of the femur and tibia. The arcuate ligament is firmly attached to the underlying popliteus muscle and tendon. The tendon of the popliteus muscle separates the deep joint capsule from the rim of the lateral meniscus.

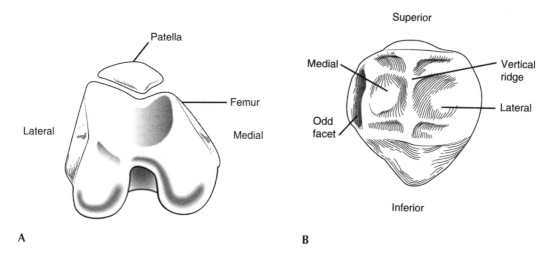

FIGURE 10-4

(A) The normal position of the patella in the intercondylar groove of the distal femur and (B) Underside of the patella with its three facets and vertical ridge. (Reprinted with permission from BC Belyea. Orthoses for the Knee: The Patellofemoral Joint. In DA Nawoczenski, ME Epler [eds], Orthotics in Functional Rehabilitation of the Lower Limb. Philadelphia: Saunders, 1997;32–33.)

PATELLOFEMORAL JOINT

The patella, a sesamoid bone embedded in the tendon of the quadriceps femoris, is an integral part of the extensor mechanism of the knee. The patella functions as an anatomic pulley, increasing the knee extension moment created by contraction of the quadriceps femoris by as much as 50%. It also guides the forces generated by the quadriceps femoris to the patellar ligament, protects deeper knee joint anatomy, protects the quadriceps tendon from frictional forces, and increases the compressive forces to which the extensor mechanisms can be subjected.[8–11]

Although the anterior surface of the patella is convex, the posterior surface has three distinct anatomic areas: The lateral and medial facets are separated by a vertical ridge, and an "odd facet" articulates with the medial condyle at the end range of knee extension (Figure 10-4). The posterior patellar surface is covered with hyaline articular cartilage, except for the distal apex, which is roughened for the attachment of the patellar tendon. Pressure between the patella and trochlear groove of the femur increases substantially as the knee flexes. During knee flexion, the patella moves in a complex but consistent three-dimensional pattern of flexion/extension rotation, medial/lateral rotation, medial/lateral tilt (also described as wavering), and a medial/lateral shift relative to the femur.[9,11] These motions occur biomechanically in the X, Y, and Z planes.

The stability of the patella is derived from the patellofemoral joint's static structural characteristics and dynamic (muscular) control. Static stability is a product of the anatomy of the patella, the depth of the intercondylar groove, and the prominent and longer lateral condyle of the femur. The sulcus angle, formed by the sloping edges of the condyles, is normally between 114 and 120 degrees; however, it can vary significantly from person to person.[12] Wiberg[13] divides the patellofemoral joint into six types based on the size and shape of facets (Table 10-1). The depth of the patellar trochlea and the facet pattern are important in patellar stability.

TABLE 10-1

Classification of Patellar Types, Listed from Most to Least Stable

Patellar Type	Description
I	Equal medial and lateral facets, both slightly concave
II	Small medial facet, both facets slightly concave
II/III	Small, flat medial facet
III	Small, slightly convex medial facet
IV	Very small, steeply sloped medial facet, with medial ridge
V (Jagerhut)	No medial facet, no central ridge

FIGURE 10-5
Structures that provide dynamic stability for the patella. (Reprinted with permission from BC Belyea. Orthoses for the Knee: The Patellofemoral Joint. In DA Nawoczenski, ME Epler [eds], Orthotics in Functional Rehabilitation of the Lower Limb. Philadelphia: Saunders, 1997;42.)

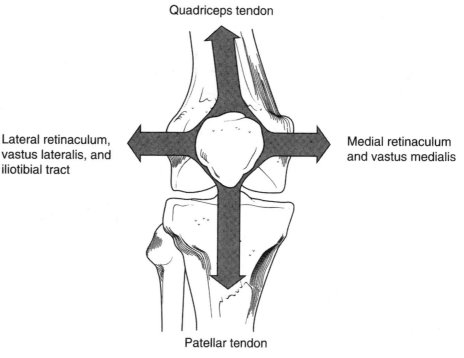

Quadriceps tendon

Lateral retinaculum, vastus lateralis, and iliotibial tract

Medial retinaculum and vastus medialis

Patellar tendon

Dynamic stability of the patellofemoral joint is derived primarily from activity of the quadriceps femoris as well as from the tensile properties of the patellar ligament (Figure 10-5). The four components of the quadriceps act together to pull the patella obliquely upward along the shaft of the femur, whereas the patellar ligament anchors it almost straight downward along the anatomic axis of the lower leg. The tibial tubercle is typically located at least 6 degrees lateral to the mechanical axis of the femur.

Because the structure of the patellofemoral articulation and the muscular/ligamentous forces that act on the patella are complex, patellar dynamics involve much more than simple cephalocaudal repositioning as the knee is flexed or extended. Van Kampen and Huiskes[11] describe the three-dimensional motions of the patella as flexion rotation, medial rotation, wavering tilt, and lateral shift. All of these patellar movements (except flexion) are influenced by the rotation of the tibia and the dynamic stabilization of the muscles that act on the patella.

BIOMECHANICS OF KNEE MOTION

The ability to evaluate and manage injuries of the knee requires an in-depth understanding of the biomechanical characteristics of the knee joint. The *kinematics of the knee* describe its motion in terms of the type and location and the magnitude and direction of the motion.[14] The *kinetics of the knee* describe the forces that act on the knee, causing movement.[14] Kinetic forces are classified as either external forces that work on the body (e.g., gravity) or as internal, body-generated forces (e.g., friction, tensile strength of soft tissue structures, muscle contraction).

Motion in the tibiofemoral joint can be best understood by separating the motion into its physiologic and accessory components. Physiologic motion can be controlled consciously, most often through voluntary contraction of muscle. Osteokinematic (bone movement) and arthrokinematic (joint surface motion) are examples of physiologic motion. Accessory motion occurs without conscious control and cannot be reproduced voluntarily. Joint play, which is elicited by passive movement during examination of a joint, is an example of an accessory motion. The magnitude and type of accessory motion possible are determined by the characteristics of a particular articulation and the properties of the tissues that surround it.

One of the important accessory component motions of the tibiofemoral joint is its "screw home" or locking mechanism. In the final degrees of knee extension, the tibia continues to rotate around the large articular surface of the medial femoral condyle. This motion cannot be prevented or changed by volitional effort; it is entirely the result of the configuration of the articular surfaces. When the knee is flexed to or beyond 90 degrees, however, conscious activation of mus-

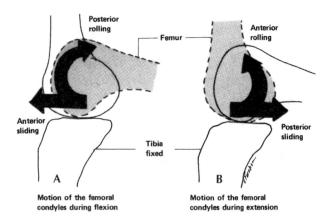

FIGURE 10-6

Diagram of femoral motion on a fixed tibia. (A) As the knee flexes, the femoral condyles roll posteriorly (curved arrow) while gliding/sliding forward (straight arrow). (B) As the knee extends, the condyles roll forward (curved arrow) while gliding posteriorly (straight arrow). (Reprinted with permission from CC Norkin, PK Levangie. Joint Structure and Function: A Comprehensive Analysis [2nd ed]. Philadelphia: Davis, 1992;355.)

cles can produce physiologic (osteokinematic) external (lateral) or internal (medial) rotation of the tibia on the femur.

Three osteokinematic motions are possible at the tibiofemoral joint. Knee flexion/extension occurs in the sagittal plane around an axis in the frontal plane (X axis). Internal/external rotation of the tibia on the femur (or vice versa) occurs in the transverse plane around a longitudinal axis (Y axis). Abduction/adduction occurs in the frontal plane around a horizontal axis (Z axis). The arthrokinematic movements of the tibiofemoral joint are rolling, gliding, and sliding (Figure 10-6). It is important to note that the roll-glide ratio is not constant during tibiofemoral joint motion: Approximately 1:2 in early flexion, the roll-glide ratio becomes almost 1:4 in late flexion.[15] Rolling and gliding occur primarily on the posterior portion of the femoral condyles. In the first 15–20 degrees of flexion, a true rolling motion of the femoral condyles occurs in concert with the tibial plateau. As the magnitude of flexion increases, the femur begins to glide posteriorly on the tibia. Gliding becomes more significant as flexion increases.[7]

From a kinematic standpoint, the ACLs and PCLs operate as a true "gear" mechanism controlling the roll-glide motion of the tibiofemoral joint. With rupture of either or both of the cruciate ligaments, the gear mechanism becomes ineffective, and the arthrokinematic motion is altered. In an ACL-deficient knee, the femur is able to roll beyond the posterior half of the tibial plateau, increasing the likelihood of damage or tear of the posterior horn of the medial or lateral meniscus.

TABLE 10-2

Examples of Commercially Available Knee Orthoses

Orthoses for the tibiofemoral joint
To immobilize the knee
  Plaster cast
  Velcro immobilizer without orthotic knee joint
  Velcro immobilizer with adjustable locking orthotic knee
  Custom-thermoplastic knee immobilizer (knee cylinder)
Rehabilitative braces (hinged knee orthoses)
  Bledsoe brace
  Donjoy ELS brace
  Donjoy IROM brace
  Donjoy system 2 brace
Functional braces (hinged knee orthoses)
  Can-Am brace
  CTi brace
  Donjoy Defiance brace
  Donjoy Goldpoint brace
  Generation II
  Lenox Hill Derotation brace
  Lenox Hill Precision Fit brace
  MKS II orthoses
  Omni Avant Guard brace
  OrthoTech
  Townsend brace
Prophylactic braces
  Anderson knee stabilizer
  McDavid knee guard
Orthoses for the patellofemoral joint
To control tracking
  Palumbo brace
  OrthoTech Tru-Pull
  Air Donjoy
To facilitate normal tracking
  On Track system
  Infrapatellar straps
  McConnel taping techniques

Because the knee has characteristics of a hinge joint and an arthodial joint, two types of motion (translatory and rotatory) can occur in each plane of motion (sagittal, frontal/coronal, transverse). For this reason, knee motion is described as having six degrees of freedom. The three translatory motions of the knee include anteroposterior translation of 5–10 mm, mediolateral translation of 1–2 mm, and compression-distraction motion of 2–5 mm. The three rotatory motions occur in flexion/extension, varus/valgus, and internal (medial)/external (lateral) rotation.[4,15]

ORTHOSES FOR THE KNEE

A sample of the many knee orthoses that are commercially available for health professionals in sports medicine is listed in Table 10-2. Some are designed to immobilize the knee after surgical repair of damaged or ruptured ligaments or menisci during the acute phases of healing. *Rehabilitative orthoses* are designed to protect the knee and allow progressive increase in active range of motion during rehabilitation. *Functional knee orthoses* provide additional protection as rehabilitation is completed and a patient returns to normal activities. A final group, *prophylactic knee orthoses*, attempt to prevent injury (or at least lessen the extent of injury) in athletes who are at risk of injury during competition. Given the complexity of the knee joint (with its polycentric axis of rotation for flexion/extension, asymmetry of the lateral and medial compartments, and the arrangement of its muscular and ligamentous attachments), most orthotic designs are unable to support, protect, or stabilize the knee with the same efficiency as its own physiologic motion.

REHABILITATION KNEE ORTHOSES

Orthoses used in the postoperative and early rehabilitation of patients who have had surgical repair of damaged ligaments are designed to control knee motion carefully to minimize excessive loading on healing tissues[3] (Figure 10-7). Although many rehabilitation knee orthoses are on the market, an effective orthosis has several important characteristics. The orthosis must be adjustable to accommodate for changes in limb girth due to edema or to atrophy. It must remain in the desired position on the limb during upright and sitting activities. It must be comfortable to wear, easy to don and doff, durable, and economical. Most physicians require an adjustable knee unit so that "free" active range of motion can be increased incrementally as the patient's condition improves. The ability to move in carefully controlled ranges of motion is thought to improve ligamentous strength and to minimize the risk of scar formation in the intracondylar notch that is associated with flexion contracture.[15]

FUNCTIONAL KNEE ORTHOSES

Use of knee orthoses as functional braces parallels the development of the discipline of sports medicine since the early 1970s.[16] In the years before 1970, orthoses that were designed for patients with neuromuscular dysfunction were adapted in an attempt to meet the needs of injured athletes with a functionally unstable knee. Typically, the adapted orthosis was cumbersome and significantly impaired the quality of the athlete's performance. To assist professional athletes in quickly and safely returning to competition, the sports medicine community explored alternative orthotic interventions to manage an unstable knee. The development of functional knee orthoses as

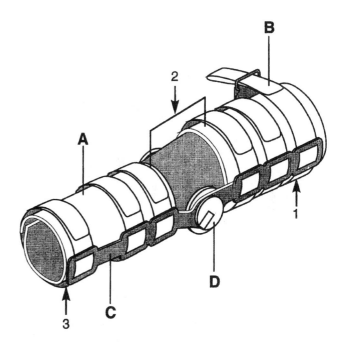

FIGURE 10-7

The components of most commercially available rehabilitation knee orthoses include (A) open cell foam interface around calf and thigh; (B) nonelastic, adjustable Velcro strap for closures; (C) lightweight metal, composite, or plastic sidebars; and (D) single-axis or polycentric hinge that can be locked or adjusted, or both, to allow motion in the desired limited range. The force systems of these orthoses apply a pair of anteriorly directed forces at the (1) proximal posterior thigh and (3) distal posterior calf, against a posteriorly directed force (2) applied over or on either side of the patella. Varus and valgus stressors are resisted by the sidebars. (Reprinted with permission from P Trautman. Lower Limb Orthoses. In JB Redford, JV Basmajian, P Trautman [eds], Orthotics: Clinical Practice and Rehabilitation Technology. New York: Churchill Livingstone, 1995;30.)

alternatives to surgery (which often sidelined athletes for considerable periods of time) was especially welcomed.[17]

Lenox Hill Derotation Orthosis

The Lenox Hill Derotation knee brace, developed by Nicholas and Castiglia of Lenox Hill Hospital in the early 1970s to protect the chronically unstable knees of football quarterback Joe Namath, was the primary design that was commercially available until the late 1970s.[18] The original orthosis has medial and lateral uprights, a single-axis orthotic knee joint with a medial fulcrum pad, a broad elastic thigh and calf cuff/strap to hold the orthosis in place, and a set of derotation straps to control movement of the tibia on the femur.

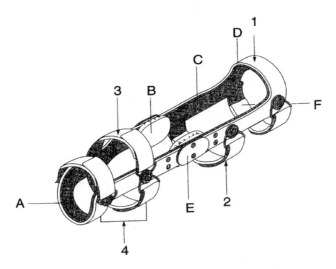

FIGURE 10-8

Components of most contemporary functional knee orthoses include (A) the calf section/cuff with its closure; (B) medial or lateral condylar pads, or both; (C) medial and lateral uprights; (D) the thigh section/cuff with its closure; (E) an adjustable knee hinge; and (F) the thigh strap. The stabilizing forces that are typically applied by the orthosis include (1) a posterior force over the anterior proximal thigh, (2) an anterior force on the distal posterior femur, (3) a posterior force at the proximal anterior tibia, and (4) an anterior force at the midshaft of the posterior tibia. (Reprinted with permission from P Trautman. Lower Limb Orthoses. In JB Redford, JV Basmajian, P Trautman [eds], Orthotics: Clinical Practice and Rehabilitation Technology. New York: Churchill Livingstone, 1995;31.)

This orthosis is intended to control mediolateral instability, rotational instability, and multiple ligament impairment.[19] Subsequent versions of the Lenox Hill orthosis are available in standard, lightweight, and ultralightweight versions; with a dial-lock option to adjust available range of motion and with protective under- and over-sleeves.

The original design has evolved considerably: More than three dozen functional braces are being manufactured in today's sports medicine market (see Table 10-2 for examples). The components of a functional knee orthosis are diagrammed in Figure 10-8. Most are based on a lightweight rigid suprastructure made from carbon composite or titanium alloy. Many use adjustable elasticized or Velcro strapping to apply a four-point stabilizing force and to hold the orthosis in position on the limb. Some have polycentric knee units; others allow variable flexion control or assisted extension. Unfortunately, systematic critical evaluation of the efficacy of functional knee orthoses has not kept pace with the development of new designs; there is a paucity of clin-

ical and laboratory research defining the indications for, roles of, or outcomes of use for these functional braces.[17]

PROPHYLACTIC KNEE ORTHOSES

In the 1990s, considerable debate took place concerning the potential benefits or effectiveness of orthoses that were designed to prevent knee injuries or to minimize the severity of injury for athletes involved in high-risk injury activities.[20-23] Most are designed to protect the integrity of medial knee structures against laterally directed forces by using a hinged lateral frame, held in place by a set of thigh and calf cuffs or straps. The hinge may be single axis or polycentric; many designs have also incorporated a hyperextension stop for further protection of the athlete's knee against forceful hyperextension injury. Prophylactic knee orthoses are available "off the shelf" or can be custom molded for the individual athlete. Clinical practice and research have not yet resolved the debate about the efficacy of prophylactic orthoses. Questions remain about the relationship between the biomechanical characteristics of the orthoses and the anatomic knee, the response of the orthosis to valgus loading, the impact of the orthosis on the continuum of locomotion (walking to running), and the ability of the orthosis to prevent injuries during activity as intended by its design.

Many of the studies that have investigated the biomechanical performance of prophylactic braces have used either cadaver knees or mechanical surrogate models of the knee. Most have concluded that protection of the MCL has been inconsistent and only borderline at best.[21,24-28] Many health care providers are concerned about how the orthosis might preload the MCL before normal physiologic loading.[24,26,27] Our understanding of the interaction between the orthosis and the tissues of the knee is based on the properties of human tissue and of brace materials under static and dynamic loading conditions.

Many manufacturers report high resistance of the braces to laterally directed impact loading; however, the research design and methodology on which these claims are based are often poor or flawed. In some cases, the braces are actually less rigid and resistant to derangement during loading than is the anatomic knee itself. The ability of a knee orthosis prepositioned in flexion to protect against major ligament damage is also being questioned.[29]

Joint line clearance during brace deformation is an additional concern. Theoretically, the prophylactic brace is designed to transmit valgus loads on the knee over the greatest possible area to dissipate the forces away from susceptible ligaments effectively.[22,26,27] The orthotic hinge forms a bridge over the joint line; its sites of attachment are best placed as far as possible on the proximal femur and distal tibia. Clearance between the hinge and the joint themselves must be adequate. Contact between the hinge and the joint creates a three-point bending system centered at the joint, inadvertently preloading the MCL.[26,27]

Prophylactic knee braces have grown in popularity over the last 20 years despite a shortage of scientific evidence of their efficacy or of any potentially detrimental effects. Researchers have evaluated the impact of lateral bracing on injury rates among high school and college football players; most have found no significant reduction in injury as a result of prophylactic bracing.[23,30-33] Researchers and athletic trainers have concerns about the risk of injury to other areas of the limb when these orthoses are worn during competition. In a two-season prospective study of potentially protective benefits of prophylactic bracing in a sample of 580 high school football players, Grace et al.[23] found a dramatic increase in the number of injuries of the ankle and foot among athletes who wore the braces. In contrast, Sitler et al.[32] found no significant difference in the frequency of ankle injuries between a knee brace group and a control group of military cadets. Additionally, the severity of MCL and ACL knee injury was not reduced with the use of unilateral-biaxial prophylactic knee braces.[32]

If prophylactic braces are intended to prevent or to reduce the severity of injury, clinicians and brace manufacturers must work to be responsible for critical evaluation of these devices to define better their appropriate use and outcomes. Clinicians who go to the research literature for evidence supporting the use of prophylactic bracing are likely to find studies that are inconclusive because of methodologic problems and limited sample size.[34-38] Many studies reported in the literature have little bearing on ultimate brace function or true physiologic application to the playing field. At the present time, clinicians must hold vendors accountable for their products, requesting well-designed and clearly reported quantitative studies to support the narrative accounts in marketing brochures about design criteria.

FUNCTIONAL KNEE ORTHOSES AND PERFORMANCE

A number of researchers have investigated the impact of functional braces on performance and endurance in non-injured and previously injured athletes. Stephens[39] found little impact on speed of running in noninjured collegiate basketball players during straight line running tasks (end line to foul line, full court) when comparing performance in two functional braces to nonbraced speed. Although these results are positive, the in-brace time and types of activity used for the study were significantly different than those of an active, full-length basketball game.

Highgenboten et al.[40] found a 3–6% increase in metabolic cost during steady-state treadmill running when functional braces were worn. Subjects also had higher ratings of perceived exertion when exercising with the brace. These effects were attributed to the weight of the brace.

Most functional knee braces weigh close to 1 pound. Despite the use of lightweight materials that are resilient to various forces, it is possible that long in-brace times can lead to fatigue or to injuries to other areas of the body that compensate for the added weight of the orthosis. This may explain the increase in injuries of the foot and ankle reported by Grace et al.[23] in athletes who wore braces. Styf et al.[41] studied changes in intramuscular pressures within the anterior compartment of the leg at rest, during exercise, and after exercise, comparing three orthoses. Intramuscular pressures at rest and muscle relaxation pressure during exercise were higher when subjects wore each of the orthoses. To evaluate whether distal strapping was responsible for this increase in pressure, distal straps were removed and subjects retested; intramuscular pressure and muscle relaxation pressure returned to levels that were similar to nonbraced levels. This study demonstrates the subtle yet potentially important impact of orthoses on muscle function that may contribute to vulnerability to injury.

FUNCTIONAL KNEE ORTHOSES FOR ANTERIOR CRUCIATE LIGAMENT INSUFFICIENCY

For more than 20 years, functional knee orthoses have been used to prevent forward subluxation of the tibia on the femur for patients with ACL insufficiency. A variety of designs have evolved to be used for partial ACL tears or for complete ACL rupture. A number of research studies have attempted to evaluate whether these orthoses are as effective as the marketing literature suggests. One strategy has been to compare forward excursion of the tibia on the femur using clinical tests of knee instability, performed on a subject with and without bracing.[16,29,42] In a high percentage of subjects, the tibia was demonstrated to be more stable in-brace, with a reduction in translation and rotation noted, when compared to out-of-brace testing. Although this evidence is encouraging, results must be carefully interpreted, because the relationship between static testing and actual physiologic loading during sport activity has not been well established. Noyes et al.[43] have demonstrated that manual examination cannot duplicate the magnitude of force that is present during activity.

Another strategy is to use cadaver models to evaluate the efficacy of functional knee orthoses for support of the ACL.[43,44] The major drawback of this type of study, however, is the difference between living and preserved tissue. Because active muscle contraction and normal soft tissue compliance contribute to strain on the ACL, the lack of active musculature and compliance changes in soft tissue around the knee limit the application of cadaver study findings. Similarly, the magnitude and sequence of muscle contraction alter the stiffness between the brace and the soft tissue of the leg. It is not possible to reproduce this interface in cadaver studies.

Although static and cadaver studies have been the first step in critically evaluating the efficacy of functional knee orthoses for patients with ACL insufficiency, the most informative research would be done in vivo. This is especially important because static and cadaver studies cannot replicate the real-life physiologic loading that occurs in the knee during activities.[43-48] The next challenge for clinical researchers is to develop methodology to evaluate functional knee orthoses during functional activities.

At this time, few studies have looked at advanced levels of testing functional knee braces. Cook et al.[49] compared the ability of subjects with absent ACLs (n = 14) to perform running and cutting maneuvers with and without a commercially available orthosis. Subjects' performance with the orthosis was objectively and subjectively better. In a similar study that compared the performance of subjects with ACL deficiency in several orthoses, Marans et al.[50] report improved performance in two of the six orthoses evaluated.

Another strategy is to evaluate muscle function when subjects with ACL deficiency use a functional knee orthosis. Branch et al.[51] found little difference in electromyographic firing patterns between in-brace and out-of-brace testing.[51] Because muscle activity was similarly reduced under both conditions (as referenced to an ACL intact limb), the researchers suggest that functional knee orthoses do not have a significant proprioceptive influence on muscle function.

A number of studies have examined the metabolic cost using dynamic analysis of orthotic use to test the validity and reliability of functional knee braces on ACL-insufficient knees.[40,52] Whether the slight increase in energy requirements noted is offset by protection and improved function while wearing the orthosis is not yet understood.

INFORMED CLINICAL DECISION MAKING

Because of the large number of functional knee orthoses currently marketed, it is very challenging and often frustrating for clinicians and surgeons to evaluate the information published in marketing literature when research support is not always available. It is also challenging to remain well informed because orthotic designs are constantly being modified and "improved." Making a sound decision about which design can best meet the stability and activity needs of a given individual can be a daunting task and must not be based on which sales representative most recently shared information or which orthosis is currently the most popular choice. Although patients may seek a functional orthosis to protect their knee or to improve their performance, many do not have the knowledge or resources to understand the specifics and idiosyncrasies of each brace. To make an informed decision, the clinician must consider the patient's specific injury and pattern of instability, the present and anticipated strength and bulk of their muscles around the injured knee, and the activities and likely mechanism of being reinjured in the patient's preferred sports activities. Decisions about orthotic options must be deliberately made, with discussion involving the patient, physical therapist or athletic trainer, orthotist, brace manufacturer, and physician. Quick decisions about a functional knee orthosis, made without carefully evaluating the match between the patient's needs and the orthotic design, lead to frustration and dissatisfaction for all involved.

In evaluating information presented about knee orthoses published in the literature, health professionals must look closely at research design and methodology and evaluate the clinical relevance of the conclusions drawn from study results. Two important questions to ask might be (1) whether the study evaluates the orthosis under static conditions or during dynamic use and (2) whether the study used cadaver models or physiologically active joints in the evaluation of orthotic performance. Many of the most frequently cited studies evaluate brace performance under static conditions, specifically the ability of particular orthoses to prevent anterior excursion of the tibia on the femur as measured by standard clinical tests for ligamentous instability (e.g., Lachman's, pivot shift, or Losee's tests). Some studies have used electronic and mechanical instrumentation to evaluate orthotic performance more precisely under similar static conditions. Although many studies demonstrate the efficacy of knee orthoses in prevention of excessive anterior excursion under static conditions, to generalize these static results to dynamic activity for patients with ACL-deficient knees is foolhardy. Because an orthosis can provide a degree of stability for the knee under static conditions does not guarantee that it can also stabilize the knee during high demand activity. The low load levels applied to knee ligaments during static or cadaver model testing do not accurately reflect load levels during functional and athletic activities. Decisions to choose a particular orthosis based on this type of research alone are not well informed.

Options: Hinge Design

Hinge options for knee orthoses range from simple single-axis (unicentric) designs to complex four-bar polycentric designs. Most commercially available "off the shelf" functional knee orthoses have hinges in one of three categories: (1) the single-axis hinge, (2) the posterior offset hinge, or (3) the polycentric or genucentric hinge.

All single-axis/unicentric hinges act as a simple hinge; a unicentric hinge becomes incongruent with the anatomic joint axis as the instantaneous axis of rotation of the knee changes with movement through the range of motion. Posterior offset designs attempt to improve the match between orthotic and anatomic axis of motion by approximating the location of the sagittal radius of curvature of the posterior femoral condyles as it articulates with the tibia in flexion.[53] Polycentric designs attempt to replicate the instantaneous axis of rotation of the anatomic knee joint, using two geared surfaces that mechanically constrain motion into a defined path.[54] Theoretically, polycentric or genucentric hinges are better able than unicentric hinge designs to match the rolling and gliding of the tibiofemoral joint as the knee flexes and extends. This closer match to physiologic motion is meant to reduce pistoning, discomfort, and slippage of the orthosis on the limb during activity.

It is important to remember, when considering which hinge design to select, that the soft tissue of the knee between the orthosis and the bone compromises the impact of any hinge on the kinematics of the knee. The most important characteristic of the hinge is its ability to transfer load during activity. Poorly designed or constructed hinges, or those made of weak or pliable materials, cannot effectively accomplish this task, and abnormal translations and rotations will not be well controlled. The work of Lew et al.[54] demonstrated greater variation in the pistoning constraint forces in a particular joint design than across designs when three orthoses were compared during specific activities.

Regalbuto et al.[55] evaluated the performance of four hinge designs fit into a custom-fit knee orthosis in three healthy subjects. Subjects wore the orthosis while performing a squat, an 8-in. step-up, a stand-to-sit activity, and an open chain knee extension exercise. The researchers found that accurate hinge placement was a more important influence on function and comfort than hinge kinematics. Differences in kinematics among the four designs were masked by the compliance of the soft tissues between the brace cuffs and the bones of the knee.

ORTHOSES FOR PATELLOFEMORAL DYSFUNCTION

Just as evidence to support prophylactic and functional orthoses for tibiofemoral joint instability is inadequate, research support for the efficacy of patellofemoral taping and bracing is lacking. Nevertheless, orthotic management of patellofemoral dysfunction has become widespread in athletic and in nonathletic practice environments. The need for well-designed clinical research studies is pressing.

Patellofemoral braces are often used as an adjunct to exercise to (1) provide pain relief and improve function for patients with patellofemoral pain syndrome, (2) prevent or control patellar subluxation or dislocation in patients with patellar tracking problems, (3) provide pain relief and support healing for patients with patellar tendonitis of the quadriceps or patellar tendon and for patients with Osgood-Schlatter disease, and (4) manage patients with chondromalacia and other symptomatic degenerative articular changes of the patellofemoral joint.[56]

Many patellofemoral braces are constructed from elasticized or neoprene type materials, with a cutout for the patella, crescent-shaped buttresses sewn in place or held by Velcro, and reinforcing straps. The purpose of the buttress and straps is to stabilize the position of the patella as it slides in the intracondylar groove during knee motion.[10] Another design uses a curved vinyl-covered strap worn snugly at the patellar tendon to support and elevate the patella during activity for more efficient tracking.[57,58] Normalization of tracking can, theoretically, minimize abnormal compressive forces on the articular surfaces, reduce the likelihood of further degenerative changes, and provide relief of symptoms.[56]

In a longitudinal study of 25 patients with unilateral retropatellar pain syndrome, Reikeras[59] found patellofemoral bracing to be minimally effective for symptom relief and for return to functional activities. In contrast, comprehensive conservative management of chondromalacia[60] and of patellofemoral pain[61] staged for acute symptom management, exercises to build flexibility and strength, maintenance exercise for eccentric control and muscular endurance, and return to activity using patellofemoral bracing were effective for 77–82% of patients. A preliminary report by Crocker and Stauber[62] demonstrated that use of a patellar stabilizing brace enabled four of five subjects to generate normal strength curves and increased power during isokinetic testing. Subjects in this study also experienced improved performance in functional and sport activities when wearing the patellofemoral brace. In a larger study, 59 of 62 patients with diagnoses of patellar subluxation, patellofemoral arthritis, or Osgood-Schlatter disease were able to perform activities that typically provoked symptoms (pivoting, running, stair climbing, and long-distance walking) when wearing a patellofemoral brace.[10]

Although these results are encouraging, the use of a patellofemoral brace as the primary intervention for patients with patellofemoral pain is not well supported. Conservative management strategies with established efficacy include activity modification, limited use of non-steroidal anti-inflammatory medications, and strengthening and flexibility exercises. Further clinical research to evaluate carefully the added benefit of patellofemoral bracing in the conservative management of patellofemoral dysfunction is necessary.

SUMMARY

In this chapter, we have reviewed the normal structure and function of the tibiofemoral and patellofemoral joints, with special attention to the role of the collateral and cruciate ligaments in the arthro- and osteokinematics of the knee joint. We have defined three types of knee orthoses for the tibiofemoral joint: rehabilitation orthoses, functional orthoses, and prophylactic orthoses. In reviewing the research literature, we have found a gap between what many of these orthoses are designed to do and evidence of their efficacy. We have described the research strategies that are most frequently used in the study of knee orthoses and have discussed problems with research design, methods, and generalizability to patients and athletes involved in dynamic activities. Similar problems exist when the role of patellofemoral orthoses in sports medicine and rehabilitation are considered.

After reading this chapter, it is hoped that health care professionals will be better able to evaluate the intent and design of knee orthoses and to ask for clinically applicable evidence of efficacy from brace designers and manufacturers. Clinicians also have an opportunity to contribute to the understanding of the contribution of knee orthoses in rehabilitation and long-term management of patients with ligamentous instability by participating in clinical research.

REFERENCES

1. Cawley PW. Is Knee Bracing Really Necessary? A Review of Current Research on Brace Function, the Natural History of Graft Remodeling, and Physiologic Implications. Carlsbad, CA: Smith & Nephew Donjoy Biomechanics Research Laboratory, 1989.

2. Trautman P. Lower Limb Orthoses. In JB Redford, JV Basmajian, P Trautman (eds), Orthotics: Clinical Practice and Rehabilitation Technology. New York: Churchill Livingstone, 1995;13–54.

3. Drez D, DeHaven K, D'Ambrosia R. Knee Braces Seminar Report. Chicago: American Academy of Orthopaedic Surgeons, 1984.

4. Norkin CC, Levangie PK. The Knee Complex. In Joint Structure and Function: A Comprehensive Analysis (2nd ed). Philadelphia: Davis, 1992;337–378.

5. Antich TJ. Orthoses for the Knee: The Tibiofemoral Joint. In DA Nawoczenski, ME Epler (eds), Orthotics in Functional Rehabilitation of the Lower Limb. Philadelphia: Saunders, 1997;57–76.

6. Terry GC, Hughston JC, Norwood LA. Anatomy of the iliopatellar band and iliotibial tract. Am J Sports Med 1986;14(1):39–45.

7. Greenfield BH. Functional Anatomy of the Knee. In BH Greenfield (ed), Rehabilitation of the Knee: A Problem Solving Approach. Philadelphia: Davis, 1993;1–42.

8. Cox AJ. Biomechanics of the patello-femoral joint. Clin Biomech 1990;5:123–130.

9. Grabiner MD, Koh TJ, Draganich LF. Neuromechanics of the patellofemoral joint. Med Sci Sports Exerc 1994;26(1):10–21.

10. Palumbo PM. Dynamic patellar brace: a new orthosis in the management of patellofemoral disorders. Am J Sports Med 1981;9(1):45–49.

11. Van Kampen A, Huiskes R. The three-dimensional tracking pattern of the human patella. J Orthop Res 1990;8(3):372–382.

12. Larson RL, Cabaud HE, Slocum DB, et al. The patellar compression syndrome: surgical treatment by lateral retinacular release. Clin Orthop 1978;34:158–167.

13. Wiberg G. Roentgenographic and anatomic studies on the femoropatellar joint: with special references to chondromalacia patellae. Acta Orthop Scand 1941;12:319–409.

14. Norkin CC, Levangie PK. Basic Concepts in Biomechanics. In Joint Structure and Function: A Comprehensive Analysis (2nd ed). Philadephia: Davis, 1992;1–56.

15. Muller W. The Knee: Form, Function, and Ligament Reconstruction. Berlin: Springer-Verlag, 1983.

16. Bassett GS, Fleming BW. The Lenox Hill brace in anterolateral rotatory instability. Am J Sports Med 1983;11(5):345–348.

17. Branch TP, Hunter RE. Functional analysis of anterior cruciate ligament braces. Clin Sports Med 1990;9(4):771–797.

18. Nicholas JA. Bracing the anterior cruciate ligament deficient knee using the Lenox Hill derotation brace. Clin Orthop 1983;172:137–142.

19. Beets CL, Clippinger FW, Hazard PR, Vaugh DW. Orthoses and the dynamic knee: a basic overview. Orthot Prosthet 1985;39(2):33–39.

20. Black KP, Raasch WG: Knee Braces in Sports. In JA Nicholas, EB Hershman (eds), The Lower Extremity and Spine in Sports Medicine (2nd ed). St. Louis: Mosby, 1995;987–998.

21. Erickson AN, Yasuda K, Beynnon B. An in vitro dynamic evaluation of prophylactic knee braces during lateral impact loading. Am J Sports Med 1993;21:26–35.

22. Garrick JG, Requa RK. Prophylactic knee bracing. Am J Sports Med 1987;15(5):471–476.

23. Grace TG, Skipper BJ, Newberry JC, et al. Prophylactic knee braces and injury to the lower extremity. J Bone Joint Surg 1988;70A(3):422–427.

24. Baker BE, VanHanswyk E, Bogosian SP, et al. The effect of knee braces on lateral impact loading of the knee. Am J Sports Med 1989;17(2):182–186.

25. Baker BE, VanHanswyk E, Bogosian SP. A biomechanical study of the static stabilizing effect of knee braces on medial stability. Am J Sports Med 1987;15:566–570.

26. France EP, Paulos LE, Jayaraman G, Rosenberg TD. The biomechanics of lateral knee bracing. Part II: Impact response of the braced knee. Am J Sports Med 1987;15(5):430–438.

27. Paulos LE, France EP, Rosenberg TD, et al. The biomechanics of lateral knee bracing. Part I: Response of the valgus restraints to loading. Am J Sports Med 1987;15(5):419–429.

28. Paulos LE, Cawley PW, France EP. Impact biomechanics of lateral knee bracing. The anterior cruciate ligament. Am J Sports Med 1991;19(4):337–342.

29. Cawley PW, France EP, Paulos LE. Comparison of rehabilitative knee braces. A biomechanical investigation. Am J Sports Med 1989;17(2):141–146.

30. Hewson GF, Mendini RA, Wang JB. Prophylactic knee bracing in college football. Am J Sports Med 1986;14(4):262–266.

31. Rovere GD, Haupt HA, Yates CS. Prophylactic knee bracing in college football. Am J Sports Med 1987;15(2):111–116.

32. Sitler M, Ryan J, Hopkinson W, et al. The efficacy of a prophylactic knee brace to reduce injuries in football. A prospective, randomized study at West Point. Am J Sports Med 1990;18(3):310–315.

33. Teitz CC, Hermanson BK, Kronmal RA, Diehr PH. Evaluation of the use of braces to prevent injury to the knee in collegiate football players. J Bone Joint Surg 1987;69A(1):2–9.

34. Borsa PA, Lephart SM, Fu FH. Muscular and functional performance characteristics of individuals wearing prophylactic knee braces. J Athletic Training 1993;28(4):336–342.

35. Liggett CL, Tandy RD, Young JC. The effects of prophylactic knee bracing on running gait. J Athletic Training 1995;30(2):159–161.

36. Osternig LR, Robertson RN. Effects of prophylactic bracing on lower extremity joint position and muscle activation during running. Am J Sports Med 1993;21(5):733–737.

37. Van Horn DA, Makinnion JL, Witt PL. Comparison of the effects of the Anderson knee stabler and McDavid knee guard on the kinematics of the lower extremity during gait. JOSPT 1988;9(7):254–260.

38. Veldhuizen JW, Koene FM, Oostvogel HJ. The effects of a supportive knee brace on leg performance in healthy subjects. Int J Sports Med 1991;12(6):577–580.

39. Stephens DL. The effects of functional knee braces on speed in collegiate basketball players. JOSPT 1995;22(6):259–262.

40. Highgenboten CL, Jackson A, Meske N. The effects of knee brace wear on perceptual and metabolic variables during horizontal treadmill running. Am J Sports Med 1991;19(6):639–643.

41. Styf JR, Nakhostine M, Gershuni DH. Functional knee braces increase intramuscular pressures in the anterior compartment of the leg. Am J Sports Med 1992;20(1):46–49.

42. Colville MR, Lee CL, Ciullo JV. The Lenox Hill brace. An evaluation of effectiveness in treating knee instability. Am J Sports Med 1986;14(4):257–261.

43. Noyes FR, Grood ES, Butler DL, Malek M. Clinical laxity tests and functional stability of the knee: biomechanical concepts. Clin Orthop 1980;146:84–89.

44. Wojtys EM, Loubert PV, Samson SY, Viviano DM. Use of a knee-brace for control of tibial translation and rotation. J Bone Joint Surg 1990;72A(9):1323–1329.

45. Beck C, Drez D, Young J, et al. Instrumented testing of functional knee braces. Am J Sports Med 1986;14(4):253–256.

46. Beynnon BD, Pope MH, Wertheimer CM, et al. The effect of functional knee-braces on strain on the anterior cruciate ligament in vivo. J Bone Joint Surg 1992;74A(9):1298–1312.

47. Jonsson H, Karrholm J. Brace effects on the unstable knee in 21 cases. A roentgen stereophotogrammetric comparison of three designs. Acta Orthop Scand 1990;61(4):313–318.

48. Mishra DK, Daniel DM, Stone ML. The use of functional knee braces in the control of pathologic anterior knee laxity. Clin Orthop 1989;April(241):213–220.

49. Cook FF, Tibone JE, Redfern FC. A dynamic analysis of a functional brace for anterior cruciate ligament insufficiency. Am J Sports Med 1989;17(4):519–524.

50. Marans HJ, Jackson RW, Piccinin J, et al. Functional testing of braces for anterior cruciate ligament–deficient knees. Can J Surg 1991;34(2):167–172.

51. Branch TP, Hunter RE, Donath M. Dynamic EMG analysis of anterior cruciate deficient legs with and without bracing during cutting. Am J Sports Med 1989;17(1):35–41.

52. Zetterlund AE, Serfass RC, Hunter RE. The effect of wearing the complete Lenox Hill derotation brace on energy expenditure during horizontal treadmill running at 161 meters per minute. Am J Sports Med 1986;14(1):73–76.

53. Gardner HF, Clippinger FW. A method for location of prosthetic and orthotic knee joints. Artif Limbs 1979;13:31–35.

54. Lew WD, Patrnchak CM, Lewis JL, et al. A comparison of pistoning forces in orthotic knee joints. Orthot Prosthet 1984;36(2):85–95.

55. Regalbuto MA, Rovick JS, Walker PS. The forces in a knee brace as a function of hinge design and placement. Am J Sports Med 1989;17(4):535–542.

56. Belyea BC. Orthoses for the Knee: The Patellofemoral Joint. In DA Nawoczenski, ME Eppler (eds), Orthotics in Functional Rehabilitation of the Lower Limb. Philadelphia: Saunders, 1997;31–56.

57. Levine J, Splain S. Use of the infrapatellar strap in the treatment of patellofemoral pain. Clin Orthop 1979;139:179–181.

58. Levine J. A new brace for chondromalacia patella and kindred conditions. Am J Sports Med 1978;6(3):137–140.

59. Reikeras O. Brace with a lateral pad for patellar pain: 2 year follow-up of 25 patients. Acta Orthop Scand 1990;61:319–320.

60. DeHaven KE, Lolan WA, Mayer PJ. Chondromalacia patellae in athletes: clinical presentation and conservative management. Am J Sports Med 1979;7(1):5–11.

61. Malek M, Mangine R. Patellofemoral pain syndromes: a comprehensive and conservative approach. J Orthop Sports Phys Ther 1981;2(3):108–116.

62. Crocker B, Stauber WT. Objective analysis of quadriceps force during bracing of the patella: a preliminary study. Aust J Sci Med Sport 1989;21:25–28.

SUGGESTED READING

Bellamy MM. Controversy faces braces. Sportcare and Fitness 1988;Sept/Oct:17–24.

Burns GS, Hull ML, Patterson HA. Strain in the anteromedial bundle of the anterior cruciate ligament under combination loading. Orthop Res 1992;10:167–176.

Cawley PW. Postoperative knee bracing. Clin Sports Med 1990;9(4):763–770.

Cawley PW, France EP, Paulos LE. The current state of functional knee bracing research. A review of the literature. Am J Sports Med 1991;19(3):226–233.

France EP, Cawley PW, Paulos LE. Choosing functional knee braces. Clin Sports Med 1990;9(4):743–750.

Fuss FK. Anatomy of the cruciate ligaments and their function in extension and flexion of the human knee joint. Am J Anat 1989;184(2):165–176.

Gray HG. Gray's Anatomy. Philadelphia: Running Press, 1974;274–276.

Henry JH. The Patellofemoral Joint. In Nicholas JA, Hershman EB (eds), The Lower Extremity and Spine in Sports Medicine (2nd ed). Philadelphia: Mosby, 1995;940–970.

Hofmann AA, Wyatt RWB, Bourne MH, et al. Knee stability in orthotic knee braces. Am J Sports Med 1984;12(5):371–374.

Houston ME, Goemans PH. Leg muscle performance of athletes with and without knee support braces. Arch Phys Med Rehabil 1982;63(9):431–432.

Liu SH, Daluiski A, Kabo JM. The effects of thigh soft-tissue stiffness on the control of anterior tibial displacement by functional knee orthoses. J Rehab Res Dev 1995;32(2):135–140.

Seebacher JR, Inglis AE, Marshal JL. The structure of the posterolateral aspect of the knee. J Bone Joint Surg 1982;64(4):536.

Sell KE. On the field again: knee bracing options. Adv Rehabil 1996;March;51–53.

Silbey MB, Fu FH. Knee Injuries. In FH Fu, DA Stone (eds), Sports Injuries. Mechanisms, Prevention, Treatment. Baltimore: Williams & Wilkins, 1994;949–976.

Terry GC. The anatomy of the extensor mechanism. Clin Sports Med 1989;8(2):163–177.

Warren LF, Marshall JL. The supportive structures and layers on the medial side of the knee. An anatomical analysis. J Bone Joint Surg 1979;61(1):56.

11

Knee-Ankle-Foot Orthoses

Thomas V. DiBello

For patients with neuromuscular or musculoskeletal impairments of the lower extremities who may require an orthosis to enhance functional mobility (gait or transfers, or both), decisions about orthotic prescription are best made in the context of an interdisciplinary team framework. This team is comprised of the patient and his or her family or caregivers, any physicians involved in his or her care (e.g., a neurologist, orthopedist, or physiatrist), the physical and occupational therapists who are likely to be involved in functional training, and the orthotist who will design, fabricate, deliver, and maintain the orthosis. Recommendations about orthotic options are based on four types of information: (1) an understanding of the patient's diagnosis and prognosis; (2) a thorough assessment of gait, muscle function and motor control, range of motion, and alignment of the limb; (3) an understanding of the patient's general medical condition and level of fitness; and (4) discussion of the patient's typical or desired vocational and leisure activities. A clear goal or set of goals for orthotic intervention is formulated based on these findings: The team might recommend a pair of knee-ankle-foot orthoses (KAFOs), for example, for a patient with paraplegia secondary to spinal cord injury who wants to pursue ambulation, if that patient requires more external stability at the knee than can be provided by a solid-ankle ankle-foot orthosis (AFO).

This team approach allows consideration of a variety of important influences on the eventual outcome of orthotic intervention, ranging from the specifics of the patient's diagnosis to the patient's preferred lifestyle and leisure activities. The importance of this discussion, which must include the patient, cannot be overstated. The use of an orthosis, a mechanical device that can enhance as well as constrain lower limb function, requires considerable adjustment on the part of the patient. Acceptance and consistent use of the orthosis depend, to a large extent, on how well the device meets the patient's specific needs or goals and how much use of the device is inconvenient or disruptive to his or her lifestyle.

An important component of orthotic intervention is assessment of the patient's preconception or expectation about the outcome of orthotic intervention. If a patient expects that the success of an orthosis depends on a return to "normalcy" in walking, he or she is certain to be disappointed with the intervention and frustrated with the device. Patient education and discussion about the likely functional outcomes of KAFO use are especially important when patient expectation and reality are mismatched. Failure to discuss and define anticipated functional status and tradeoffs of orthotic use early in the process often leads to difficulties with or rejection of the orthosis.

ROLE OF THE MEDICAL DIAGNOSIS

It is important for the team to consider carefully the diagnosis that makes prescription of an orthosis necessary, including its etiology and prognosis. Is the patient's musculoskeletal or neuromuscular status stable and likely to remain the same over time? Does the patient's disease typically have a progressive course, such that decline in function is anticipated over time? Or, as in the case of traumatic injury, will the patient's condition and functional ability improve with time as healing occurs? Diagnosis also helps the team to define what might be expected in terms of muscle function and strength, range of motion and joint function, and functional mobility and gait. All of these factors must be accounted for in the design of the orthosis.

GAIT ASSESSMENT

An effective assessment of the lower limb function is based on a thorough understanding of the intricacies of normal stance and swing phase biomechanics.[1] Assessment

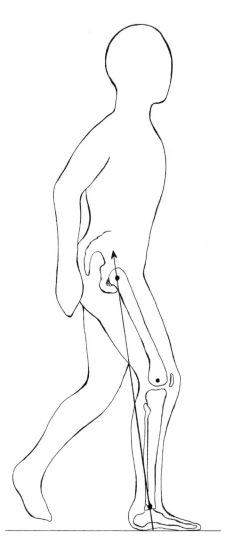

FIGURE 11-1

The ground reaction force passes through the ankle, behind the knee, and through the hip as loading response moves toward midstance, creating an external flexion moment at the knee. To achieve stability, muscle activity of the quadriceps, hamstrings, and gastronemius/soleus combine to create an internal extension moment to counterbalance the flexion moment of the ground reaction force.

of gait includes quantitative kinematic measures (such as gait speed, stride and step length, cadence, and double support time) and an observational gait analysis that assists the team in identifying primary problems in the context of the gait cycle as well as possible compensatory strategies.[1–3] For patients with complex gait problems, videotaping or computerized gait analysis may be a valuable tool for the team in appreciating what is happening during stance and swing. Clear definition and quantification

of gait deviations assist the team in determining the level of orthotic intervention that is necessary to achieve the specified goals.

KAFOs are considered when excessive movement occurs at the knee during stance phase. Excessive flexion may be present so that stance phase stability is compromised. The patient may have hyperextension or recurvatum that jeopardizes the structural integrity of the joint and, if unchecked, will threaten stance phase stability. Abnormal or excessive varus or valgus angulation may be present when the limb is loaded in stance, which compromises joint function and structure and can further alter biomechanical function over time to compromise the patient's ability to walk in the future.

It is very important that assessment of knee function does not occur in isolation but is instead evaluated in the context of a closed chain or system: Position of and muscular action around the ankle and the hip have an impact on knee function throughout stance and swing phases. Ankle position affects the position of the knee in relation to the ground reaction forces. In normal gait, as loading response transitions toward midstance, the foot has moved into a foot-flat position so that the ankle is in slight plantar flexion. Concurrently, knee flexion is controlled to approximately 15 degrees to "absorb shock" as the limb is loaded; this is quickly followed by knee extension. The hip is supported in 30 degrees of flexion and begins to extend with forward progression, and the hip abductors work to keep the pelvis level. In this early stance period, the ground reaction force passes through the ankle, behind the knee, and through the hip, creating an external flexion movement at the knee (Figure 11-1). To counteract this ground reaction force–derived external flexion moment, the quadriceps must contract to prevent the knee from collapsing into further flexion. In addition, the hamstrings contract to stabilize hip position, and the gastrocnemius begins to contract eccentrically to control forward progression of the tibia. This combination of muscle activity provides an internally generated knee extension moment that balances the external flexion moment at the knee generated by the ground reaction force.

If position or muscle function at the hip, knee, or ankle is altered or disturbed in any way, the system is thrown out of equilibrium, and gait will be less efficient or compromised.[4] If ankle position changes, the relative position of the ground reaction force will also change, altering the magnitude of the moment generated at the knee. If the strength or motor control of any of the involved musculature is impaired, the patient's ability to generate the appropriate internal extension moment to balance the external flexion moment may be compromised. When significant hypertonicity (spasticity) is present, excessive muscle activity often occurs that overpowers the external moment or alters the sequencing of muscle action.[5] The magnitude of disruption of the equilibrium between externally and internally generated moments determines whether the patient will be able to recover from or compensate for the imbalance. The magnitude of disruption and the resultant impact on gait also determine the level of orthotic intervention that is necessary to achieve the specified goal. When the evaluation of lower extremity function indicates that an AFO cannot effectively influence the position of the ground reaction force as it crosses the knee, a KAFO is likely to be the appropriate orthosis.

An orthosis of any kind does three things: It protects the joints of the limb that it crosses, it provides stance phase stability when structural integrity or motor control is impaired, and it has an impact on the patient's ability to function (i.e., functionality). The relationship between functionality and stability/protection in lower extremity orthoses is somewhat inverse: Any orthosis that provides stance phase stability for patients with lower limb weakness due to a neuromuscular disorder or protection for a patient who is in rehabilitation after traumatic injury has an impact on mobility in swing and limb movement during other functional activities. Improved function does not imply normalcy. The goals of stability and protection would provide patients improved function as compared to ambulation without an orthosis, but gait cannot be restored to normal.

When protection or stability of the knee is the primary goal of treatment, an AFO may not be sufficient, and a KAFO may be indicated.[6] When the desired control is for reduction of knee joint hyperextension or mild to moderate varus or valgus angulation is present, the KAFO can be built with a nonlocking knee joint. When hyperflexion (the tendency to "buckle" under body weight) or severe varus or valgus angulation is present, a locking orthotic knee joint is incorporated into the KAFO. When the orthosis locks the limb in extension, stance phase stability is enhanced, but swing phase clearance is compromised. The decision to use a nonlocking or locking orthotic knee joint is based on each patient's available range of motion and muscle strength and function. A KAFO can be used to support one impaired limb, for example, after trauma injury or after stroke. Bilateral KAFOs are often prescribed for patients with paraplegia or with traumatic injury of both lower extremities. A patient with bilateral locked-knee KAFOs most often requires an assistive device (crutches or a walker) for external support during ambulation. The most efficient gait pattern is determined by hip function: Most patients who use bilateral KAFOs develop a swing-to or swing-through gait pattern. Some may be able to use a reciprocal pattern if sufficient muscle function is present at the hip (minimally, volitional control of hip flexion).[7]

EVALUATION AND MEASUREMENT

The evaluation process includes assessment of the patient's height and weight, the status of circulation and sensation in the affected lower extremity, the condition and integrity of the patient's skin, soft tissue density and bony prominences, and the patient's living or working environment. Specific measurements of range of motion and fixed contractures, muscle strength and tone, and leg length and limb girth are also made. This information, when combined with functional assessment of gait and mobility tasks, helps the team to define the appropriate orthosis. Several critical decisions regarding specific aspects of the orthotic design must be made about materials and components. The orthotist must first select the appropriate type and gauge of plastic or metal to use. Decisions about whether reinforcing materials will be necessary, which to choose, and where to place the reinforcements must be made. The extent of contact that the orthosis will make with the patient's body must also be carefully considered; although intimate fit provides optimal control, one must protect areas that are vulnerable to pressure and account for potential variations in limb volume. The choices made in this planning stage ultimately define the success or failure of a particular orthosis.[6] The orthotist calls on his or her knowledge and understanding of material characteristics to decide on the appropriate materials and the most effective way to implement them. Blending combinations of plastic, metal, and composite materials permits the orthotist to provide an orthosis that is flexible where needed but rigid and stiff in other areas. In this way, a skilled clinician can maximize control while minimizing the orthosis' impact on function.

The most critical component of assessment and orthotic prescription is a clear understanding of the sequential deviations in the patient's gait pattern. This knowledge enables the orthotist to provide the maximum amount of correction without causing discomfort. As the orthotist measures the limb (for a conventional metal, double upright orthosis) or takes an impression by casting the limb (to make a positive model for a thermoplastic orthosis), he or she must position the limb in optimal alignment, given that patient's neuromuscular or musculoskeletal impairments and functional limitations. The orthotist uses a series of overlapping three-point force systems, beginning at the foot and moving proximally, to achieve this opti-

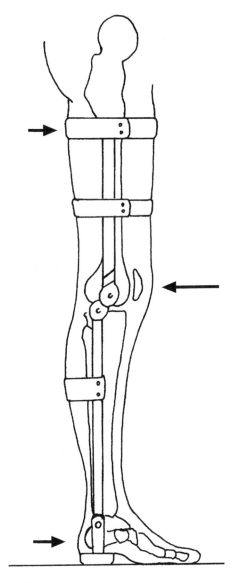

FIGURE 11-2
Schematic diagram of the components and sagittal plane force system acting at the knee in a conventional knee-ankle-foot orthosis.

sion throughout stance; another will address valgus, and a third will target midfoot control to minimize the abnormal pronation. The impact of each on the others as the stance phase progresses must also be considered.

DESIGN OPTIONS

Two KAFO designs are being used in contemporary clinical practice. A *conventional* (metal and leather) KAFO is attached to the patient's shoe via a stirrup and can be worn either under or external to clothing. A *molded thermoplastic* KAFO fits within the patient's shoe and is designed to have an intimate fit so that it can be worn under clothing. Any orthosis, as an external device applied to the patient's limb, in some ways facilitates and in others inhibits function: What is advantageous for one patient may be disadvantageous to another. A design that is very effective in meeting the needs of one patient may be contraindicated for patients with different physical characteristics or medical conditions. In choosing materials, components, and orthotic design, the orthotist must consider many factors: durability and weight of the materials, the preciseness of control that is possible across all planes of motion, the ease of donning and doffing the device, the ease of adjustability and of maintenance, and the overall cosmesis of the finished orthosis. The decision to prescribe a conventional or thermoplastic KAFO is founded on the needs and characteristics of the individual patient.

Conventional Knee-Ankle-Foot Orthoses

A conventional KAFO has a metal frame (double uprights) that is attached to a shoe via a stirrup system and leather coverings over the calf and thigh bands (Figure 11-2). Typically, a pair of orthotic ankle joints is used to connect the stirrup to the distal (lower) metal uprights, and a pair of orthotic knee joints connects the distal (lower) and proximal (upper) metal uprights, as determined by the patient's specific needs. The uprights are most often stainless steel or aluminum. The length and contour or the uprights are based on a tracing (delineation) of the limb and on girth measurements. The uprights and joints form a rigid structure or cage around the limb. The orthosis contacts the patient's limb at the leather-covered posterior bands and the anterior straps that are used to hold the limb within the orthosis. An anterior kneepad can be added as an additional contact point. A three-point pressure system stabilizes the knee in the sagittal plane to control flexion/extension: Two anteriorly directed forces (applied by the posterior thigh band proximally and the

mal alignment in the design of the orthosis.[8] The orthotist must assess range of motion at each joint and then design the orthosis to reduce or eliminate each deviation in sequence through the application of appropriate three-point force systems. Consider a patient who presents with hyperextension at the right knee while transitioning from initial contact to loading response, excessive pronation of the midfoot during midstance, and hyperextension with valgus at the knee throughout the stance phase. For this patient, one force system will control knee hyperexten-

TABLE 11-1

Comparison of Advantages and Disadvantages
of Conventional Knee-Ankle-Foot Orthoses

Advantages
  Very strong
  Most durable
  Easily adjusted
Disadvantages
  Heavy
  Must be attached to shoe or shoe insert
  Less cosmetic
  Fewer contact points reduce control
Indications
  When maximum strength and durability are needed
  For patients with significant obesity
  For patients with uncontrolled or fluctuating edema (e.g.,
    congestive heart failure, dialysis)
Contraindications
  When issues of energy expenditure make weight of the
    orthosis a factor
  When control of transverse plane motion is important

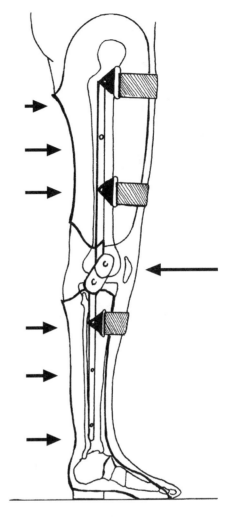

FIGURE 11-3

Schematic diagram of the components and sagittal plane force
systems that are necessary to control knee flexion/extension.
Because the point of force application is distributed over the entire
posterior surface of the intimately fitting orthotic shell, more pre-
cise and more comfortable control of the limb is possible.

shoe and posterior calf band distally) are opposed by a
single posteriorly directed force (applied by the anterior
kneepad or by anterior thigh and calf straps, or both).[9]
Theoretically, additional force systems (a pair of proxi-
mal/distal forces opposing a central force) act in the
frontal plane to control varus and valgus at the knee. The
less than intimate fit of this orthosis reduces the efficacy
of varus/valgus control systems. Although conventional
KAFOs are quite durable and easily adjusted, they tend
to be heavier and less cosmetically pleasing than thermoplastic versions. The advantages/disadvantages and
indications/contraindications of conventional KAFOs
are summarized in Table 11-1.

Thermoplastic Knee-Ankle-Foot Orthoses

In the thermoplastic KAFO (Figure 11-3), a shell is vacuum formed over a positive model of the patient's limb.
The distal shell, which fits intimately over the foot, ankle,
and lower leg, is basically an AFO with a proximal anterior strap (usually Velcro) closure. Depending on the
patient's needs, this distal component may be either a
solid-ankle or articulating design. The proximal shell
encases the thigh from the greater trochanter to just above
the femoral condyles and typically has a pair of anterior
straps (again usually Velcro) for closure. Metal knee
joints and sidebars (made of stainless steel, aluminum,
or titanium) connect the proximal and distal shells. The
type of plastic chosen for the shell determines the rigidity of the orthosis. The key feature of this orthosis is its

intimate total contact fit and resultant potential to control the limb. Covering and encompassing a large surface area with the plastic reduces the force per unit area
that is required for stabilization or control of the limb,
diminishing the likelihood of discomfort or skin irritation, which is associated with high or excessive pressure.
On the other hand, if the fit is less than optimal such that
pistoning occurs within the orthosis during gait or tissue is excessively compressed where the fit is too tight,
patients will complain of discomfort, and skin problems
are likely to occur.

In this design, a series of overlapping three-point force
systems is possible. The force system for control of flex-

TABLE 11-2

Comparison of Advantages and Disadvantages
of Thermoplastic Knee-Ankle-Foot Orthoses

Advantages
  Lightweight
  Interchangeability of shoes
  Greater cosmesis worn under clothing
Disadvantages
  Can be hot to wear
Indications
  Intimate/total contact fit makes maximum
    limb control possible
  When energy expenditure makes weight
    of the orthosis an issue
  When control of transverse plane
    motion is needed
Contraindications
  Intimacy of fit is difficult when the patient
    is significantly obese
  Intimacy of fit is compromised when the
    patient has uncontrolled or fluctuating edema

ion/extension in the sagittal plane is essentially the same as that of a conventional KAFO, although the posterior force is distributed over a wider surface area. As a result of the total contact design of the shells, a more precise control of the limb is possible, in both the frontal and transverse planes; this is particularly important when dealing with segmental deviations secondary to transverse plane rotational problems.[10] Because of the multiplanar characteristics of the knee joint, varus or valgus deviations at the knee typically include a rotatory component. Controlling this is more easily accomplished with the total contact design of the thermoplastic KAFO than with the double upright system of a conventional KAFO. The intimate fit of the thermoplastic KAFO may be problematic, however, for patients with fluctuating limb volume secondary to edema or cyclical weight gain or loss. Many patients enjoy the ability to wear a variety of shoes (as long as heel height is the same) and the cosmesis afforded by wearing the thermoplastic orthosis under their clothing. As lightweight as this orthosis is, the large contact area may make it difficult to dissipate body heat, so that the orthosis is uncomfortably warm for patients who are very active or who live in hot climates. Advantages and disadvantages are summarized in Table 11-2.

CONTROL OF THE ANKLE IN KNEE-ANKLE-FOOT ORTHOSES

The ankle joints used in KAFOs are the same as those that are available for AFOs. The orthotist can choose among three types of orthotic ankle joints: (1) a nonarticulating or fixed-ankle design (as in a solid-ankle AFO); (2) an articulating design that allows dorsiflexion (for forward progression of the tibia over the foot in stance) but blocks plantar flexion, or provides dorsiflexion assistance (to enhance swing phase clearance); or (3) a single-axis articulating design that allows free dorsiflexion and plantar flexion within a specific range of motion. What is important to consider, however, is how the ankle configuration and ground reaction force influence knee function and forward progression during gait.

If a patient's condition requires a KAFO with a locked knee joint, the impact of the ground reaction force on the knee is negated.[2,11] Using an ankle joint that permits movement of the ankle through a specific range of motion is beneficial in improving the patient's level of function when the knee is locked, enhancing forward progression of the body over the foot during stance. Ambulation with both a locked knee and a locked ankle becomes very difficult. Locking the ankle precludes progression through the stance phase rockers found in normal gait; forward progression over the foot in stance is significantly compromised. Additionally, clearance in swing is compromised by the locked knee. Patients must use compensatory strategies for functional gait: They may have uneven stride length and stance times because of difficulty with forward progression and may vault or circumduct to enhance swing clearance of the limb in the orthosis.

When motion at the ankle must be eliminated to protect the joint or to control the impact of abnormal tone, and the knee joint must remained locked for stance phase stability, the orthotist often places a rocker sole on the patient's shoe.[12] This rocker sole simulates the normal rockers of gait, enhancing forward progression by reducing the toe lever of the orthosis, improving the smoothness of the patient's gait and reducing the likelihood of compensatory gait deviations.

Ideally, if a patient's condition or level of function requires that the orthotic knee joint remain locked during ambulation, the orthotist is able to use an articulating ankle joint so that some ankle motion is possible. The ability to move into plantar flexion enhances the transition from initial contact to loading response (although the locked knee may compromise the shock absorption function of loading response). The ability to move into dorsiflexion enhances the forward progression of the limb over the fixed foot, especially in the transition from midstance toward terminal stance. The design characteristics of the orthotic ankle joint (whether metal or plastic, allowing free or limited motion) must be consistent with the overall design of the KAFO. In those instances in which ankle control is not particularly influenced by the desired knee control, the type of ankle joint and ankle position is determined by the patient's particular musculoskeletal and neuromuscular function or needs at the ankle.

ORTHOTIC KNEE JOINTS

A wide variety of orthotic knee joints are available for use in KAFOs in current clinical practice. In this chapter, we discuss the designs that are most often encountered by rehabilitation professionals involved in functional gait training. When a patient has a special need, the orthotist uses knowledge of mechanics and product availability to tailor a joint to the specific needs of that patient.

Single-Axis Knee Joints

The single-axis knee, also known as a *straight knee joint without drop lock* or a *free knee*, permits unrestricted flexion and extension to neutral in the sagittal plane (most designs prevent hyperextension) while providing mediolateral stability (Figure 11-4A). The joint is designed to pivot around a single point or axis, like a simple hinge. The orthotist positions the axis of this orthotic joint medially along the midline of the extended leg at a point approximately one-half the distance between the adductor tubercle and the medial tibial plateau. The lateral joint is also positioned at the approximate axis of the anatomic knee joint. Although some degree of torque is created by the mismatch between the single-axis orthotic knee joint and the polycentric anatomic knee joint, for most patients this is not problematic. The free, single-axis knee is appropriate for patients who have enough muscle function to ensure knee stability in stance but who tend to move into recurvatum, have significant structural (mediolateral) instability of the knee joint, or fall into excessive varum or valgus in stance.[13,14]

Single-Axis Locking Knee

With the addition of a locking mechanism, such as a ring or drop lock, the single-axis or locked knee provides rigid stability to the knee in all planes (Figure 11-4B). Its alignment is the same as that of the single-axis free knee. Although a drop (ring) lock is the most commonly used locking mechanism, a variety of other locking mechanisms are also available, depending on the patient's functional requirements. This type of orthotic knee joint is appropriate for patients who are unable to control the knee effectively during stance phase, requiring additional external stability to prevent or restrain excessive knee flexion as body weight is transferred onto the limb.[15]

Offset Knee Joint

The offset knee joint is also known as a *posteriorly offset, free knee* (Figure 11-4C). This design is aligned with its axis of rotation behind the midline of the leg, posterior to the axis of the anatomic knee. In early stance, during the period of double support, the ground reaction passes closer to the center of the axis of the orthotic joint, reducing the magnitude of the external flexion moment that is acting to flex the limb. With continued forward progression, the ground reaction force quickly moves anterior to the orthotic joint, creating an extensor force that mechanically augments stance phase stability during single limb support.[16,17] When used properly, this joint permits the orthotist to design a device that allows stability in the knee from initial contact through midstance; however, alignment of the knee and ankle must be precise if it is to be effective. A drop lock or other locking mechanism can be added to stabilize the knee in an extended position when the patient will be standing for long periods of time or when additional stability is advisable (e.g., when the patient is walking on uneven ground). This option is valuable for patients with limited knee control due to lower motor neuron disease, such as polio, or low thoracic–upper lumbar spinal cord injury.

Variable Position Orthotic Knee Joint

The variable position locking orthotic knee joint is also known as a *dial lock* or as an *adjustable locking knee joint* (Figure 11-4D). This design is intended for patients who are unable to achieve full extension due to knee flexion contracture. With flexion contracture, the position of the ground reaction force stays posterior to the anatomic knee joint; it may be difficult or impossible for the patient with weakness or motor control impairment to develop or maintain the necessary counteractive muscle force for stance stability. Instead, the variable position orthotic knee joint is locked in the most extended position possible, providing an external mechanical stability.[8,15] In addition to being used to accommodate a fixed knee flexion contracture, the variable position joint can be gradually adjusted into extension to assist elongation of soft tissue contracture as a patient's function improves and range of motion increases.[18]

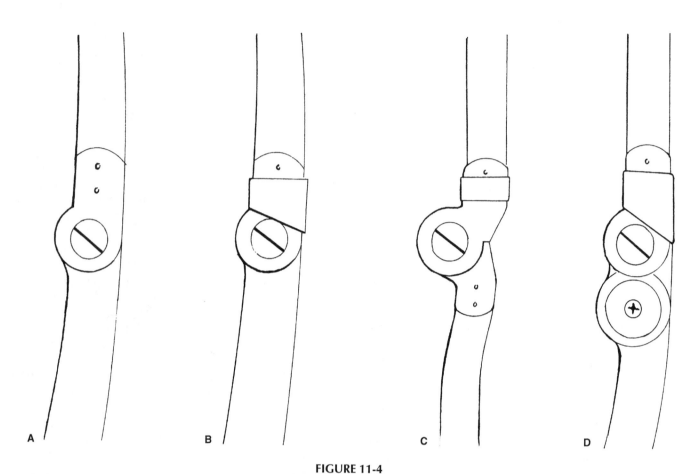

FIGURE 11-4

*Orthotic knee joints most often used in knee-ankle-foot orthoses. **(A)** A single-axis, or free, knee allows full flexion and extension while providing mediolateral stability to the knee joint. **(B)** A locked knee is typically locked while the patient is standing, providing stability in all planes, and unlocked to permit knee flexion in sitting. **(C)** The axis of the offset orthotic knee joint is positioned behind the anatomic knee axis, increasing the biomechanical stability of the orthosis. It is available with and without a locking mechanism. **(D)** A variable position, or adjustable, orthotic knee joint permits the orthotist to accommodate for changing range of motion or for fixed contracture at the knee.*

Locking Mechanisms

The most commonly used locking mechanism is the ring or drop. This very simple design "captures" the male and female halves of the orthotic joint when it is fully extended, blocking subsequent movement into flexion or hyperextension. A small ball bearing incorporated into the upright ensures that the drop lock stays in the desired position until the patient purposefully unlocks or locks the orthosis. Although this mechanism is simple, durable, strong, and safe, the knee must be fully extended for the lock to be engaged or disengaged. Most KAFOs have a medial and a lateral upright. For optimal safety, a drop or ring lock should be engaged on both uprights. Having to manage drop locks on both sides of the orthosis simultaneously to engage or disengage the lock mechanism may be challenging for patients with limited hand function, significant lower extremity spasticity or contracture, or difficulty in balancing on one crutch while using a hand to work the locking mechanism.[18]

For patients who have difficulty managing drop locks, an alternative mechanism may be a spring-loaded bail lock (Figure 11-5). This is essentially a lever system, which connects the medial and lateral locks of a KAFO, permitting them to be engaged or disengaged simultaneously. Other locking mechanisms that use lever systems to manage the lock include pawl locks, cam locks, or Swiss locks.[8,18] To use a bail lock, the patient backs up against the edge of the seating surface (e.g., wheelchair, mat table, kitchen or desk chair); pressure against the posterior bar activates the bail's mechanism to disengage the lock, and the patient is able to sit with knee

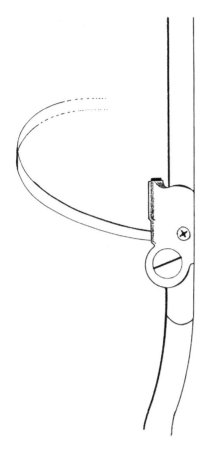

FIGURE 11-5

A bail-locking mechanism allows the medial and lateral locks to be disengaged at the same time by a posterior pressure, as against the edge of the seating surface. This mechanism is often used for patients with paraplegia who must maintain bilateral upper extremity support via crutches for stability.

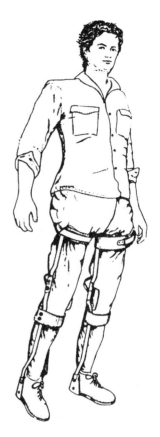

FIGURE 11-6

The Craig-Scott orthosis is a modified version of a conventional knee-ankle-foot orthosis, designed to be as lightweight as possible and to capitalize on alignment stability to enhance ambulation and upright activities in patients with low thoracic and lumbar spinal cord injury. (Reprinted with permission from DG Shurr, TM Cook. Prosthetics and Orthotics. Norwalk, CT: Appleton & Lange, 1990;141.)

flexion. Although theoretically convenient and easy to use, this type of lock mechanism is most appropriate for patients with enough upper body strength and coordination to control the descent into sitting or for those who have previous experience with its use. If the exposed bail passing behind the knee is inadvertently bumped, the locks may disengage unexpectedly, and the patient may fall. Although the posterior edge of a properly contoured bail is angled downward to reduce the likelihood of unexpected unlocking, an upwardly directed force would still unlock these joints.

Special Knee-Ankle-Foot Orthoses Designs

Conventional and thermoplastic KAFO designs have been adapted or modified to meet the needs of groups of patients with special needs. For growing children with muscular dystrophy, a modular system that allows the orthotist to adjust the length of the uprights and quickly replace outgrown thigh or calf supports has been developed.[19] A pair of lightweight long-leg calipers with no knee joint have traditionally been used to facilitate function in standing for adults with spinal cord injury; however, calipers are currently being replaced by a standing frame.[20] A Craig-Scott orthosis, also known as a *double-bar hip-stabilizing orthosis* (Figure 11-6), is a lightweight variation of a traditional KAFO that was designed for patients with paraplegia.[21] This orthosis is designed to maximize stability in stance with the minimal amount of bracing. A single thigh band and anterior strap are positioned just below the ischial tuberosity at the level of the greater trochanter; a single calf band and support are positioned just below the knee. Patients without active hip control are stable in standing, assisted by the orthotic's dorsi-assist ankle joints and offset locking knee joints and in a position of hip hyperextension and exaggerated lumbar lordosis. With this combination of orthotic and posture, the ground reaction force passes just anterior to the knee and posterior to the hip, so that little or no muscular counterforce is necessary. Conventional KAFOs are also being used in conjunction with functional electrical stimulation protocols for ambulation in patients with spinal cord injury. A variety of braking orthotic knee joints have been developed to augment stance stability when muscle fatigue from repeated electrical stimulation is problematic.[22]

CHOOSING THE APPROPRIATE DESIGN AND COMPONENTS

The choice of a specific orthotic design and of a particular knee joint is based on a careful assessment of the patient's neuromuscular and musculoskeletal impairments, present and potential level of function, and a clear definition of key goals. The orthotist, after discussion with the patient and the clinic team, designs an orthosis that can most effectively achieve the desired goals. A set of general guidelines for choosing the orthotic knee joints that can best achieve desired knee control is presented in Table 11-3. This framework may need to be modified to meet specific or unique patient characteristics or circumstances.

DELIVERY AND FUNCTIONAL TRAINING

After the orthosis has been fabricated, the orthotist inspects the device to ensure that components work properly and that the thigh and calf bands or thermoplastic shells have been contoured appropriately, that plastic edges have been smoothed and rounded, and that metal surfaces have been buffed or coated. The orthotist then examines the fit of the orthosis to the patient's limb, in the intended functional, weight-bearing position (Table 11-4). The contours of cuffs or shells are reassessed in this position of function, with particular attention to vulnerable areas of skin or soft tissue. The overall length of the uprights and positions of the cuffs/shells and orthotic joints are inspected. Alignment of the components of the KAFO is also carefully evaluated. Ideally, the patient is able to stand comfortably, without skin irritation or pain. If minor problems with fit are identified, simple adjustments of fit and alignment can be made to address them. The orthotist and other members of the team then assess the effectiveness of the orthosis in meeting the defined functional goals, observing the degree of correction that is possible in quiet standing and during gait.

The orthotist carefully assesses any corrections that the orthosis is able to achieve, comparing posture and alignment to preorthotic assessment findings. Consider a patient who initially presented with 20 degrees of genu valgum in weight bearing that was correctable to 10 degrees when unweighted. The orthotist would reassess the amount of genu valgum that is present in standing, anticipating that the limb will be supported in the corrected 10-degree position.

If the orthosis fits appropriately and achieves its intended goals of protection, stability, or mobility, the patient must learn how to use the device. The patient and caregivers must understand how to don and doff the orthosis, including the way in which the limb is best positioned within the orthosis and the appropriate adjustment of stabilizing straps. They must learn about the locking mechanism at the knee, practicing the mechanics of locking and unlocking the joint several times. Patients and caregivers must be instructed in the care and maintenance of the orthosis, including keeping it clean and routinely inspecting components for wear and tear. An orthosis, as a mechanical device with moving parts, requires regular cleaning and occasional lubrication of its mechanical parts.

In most cases, especially if a patient is new to the use of an orthosis, a wearing schedule is developed, tailored to the patient's specific needs and physical condition, in which the patient gradually increases to full-time wear.

Gait training begins once any adjustments to alignment or fit have been completed. Initial gait training activities might begin with weight shifting from the intact toward the involved limb (for patients with unilateral deficits) and progress to controlled stance on the orthosis while the intact limb is in swing. Training may initially occur in the stable environment of the parallel bars but must progress to functional ambulation using the assistive device and gait pattern that are most appropriate for the individual patient, within the confines of stability necessary for safe ambulation. Often, the orthotist reevaluates the fit and function of the orthosis once a patient has developed a comfortable pattern of ambulation to fine tune alignment so that the most biomechanically sound and energy efficient gait pattern is possible. Advanced gait training activities include ambulation on uneven terrain, ramps, and stairs. It is also important to assist patients in developing strategies to manage unexpected falls; patients with sufficient upper extremity function and motor control may benefit from practicing getting up and down from the floor.

TABLE 11-3
Indications and Contraindications for Orthotic Knee Joint Designs

Desired Knee Control	Orthotic Knee Design				
	Single Axis, Unlocked	Single Axis, Locked	Offset, Unlocked	Offset, Locked	Variable Position, Locked
Stabilization of flail knee with knee extension moment and free knee joint motion	Contraindicated	Contraindicated	**Indicated**	Contraindicated	Contraindicated
Stabilization of flail knee without use of knee extension moment and free knee joint motion	Contraindicated	**Indicated**	Contraindicated	**Indicated**	Unnecessary
Control of genu recurvatum	Contraindicated	**Indicated** if orthosis will only be used locked when ambulating	**Indicated**	**Indicated** when patient will lock knee intermittently	Contraindicated
Reduction of knee flexion contracture	Contraindicated	Lacks adjustability	Contraindicated	Lacks adjustability	**Indicated**
Control of genu valgum	**Indicated**	**Indicated** Use of lock optional	**Indicated**	**Indicated** Use of lock optional	Unnecessary
Control of genu varum	**Indicated**	**Indicated** Use of lock optional	**Indicated**	**Indicated** Use of lock optional	Unnecessary

Source: Modified with permission from Dallas Short Course in Orthotics and Prosthetics—Course Manual. 1993;18–22.

TABLE 11-4
*Guiding Questions for Delivery and Fitting
of a Knee-Ankle-Foot Orthosis*

Is the orthosis consistent with the design criteria or prescription?

Is the craftsmanship acceptable?

Is the general appearance of the orthosis acceptable?

Are the mechanisms for closure (Velcro straps or buckles) of adequate length and in the appropriate position to stabilize the limb in the orthosis?

Will the patient be able to don/doff the orthosis independently (after functional training)?

Is clearance or pressure relief sufficient around bony prominences or areas of fragile skin and soft tissue?

Are the mechanical knee and ankle joints properly aligned with respect to the axis of the anatomic joints?

Do all the mechanical parts (joints and locks) function smoothly?

If the orthosis is of conventional design, are the uprights and cuffs the proper length and in an optimal position for the desired degree of control?

If the orthosis is thermoplastic, is the total contact and surface area appropriate for distribution of force and the desired control of the knee and limb segments?

SUMMARY

The decision to prescribe a KAFO for a patient with musculoskeletal or neuromuscular impairments is often made when knee instability cannot be adequately managed by an AFO design. A KAFO is often chosen when genu valgum or varum is problematic or when structural instability of ligaments of the knee is present. The orthotist, therapist, and other members of the team involved in the patient's care choose the most appropriate orthotic design and components based on clearly defined functional goals, after careful evaluation of the patient's limb condition, motor control, and gait.

KAFOs provide an external stabilization to counteract the flexion moment that is created when the ground reaction force passes posterior to the knee in early stance. Conventional and thermoplastic KAFOs use a three-point force system to control the knee motion in sagittal, frontal, and transverse planes. The intimately fitting thigh and distal shells of thermoplastic KAFOs are better able to control forces in the transverse plane than are conventional designs. Although any of the ankle joint or AFO designs can be incorporated into a KAFO, an articulating orthotic ankle joint, which allows dorsiflexion, enhances forward progression over the foot during the stance phase of gait. A number of options for orthotic knee joints are available, some locking and others unlocking; the choice of orthotic knee joint is determined by how well the patient is able to control motion actively at the knee.

After the KAFO has been fabricated, its fit and function are carefully evaluated by the orthotist, therapist, and other members of the team. The orthosis must be comfortable to wear and effectively achieve its functional goals if the patient is to accept and use the device. Once any necessary adjustments to alignment and fit have been made, an initial wearing schedule is developed to gradually bring "time in brace" up to full-time use. A period of gait training, including instruction and practice with the appropriate assistive device and ambulation on level and uneven surfaces, ramps, and stairs, is begun. The patient and caregivers also need to understand how to clean and maintain the orthosis; regularly scheduled rechecks with the orthotist ensure continued effectiveness of and satisfaction with the orthosis.

REFERENCES

1. Inman VT, Ralston HJ, Todd F. Human Walking. Baltimore: Williams & Wilkins, 1981.

2. Perry J. Gait Analysis: Normal and Pathological Function. Thorofare, NJ: Slack, 1992.

3. Rancho Los Amigos Observational Gait Handbook. Los Amigos Research and Education Institute, Rancho Los Amigos Medical Center, Downey, CA 1989.

4. Smith LK, Weiss EL, Lehmjuhl DL. Brunnstrom's Clinical Kinesiology (5th ed). Philadelphia: Davis, 1996.

5. Gage JR. Gait Analysis in Cerebral Palsy. London: Mackeiht, 1991;61–130, 177–182.

6. Cary JM, Lusskin R, Thompson RG. Prescription Principles. In WH Bunch, Atlas of Orthotics: Biomechanical Principles and Application. St. Louis: Mosby, 1985;3–6.

7. Somers MF. Ambulation. In Spinal Cord Injury: Functional Rehabilitation. Norwalk, CT: Appleton & Lange, 1992; 231–268.

8. Trautman P. Lower Limb Orthoses. In JB Redford, JV Basmajian, P Trautman (eds), Orthotics: Clinical Practice and Rehabilitation Technology. New York: Churchill Livingstone, 1995;13–55.

9. Perry J, Hislop HJ (eds). Principles of Lower Extremity Bracing. Alexandria, VA: American Physical Therapy Association, 1967.

10. Moore TJ. Lower Limb Orthoses. In B Goldberg, JD Haus (eds), Atlas of Orthoses and Assistive Devices (3rd ed). St. Louis: Mosby, 1997;377–463.

11. Fishman S. Lower Limb Orthoses. In WH Bunch (ed), Atlas of Orthotics: Biomechanical Principles and Application. St. Louis: Mosby, 1985;199–237.

12. Shoe Modifications and Foot Orthoses. In Berger N, Edelstein JE, Fishman S, et al. (eds), Lower Limb Orthotics. New York: New York University Medical Center, Post Graduate Medical School, Prosthetics and Orthotics, 1986; 110–128.

13. Edelstein JE. Orthotic Assessment and Management. In SB O'Sullivan, TJ Schmitz (eds), Physical Rehabilitation: Assessment and Treatment (3rd ed). Philadelphia: Davis, 1994; 655–684.

14. Lunsford T. Orthotic Principles. In Rancho Los Amigos Medical Center Prosthetics and Orthotics Course Syllabus: Critical Decisions in Patient Management. Downey, CA: Professional Staff Association, 1985;6:1–9.

15. Zablotny CM. Use of Orthoses for the Adult with Neurological Involvement. In DA Nawoczenski, ME Eppler (eds), Orthotics in Functional Rehabilitation of the Lower Limb. Philadelphia: Saunders, 1997;205–243.

16. Clark D. Knee-Ankle-Foot Orthosis Design for Polio. In Rancho Los Amigos Medical Center Prosthetics and Orthotics Course Syllabus: Critical Decisions in Patient Management. Downey, CA: Professional Staff Association, 1985;6:60–62.

17. Hahn HR. Lower extremity bracing in paraplegics with usage follow-up. Paraplegia 1970;8(3):147–153.

18. Ankle, Knee, and Hip Orthoses. In Berger N, Edelstein JE, Fishman S, et al. (eds), Lower Limb Orthotics. New York: New York University Medical Center, Post Graduate Medical School, Prosthetics and Orthotics, 1986; 129–164.

19. Taktak DM, Bowker P. Lightweight modular knee-ankle-foot orthosis for Duchenne muscular dystrophy: design, development, and evaluation. Arch Phys Med Rehabil 1995;76(12):1156–1162.

20. Hawran S, Biering-Sorensen F. The use of long leg calipers for paraplegic patients: a follow up study of patients discharged 1973–1982. Spinal Cord 1996;34(11): 666–668.

21. Hahn HR. Lower extremity bracing in paraplegics with usage follow-up. Paraplegia 1970;8(3):147–153.

22. Goldfarb M, Durfee WK. Design of a controlled brake orthosis for FES aided gait. IEEE Transactions on Rehabilitation Engineering 1996;4(1):13–24.

12

Hip-Knee-Ankle-Foot Orthoses

JAMES H. CAMPBELL

The clinical decision to provide any individual, whether a child or an adult, with a hip-knee-ankle-foot orthosis (HKAFO) is based on careful consideration of the relative advantages and disadvantages of such an orthosis with respect to its impact on function, mobility, and energy cost. Clear indications for bracing the hip and trunk for patients with significant neuromuscular or musculoskeletal impairments have not been well documented. An HKAFO is a cumbersome device, and donning and doffing are often quite difficult. The additional control of joint motion achieved by going above the hips must be balanced against the practical challenges that the individual patient will undoubtedly face when using the orthosis.

Prescription of an HKAFO must be based on biomechanical deficits, independent of specific conditions, and on an appropriate orthotic design. A thorough understanding of specific pathologies and individual patient requirements, however, is necessary if patient acceptance of the device and compliance with its use are to be successful. In this chapter, we describe the most commonly used components and designs of HKAFOs and explore their use in the management of mobility dysfunction for patients with neuromuscular impairments. We begin with a discussion of traditional (conventional) HKAFOs, investigate the clinical use of the parapodium and standing frames, and finally explore orthotic options for reciprocal gait for patients with neuromuscular disease or disability.

TRADITIONAL/CONVENTIONAL HIP-KNEE-ANKLE-FOOT ORTHOSES

The traditional or conventional HKAFOs that were commonly prescribed for patients with polio, spinal cord injury, myelomeningocele, or spastic quadriplegic cerebral palsy before the 1980s were typically manufactured from a combination of metal and leather materials (Figure 12-1A). Most often, they were applied bilaterally; occasionally, a single HKAFO was used to control the motion of just one extremity. The high energy cost of gait associated with these orthoses often limited their functional use. Just as thermoplastic materials and lighter but durable metals have become materials of choice for ankle-foot orthoses (AFOs) and knee-ankle-foot orthoses, they have been incorporated into the manufacture of HKAFOs (Figure 12-1B). Today, custom-fit and custom-fabricated thermoplastic HKAFOs are much lighter in weight. Because of the intimacy of their fit on the lower extremity, thermoplastic HKAFOs may also provide better biomechanical control of the limb.

Orthotic Hip Joints and Pelvic Band

An orthotist can choose from a variety of commercially available orthotic hip joints to control hip joint motion (Figure 12-2). Most designs have a single mechanical axis; some allow free flexion/extension when unlocked, and others can be set to allow motion only within a desired, more limited range. Single-axis hip joints inherently restrict motions of abduction/adduction and rotation. Although dual-axis hip joints with separate mechanical control systems for flexion/extension and for abduction/adduction are also available, the single-axis joint provides the desired control for the majority of patients who require HKAFO systems for standing and mobility.

The orthotist selects the appropriate joint after considering the patient's functional disability, the treatment objectives, and the specific joint control that is required. He or she can choose a joint that is designed to allow free motion, to assist or resist motion, to stop motion at a particular point in the range of motion, or to hold or eliminate all motion in the prescribed plane. The mechanical joint that best meets

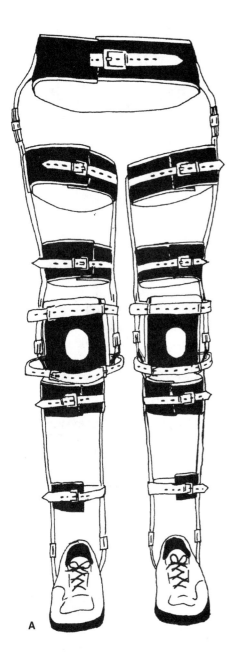

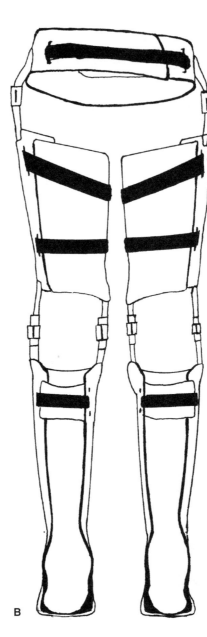

A   B

FIGURE 12-1
(A) Example of a traditional metal and leather hip-knee-ankle-foot orthosis (HKAFO), with its pelvic band, orthotic hip joints and locks, proximal and distal thigh bands, orthotic knee joints and stabilization pads, proximal and distal calf bands, ankle joints, and stirrups. (B) Themoplastic HKAFOs, typically lighter in weight than conventional HKAFOs, also have a pelvic band and orthotic hip and knee joints. Because they distribute forces over a wider thigh and calf band, an anterior knee stabilization pad may not be necessary. Many incorporate a solid-ankle or articulating ankle ankle-foot orthosis design, fitting inside the shoe rather than in an external stirrup.

the patient's needs is attached proximally to a metal pelvic band, positioned between the trochanter and iliac crest (Figure 12-3). The center of the mechanical joint (axis of motion) is positioned just proximal and anterior to the greater trochanter. Distal stabilization is achieved by the attachment of the distal arm of the joint to the thigh cuff/upright.

Traditional Hip-Knee-Ankle-Foot Orthoses for Adults with Spinal Cord Injury

Most adults with paraplegia after lower thoracic or lumbar spinal cord injury have the potential to use

bilateral knee-ankle-foot orthoses to provide the external stabilization of the knee and ankle that is required for upright activities and swing-through gait with crutches.[1] This is possible, despite weakness of the hips and trunk, by standing with an exaggerated lumbar lordosis. In this position, the center of gravity (weight line) falls posterior to the hip joint, creating an extension moment at the hip, achieving stability by alignment. Although, theoretically, HKAFOs (which add hip joints and pelvic band, with or without thoracic extensions) would provide stability for patients with high thoracic spinal cord injury, little evidence has

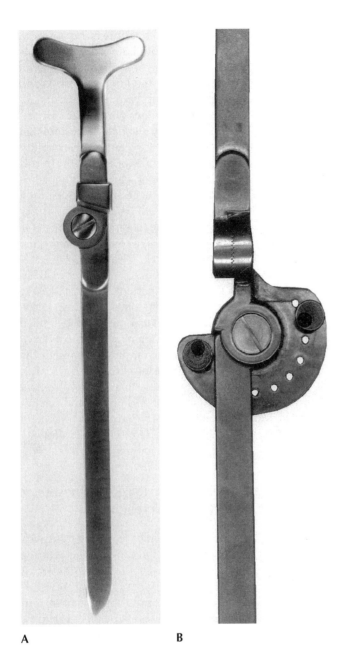

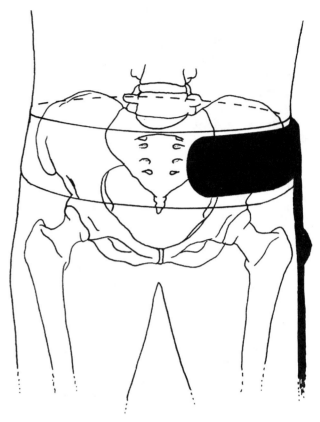

FIGURE 12-3

For effective control of hip motion, the pelvic band is positioned between the greater trochanter of the femur and the crest of the ilium. The orthotic hip joint is placed slightly proximal and anterior to the greater trochanter of the femur.

A　　　　　**B**

FIGURE 12-2

(A) Examples of a single-axis hip joint. A drop lock holds the hip in extension in standing but allows free hip flexion for sitting when disengaged. (B) Another type of hip joint allows controlled flexion and extension within a limited range of motion while limiting abduction/adduction and rotation.

been found that the addition of hip joints and pelvic band is functionally beneficial.[1]

Traditional Hip-Knee-Ankle-Foot Orthoses for Children with Myelomeningocele

The primary goal of rehabilitation for children with myelomeningocele (spina bifida) is to facilitate the developmental process (motor and cognitive), striving for as close to "normal" development as the child's neuromuscular and musculoskeletal impairments allow.[2] To achieve this goal, orthopedic and orthotic management of the child's spine and lower limbs focuses on achieving a stable upright posture. This can only be accomplished, however, if the child's lower extremities can be positioned in hip and knee extension: Prevention of flexion contracture or deformity of the hips and knees is paramount. The level of motor and sensory impairment in the child's lower extremities is an important consideration in the process of orthotic prescription and fitting. Rehabilitation interventions are designed to simulate or approximate normal developmental activities: Achieving trunk control in sitting is often the therapeutic focus for infants between 6 and 8 months of age; supported standing and locomotion activities are encouraged for children between 1 and 2 years of age. The relationship between motor and cognitive development has been clearly established; orthopedic, surgical, and orthotic management support rehabilitation interventions that target age- and neurosegmental level–appropriate activities for the child.[2–4]

If children with myelomeningocele also develop hydrocephalus, the potential to become independent in locomotion is further challenged. Any additional postural instability and intellectual impairment associated with hydrocephalus may make it more difficult for the child to learn to use the limbs or an orthosis effectively. Some children with myelomeningocele have bony deformity (such as malformation of vertebrae) that, along with their paralysis, places them at risk for development of secondary musculoskeletal impairments. Some of the most commonly encountered musculoskeletal problems include scoliosis and kyphosis, abnormalities of the ribcage, hip dislocation, osteoporosis and risk of fracture, and development of contracture or fixed limb deformities, or both, especially of the ankle and knee.

Orthopedic and surgical management of children with myelomeningocele has three goals[5]:

1. To correct the primary deformity, maintain the correction, prevent its recurrence, and avoid the production of secondary deformities or musculoskeletal impairments
2. To obtain the best possible locomotor function
3. To prevent or minimize the effects of sensorimotor deficiency

It is critically important that orthotic management work toward these same goals.

Orthotists often become active members of the interdisciplinary rehabilitation team when a child is ready to begin standing activities, usually between 12 and 18 months of age. In the 1960s and 1970s, conventional HKAFOs were the primary orthotic option for these children. Currently, there is considerable controversy and difference of opinion with regard to the advantages of fitting such children with this orthotic design. Providing for stability of the pelvis and hip has been problematic for children who have an imbalance of muscle power around the hip joint.[6,7] Many children with myelomeningocele may have some ability to activate hip flexor muscles (inner-

vated by L2 and L3 nerve roots) but little or no power in hip extensors (innervated below L3 root levels). This imbalance of muscle tone and power often results in an exaggerated anterior pelvic tilt and lumbar lordosis and the development of significant hip flexor tightness or contracture.[7] Although some clinicians argue that conventional HKAFOs provide stability and reduce the potential for hip flexion contracture, others question their ability to prevent lumbar lordosis and flexor tightness. In this author's experience, a pelvic band can provide mediolateral hip stability but is not successful in controlling anterior pelvic tilt.[8]

Until reciprocating gait orthoses became available in the 1980s, conventional HKAFOs were routinely prescribed for children with myelomeningocele. Wearing the HKAFO, children were taught to ambulate using walkers or crutches in a pivot or swing-through gait pattern.[9,10] Most of these early HKAFOs had single-axis hip joints with drop locks, which attempted to stabilize a weak hip in an extended position and to prevent the hips from falling into a flexed position while the patient was standing. Although the HKAFO design does stabilize the lower extremities for stable stance, most have been unable to effectively control the position of the lumbar spine and pelvis biomechanically. Orthotists sought alternative strategies to control trunk and pelvic stability more effectively while allowing enough hip motion for a functional step.[11]

Traditional Hip-Knee-Ankle-Foot Orthoses for Children with Cerebral Palsy

Few areas of orthotic management have attracted as much attention during the last several decades as the orthotic management of cerebral palsy. The routine practice of prescribing and fitting conventional HKAFOs for children with spastic quadriplegia or diplegia has been supplanted by more effective and less expensive forms of orthotic management. The current approach to the management of children with cerebral palsy better integrates therapeutic, orthotic, and surgical interventions, based on the severity of the child's neuromuscular deficit, potential for functional mobility, and current motor and cognitive developmental status. Custom-molded AFOs of a variety of designs have been found to be effective in providing just enough external sagittal plane stability for effective upright posture in children who have the potential to become functional ambulators. It must be noted that AFOs do not influence hip position or motion in the frontal or transverse planes. HKAFOs or hip orthoses are sometimes used to protect or maintain hip position after orthopedic surgery to correct bony deformity (e.g., correction of femoral anteversion or derotation osteotomy) or after lengthening procedures of hip adductors or hamstrings.

PARAPODIUMS, STANDING FRAMES, AND SWIVEL WALKERS

Attempts to improve orthotic options for children with lower extremity neuromotor dysfunction have led to the commercial development of a variety of parapodiums, standing frames, and swivel walkers. Although most of these orthoses include proximal components to control the thoracic and lumbar spine (and can most accurately be defined as thoracolumbar HKAFOs), most are classified within the HKAFO family. These orthotic options were developed with the goal of improving function and encouraging independence for patients whose needs could not be adequately addressed by conventional HKAFOs.[4,9] Most allow the child (or adult) who is using them to function in standing and in limited ambulation with significantly less energy cost. Most can be used without a walker or crutches, leaving the hands free for functional activities. Because most designs are available in a kit form, the cost of fabrication and fitting is significantly less than that for conventional HKAFOs.

All of these orthoses provide stability in standing, and some allow limited mobility as well. The earliest versions (Figure 12-4) were designed to facilitate the ability to stand; however they did not always meet the stability needs of timid or apprehensive children who were fearful of falling. Active patients discovered that a frame's structural strength, although sufficient for quiet standing, was compromised or failed during more adventurous activities such as swing-through gait with crutches or independent transfers. Standing frames and similar orthoses are very useful in the classroom, where the ability to stand at the same eye level as one's peers and to function with the hands free enhances participation and empowers students with disability to participate more fully in academic and social activities. Although many therapists acknowledge the advantages of these orthoses, others complain about the difficulty of donning and doffing the device and of the child's inability to move to and from the floor while wearing it.

From this author's clinical experience, the parapodium designed at Ontario Crippled Children's Center in Toronto[9] and the swivel walker designed at the Orthotic Research and Locomotor Assessment Unit in Oswestry, England[12] (Figure 12-5), are valuable orthotic options

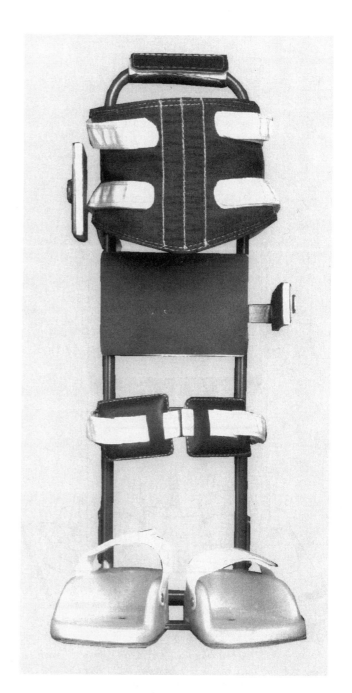

FIGURE 12-4
Standing frame orthosis developed at Gillette Children's Hospital. Note that the tubular frame has no hip, knee, or ankle joints. The fulcrum of the three-force system used to ensure hip extension is the broad posterior pelvic pad (at the center, without Velcro straps), with counterforces delivered by the anterior thoracic corset and the anterior kneepads.

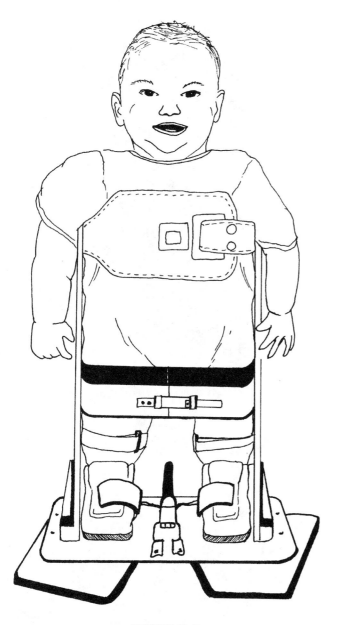

FIGURE 12-5

A young child with myelomeningocele, upright in an Orthotic Research and Locomotor Assessment Unit swivel walker. The ankles are stabilized in a neutral position against the foot plate, knees in extension by a padded anterior bar, hips in extension by a broad pelvic band, and the trunk supported by a broad chest strap. Some versions have orthotic joints at the knee and hip that allow the child to sit but lock when the child is assisted into standing. The child learns to use reciprocal movement of the arms to shift weight from side to side, alternately advancing one of the swivel pads under the foot plate.

to consider when managing the child who has significant neuromuscular or skeletal deficit. Standing frames and swivel walkers are also available in adult sizes but are not used as often for adults as they are for children. They hold the same advantages for adults with paraplegia and other neuromuscular disorders who are required to sustain a hands-free upright posture for vocational, therapeutic, or practical purposes.

HIP-KNEE-ANKLE-FOOT ORTHOSES DESIGNED FOR RECIPROCAL GAIT

Two additional lumbosacral-HKAFO systems have been developed for persons with paraplegia; both use a simple lateral weight shift from one limb to the other as the basis for orthotic-assisted reciprocal gait. The hip guidance orthosis (HGO or parawalker) was developed at the Orthotic Research and Locomotor Assessment Unit,[4,11,13,14] and the reciprocal gait orthosis (RGO) was developed at Louisiana State University (LSU).[15] Both of these systems were designed for patients with high-level spinal cord dysfunction (congenital or traumatic) who would not otherwise be candidates for ambulation. The similarities and differences in the design and use of these orthoses have been the focus of intense research in the last decade.

Hip Guidance Orthosis

Whittle and Cochrane[16] suggest that the most important design aspect of the HGO or parawalker (Figure 12-6) is its rigidity in single limb support, which enhances the patient's ability to clear the contralateral limb as it advances in swing. The work of Jefferson and Whittle[17] demonstrates that, in an HGO, the lower limbs remain essentially parallel in the coronal plane, providing for better ground clearance of the limb in swing.

The HGO enables patients with paraplegia to walk independently with a reciprocal gait pattern.[18] Theoretically, this orthosis also reduces the energy cost of walking because the patient does not have to lift body weight off the ground, as is necessary with a swing-through gait using conventional HKAFOs and crutches. Studies that compared the physiologic cost of walking in the HGO and conventional HKAFOs in children with myelomeningocele demonstrated an 87% increase in gait speed and 10 beats per minute reduction in heart rate when using the HGO.[14] Watkins et al.[18] report that the HGO works effectively to enable individuals with complete thoracic level spinal cord injury to undertake therapeutic walking, based on approximately 200 fittings of the orthosis.[18] The HGO system has also been successful in adult patients with complete spinal cord lesions ranging from C-8 to T-12 levels, with more than 85% of those fitted with an HGO continuing to use their orthosis on a regular basis at the 20-month follow-up interview.[19] Many of those who learn to use an HGO achieve independent use of the orthosis and low energy ambulation indoors and outdoors and on a variety of floor or ground surfaces.

Hip Guidance Orthosis for Children with Myelomeningocele

The HGO was originally developed for children with myelomeningocele.[18] The goal of the HGO is to provide the opportunity for functional independent ambulation. Rose et al.[14] define three criteria for independent orthosis-supported ambulation for these children. First, energy cost must be low at a reasonable speed of ambulation (30–60% of normal speed for the child's age-matched peers). Second, the child must be able to transfer independently from sitting (chair) to walking and vice versa. Third, the child must be able to don and doff the orthosis independently, within a reasonable amount of time without unreasonable effort. Researchers at the Orthotic Research and Locomotor Assessment Unit tracked 27 children who had used the HGO for at least 6 months to evaluate the outcomes of its use. Their work has identified that stability of the trunk (the ability to sit with the arms raised above the head for a prolonged period without support) is an important predictor of HGO success.[14] The HGO is able to provide, at low energy cost, reciprocal ambulation for children with low thoracic and high-level lumbar lesions. Twenty-five of 27 children had to be upright in another orthosis before using an HGO. Only 2 of 27 (7.6%) children had scoliosis.[20] Further work is required to investigate how this extraordinarily low incidence of scoliosis is related to the use of an HGO or a conventional HKAFO.

Reciprocal Gait Orthoses

Douglas et al.[15] describe the LSU RGO (Figure 12-7) as a lightweight bracing system that gives structural stance phase support to the lower trunk and lower limbs of the patient with lower extremity paralysis; it uses a cable-coupling system to provide hip joint motion for swing phase. In the RGO, via its cable system, flexion of one hip (in swing) results in extension of the other hip (concurrently in stance). The hip joints of the orthosis are coupled together using two Bowden cables to transmit the necessary forces (although the original design used a single cable, functional problems and subsequent revisions evolved into the use of a second cable). This reciprocal coupling has the added

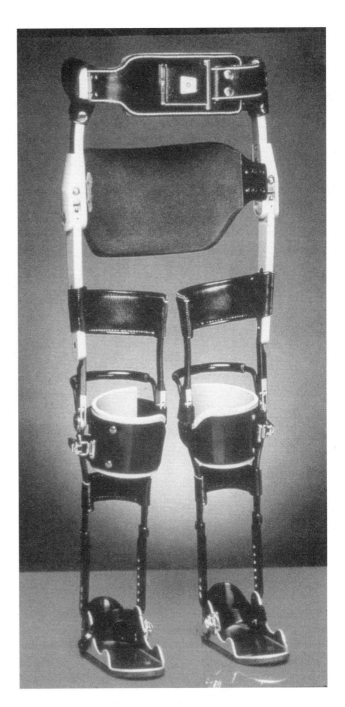

FIGURE 12-6

The hip guidance orthosis, usually worn over clothing, provides a rigid support system for the stance limb. Advancement of the swing limb occurs with its unweighting when the patient leans or shifts laterally onto the stable stance limb.

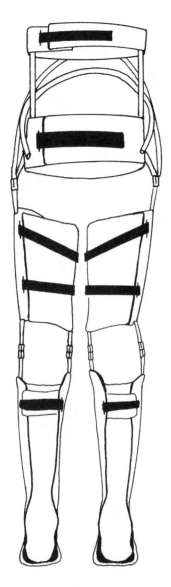

FIGURE 12-7

The reciprocal gait orthosis uses a dual cable system to couple flexion of one hip with extension of the other. This coupling assists forward progression of the swing limb while ensuring stability of the stance limb.

TABLE 12-1

Diagnoses of Patients Who Successfully Used a Reciprocal Gait Orthosis (RGO)

Patient Diagnosis	Number of Patients Fitted with an RGO
Myelomeningocele	95
Traumatic paraplegia	18
Muscular dystrophy	15
Cerebral palsy	8
Multiple sclerosis	1
Sacral agenesis	1

Source: Adapted from R Douglas, PF Larson, R D'Ambrosia, RE McCall. The LSU reciprocation gait orthosis. Orthopedics 1983;6:834–839.

benefit of eliminating simultaneous hip flexion and reducing the risk of "jackknifing" during ambulation. Douglas et al.[15] have used the RGO for patients with a variety of neuromuscular disorders (Table 12-1) and report that long-term bracing with RGO, and the early ambulation this makes possible, decreases the potential for development of secondary deformity. In a group of 100 adults with paraplegia fitted with an RGO, seven were able to ambulate 100 feet with no more than two 30-second rest periods. For many patients, up to 45 hours of training were necessary to achieve functional gait with an RGO. Although the RGO has clearly been shown to be an effective intervention for reciprocal gait in adults and children with paraplegia, some extravagant claims about its success have resulted in uncertainty about prescription criteria.[21]

Reciprocal Gait Orthoses for Children with Myelomeningocele

The RGO was initially designed to afford an upright posture and reciprocal gait pattern for children with myelomeningocele and has been used routinely for such patients during the past 20 years.[8] Little has been published, however, to substantiate its effectiveness for this group, and it is reasonable to suggest that considerably more attention has been given to its suitability for the adult paraplegic population than to the group for whom it was designed. Yngve et al.[22] analyzed the effectiveness of the RGO in children with myelomeningocele who had absence or weakness of the hip extensor mechanism. Patients ranged in age from 18 months to 15 years. The function and potential benefit of three configurations of the reciprocating mechanism were evaluated. In the first configuration, ambulation was tested with the reciprocating mechanism engaged to allow hip flexion with contralateral hip extension. The first configuration represents the normal settings for the RGO. In the second configuration, the reciprocating mechanism was released to provide free flexion and extension at the hips, representing a conventional HKAFO with unlocked hip joints. In the third configuration, the hip joints were locked to eliminate hip motion, representing a conventional HKAFO with restricted hip motion.

Each child ambulated at his or her maximum velocity for 15–31 m in each of the three configurations. The distance that the child walked was determined by individual strength and ability. The number of steps taken and the time to complete their distance were recorded, and velocity and step length were calculated. Although 17 children were included in the study sample, gait characteristics of only 8 children were analyzed. In five of these eight children, gait speed was significantly faster in the RGO than in the other configurations. It is important to note that 75% of the children in the sample had motor function at the L-3 level and that only 18% had complete paralysis of hip musculature. The authors also did not provide information about how and why data from a subsample were used in analysis. Given these concerns, it is not possible to draw any meaningful conclusions about function and neurosegmental level while a patient is wearing an RGO.

McCall et al.[3] fit a group of 29 children with neurologic deficiencies (age range, 1–16 years) with the RGO at Shriners Hospital, Shreveport Unit, between 1981 and 1982. They report that the RGO offered improved standing and ambulatory potential in these neurologically deficient children, while preventing development of deformity and increasing patient independence. Mazur et al.[23] further investigated differences in functional characteristics of reciprocal gait and swing-through gait using the technology of a gait laboratory. In a sample of three children with thoracic level myelomeningocele, reciprocal gait with an RGO was modestly more efficient than a conventional HKAFO.

Guidera et al.,[24] in a retrospective review, evaluated the long-term usage pattern of patients fitted with reciprocating gait orthoses at the Shriners Hospital for Crippled Children in Tampa, Florida. Twenty-one children (13 boys, 8 girls; mean age, 8.75 years) were reevaluated 2 years after receiving their RGO. Nine of the children had thoracic level lesions with no active hip flexion; 12 children had lumbar level lesions. All of the children had required surgical correction of lower limb or spinal deformities before or during the bracing period, and 17 exhibited residual contracture. Eleven patients required additional orthotic support of the spine. When questioned about their use of the RGO, all patients reported problems with donning and doffing, wear and tear on clothing, heat, having multiple repairs, and down time. Almost half of the children were still using the RGO, but only four were community ambulators. The RGO was typically used at school rather than at home. The authors examined energy efficiency of three patients who used the RGO consistently: All were more energy efficient, and two were faster with a swing-through gait pattern as compared to the reciprocating pattern. Despite this, patient preference was to reciprocate.

Guidera et al. then evaluated various factors that may contribute to the long-term success or failure of the RGO. Discontinuance occurred more often in children with a thoracic level lesion, in the presence of obesity, when there was a lack of patient or family support, and if the patient had spinal deformity, mental retardation, knee flexion contracture of more than 30 degrees, or hip flexion contracture of more than 45 degrees. Other negative factors included spasticity, trunk and upper extremity weakness, asymmetric hip dislocation or motor function, and lack of prior standing or walking in a parapodium or other type of orthosis. These factors, especially in combination, have an adverse impact on long-term use and effective ambulation in an RGO.

Rogowski et al.,[25] at Newington Children's Hospital, evaluated the outcomes of fitting with RGOs for children with thoracic and high lumbar level of paralysis. They were especially interested in the criteria or indicators for fitting with an RGO, as well as the use and acceptance of the orthosis, using data from 48 consecutive cases fit between 1982 and 1991. The average time spent in the orthosis for their sample was 6.3 hours a day. Many of the children in the Newington study discontinued brace use between the ages of 7.5 and 11.5 years. In this study of children with paraplegia, the most important determinants of RGO use were age and level of paralysis.

Comparison of the Hip Guidance Orthosis and the Reciprocal Gait Orthosis

The HGO and the RGO enable patients with paraplegia that results from traumatic or congenital spinal cord dysfunction to ambulate using a reciprocal gait pattern. Studies have begun to compare these orthoses in terms of energy expenditure.

Banta et al.[26] determined relative oxygen cost (ml/kg/m) of gait with an HGO (parawalker) and an RGO in five subjects (four adults and one child) with paraplegia. An oxylog was used to record oxygen consumption while the subjects ambulated during steady state. Although all of the subjects trained and used the orthoses for varying amounts of time, the data suggest that the HGO enables a more energy-efficient gait: On average, the oxygen cost while using the parawalker was 27% less than that of the RGO, with reductions of between 12% and 42%. Subjects also ambulated faster with the HGO, with a mean increase in gait speed of 33%. These preliminary results indicate that the HGO may be a more efficient orthosis for level ambulation for patients with paraplegia.

In 1989, the Department of Health and Social Security in the United Kingdom commissioned an extensive comparative trial of both orthoses.[16,27] Twenty-two patients with paraplegia from the Nuffield Orthopedic Centre in Oxford, England (18 men, 4 women), used each orthosis for 4 months in a crossover study. Clinical, ergonomic, biomechanical, psychological, and economic assessments were repeated over the course of the study. Of the individuals in the sample, 15 were able to use both orthoses, 5 were unable to use either of the orthoses, and 2 were able to use the HGO but not the RGO. At the conclusion of the trial, 12 subjects chose to keep the RGO, 4 preferred the HGO, and 6 discontinued use of both orthoses. Those who chose the RGO preferred its appearance. Those who chose the HGO appreciated how quickly the orthosis could be donned and doffed. Although Jefferson and Whittle[17] found that intersubject differences were much larger than interorthosis differences, biomechanical assessment demonstrated that the patterns of movement were not identical in the two orthoses. One limitation of the study was the composition of the sample: No children were included, although both systems were designed for the pediatric patient with paraplegia. As a result, no conclusions about the benefits or drawbacks for children with paraplegia can be drawn.

In a single case design study that involved a 33-year-old with a complete traumatic paraplegia at the T-5 level who was a proficient user of HGO and RGO systems, very few differences in general gait characteristics were identified.[17] The results of this study were based on measurements taken from videotape and the VICON gait analysis system (Oxford Metrics Ltd, Oxford, UK) data. Although stride length was similar with both orthoses, a smaller range of pelvic motion as well as a more fluent gait occurred with the HGO. In the sagittal plane, less hip extension was noted when the patient ambulated with the HGO as compared to the RGO. In the coronal plane, more hip abduction occurred with the HGO than the RGO. This important difference is attributed to lower extremities that remain essentially parallel during walking, which leads to a more efficient toe clearance during swing. The major contribution of this study is a clearer understanding of the biomechanics of movement (based on objective measurement) of these two orthoses when used by an adult with paraplegia who is free of existing deformity or contracture. One of the limitations of a single case design is the ability to apply these results to the population of those with paraplegia: In children with tightness of hip flexors, contracture has a considerable influence on pelvic measurements and stride length.

Other Types of Reciprocal Gait Orthoses

The advanced reciprocating gait orthosis, developed by Hugh Steeper Limited of London, is best described as a modified LSU RGO. A single push-pull cable links the mechanical hip joints. The most appreciated improvement reported by investigators who have examined this design is the ease it confers on rising from a sitting position and on sitting down again after standing. This improvement is the result of a cable link between orthotic hip and knee joints and the addition of pneumatic struts to assist knee extension. The arrangement assists patients in standing directly from a sitting position in which the knees are typically flexed, without prior manual straightening and locking of the knees.

The isocentric reciprocating gait orthosis is a further modification of the LSU RGO. In this variant, the two crossed Bowden cables are replaced by a centrally pivoting bar and tie rod arrangement.

SUMMARY AND CONCLUSION

For children and adults with paraplegia, evidence suggests that the HGO/parawalker provides better ground clearance and a smooth gait pattern. These benefits are possible because of the mechanical rigidity of the orthosis; however, they are achieved only with significant cosmetic deficit. In many instances, the improved cosmesis of the RGO is much preferred by patients. The mechanical reliability of the RGO, however, has been questioned in the literature. In more recent developments, an advanced reciprocating gait orthosis design enhances the patient's ability to rise to standing up and to sitting down without having to lock or unlock orthotic knee joints. The isocentric reciprocating gait orthosis attempts to combine the mechanical advantages of the HGO with the cosmetic and therapeutic advantages of other RGOs. Perhaps the most important finding across most of the studies comparing RGOs and HGOs relate to general gait parameters: Functional differences among the contemporary orthotic options are small.[1]

Despite the considerable activity and associated expense within this subject area, research and clinical experience indicate that most individuals with paraplegia opt for wheelchair mobility after discharge to the community because this provides a faster, safer, and more practical means of mobility with considerably less energy expenditure.

The ability to walk remains an important objective for many children who are paraplegic, as well as for their parents. The ability to reach the goal of functional ambulation depends on many factors, including the cause of the paraplegia, the level of the neuromuscular lesion, the presence of hydrocephalus, the strength of the upper limbs, the availability and effectiveness of parental support, and the child's own coordination and motivation. The ability to ambulate is also dependent on the prescription and fitting of an appropriate orthosis. The literature indicates that contemporary forms of orthotic management, specifically the HGO and the RGO, improve function for many children with paraplegia. This claim has been supported by this author's research and clinical experience.[8] What remains unclear, however, is the influence of these accepted designs on the development of joint contracture and the progression of deformity. The problem of progressive deformity in children with paraplegia is significant. Often a spinal deformity appears within the first decade and progresses to skeletal maturity; the most common deformity is an increased lumbar lordosis. For children with a neurologic level of lesion at T-12 or higher, the incidence of spinal deformity is almost 100%. The impact of fitting of an HKAFO, especially of the HGO and RGO, on the prevention of spinal deformity requires much more scholarly attention and study.

REFERENCES

1. Goldberg B, Hsu JD. Atlas of Orthoses and Assistive Devices. American Academy of Orthopaedic Surgeons. St. Louis: Mosby, 1997;391–399.
2. Menelaus MB. The Orthopaedic Management of Spina Bifida Cystica. Edinburgh, UK: Churchill Livingstone, 1980.
3. McCall RE, Douglas R, Rightor N. Surgical treatment in patients with myelodysplasia before using the LSU reciprocation gait system. Orthopedics 1983;6:843–848.
4. Rose GK. Orthoses for the severely handicapped; rational or empirical choice. Physiotherapy 1980;66(3):76–81.
5. Sharrard WJW. Long term follow-up of posterior iliopsoas transplantation for paralytic dislocation of the hip. Dev Med Child Neurol 1969;(Suppl 1):96.
6. Glancy J. Dynamics and the L3 through L5 myelomeningocele child. Clin Prosthet Orthot 1984;8(3):15–23.
7. Lehneis HR. Orthotic pelvis control in spina bifida. Clin Prosthet Orthot 1984;8(3):26–28.
8. Campbell JH. The Orthotic Management of the Paraplegic Child; Clinical and Biomechanical Analysis. Ph.D. thesis, University of Strathclyde, Glasgow, Scotland, 1996.
9. Motlock W. The parapodium: an orthotic device for neuromuscular disorders. Artif Limbs 1971;15:37–47.
10. Rose GK. Splintage for severe spina bifida cystica. J Bone Joint Surg. 1970;52(1):178–179.
11. Rose GK. The principles and practice of hip guidance articulations. Prosthet Orthot Int 1979;3(1):37–43.
12. Rose GK, Henshaw JT. Swivel walkers for paraplegics—considerations and problems in their design and application. Bull Prosthet Res 1973;10(20):62–74.
13. Major RE, Stallard J, Rose GK. The dynamics of walking using the hip guidance orthosis (HGO) with crutches. Prosthet Orthot Int 1981;5(1):19–22.
14. Rose GK, Stallard J, Sankarankutty M. Clinical evaluation of spina bifida patients using hip guidance orthosis. Dev Med Child Neurol 1981;23(1):30–40.
15. Douglas R, Larson PF, D'Ambrosia R, McCall RE. The LSU reciprocation gait orthosis. Orthopedics 1983;6:834–839.
16. Whittle MW, Cochrane GM. A Comparative Evaluation of the Hip Guidance Orthosis (HGO) and the Reciprocating Gait Orthosis (RGO). Health Equipment Information No.192. London: National Health Service Procurement Directorate, 1989.
17. Jefferson RJ, Whittle MW. Performance of three walking orthoses for the paralyzed: a case study using gait analysis. Prosthet Orthot Int 1990;14(3):103–110.
18. Watkins EM, Edwards DE, Patrick JH. Parawalker paraplegic walking. Physiotherapy 1987;73(2):99–100.
19. Summers BN, McClelland MR, Masri WS. A clinical review of the adult hip guidance orthosis (parawalker) in traumatic paraplegics. Paraplegia 1988;26(1):19–26.
20. Rose GK, Sankarankutty M, Stallard J. A clinical review of the orthotic treatment of myelomeningocele patients. J Bone Joint Surg 1983;65(3):242–246.
21. Patrick JH. Developmental research in paraplegic walking. Br Med J 1986;292(6523):788.
22. Yngve DA, Roberts JM, Douglas R. The reciprocating gait orthosis in myelomeningocele. J Pediatr Orthop 1984;4(3):304–310.
23. Mazur JM, Sienko-Thomas S, Wright N, Cummings U. Swing-through vs reciprocating gait patterns in patients with thoracic level spina bifida. Z Kinderchir 1990;45(Suppl 1): 23–25.
24. Guidera KJ, Raney E, Ogden JA, et al. The use of reciprocating gait orthosis in myelodysplasia (abstract). J Pediatr Orthop 1993;13(3):341–348.
25. Rogowski EM, Fezio JM, Banta W. Long term clinical experience with the reciprocating gait orthotic system. J Assoc Child Prosthet Orthot Clin 1992;27:54.
26. Banta JV, Bell KJ, Muik EA, Fezio JM. Parawalker: energy cost of walking. Eur J Pediatr Surg 1991;1(Suppl 1):7–10.
27. Whittle MW, Cochrane GM, Chase AP, et al. A comparative trial of two walking systems for paralyzed people. Paraplegia 1991;29(2):97–102.

SUGGESTED READING

Kirtley C, Whittle MW, Jefferson R. Influence of walking speed on gait parameters. Biomed Eng 1985;7(4):282–288.

Moore PM. The parawalker: walking for thoracic paraplegics. Physiotherapy Pract 1988;4:18–22.

Ogilvie C, Messenger N, Bowker P, Rowley DI. Orthotic compensation for non-functioning hip extensors. Z Kinderchir 1988;43(Suppl 2):33–35.

Rose GK, Henshaw JT. A swivel walker for paraplegics: medical and technical consideration. Biomed Eng 1972;7: 420–425.

13

Hip Orthoses

WILLIAM J. BARRINGER

The study of orthotics for management of the hip has often been overshadowed by more glamorous aspects of orthotic care in sports medicine rehabilitation, in stabilization of the spine, in the management of cerebral palsy and other neuromuscular pathologies, and in the management of fractures. Students in the fields of medicine or rehabilitation may be introduced to a few orthoses associated with specific pathologies of the hip and their basic fitting principles. Although this may be adequate for the general health care practitioner, those who work with children need more in-depth education about orthotic management of hip dysfunction. Orthopedic surgeons, physical therapists, and orthotists who are working with children should be well aware of the indications and limitations of a variety of hip orthoses, the biomechanical principles involved in their use, and the functional outcomes associated with each. The ability to explain the rationale and wearing requirements to family members and other caregivers is also critical to successful orthotic management of hip pathologies.

This chapter provides a general guideline and reference for the appropriate use of hip orthoses. The two most common childhood pathologies that are managed with hip orthoses—developmental dysplasia of the hip (DDH) and Legg-Calvé-Perthes disease—are discussed. The use of hip orthoses for postoperative management of elective orthopedic surgery is also addressed. The chapter focuses on the issues that are most relevant to the rehabilitation team, including clinical decision making, biomechanical principles, and outcome expectations, rather than on the technical aspects of orthotic fabrication.

HIP STRUCTURE AND FUNCTION

The hip (coxofemoral) joint is a synovial joint formed by the concave socket-like acetabulum of the pelvis and the rounded ball-like head of the femur (Figure 13-1). Because of the unique bony structure of the hip joint, movement is possible in all three planes of motion: flexion/extension in the sagittal plane, abduction/adduction in the frontal plane, and internal/external rotation in the transverse plane. Most functional activities blend movement of the femur on the pelvis (or of the pelvis on the femur) across all three planes of motion. The hip joint has two important functions. First, it must support the weight of the head, arms, and trunk during functional activities (such as erect sitting and standing, walking, running, and stair climbing, and during transitional movements in activities of daily living). Second, it must effectively transmit forces from the pelvis to the lower extremities during quiet standing, gait, and other closed chain activities.[1]

The acetabulum is formed at the convergence of the pubis, ischium, and ilium. Its primary orientation is in the vertical, facing laterally, but it also has a slight inferior and anterior tilt. Developmentally, the depth of the acetabulum is dynamically shaped by motion of the head of the femur during leg movement and weight bearing. The acetabulum is not fully ossified until late adolescence or early young adulthood. The *articular surface of the acetabulum* is a horseshoe-shaped, hyaline cartilage–covered area around its anterior, superior, and posterior edges. A space along the inferior edge, called the *acetabular notch*, is nonarticular and has no cartilage covering. The *acetabular labrum* is a fibrocartilaginous ring that encircles the exterior perimeter of the acetabulum, increasing joint depth and concavity. The center of the acetabulum, the *acetabular fossa*, contains fibroelastic fat and the ligamentum teres, and is covered by synovial membrane.

The femoral components of the hip joint include the femoral head, the femoral neck, and the greater and lesser trochanters. The spherical articular surface of the femoral head is covered with hyaline cartilage. Because the femoral

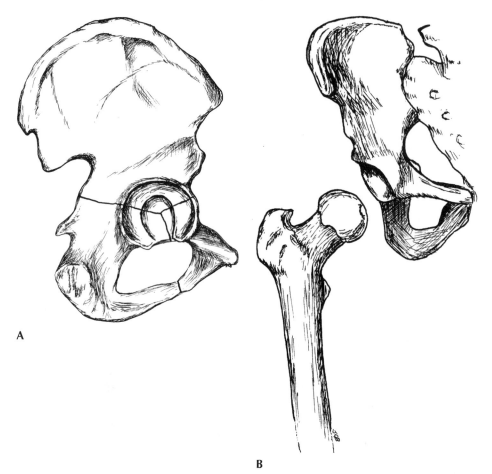

FIGURE 13-1
*Anatomy of the hip joint. **(A)** The articular surface of the socket-like acetabulum, a horseshoe-shaped area covered by hyaline cartilage, is extended by the acetabular labrum. **(B)** The proximal femur is angled to seat the femoral head optimally within the acetabulum, to support the upper body and to transmit loading forces to or from the lower extremity.*

A

B

head is larger and somewhat differently shaped than the acetabulum, a portion of its articular surface is exposed in any position of the hip joint. The femur and acetabulum are most congruent when positioned in a combination of flexion, abduction, and external rotation. The proximal femur, comprised of trabecular bone, is designed to withstand significant loading while also permitting movement through large excursions of range of motion. The orientation of the femoral head and neck in the frontal plane, with respect to the shaft of the femur, is described as its *angle of inclination* (see Figure 6-3). In infancy the angle of inclination may be as much as 150 degrees but decreases during normal development to approximately 125 degrees in midadulthood and to 120 degrees in later life.[2] The orientation of the proximal femur to the shaft and condyles in the transverse plane, called the *angle of anteversion*, is also a key determinant of hip joint function (see Figures 6-4 and 6-5). Anteversion may be as much

as 40 degrees at birth, decreasing during normal development to approximately 15 degrees in adulthood.[2] These two angulations determine how well the femoral head is seated within the acetabulum and, in effect, the biomechanical stability of the hip joint. The functional stability of the hip joint is supported by a strong fibrous joint capsule and by the iliofemoral and pubofemoral ligaments. Fibers of the capsule and ligaments are somewhat obliquely oriented, becoming most taut when the hip is in an extended position.

Most nontraumatic hip joint dysfunction or pathology occurs either in childhood or in late adult life and frequently is related to one or more of the four following factors:

1. Inadequate or ineffective development of the acetabulum and head of the femur in infancy

2. Avascular necrosis of the femoral head associated with inadequate blood supply during childhood

3. Loss of cartilage and abnormal bone deposition associated with osteoarthritis
4. Loss of bone strength and density in osteoporosis

Orthotic intervention is an important component in the orthopedic management of many of these conditions. Most often, hip orthoses are used to protect or position the hip joint by limiting motion within a desirable range of flexion/extension and abduction/adduction. It is important to note that hip orthoses alone are not effective in controlling internal/external rotation of the hip joint. If precise rotational control is desired, a hip-knee-ankle-foot orthosis (HKAFO) must be used.

ORTHOTIC MANAGEMENT IN DEVELOPMENTAL DYSPLASIA OF THE HIP

DDH is the current terminology for a condition previously called *congenital dislocation of the hip*. This new term includes a variety of congenital hip pathologies, including dysplasia, subluxation, and dislocation. This inclusive terminology is preferred, as it includes those infants with normal physical examination at birth who later are found to have a subluxed or dislocated hip, in addition to those who are immediately identified as having hip pathologies.[3]

Incidence and Etiology of Developmental Dysplasia

Instability of the hip due to DDH occurs in 11.7 of every 1,000 live births, with most of these classified as hip subluxation (9.2/1,000), followed by true dislocation (1.3/1,000) and dislocatable hips (1.2/1,000).[4] Hip dislocation is more common in girls (70%) than in boys, and among white than among black newborns. Approximately 20% of all hip dislocations are associated with breech presentation, although the incidence of breech presentation in the normal population is approximately 4%.[5] A familial tendency is also found: DDH is much more likely to occur when an older sibling has had congenital subluxation or dislocation. The risk of dysplasia increases with any type of intrauterine malpositioning leading to extreme flexion and adduction at the hip. This occurs more commonly during first pregnancies, if and when tightness of maternal abdominal or uterine musculature is present, when the infant is quite large, or when insufficient amniotic fluid restricts intrauterine motion.[6] A higher incidence of DDH is also found among new-borns with other musculoskeletal abnormalities, including torticollis, metatarsus varus, clubfoot, or other unusual syndromes. The most common clinical sign of DDH is limitation in hip abduction.[7]

At birth, the acetabulum is quite shallow, covering less than half of the femoral head. In addition, the joint capsule is loose and elastic. These two factors make the neonate hip relatively unstable and susceptible to subluxation and dislocation. Normal development of the hip joint in the first year of life is a function of the stresses and strains placed on the femoral head and acetabulum during movement. In the presence of subluxation or dislocation, modeling of the acetabulum and femoral head is compromised. The goal of orthotic management in developmental dysplasia is to achieve optimal seating of the femoral head within the acetabulum while permitting the kicking movements that facilitate shaping of the acetabulum and femoral head for stability of the hip joint.[8] This is best achieved if the child is routinely positioned in flexion and abduction at the hip. If DDH is recognized early, and appropriate intervention initiated, the hip joint is likely to develop normally. If unrecognized and untreated, DDH often leads to significant deformity of the hip as the child grows, resulting in compromised mobility and other functional limitations.

Early Orthotic Management of Developmental Dysplasia: Birth to 6 Months

In 1958, Professor Arnold Pavlik of Czechoslovakia described an orthosis for the treatment of dysplasia, subluxation, and dislocation of the hip. This orthosis, which now bears his name, the Pavlik harness, relies on hip flexion and abduction to stabilize the hip at risk. In the United States it has become widely accepted as an effective treatment for the unstable hip in neonates from birth to 6 months of age.

Pavlik Harness
At first glance, the Pavlik harness seems a confusing collection of webbing, Velcro, padding, and straps. In reality, this dynamic orthosis (Figure 13-2) has three major components: (1) a shoulder and chest harness that provides a proximal anchor for the device, (2) a pair of booties and stirrups used as the distal attachment, and (3) anterior and posterior leg straps between chest harness and booties used to position the hip joint optimally. The anterior strap allows flexion but limits extension, whereas the posterior strap allows abduction but limits adduction. The child is free to move into flexion and abduction, the motions that are most likely to facilitate functional shaping of the acetabulum in

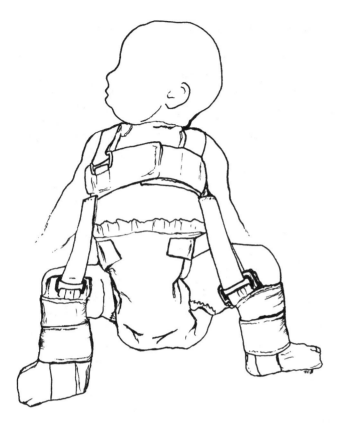

FIGURE 13-2

A Pavlik harness positions the infant's lower extremities in hip flexion and abduction, in an effort to position the femoral head optimally within the acetabulum, facilitating normal bony development of the hip joint. The anterior leg straps allow hip flexion but limit hip extension; the posterior straps allow abduction but limit adduction.

the months after birth.[9] To be effective, however, the fit of the harness must be accurately adjusted for the growing infant, and the orthosis must be properly applied. Because of this, the family caregiver must be involved in an intensive education program when the newborn is being fit with the Pavlik harness. Nurses, physical and occupational therapists, pediatricians, and orthopedic residents who work with newborns also need to understand the function and fit of this important orthosis.

The guidelines for properly fitting a Pavlik harness include the following key points:[10]

1. The shoulder straps cross in the back to prevent the orthosis from sliding off the infant's shoulders.

2. The chest strap is fit around the thorax at the infant's nipple line.

3. The proximal calf strap on the bootie is fit just distal to the knee joint.

4. The anterior leg straps are attached to the chest strap at the anterior axillary line.

5. The posterior leg straps are attached to the chest strap just over the infant's scapulae.

In a correctly fit orthosis, the lower extremity is positioned in 100–120 degrees of hip flexion, as indicated by the physician's evaluation and recommendation. The limbs are also positioned in 30–40 degrees of hip abduction. The distance between the infant's thighs (when the hips are moved passively into adduction) should be no more than 8–10 cm. In a well-fit orthosis, extension and adduction are limited, whereas flexion and abduction are freely permitted: The infant is able to "kick" actively within this restricted range while wearing the orthosis. This position and movement encourage elongation of adductor contractures, which in turn assists in the reduction of the hip and enhances acetabular development.

Three common problems indicate that the fit of the harness requires adjustment:

1. If the leg straps are adjusted too tightly, the infant is unable to kick actively.

2. If the anterior straps are positioned too far medially on the chest strap, the limb is positioned in excessive adduction rather than the desired abduction.

3. If the calf strap is positioned too far distally on the lower leg, it does not position the limb in the desired amount of hip flexion.

Clinical Concerns

Optimal outcomes in infants with DDH are associated with early aggressive intervention of the unstable hip using the Pavlik harness. It is essential that families and health care professionals seek proper orthopedic care to avoid misdiagnosis and mistreatment. One of the most common misdiagnoses is mistaking dislocation for subluxation and implementing a triple- or double-diapering strategy for intervention. Although this strategy does position the infant's hip in some degree of flexion and abduction, bulky diapers alone are insufficient for reducing dislocation.

Initially, most infants wear the Pavlik harness 24 hours a day. The parents can be permitted to remove the harness for bathing, at the discretion of the orthopedist. It is important, especially early in treatment, that the fit and function of the orthosis be reevaluated frequently to ensure proper position in the orthosis.

Families must be instructed in proper skin care and in bathing the newborn or infant wearing the orthosis. Initially, they may be advised to use diapers, but not any type of shirt, under the orthosis. The importance of keeping regularly scheduled recheck appointments for effective monitoring of hip position and refitting of the orthosis as the infant grows cannot be over-stressed to the parents or caregivers. Missed appointments often result in less than optimal positioning of the femoral head with respect to the acetabulum, a less than satisfactory outcome of early intervention, and the necessity of more involved treatment procedures as the child grows.

The many straps of the Pavlik harness can be confusing to the most caring of families. The proper donning and doffing sequence should be thoroughly explained and demonstrated to the family. Additional strategies to enhance optimal reduction of the hip, such as prone sleeping, need to be encouraged.

Over time, when hip development is progressing as desired, the wearing schedule can be decreased to night and naptime wear. This often welcomed change in wearing time can begin as early as 3 months of age if x-ray and physical examination demonstrate the desired bone development. When the orthopedist determines the hip to be normal according to radiographs and is satisfied with the clinical examination, the orthosis can be discontinued. If development of the hip is slow or the infant undergoes rapid growth, it may be advisable to continue the treatment with another type of hip abduction orthosis designed for older and larger babies, to maintain the position of flexion and abduction for a longer period of time.

Management of Developmental Dysplasia: 6 Months and Beyond

For older infants and toddlers (6–18 months) whose DDH was unrecognized or inadequately managed early in infancy, intervention is often much more aggressive and may include traction, open or closed reduction, and hip spica casting. For infants who are growing quickly or whose bone development has been slow, an alternative to the Pavlik harness is necessary. After the age of 6 months, especially as the infant begins to pull into standing in preparation for walking, the Pavlik harness is no longer able to provide the desired positioning for reduction. Often, the infant is simply too large to fit into the harness. By this time, families who have been compliant

with harness application and wearing have grown to dislike it and are ready for other forms of treatment.

Hip Abduction Orthosis

A custom-fit prefabricated thermoplastic hip abduction orthosis is often the next step in orthotic management of DDH. This orthosis consists of a plastic frame with waist section and thigh cuffs, waterproof foam liner, and Velcro closures. The static version is fixed at 90 degrees of hip flexion and 120 degrees of hip abduction (Figure 13-3). An adjustable joint can be incorporated into the abduction bar; however, hip flexion is maintained at 90 degrees. This orthosis appears to be static, but the child is able to move within the thigh sections while the "safe zone" for continued management of hip position is maintained.

Many families view the hip abduction orthosis as an improvement over the Pavlik harness: The caregivers and the infant are free from cumbersome straps, the orthosis is easily removed and reapplied for diaper changing and hygiene, and the orthosis itself is waterproof and easier to keep clean. Parents and caregivers are able to hold the infant without struggling with straps, and the baby is able to sit comfortably for feeding and play.

Because most hip abduction orthoses are prefabricated, the knowledge and skills of an orthotist are necessary to ensure a proper custom fit for each child. To determine what the necessary modifications are, the orthotist evaluates three areas:

1. *The length of the thigh cuffs.* Thigh cuffs are trimmed proximal to the popliteal fossae. Cuffs that are too long can lead to neurovascular compromise if the child prefers to sleep in a supine position, as the risk of compression of the legs against the distal edge of the cuffs is present.

2. *The width of the anterior opening of the waist component.* Although the plastic is flexible, the opening may need to be enlarged for heavy or large-framed infants.

3. *The foam padding of the thigh and waist components.* All edges must be smooth to avoid skin irritation or breakdown, and the circumference of the padding should fit without undue tightness.

Modifications may require reheating or trimming of the plastic or foam padding. Usually this fitting takes place in the orthotist's office or the clinic setting where the necessary tools are readily available. Once the fit is evaluated and modified as appropriate for the individual child,

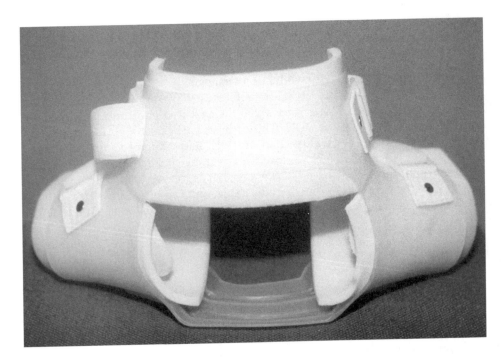

FIGURE 13-3
A posterior view of a static hip abduction orthosis, which positions the infant in 90 degrees of hip flexion and 120 degrees of abduction.

the parents or caregivers are instructed in proper donning/doffing and orthotic care.

Clinical Concerns

The static hip abduction orthosis is used in either of two ways. First, the orthosis may be a continuation of the course of treatment established by the Pavlik harness, as determined by the orthopedist's evaluation of the child's hip. As a continuation of treatment, the orthosis can be worn for day and nighttime wear; most often, however, it is reserved for nighttime use while the child is sleeping. The use of the orthosis at night is believed to facilitate development of acetabular growth cartilage.[10] If the orthosis is consistently worn for several months and evidence of effective reduction and reshaping of the joint is present, it is less likely that more aggressive forms of treatment will be necessary as the child grows.

The second application for the hip abduction orthosis is for follow-up management for children with DDH who require an orthopedic intervention, such as traction, surgical reduction, or casting. In this case, the orthosis provides external stability to the hip during the postoperative weeks and months, while the baby regains range of motion and continues to grow and progress through the stages of motor development. This extra stability reduces parental and physician concern about dislocation and other undesired outcomes of the orthopedic procedure.

The static hip abduction orthosis has obvious advantages over plaster or synthetic hip spica casts, including greater ease in diaper hygiene and bathing, and is often welcomed by families as a positive next step in treatment. Fitting requires the knowledge and skills of an orthotist familiar with proper fitting techniques, who is able to manage potentially irritable babies just freed from a confining hip spica cast.

Goals of Orthotic Intervention for Children with Developmental Dysplasia of the Hip

To be effective, orthotic intervention for DDH must have a set of clearly described treatment objectives against which success can be measured. The components necessary for effective orthotic interventions for children with DDH include

1. Clearly presented verbal, psychomotor, and written instructions for the child's family or caregivers, with an additional goal of minimizing stress in an already stressful situation.

2. Effective communication among members of the health care team about the appropriate use and potential pitfalls of the orthosis. This often includes education about the orthosis provided by the orthotist and careful monitoring of family compliance and coping by all members of the team (orthotists, orthopedists, pediatricians, therapists, nurses, and other health professionals who may be involved in the case).

3. Safe and effective hip reduction to minimize the necessity of more aggressive casting or surgery. This

requires proper orthotic fit and adjustment, as well as consistency in wearing schedules.

The ultimate goal is to facilitate normal development of the hip joint, providing the child with a pain-free, stable, functional hip that will last throughout his or her lifetime.

ORTHOTIC MANAGEMENT OF LEGG-CALVÉ-PERTHES DISEASE

Legg-Calvé-Perthes disease is a hip pathology that affects otherwise healthy school-aged children. Although the clinical signs and symptoms of Legg-Calvé-Perthes disease, as they differ from tuberculosis involving the hip, were first described by Arthur T. Legg in 1910,[11] the etiology of this condition is not clearly understood, and its treatment and orthopedic management continue to be controversial. The hallmark of Legg-Calvé-Perthes disease is a flattening of the femoral head, most likely associated with avascular necrosis. Left untreated, Legg-Calvé-Perthes disease leads to permanent deformity and osteoarthritis in the adult hip. The disease is four times as common in boys between the ages of 4 and 8 years old than in girls.[12,13] It generally involves only one hip; only approximately 12% of the cases are bilateral. It is rare within the black population. Several options for orthotic management of Legg-Calvé-Perthes disease have evolved over time. All are designed to help maintain a spherical femoral head and normal acetabulum.

Etiology of Legg-Calvé-Perthes Disease

The etiology of Legg-Calvé-Perthes disease remains controversial even 90 years after it was first described. Most researchers believe that Legg-Calvé-Perthes is a result of some event or condition that compromises blood flow to the femoral head and leads to avascular necrosis. The exact mechanism that triggers this compromise is unknown. Some theories focus on an acute trauma that damages the vascular system of the femoral head, whereas others suggest that repeated episodes of a transient synovitis may compromise blood flow.[7,12] A genetic predisposition to delayed bone age that exposes vessels to high rates of compression as they pass through cartilage to the bony head has also been suggested. Although the exact etiology of Legg-Calvé-Perthes remains a mystery, it is certainly linked to episodes of avascular necrosis in the femoral head. The goal of intervention in children with Legg-Calvé-Perthes is to facilitate revascularization of the femoral head and to restore normal anatomic shape and alignment of the hip joint.

Evaluation and Treatment of Legg-Calvé-Perthes Disease

Three characteristic symptoms are associated with development of Legg-Calvé-Perthes disease in children: (1) a noticeable limp, often with a positive Trendelenburg's sign; (2) pain in the hip, groin, and/or knee; and (3) loss of range of motion of the hip joint. When these symptoms are present, radiographic studies of the hip are used to confirm the diagnosis of Legg-Calvé-Perthes disease. These studies are used by the orthopedist to determine severity and progression of the disease. Various systems are being used to describe and classify the severity of Legg-Calvé-Perthes. The reader is referred to a text on orthopedic conditions in pediatrics for further information about classification.[14] Legg-Calvé-Perthes disease is a self-limiting process that often resolves in 1–3 years. The disease progresses through three stages: (1) avascular necrosis, (2) resorption of damaged bone, and (3) eventually a final reparative stage with revascularization, reossification, and bony remodeling. Factors that influence the eventual outcome of the disease include age at onset, severity of damage to the femoral head and epiphysis, and quality of congruency of the acetabulum and femoral head.[7,13]

Because the disease process is self-limiting, the optimal intervention strategy is controversial. The three most commonly used avenues of treatment for Legg-Calvé-Perthes disease are observation, surgical intervention, and conservative orthotic management. Decisions about treatment are often guided by age of the child, extent of femoral head deformity, and severity of incongruency between the femoral head and acetabulum.[13]

For children with minimal bony deformity, observation and exercise may be the most appropriate intervention. Because the child is likely to continue to limp until sufficient revascularization and remodeling have occurred (which may require several years) parents may be uneasy, preferring instead a more aggressive intervention. Parents are reassured when close clinical follow-up is performed, with periodic reexamination by x-ray evaluation to monitor progression of the disease process.

Surgical intervention is based on the principle of containment, optimally positioning the femoral head within the acetabulum. Proximal femoral derotation osteotomy is used to decompress and center the femoral head within the acetabulum for more functional weight bearing in an extended position.[15] A pelvic osteotomy, which repositions the acetabulum over the femoral head, is sometimes necessary when a significantly enlarged or subluxed femoral head cannot be effectively repositioned by femoral derotation osteotomy. The outcome of surgery is likely to be most positive for children who have full hip range of motion

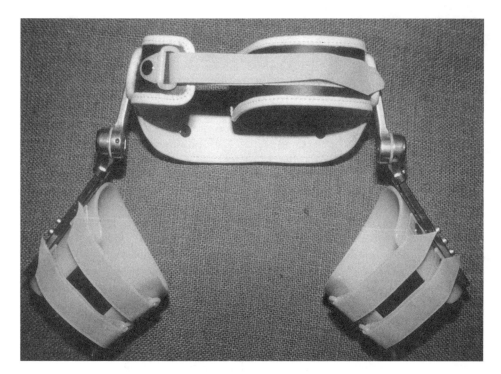

FIGURE 13-4
Scottish-Rite hip abduction orthosis (anterior view), used in the conservative management of Legg-Calvé-Perthes disease. This orthosis has three components: the pelvic band, the free-motion hip joints, and the thigh cuffs. An abduction bar can be placed between the thigh cuffs to provide extra stability in the desired position of 45 degrees of hip abduction.

preoperatively. It is important that parents understand the goals and the risks of the surgical procedure and that they are actively involved in postoperative rehabilitation efforts.

The goal of conservative orthotic management of Legg-Calvé-Perthes disease is similar to that of surgical intervention: to contain the femoral head within the acetabulum during the active stages of the disease process so that optimal remodeling can occur. Much debate has taken place concerning which intervention is most efficacious. If both are viable methods of treatment, the end result should be the same: a well-shaped femoral head and pain-free hip. Comparing the efficacy of surgical versus orthotic management of Legg-Calvé-Perthes disease is challenging because of differences in study design and definition of control for variables such as age of onset, duration of the disease, sex, and inadequate interobserver reliability of classification systems.[16] Although two reports published in 1992 question the efficacy of orthotic treatment,[17,18] other studies advocate orthotic treatment even in very severe cases of the disease. Because studies have reported success as well as lack of success for all three types of intervention (noncontainment/observation, surgery, and the use of orthoses), the most appropriate management of Legg-Calvé-Perthes disease has not been clearly determined. A multicenter study now in progress, designed to compare these different strategies using valid scientific controls, will shed new light on the treatment and better define the role of orthoses in managing Legg-Calvé-Perthes disease.

Orthotic Management: Scottish-Rite Hip Abduction Orthosis

The most commonly used orthosis in the nonoperative management of Legg-Calvé-Perthes disease is the Scottish-Rite hip abduction orthosis (Figure 13-4). The design of this orthosis allows the child to walk and be involved in other functional activities while containing the femoral head in the acetabulum with abduction of the hips. The Scottish-Rite orthosis has three components: a pelvic band, a pair of single-axis hip joints, and a pair of thigh cuffs. An abduction bar may also be included, interconnecting the thigh cuffs with a ball-and-socket joint as an interface. The Scottish-Rite orthosis holds each hip in approximately 45 degrees of hip abduction, permits flexion and extension of the hip, and can be worn over clothing. While in the orthosis the hips are abducted and flexed, but the patient has no limitation in knee range of motion and therefore can sit or walk without difficulty. The orthosis is not designed to control internal rotation of the hip.

The Scottish-Rite orthosis is most effective if the child who is wearing it has close to normal range of motion at the hip joint. Limitations in range of motion cause the child to stand asymmetrically in the orthosis, which effectively reduces the amount of abduction and containment of the femoral head.

If the disease process progresses and the hip begins to lose additional range of motion, the orthotist may be the first to recognize this problem. The parents may bring the child to the clinic for an orthotic adjustment because the thigh cuffs have become uncomfortable. If loss of additional range of motion is noticed by parents or by therapists who are working with the child, an immediate referral to the orthotic clinic or physician is necessary. The Scottish-Rite orthosis is not designed to increase range of motion; its primary function is to hold the hips in abduction comfortably. Using the orthosis to restore range of motion defeats the purpose of the orthotic design and compromises treatment principles.

Communication between the orthopedist, orthotist, therapist, and family is essential. Parents must understand that this is a demanding form of treatment. Typically, the orthosis is worn continually for 12–18 months. Once radiographic evidence of femoral head reossification is seen, time in the orthosis is gradually reduced.

Absolute compliance with the wearing schedule is necessary for maximum effectiveness: A well-designed and well-fit orthosis can only work if it is being used. The first few days and weeks in the orthosis are often stressful for the parent and the child. With the hips held in an abducted position, routine tasks, including walking, may require assistance until the child learns effective adaptive strategies. Physical therapists may work with the child on crutch-walking techniques on level surfaces, stairs, inclines, and uneven surfaces. They may make suggestions for adaptation of the home and school environments so that sitting and transitions between floor, chairs, and standing quickly become manageable. If family education and support efforts are effective, so that parents and children weather this difficult initial stage in orthotic management well, the likelihood of compliance in the remaining months of intervention is significantly enhanced.

HIP ORTHOTICS IN POSTOPERATIVE CARE

Numerous musculoskeletal and neuromuscular conditions, in addition to Legg-Calvé-Perthes disease and developmental dysplasia, may necessitate surgical intervention for children with hip and lower extremity dysfunction or deformity. Orthoses that control hip and leg position are often used in the weeks and months after surgery as an alternative to traditional plaster casts or as a follow-up strategy once casts are removed. Although a cast may be applied in the operating room for immediate postoperative care, orthoses are often fit soon afterward and effectively shorten the time that a child spends in a cast. Hip orthoses are used when immobilization and support will be required for a long period of time, when complications arise, or when a child's special needs demand their use.

One of the major benefits of an orthosis (as compared to a plaster cast) is in regard to hygiene, especially for children who have not yet developed consistent bladder and bowel control. Additional benefits of postoperative hip orthoses include the following:

1. Being much lighter than traditional casts, hip orthoses reduce the burden of care for parents and caregivers who must lift or carry the child.
2. Hip orthoses can be removed for inspection of surgical wounds and for bathing and skin care.
3. Hip orthoses can be removed for physical therapy, range of motion, mobilization, strengthening, or other appropriate interventions.
4. Thermoplastic orthoses are waterproof; therefore, residues of perspiration or urine can be easily cleaned and sanitized with warm soap and water.
5. A well-fit orthosis is less likely to cause skin irritation or breakdown and, unlike a cast, can often be adjusted if areas of impingement do develop.
6. The position and amount of abduction can be easily adjusted.
7. A hip orthosis can be custom designed to meet the needs of a patient with complicated needs, especially those who have had multiple surgical procedures.

Postoperative Hip Orthoses

Two basic designs are available for children's postoperative orthoses. The first is composed of thigh cuffs that fit between the knee and hip joint, an abduction bar, and Velcro closures (Figure 13-5). This orthosis can be fabricated from measurements taken before surgery and fit with no delay as soon as the cast is removed. It can also be fit in lieu of a cast if the surgical procedure was minor or when static positioning of the hip is required. This type of orthosis is commonly used after adductor release or varus osteotomy with adductor release, or for the management of a septic hip. A postoperative hip orthosis is most often used for extended periods of nighttime-only wear but in some circumstances can also be worn during the day.[19] In our clinic this orthosis is most commonly used after hip procedures in patients with cerebral palsy.

Patients and caregivers find the postoperative hip orthosis a welcome relief from a cast. Despite its simple appearance, families should be given special instructions about how the orthosis is worn and cared for. It can be worn over clothing or pajamas, or next to the skin if necessary. It should not cause skin irritation or discomfort on either side of the hip joint. If the patient experiences any hip joint pain, the orthotist should consult with the orthopedist to determine if the angle of abduction can be safely adjusted. Overzealous attempts to abduct the hip can cause pain and reduce com-

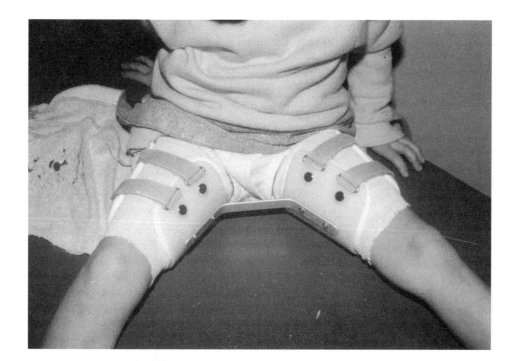

FIGURE 13-5

A postoperative hip abduction orthosis has two components: a pair of thigh cuffs held in position by an abduction bar.

pliance. Occasionally, this orthosis may be difficult to keep in place even though it has been properly fit: A simple suspension belt can be added to ensure optimal positioning.

The second option for postoperative care is a modification of a knee-ankle-foot orthosis. This orthosis is composed of two thermoplastic knee-ankle-foot orthoses without knee joints but with an abduction bar and Velcro closures (Figure 13-6). Fabrication of this type of orthosis requires that plaster impressions be taken: Simple length and circumferential measurements are not adequate to ensure proper fit. Ideally, these impressions are taken at the first postoperative cast change, the orthosis is then fabricated, and fitting occurs during the next clinic appointment. It is not advisable to take the impressions before surgery: Postoperatively, each joint will be at a new angle, compromising the fit of the orthosis based on preoperative impressions. This type of orthosis is recommended for patients who have had bony procedures around the hip as well as extensive soft tissue procedures, such as hamstring or heel cord release, which require protection in the early stages of healing. In our clinic, this orthosis is most often used for patients with cerebral palsy or myelomeningocele. In some circumstances, when more precise control of the hip joint is desirable, the orthosis can be extended upward to include the pelvis.

Because of the intimate fit of this orthosis, parents and caregivers must be given careful education concerning proper fit and cleaning. It is especially important to include careful inspection of the posterior aspect of the calcaneus: This area is vulnerable to skin breakdown from prolonged pressure and may be overlooked during skin checks that focus on the healing surgical wounds. Because the foam lining and thermoplastic material do not "breathe," perspiration cannot effectively evaporate. The orthosis should be removed periodically for cleaning to minimize the risk of skin maceration or infection from microorganisms that thrive in warm moist environments.

The postoperative orthosis has proved to be very useful in the overall orthopedic management of children with musculoskeletal or neuromuscular diseases. The orthosis is an effective substitute for heavy casts, especially when skin irritation and incontinence are concerns. The postoperative hip orthosis helps to ensure healing in the optimal joint position and reduces the likelihood of recurrence of the deformity that prompted surgical intervention.

HIP ORTHOSES IN THE MANAGEMENT OF THE ADULT HIP

Orthotic intervention for the hip in the adult population is limited, focusing on two groups of patients. Hip orthoses are most commonly used as postsurgical and postcast care of adult patients who have sustained a complex hip or proximal femoral fracture from a traumatic event, such as a motor vehicle accident, industrial accident, or fall. In some circumstances, a hip orthosis can be used for older adults after a total hip procedure, revision of a total hip, or fracture associated with total hip arthroplasty. Although injury that affects the hip can occur at any point in the life span, most adults with trauma-related fractures who are

FIGURE 13-6

For postoperative management of children after extensive bony and soft tissue surgery, knee-ankle-foot orthoses with the addition of an abduction bar are often used subsequent to cast removal. Rotation of the hip is well controlled by the intimate fit of the orthosis, including the ankle-foot complex. When precise control of the hip is necessary, the postoperative hip abduction orthosis encompasses the pelvis as well.

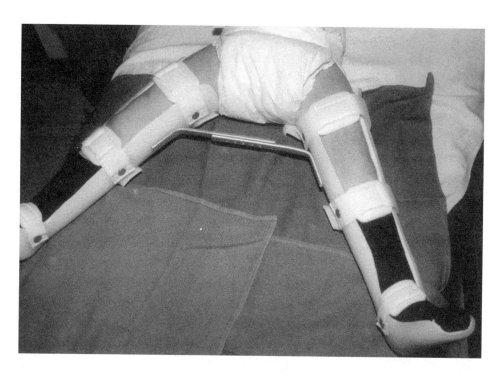

managed with hip orthoses are young and middle-aged, and many of those who are undergoing a new or revised total joint arthroplasty are 65 years or older. It is important to note that as the number of older adults increases in the US population so will the number of hip fractures: One estimate suggests that as many as 512,000 hip fractures will occur in the United States by the year 2040.[20]

In both of these circumstances, stabilization of the orthopedic injury and rehabilitation planning are important issues. Patients with this type of injury of the hip often require extensive physical therapy programs. Clinicians must understand age-related pathophysiologic changes that affect the healing musculoskeletal system, the impact and detrimental effects of prolonged bed rest, and the optimal point at which an orthosis should be integrated into the overall treatment plan

Use of Orthoses in Total Hip Arthroplasty

Although a hip orthosis is usually not indicated in most simple, elective total hip arthroplasties, in some circumstances this orthosis can facilitate healing and rehabilitation. Hip orthoses can be used for patients with significant osteoporosis in whom femoral fracture occurs during total joint surgery or for those who require emergency total joint replacement as a result of trauma. Hip orthoses are also used for patients who are undergoing revision of a total hip replacement as a consequence of recurrent dislocation or of aseptic loosening of the femoral component. If control of rotation is desired, an HKAFO can be prescribed to provide additional support and protection to healing struc-

tures. Most HKAFOs have a pelvic band and belt and an adjustable hip joint that can be locked, allow free motion, or limit motion within a specific range (Figure 13-7). An adjustable anterior panel can be added to the thigh section if a fracture has occurred during the surgical procedure and requires additional protection. The knee joint can also be locked, free motion, or adjustable for specific ranges of motion, depending on the patient's need. The ankle-foot orthosis component is necessary to provide maximum control of unwanted rotation of the hip.

At our institution HKAFOs are custom fabricated, based on an impression of the patient's limb. We believe that this increases our ability to provide an optimal fit and allows customization of the orthosis to meet the specific needs of the patient. If this approach is not amenable to certain health care environments, prefabricated custom-fit HKAFOs and hip orthoses are available as alternatives to custom-molded orthoses.[21] These orthoses are fabricated from components that are then custom fit based on the patient's limb measurements. Most postoperative hip orthoses are designed to limit flexion and adduction of the hip joint (Figure 13-8). They try to prevent dislocation by supporting the optimal position of the hip joint within a safe range of motion and by providing a kinesthetic reminder when patients attempt to move beyond these ranges.[21] It should be noted that many of the prefabricated hip orthoses that are commercially available are unable to provide maximum control of rotation because they do not encompass the foot. Careful evaluation of the patient is required to determine which alternative is most appropriate. In both cases, the orthosis is worn when-

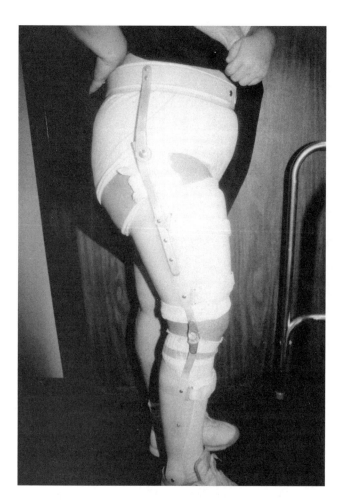

FIGURE 13-7
Lateral view of a heel-knee-ankle-foot orthosis, prescribed for postoperative management after a complex total hip arthroplasty. Note the pelvic band, free hip joint, supportive thigh cuff, and free knee joint. The ankle-foot orthosis component is necessary for effective control of rotatory forces through the femur and hip joint.

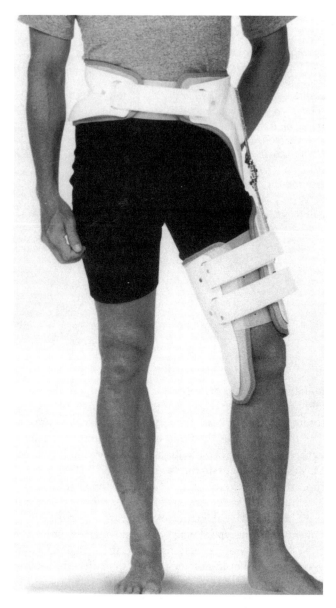

FIGURE 13-8
A postoperative hip abduction orthosis has three components. The proximal component is a padded pelvic band with a lateral extension and anterior closure that fits snugly around the upper pelvis. The distal component is a thigh cuff with a medial extension across the medial knee joint. These two pieces are connected by uprights and an adjustable hip joint, angled toward hip abduction and adjusted to limit hip flexion or extension. (Reprinted with permission from Orthomerica Newport. JPO 1995;7[1]:advertisement on front cover.)

ever the patient is out of bed and, in some instances, while the patient is in bed as well. The orthosis is usually worn for at least 8 weeks after total hip revision.

Clinical Concerns

Because lower extremity orthoses add weight to a lower extremity that is already compromised, orthotists must be sensitive to the selection of lightweight materials and components. This is especially true for older patients, who may have limited endurance because of cardiac or respiratory disease. Although the initial orthosis may restrict joint motion to provide external stability to a vulnerable hip joint, the orthotic hip, knee, and ankle joints

can be adjusted to meet the patient's needs as the rehabilitation program progresses. Hip orthoses and HKAFOs may be important adjuncts for rehabilitation in the following ways:

FIGURE 13-9
A postoperative custom-molded hip orthosis is sometimes used instead of a plaster hip spica cast when complete immobilization of the hip joint is required.

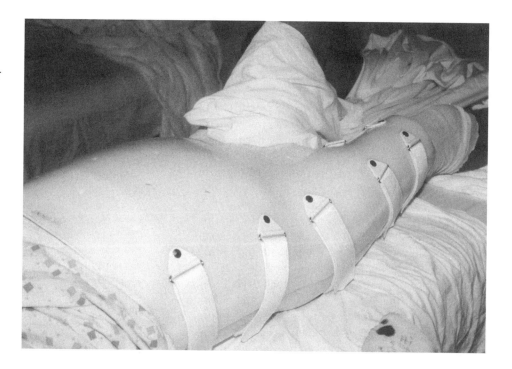

1. A well-fit hip orthosis provides protection against dislocation in patients who are predisposed to this problem.

2. Hip orthoses protect and support healing fracture sites, often allowing earlier mobility and gait training than would otherwise be possible.

3. Early and safe weight bearing for older patients with dislocation or fracture reduces the risk of secondary complications associated with prolonged bed rest or immobility.

4. The orthotic hip, knee, and ankle joints can be adjusted to restrict or permit motion to match the patient's specific needs at initial fitting and as the treatment program progresses.

Following surgical intervention after fracture or total joint arthroplasty, the focus of the rehabilitation program shifts to mobility training, strengthening, flexibility, and endurance. The decision to recommend a hip orthosis is very individual, influenced by the severity of the musculoskeletal problem, the patient's particular circumstances, and the experience and preferences of the health professionals involved in postoperative care. Few definitive guidelines or documentation are available concerning the efficacy of hip orthoses in the postoperative management of hip fracture or arthroplasty. An orthosis is best used to augment the goals of rehabilitation, including the return to preoperative ambulatory status, safe and protected weight bearing during activities of daily living, facilita-

tion of union of the fracture site, and ultimately return to presurgical social and self-care independence.

Hip Orthoses in Post-Trauma Care

The other group of patients who may benefit from hip orthoses are those who have experienced traumatic fractures of the femur, hip, or pelvis as a result of motor vehicle accidents, industrial accidents, or falls from great heights. Most of these patients are fit with their orthosis after stabilization of the fracture with internal fixation. The HKAFO is similar in design to the orthosis described for older patients after hip fracture or arthroplasty. Depending on the need for external support and stability, the hip joint can be locked to prevent flexion and extension or may allow motion within a limited range. For some patients, it may be necessary to incorporate a lumbosacral spinal orthosis to achieve the desired control of pelvic and hip motion. The ankle-foot orthosis component provides control of hip rotation in the transverse plane.

When complete immobilization is warranted after orthopedic trauma of the lower spine, pelvis, and hip, a custom-molded thermoplastic version of a hip spica cast can be fabricated (Figure 13-9). This hip orthosis has anterior and posterior components, extending from the mid- to lower thoracic trunk to just above the femoral condyles of the fractured extremity and to the groin of the intact extremity. This design provides maximum stability and can be used in lieu of or after casting. The position of the lower extremity within the orthosis is determined by the type and extent of the surgical repair. When the patient is lying in the supine position, the anterior component can be removed for skin inspection and personal care. Similarly, the posterior component can be removed when the patient is prone. This is an advantage for patients with open wounds or difficulty with continence and is especially appreciated if immobilization will be required for an extended period.

Many patients who are recovering from musculoskeletal trauma involving the pelvis and hip joint require physical therapy for gait and mobility training after surgery and an intensive rehabilitation program to regain preinjury muscle strength, range of motion, and functional status. It is important that the orthopedic surgeon and therapists, as well as the patient and family, clearly understand the advantages provided and the mobility limitations imposed by postsurgical hip orthoses. An optimal orthosis can facilitate rehabilitation if fabricated with lightweight but durable components that can be adjusted as the patient progresses, while meeting the individual patient's need for stability or supported mobility of the hip. An appropriate hip orthosis also enhances early mobility and protected weight bearing, reducing the risk of loss of function related to bed rest and deconditioning.

SUMMARY AND CONCLUSION

Hip orthoses are important in management of hip disorders in infants and children, as well as in the postsurgical care of children and adults. An understanding of the designs of and indications for the various hip orthoses is essential for physicians and rehabilitation professionals working with patients who have orthopedic problems of the pelvis, hip joint, or proximal femur. For children with DDH or Legg-Calvé-Perthes disease, hip orthoses are the primary intervention for prevention of future deformity and disability. Hip orthoses are essential elements of postoperative care and rehabilitation programs for children who have had surgical intervention for bony deformity or soft tissue contracture and for adults who have had repair of a traumatic injury or revision of a total hip arthroplasty. The efficacy of orthotic intervention is also influenced by patient and caregiver compliance: The key to successful use of these orthoses is clear and open communication between the physician, therapist, orthotist, and family concerning the primary goals of the orthosis, its proper application and wearing schedule, and the possible difficulties that may be encountered. Positive health care outcomes and happy patients and families are contingent on the ability of the health care team to communicate.

REFERENCES

1. Norkin CC, Levangie PK. The Hip Complex. In Joint Structure and Function: A Comprehensive Analysis (2nd ed). Philadelphia: Davis, 1992;300–336.
2. Steinberg ME (ed). The Hip and Its Disorders. Philadelphia: Saunders, 1991.
3. Ilfeld FW, Westin GW, Makin M. Missed or developmental dislocation of the hip. Clin Orthop 1986;Feb(203):276–281.
4. Mubarik SJ, Leach JL, Wenger DR. Management of congenital dislocation of the hip in the infant. Contemp Orthop 1987;15:29–44.
5. MacEwen GD, Ramsey PL. The Hip. In RB Winter, WW Lovell (eds), Lovell and Winter's Pediatric Orthopaedics (1st ed). Vol 2. Philadelpha: Lippincott, 1978;724.
6. Hesinger RN. Congenital dislocation of the hip; treatment in infancy to walking age. Orthop Clin North Am 1987;18(4):597–616.
7. Leach J. Orthopedic Conditions. In SK Campbell (ed), Physical Therapy for Children. Philadelphia: Saunders, 1995;353–382.
8. Walker JM. Musculoskeletal development: a review. Phys Ther 1991;71(12):878–889.
9. Pavlik A. The functional method of treatment using a harness with stirrups as the primary method of conservative therapy for infants with congenital dislocation of the hip. Clin Orthop 1992;Aug(281):4–10.
10. Wenger DR, Rang M. Developmental Dysplasia of the Hip. In DR Wenger, M Rang (eds), The Art and Practice of Children's Orthopaedics (1st ed). New York: Raven, 1993;272–280.
11. Legg AT. An obscure affection of the hip joint. Boston Med Surg J 1910;162–202.
12. Canale ST. Osteochondroses. In ST Canale, JH Beatty (eds), Operative Pediatric Orhtopedics. St. Louis: Mosby–Year Book, 1991;743–776.
13. Catterall A. The natural history of Perthes disease. J Bone Joint Surg 1971;53B(1):37–53.
14. Tachdjian MO. Pediatric Orthopedics (2nd ed). Philadelphia: Saunders, 1990.
15. Wenger DR, Ward WT, Herring JA. Current concepts review: Legg-Calvé-Perthes disease. J Bone Joint Surg 1991;73(5):778–788.
16. Herring JA. Current concepts review. The treatment of Legg-Calvé-Perthes disease; a critical review of the literature. J Bone Joint Surg 1994;76A(3):448–458.
17. Martinez AG, Weinstein SL, Deat FR. The weight bearing abduction brace for the treatment of Legg-Perthes disease. J Bone Joint Surg 1992;74A(1):12–21.
18. Meehan TL, Angel D, Nelson JM. The Scottish-Rite abduction orthosis for the treatment of Legg-Perthes disease. A radiographic analysis. J Bone Joint Surg 1992;74A(1):2–12.
19. Drennan JC. Orthopaedic Management of Neuromuscular Disorders (1st ed). Philadelphia: Lippincott, 1983;278.
20. Cummings SR, Rubin SM, Black D. The future of hip fractures in the United States: numbers, costs, and potential effects of postmenopausal estrogen. Clin Orthop 1991;March(252):163–166.
21. Lima D, Magnus R, Paprosky WG. Team management of hip revision using a post-op hip orthosis. JPO 1994;6(1):20–24.

14

Spinal Orthoses

Patrick Flanagan, Thomas M. Gavin, Donna Q. Gavin, and Avinash G. Patwardhan

Management of spinal dysfunction with an orthosis or brace is not new or unique to the twentieth century medical profession. In 1743, Nicholas Andry, a professor of medicine in Paris, suggested in his book, *Orthopaedia*,[1] the following strategy to straighten the spine in children:

> If the spine be crooked in the shape of an S, the best method you can take to mend it is to have recourse to the whale bone bodice, stuffed parts shall exactly answer to those protuberances which ought to be repressed, and these bodices must be renewed every three months at least.

Even earlier in history, in the second century, Galen (131–201 AD) first used the terms *scoliosis, lordosis,* and *kyphosis* and used dynamic bracing and an exercise program to treat spinal deformity. The evidence from prehistoric bone findings is that humans began to use splints for weak limbs and broken bones as early as 9000 BC in the Paleolithic age. Crude lumbar supports constructed from tree bark have been recovered from the cliff dwellings of the pre-Columbian Indians.[2] The use of mechanical devices to treat pathologic conditions of the spine has a long and rich history.

The principles of current orthotic treatment for spinal deformities can be traced to the development of the Milwaukee brace by Drs. Blount and Schmidt in the late 1940s.[3] The Milwaukee brace was initially developed as a postoperative alternative to plaster of Paris casts after corrective surgery for patients with scoliosis. Soon afterward, the Milwaukee brace began to be used as the primary therapy in conservative nonoperative management of scoliosis.[4] Biomechanical analysis of this orthosis in the 1970s led to a better understanding of the mechanisms of action and of the primary and secondary functions of spinal orthoses.[5] The information gained from the early versions of the Milwaukee brace, and the development of

new thermoplastic materials, led to the design of shorter profile orthoses that are able to stabilize the spine without the cervical components of the Milwaukee brace.

The efficacy of spinal orthoses in the management of spinal dysfunction has been the focus of many recent research efforts. The effectiveness of orthotic intervention for spinal deformity or fracture has been supported, whereas the evidence for the role of orthotic intervention in the management of low back pain or postoperative protection of spinal implants is less clear.

NOMENCLATURE OF SPINAL ORTHOSES

Since the appearance of the Milwaukee brace in the late 1940s, many different types of spinal orthoses have been developed, each to manage a particular spinal pathology. Most were named for the orthotist or physician who first designed the orthosis or the city where it was developed. The lack of consistency in naming orthoses led to much confusion in describing their actual function. In 1973, the American Academy of Orthopaedic Surgeons charged a commission of practitioners to develop standardized orthotic terminology. Spinal orthoses are named by the regions of the thorax and back that are encompassed by the orthosis (Table 14-1).

A variety of orthotic designs are available in each of the categories of spinal orthoses. Common to all designs, regardless of name or appearance, are three basic functions. Spinal orthoses are designed to do one or more of the following:

1. Immobilize gross spinal motions (limit motion of the torso in all degrees of freedom)
2. Immobilize individual motion segments (reduce range of motion of an intervertebral segment)

TABLE 14-1
Nomenclature for Spinal Orthoses

SIO	*Sacroiliac orthoses* encompass the sacral and iliac regions of the lower spine and pelvis.
LSO	*Lumbosacral orthoses* encompass the lumbar and sacral regions of the lower spine.
TLSO	*Thoracolumbosacral orthoses* encompass the thoracic (ribs), lumbar, and sacral regions of the spine.
CTLSO	*Cervicothoracolumbosacral orthoses* encompass the cervical (neck), thoracic, lumbar, and sacral regions of the spine.
CO	*Cervical orthoses* encompass the cervical spine region.
CTO	*Cervicothoracic orthoses* encompass the cervical and thoracic regions of the spine.

3. Apply external forces to correct deformity or to prevent progression of deformity

A spinal orthosis can be designed to control gross movement of the trunk and intersegmental motion of the vertebrae in one or more of the three planes of motion: lateral flexion (side bending) in the coronal/frontal plane, flexion (forward bending) or extension (backward bending) in the sagittal plane, and axial rotation (twisting) in the transverse plane.

Health professionals caring for patients who require a spinal orthosis must understand the function of the orthosis and the planes of motion that are being controlled and incorporate these orthotic goals into the rehabilitation process. Successful orthotic treatment for spinal deformity, for traumatic injury of the spine, for low back pain, and for postoperative protection mandates a thorough knowledge of the orthosis' biomechanical mechanisms of action. Success also depends on sound clinical procedure for fabrication and fitting, adequate follow-up, effective patient instruction, and physical therapy as an adjunct to the orthosis.

An orthosis can be worn for one or more of the following reasons: to provide support to the abdomen and spine, to control motion of the trunk, and to manage pain. Trunk support is indicated when patients have weakened spinal or abdominal musculature that results in acute back pain or the likelihood of deformity. Motion control is necessary when stability after spinal fracture or surgery would be compromised or when other pathology would be aggravated by motion. When functional capabilities are impeded by spinal pain, an orthosis can be tried to reduce the intensity of the pain.[6-11] In this chapter we explore the role of spinal orthoses in the management of low back pain, after traumatic vertebral injury and fracture, and in the nonsurgical and the postoperative care of patients with spinal deformity or instability. We consider the indications for specific spinal orthotic designs, their biomechanical mechanisms of action, their technical parameters, and their intended treatment outcomes.

ORTHOTICS IN THE TREATMENT OF LOW BACK PAIN

The prevalence of low back pain in the United States is extremely high: 80% of the population will experience significant low back pain at some time in their lives.[12] The primary goal of an orthosis in the management of low back pain is to decrease pain: Most designs accomplish this by (1) limiting motion of the lumbar spine and by (2) providing greater abdominal support. Optimal lumbar posture has been identified as an important contributor to reduction of pain.[6,13] An orthosis that supports the lumbar spine in optimal posture may be an effective conservative treatment modality for low back pain. A wide variety of orthotic designs are used to meet this goal, ranging from lumbosacral (LS) corsets to rigid thermoplastic thoracolumbosacral orthoses (TLSOs).

Lumbosacral Corsets

The LS corset is the most frequently prescribed supporting orthosis for patients with low back pain (Figure 14-1). Corsets are made from soft canvas or Dacron materials, fortified with rigid and flexible stays. These stays can be contoured to accommodate a deformity or can be straight to encourage postural correction. When donned properly, the LS corset can effectively limit much, but not all, motion of the lumbar spine; it cannot, however, achieve the same degree of gross and segmental immobilization of the spine as a rigid TLSO.[14]

LS corsets encompass the abdomen and the pelvis. In exerting circumferential pressure, they increase intracavitary pressure in the abdomen and transmit a three-point pressure system to the lumbar spine. Typically, the anterior borders of the LS corset are superior to the symphysis pubis and inferior to the xiphoid process. The posterior borders extend between the sacrococcygeal junction of the pelvis and the inferior angle of the scapulae.

Fabric LS corsets, sacroiliac orthoses, and thoracolumbar (dorsolumbar) corsets primarily function to reduce overall gross trunk motion. A snugly fit nonelastic LS or thoracolumbar corset compresses fluid and tissues of the abdomen and abdominal cavity, theoretically reducing axial loading of vertebral bodies. Pain that results from muscle strain is effectively managed with a corset because the activity of spinal and abdominal muscles is reduced while the corset is being worn. It is important to note that long-term corset use can lead to muscle atrophy, ultimately increasing the chance of reinjury. For this reason, corsets are best used only during the acute phase of back pain.

LS corsets are most often used to manage acute low back pain; their efficacy in chronic low back pain is questionable. Corsets are designed to support the trunk in lumbar extension, as this position seems to be effective in reducing the pain that results from bulging or herniation of lumbar disks above the level of the L5–S1 junction. For disk-related pain at the level of L5–S1, other interventions are more effective. A bay cast spica was shown to provide nearly complete symptomatic relief of discogenic pain at the L5–S1 junction.[6] Patients with low back or leg pain secondary to spondylolysis or spondylolisthesis often have better pain relief with a TLSO fitted in lumbar flexion.[7]

Willner's Instruments for Spinal Stabilization

An important study reported by Willner[8] found that a rigid orthosis prescribed randomly and independently of diagnosis for patients with chronic low back pain was effective only approximately 50% of the time. In a subsequent study Willner[15] predicted the likelihood that a rigid orthosis would be a successful intervention for low back pain with reasonable accuracy based on pain relief provided by a testing orthosis that stabilized the spine. Based on his findings, a program for management of chronic low back pain with Willner's instrument for spinal stabilization (WISS) test orthosis has been developed.[6,15] The WISS is an adjustable TLSO that can either extend or flex the lumbar spine, based on the initial setting of the posterior pad in extension, neutral, or flexion. The anterior panel is also adjustable and provides abdominal support while helping to keep the orthosis in place.

Gavin et al.[6] conducted a prospective study to determine whether a 5-day trial wearing of the WISS would predict the outcome of orthotic treatment for chronic low back pain. Patients enrolled in the study had back pain for at least 6 months that had not been relieved by conventional treatment. Patients were fit with the WISS and wore the device for a 5-day trial. For patients with disk herniation, multiple level disk bulging, degenerative disk disease (excluding those with L5–S1 pathologies), the WISS was set at maximum lumbar extension. For those with lumbar instability spondylolisthesis, lumbar stenosis, or facet syndrome, the WISS was set in maximum lumbar flexion. Preliminary results suggest that patients with long-standing low back pain that was unrelieved by conventional treatment obtain pain relief by orthotic treatment when prescribed after a successful 5-day trial with the WISS orthosis.

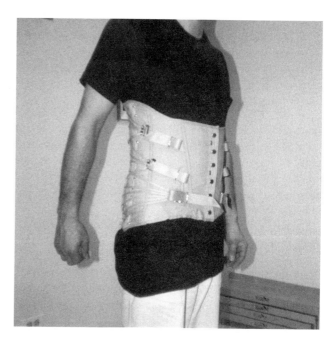

FIGURE 14-1

Lumbosacral corsets are used for patients with acute low back pain. Made from soft canvas, the anterior openings are secured with Velcro, hook-and-eyelet, or zipper closures. The corset has stays of various stiffnesses that are sewn in to support the trunk. Most also have a mechanism to tighten the corset to fit snugly to the patient's trunk. A lumbosacral corset limits motion of the lumbar spine and provides external support for the abdomen.

Pelvic Position in Lumbosacral Muscle Strain versus Disk Herniation

Reduction of lumbar lordosis has been recommended in the management of back pain that results from LS muscle strain.[8,9,16,17] Reduction in lumbar lordosis combined with increased intra-abdominal cavitary pressure can relieve pain caused by LS muscle strain. Theoretically, the flexed spine allows vertical transmission of the body weight through the vertebra and reduces the necessity for muscle activity. Patients with disk herniation may be more comfortable with orthoses that maintain or increase LS lordosis.[6] An orthosis that increases lordosis can, theoretically, facilitate the opening of intervertebral spaces and the closing of facet joints. This postural alteration is helpful for pathologies such as herniation of the nucleus pulposa.[18] Most orthotists recommend that spinal orthoses be fabricated in the posture that most effectively reduces pain or best accommodates a rigid deformity. It is important to note that, although all LS spinal orthoses reduce gross trunk motion, not all are equally effective in reducing intersegmental motion of the vertebral column.[14,19-26] Motion reduction of gross overall trunk motion and of intersegmental motion is necessary as the primary mechanism for effective pain management and for postoperative immobilization and fracture healing.[6,27]

Sacroiliac and Thoracolumbar Corsets

Sacroiliac corsets are meant to support only the sacroiliac joint. With end points inferior to the waist and superior to the pubis, these garments encompass the pelvis but not the lower trunk. Sacroiliac corsets increase in abdominal circumferential pressure only slightly and are best used for patients with mild sacroiliac dysfunction. Because they are so narrow, sacroiliac corsets do not provide significant support to the spine.

Because the thoracolumbar (dorsolumbar) corset encompasses much of the thoracic spine, leverage of the corset system is increased to control motion and to support the trunk. The inferior borders of a thoracolumbar corset are the same as those of an LS corset. The superior posterior border terminates just inferior to the scapular spine. Shoulder straps create a posteriorly directed force aimed at facilitating extension of the thoracic spine. Although the thoracolumbar corset encloses much of the thoracic spine, its leverage is insufficient to prevent thoracic spinal motion. The corset serves primarily as a kinesthetic reminder to control such motion. Thus, thoracolumbar corsets provide trunk support but do not significantly control intersegmental motion.

TRADITIONAL SPINAL ORTHOSES

Traditional metal and leather spinal orthoses provide motion control and trunk support because they are custom fabricated to fit specific anatomic landmarks so that the orthoses have the best possible leverage against the trunk. Most designs for traditional spinal orthoses have a pelvic and a thoracic band and a set of lateral and/or paraspinal bars. These bands and bars are made from radiolucent aluminum alloys that are malleable yet stiff enough to hold their shape.

The *pelvic band* is fit closely at the posterior midline, with its inferior edge against the sacrococcygeal junction. The band is contoured or curved downward to contain the gluteal muscles on either side of the midline and to create the maximum possible leverage for control of the pelvis. The pelvic band wraps around the pelvis laterally, terminating just anterior to the midaxillary trochanteric line (MATL). A design variation proposed by Norton and Brown[23] has inferior projections from the lateral bars, terminating in disks over the trochanters, in an effort to improve motion control at the LS junction.[3] A strap that fastens in the front connects to these disks to achieve additional leverage in the sagittal plane. The position of the disks also improves leverage for control of motion in the coronal plane.

The upper edge of the *thoracic band* is usually placed 24 mm below the inferior angle of the scapulae. The thoracic band is high and horizontal at the posterior midline and curves inferolaterally to provide relief for the scapulae. The thoracic band also wraps around the trunk laterally, ending just in front of the MATL at the lateral midline of the body.

When an orthotic design includes *paraspinal bars*, they are placed on either side of the posterior midline over the paraspinal muscle mass. Paraspinal bars on LS orthoses (LSOs) are vertical, spanning from the pelvic band to the thoracic band. For traditional TLSOs, the paraspinal bars end just inferior to the spine of the scapulae. If the orthosis has *lateral bars*, they are placed at the lateral midline of the trunk, following the MATL from the inferior edge of the pelvic band to the superior edge of the thoracic band. If the orthosis has an interscapular band, it is positioned within the lateral borders of the scapulae, with a bottom edge placed just above the inferior border of the scapulae.

Most traditional metal and leather spinal orthoses have a corset front or anterior panel that is closed by laces, buckles, or Velcro straps. The anterior panel, if fastened correctly, increases abdominal intracavitary pressure in the same way that LS corsets do.

Sagittal Control Lumbosacral Orthoses: The Chairback Orthosis

A spinal orthosis that is designed to control motion in the sagittal plane is the chairback LSO, which has a thoracic and pelvic band connected by two paraspinal bars. A full-trunk corset is attached to the paraspinal bars. This orthosis is prescribed when the patient's condition requires reduction of gross and intersegmental flexion and extension motion of the trunk. Motion into forward trunk flexion is limited by a pair of posterior-directed forces applied by the anterior corset, one at the xiphoid level and the other at the pubis. These forces oppose a single anterior-directed force applied at the midpoint of the paraspinal bars. The force system for restriction of extension has two anterior-directed forces applied across the thoracic and pelvic bands that oppose a posterior-directed force applied at the midpoint of the corset panel. Increased intercavitary pressure can act to unload the spine and its disks by transmitting load onto soft tissue of the trunk. This orthosis is used primarily for pain management and as a kinesthetic reminder to limit motion for patients with low back pain. The orthosis does not limit motion enough to stabilize the trunk for patients with spinal fractures.[28] The chairback design can be made as a TLSO by increasing the proximal length of the paraspinal bars and by the addition of shoulder straps.

Sagittal-Coronal Control Lumbosacral Orthoses: The Knight Orthosis

When a pair of lateral bars is added to the orthosis, control of spinal motion is possible in the coronal (frontal) as well as the sagittal plane. This orthosis, also known as a *Knight spinal orthosis,* has thoracic and pelvic bands connected by a set of paraspinal bars and a set of lateral bars, with an anterior half-corset closure (Figure 14-2). Control of flexion/extension is achieved by the same three-point force systems described for the chairback LSO. Lateral flexion of the trunk is controlled by medially directed forces at the edges of thoracic and pelvic bands, opposing a force at the midpoint of the opposite lateral bar. This orthosis was originally designed for patients with tuberculosis of the spine but is now used primarily in the management of low back pain.[28] It is sometimes prescribed for patients with stable noncompression fractures of the lumbar spine; however, this orthosis does not sufficiently control the pelvis or thorax when compression fractures or complex spinal injuries require more complete limitation of motion or total immobilization.[29] The Knight orthosis can also be fabricated as a TLSO if more support of the thoracic spine is necessary.

Extension-Coronal Control Lumbosacral Orthoses: The Williams Orthosis

The Williams LSO is a dynamic orthosis that has a thoracic and a pelvic band, a pair of lateral bars, and a set of oblique bars positioned between the lateral bars and pelvic band. The attachments between the thoracic band and lateral bars are mobile; structural integrity is achieved by the firmly attached oblique bars. The articulation between the thoracic band and lateral bars allows the patient to move into some trunk flexion in the sagittal plane. The nonarticulating connections between lateral bars and pelvic band, reinforced by the oblique bars and a snugly fit, inelastic pelvic strap, limits trunk extension. The Williams LSO was originally designed as a treatment for spondylolisthesis[30] and continues to be used in its management today.[31,32] Although flexion orthoses have been used for patients with lumbar disk herniation in the past, recent work suggests that lordosis (lumbar extension) is more comfortable for patients and physiologically appropriate for reduction of herniation, so that flexion orthoses are not suitable for this population.[8]

Flexion Control Thoracolumbosacral Orthoses: The Jewitt and Cash Orthoses

When compression fracture of the lumbar or low thoracic spine has occurred, it is very important to limit trunk flexion during the healing process. Two orthoses

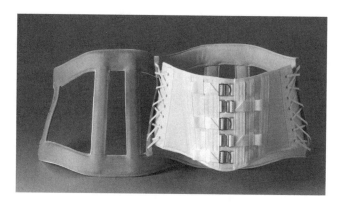

FIGURE 14-2

When a pair of lateral bars is added to a chairback orthosis, control of lateral flexion becomes possible. This Knight spinal orthosis is used when limitation of sagittal and coronal plane motion is required. (Courtesy of J. A. Sankey, C.P.O., Central Brace Co., Hickory Hills, IL.)

that are designed specifically to limit flexion while encouraging trunk hyperextension are the Jewitt TLSO flexion control orthosis and the Cash hyperextension orthosis (Figure 14-3). Both of these orthoses are available in various styles and sizes from a number of manufacturers. The Jewett orthosis has an anterolateral aluminum frame with pads at the pubis, sternum, and lateral midline of the trunk and a posterior lumbar pad. Trunk flexion is limited by a single three-point pressure system, with posterior-directed forces applied at the sternum and the pubis, which oppose an anterior-directed force applied by the posterior lumbar pad. When the orthosis is well fitting, this force system prevents flexion of the spine but allows active hyperextension. The Cash orthosis (cruciform anterior hyperextension orthosis) has an adjustable-length anterior cross with sternal and pelvic pads at the ends of the vertical bar as well as lateral pads and a posterior belt. The Cash orthosis uses the same three-point pressure system to control trunk flexion as the Jewett design.

Sagittal Control Thoracolumbosacral Orthoses: The Taylor Orthosis

The Taylor orthosis has a pelvic band, two paraspinal bars, an interscapular band, and a pair of axillary straps. The orthosis is designed to limit flexion and extension of the thoracic and lumbar spine. An anterior-directed force is applied at the interscapular band to resist extension. The axillary straps apply posterior-directed forces, which function to limit trunk flexion.

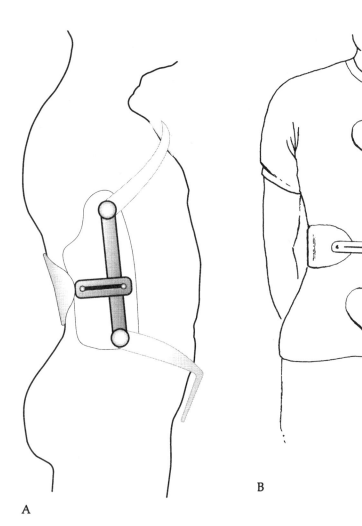

A

B

Sagittal-Coronal Control Thoracolumbosacral Orthoses: The Knight-Taylor Orthosis

The sagittal-coronal control TLSO is a hybrid of the Knight LSO and the Taylor TLSO, which has a pelvic and a thoracic band, lateral bars, paraspinal bars that reach the spine of the scapula, an interscapular band, and a pair of axillary straps. With this combination of components, the orthosis resists extension, flexion, and lateral flexion of the thoracic and lumbar spines.

Thoracolumbosacral Orthoses with Triplanar Control: The Subclavicular Orthosis

The components of the subclavicular orthosis include the traditional pelvic band, sidebars, paraspinal bars, and

thoracic band. What makes this design unique is a set of subclavicular extensions that wrap upward around the anterior of the trunk from the thoracic band (hence its description as a "cowhorn" orthosis). With the addition of these subclavicular extensions, this orthosis is able to limit trunk rotation (motion in the transverse plane) in addition to flexion/extension (sagittal plane motion) and lateral flexion (coronal/frontal plane motion). As rotation to the right is attempted, for example, counterforces that limit that direction of motion are applied by the left subclavicular extension and the right sides of the thoracic and pelvic bands. This orthosis is a metal alternative to a custom-molded thermoplastic "body jacket" TLSO for low thoracic and lumbar injuries. Other conventional metal TLSOs that attempt to provide triplanar control are Arnold, Magnusen, and Steindler custom designs.

THERMOPLASTIC SPINAL ORTHOSES

Molded thermoplastic orthoses that encase the trunk are prescribed when the therapeutic goal is immobilization of the spine in all three planes of motion. These orthoses are indicated when instability or dysfunction is present at several vertebral levels or for patients with significant instability after a burst vertebral fracture. They are often used in the postoperative care of patients with traumatic vertebral fracture or spinal cord injuries, and patients with spinal deformity who have had fusion or instrumented surgeries at the thoracolumbar level. Rigid thermoplastic spinal orthoses may be necessary for patients whose size, shape, or condition precludes the use of a traditional LSO or TLSO. Some rigid thermoplastic spinal orthoses are custom fit from prefabricated blanks; others are custom molded over a positive model of the patient's trunk. Many are made from perforated materials to release body heat that is generated during activity. Some are lined with closed cell foam to increase patient comfort and to minimize the risk of pressure-related skin problems. Most patients wear a lightweight T-shirt under the orthosis, to wick perspiration away from the skin and to minimize friction and the potential for skin irritation. Typically, the superior trimlines of LSO are at the level of the xiphoid process; the superior trimline of a TLSO extends upward to the notch of the sternum. Thermoplastic LSOs and TLSOs are carefully shaped to envelop the pelvis; most have an anteroinferior trimline at the groin.

Raney Flexion Lumbosacral Orthoses

The custom-fit or molded Raney flexion LSO is the thermoplastic version of the traditional Williams flexion orthosis (Figure 14-4). Because it encases the pelvis entirely, the Raney is better able to hold the LS spine in a flexed position (posterior tilt) during activity than is its traditional counterpart. The major difference between these two devices is that, although the dynamic design of the Williams LSO allows flexion while preventing extension, the Raney jacket is rigid, holding the pelvis in a static position. More abdominal compression occurs with the semirigid plastic anterior shell of the Raney jacket than is possible with the flexible anterior corset of the Williams LSO. The Raney orthosis is often used in the management of spinal instability and pain in patients with spondylosis and spondylolisthesis.

Boston Overlap Braces

For patients who require immobilization in a neutral pelvic position or in lordosis (lumbar extension), the Boston overlap brace (BOB) is often prescribed. Prefabricated shells are custom fit to meet the patient's individual positioning

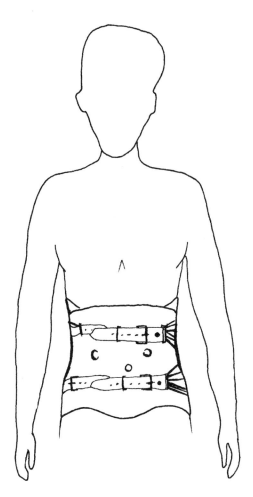

FIGURE 14-4
Custom-fit Raney flexion orthosis.

needs. The posterior shell encloses the trunk from the inferior angle of the scapula to the sacrococcygeal level and the anterior shell from the xiphoid process of the sternum to the pubis. These trimlines ensure that the BOB effectively controls motion in the sagittal and coronal planes. The BOB is often used for patients with stable, nondisplaced fractures of the mid and lower lumbar spine, spondylolysis, or spondylolisthesis. Patients with fractures of L1 and L2 are better managed with a molded TLSO.

Molded Thoracolumbosacral Orthoses: Body Jackets

Molded TLSOs are most commonly used in the postsurgical management of patients with fracture or spinal deformity of the thoracic and upper lumbar spine. The total contact design maintains spinal alignment and limits movement of the trunk in all three planes of motion (Figure

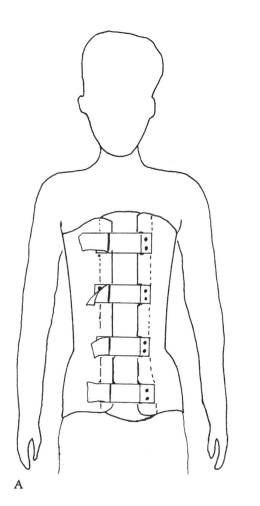

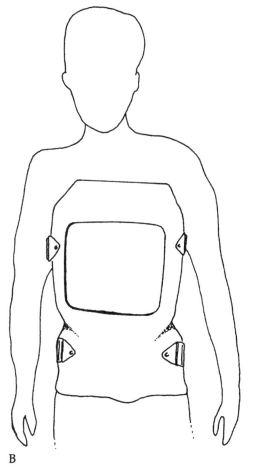

A   B

FIGURE 14-5
*Molded thoracolum-
bosacral orthoses (body
jackets) use a total con-
tact design to control flex-
ion/extension in the sagittal
plane, lateral flexion/side
bending in the frontal
plane, and trunk rotation in
the transverse plane. They
can be fabricated as a single
unit (A) with an anterior
opening or in a bivalve
design (B) with an anterior
and a posterior shell and
lateral closures.*

14-5). The orthosis can be fabricated as a single piece with an anterior opening or in a bivalve design with an anterior and a posterior shell. In both versions, the superior anterior trimline of the orthosis is just below the clavicle. Shoulder flanges or extensions can be added to enhance motion control of the spine as patients use the upper extremities during daily activities. The superior posterior trimline falls just below the spine of the scapula. The anteroinferior edge of the orthosis is trimmed at the distal pubis and arches slightly upward laterally to accommodate the thigh in sitting. The inferior edge of the posterior shell is trimmed low at the sacrococcygeal junction.

If a patient has upper thoracic instability or significant thoracic kyphosis, it is often necessary to add a cervical component, such as a sterno-occipito-mandibular immobilizer (SOMI), four-poster, or C. D. Denison cervical orthosis (C. D. Dennison Orthopaedic Appliance Co., Baltimore, MD), to the TLSO to achieve the desired control of motion. Similarly, if the goal of orthotic intervention is immobilization at the LS junction, the body jacket LSO

or TLSO must be extended, via an orthotic hip joint and thigh cuff, to limit the pelvic motion that normally accompanies extension of the hip.

ORTHOTICS IN SPINAL DEFORMITY: SCOLIOSIS

Scoliosis, also known as *curvature of the spine*, is a three-dimensional, progressive deformity of the spine. The Milwaukee brace, a cervicothoracolumbosacral orthosis (CTLSO) with a snugly fit pelvic component, anterior and paraspinal bars, corrective pads, and neck ring, was developed in the 1950s as a nonoperative intervention in an attempt to prevent progression of the curve for patients who had not yet reached skeletal maturity. In recent years, low-profile TLSO designs (e.g., the Boston, Miami, Rosenberger, Lyon, Wilmington, and Charleston orthoses), more cosmetic without a cervical ring, have supplanted the Milwaukee brace in the nonoperative management of scoliosis (see Figure 15-2). Scoliosis can be classified into three etiologic categories. *Idiopathic scoliosis* (etiology unknown) is by far the most common. *Neuromuscular* ("paralytic") *scoliosis* is the result of muscular imbalance secondary to a neuromuscular disease. *Congenital scoliosis* occurs when a congenital anomaly or malformation of the spine has occurred.

For curves that are detected during childhood, the risk of rapid progression of the curve during the adolescent growth spurt is very high.[33] The risk of curve progression is inversely related to age: the younger the child at the time of diagnosis, the greater the progression because of the longer period of growth remaining. The magnitude is also related to the risk of progression: the larger the curve at diagnosis, the greater the likelihood of curve progression. Prospective studies suggest that curve progression will occur in children diagnosed before the age of 10 with curves of 20 degrees or more; the incidence of curve progression in children with curves of less than 20 degrees is 50%.[34]

Biomechanical mathematical models aid our understanding of the risk of progression of spinal curvatures, their patterns of instability, and how an orthosis may be able to stabilize the curve. Curve progression has been explained using Euler's theory of elastic buckling of a slender column.[35] A slender column (spine) that is fixed at the base (pelvis) and subject to a normal biological axial compressive force (gravity + weight of head and upper torso) will buckle when this force reaches a certain magnitude (Figure 14-6). The magnitude of load that leads to buckling (critical load) depends on the flexibility, length, and end support conditions of the column (spine). This model assumes an elastic column, such that the load at

buckling will not vary as the magnitude of the curve increases, that the column will suddenly collapse when this buckling load is reached, and that it will return to its original state in the absence of axial load.

The curve progressions of scoliosis are not well explained by this model, however. Curve progression is a slow plastic deformation that occurs even in the absence of axial loading. The axial load that is required to cause this permanent increase in the initial spine curvature is termed the *critical load* of the column.[36] As the curve magnitude of the spine increases, its ability to carry a load without further deformation decreases as the magnitude of critical load decreases. When curves are greater than 60 degrees, the load carrying ability of the spine is critically and severely compromised.

Biomechanics of Action

Orthoses that are designed for management of scoliosis use three principles (end-point control, transverse loading, and curve correction) to prevent curve progression and to stabilize the spine. *End-point control* is the fixation that occurs as a result of the mechanical constraints of the orthosis as it is worn on the trunk. In low-profile TLSO scoliosis designs and in the Milwaukee brace CTLSO, the pelvic interface fixes the orthosis rigidly to the base of the spine. In a Milwaukee brace, the neck ring attempts to fix the head and neck over the center of the pelvis. End-point control substantially improves the stability of the spine, increasing the critical load that it is able to support without further deformation.

FIGURE 14-6
Patterns of elastic buckling (carrying capacity) of a straight column when one end is fixed and the other is free (A), one end is fixed and the other is pinned (B), and both ends are fixed (C). P = buckling load of a slender elastic column of uniform material properties and cross sectional geometry. (Reprinted with permission from TM Gavin, AG Patwardhan, WH Bunch. Principles and Components of Spinal Orthosis. In B Goldberg, JD Hsu [eds], Atlas of Orthoses and Assistive Devices. St. Louis: Mosby, 1997.)

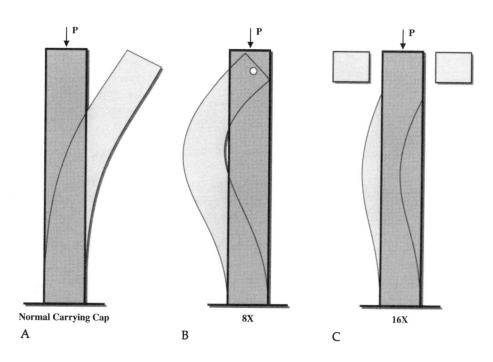

Normal Carrying Cap

A

8X

B

16X

C

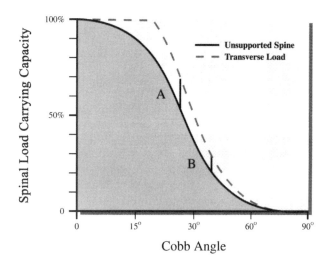

FIGURE 14-7

All scoliosis orthoses provide some form of a transversely directed load to the curvature of the spine. (A) indicates that the transverse support of a 25–30 degree curve by a brace raises the critical load-bearing capacity of the spine from approximately 50% of normal to 70% of normal. With increasing curvature, the effect of transverse support is less. (B) indicates that a curve of 45 degrees only has its critical load increased from 20% of normal to 30% of normal, which may not be adequate for prevention of curve progression. (Reprinted with permission from TM Gavin, AG Patwardhan, TM Bunch. Principles and Components of Spinal Orthosis. In B Goldberg, JD Hsu [eds], Atlas of Orthoses and Assistive Devices. St. Louis: Mosby, 1997.)

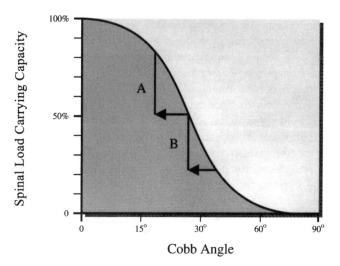

FIGURE 14-8

Curve correction in the orthosis has the greatest effect on the critical load capacity of the spine. (A) indicates that reducing a curve of 30 degrees to 20 degrees in an orthosis increases the stability of the curve from 50% to 80%. (B) indicates reducing a 45 degree curve down to 30 degrees increases the critical load from 20% to 50% of normal. (Reprinted with permission from TM Gavin, AG Patwardhan, WH Bunch. Principles and Components of Spinal Orthosis. In B Goldberg, JD Hsu [eds], Atlas of Orthoses and Assistive Devices. St. Louis: Mosby, 1997.)

Transverse loading applied at the apex of the curve also increases the critical load of the spine (Figure 14-7). For curves of less than 25 degrees, application of a nontranslatory transverse support raises the critical load from 50% to 70% of normal; this increase may be enough to prevent further curve progression. In curves of 45 degrees, although application of transverse support raises critical load from 20% to 30% of normal, this is not sufficient for prevention of progression even in an orthosis.

Correction of the curve increases critical load beyond the level provided by transverse support (Figure 14-8). When an initial curve of 45 degrees is reduced to a corrected curve of 30 degrees, the load-carrying capacity of the spine is increased from 20% to 50% of normal capacity. The larger the initial curve, the greater the need to reduce its magnitude by curve correction if the goal of preventing curve progression is to be met. The combination of endpoint control, application of transverse loading, and curve correction enhances the orthosis' ability to stabilize the scoliotic spine and prevent further curve progression.

Successful outcomes of orthotic intervention vary somewhat by the etiology or category of scoliosis. For patients with idiopathic scoliosis, an orthosis may prevent curve progression enough that surgery becomes unnecessary. For patients with neuromuscular scoliosis, a successful orthotic program provides stability for function in sitting and may delay the need for spinal fusion. For patients with congenital curves, the orthosis helps to control development of compensatory curves but cannot correct the congenital anomaly itself. For those with congenital scoliosis, another important orthotic goal is the reduction of spinal decompensation, so that the vertebra at T1 is centered over the sacrum in the coronal plane.

Orthotic Options for Patients with Scoliosis

The effectiveness of the Milwaukee brace as an orthotic intervention for spinal deformities in children is well documented.[4,37–40] The biomechanical effectiveness of the more cosmetic, "underarm" TLSOs, often prescribed by subjective preference of the practitioner, patient, and family, is not as well supported. In some cases, a CTLSO may provide more stability to curvature than the TLSO. In a biomechanical comparison of mechanical stabilization provided by the Milwaukee CTLSO and low-profile TLSO as interventions for idiopathic scoliosis, Patwardhan et al.[41] found that both designs were effective in stabilizing lumbar primary curves but that the TLSO was 25% less effective in stabilizing primary thoracic curves. Their findings also highlight the importance of proper pad placement and placement of counterforce and trimlines. In a primary thoracic curve with an upper end point at T5, for example, maximum spinal stability and curve correction are achieved with the trimline/counterforce at T5–6 and a pad at the apex (most laterally displaced, nontilted vertebrae or disk space) of the thoracic curve. If the trimline is below the T5–6 end point, the orthosis is less able to correct the curve, and spinal stability decreases as much as 20% for each vertebral level below the end point that the trimline falls. Misplacement of the apical pad, both above and below the apex of the thoracic curve, also results in loss of stability. Misplacement of pad location and counterforce/trimlines has similar effects when the primary curve is in the lumbar spine. These results underscore the sensitivity of the curve to pad height placement and suggest that frequent clinical adjustments of pad placement are necessary as the child grows.

Outcome differences have been reported when different styles of low-profile orthoses for scoliosis are compared. In a comparison of the Boston TLSO (see Figure 15-2) and the Charleston bending TLSO (Figure 14-9), both orthoses were successful in prevention of curve progression and spinal surgery for patients with single curves of less than 35 degrees, but the Boston TLSO was more effective in managing curves between 36 and 45 degrees or if multiple curves were present.[42] The Charleston TLSO is designed to unbend the curve and is worn overnight while the patient is sleeping, whereas the Boston TLSO is worn full time for 18–23 hours. Although acceptable outcomes have been reported for both orthotic designs, more research is needed to provide clinical guidelines to match type and magnitude of curve to the appropriate orthosis.[43,44] Development of an accurate measurement for patient compliance is also needed, to develop guidelines for optimal wearing time.

There is some evidence that holding the curve as is may not be sufficient to prevent surgery, especially when magnitude of the curve is large. Greater correction of the curve in the orthosis appears to be needed if the spine is to approach nearly normal critical load bearing such that curve progression is minimized and surgery is avoided.[39,41] In a study aimed at identifying accurate prognostic indicators for final outcome of orthotic intervention, reduction of the Cobb angle (degree of curvature) and vertebral rotation on radiography 1–2 months after initial brace wear was necessary for a good nonsurgical outcome when brace wear was discontinued at skeletal maturity.[45]

ORTHOTIC INTERVENTION FOR SPINAL DEFORMITY: KYPHOSIS

Kyphosis, a hyperflexion of the spine (round back), can be the result of neuromuscular impairment, congenital anom-

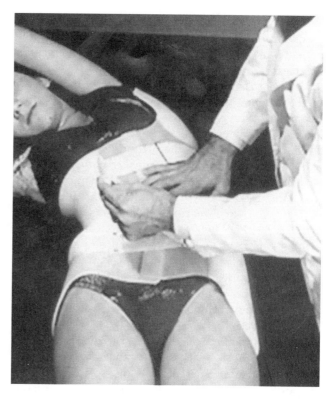

FIGURE 14-9
The Charleston bending brace applies corrective forces to unbend the scoliotic curve while the patient sleeps. End-point stabilization occurs at the pelvis, and transverse loading combined with curve correction realigns the spine to minimize the primary curve. (Reprinted with permission from TM Gavin, AG Patwardhan, WH Bunch. Principles and Components of Spinal Orthosis. In B Goldberg, JD Hsu [eds], Atlas of Orthoses and Assistive Devices. St. Louis: Mosby, 1997.)

alies, or degenerative changes in the spine, such as Scheuermann's disease. In Scheuermann's disease, osteochondrosis of the thoracic spine occurs as a result of a disturbance in the anterior epiphyseal growth plates, which leads to anterior wedging of one to three consecutive vertebrae and a kyphotic curve (measured by the Cobb method) of 45 degrees or more. Orthotic intervention is more successful in managing kyphosis that results from Scheuermann's disease than that caused by other etiologies.

The Milwaukee orthosis for kyphosis is most often prescribed when the apex of the kyphotic curve is above the T8 vertebra. In the orthosis, a three-point triangulation of force "opens" the vertebrae that have become wedged to allow bony remodeling. Because the anterior-directed force applied by the kyphosis pads is high, patients have a tendency to lean on the throat mold in an effort to be comfortable. Patients whose kyphosis is being managed by the Milwaukee brace benefit tremendously from a physical therapy exercise program that emphasizes thoracic hypertension and posterior lumbar tilt. This type of exercise program improves posture within the brace and assists the patient in developing an active muscle-generated counterforce that opposes the kyphosis pads. Low-profile TLSOs are prescribed when the apex of the kyphotic curve is below the T8 vertebra. In lower curves, the sternum can be used as a point of force application so that the triangulating force system can be effective in correcting the curve.

The primary goal in the orthotic management of Scheuermann's kyphosis is bony remodeling of the wedged vertebrae for an overall reduction of curvature. In a comparison study, the mean curve reduction for patients who were wearing a Boston lumbar kyphosis orthosis was 27%, whereas those who wore a modified Milwaukee orthosis had a mean curve reduction of 35%.[46] The Milwaukee orthosis was more effective in treatment of patients with curves of 70 degrees or more. The Boston brace may be an acceptable (and better received) intervention for patients with curves of less than 70 degrees.[46]

Orthotic wear time can be reduced gradually (weaning out of the orthosis) when bony remodeling has resulted in a measurable change of at least 5 degrees in the wedged vertebrae. Significant risk of loss of curve correction (up to 15 degrees) is present, even after 4–6 months of orthotic intervention, if brace wear is discontinued prematurely.[47]

ORTHOTICS FOR TREATMENT OF SPINAL FRACTURES

The primary function of orthoses in the management of patients with spinal fracture is to provide biomechanical stability. Spinal orthoses are used in nonoperative and postoperative care of patients with thoracolumbar injuries. An orthosis can stabilize the spine in one or more of the following ways:

1. Limitation of gross motion of the trunk to reduce movement and sway of the vertebral column during activities of daily living. It is important to note that restriction of gross trunk motion cannot limit segmental motion of the spine: Reduction of gross motion provides stability to the vertebral column by minimizing bending moments.

2. Reduction of segmental motion of the spine itself, which is necessarily accompanied by reduction of gross motion.

3. Positioning of the spine in hyperextension using a three-point force system to permit optimal bony healing, used primarily in nonoperative management of thoracolumbar injury.

Orthotic Design and Restriction of Gross Motion

A variety of orthotic designs are available when limitation of gross trunk motion (flexion/extension, lateral flexion/side bending, and axial rotation) is the primary goal. In a study comparing the effectiveness of four spinal orthoses (the Raney jacket, a custom-molded polypropylene TLSO, a Camp canvas LS corset [Camp International, Inc., Jackson, MI], and an elastic corset) in restricting gross motion of the lumbar spine, motion was most effectively limited by the Raney jacket and molded TLSO; the Camp canvas corset was moderately restrictive, and the elastic corset was minimally restrictive.[20] All of the orthoses restricted lateral flexion/side bending more effectively than lumbar flexion/extension.

Lantz and Schultz[21] compared restriction of gross body motion (flexion/extension, lateral bending, and torsion/rotation) during sitting and standing, using an LS corset, a chairback orthosis, and a custom-molded TLSO. As might be anticipated, the custom-molded TLSO restricted motion most effectively, and the LS corset was least effective, especially for upper trunk and body motion.

Orthotic Design and Segmental Immobilization

Nagel et al.[22] investigated the ability of three orthoses (a three-point hyperextension orthosis, a Taylor-Knight TLSO, and a body cast) to provide segmental immobilization by evaluating the effect of a seat belt type injury at L1–2 of the spines of human cadavers. Joint space range of motion was measured in flexion/extension, lateral bending, and axial rotation before and after orthotic intervention. The three-point hypertension orthosis was able to limit flexion/extension motion but did not prevent vertebral motion in lateral bending or axial rotation. The Taylor-Knight orthosis was effective in limiting vertebral motion in lateral bending and, to a lesser extent, in flexion/extension but had little effect on limiting axial rotation. The body cast was able to limit segmental motion in all three motions.

Norton and Brown[23] evaluated the ability of an orthosis to limit motion at different vertebral levels. None of the orthoses that they evaluated was particularly effective in limiting segmental motion, with most better able to reduce motion at upper than at lower levels. At times, increased motion was observed at the LS joint. Lumsden and Morris[24] confirmed this observation for axial rotation at the LS joint, noting that a chairback orthosis was more effective than a corset and that the orthoses in general were most effective at immobilizing upper levels and least effective at the LS joint.

Fidler and Plasmans[48] compared the effectiveness of the canvas corset, Raney jacket, baycast, and baycast spica on limiting segmental motion in flexion in normal adults. In their study, segmental motion at midlumbar levels was reduced by one-third when subjects wore a canvas corset and by two-thirds when subjects wore a Raney jacket or baycast. Only the baycast with spica limited motion at the lower lumbar levels.

Orthotic Design and Hyperextension of the Spine

Patwardhan et al.[29] studied the effectiveness of the Jewett hyperextension orthosis for patients with single- and with two-level injuries of the spine. For single-level injuries with a 50% loss of segmental stiffness, the Jewett orthosis effectively restored stability under normal gravitational load and when large flexion loads were imposed. For patients with severe two-level injuries with loss of stiffness between 50% and 85% of normal, the Jewett orthosis restored stability as long as the patient's activity level was restricted. For patients with more than 85% loss in segmental stiffness, the orthosis alone was not effective in preventing progression of deformity.

Other Strategies to Evaluate Orthotic Effectiveness

Other methods used to investigate the effectiveness of spinal orthoses include evaluation of myoelectric activity in the paraspinal musculature, assessing change in intradisk pressure, and assessing change in intra-abdominal cavity pressures. Although Morris and Lucas[49] found a reduction of the myoelectric activity of abdominal muscles during brace wear, they saw little change in intraabdominal or intrathoracic pressures. Waters and Morris compared myoelectric activity of the trunk muscles during level walking at different speeds when the subject wore a chairback LSO and an LS corset.[17] Although little change occurred in muscle activity during quiet standing or at comfortable gait speed, muscle activity of the paraspinal muscles, but not of the abdominal muscles, increased during fast gait in a chairback orthosis.

Lantz and Schultz[50] compared the myoelectric activity of the paraspinal and abdominal muscles during isometric tasks that involved exertion when subjects wore an LS corset, a chairback orthosis, and a custom-molded TLSO. None of the orthoses was consistently effective in reducing measured myoelectric activity: The chairback orthosis reduced myoelectric activity during symmetric anterior weight-holding tasks, and the TLSO was most effective in the lateral bending and torsion resisting tasks.

Nachemson and Morris[51] measured the effect of an inflatable LS corset on intradiscal pressures in the lumbar spine. Minimal difference in intradiscal pressures was found when subjects wore no corset and the noninflated corset, but disk pressures decreased by 25% when the corset was inflated. In a subsequent study, Nachemson et al.[25] monitored intradiscal pressures, intra-abdominal pressures, and myoelectric activity of trunk muscles while normal subjects performed eight different activities wearing Jewett and Cash hyperextension orthoses. In some subjects myoelectric activity of the erector spinae and abdominals decreased, whereas in others myoelectric activity increased. Krag et al.[52] measured intra-abdominal pressure and myoelectric activity in the erector spinae muscles in normal subjects performing isometric extension pulls in upright and flexed postures with no orthosis under three orthotic conditions: wearing a Camp LS corset, wearing a Raney flexion jacket, and without an orthosis. Intraabdominal pressure increased slightly when subjects wore the orthoses; however, myoelectric activity of back musculature did not decrease as expected, even when subjects voluntarily attempted to increase intra-abdominal pressure above normal levels.

Although these researchers have attempted to demonstrate the effect of orthotic wear on the activity of trunk muscles, on abdominal cavity pressure, and on intradiscal pressure, methodologic problems and inconsistent results prevent us from understanding these effects at this time.

ORTHOTICS FOR THORACOLUMBAR FRACTURE

Most stable thoracolumbar fractures without signs of neurologic compromise do not require surgery and are managed with an orthosis that holds the trunk in sagittal hypertension until bony healing has occurred. Complex and unstable spinal fractures typically require surgical repair, possible with internal fixation or fusion, followed by immobilization in a custom TLSO or body cast. Guidelines for deciding which fractures require surgical intervention and which do not are not well established. Several clinical studies have compared operative and nonoperative management of burst fractures and fracture dislocations of the spine, but the results have been equivocal.

In a study of traumatic burst vertebral fractures of the thoracolumbar spine without neurologic deficit treated nonoperatively by application of a body cast, wearing of an orthosis, or bed rest, Weinstein et al.[53] reported that all three methods had acceptable long-term results. Effective outcomes have been reported when spinal fractures caused by lap/seat belts were managed by hyperextension orthosis wear. Similarly, Gertzbein and Court-Brown[54] suggest that flexion distraction injuries of the thoracolumbar spine without neurologic injuries can be managed effectively without surgery by hypertension orthosis. In a study by McEvoy and Bradford,[55] patients with burst fractures of the thoracic or lumbar spine were treated nonoperatively by application of a body cast or by wearing a polypropylene body jacket (mean immobilization time, 4.5 months, with a range of 2–6 months). Casts were removed or orthoses discontinued at the physician's discretion; radiographs typically demonstrated stability and healing. Two additional studies by Willen et al.[56] and by Davies et al.[57] support the use of a hypertension orthosis brace as an effective alternative to surgery for patients with fractures of the thoracolumbar region. Hyperextension casts have been used effectively as a conservative alternative to surgery for reduction of moderate to severe wedge compression fractures.[58] The results of these clinical studies are supported by the finite element model of progression of deformity proposed by Patwardhan et al.[29]

Criteria for orthotic design in the nonoperative treatment of spinal injury must be based on an understanding of the biomechanical deficit that has resulted from the injury and the impaired spine's vulnerability to progression of deformity. When any evidence of progression of deformity during nonoperative orthotic intervention is present, a careful reevaluation must be made to determine whether continued conservative orthotic treatment will place the patient at risk of developing neurologic deficit. Patient compliance is essential as well: The ideal orthosis will be ineffective if it is worn improperly or inconsistently.

POSTOPERATIVE ORTHOTIC TREATMENT FOR THORACOLUMBAR INJURY

The Milwaukee brace and body cast worn postoperatively reduce axial force on the Harrington rod (spinal instrumentation) in patients with idiopathic scoliosis during standing and walking.[59] Postoperative orthoses act to restrict motion, protecting injured segments from motion and theoretically reducing loads on the surgical constructs until solid fusion occurs.[60] With advances in surgical instrumentation, however, it is not well documented just how effective postoperative orthoses are in reducing stresses on any particular implant. The role of an orthosis for postoperative immobilization after spinal fusion for low back pain remains controversial. A custom-molded TLSO in neutral sagittal alignment is the standard of postoperative immobilization for patients with significant thoracolumbar injuries. In these cases, the goal of surgery (with

instrumentation, bone graft, and/or fusion) is to restore segmental stability; the role of postoperative orthosis is to protect the surgical construct from the planes of motion that make it vulnerable to failure. Typically, motions to be guarded against in the immediate postoperative period are trunk flexion and trunk torsion/rotation.

To be effective, the TLSO must have enough anterior height to resist forward bending at the sternum, as well as firm end-point stabilization of the pelvis. The distal trimlines often must extend into the groin to capture the pelvis firmly, which may interfere somewhat with the patient's ability to sit comfortably and to perform lower extremity activities of daily living. Although this may make rehabilitation challenging for a short period of time, the goal of spinal stabilization takes precedent in the postoperative period. The orthotist is also careful with upright alignment to ensure that the orthosis holds the trunk in a neutral position, avoiding the application of a flexion or extension load to the torso to minimize the translation of stresses onto surgical instruments.

A thigh extension with an orthotic hip joint is added to the postoperative custom-molded TLSO of patients with spinal fusion at L5–S1 to immobilize the LS joint effectively. A TLSO without this thigh extension may have no effect or may actually increase LS motion.[23,24] For patients with mid- to upper thoracic injury or injury at multiple levels, an orthosis that is designed to immobilize the cervical spine can be added to the TLSO.

A design of the spinal orthosis for thoracolumbar injury is based on an understanding of its biomechanical mechanism of action, clinical intuition, and patient assessment. Use of a brace that provides too much or too little stabilization compromises desired surgical and functional outcomes. Many trauma centers have established criteria for selection of an orthosis. Patient and caregiver education about the purpose and design of the orthosis and the consequences of noncompliance is another important component to ensure that the desired outcome is achieved.

ORTHOTICS IN CERVICAL SPINE INSTABILITY

The cervical spine is complex, and knowledge of its anatomy and arthrokinematics provides the foundation for understanding the role of the many orthoses that are designed to manage cervical spine instability. The seven cervical vertebrae and their surrounding soft tissues constitute the most mobile segment of the spine. Anatomically unique, the atlantoaxial complex (occiput, C1, C2) can be considered and examined separately from the rest of the cervical spine.[58]

TABLE 14-2
Comparison of Restriction of Cervical Motion Accomplished by Five Cervical Orthoses, Measured as Percent Normal Cervical Motion Allowed

	Motion				
Orthosis	Flexion Only	Extension Only	Flexion and Extension	Rotation	Lateral Tilt
Aspen collar	41%	36%	38%	62%	69%
Philadelphia collar	33%	41%	37%*	52%	66%
Stiffneck collar	25%	35%	30%	43%	50%
Miami J collar	24%*	29%	27%	35%	49%*
NecLoc collar	17%	23%	20%	27%	40%

Note: Differences in restriction of motion were evaluated by paired t test, with each collar compared to the one listed above. All were significantly different ($p < .05$) except for those marked with *.
Source: Adapted with permission from V Askins, FJ Eismont. Efficacy of Five Cervical Orthoses in Restricting Cervical Motion: A Comparison Study. Proceedings of the tenth annual meeting of the North American Spine Society, Washington, DC, October 1995.

The cervical spine rotates in the transverse plane for a total excursion of 160 degrees. Approximately one-half of this rotation occurs at the C1 and C2 level, with the remainder occurring across the joints below this level.[61] Although movements of flexion and extension occur at all cervical levels, the greatest range of these motions happen at the C5-6 level. Lateral flexion occurs in the more caudal (C3–7) levels of the cervical spine.

Examination of the complete cervical spine requires several strategies. Anterior surfaces of the first and second vertebrae (C1, C2) are best viewed through an open mouth. Palpation of the Adam's apple (thyroid cartilage) approximates the levels of C4–6. Maximal forward flexion of the head and neck exposes the bony spinous processes of the C7 and T1 vertebrae.

Cervical orthoses can be classified or grouped in several ways. One strategy is to divide orthoses by the mechanism of control into two groups: skin contact orthoses and skeletal devices. Another is to classify orthoses by the magnitude of motion control that they provide, into a minimum control group and an intermediate control group.[58] In this chapter, we use Nachemson's[28] classification of cervical orthoses into three groups (soft, reinforced, rigid) based on material construct.

Cervical orthoses are designed to minimize the physiologic loads and motions between the head and thorax. Several studies have assessed the ability of different orthoses to restrict motion of the cervical spine, enabling the orthotist to classify orthoses from least to most restrictive[62,63] (Table 14-2). Control of flexion/extension motion in the sagittal plane is the most efficiently accomplished; restriction of rotation and lateral tilt is much more challenging. Our discussion begins with orthoses that provide the least restriction of motion, moving to those that provide the most motion control of the cervical spine.

Soft Collars

Although patients find a soft collar quite comfortable to wear, this type of cervical orthosis does little to restrict motion in any plane (Figure 14-10). This device is used primarily as a kinesthetic reminder for patients with mild whiplash injury or neck pain to restrict their cervical motion. Because this orthosis is not stabilized against the upper trunk or occiput, wearing it does not guarantee optimal cervical alignment. The collar is usually a narrow block of foam rubber material covered with stockinet or knitted material, and it is closed around the neck with Velcro.

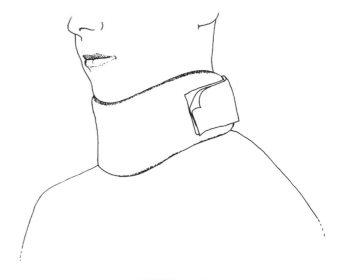

FIGURE 14-10
A soft collar reminds the patient to limit motion of the neck but provides little stability for the cervical spine.

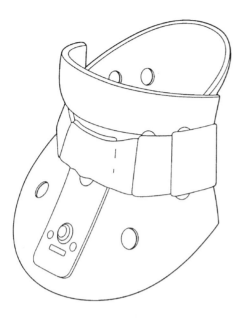

FIGURE 14-11

Philadelphia collar, with an anterior opening for respiratory apparatus and tracheostomy care. (From DG Shurr. Prosthetics, Orthotics and Orthopaedic Rehabilitation. In CR Clark, M Bonfiglio [eds]. Orthopaedics: Essentials of Diagnosis and Treatment. New York: Churchill Livingstone, 1994:340)

Reinforced Cervical Collars

To provide more stability than is possible in a soft cervical collar, a variety of commercially manufactured reinforced collars are available. A reinforced collar has an outer plastic/semirigid frame and an inner soft pad or closed cell foam shell that interfaces with the skin. Many have anterior openings to accommodate respiratory apparatus fixation. The Philadelphia collar is the most recognized reinforced collar (Figure 14-11). Most reinforced collars have an anterior shell that supports the chin and a posterior shell that supports the occiput of the skull, attached firmly together by Velcro closure. Although the Philadelphia collar does provide some support for the weight of the head in the sagittal plane, because of its low trimlines, this collar cannot effectively immobilize the cervical spine enough to prevent lateral bending or rotation.

Other reinforced collars (e.g., the Newport, Miami J, or Aspen collars) are designed with higher trimlines in an attempt to provide more motion control. The semirigid frame of these orthoses tends to be longer than that of the Philadelphia collar. The distal trimline and padding typically lie against the manubrium of the sternum anteriorly and the spinous processes of the first several thoracic vertebrae posteriorly. The proximal trimline and padding encompass the lateral surface and underside of the mandible anteriorly and fit snugly against the lateral and posterior

surface of the skull. Like the Philadelphia collar, these cervical orthoses are held in place by Velcro closures.

Guidelines for Reinforced Cervical Collars and Cervicothoracic Orthoses

Several important points should be remembered if a reinforced collar or a cervicothoracic orthosis (CTO) is to be as effective as possible during rehabilitation: a snug fit, pressure relief and skin care, and neutral alignment. The key to success is centered on patient and caregiver understanding of the design and purpose of the collar and on consistent wearing of the device.

Snug Fit

Patients and caregivers are often tempted to loosen the straps of the collar in an effort to be more comfortable. The effectiveness of the collar worn less tightly closed than in the original fitting, however, is equivalent to being out of the collar completely.[64] The superior edge of a well-fit collar is in total contact against the mandible and occipital areas; the inferior edge rests against the sternum, muscle belly of the upper trapezius, and upper thoracic spine. When adjusted correctly, neck motion within the collar is at a minimum.

Pressure Relief and Skin Care

Because of the firm fit and total contact of reinforced cervical collars on the mandible, posterior skull, and superior trunk surfaces, patients who wear them are at risk of skin irritation or breakdown, especially if the contact pressure of the orthosis reaches or exceeds the amount of pressure that would cause capillary closure. Plaisier et al.[65] compared craniofacial pressures exerted by four different reinforced collars. The Stiffneck extraction collar, often used by emergency medical technicians as a means of immobilization when cervical spinal cord injury is suspected, exceeded capillary closing pressure at most contact points. This suggests that extraction type collars are best used for a short duration and are not appropriate for long-term use during rehabilitation. It is also important that patients and caregivers establish a routine for skin care and shaving and that care is taken to keep the mandibular and chin support of the anterior shell clean and free of food or debris that can become entrapped at mealtime.

Neutral Alignment

Most reinforced cervical collars are designed to hold the head and neck in as close to a neutral position as possible. If a patient wears the collar when supine in bed, care must be taken that neutral position is maintained. Optimally, only a single pillow placed under the upper back (scapula), neck, and head is used for sleeping. When several pillows are placed under the patient's head and neck, a large flexion moment is created, which, in turn, creates areas of high-pressure contact with the skin, increasing discomfort and the risk of skin breakdown. The Philadelphia collar, for example, exerts acceptable pressures in the upright position but greater than capillary closure pressure when the patient is supine, even if no pillows are used.[65] It is equally important to limit exercises that cause cervical motion while the collar is worn, so that neutral alignment is not inadvertently compromised.

Cervicothoracic Orthoses

At times nonoperative and postoperative care of cervical spine injuries requires more stability or better immobilization than is possible with reinforced cervical collars. To provide greater motion control, the distal end-point control must encompass at least the upper thoracic spine and trunk. A variety of "poster" orthotic designs that have thoracic components are connected to occipital and mandibular pieces by two or four uprights or posts. A variety of thermoplastic bivalve designs encase the upper trunk, neck, and chin and occiput. Control of sagittal plane flexion and extension is enhanced by the stabilizing effect of the thoracic extension in both of these CTO designs. Although control of lateral flexion and rotation is often better than that achieved by a reinforced collar, these motions cannot be completely limited by poster style or rigid cervicothoracic orthoses. The only orthosis that guarantees complete immobilization is a "halo" cervical device.

Sterno-Occipito-Mandibular Immobilizers

The SOMI is a metal and thermoplastic orthosis that is most often chosen for patients with instability at or above the C4 vertebral level[62] (Figure 14-12). The SOMI has a T-shaped yoke worn over the shoulders and anterior chest that connects to the occipital support via a U-shaped metal rod. The distal end of the yoke is anchored by a strap that wraps around the patient's midtrunk. The mandibular support is attached to the yoke by a single flat post and to the occipital support by lateral straps. An alternate configuration uses a headband to stabilize the head in the device rather than the mandibular support, which makes feeding and oral care less problematic. The SOMI is especially effective in controlling flexion. The metal support rods can be adjusted to position the neck in neutral, extended, or flexed position, for optimal positioning given the nature of the patient's injury or surgical repair. The device is relatively simple to fit and can be easily donned and doffed when the patient is supine.

Yale Cervicothoracic Orthoses

The Yale CTO is a thermoplastic device designed to stabilize the lower cervical spine; it is used in patients with

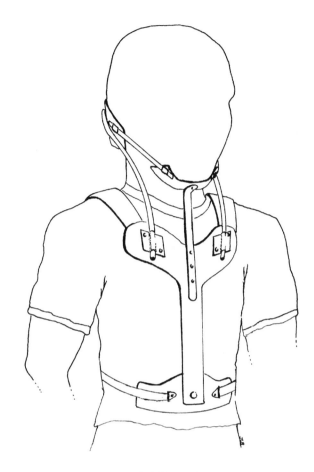

FIGURE 14-12

The sterno-occipito-mandibular immobilizer is used to stabilize the upper cervical spine. The U-shaped metal support rods can be adjusted to match the particular positioning requirements of the patient's condition.

spinal instability or injury below the C4 vertebral level (Figure 14-13). The Yale orthosis is basically a snugly fit reinforced cervical collar with anterior and posterior extensions attached to a thoracic band. The extensions and thoracic band create a longer lever arm for more effective control of spinal motions. Although the device effectively limits flexion/extension, patients are able to rotate through a limited range of motion.

Minerva Cervicothoracic Orthoses

The Yale CTO was designed as a lighter-weight and less care-intensive version of the Minerva CTO. The Minerva is a custom-molded thermoplastic orthosis with an anterior and posterior shell (bivalve design) encasing the patient's neck and upper chest from jaw to umbilicus on the anterior surface and from occiput to midback on the posterior surface (Figure 14-14). The shells of the Min-

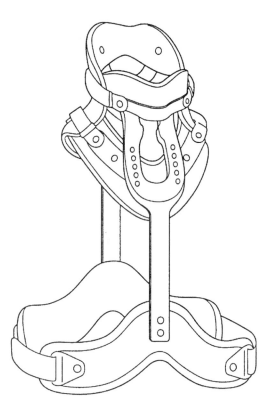

FIGURE 14-13

The chest extensions of a Yale cervicothoracic orthosis provide better leverage for control of lower cervical and upper thoracic vertebral motion than is possible with other reinforced collars. (From DG Shurr. Prosthetics, Orthotics and Orthopaedic Rehabilitation. In CR Clark, M Bonfiglio [eds]. Orthopaedics: Essentials of Diagnosis and Treatment. New York: Churchill Livingstone, 1994:341)

erva are held snugly in place around the trunk and neck by Velcro closures. Although this rigid orthosis provides more aggressive control of gross and intersegmental motion of the cervical and upper thoracic spine than is possible with other CTO designs, several disadvantages must be considered as well. The Minerva can be very difficult to apply and take off. It is very hot to wear and is not well tolerated by patients in warm climates. It is also associated with a higher incidence of skin irritation and pressure sores when compared to other CTO designs.[66]

Other Cervicothoracic Orthosis Designs

A number of other poster CTO designs are available for patients with serious spinal injuries or surgeries. The C. D. Denison design uses an anterior and posterior bar placed at the midline to support the weight of the head on a yoked thoracic component. In four-poster designs, two anterior and two posterior posts connect the lateral undersurface of the mandibular support and occipital support to the tho-

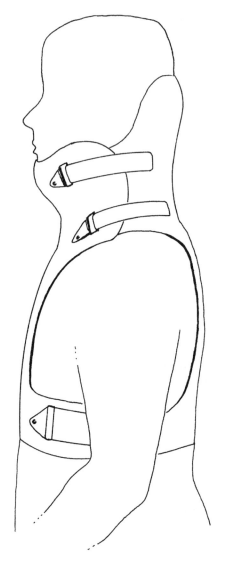

FIGURE 14-14

The Minerva cervicothoracic orthosis encases the cervical and upper thoracic spine.

racic component. These orthoses are more restrictive than reinforced cervical collars but may not restrict motion as well as the Yale CTO or the Minerva design. These designs are often incorporated into a TLSO for patients with multiple injuries or extensive spinal surgery that require protection of the cervical, thoracic, and lumbar spine.

Halo

When complete control of the cervical and upper thoracic spine in all three planes of motion is required, the orthosis of choice is the halo[62] (Figure 14-15). The halo was first used as an extension of a body jacket for immobilization of patients with severe poliomyelitis and paralysis of the cervical musculature.[67] In current practice, the halo is used in three ways. If applied before surgery, it minimizes movement and protects the spinal cord during surgical procedures. If applied immediately after open reduction–internal fixation or fusion surgery, the halo controls cervical motion until adequate healing and bony union have been achieved at the surgical site. The halo is also used in conservative nonoperative management of nondisplaced upper cervical vertebral fractures.

The halo has three components: the ring and skull pins that surround the skull, a vest worn around the thorax, and the suprastructure that fixates the ring to the vest.

Ring and Skull Pins

The ring of the halo is positioned approximately 1 cm above the eyebrow and the tip of the ears, with at least 1 cm clearance between the ring and skin surface. Four pins are inserted ⅛ in. into the outer bony layer (table) of the skull with 6 to 8 pounds/inch^2 of torque. The anterior pins are placed in the lateral one-third of the eyebrow to avoid the frontal sinus, supraorbital and subtrochlear nerves, and temporalis muscle. Posteriorly, pins are placed 1–2 cm posterior to the ear in diagonal opposition to the anterior pin site. This arrangement places the ring below the greater equator of the skull, in areas that are most likely to have the thickest bone mass.[68] Optimally, pins are inserted perpendicular to the skull to maximize the ultimate load and minimize deformation of the pin bone complex to reduce the risk of failure.[69] Additional pins inserted with less torque are used for children with incompletely developed skulls, for patients with skull fracture, for those with sloping brows, and for patients who are in traction before application of the halo. Halo rings are available in open and in closed configurations. Although open rings can facilitate fitting, increased pain and pin problems can occur when an open ring is used.[70]

Halo Superstructure

The superstructure of the halo orthosis is available in several designs. In one design, two anterior and two posterior metal rods rigidly link the ring apparatus to the vest. In another, a pair of lateral rods rise toward the ring from a metal yoke that arches over the shoulders and is anchored to the vest. The purpose of the superstructure is to fixate the ring to the vest. Most superstructures can be adjusted so that the patient's head and neck can be held in the position or plane necessary for the particular injury or surgical procedure that warrants a period of immobilization.

Vest

The vest is the foundation and point of stability for the halo system. A halo vest is usually fabricated from flexible thermoplastic and has a removable liner made from

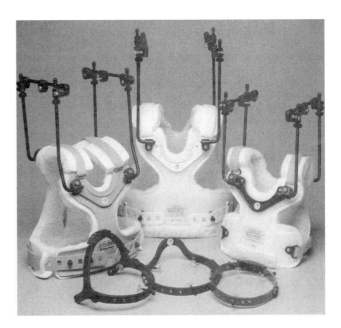

FIGURE 14-15
The halo orthosis is the only device that immobilizes the cervical spine effectively in all three planes of motion. The head is stabilized within an open ring (left foreground) or closed ring (right foreground) by a set of pressure pins. The ring is anchored to the stabilizing thoracic vest by the halo's metal superstructure. (Courtesy of Bremmer Medical, Acromed Corp., Jacksonville, FL.)

lamb's wool or a similar material. With the patient supine, the anterior shell of the vest can be opened without compromising stability for hygiene. This feature is also important if emergency respiratory access is needed. In most halo vests, the distal trimline is at or slightly above the inferior costal margin of the last rib; extending it beyond this provides no additional cervical stability.[71]

Avoiding Complications

A number of potentially serious problems are associated with the halo orthosis, including loosening of pins, pin site infection, pin discomfort, ring migration, pressure sores, nerve injury, prolonged bleeding at pin sites, and puncture of the dura.[72] Caregivers and health care providers who work with patients in a halo during rehabilitation must be watchful for signs that these problems may be developing and notify the physician or orthotist promptly so that appropriate intervention or adjustment can occur. The risk of problem development is minimized when a routine of halo care is in place.

Daily pin care requires cleansing of each pin site with its own cotton swab that has been soaked in one-half strength peroxide and normal saline solution, followed by an application of povidone-iodine (Betadine) solution. Two important signs of impending infection are soreness or oozing at a pin site and extreme sensitivity to touch during routine care. Pin site or headache pain that persists beyond the third day "in halo" should also be reported to the physician.

A well-fit vest should not create undue pressure over any body prominence. Patient complaints about point pressure, tightness, or irritation over the scapulae, ribs, clavicles, or other areas covered by the vest often suggest that vest adjustment is necessary. It is not unusual for patients to complain of itchiness under the vest; relieving this itch should be accomplished with lotion or with a blunt object used in a gentle fashion.

Halo in Rehabilitation

The added mass of a halo orthosis changes the position of the center of gravity within the trunk. Initially, patients may experience this extra mass as being "top-heavy." For patients without neurologic deficit who are able to ambulate while in the halo, a posture that accommodates this added mass is slight forward flexion of the trunk. Some patients might require a cane or walker until postural control adapts to the halo. Patients with cervical spinal cord injury who begin their rehabilitation with a halo may have to readjust their postural control strategies in sitting when the halo is discontinued later in their rehabilitation, because their center of mass shifts back to its normal position.

If a patient in a halo has a fall, pin sites should be examined for loosening or bleeding. If the apparatus appears to be less stable after a fall, it is best to have the patient remain supine until the physician or orthotist evaluates and adjusts the device.

SUMMARY

The selection of the appropriate spinal orthosis for a given patient is based on a variety of objective and clinically informed subjective factors. These include the type and severity of the disorder, the age and size of the patient, the availability of assistance and support in the home and community, and the desired mechanisms of action of the orthosis. These factors are best evaluated and orthotic decisions are most effectively made in the context of a multidisciplinary team. Effective teams share information about the nature of a patient's condition, the reason that an orthosis is necessary, and the factors (positive and negative) that will influence the eventual outcome of the orthotic intervention. Communication is the foundation for effective teaming.

The orthotist is responsible for recommending and providing the ideal orthosis to treat a patient's spinal condition. A properly fitted spinal orthosis does not inflect pain or cause skin breakdown. Patients and caregivers, as members of the team, must clearly understand why an orthosis is being prescribed and what impact the orthosis will have on daily function and mobility. Regularly scheduled follow-up appointments are necessary so that the orthotist can adjust the orthosis should technical errors come to light or the patient's status change over time. Recognition of potential problems before they develop can only enhance outcome.

Rehabilitation professionals who are working with patients using spinal orthoses are responsible for creating rehabilitative programs that respect and facilitate the use of spinal orthoses. To accomplish this, therapists must understand how the orthosis is designed to stabilize or support the spine. Open communication between rehabilitation professionals and the orthotist is essential, so that the goals of the orthosis and of rehabilitation are supportive and any problems or questions are quickly addressed.

Consistent clinical evidence has shown that spinal orthoses are effective in the nonsurgical and postoperative care of many types of spinal disorders. Research in biomechanical design and engineering has advanced our understanding of how spinal orthoses work, why they work, and how their use can be optimized. Comparative studies have begun to identify differences in efficacy and outcomes of various LSO, TLSO, cervical orthotic, and CTO devices. The design of spinal orthoses will be refined and improved as research continues in this important area.

The natural history of many of the spinal disorders managed with orthoses is not well understood and warrants further epidemiologic study. The impact of orthoses on the progression or resolution of the disorder also requires further clinical study. The results of these types of studies can only enhance the clinical team's confidence in their recommendations and their ability to predict outcomes of orthotic treatment. Clinicians should be aware that, among the many orthoses that are currently produced and mass marketed, some devices are not well supported by scientific research. Rehabilitation professionals, as advocates for their patients, should be informed and critical consumers.

In this chapter, we have provided an overview of the major types of spinal orthoses that may be encountered by health professionals who work in acute care and various rehabilitation settings. We have also discussed many factors that facilitate and inhibit successful orthotic outcome. Recognition of the importance of fit, of proper donning technique, of the need for follow-up and maintenance, and of the importance of patient education and compliance can only enhance the success of orthotic intervention. Failure to recognize and act on these issues compromises the rehabilitation process and can lead to serious secondary problems, complications, or surgical failure, as if the patient with spinal disorder or injury had no orthosis at all.

REFERENCES

1. Andry N. Orthopaedia. Philadelphia: Lippincott, 1961. (Facsimile reproduction of the 1st ed in English, London, 1743.)

2. Atlas of Orthopaedic Appliances, American Academy of Orthopaedic Surgeons. Ann Arbor, MI: Edwards Bros., 1952.

3. Blount WP, Schmidt AC, Keever ED, Leonard ET. Milwaukee brace in the operative treatment of scoliosis. J Bone Joint Surg 1958;40A:511–525.

4. Blount WP, Moe JH. The Milwaukee Brace. Baltimore: Williams & Wilkins, 1973.

5. Andriacchi TP, Schultz AB, Belytschko TB, DeWald RL. Milwaukee brace correction of idiopathic scoliosis. J Bone Joint Surg 1976;58A(6):806–815.

6. Gavin TM, Boscardi JB, Patwardhan AG, et al. Preliminary results of orthotic treatment for chronic low back pain. J Prosthet Orthot 1993;5(1):25–29.

7. Micheli LJ, Hall JE, Miller ME. Use of the modified Boston brace for back injuries in athletes. Am J Sports Med 1980;8(5):351–356.

8. Willner S. Effect of a rigid brace on back pain. Acta Orthop Scand 1985;56(1):40–42.

9. Salter RB. Textbook of Disorders and Injuries of the Musculoskeletal System (2nd ed). Baltimore: Williams & Wilkins, 1983.

10. Spinal Orthotics. New York University: Post Graduate Medical School, Prosthetics and Orthotics, 1973.

11. Thompson A. Appliances for the Spine and Trunk. In American Academy of Orthopaedic Surgeons: Orthopedic Appliance Atlas, vol I. Ann Arbor, MI: Edwards Bros, 1952.

12. Anderson JAD. Back Pain and Occupation. In MIV Jayson (ed), The Lumbar Spine and Back Pain. New York: Churchill Livingstone, 1987;16.

13. Fishman S, Berger N, Edelstein JE, Springer WP. Spinal Orthoses. In WH Bunch (ed), American Academy of Orthopaedic Surgeons: Atlas of Orthotics; Biomechanical Principles and Applications (2nd ed). St. Louis: Mosby, 1985:238–258.

14. Fidler MW, Plasmans CMT. The effect of four types of support on the segmental mobility of the lumbosacral spine. J Bone Joint Surg 1983;65A(7):937–943.

15. Willner S. Test instrument for predicting the effect of rigid braces. Prosthet Orthot Int 1990;14(1):22–26.

16. Lucas D, Jacobs RR, Traukman T. Spinal Orthotics for Pain and Instability. In Redford GB, Orthotics Etcetera (3rd ed). Baltimore: Williams & Wilkins, 1986.

17. Waters RL, Morris JM. Effects of spinal supports on the electrical activity of muscles of the trunk. J Bone Joint Surg 1970(1);52A:51–60.

18. Hampton D, Laros G, McCarron R, Franks D. Healing potential of the annulus fibrosis. Spine 1989;14(4):398–401.

19. Perry J. The use of external support in the treatment of low back pain. J Bone Joint Surg 1970;52A(7):1440–1442.

20. Buchalter D, Kahanovitz N, Viola K, Dorsky S, et al. Three-dimensional spinal motion measurements. Part 2: A non-invasive assessment of lumbar brace immobilization of the spine. J Spinal Dis 1988;1(4):284–286.

21. Lantz SA, Schultz AB. Lumbar spine orthosis wearing. I: Restriction of gross body motions. Spine 1986;11(8):838–842.

22. Nagel DA, Koogle TA, Piziali RL, Perkash I. Stability of the upper lumbar spine following progressive disruptions and the application of individual internal and external fixation devices. J Bone Joint Surg 1981;63(1):62–70.

23. Norton PL, Brown T. The immobilizing efficiency of the back braces; their effect on the posture and motion of the lumbosacral spine. J Bone Joint Surg 1957;39A:111–139.

24. Lumsden RM, Morris JM. An in vivo study of axial rotation and immobilization at the lumbosacral joint. J Bone Joint Surg,1968;50(8):1591–1602.

25. Nachemson A, Schultz AB, Andersson GBJ. Mechanical effectiveness studies of lumbar spine orthoses. Scand J Rehabil Med 1983;(Suppl):9:139–149.

26. Gilbertson LG, Goel VK, Patwardhan AG, et al. The Biomechanical Function of "Three Point" Hyperextension Orthoses. Proceedings of the American Society of Mechanical Engineers 112th winter annual meeting, Atlanta, 1991.

27. Schimandle JH, Weigel M, Edwards CC. Indications for Thigh Cuff Bracing following Instrumented Lumbosacral Fusions. Proceedings of the 8th annual meeting of the North American Spine Society, San Diego, 1993.

28. Nachemson AL. Orthotic treatment for injuries and diseases of the spinal column. Phys Med Rehabil 1987;1:22–24.

29. Patwardhan AG, Li SP, Gavin T, et al. Orthotic stabilization of thoracolumbar injuries—a biomechanical analysis of the Jewett hyperextension orthosis. Spine 1990;15(7):654–661.

30. Williams PC. Lesions of the lumbosacral spine-lordosis brace. J Bone Joint Surg 1937;19:702.

31. Kim SS, Denis F, Lonstein JE, Winter RB. Factors affecting fusion rate in adult spondylolisthesis. Spine 1990;15(9):979–984.

32. Luskin R. Pain patterns in spondylolisthesis. Clin Orthop 1965;40:125–136.

33. Duval-Beaupere G. Pathogenic Relationship between Scoliosis and Growth. In PA Zorab (ed), Proceedings of the Third Symposium on Scoliosis and Growth. Edinburgh: Churchill Livingstone, 1971;58.

34. Lonstein JE, Carlson M. The prediction of curve progression in untreated idiopathic scoliosis during growth. J Bone Joint Surg 1984;66(7):1061–1071.

35. Lucas DB. Mechanics of the spine. Bull Hosp Jt Dis Orthop Inst 1970;31(2):115–131.

36. Patwardhan AG, Bunch WH, Meade KP, et al. A biomechanical analog of curve progression and orthotic stabilization in idiopathic scoliosis. J Biomech 1986;19(2):103–117.

37. Carr WA, Moe JH, Winter RB, Lonstein J. Treatment of idiopathic scoliosis in the Milwaukee brace: long-term results. J Bone Joint Surg 1980;62(4):599–612.

38. Edmonsson A, Morris J. Follow-up study of Milwaukee brace treatment in patients with idiopathic scoliosis. Clin Orthop Jul-Aug 1977;(126):58–61.

39. Lonstein JE, Winter RL. Milwaukee brace treatment of adolescent idiopathic scoliosis—review of 1,027 patients. J Bone Joint Surg 1994;76(8):1207–1221.

40. Nachemson AL, Peterson LE. Effectiveness of treatment with a brace in girls who have adolescent idiopathic scoliosis. A prospective, controlled study based on data from the brace

study of the Scoliosis Research Society. J Bone Joint Surg 1995;77(6):815–822.

41. Patwardhan AG, Gavin TM, Bunch WH, et al. Biomechanical comparison of the Milwaukee Brace and the TLSO for treatment of idiopathic scoliosis. J Prosthet Orthot 1996;8(4):115–122.

42. Katz DE, Richards BS, Browne R, Herring JA. A comparison between the Boston brace and the Charleston bending brace in adolescent idiopathic scoliosis. Spine 1997;22(12):1302–1312.

43. Wilhemy JK, Farrow B, Zeller JL. Five Year Study Evaluating the Use of the Charleston Night Brace for the Treatment of Idiopathic Scoliosis. Proceedings of the 25th annual meeting of the Scoliosis Research Society, Honolulu, HI, 1990.

44. Mitchell TM, Smith BG, Thomson JD. Effectiveness of the Boston Brace in the Treatment of Large Curves in Adolescent Idiopathic Scoliosis. Proceedings of the 31st annual meeting of the Scoliosis Research Society, Ottawa, Canada, October 1996.

45. Upadhay SS, Nelson IW, Ho EK, et al. New prognostic factors to predict the final outcome of brace treatment in adolescent idiopathic scoliosis. Spine 1995;20(5):537–545.

46. Gutowski WT, Renshaw TS. Orthotic results in adolescent kyphosis. Spine 1988;13(5):485–489.

47. Montgomery SP, Erwin WE. Scheuermann's kyphosis—long-term results of Milwaukee brace treatment. Spine 1981;6(1):5–8.

48. Fidler MW, Plasmans CMT. The effect of four types of support on the segmental mobility of the lumbosacral spine. J Bone Joint Surg 1983;65(7):943–947.

49. Morris JM, Lucas DB. Physiological considerations in bracing of the spine. Orthop Prosthet Appl 1963;37:44.

50. Lantz SA, Schultz AB. Lumbar spine orthosis wearing. II: Effect on trunk muscle myoelectric activity. Spine 1986;11(8): 838–842.

51. Nachemson A, Morris JM. In vivo measurements of intradiscal pressure. J Bone Joint Surg 1964;46A:1077–1092.

52. Krag MH, Byrne KB, Pope MH, Bayliss D. The effect of back braces on the relationship between intra-abdominal pressure and spinal loads. Adv Bioengineering 1986;22–23.

53. Weinstein JN, Cellalto P, Lehmann TR. Thoracolumbar "burst" fractures treated conservatively: a long-term follow-up. Spine 1988;13(1):33–38.

54. Gertzbein SD, Court-Brown CM. The Rationale for Management of Flexion/Distraction Injuries of the Thoracolumbar Spine Based on a New Classification. Proceedings of the 22nd annual meeting of the Scoliosis Research Society, Vancouver, Canada, September 1987.

55. McEvoy RD, Bradford DS. The management of burst fractures of the thoracic and lumbar spine—experience in 53 patients. Spine 1985;10(7):631–637.

56. Willen J, Lindahl S, Nordwall A. Unstable thoracolumbar fractures—a comparative clinical study of conservative treatment and Harrington instrumentation. Spine 1985;10(2): 111–112.

57. Davies WE, Morris JH, Hill V. An analysis of conservative (nonsurgical) management of thoracolumbar fractures and fracture dislocations with neural damage. J Bone Joint Surg 1980;62(8):1324–1328.

58. White A, Panjabi M. In AA White, MM Panjabi (eds), Clinical Biomechanics of the Spine (2nd ed). Philadelphia: Lippincott, 1990;235–255.

59. Nachemson A, Elfstrom G. Intravital wireless telemetry of axial forces in Harrington distraction rods in patients with idiopathic scoliosis. J Bone Joint Surg 1971;53(3):445–465.

60. Lorenz MA, Patwardhan AG, Zindrick MR. Instability and Mechanics of Implants and Braces for Thoracic and Lumbar Fractures. In T Errico (ed), Spinal Trauma. Philadelphia: Lippincott, 1990;271–280.

61. Bland JH. Disorders of the Cervical Spine (2nd ed). Philadelphia: Saunders, 1994.

62. Johnson RM, Hart DL, Simmons EF, et al. Cervical orthoses: a study comparing their effectiveness in restricting cervical motion in normal subjects. J Bone Joint Surg 1977;59(3):332–339.

63. Askins V, Eismont FJ. Efficacy of five cervical orthoses in restricting cervical motion: a comparison study. Spine 1997;22(11):1193–1198.

64. Fisher SV. Proper fitting of the cervical orthosis. Arch Phys Med Rehabil 1978;59(11):505–507.

65. Plaisier B, Gabram SG, Schwartz RJ, Jacobs LM. Prospective evaluation of craniofacial pressure in four different cervical orthoses. J Trauma 1994;37(5):714–720.

66. King A. Spinal Column Trauma. In MH Myers (ed), The Multiply Injured Patient With Complex Fractures. Philadelphia: Lea & Febiger 1984;46.

67. Perry JP, Nickel VL. Total cervical spine fusion for neck paralysis. J Bone Joint Surg 1959;41A:37–60.

68. Garfin SR, Botte MJ, Centeno RS, Nickel VL. Osteology of the skull as it affects halo pin placement. Spine 1985;10(8): 696–698.

69. Triggs KJ, Ballock RT, Lee TQ, et al. The effect of angled insertion on halo pin fixation. Spine 1989;14(8):781–783.

70. Wetzel FT, Dunsieth NW, Kuhlengel KR, Paul EM. The effectiveness of the cervical halo: open versus closed ring. A preliminary report. Paraplegia 1995;33(2):110–115.

71. Wang GJ, Moskal JT, Albert T, et al. The effect of halo-vest length on stability of the cervical spine. J Bone Joint Surg 1988;70(3):357–360.

72. Botte MJ, Byrne TP, Abrams RA, Garfin SR. The halo skeletal fixator: current concepts of application and maintenance. Orthopedics 1995;18(5):463–471.

15

Orthotics and Exercise in the Management of Scoliosis

Thomas M. Harrigan

The goal of this chapter is to provide insight into the diagnosis and treatment of idiopathic and neuromuscular scoliosis. A thorough knowledge of the natural history of this disease is critical if health professionals are to understand fully the process of orthotic prescription for patients with scoliosis. We discuss the roles of the orthotist and therapist, as well as the goals of bracing and exercise. We also explore the process of evaluation and the options for conservative and surgical treatment options for management of patients with scoliosis.

HISTORICAL PERSPECTIVE: SPINAL TRACTION AND THE ADVENT OF BRACING

With all the advances in medical technology, it is easy to forget that many of today's most common ailments have been identified and treated for thousands of years. Hippocrates (born 460 BC) first described the signs and symptoms of scoliosis 2,400 years ago and noted that curvature of the spine occurred even in individuals who were in apparently good health.[1] Hippocrates also described the use of spinal traction to straighten the spine in scoliosis, a concept that may have its roots in ancient Egypt. The use of traction for spinal problems has led to numerous surgical and nonsurgical treatment approaches. Galen (131–200 AD) was the first to use the terms *scoliosis*, *kyphosis*, and *lordosis*; he also used traction in the treatment of this deforming condition.

Sayre, in 1874, first applied a cast to a patient with spinal deformity who was under traction. In 1895, Brackett and Bradford developed a distraction frame that was the precursor to the currently used Risser casting frame.[2,3] Hibbs and Risser developed and used hinged or turnbuckle casts in the 1920s.[4] In 1944, the Milwaukee brace was developed by Drs. Blount and Schmidt (Figure 15-1). This brace, a cervicothoracolumbosacral orthosis (CTLSO), was initially used as a postoperative modality, but it soon found a more important role. Since 1954, it has been used in the nonoperative treatment of idiopathic scoliosis.[5] The initial design incorporated distraction; however, this has since been modified secondary to problems with malocclusion of the jaw.[6]

Subsequent to the Milwaukee brace, a variety of low-profile thoracolumbosacral orthoses (TLSOs) have been introduced. Most of these spinal orthoses are named for the city where they were developed; the Boston brace, the Miami orthosis, the Wilmington brace, and the Lyon brace are examples among many. These spinal orthoses share one characteristic: All control the alignment of the thoracolumbosacral spine but have no superstructure for the cervical spine. The Boston brace was developed in the 1970s by Hall and Miller.[7] Although other biomechanically sound brace systems function well in controlling curve progression, the Boston brace system is more globally accepted (Figure 15-2). As a result of its frequent use, far more long-term data are available to substantiate the merits of the Boston brace than are available for other orthoses.[8-10] Despite the confusion regarding the brace name and style, most TLSOs that are designed for patients with scoliosis follow similar principles of prescription, wearing schedules, and discontinuance.

TERMINOLOGY AND CLASSIFICATION OF SCOLIOSIS

The Scoliosis Research Society has adopted a set of terms and definitions to describe the multitude of spinal conditions that can lead to scoliosis.[11-13] Curves can be described either by etiology of the structural changes (summarized in Table 15-1) or by the spinal level of the anatomic apex of the curve.

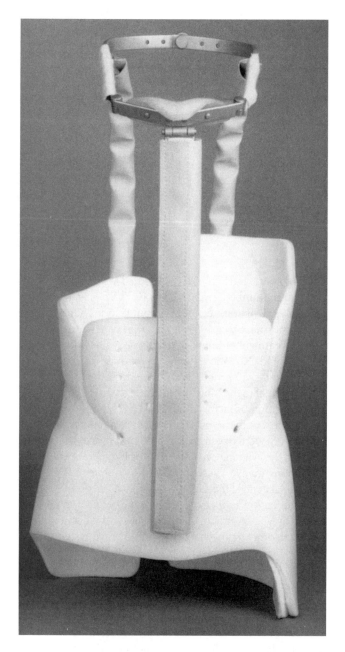

FIGURE 15-1

Milwaukee brace. Note the tightly fitting pelvic section and the suprastructure with its ring-like chin and occipital supports.

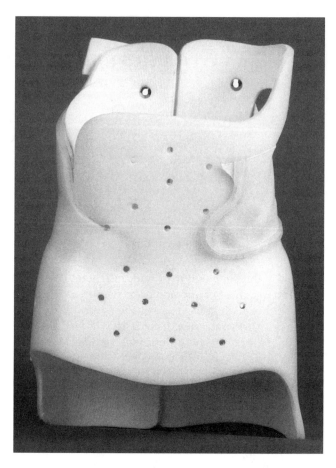

FIGURE 15-2

An example of the Boston brace, designed for patients with a thoracic curve.

liosis, and are summarized in Table 15-2. These standards and definitions are used in the discussion of management of scoliosis throughout this chapter.

IDIOPATHIC SCOLIOSIS

The etiology of idiopathic scoliosis is unclear even though many theories have been raised and many studies have investigated potential contributing factors. The possible role of genetic factors, growth velocity, musculoskeletal irregularities such as ligamentous imbalances across vertebral segments, muscle strength imbalances, vestibular and central nervous system dysfunction, and biochemical factors have all been explored, but no explanatory model has evolved.[14–22] Lonstein[23] suggests that the etiology of scoliosis must be multifactoral, with two underlying mechanisms at work, one related to the curve development and the second related to curve progression.

In a cervical scoliosis, the apex of the curve is at or between the vertebral body of C1 and C6. In a cervicothoracic curve, the apex is at C7, C8, or T1. A thoracic curve has an apex at or between T2 and T11. A thoracolumbar curve reaches its apex at the T12 or L1 vertebral body. A lumbar curve occurs at L2, L3, or L4, whereas a lumbosacral curve reaches its apex at L5 or S1. A number of descriptive terms are also used in the diagnosis, evaluation, and management of sco-

It is likely that each of the many potential contributors that have been investigated (growth, genetic, chemical, biomechanical, and neuromuscular) may be involved and that the interrelationship of these factors determines whether a curve is progressive or nonprogressive.[23]

Prevalence and Natural History of Idiopathic Scoliosis

Effective intervention and management of scoliosis are founded on an understanding of the prevalence and the natural history of the disease. Idiopathic scoliosis has been studied and documented for many years. Epidemiologic studies have documented that, with few exceptions, the prevalence of scoliosis is constant worldwide.[24] Prevalence does vary by age group, type of scoliosis, and magnitude of curve. In their examination of school-aged children, Lonstein et al.[25] reported that a structural scoliosis was identified in 1.1% of subjects.[25] In looking at the distribution of idiopathic scoliosis in a group of patients categorized by age at onset, Risenborough and Wynne-Davies[26] report that 0.5% were classified as having infantile scoliosis, 10.5% had juvenile onset, and 89% had onset in adolescence. It is likely that the juvenile group is under-represented, because many children are not carefully evaluated until they become adolescents. The distribution of curve magnitude also varies: The prevalence of "small" curves (between 10 and 20 degrees) is 20–30 per 1,000, the prevalence of moderate curves (between 20 and 30 degrees) is 3–5 per 1,000, and the prevalence of large curves (more than 30 degrees) is 2–3 per 1,000 people.[21]

Studies of the *infantile idiopathic scoliosis* population (with onset between birth and 3 years of age) suggest a genetic tendency in the development of scoliosis. A gender difference is also seen in infantile scoliosis, with a greater incidence among male than female infants. The most common pattern is a left thoracic curve. Fortunately, the condition is quite rare and is usually self-limiting, with 80–90% of the infantile scoliosis curves resolving spontaneously.[27,28] Infantile scoliosis can be divided into two types: a resolving or a progressive curve. In 1972, Mehta[29] observed that the progressive and resolving curves could be differentiated by examining the rib vertebral angle difference (RVAD). In a normal spine, no difference is found between the left and right angles, and the relationship between rib and vertebra is symmetric. A child with scoliosis has asymmetry, and the RVAD is measured as the difference between the rib vertebral angle of the concave and convex ribs of the apical vertebra. Mehta also describes two phases of rib deformity. In phase I, the convex rib head does not overlap the vertebral body, whereas in phase II an overlap can be seen. Resolving curves are found to have a phase I configuration and an RVAD of less than 20 degrees.

TABLE 15-1
Classification System for Structural Scoliosis

Idiopathic
Infantile (0–3 yr)
Resolving
Progressive
Juvenile (3–10 yr)
Adolescent (>10 yr)
Neuromuscular
Neuropathic
Upper motor neuron
Cerebral palsy
Spinocerebellar degeneration
Friedreich's ataxia
Charcot-Marie-Tooth disease
Roussy-Lévy disease
Syringomyelia
Spinal cord tumor
Spinal cord trauma
Other
Lower motor neuron
Poliomyelitis
Other viral myelitides
Trauma
Spinal muscular atrophy
Werdnig-Hoffmann disease
Kugelberg-Welander disease
Myelomeningocele (paralytic)
Dysautonomia (Riley-Day syndrome)
Other
Myopathic
Arthrogryposis
Muscular dystrophy
Duchenne's (pseudohypertrophy)
Limb-girdle
Fiber-type disproportion
Congenital hypotonia
Myotonic dystrophica
Other

Juvenile idiopathic scoliosis manifests between the ages of 4 and 10 years and accounts for between 11% and 16% of all idiopathic scoliosis. Prevalence varies by gender across age subgroups: Distribution is fairly equal among male and female children between 4 and 6 years, whereas it is more frequent in girls between 7 and 10 years of age. The most commonly observed pattern in juvenile idiopathic scoliosis is a right thoracic curve.[30]

In *adolescent idiopathic scoliosis*, the curve manifests after the age of 10 years. This is a fairly common condition, affecting approximately 1% of all children.[21,25] The prevalence of curves progressively increases in girls as the curve magnitude increases: The overall female-male ratio within this group is 3.6:1.0, but it increases to 6.4:1.0 when curve magnitude is 20 degrees or more.[24] The single right thoracic curve is the most common pattern among adolescents with idiopathic scoliosis.[31]

TABLE 15-2

Glossary and Definitions of Terms in Scoliosis

Term	Definition
Adolescent scoliosis	Spinal curvature presenting at or about the onset of puberty and before maturity
Adult scoliosis	Spinal curvature that develops after skeletal maturity
Angle of thoracic inclination	With the trunk flexed 90 degrees at the hips, this is the angle between the horizontal plane and a plane across the posterior rib cage at the greatest prominence of a rib hump
Apical vertebra	The most rotated vertebra in a curve; the most deviated vertebra from the vertical axis of the patient
Body alignment	(1) Alignment of the midpoint of the occiput over the sacrum in the same vertical plane as the shoulders over the hips; (2) in radiography, when the sum of the angular deviations of the spine in one direction is equal to that in the opposite direction (also described as balance or compensation)
Café au lait spots	Light-brown, irregular areas of skin pigmentation; if they are sufficient in number and have smooth margins, they suggest neurofibromatosis
Cobb angle or method (curve measurement)	On x-ray, the uppermost and lowermost vertebrae in the curve are identified; a perpendicular line is drawn from the transverse axes of these vertebrae, and the angle formed at their intersection (Cobb angle) measures the severity of the curve; if vertebral end plates are poorly visualized, a line through the bottom or top of the pedicles can be used
Compensatory curve	A curve, which can be structural, above or below the major curve that tends to maintain normal body alignment
Congenital scoliosis	Scoliosis due to congenitally anomalous vertebral development
Double major scoliosis	Scoliosis with two structural curves
Double thoracic curves	Two structural curves within the thoracic spine
End vertebra	(1) Uppermost vertebra of a curve, the superior surface of which tilts maximally toward the concavity of the curve; (2) the most caudal vertebra, the inferior surface of which tilts maximally toward the concavity of the curve
Fractional curve	Compensatory curve that is incomplete because it returns to the erect; its only horizontal vertebra is its caudad or cephalad one
Full curve	Curve in which the only horizontal vertebra is at the apex
Gibbus	Sharply angular kyphos
Hyperkyphosis	Sagittal alignment of the thoracic spine in which more than the normal amount of kyphosis is present (a kyphos)
Hypokyphosis	Sagittal alignment of the thoracic spine in which less than the normal amount of kyphosis is present but not so severe as to be lordotic
Hysterical scoliosis	Nonstructural deformity of the spine that develops as a manifestation of a conversion reaction
Idiopathic scoliosis	Structural spinal curvature for which no cause is established
Iliac epiphysis or apophysis	Epiphysis along the wing of an ilium
Inclinometer	Instrument used to measure the angle of thoracic inclination or rib hump
Infantile scoliosis	Spinal curvature that develops during the first 3 yr of life
Juvenile scoliosis	Spinal curvature that develops between the skeletal age of 3 yr and the onset of puberty (10 years)
Kyphos	Change in alignment of a segment of the spine in the sagittal plane that increases the posterior convex angulation; an abnormally increased kyphosis
Kyphoscoliosis	Spine with scoliosis and a true hyperkyphosis; a rotatory deformity with only apparent kyphosis should not be described by this term
Kyphosing scoliosis	Scoliosis with marked rotation such that lateral bending of the rotated spine mimics kyphosis
Lordoscoliosis	Scoliosis associated with an abnormal anterior angulation in the sagittal plane
Major curve	Term used to designate the largest structural curve
Minor curve	Term used to refer to the smallest curve, which is always more flexible than the major curve
Nonstructural curve	Curve that has no structural component and that corrects or overcorrects on recumbent side-bending radiographs
Pelvic obliquity	Deviation of the pelvis from the horizontal in the frontal plane; fixed pelvic obliquities can be attributable to contractures either above or below the pelvis
Primary curve	First or earliest of several curves to appear, if identifiable
Risser sign	Rating system used to indicate skeletal maturity, based on degree of ossification of the iliac epiphysis
Rotational prominence	In the forward-bending position, the thoracic prominence on one side is usually due to vertebral rotation, causing rib prominence; in the lumbar spine, the prominence is usually due to rotation of the lumbar vertebrae
Skeletal age (bone age)	Age obtained by comparing an anteroposterior radiograph of the left hand and wrist with the standards of Gruelich and Pyle's atlas[52]
Structural curve	Segment of the spine with a lateral curvature that lacks normal flexibility; radiographically, it is identified by the complete lack of a curve on a supine film or by the failure to demonstrate complete segmental mobility on supine side-bending films

Term	Definition
Vertebral end plates	Superior and inferior plates of cortical bone of the vertebral body adjacent to the intervertebral disk
Vertebral growth plate	Cartilaginous surface covering the top and bottom of a vertebral body, which is responsible for linear growth of the vertebra
Vertebral ring apophyses	Most reliable index of vertebral immaturity, seen best in lateral radiographs or in the lumbar region in side-bending anteroposterior views

Three important predictors for curve progression have been identified: curve pattern, age, menarche status, and a positive Risser sign.[32-34] Curve flexibility and decompensation may be important, although the evidence is not conclusive. Lonstein and Carlson's work[32] examining the natural history of this condition has furthered our ability to predict the likelihood of progression (Tables 15-3 and 15-4). Risk for progression increases if the initial curve occurs before the onset of menstruation, as the magnitude of the curve increases, the younger the age at diagnosis, and if a double curve pattern is present. Patients whose curves measure less than 30 degrees at skeletal maturity tend not to progress regardless of curve pattern. The amount of vertebral rotation appears to be related to further progression into adulthood. Curves of more than 30 degrees with apical vertebral rotation greater than 25% are twice as likely to progress. Thoracic curves that measure between 50 and 75 degrees progress the most rapidly, at a rate of 0.75–1.0% per year.[35]

TREATMENT OF IDIOPATHIC SCOLIOSIS

The preceding information about the natural history of scoliosis assists the clinician in answering two important questions: (1) Is the curve likely to progress in a patient who has not yet reached skeletal maturity? (2) If a patient has reached skeletal maturity, will the curve progress into adulthood? Based on the answer to these questions, the physician, orthotist, and therapist can choose one of three options: (1) to observe the curve's status carefully over time, (2) to manage the patient's scoliosis nonoperatively with a spinal orthosis and exercise, or (3) to intervene surgically to correct the curve.

For patients with curves of less than 25 degrees, careful observation is recommended. Typically, patients are reevaluated every 6 months, including recording height and weight, using radiography (x-ray) to measure curve progression accurately, and estimating time until skeletal maturity might be reached.

When a patient's curve progresses beyond 25 degrees, or if the curve has increased 5 or more degrees over the 6-month interval, a spinal orthosis is prescribed and an exercise program is implemented. All skeletally immature children who initially present with a curve between 30 and 45 degrees are managed with an orthosis and exercise. Bracing is usually contraindicated for skeletally mature individuals, as well as for those who present with curves of more than 45 degrees or less than 25 degrees without documented progression. Use of an orthosis is also contraindicated in the presence of thoracic lordosis.[23] Depending on the location of the curve(s), the orthotist will recommend either a Milwaukee brace (CTLSO) or a low-profile TLSO style orthosis, such as the Boston brace.

Although the efficacy of orthoses in the management of idiopathic scoliosis has been controversial, long-term and multicenter studies suggest that bracing is an effective intervention. In 1994, an important report by Lonstein and Winter[36] documented their experience in treating adolescent

TABLE 15-3

Incidence of Progression as It Relates to the Magnitude of the Curve and Risser Sign

	Percentage of Curves That Progressed	
Risser Sign	5- to 19-Degree Curves	20- to 29-Degree Curves
Grade 0 or 1	22	68
Grade 2, 3, or 4	1.6	23

Source: Reprinted with permission from JE Lonstein, M Carlson. Prediction of curve progression in untreated scoliosis during growth. J Bone Joint Surg 1984;66A:1061–1071.

TABLE 15-4

Incidence of Progression as Related to Magnitude of the Curve and the Age of the Patient When First Seen

	Percentage of Curves That Progressed[a]	
Age when First Seen (yr)	5- to 19-Degree Curves	20- to 29-Degree Curves
10 and younger	45 (38)	100 (10)[b]
11–12	23 (147)	61 (61)
13–14	8 (201)	37 (119)
15 and older	4 (67)	16 (84)

[a]Numbers in parentheses indicate the number of patients in each group.
[b]Note that this figure of 100% is based on only 10 patients.
Source: Reprinted with permission from JE Lonstein, M Carlson. Prediction of curve progression in untreated scoliosis during growth. J Bone Joint Surg 1984;66A:1061–1071.

idiopathic scoliosis with Milwaukee bracing and compared their orthoses-based outcome to those of previously published natural history studies. Unsuccessful orthotic outcome (rate of failure) was defined as a curve progression of 5 degrees or more at final follow-up or progression to surgery. In Lonstein and Winter's sample, 40% of patients with initial curves of less than 30 degrees and Risser signs of 0 and 1 "failed," as compared to 68% in the natural history studies. For patients with Risser signs of 2 or more, the failure rate with the Milwaukee brace was 10%, as compared to 23% in the natural history studies. Rates of failure were found to be less in the 30- to 39-degree group as well.[36]

Nachemson et al.,[9] in 1995, reported the results of a multicenter prospective study of brace efficacy that compared the effect of treatment with observation only versus underarm TLSO on skeletally immature girls with adolescent idiopathic scoliosis.[9] Patients in the study had right thoracic or thoracolumbar curves of 25–35 degrees. The rate of failure for those who wore the orthosis was 19%, versus 50% in the observation-only group. Overall, the use of the orthosis was 40% more effective than treatment with observation alone. Montgomery and Willner[34] report an almost 300% greater risk of failure among patients when orthotic intervention was initiated after the curve had progressed 45 degrees or more, as compared to interventions initiated when curves measured between 25 and 35 degrees. No other nonoperative treatment besides bracing has been shown to alter the natural history of idiopathic scoliosis. Nachemson's multicenter study also examined transcutaneous electrical stimulation versus observation only and found that the curves treated with transcutaneous electrical stimulation only progressed to surgery at a rate equal to those that were observed only.[9] The brace wear group was the only group that demonstrated a significant change from the natural history.

Goals of Orthotic Intervention

The primary goal of orthotic intervention in idiopathic scoliosis is prevention of further progression. Orthotic intervention does not result in permanent correction of spinal alignment. The orthosis is designed to stabilize the curve through growth until skeletal maturity is reached. Most studies report that the curve magnitude after bracing is approximately the same as the prebracing curve; the important outcome is arresting or forestalling progression of the curve.[8,37–39]

In-Brace Curve Correction

Most orthotists strive to fabricate an orthosis that is able to achieve as much curve correction as possible while the patient is wearing it. This goal is based on the premise that passive curve reduction lessens abnormal forces acting on the spine and that this external stability minimizes the likelihood of curve progression. Ideally, the goal is 100% correction within the brace. In reality, factors such as inflexibility of the curve and skin tolerance to pad pressure limit complete correction. An important predictive factor for successful orthotic outcome is degree of initial in-brace correction.[40,41] Fifty percent initial in-brace correction appears to be the minimum necessary to achieve the desired long-term orthotic outcome.[8,39]

Spinal Balance

Little clinical evidence has supported the need to achieve complete spinal balance or compensation while the brace is being worn. It seems that bending movements would be decreased when the head and mass of the body are centered over the pelvis. Biomechanical modeling demonstrates that decompensation does have a destabilizing effect.[42] For this reason, attention to spinal balance is important in brace design and fitting. Additional components, such as an axillary sling on a Milwaukee brace or an axillary extension on a Boston brace, may effectively address this issue.

Derotation

Correction of the abnormal rotation of spinal segments is an additional goal of orthotic intervention in scoliosis. It is important to note that the relationship of lateral curvature to rotation is not 1:1. Because of the three-dimensional nature of scoliosis deformity, when lateral curvature is reduced, the magnitude of the rotation deformity is also reduced. The goal of orthotic intervention is to reduce the rotational deformity to zero while the patient is wearing the brace. The Boston brace system that is used to manage thoracic curves may incorporate posterolaterally positioned derotational pads to provide sagittal and coronal plane corrective forces. Such forces act to reduce lateral curvature and abnormal rotation of the vertebrae.

One of the problems associated with idiopathic scoliosis is hypokyphosis. Some evidence has been found that use of an orthosis may be a contributor to this limitation.[43,44] Because of the risk of further loss of kyphosis in the spine that is already hypokyphotic, the posterior component of the thoracic pad has been eliminated in most brace designs. Although forces are aimed at achieving lateral correction, any decrease in Cobb angle also results in a decrease in the rotational deformity.[45] Because spinal rotation is so difficult to measure, however, the efficacy of these techniques cannot be fully evaluated. One method that is used to approximate measurement of vertebral rotation is assessment of trunk shape. It appears that rib hump deformity associated with vertebral rotation is not greatly influenced by the brace, although cosmetic appearance can be improved.[45,46]

Delaying Surgical Spinal Fusion

For children and adolescents with significant or large curves, the goal of orthotic intervention is to minimize the risk of rapid curve progression and to delay the need for surgical intervention. This delay is important so that the child can achieve as much height (trunk height) as possible before spinal fusion. Because only 80% of trunk stature is achieved by age 10, this delay is especially important in very young patients, so that skeletal growth can continue as long as possible.[47] Orthotic intervention is important, even when future surgical correction is predicted; efficacy of surgical correction of the curve may be enhanced when less soft tissue contracture and vertebral deformity are present in small presurgical curves.

Prevention of Curve Progression

The primary goal of any orthosis used in the treatment of idiopathic scoliosis should be prevention, or at least minimization of curve progression for patients with skeletal immaturity, through the entire growth period until skeletal maturity can be documented.

The risk of curve progression is best understood from a biomechanical perspective. The spine functions as a flexible column. All flexible structures have an upper load limit; when this limit is exceeded, plastic deformation begins to occur. Unlike a straight or rigid column that quickly reaches the point of failure and rapidly collapses when overloaded, the spine slowly bends as it collapses; that is, a plastic deformation of the spinal column occurs. Critical load is the point at which the spine begins to bend and deformation commences. As curve magnitude increases, magnitude of critical loading is reduced, and deformation becomes more likely. Critical load rapidly drops as curves progress past 25 degrees; as a result, the rate of curve progression increases as the magnitude of the curve increases. An orthosis is designed to stiffen the spine artificially, reducing the curve, raising the critical load, and substantially reducing the likelihood of additional plastic deformation. Consider a curve with an initial deformity of 30 degrees: With orthotic correction (reduction) of this curve to 20 degrees, critical load increases from 50% to 80% of normal (erect stance). For patients with large and less correctable curves, however, critical load is not sufficiently influenced by the orthosis. In curves of 45 degrees, critical load is approximately 20% of normal. Unless the curve can be reduced at least 50% by wearing the orthosis, the minimal improvement in critical load will be insufficient to forestall further deformation and progression of the curve.[42]

The Milwaukee brace and most of the low-profile orthoses that are used to treat idiopathic scoliosis (e.g., Boston or Miami braces) use similar biomechanical principles to achieve the goals of end-point control, curve correction, and continuous transverse support.[48] The degree of correction is dependent on four factors: the positioning of the pad, the magnitude of the corrective force applied by the pad, the direction of the applied force, and the duration that these forces are applied. The effectiveness of the pads is limited by the physical characteristics of the underlying tissue, specifically the tissue's ability to transmit and tolerate the forces that are necessary for curve correction. The location of the apex of the curve is the critical determinant of which style of orthosis is prescribed. Curves with an apex at or above the seventh thoracic vertebra most often require the Milwaukee style CTLSO, whereas curves below the seventh thoracic vertebra are effectively managed with a TLSO. Factors that must also be considered in orthotic prescription include skeletal age and curve magnitude. For primary thoracic curves, maximum stability is achieved with the CTLSO; the TLSO is as much as 25% less effective.[48] For patients at high risk of curve progression (e.g., a patient with an idiopathic juvenile scoliosis curve of 40 degrees or more), the CTLSO is often a better choice because of its biomechanical advantage for in-brace curve correction when compared to a TLSO. The likelihood of compliance or orthotic acceptance by the child and parents must be weighed against optimal biomechanics: A Milwaukee brace that achieves excellent correction but is worn sporadically because of compromised cosmesis will not be an effective intervention. In this case, the slightly less efficient TLSO may be preferable if it will be worn consistently.

SURGICAL MANAGEMENT OF IDIOPATHIC SCOLIOSIS

For a number of patients with scoliosis, the curve progresses despite compliant brace wear. For those patients in whom nonoperative treatment has not been successful, surgical management of the curve must be considered. Curves that progress beyond 40 degrees in skeletally immature patients and beyond 50 degrees in those who have reached full skeletal maturity typically require surgery.[35] Surgery for scoliosis has four goals: to achieve the maximally prudent curve reduction, to achieve spinal balance postoperatively, to provide spinal stabilization by arthrodesis, and to arrest further curve progression at the fusion site. The first successful spine surgery for scoliosis was performed by Hibbs in 1911. Since then, surgical technique and instrumentation have advanced significantly. Harrington distraction and compression rods, first used in 1962, became the standard for operative intervention for patients with scoliosis. Other surgical techniques and procedures can also be

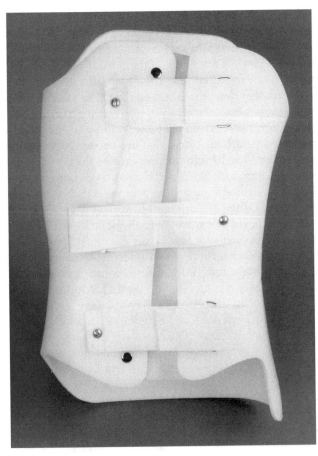

FIGURE 15-3

Example of a postoperative, anterior-opening, total contact thoracolumbosacral orthosis. The shell of this particular orthosis is polyethylene, with a foam lining. This type of orthosis is prescribed when passive rigid control is desired.

used in surgical management of scoliosis, such as the Luque segmental, Cotrel and Duboussett, and Texas Scottish-Rite techniques. A study by McMaster[49] compared the Harrington and Luque techniques; frontal correction was found to be similar in the two groups, but those who received Luque segmental instrumentation demonstrated better sagittal contouring and less loss of correction. These newer types of instruments, combined with increased attention to the improvement of sagittal contouring, have resulted in better postoperative outcomes.

Orthoses and Physical Therapy in Surgical Management

Many children are managed postoperatively with a custom-fit, total contact TLSO (Figure 15-3). These orthoses serve a protective function; the goal is to limit gross move-

ment of the trunk, thereby reducing stress on the new surgical hardware and bony implants. The orthotist usually measures or casts the patient for the orthosis on the first or second postoperative day. Unless significant asymmetries are present in the trunk and pelvis, a TLSO can be fabricated from accurate circumferential and length measurements of the patient's trunk. In the presence of significant asymmetry, however, the patient must be molded with plaster of Paris to achieve a comfortable and well-functioning orthosis.

It is helpful if the physical therapist is able to complete a preoperative assessment of posture, range of motion (ROM), strength, and respiratory function. Preoperative review of breathing exercises, postural drainage positions, effective coughing techniques, and use of proper body mechanics can be helpful in lessening postoperative morbidity. In many settings, however, referral to physical therapy occurs after surgery, and the therapist becomes involved in the early postoperative management of these patients. Instruction in breathing exercises, effective coughing, and (if necessary) postural drainage, as well as practice of proper body mechanics and mobility training, is typically part of early postoperative physical therapy management. In many settings, patients begin to get out of bed and resume limited functional activities within 2–3 days after surgery, and discharge occurs within a week after operation. Physical and occupational therapists also assess the need for adaptive equipment, potential architectural barriers to mobility, and the need for additional services at home.

EVALUATION STRATEGIES

When a patient with scoliosis is referred to an orthotist or physical therapist, the first step in the evaluation process is a thorough history, which includes the following: (1) when the curve was first noticed (onset of the curve); (2) who made the initial diagnosis and what circumstances led to its diagnosis; (3) which, if any, tests have been performed; (4) the family's health history, especially related to spinal dysfunction; and (5) the patient's current age, physical maturity, and overall health. Information about previous interventions (treatment history) and their outcomes should be collected. Finally, the presence of pain must be determined, including its nature, location, and management strategies.

Clinical Evaluation

Clinical evaluation of patients with scoliosis begins with a careful examination of posture. With the patient standing in a relaxed or typical posture, the orthotist or therapist notes frontal plane symmetry/asymmetry and alignment of the trunk, the patient's typical head and neck position, shoulder height, and scapular alignment. The fullness or relative muscle bulk in the muscles of the shoulder girdle and of the paraspinal muscle groups is noted, as is the shape of the chest wall. Symmetry/asymmetry of the pelvis is indicated by comparing positions of the height of posterosuperior iliac spines and iliac crests. Leg length is assessed by observing symmetry of left and right popliteal creases while both knees are fully extended and the feet are flat on the floor. Postural assessment in the sagittal plane includes observation and measurement of cervical and lumbar lordosis as well as thoracic and sacral kyphosis.

Truncal decompensation (trunk balance) describes the relative position of the head with respect to the sacrum: the horizontal distance between a plumb line dropped from the center of the occiput and a plumb line dropped from the spinous process of the first sacral vertebra (Figure 15-4). The Adams test, which assesses rotation deformity, is another important component of the evaluation. In this functional test, the patient begins in standing with the knees straight, feet together, and hands together with palms and fingers in opposition and then bends forward from the waist (Figure 15-5). The examiner views the spine from anterior, posterior, and lateral points of view, so that symmetry/asymmetry and rotation of the cervical, thoracic, and lumbar spine can be fully assessed. A scoliometer is a tool that, when placed at the point of maximal prominence, measures the degree of rotational deformity when it is placed at the position of maximal prominence (Figure 15-6).

The flexibility of the spinal deformity is also assessed in the Adams test maximum trunk flexion position. The examiner stabilizes the patient's pelvis and then asks the patient to side bend to the left and then to the right, applying a gentle passive force at the end of the active range. This provides information about the extent of unbending and derotation that may be possible for the patient's particular curve. The relative stiffness of the curve provides information about the structural features of the deformity. It is important to note that the accuracy of the forward bend test can be influenced by limitations in muscle length, especially if hamstring or erector spinae tightness is present.[50] It is important, therefore, to include assessment of lower extremity ROM as part of the evaluation, including special tests (e.g., the Thomas test for hip flexion tightness or contracture and straight leg raise testing for hamstring length). Limitations in normal ROM of the lower extremities often influence brace wear and comfort. For example, the pelvic modules for the Milwaukee or Boston braces are fabricated with 15 degrees of lordosis and position the pelvis during wearing in a posterior pelvic tilt. If significant tightness of the iliopsoas muscle is present, patients

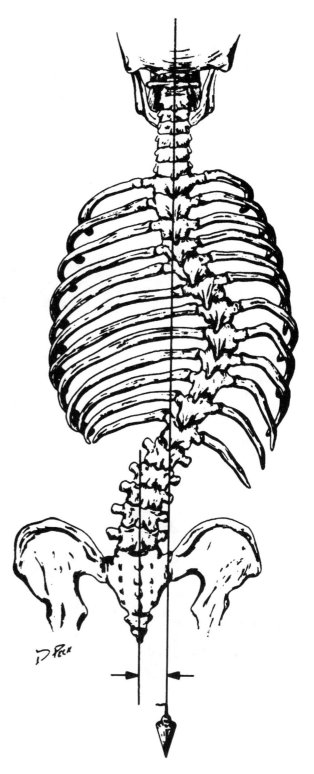

FIGURE 15-4

In this diagram of a right thoracic curve, the occiput is aligned well to the right of the first sacral spinous process. Because of its relative position to the right with respect to S1, the patient would be described as being decompensated to the right.

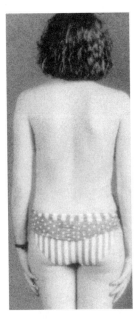

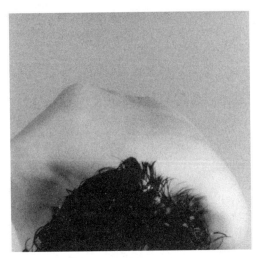

FIGURE 15-5

In the Adams test of maximum trunk flexion, the patient bends forward from the waist, keeping the knees straight and feet flat on the floor. Note that a spine that appears relatively symmetric in quiet standing is obviously asymmetric once the patient with idiopathic scoliosis bends forward. Rib hump is a consequence of abnormal rotation of the involved vertebral bodies. The examiner determines the point of maximum prominence by observing from the front, from behind, and from each side.

may not be able to achieve the desired pelvic position with a comfortable erect standing posture. Instead, they will stand with slight knee flexion to relieve tension on the hip flexor group and then attempt to align their center of mass by extending their trunk over the superior/posterior edge of the brace. In addition to being uncomfortable, it is possible that this posture within the orthosis could be inducing hypokyphosis.[44]

Other measurements that are taken during the initial evaluation include leg length, muscle girth, muscle strength of the trunk and lower extremities, and neurologic assessment, including a check of abdominal reflexes. Absent or diminished reflexes may be a sign of intraspinal pathology.[23] Evaluation of the skin and soft tissue is also necessary to determine if underlying neurologic conditions, such as neurofibromatosis or myelodysplasia, which present with a variety of skin irregularities, such as café au lait skin pigmentation and hair patches over the spine, are present.

Radiographs

The radiograph, or x-ray, is an essential clinical tool in diagnosis and treatment of idiopathic scoliosis. It is used to determine specifically the type and location of the curve and to quantify its magnitude and the degree of rotation. The radiograph is also used to assess trunk balance or decompensation and to determine skeletal age based on either the Risser sign or wrist/hand bone age. Congenital spinal malformations are detected by close inspection of the films. Radiographs taken while the patient is in the orthosis allow the clinician to determine immediately the appropriateness of pad positions and overall efficacy in terms of curve reduction.

Several important prognostic indicators for curve progression in scoliosis are based on radiographs. The Risser sign describes skeletal maturity based on the degree of ossification of the epiphysis of crest of the ilium. Ossification begins at the anterosuperior iliac spine and progresses posteriorly. The iliac crest is divided into four quarters, and

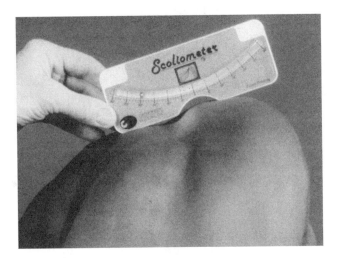

FIGURE 15-6

A scoliometer can be used to measure the degree of rotation of thoracic or lumbar curves. The device is placed on the most rotated part of the curve, as determined by observation in the Adams test of maximum trunk flexion. The scoliometer is a gauged device that functions similar to a builder's level.

the excursion or stage of maturity is designated as the amount of progression from the anterosuperior to the posterosuperior iliac spine. The curve magnitude is often measured using the Cobb technique (Figure 15-7). Bone age can be accurately determined by comparing the left wrist/hand radiograph to that of Gruelich and Pyle's atlas,[51] and vertebral rotation can be graded using a system described by Nash and Moe[52] (Figure 15-8).

Other tests, such as magnetic resonance imaging (MRI), are not routinely used in assessment of patients with scoliosis, unless evaluative findings are inconsistent or complex. One indication for MRI or other special testing is a finding of asymmetric or diminished lower extremity and abdominal reflexes; another is a suspicious or very unusual curve pattern. Patients with left thoracic curve patterns may be referred for MRI because this group of patients has a 20% incidence of intraspinal pathology (e.g., Arnold-Chiari malformation).[53]

ROLE OF EXERCISE

Exercise programs have long been used and recommended in the treatment of idiopathic scoliosis.[54] Historically, exercise has had an important role as an adjunct to the prescription of the Milwaukee brace as a form of non-surgical management of scoliosis.[37,38,55] Treatment with the Boston brace and other low-profile TLSOs such as the Wilmington, Miami, or Cuxhaven also uses exercise protocols.[8,44,56-58] Although exercise programs vary between institutions and the type of brace, exercise alone does not have a significant influence on the natural history of idiopathic scoliosis.[59,60] Because no conclusive studies have justified the efficacy of exercise, some physicians believe that ordering exercise programs as part of a routine protocol is unnecessary. Underlying this approach are beliefs that compliance to prescribed exercise protocols is usually poor, and muscle strength, ROM, and respiratory capacity can be maintained without specific exercise with the encouragement of a high-level activity for out-of-brace time. Many physicians, therapists, and orthotists recognize the importance of the role of exercise as an adjunct to nonoperative treatment with an orthosis in the management of patients with scoliosis. Typically, a physical therapist performs a comprehensive evaluation of muscle function, posture, respiratory function, and daily activities and, based on findings, identifies existing and potential problems, establishes functional and preventative goals, and formulates a plan of care. The exercise program is created to target impairments or functional limitations for each individual patient with scoliosis. Exercise programs must be concise, reasonable, and simple to perform

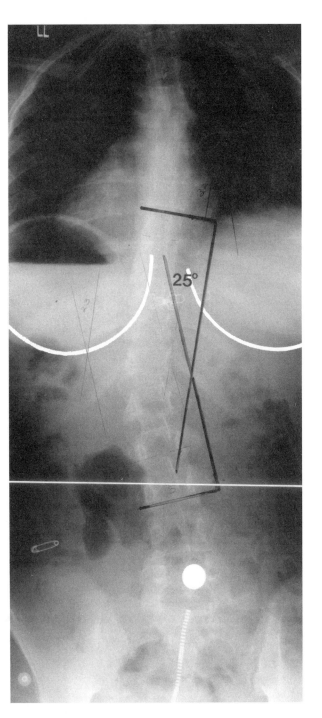

FIGURE 15-7

In the Cobb method of measuring curvature, a perpendicular line is drawn from the upper edge of the topmost vertebra that inclines most toward the concavity. A similar line is drawn from the inferior edge of the lowest vertebra with the most angulation toward the concavity. The angle at which these perpendicular lines intersect forms the Cobb angle. The apical vertebra does not enter into the measurement. The Cobb angle is usually measured directly on the radiograph.

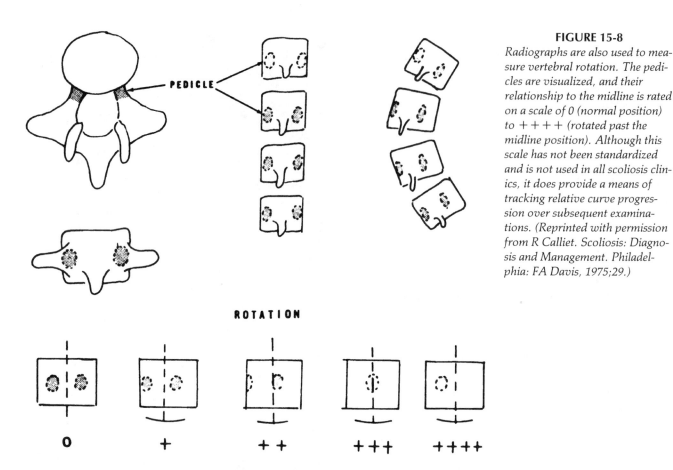

ROTATION

FIGURE 15-8
Radiographs are also used to measure vertebral rotation. The pedicles are visualized, and their relationship to the midline is rated on a scale of 0 (normal position) to + + + + (rotated past the midline position). Although this scale has not been standardized and is not used in all scoliosis clinics, it does provide a means of tracking relative curve progression over subsequent examinations. (Reprinted with permission from R Calliet. Scoliosis: Diagnosis and Management. Philadelphia: FA Davis, 1975;29.)

so that the potential for noncompliance can be minimized. Typically, patients and their families may be seen by the physical therapist for initial instruction and then for follow-up visits scheduled over a longer period of time so that progress and compliance can be more easily ascertained. The overall goals of an exercise program for patients with scoliosis are summarized in Table 15-5.

One of the ways that exercise enhances the efficacy of nonsurgical management of scoliosis is by focusing atten-

TABLE 15-5
Summary of Goals of Exercise Programs for Patients with Scoliosis

To develop or enhance the patient's awareness of his or her posture
To augment the function of the orthosis through active exercises done while in the brace
To enhance respiratory function and chest mobility
To improve trunk muscle strength and function
To improve, or prevent further loss, of range of motion of the spine and lower extremities
To enhance proper body mechanics and activities of daily living while wearing the orthosis

tion on building the patient's awareness of posture and alignment. Instruction in postural self-correction exercises is an important part of the treatment plan. Structural curves often create asymmetric postures, resulting in decompensation of the trunk. Patients need to understand their particular curve pattern and how it changes their normal postural alignment. Based on this understanding, they then learn which "self-correcting" movements can enhance symmetry. Often, use of a mirror for visual feedback facilitates the patient's ability to self-correct in the early stages of learning these exercises.

Brace design dictates whether in-brace exercise should be performed. For patients who are fitted with an active orthotic design, which has relief areas incorporated, self-correcting exercise programs will be most successful if the patient is able to perform these self-correcting exercises both while out of the orthosis and while wearing it. Consider the design of the Boston brace: Its most important biomechanical corrective feature is pelvic control. When the pelvis is stabilized, pads strategically placed within the orthosis can deliver effective derotation and lateral corrective forces on this stable base. The function of this orthosis is enhanced when the patient learns to perform

TABLE 15-6
Examples of Exercises for Patients with Scoliosis

Exercises to address muscle function and flexibility of the
    trunk and pelvis
        Posterior pelvic tilts, in multiple functional positions
        Abdominal exercises for upper, lower, and oblique
            muscle groups
        Anterior chest wall stretches
        Spinal stabilization and stretching into the curve
            convexity
Exercises to address the lumbopelvic relationship and lower
    extremity musculature
        Hip flexor stretches and strengthening
        Hamstring stretches and strengthening
        Iliotibial/tensor fascia latae stretches and strengthening
        Erector spinae stretches and strengthening

TABLE 15-7
*Prevalence of Spinal Deformities in Various
Neuromuscular Disorders*

Neuromuscular Disorder	*Percent with Spinal Disorder*
Cerebral palsy	25
Myelomeningocele	60
Infantile quadriplegia	100
Preadolescent quadriplegia	90
Duchenne's muscular dystrophy	95
Spinal muscular atrophy, types I, II, III	100
Friedreich's ataxia	95

Source: Reprinted with permission from JE Lonstein, TS Renshaw. Neuromuscular spine deformities. Instructional course lectures. Am Acad Orthop Surg 1987;36:285–304.

active correction of the lateral and rotatory deformity. These active exercises also serve to maintain strength and ROM of the trunk and pelvis. Patients who are fitted with passive orthotic designs typically perform self-correcting exercises only during out-of-brace times. Exercises that target muscle function, soft tissue excursion and flexibility, and postural alignment are added to the self-correcting movements as well (Table 15-6).

The effects of long-term use of an orthosis on trunk muscle strength, ROM, chest mobility, and respiratory capacity are not well documented. It seems that the prolonged use of an orthosis that encompasses much of the trunk would induce dysfunction. Although some degree of pulmonary limitation occurs even with mild to moderate curves,[61-64] decreased maximum oxygen uptake appears to be the consequence of deconditioning and lack of regular aerobic exercise and not necessarily the orthosis or the scoliosis itself.[65,66] Poor perception of health and of body image, as well as fear of injury, may contribute to inactivity and the resultant decrease in aerobic capacity.[67,68] Refsum et al.[69] suggest that, although some loss of respiratory capacity occurs while the patient is in brace in the early weeks of orthotic wear, adjustment to the orthosis appears to take place: At 6 months no significant differences were seen in cardiopulmonay function when in-brace and out-of-brace tests were compared. The lack of adequate normative data for children and adolescents describing normal ventilatory response to hypercapnia and hypoxia is problematic.

NEUROMUSCULAR SCOLIOSIS

The underlying conditions that contribute to the progressive nature of most neuromuscular curves are vastly different from those of idiopathic curves. Neuropathic curves are the result of either muscle or neurologic disease that affects the function of the muscles supporting the trunk and pelvis. Flaccidity, hypotonicity, hypertonicity, rigidity, or athetosis can create asymmetry or compromise postural stability. The prevalence of neuromuscular scoliosis varies depending on the underlying etiology (Table 15-7). Unlike idiopathic scoliosis, which typically presents in adolescence, neuromuscular scoliosis most often develops at an early age, because the neurologic or muscular diseases that underlie it are present in early childhood. Also unlike idiopathic scoliosis, most neuromuscular curves, even small ones, are progressive in nature, often increasing in severity throughout adulthood.[42,70] Curves are most likely to progress rapidly and be difficult to manage in very young patients, who will grow with compromised muscle function or abnormal tone; in patients with truncal and pelvic muscle tone asymmetries; and when progressive or severe paralysis of trunk musculature is present.

Etiology

The stiffness of the curve and its length are the most important biomechanical factors that influence curve progression of neuromuscular curves. The load-carrying capacity of a scoliotic spine decreases as stiffness of the spine decreases and length of the curve increases. The normal passive and active stiffening that affects muscles, ligaments, and disks on the spine is absent, diminished, or asymmetric in neuromuscular disorders. As a consequence, these less stiff spines are more susceptible to curvature and curve progression. As

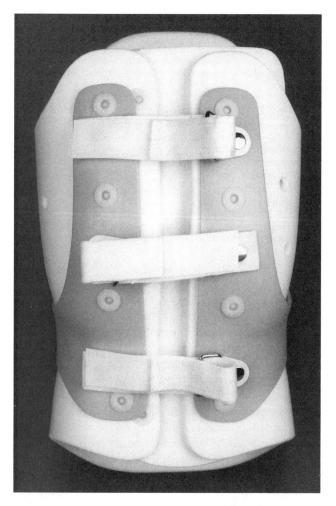

FIGURE 15-9

This accommodative, passive, total contact thoracolumbosacral orthosis, with its Aliplast (AliMed, Inc, Boston, MA) foam lining and high-density polyethylene frame, has an anterior opening and is designed to support the trunk and spine of a patient with neuromuscular scoliosis.

curve magnitude increases beyond 30 degrees, loss of stability is even more rapid. The combination of factors, such as increasing curve magnitude, trunk height, and loss of stiffness, create a situation in which curves can quickly progress.[47]

Management of Neuromuscular Scoliosis

The management of patients with neuromuscular scoliosis is, in many respects, similar to that of patients with idiopathic scoliosis, including careful observation and monitoring of curve status. Changes in curve magnitude beyond 30 degrees or changes in function indicate the need for orthotic or surgical intervention. Two important functional indicators of progression of spinal deformity are changes in the patient's ability to walk or to sit upright during functional activities.[70] Orthoses are often indicated for all neuromuscular curves that have progressed to 30 degrees or beyond. The goal of orthotic treatment is to slow the progression of the deformity and allow for continued maximal trunk height growth until surgical stabilization is indicated.

The degree of volitional trunk control is one of the determinants of orthotic design. Patients with poor trunk control most often benefit from a passive supportive orthosis, whereas those with better trunk control may benefit from an active orthosis. The passive orthosis is a total contact orthosis, based on a three-point force system in which the walls of the orthosis provide the forces that act on the spine (Figure 15-9; see Figure 15-3). These orthoses can be more or less flexible depending on the patient's skin tolerance and weight, as well as the flexibility and degree of deformity of the spine. An alternative approach is a thoracic suspension orthosis, a TLSO suspended by hooks from a seating system (Figure 15-10). This suspension creates a distractive effect on the spine as well as an unweighting of the ischial tuberosities and sacrum. This type of orthosis is most often prescribed for patients with recurrent or nonhealing sacral or ischial decubitus ulcers or for patients with significant respiratory compromise because of their underlying neuromuscular disease. Unfortunately, patients who weigh more than 40 lb are often not able to tolerate the skin pressures associated with suspension.

An active orthosis induces curve correction by passive and active forces; the walls of the orthosis act in conjunction with the patient's own muscle contractions to effect correction. Reliefs are provided in the orthosis opposite to the convexity so that rib excursion and resultant curve reduction are possible. Children with neuromuscular scoliosis are prescribed the same Boston and Milwaukee orthoses worn by those with idiopathic scoliosis if trunk function permits active correction as a component of nonsurgical management of their curves (see Figures 15-1 and 15-2).

Custom-molded seating is an orthotic alternative for individuals with neuromuscular pathologies who demonstrate poor or absent sitting and head control and for those who may be at high risk for skin breakdown. Many individuals can be effectively fit into a prefabricated, custom-fit system. Seating is often augmented by use of a TLSO: Curve management is addressed by the TLSO, and function issues are addressed with the seating. In many seating clinics, a multidisciplinary team of physical and occupational therapists, physicians, orthotists, and wheelchair vendors work with the family to create the most functional and beneficial seating arrangement. Postures assumed in the wheelchair must be carefully analyzed. It is especially important to consider weight distribution carefully to prevent skin irritation and pressure ulcer formation. Weight distribution in supported sitting is impacted by foot rest position, seat depth, chair back angulation, and altered alignment or positions when an orthosis is worn. Many of the children who require custom-fit or custom-molded seating use joystick or microswitch systems for independent mobility; joystick or microswitch position also plays a role in improving sitting posture.

Surgical Management of Neuromuscular Scoliosis

The goal of surgery is to achieve a stable well-balanced spine. The need for spinal surgery varies with the underlying neuromuscular pathology. For children with cerebral palsy, for example, the decision to operate is influenced by many factors. Children with cerebral palsy who have normal or mildly impaired cognitive function can be managed with orthotic and exercise protocols similar to those of children with idiopathic curves. Children with spastic quadriplegic cerebral palsy can be evaluated for spinal surgery when their curve impairs their ability to be functional in sitting. The nature of the curve determines surgical indications and technique, for example, the extent of spinal fusion and the use of internal fixation devices. Postoperatively, many children are placed in casts until the fusion mass solidifies. After the cast is removed, most use a TLSO for up to 1 year to protect the spine during functional activity. Early mobilization by the physical therapy team is crucial because in many cases the preoperative health and vitality of these individuals is already precarious.

SUMMARY

In this chapter we have explored the etiology of idiopathic and neuromuscular scoliosis and the biomechanical factors that contribute to curve progression. We have described a strategy for evaluation of curve severity and the special tests and measurements used in assessment of patients with scoliosis. We have discussed the use of orthoses in the nonoperative management of scoliosis, differentiating between orthoses that incorporate the cervical spine, such as the Milwaukee brace, and those that have a low-profile TLSO design, such as the Boston or Miami brace. We have discussed the role of exercise as an important adjunct to orthotic management, with the goal of facilitating self-correction of the curve and improved postural awareness, as well as prevention of secondary functional and cardiopulmonary impairments related to inactivity imposed by long-term orthotic wear. We have provided an overview of indications for surgery and the role of orthoses, exercise, and functional training in the postoperative care of patients

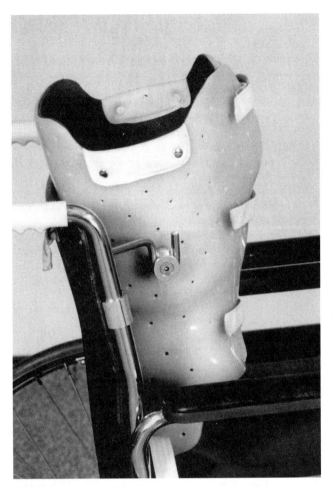

FIGURE 15-10

A thoracic suspension orthosis is suspended on this wheelchair by lateral posts, which rest on hooks attached to the wheelchair. This suspension unweights the ischial tuberosities and sacrum and distracts the spine, resulting in improved sitting and breathing in children with little or no trunk function secondary to their underlying neuromuscular disease.

with scoliosis. Optimal management of patients with scoliosis is best achieved when a multidisciplinary team of health professionals who understand the complexities of scoliosis contribute their special skills to the patients' care.

REFERENCES

1. Hippocrates. The Genuine Works of Hippocrates. Translated by Francis Adams. New York: WM Wood, 1849.
2. Bradford EH, Brackett EG. Treatment of lateral curvature by means of pressure correction. Boston Med Surg J 1893;128:463.
3. Risser J. The application of body casts for the correction of scoliosis. Instructional course lectures. Am Acad Orthop Surg 1955;12:255.

4. Hibbs RA, Risser JC, Ferguson AB. Scoliosis treated by fusion method. An end result study of 360 cases. J Bone Surg 1931;13:91.

5. Blount WP, Schmidt AC, Keever ED, Leonard ET. Milwaukee brace in the operative treatment of scoliosis. J Bone Joint Surg 1958;40A:511.

6. Logan WR. The Effect of Milwaukee Brace on the Developing Dentition. In Transaction of the British Society for the Study of Orthodontics. London: 1962;1–8.

7. Hall J, Schumann W, Stanish W. A refined concept in the orthotic management of scoliosis: a preliminary report. Prosthet Orthot Int 1975;29:7–13.

8. Emans JB, Kaelin A, Bancel P, Hall JE. Boston brace treatment of idiopathic scoliosis. Follow up results in 295 patients. Spine 1986;11(8):792–801.

9. Nachemson AL, Peterson LE, Brace Study Group SRS. Effectiveness of treatment with a brace in girls who have adolescent idiopathic scoliosis. J Bone Joint Surg 1995;77A(6):815–821.

10. Weinstein SL, Ponseti IV. Curve progression in idiopathic scoliosis. J Bone Joint Surg 1983;65A:(4);477–455.

11. Goldstein LA, Waugh TR. Classification and terminology of scoliosis. Clin Orthop June 1973;(93):10–22.

12. McAlister WH, Shackelford GD. Classification of spinal curvatures. Radiol Clin North Am 1975;13(1):93–112.

13. Terminology Committee, Scoliosis Research Society. A glossary of scoliosis terms. Spine 1976;1:57–58.

14. Cowell HR, Hall JN, MacEwen GD. Genetic aspects of idiopathic scoliosis. Clin Orthop 1972;86:121–131.

15. Willner S. A study of height, weight, and menarche in girls with idiopathic structural scoliosis. Acta Orthop Scand 1975;46(1):71–78.

16. Waters RL, Morris JM. An in vitro study of normal and scoliotic interspinous ligaments. J Biomech 1973;6(4):343–348.

17. Riddle HV, Roaf R. Muscle imbalance in the causation of scoliosis. Lancet 1975;1:1245–1247.

18. Yekutiel M, Robin GC, Yarom R. Proprioceptive function in children with adolescent idiopathic scoliosis. Spine 1981;6(6):560–566.

19. Herman R, Maulucci R, Stuyek J, et al. Vestibular functioning in idiopathic scoliosis. Orthop Trans 1979;3:218.

20. Sahlstrand T, Petruson B. A study of labyrinth function in patients with adolescent idiopathic scoliosis. Acta Orthop Scand 1979;50(6, pt. 2):759–769.

21. Willner S, Uden A. Prospective prevalence study of scoliosis in southern Sweden. Acta Orthop Scand 1982;53(2):233–237.

22. Hagglund G, Karlberg J, Willner S. Growth in girls with adolescent idiopathic scoliosis. Spine 1992;17(1):108–111.

23. Lonstein J. Idiopathic Scoliosis. In JE Lonstein, DS Bradford, RB Winter, JW Ogilvie (eds), Moe's Textbook of Scoliosis and Other Spinal Deformities. Philadelphia: Saunders, 1995.

24. Weinstein SL. Natural history of adolescent idiopathic scoliosis. Semin Spine Surg 1991;3:196–201.

25. Lonstein JE, Bjorkland S, Wanninger MH, Nelson R. Voluntary school screening for scoliosis in Minnesota. J Bone Joint Surg 1982;64A(4):481–488.

26. Risenborough EJ, Wynne-Davies R. A genetic survey of idiopathic scoliosis in Boston, Massachusetts. J Bone Joint Surg 1973;55A(5):974–982.

27. Wynne-Davies R. The aetiology of infantile idiopathic scoliosis. J Bone Joint Surg 1974;56B:565.

28. Scott JC, Morgan TH. The natural history and prognosis of infantile idiopathic scoliosis. J Bone Joint Surg 1955;37B:400–413.

29. Mehta MH. The rib vertebral angle in the early diagnosis between resolving and progressive infantile scoliosis. J Bone Joint Surg 1972;54B(2):230–243.

30. Figueiredo UM, James JIP. Juvenile idiopathic scoliosis. J Bone Joint Surg 1981;63B(1):61–66.

31. Duval-Beaupere G, Lamireau T. Scoliosis at less than 30 degrees. Properties of the evolutivity (risk of progression). Spine 1985;10(5):421–424.

32. Lonstein JE, Carlson JM. Prediction of curve progression in untreated idiopathic scoliosis during growth. J Bone Joint Surg 1984;66A(7):1061–1071.

33. Weinstein SL. Adolescent Idiopathic Scoliosis: Prevalence and Natural History. Instructional course lecture 38. St. Louis: Mosby, 1989.

34. Montgomery F, Willner S. Prognosis of brace treated scoliosis; comparison of the Boston and Milwaukee method in 244 girls. Acta Orthop Scand 1989;60(4):383–385.

35. Kehl DK, Morrissy RT. Brace treatment in adolescent idiopathic scoliosis. An update on concepts and technique. Clin Orthop April 1988;229:34–43.

36. Lonstein JE, Winter RB. The Milwaukee brace for treatment of adolescent idiopathic scoliosis. A review of one thousand twenty patients. J Bone Joint Surg 1994;76(8):1207–1221.

37. Moe JH, Kettleson DN. Idiopathic scoliosis. J Bone Joint Surg 1970;52A(8):1509–1533.

38. Keiser RP, Shufflebarger HL. The Milwaukee brace in idiopathic scoliosis. Clin Orthop July Aug 1976;(118):19–24.

39. Willers U, Normelli H, Aaro S, et al. Long term results of the Boston brace treatment on vertebral rotation in idiopathic scoliosis. Spine 1993;18(4):432–435.

40. Olafsson Y, Saraste H, Soderlund V, Hoffsten M. Boston brace in the treatment of idiopathic scoliosis. J Pediatr Orthop 1995;15(4):524–527.

41. Carr WA, Moe JH, Winter RB, Lonstein JE. The treatment of idiopathic scoliosis in the Milwaukee brace. J Bone Joint Surg 1980;62A(4):599–612.

42. Bradford DS, Hu SS. Neuromuscular Spinal Deformity. In JE Lonstein, DS Bradford, RB Winter, JW Ogilvie (eds), Moe's Textbook of Scoliosis and Other Spinal Deformities. Philadelphia: Saunders, 1995.

43. Tanner JM, Whitehouse RH. Clinical longitudinal standards for height, weight, height velocity, and stages of puberty. Arch Dis Child 1976;51(3):170–179.

44. Emans JB, Cassella MC. Boston Brace Instructional Course. Boston Brace International, Avon, MA, 1996.

45. Weisz I, Jefferson RJ, Carr AJ, et al. Back shape in the treatment of idiopathic scoliosis. Clin Orthop March 1989;(240):157–163.

46. Raso VJ, Russell GG, Hill DL, et al. Thoracic lordosis in idiopathic scoliosis. J Pediatr Orthop 1991;11(5):599–602.

47. Bunch WH, Patwardhan AG. Scoliosis: Making Clinical Decisions. St. Louis: Mosby, 1989;50–65.

48. Patwardhan AG, Gavin TM, Bunch WH, et al. Biomechanical comparison of the Milwaukee brace (CTLSO) and the TLSO for the treatment of idiopathic scoliosis. J Prosthet Orthot 1996;8(4):115–122.

49. McMaster M. Luque rod instrumentation in the treatment of adolescent idiopathic scoliosis; a comparative study with Harrington instrumentation. J Bone Joint Surg 1991;73B(6):982–989.

50. Kendall FP, McCreary EK, Provance PG. Muscles, Testing and Function (4th ed). Baltimore: Williams & Wilkins, 1993.

51. Greulich WW, Pyle SI. Radiographic Atlas of Skeletal Development of the Hand and Wrist (2nd ed). Stanford, CA: Stanford University Press, 1959.

52. Nash C, Moe J. A study of vertebral rotation. J Bone Joint Surg 1969;51A(2):223–229.

53. Winter RB, Lonstein JE, Denis F. The prevalence of spinal canal or cord abnormalities in idiopathic, congenital, or neuromuscular scoliosis. Othop Trans 1992;16:135.

54. Lovett RW. Lateral Curvature of the Spine and Round Shoulders. Philadelphia: P Blakiston's Son and Co, 1907.

55. Moe JH. The Milwaukee brace in the treatment of scoliosis. Clin Orthop 1971;77:18–31.

56. Faraday J. Current principles in the nonoperative management of structural adolescent idiopathic scoliosis. Phys Ther 1983;63(4):512–523.

57. Bassett GS, Bunnell WP, MacEwen GD. Treatment of idiopathic scoliosis with the Wilmington brace. Results in patients with twenty to thirty-nine degree curve. J Bone Joint Surg 1986;68A(4):602–605.

58. Edelmann P. Brace treatment in idiopathic scoliosis. Acta Orthop Belg 1992;58(suppl 1):85–90.

59. Hungerford DS. Spinal deformity in adolescence. Early detection and nonoperative management. Med Clin North Am 1975;59(6):1517–1525.

60. Stone B, Beekman C, Hall V, et al. The effect of an exercise program on change in curve in adolescents with minimal idiopathic scoliosis. A preliminary study. Phys Ther 1979;59(6):759–763.

61. Kearon C, Viviani GR, Killian KJ. Factors influencing work capacity in adolescent idiopathic scoliosis. Am Rev Respir Dis 1993;148(2):295–303.

62. DiRoccoc PJ, Vaccaro P. Cardiopulmonary functioning. I. Adolescent patients with mild idiopathic scoliosis. Arch Phys Med Rehabil 1988;69(3, part 1):198–203.

63. Smyth RJ, Chapman KR, Wright TA, et al. Ventilatory patterns during hypoxia, hypercapnia, and exercise in adolescents with mild scoliosis. Pediatrics 1986;77(5):692–697.

64. Kennedy JD, Robertson CF, Hudson I, Phelan P. Effect of bracing on respiratory mechanics in mild idiopathic scoliosis. Thorax 1989;44(7):548–553.

65. Kesten S, Garfinkel SK, Wright T, Rebuck AS. Impaired exercise capacity in adults with moderate exercise. Chest 1991;99(3):663–666.

66. MacLean WE, Green NE, Pierre CB, Ray DC. Stress and coping with scoliosis: psychological effects on adolescents and their families. J Pediatr Orthop 1989;9(3):257–261.

67. Goldberg MS, Mayo NE, Poitras B, et al. The Ste-Justine Adolescent Idiopathic Scoliosis Cohort Study. Spine 1994;19(14):1562–1572.

68. Valentine LE. Alteration of Body Image of Adolescent Females Braced as a Treatment for Adolescent Idiopathic Scoliosis. Thesis. Washington, DC: Catholic University, 1991.

69. Refsum HE, Naess-Anderson CF, Lange JE. Pulmonary function and gas exchange at rest and exercise in adolescent girls with mild idiopathic scoliosis during treatment with Boston thoracic brace. Spine 1990;15(5):420–423.

70. Lonstein JE, Renshaw TS. Neuromuscular Spine Deformities. Instructional Course, vol 36. St. Louis: Mosby, 1987.

16

Principles of Splinting for the Hand

SHEILA A. MACGREGOR

Two relatively interchangeable terms, *splints* and *orthoses*, are used to describe any device applied to the upper extremity that is designed to restore function or prevent deformity. To accomplish these important goals, an upper extremity splint or orthosis may immobilize or mobilize a joint, hold it in optimum alignment or position, or protect it to restore function.[1] A splint is most often used as a short-term treatment intervention, to be worn for several weeks or a few months. Splints are fabricated by occupational or physical therapists of low-temperature thermoplastic materials. An orthosis is a more permanent version of a splint, indicated for patients with long-term problems that require protection or immobilization. Orthoses are most often custom made or fit by an orthotist and are fabricated from more durable high-temperature thermoplastics. Splints and orthoses are used in conservative nonoperative management of hand, wrist, or elbow injuries or dysfunction, as well as in preoperative and postoperative care of upper extremity disabilities.

In this chapter, we review the anatomy and kinesiology of the hand and arm and identify the specific goals of splinting. We use a problem-solving approach to choosing the appropriate splint design and apply our knowledge of splinting using clinical case studies. An in-depth knowledge of the biomechanical principles of the upper extremity and a concrete method of problem solving, based on accurate evaluation of the patient, are necessary for selection and fabrication of the optimal splint.

Dr. Paul Brand, an orthopedic surgeon who specializes in hand rehabilitation, describes splinting of the upper extremity as both "an art and a science."[2] The therapist and orthotist must consider the science of anatomy and force application as well as the specific physical and psychosocial characteristics of the patient when deciding which type of splint or orthosis best matches overall treatment objectives. No two patients have identical splinting requirements, regardless of similarities in diagnosis. The factors contributing to such individual differences among patients include underlying pathology, physiologic function of the injured part, psychosocial factors affecting the patient, and physical principles that govern the design of the splint.

BASELINE KNOWLEDGE: ANATOMY AND KINESIOLOGY OF THE UPPER EXTREMITY

The complex structure of the upper extremity permits us to use our hand and arm in a wide variety of functional tasks. Injury or dysfunction to one or more of its joints, supporting soft tissue structures, muscles, or nerves often has a significant impact on the ability to use the hand in daily activities, leading to functional limitations or disability. If a splint is to be effective as an interventional tool, its design must match the bony architecture and arthrokinematics of the hand and wrist. It must be based on knowledge of the functional anatomy of muscles and their tendons and the kinetics of normal movement.

The masterful architectural design of the upper limb and hand allows movement in multiple planes of motion and permits us to perform intricate movements as well as have a powerful grasp. The forearm and hand have four structural units: the ulna and radius of the forearm, the seven carpal bones at the wrist, the five metacarpals of the palm, and the phalanges (the fingers). Each is important for the smooth operation of the hand in functional activities.

Bony Prominences of the Wrist and Hand

The shapes of the distal radius and ulna, the carpals, the metacarpals, and the phalanges, combined with the minimal amount of soft tissue and muscular "padding" around the wrist, create areas of bony prominence that are vulnerable to pressure when a splint is worn (Figure 16-1). The

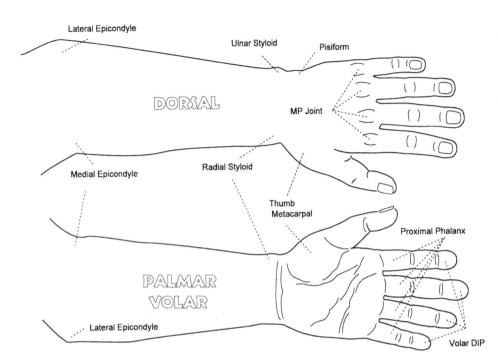

FIGURE 16-1
Bony prominences and other soft tissue structures, which are areas that are vulnerable to pressure. When splints are fabricated and fitted, care must be taken to trim or pad them adequately over these areas. DIP = distal interphalangeal; MP = metacarpophalangeal. (Courtesy of L. MacGregor, Grovetown NH; Practical Images, 1996.)

areas that are most vulnerable to discomfort and skin breakdown as a result of pressure include the dorsal metacarpophalangeal (MP) joints, the palmar surface of the MP joint of the thumb and index finger, the palmar surface of the distal joints of the fingers, the dorsal surface of the proximal phalanges of each finger, and the dorsal MP of the thumb. Other vulnerable areas include the pisiform bone of the wrist, radial and ulnar styloids, and lateral and medial epicondyles of the elbow. A splint that is designed to control motion at these joints must be adequately trimmed or padded for comfort and protection of the skin over bony prominences.

When a patient is fit with a splint, it is important to monitor carefully the areas that are vulnerable to pressure: The splint should be removed after 30 minutes of wearing time and the skin carefully inspected. Skin areas that have reddened during wear should return to normal color within 20 minutes. Persistent redness is a sign of excessive pressure and indicates that further modifications of the splint are necessary to ensure comfortable fit and avoid skin breakdown. This is a vital concern for patients with fragile skin, such as the elderly, who are most prone to the development of pressure sores.

Muscles of the Forearm and Hand

The therapist or orthotist who fabricates upper extremity splints must have a thorough understanding of the anatomy of the hand before making any type of splint that may alter its structures. Table 16-1 provides a review of the muscles of the hand and their nerve supply. For a more extensive review, the reader is referred to Fess and Phillips,[1] Wynn Parry,[3] Cailliet,[4] or Hunter et al.[5]

The muscles that act on the hand are classified as either extrinsic muscles (when the muscle belly is in the forearm) or intrinsic muscles (when they originate distal to the wrist joint).[1] The integrated function of these two muscle groups enables the hand to perform many activities. Digital extension results from a combination of the contribution of extrinsic and intrinsic tendons.

Extrinsic flexor muscles include a superficial group (pronator teres, flexor carpi ulnaris, flexor carpi radialis, palmaris longus), an intermediate group (flexor digitorum superificialis), and a deep group (flexor digitorum profundus, flexor pollicis longus). Extension of the wrist and fingers is produced by the extrinsic extensor muscle tendon system (extensor carpi radialis longus and brevis, extensor carpi ulnaris, extensor digitorum communis, extensor digiti minimi).[1] Another group of extrinsic muscles, the extensor pollicis longus and brevis and the abductor pollicis longus, extend and radially abduct the thumb.

The hand has three groups of intrinsic muscles. The thenar group (abductor pollicis brevis, flexor pollicis brevis, opponens pollicis, adductor pollicis) positions the thumb in opposition for prehension tasks. The hypothenar

TABLE 16-1
Hand Musculature Actions and Nerve Supply

Muscle	Action	Nerve
Flexor carpi radialis	Wrist flexion and radial deviation	Median
Palmaris longus	Wrist flexion and tensing of palmar fascia	Median
Flexor carpi ulnaris	Wrist flexion and radial deviation	Ulnar
Extensor carpi radialis longus	Wrist radial deviation and extension	Radial
Extensor carpi radialis brevis	Wrist extension and radial deviation	Radial
Extensor carpi ulnaris	Wrist ulnar deviation and extension	Radial
Flexor digitorum superficialis	Finger PIP flexion	Median and Ulnar
Flexor digitorum profundus	Finger DIP flexion	Median
Extensor digitorum communis	Finger MP extension	Radial
Extensor indicis proprius	Index finger MP extension	Radial
Extensor digiti minimi	Little finger MP extension	Radial
Dorsal	Finger MP abduction	Ulnar
Palmar	Finger MP adduction	Ulnar
Lumbricals	Finger MP flexion and IP extension	Ulnar and Median
Abductor digiti minimi	Little finger MP abduction	Ulnar
Opponens digiti minimi	Little finger opposition	Ulnar
Flexor digiti minimi	Little finger MP flexion	Ulnar
Flexor pollicis longus	Thumb IP flexion	Median
Flexor pollicis brevis	Thumb MP flexion	Median and Ulnar
Extensor pollicis longus	Thumb IP extension	Radial
Extensor pollicis brevis	Thumb MP extension	Radial
Abductor pollicis longus	Thumb radial abduction	Radial
Abductor pollicis brevis	Thumb palmar abduction	Median
Adductor pollicis	Thumb adduction	Ulnar
Opponens pollicis	Thumb opposition	Median

DIP = distal interphalangeal; IP = interphalangeal; MP = metacarpophalangeal; PIP = proximal interphalangeal.
Source: Reprinted with permission from BM Coppard, H Lohman. Introduction to Splinting: A Critical-Thinking and Problem-Solving Approach. St. Louis: Mosby–Year Book, 1996;26.

group (abductor digiti minimi, flexor digiti minimi, opponens digiti minimi) assists in the opposition of the fifth finger. The final group includes the dorsal and palmar (ventral) interossei for finger adduction and abduction and the lumbricals, which work with the interossei for MP flexion while the proximal interphalangeal (PIP) and distal interphalangeal (DIP) joints are extended.

When resting tone is normal in the extrinsic and intrinsic muscle groups of the forearm and hand, the wrist and digital joints are maintained in a balanced position.[1] Problems arise when an imbalance in tone or power occurs among the muscle groups. With intrinsic denervation (intrinsic minus position; Figure 16-2), the ability to flex at the MP joint while extending at the PIP and DIP joints is lost. Because extrinsic extensors are unopposed, the MP joints hyperextend. Unopposed tension of the extrinsic flexors causes the interphalangeal joints of the ring and little fingers to curl in flexion.

Innervation of the Upper Extremity

Motor neurons from the cervical spinal cord are reorganized as they travel through the brachial plexus into the three major peripheral nerves (radial, median, ulnar) that innervate muscles of the forearm, wrist, and hand. The ulnar nerve enters the hand through Guyon's canal at the wrist, passing between the volar carpal ligament and deep transverse carpal ligament, and between the pisiform and hook of the hamate. The ulnar nerve innervates extrinsic and intrinsic muscles that flex the wrist and fingers and adduct the thumb. The median nerve enters the hand through the carpal tunnel; it may pass deep to or superficial to the volar carpal ligament. The median nerve innervates extrinsic and intrinsic muscles that flex the wrist and fingers, as well as most of the thenar muscles that act to abduct and oppose the thumb. The radial nerve innervates the dorsal extrinsic musculature of the forearm that extends

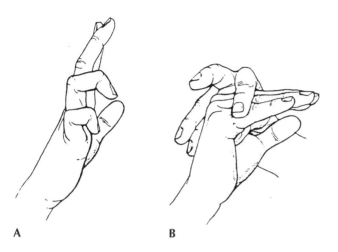

FIGURE 16-2

(A) Intrinsic minus position is a result of ulnar nerve palsy. (B) When intrinsic flexion at the metacarpophalangeal joint is restored through positioning, extension of the proximal and distal interphalangeal joints is restored. (Reprinted with permission from EE Fess, CA Phillips. Hand Splinting Principles and Methods [2nd ed]. St. Louis: Mosby, 1987;111.)

the wrist and supinates the hand. The radial nerve enters the hand at the dorsum of the wrist, dividing into deep and superficial branches.

All three of these peripheral nerves also carry sensory information from the hand and arm back through the brachial plexus to the cervical spinal cord. The radial nerve covers the dorsal surface of the thumb to the middle of the dorsum of the hand. The median nerve carries sensation from the palmar thumb to the midline of the fourth digit and dorsal index and middle fingers. The ulnar nerve carries information from the palmar and dorsal surface of the lateral half of the fourth digit and all of the fifth digit.

Soft Tissue Structures of the Hand

The joints of the wrist and hand are enclosed in a fibrous capsule composed of irregular, dense connective tissue. During normal movement, this joint capsule accepts stress and permits stretch in all directions of that joint's movement.[6] If the hand has been injured and is immobilized during the acute stage of healing or after surgical repair, the joint capsules of the immobilized joints adaptively shorten in the immobilized position, altering the joint's ability to move through its normal range and limiting functional use of the hand. Wrist and hand splints must be carefully designed to minimize unwanted deformity. Dynamic splints are often used to improve joint mobility as tissues heal.

The volar plate is another soft tissue structure important for stability of the hand and fingers. This fibrocartilaginous structure serves as an articulating surface, an attachment for ligaments, an additional confining structure for synovial fluid, and an inhibitor for dorsal dislocation during MP extension.[6] Conditions such as rheumatoid arthritis can alter the structure of the volar plate, resulting in joint laxity or deformity.

The transverse intermetacarpal ligament helps to support and stabilize the hand as part of the distal transverse arch and is important for grasping and prehensile activities. Collateral ligaments provide joint stability for the fingers and thumb. When trauma to the hand occurs, splint designs often position the MP joint in flexion to maintain the length of these important ligaments.[6]

Arches of the Hand

The many functions of the hand are dependent on a set of three bony arches: the distal transverse arch, the proximal transverse arch, and the longitudinal arch (Figure 16-3). The intrinsic muscles of the hand are responsible for the maintenance of the arches and for manipulative functions. When

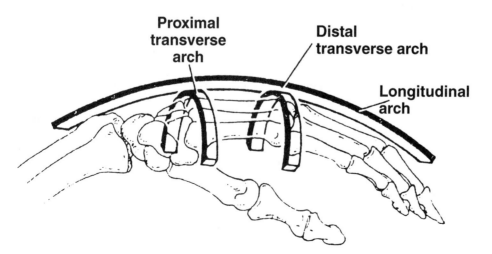

Proximal transverse arch

Distal transverse arch

Longitudinal arch

FIGURE 16-3

Arches of the hand. The proximal transverse arch is set by the alignment of the distal row of carpals, and the more flexible distal transverse arch encompasses the second to fifth metacarpal heads. The shallower longitudinal arch includes each of the digits and its corresponding metacarpal, as well as the carpals. (Reprinted with permission from EE Fess, CA Phillips. Hand Splinting Principles and Methods [2nd ed]. St. Louis: Mosby, 1987;5.)

intrinsic paralysis or orthopedic trauma alters the alignment of the arch system, the ability to use the hand in daily living is significantly compromised. Patients with a "flat hand" are unable to hold a pencil, grasp a doorknob, hold a cup, or effectively manipulate objects with the fingers.

The concave distal transverse arch enables the thumb and other fingers to oppose and to make a cupping motion of the hand for holding objects and is supported by intermetacarpal ligaments and MP volar ligaments. The proximal transverse arch at the wrist is supported by the annular ligaments and the carpal bones. The keystone of this proximal arch is the capitate bone. These arches provide stability to the hand and wrist and act as a fulcrum by providing a mechanical advantage to the tendons of the finger flexors.

The longitudinal arch, which lies perpendicular to the other arches, is formed by the length of the carpal, metacarpal, and phalanges of each digit of the hand. This longitudinal arch is the basis for the three-jaw chuck position of the hand. It also maintains full mobility of the phalanges. The longitudinal arch is most prominent at the second and third fingers. The function of the longitudinal arch is compromised by paralysis of the intrinsic muscles, poor positioning of the hand, edema, dorsal scarring, adherent extensor tendons, and the bony obstructions that are common in arthritis.[7]

Flexion Creases of the Palm and Fingers

Flexion creases in the palmar surface of the hand are anatomic landmarks that are used as a functional "road map" for splinting. They include distal, middle, and proximal creases of the phalanges; distal and proximal creases of the palm; distal and proximal creases at the wrist; and thenar, proximal, and distal creases of the thumb. Splints or orthotics that cover a flexor crease limit the motion of the underlying joint. If mobility of the joint is desired, the splint should be trimmed proximal to the crease. If full MP flexion is desired, for example, trimlines must not obscure any portion of the distal palmar crease.[7] For full mobility and use of the thumb, the thenar crease must be clear.

Dual Obliquity of the Hand

An object held in the closed hand is neither parallel nor perpendicular to the long bones of the radius and ulna but is held at an oblique angle to the radius and ulna. This is the result of two factors. First, the metacarpals differ in length, becoming progressively shorter toward the ulnar side of the hand. Second, the first, fourth, and fifth metacarpals are more mobile than the centrally placed second and third metacarpals. As a result of these characteristics, two oblique angles are evident (Figure

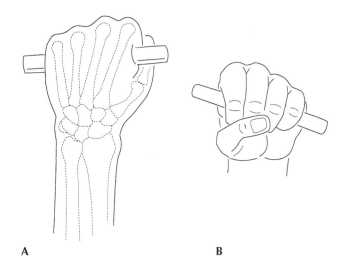

A   **B**

FIGURE 16-4

*Dual obliquity of the hand can be illustrated by gripping a pencil in a flexed hand. (**A**) The pencil is held at a slightly oblique angle to the plane of the forearm because of progressive shortening of the metacarpals. (**B**) Radial-to-ulnar metacarpal head descent also creates an oblique angle, so that the pencil is higher on the radial side than on the ulnar side of the hand. (Redrawn with permission from RM Duncan. Basic principles of splinting the hand. Phys Ther J 1989;69:116; courtesy of L. MacGregor, Grovetown NH; Practical Images, 1996.)*

16-4). The radial side of the splint must be somewhat longer and higher than the ulnar side to capture the hand's obliquity.

COMPONENTS OF FUNCTIONAL MOVEMENT

The primary role of the upper limb is to place the hand in its proper position of function.[4] The elbow, which connects the upper arm to the forearm, plays an important role, bringing items toward the body or reaching out for objects by positioning the hand in space. To bring the hand to the mouth, the elbow must flex up to 150 degrees. Forearm pronation and supination during elbow flexion or extension place the hand in the desired position of function.

The primary function of the hand is to carry out prehensile activity (grasp, manipulation, and release of objects).[8] Four basic components of hand movement have been identified[9]:

1. Mobility of the thumb for opposition
2. Alignment and mobility of the index and middle fingers for precision pinch

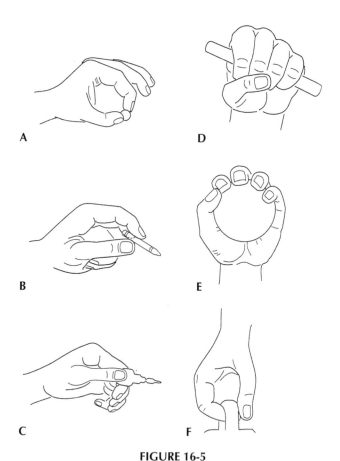

FIGURE 16-5

Prehension patterns. Pinch prehension has three variations: (A) tip to tip, (B) three-jaw chuck, and (C) lateral pinch. Grasp has two variations: (D) cylindrical and (E) spherical. A hook pattern (F) is used to carry heavy objects. (Courtesy of L. Mac-Gregor, Grovetown NH; Practical Images, 1996.)

3. Functional stability provided by the fourth and fifth fingers to enhance the power of grasp
4. The "backbone" of the hand (formed by the carpals and transverse carpal arch, the longitudinal arch along the second and third metacarpals, and the radiocarpal joint) is the fixed point around which the other three components occur; it is important to note that hand and wrist stability are both dependent on the radiocarpal joint

Prehension Patterns

The hand is used in three ways during functional activities: to pinch, to grasp, or to hook objects (Figure 16-5). Pinch patterns are used to hold or manipulate small objects between the thumb and first two fingers. A tip-to-tip pinch pattern is used to pick up small objects such as pins and to fasten buttons. The three-jaw chuck pinch uses the thumb

and the pads of the index and middle fingers. In the lateral pinch, the thumb holds an object against the side of the index finger. When using a cylindrical grasp, the palm serves as an opposition platform as the fingers close over an object such as a railing, hammer, or can of soda. When a ball grasp is used to hold spherical objects, the fingers rotate around the object as it is held against the palm. When carrying heavy objects, such as a suitcase, a hook pattern is most efficient. This is accomplished with flexion of the interphalangeal joints; the wrist and MP joints are stabilized in neutral.

GOALS OF SPLINTING

Wrist and hand splints are appropriate for a wide variety of patient problems. The type of splint chosen for a particular patient is determined by the objectives of the therapeutic intervention. A splint or orthosis for the wrist and hand can be designed to accomplish one or more of the following objectives[10]:

1. To prevent deformity by maintaining normal tissue length, balance, and excursion
2. To immobilize and stabilize an injured or unstable hand
3. To protect healing tissues
4. To correct deformity or dysfunction by reestablishing normal tissue length and excursion
5. To control and modify scar formation
6. To improve function by substituting for dysfunctional structures or tissues
7. To provide an opportunity to exercise

A wide variety of static and dynamic splint designs are currently in use. The American Society of Hand Therapists uses a descriptive classification system for upper extremity splints based on their anatomic focus, kinematic direction, primary purpose, and inclusion of secondary joints.[11] A well-designed wrist and hand splint maintains the normal transverse and longitudinal arches, preserves the normal axis of joint motion, and permits balanced function of unaffected muscles. It also provides the most practical prehension pattern and allows for mobility and use of the hand while ensuring optimal stability. Much of the palmar surface and digits are open for optimal sensory and perceptual function.[7] Adequate trimlines, flared edges, and appropriate relief areas protect bony prominences and vulnerable soft tissue. Forces applied over large surface areas make the splint more comfortable to wear and reduce the risk of pressure-related skin breakdown. Corrective forces are adjusted for prolonged gentle elongation of tissues when correction of the deformity is desired.

Splinting Positions

The main functions of the fingers are to grasp, hold, and release objects. When splints are designed, the normal transverse arches must be preserved to protect the functions of the hand. It is important that the web space between the thumb and index finger be maintained at 35 degrees to allow three-jaw chuck and lateral pinch. A functional thumb needs a mobile web space to pick up varying sizes of items. Flexion of the first carpometacarpal joint allows for opposition of the thumb for tip-to-tip prehension. Extension of the metacarpal and interphalangeal joints aids in stabilization of the thumb as a post for opposition. The key joint for effective grasp is the metacarpal joint.

Splints can be designed to place the hand in a functional hand position, in a resting hand position, or in an intrinsic plus position, depending on the needs of the patient. In the *functional position* (Figure 16-6A), the wrist is held in 30 degrees of extension. For effective thumb opposition and the ability to use pinch prehension, the MP joints require 35–40 degrees of flexion, the PIP joints flex to 45 degrees, and the DIP joints flex to between 5 and 10 degrees. When splinting for the purpose of *resting* the joints (Figure 16-6B), the forearm is positioned midway between pronation and supination. The wrist is positioned at approximately 20 degrees of extension, the phalanges are slightly flexed, and the thumb is held in partial opposition. *Resting position* ensures balance of the long extensors, the long flexors, and the intrinsic muscles of the hand. An *intrinsic plus* splint holds the MP joints in flexion, with the PIP and DIP joints in full extension.

For patients with weakness of the wrist and fingers, functional grasp can be achieved by tenodesis action. When the wrist is flexed, elongation of the finger extensor tendons make it difficult to flex the fingers into a fist. When the wrist is extended, the finger flexors become elongated, and the fingers are naturally drawn into a position of flexion. For patients with quadriplegia who are able to extend the wrist, allowing adaptive shortening of finger flexors may permit them to use tenodesis to enhance hand function in the absence of volitional control of the fingers.

Important Considerations in Splinting

In the design and fabrication of a splint, five considerations or precautions must be kept in mind.[12] First, care must be taken to avoid applying pressure over bony prominences, especially the ulnar styloid, radial styloid, pisiform, and epicondyles of the metacarpals. Second, the splint must not compress the superficial radial sensory nerve and cutaneous branch of the ulnar nerve as they travel into the hand. Third, the splint base must be of adequate length to distribute the forces and counter-

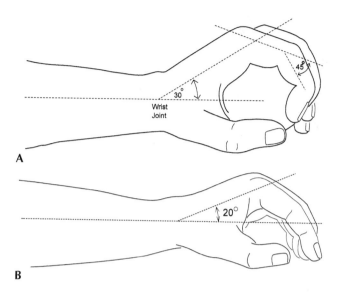

FIGURE 16-6
*Comparison of the functional position (**A**) and resting position (**B**) for splinting of the hand. (Courtesy of L. MacGregor, Grovetown NH; Practical Images, 1996.)*

forces over the forearm comfortably. As a general rule, most forearm-based splints are at least two-thirds the length of the forearm. Fourth, special care should be taken when splinting patients with an insensate hand, open wound or grafts, or vascular insufficiency. Fit is especially important for very young and very old patients, whose skin may be vulnerable to irritation or breakdown. Finally, newly fabricated splints require careful monitoring for onset of joint pain, joint stiffness, areas of skin irritation or pressure, edema or pooling, sensory changes, temperature changes, and vascular changes that indicate developing problems. The patient's attitude toward and acceptance of a splint must also be considered if it is to be effective.

In addition to assuring that the splint fits appropriately, one must monitor its effectiveness in meeting the therapeutic goals, especially if the patient's condition is changing. Patients and their caregivers must understand how to don and doff the splint, how to keep it clean, when to wear or not wear the splint, and how and why the splint meets their particular needs. It is important to provide written information as well as demonstration and verbal instruction regarding the proper care and wearing of the splint.

STATIC SPLINTS

Static splints are used when it is necessary to maintain a joint in one position. When in a static splint, tissues

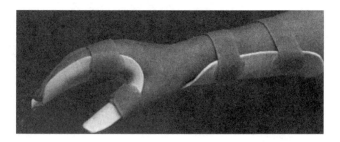

FIGURE 16-7
The resting hand splint can be used to maintain the hand and wrist in a position of function. (Reprinted with permission from BM Coppard, H Lohman. Introduction to Splinting: A Critical Thinking and Problem-Solving Approach. St. Louis: Mosby–Year Book, 1996;97–98.)

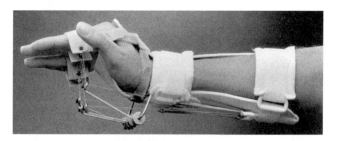

FIGURE 16-8
This dynamic splint with its outrigger is designed to mobilize stiff metacarpophalangeal joints and elongate shortened finger extensors and their tendons. (Photo courtesy of Smith & Nephew Rolyan, Inc., Germantown, WI.)

can be positioned at resting length (Figure 16-7) or can be placed under gentle tension if the joint is held in its elongated range. Static splints are used to prevent or correct an existing deformity by maintaining the normal balance of the upper extremity. They can be used to reduce stress on a joint or to protect a painful, inflamed, or insensate hand. Static splints can be used to improve hand or wrist function by substituting for a weak muscle. They are used in serial stretching to increase or maintain range of motion for patients with soft tissue contracture. Static splints are often used to control or modify scar formation after flexor tendon repairs or serious burns of the upper extremity.[10] Additionally, static splints can be used to provide the immobilization that is necessary to minimize inflammation or to promote vascularization of skin or bone grafts and to protect healing bone or newly repaired structures.

DYNAMIC SPLINTS

In a dynamic splint design, an outrigger or elastic pulley system is added to a static splint base to apply gentle force in a specific direction (Figure 16-8). Dynamic splint designs are used to mobilize stiff joints; to elongate skin, soft tissues, tendons, or adhesions; to maintain optimal joint alignment; to substitute for absent muscle power or assist weak muscles; or to provide an opportunity for exercise for a healing or impaired hand. Dynamic splints can be prescribed after the inflammatory phase of wound healing to optimize alignment of collagen during fibroplasias.[13] Dynamic splints are also used later in wound healing to enhance outcomes of scar maturation.[13]

Dynamic splints are chosen if the therapeutic goal is to minimize limitations of range of motion when the

impaired joint has a soft "end feel." They can also substitute for weak or denervated muscles to enhance hand function. Dynamic splints can be designed to provide strengthening of specific muscles while controlling proximal joints, length of muscle tendons during contraction, force magnitude, and line of pull after injury or surgical repair. They are also used to lengthen adhesions by applying gentle elongation proximally and distally. These splints also are used to provide controlled excursion for healing tendons.[10]

The goal of dynamic splinting is to provide a low-amplitude force over a prolonged period of time to influence the remolding of new and healing tissue.[10] Because tissue remodeling is itself a dynamic process, the fit and effectiveness of the dynamic splint must be reassessed and readjusted on an ongoing basis. Often, measurable gains are recorded within one or two treatment sessions. Wearing schedules for dynamic splints are dependent on two factors: the tolerance of the targeted soft tissue to elongation and stretch and the patient's tolerance and willingness to comply with the treatment protocol.

Biomechanical Principles of Splinting

Whether a splint is static or dynamic in design, it is founded on a first-class lever system, with three points of pressure acting on the extremity.[14] In a volar wrist splint, for example (Figure 16-9), the primary point of pressure is applied at the axis of the wrist joint by the dorsally placed wrist strap. A proximal counterforce (force arm of the lever system) is applied to the forearm, where it is stabilized in the forearm trough. As the length of the forearm trough increases, the amount of pressure required as counterforce decreases. The distal counterforce (resistance arm

FIGURE 16-9
Most wrist and hand splints act as a first-class lever system with three points of pressure. In this volar splint design, the axis is at the wrist joint, with proximal and distal counter-forces. (Redrawn from RM Duncan. Basic principles of splinting the hand. Phys Ther J 1989;69:113; courtesy of L. MacGregor, Grovetown NH; Practical Images, 1996.)

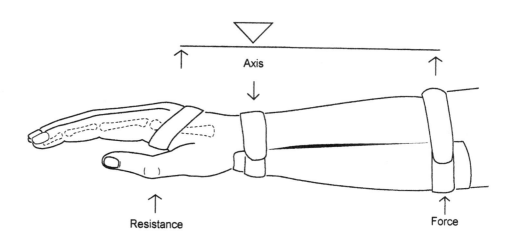

of the lever system) acts at the palmar aspect to the weight of the hand.[8,14]

The strength of the splint base, for both static and dynamic designs, can be enhanced by the contours in splinting material as it is shaped during fabrication. Careful molding of the arches within the forearm trough and hand segment minimizes distal migration of the splint on the extremity. Many splint designs use a pattern for a forearm trough that is two-thirds the length and width of the forearm.

Dynamic Splint Forces

The force that is applied to soft tissues by a dynamic wrist or hand splint must be gentle; excessive force can lead to pain, inflammation, and further injury, increasing the likelihood of problematic scar formation. Cell formation is encouraged through slow stretching for eventual elongation. Because soft tissue is viscoelastic, fairly low forces applied over long periods promote remodeling and increase tissue length. The forces applied by a dynamic splint can be measured using a spring tension gauge. Most patients are able to tolerate forces between 100 and 300 g. In many instances, the tension of dynamic splints is adjusted to be less forceful when a splint is worn overnight. Variations in diagnosis and physiologic timing play a part in determining what range of force is to be applied.[11]

Brand[15] poses a series of key questions to consider when fitting a patient with a dynamic splint. Given the therapeutic goals of the splint and the condition/status of the patient's tissues, how much force should be applied? Through what surfaces of the limb? How long should the force be applied? What structures are targeted by the application of the force? What is the leverage of force application? What are the reactive and the stabilizing forces in the lever system? How closely does the dynamic design address the therapeutic goals or purpose of the splint?

How will the effect of the force application be assessed or measured? Do the splint design and force application avoid secondary tissue injury or harm?

A dynamic splint applies a correcting or elongating force to a limb segment and its soft tissue. When the goal is to correct joint deformity, the angle of pull must be perpendicular (90 degrees) to the long axis of the targeted structure to be most effective. When the angle of pull is less than 90 degrees, compression of the joint occurs; when the angle of pull is more than 90 degrees, distraction of the joint results.

Rubber bands or elastic cords are often used as traction devices. In most instances, they are arranged to pull toward the scaphoid or base of the third metacarpal as a center point.[9] This is especially important when traction is applied to achieve finger flexion, so that the fingers are pulled toward the palm in the obliquity that is necessary for normal hand function.

Many dynamic splint designs incorporate an outrigger frame and nylon lines or filaments to connect the traction device and the anchor loops around the fingers. Preformed outrigger kits are available from several manufacturers. A dynamic splint can have a high or low profile, depending on the height of the outrigger and the method used to apply force (Figure 16-10). A high-profile dynamic splint has a direct line of pull between the outrigger and the involved limb segment.[13] The outrigger must be high enough to maintain the 90-degree angle of pull and to exert a constant force. A high-profile outrigger often interferes with daily tasks; many patients find high-profile splints unacceptable cosmetically. Low-profile dynamic splints use a pulley system to redirect the line of pull between the outrigger and the finger so that the traction device and the outrigger line are parallel to the splint base. This low profile improves splint cosmesis because the outrigger is positioned as close as possi-

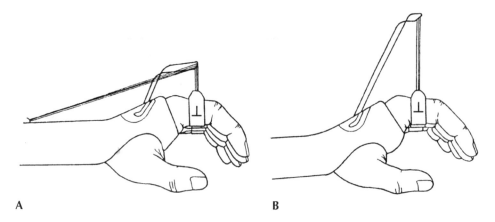

A   B

FIGURE 16-10
(A) In a low-profile dynamic splint, the traction system is parallel to the splint base, and a pulley system ensures a perpendicular line of pull. (B) In a high-profile dynamic splint, the traction system is attached to an outrigger, with a direct perpendicular line of pull. (Reprinted with permission from BM Coppard, H Lohman. Introduction to Splinting: A Critical Thinking and Problem-Solving Approach. St. Louis: Mosby–Year Book, 1996;146.)

ble to the finger that is being mobilized. Low-profile designs also simulate normal tendon glide; the traction device is like a muscle belly, whereas the outrigger line is like a tendon.[13]

For a more in-depth overview on the mechanics of splinting, the reader is referred to Fess and Phillips (pp 125–162).[1]

Precautions with Dynamic Splints

Dynamic splints are most often chosen when a prolonged and gentle force is needed to mobilize stiff finger or wrist joints.[11] The potential problems to watch for when using a dynamic splint include

1. Excessive pressure, which can lead to vascular compromise of affected tissues
2. Excessive torque forces, which cause unstable forces to act on a joint or the extremity
3. Incorrect alignment: Although forces applied at a 90-degree angle ensure "balance" around the joint and appropriate force distribution within the splint, those applied at more or less than 90 degrees result in rotational forces and unequal pressure distribution; it is important to make ongoing adjustments as the range of motion of the digits changes
4. Stress to adjacent joints, which can often be minimized by including other fingers within the splint
5. Skin irritation: High shear effects can be avoided by rounding splint edges, by keeping pressures low, and by eliminating unwarranted motion and friction[11]
6. Immobilization: Splints must be designed to apply corrective forces to only those joints that lack pas-

sive motion, avoiding unwanted immobilization of nontargeted joints

FREQUENCY AND DURATION OF SPLINTING

Schultz-Johnson[10] suggests the following guidelines for therapists and patients when developing an intervention plan based on the use of upper extremity splints. The first principle considers the tension applied by the splint: Light-tension splinting over many hours typically yields better results (and is better tolerated by patients) than high-tension splinting over a shorter period. The second principle concerns the condition of the joint being targeted: Joints with passive range of motion limitations that have a hard end feel often require many more hours of splinting than do those with a soft end feel. In some cases serial splinting or casting may be an option to consider. The third guideline considers patient activity level: Although dynamic splints are effective when a patient is active and functioning during the day, most patients better tolerate a static splint while sleeping. This implies that it may be necessary to fabricate a static splint for sleeping for patients who wear a dynamic splint during the day. Finally, the best-accepted wrist or hand splint is one that allows the patient to use the hand in an active functional way as much as possible.

Wrist and hand splints are prescribed after soft tissue injury or surgical repair of musculoskeletal or neuromuscular impairments, or both. If splinting after surgery, the therapist need to be knowledgeable about the surgical procedure itself and the stages of wound healing when making decisions about the timing of immobilization or protection of joints and about when to begin application of forces to the joint.[16] These factors also influence when postoperative passive or active range of motion exercises can begin. Some postoperative, passive range of motion protocols for tendon repair, for example, can begin within the first several days after surgery, with the approval of the referring physician. Intervention of dynamic splinting should always follow the prescription of the physician.

Although postoperative protocols vary by the type and extent of repair, some general guidelines should be considered.[16] For patients who have had surgical repair of nerve damage, bulky dressings and static splints are often used for up to 6 days after operation when gentle, passive range of motion may begin to minimize the risk of adhesion. For patients with tendon repairs, the limb is generally protected for up to 7 days, although gentle, protected (midrange) passive range of motion may begin earlier. For patients with unstable fractures, immobilization in a cast or fracture brace is usually preferred for at least 4–6 weeks until evidence of bony union is seen. The limb can be supported by a static splint once the cast has been removed. In some instances (as long as the fracture site appears to be stable) a light-tension dynamic splint can be used to mobilize joints that have become stiff during immobilization. When a bone graft has been performed after nonunion of a fracture site, the limb is typically immobilized until the graft is deemed intact for motion. Upper extremity splinting can be used to support and protect the graft site during function once healing has occurred. For patients with an acute edema after trauma or surgical repair, the fit and suspension of splints must be frequently reassessed and adjusted. Patients with acute edema can also be managed with elevation of the limb, use of a compression wrap or garment, or manual lymph drainage or massage. The decision to use a static or dynamic splint design is also determined by the condition or status of the patient's soft tissue and phase of healing (inflammatory, fibroplastic, or maturation of the scar).

Most hand therapists would agree that a splint is best worn intermittently, for no more than 10–12 hours at a time, depending on the goals of the splint prescription. For patients who have just been fitted with a splint, it is important to evaluate fit and pressure application frequently (every 2 hours) to avoid secondary skin or healing problems.

PROBLEM-SOLVING APPROACH TO SPLINTING

When designing a splint for a particular patient, the therapist must consider the basic principles of splinting and must gather the additional important information from the referring physician and the patient. Open communication between the therapist and the physician regarding the purposes and goals for the splint is essential. A true understanding of the diagnosis and the biomechanics involved with the injury or surgical repair is necessary when designing an appropriate splint. Insufficient information can lead to incorrect fitting of the splint and confusion about its purpose and goals. Referral information must include (1) the patient's diagnosis; (2) the date of injury, onset of the problem, or date of surgery; (3) the type of splint desired by the physician; (4) clearly stated goals for the desired splint; and (5) the anticipated frequency and duration of wear.[10] Discussion between the referring physician and therapist often clarifies which design options will most effectively meet the therapeutic goals for a given patient.

Problem Identification

When a patient has been referred for splinting, the therapist collects additional information to determine the degree of impairment, to identify the primary problems to be addressed by the splint, to evaluate the likely tolerance of the tissues for splint application, and to anticipate outcomes of splinting. A variety of assessments or evaluations are used to collect the data that will guide splint design and fabrication.[10] These include, but are not limited to, the following:

1. Measurement of active and passive range of motion
2. Muscle function and strength testing
3. Sensory testing
4. Evaluation of the condition of tendons and ligaments
5. Assessment of skin and wound (scar) condition
6. Evaluation of limb volume or girth for possible edema
7. Evaluation of joint integrity
8. Assessment of soft tissue condition and elasticity
9. The patient's experience of pain
10. The present functional status of the limb
11. The patient's neuromuscular control of the limb

The data generated by this assessment are used by the therapist to clearly define the current problem or combination of problems (problem set). Proper interpretation of this information helps the therapist to anticipate (and avoid) future problems of the involved extremity and to estimate the rehabilitation potential of the injured hand. Periodic reassessments are necessary to track the patient's progress, provide incentives to the patient, and monitor the effectiveness of the splinting regime.

TABLE 16-2

Problem Sets*

I: TISSUE STATUS
   Are all tissues in continuity?
   Will active motion, passive motion, or the engagement of
      resistance jeopardize tissue continuity?
   Are all tissues of normal length, strength, and density?
   Is inflammation present?
II: COMPONENTS OF FUNCTION
   Is active motion normal? If not, why not?
   Is passive motion normal? If not, why not?
   Is strength normal? If not, why not?
   Is sensation normal? If not, why not?
III: SCAR
   Is the scar soft and supple?
   Is the scar much higher than the surrounding skin?
   Does the observable scar move when the tendon beneath it
      moves?
   Are the superficial and deep scars long enough to allow
      normal motion?
   Is the deep scar too attenuated to allow normal motion?
IV: PAIN
   Does the patient experience pain in conjunction with this
      pathology that compromises function or treatment com-
      pliance?
V: FUNCTION
   Can this patient perform activities of daily living?
   Is the patient's ability to prehend and manipulate objects
      affected?
   Is the patient's fine or gross motor coordination affected?

*Problem sets include evaluation of tissue status, components of func-
tion, scar, pain, and functional activities of the patient.
Source: Reprinted with permission from K Schultz-Johnson. Splinting—A Problem-Solving Approach. In BG Stanley, SM Tribuzi (eds),
Concepts in Hand Rehabilitation. Philadelphia: FA Davis, 1992;242.

Problem Sets

A well-defined problem set helps to identify splinting concerns and enables the therapist to consider the best splinting option for the patient's problem (Table 16-2). Four
diagnostic questions are helpful in defining a problem set
for a given patient.[10]

1. What are the implications of this patient's diagnosis?
2. What tissues have been damaged or repaired?
3. How do these tissues normally relate to the surrounding tissues and structures?
4. How did the pathology occur?

The answers to these questions, when combined with the
therapist's knowledge of normal hand structure and function, the biological basis of wound healing, and the
response of normal and healing tissue to stress, guide splint
design and intervention.

Patient Characteristics

The functional outcome of upper extremity splinting is
also influenced by several important patient-related factors, such as the patient's cognitive abilities, personality,
tolerance of frustration or pain, and attitudes and expectations about healing and the rehabilitation process.[10] It
is important to consider the following questions before fitting a patient with a splint:

1. How will the patient interact with the splint?
2. What are the possible compliance issues that will have
   an impact on whether the patient will wear the splint
   in the recommended regime?
3. What impact will the patient's physical and cognitive abilities and attitudinal and motivational factors
   have on splint wearing (donning/doffing, wearing
   schedule), splint care and upkeep, and any necessary
   home exercises?
4. Will the patient's health insurance cover fitting,
   fabrication, and follow-up for the splint? What are
   the anticipated out-of-pocket expenses for the
   patient? How will these factors influence splint
   design and material choices and scheduling of follow-up visits?
5. How far does the patient live from the site of care?
   Will it be necessary to adjust the number of visits due
   to the constraints of travel?
6. Will compliance with the splint regime improve with
   written instructions, ease of application of the splint,
   or cosmesis of the splint? Will the patient need the
   assistance or supervision of another to use the splint
   as intended?
7. In what ways will the patient's usual function (activities of daily living, work, leisure) be affected by the
   splint? Will it be necessary to use a low-profile
   approach to enhance compliance without compromising function in activities of daily living?
8. How adept is the patient at using the noninvolved
   hand and arm? Will the patient be able to don and
   doff the splint independently? Would independence
   be possible with special adaptations or straps?
9. If the patient will be returning to work with the
   splint, how will splint design and materials need to
   be adjusted with respect to the stresses or demands
   of the patient's work activities and roles? This is
   especially important to consider for those who
   operate equipment or machinery: The danger of
   having a splint caught in the machinery must be
   minimized.

SPLINTING MATERIALS

Splinting materials are available from a number of different manufacturers and with a wide variety of characteristics (such as how conforming the material is when heated, its "memory" to resist deformation, and its durability). Although many lower extremity orthoses are fabricated from high-temperature thermoplastics, hand and wrist splints are made with low-temperature thermoplastics for several reasons. Because low-temperature thermoplastics become moldable when heated between 130° and 180°F, most can be molded directly on the patient's limb, without the need for casting and the making of a positive model. They also cool and set much more quickly than do high-temperature materials, so that the splint can often be designed, fabricated, and delivered in a single visit. Similarly, the fit of splints made from low-temperature thermoplastic can be quickly and easily adjusted by spot reheating with a heat gun. Typically low-temperature thermoplastics are also less expensive to purchase than are high-temperature materials.

To select the thermoplastic material which best addresses the goals of a given splint design, the therapist considers the characteristics of the material, including its memory, drapability, resistance to drape, rigidity, and self-adherence. The handling characteristics of a material determine how easily it molds to the patient's limb. A material with good memory returns to its preheated shape and size when reheated. Rigidity refers to how strong and resistant to stress the material will be after cooling and hardening. This is particularly important when molding material with controlled stretch for large splints. *Drapability* refers to how easily the material molds to the contours of the body without assistance. A highly moldable material is used when intimate skin contact is desired but usually must be handled carefully during the fabrication process. Materials with a resistance to draping can be handled more aggressively and may be better suited to patients who have abnormal tone, weakness, or other reasons that make it difficult for them to cooperate during the fabrication process. Self-adherence refers to the ability of the material to bond to itself when heated. Materials can be coated to prevent self-sticking if this characteristic is not desired. Some low-temperature materials (manufactured by Smith & Nephew Rolyan, Inc, Germantown, WI and by North Coast Medical, Inc, San Jose, CA) are grouped by their characteristics in Table 16-3.

Strap Placement Considerations

Velcro hook and loop tape is the most frequently chosen method for securing the splint to the upper extremity.

TABLE 16-3
Thermoplastic Materials Property Guideline

Characteristic	Material	Heating Temperature (°F)
Memory	Aquaplast-T	160–170
	Watercolors	160–170
	Aquaplast Blue Stripe	160–170
	Aquaplast Green Stripe	160–170
	NCM Spectrum	140–145
	Orfit Soft	135
	Orfit Stiff	135
Rigidity	Ezeform	160–170
	NCM Clinic	160
	NCM Clinic D	160
	NCM Preferred	160
	Polyform	150–160
Conformability and drapability	Aquaplast Blue Stripe	160–170
	Contour form	140–145
	Ezeform	160–170
	NCM Clinic	160
	NCM Clinic D	160
	Polyform	150–160
	Polyform Light	150–160
	Polyflex II	150–160
	Polyflex Light	150–160
	Orfit Soft	135
	Orthoplast II	150–160
Moderate drapability	Aquaplast-T	160–170
	Ezeform	160–170
	Ezeform Light	150–160
Resistance to drape	Aquaplast Green Stripe	160–170
	Caraform	140–145
	Synergy	160–170
Self-adherence	Aquaplast	160–170
	Contour colors	140–145
	Contour form	140–145
	Ezeform	160–170
	NCM preferred	160
	Orfit Soft	135
	Orfit Stiff	135
	Spectrum	160
	Synergy	160–170

NCM = North Coast Medical.
Source: Reprinted with permission from BM Coppard, H Lohman. Introduction to Splinting: A Critical Thinking and Problem-Solving Approach. St. Louis: Mosby–Year Book, 1996;8.

Other options include strapping made of elastic, webbing, or loop tape composites. Sometimes a strap is riveted to the splint to reinforce it at a point of stress. Straps must be placed carefully to ensure that the splint is held in place with an even pressure. Straps that are too tightly adjusted can lead to a "windowpane" edema of the areas on either side of the strapping.

Prefabricated Splints

A variety of prefabricated splints which can be modified to fit the patient properly are commercially available. Because modification is less time consuming than fabrication of a splint, prefabricated splints are often more cost effective when time and expense of materials are factors. It is imperative to assess the fit, function, and comfort of any "off the shelf" splint provided to a patient as carefully as if the splint were being custom fit and fabricated. Therapists must strive to fit a prefabricated splint to the patient's hand rather than attempting to fit the patient's hand to the splint.[8] Commercially manufactured prefabricated splints are made from a variety of materials; they may use metal bands as reinforcers and screws or springs to apply even tension, and they may provide compression and support for joints and soft tissues using materials such as neoprene.

CASE STUDIES

Hand and wrist splints are used in the management of many types of injuries and surgical repairs, to protect joints and assist function in a variety of orthopedic or neuromuscular conditions and to manage abnormal muscle tone (spasticity) in the hand and fingers. The following case studies are meant to assist the reader in understanding the evaluative process and applying basic principles of splint-ing in prescription of a splint. In each case study, we use a problem-solving process to identify the most salient problems to be addressed with splinting, and we describe how a particular splint design meets the goals and purposes of that patient's problem.

Patient with Laceration of the Ulnar Nerve

A 29-year-old steelworker fell with an outstretched hand on a hard, jagged metal surface, resulting in a laceration of the ulnar nerve at the wrist. Patients with ulnar nerve injury at the wrist (a low ulnar nerve lesion) lose innervation of the intrinsic muscles of the hand. Without the activity of the lumbrical muscles (innervated by the ulnar nerve), the action of the extensor digitorum communis is unopposed, and there is hyperextension of the MP joint of the fourth (ring) and fifth (little) finger. This is often referred to as a *claw hand deformity* or an *intrinsic minus hand* (see Figure 16-2A). Patients with this type of impairment are unable to open the fingers of the hand effectively enough to grasp large objects (Figure 16-11).

A splint is used for patients with peripheral nerve injury for four reasons.[17] It can be used to

1. Prevent overelongation of denervated muscles due to unopposed activity of intact muscles or the effects of gravity

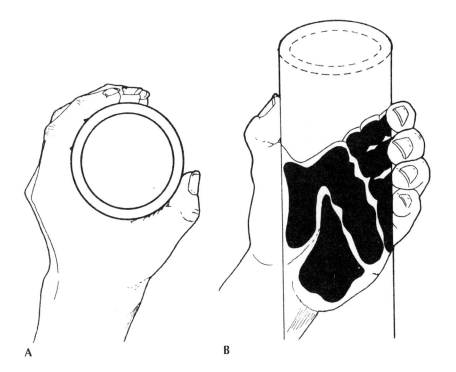

A   **B**

FIGURE 16-11
(A) In a hand with intact innerva-tion, contact between palm and finger surfaces is uniform around the cylinder. (B) After ulnar nerve injury at the wrist or in an intrinsic minus hand, a patient has diffi-culty opening the hand for grasp, and the area of contact is limited to the fingertips and the metacarpal heads. (Reprinted with permission from PW Brand, A Hollister. Clin-ical Mechanics of the Hand [2nd ed]. St. Louis: Mosby–Year Book, 1993;39.)

2. Prevent joint contractures because of abnormal positioning of the hand that result from muscle imbalance

3. Minimize the evolution of abnormal "substitution" patterns of movement as the patient attempts to be functional despite the injury

4. Maximize use of the hand by supporting the limb in a functional position, or by substituting for the action of the denervated muscles

For patients with low ulnar nerve damage (palsy), the primary goal for splinting is to prevent overstretching of the denervated intrinsic muscles of the ring and little fingers. An "anticlaw" splint is designed to block MP joint hyperextension while allowing the extensor digitorum communis tendon to extend the PIP joints (Figure 16-12). A dorsal, protective static splint that allows full finger flexion range with minimal coverage at the palmar surface is often successful, facilitating use of the hand.

Patient with Rheumatoid Arthritis

A 51-year-old woman with rheumatoid arthritis who greatly enjoys gardening as a hobby has found that gardening activities now lead to red, hot, and painfully swollen joints in her hand. She has also noted an increasing degree of ulnar drift of her MP joints. Her doctor has advised her to rest her hand and wrist to quiet the inflammation that developed after her most recent attempt at gardening.

The goals of splinting for patients with rheumatoid arthritis are different from those for ulnar nerve laceration. In rheumatoid arthritis, splints are used to[18]

1. Reduce inflammation during acute flare-ups of the rheumatoid arthritis

2. Rest and support weakened structures during acute flare-ups, as well as during function between flare-ups

3. Properly position joints to minimize microtrauma and enhance function

4. Minimize development of fixed joint deformity

5. Improve functional use of the hand in activities that are important to the patient

The inflammation during an acute episode of rheumatoid arthritis is responsible for the destruction of joints, especially of the hand and wrist. Splinting helps to protect joints during the inflammatory process. Through use of a resting hand splint, joints of the wrist and fingers can be held in a protective resting posture, until pain and swelling decrease. Most resting splints for

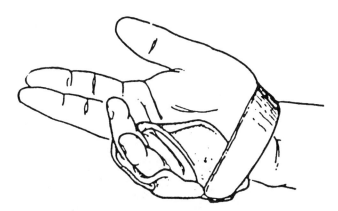

FIGURE 16-12

A metacarpophalangeal flexion splint design can be an effective "anticlaw" splint for patients with an ulnar nerve injury. Note that metacarpophalangeal joint hyperextension is prevented by the splint and that most of the palmar surface of the hand is uncovered for optimal sensory and prehensile function. (Reprinted with permission from American Society of Hand Therapists. Splint Classification System. American Society of Hand Therapists; Garner, NC, 1992;42.)

patients with inflammation of the wrist and hand provide volar support with the wrist positioned in neutral position (10–15 degrees of wrist extension) with slight flexion (up to 25 degrees) of the MP joints (see Figure 16-7). When the joints of the thumb are inflamed, the recommended thumb position is in abduction, to maintain an open web space.

Once the inflammatory stage has subsided, the focus of the splint becomes promotion of optimal joint alignment during daily activities. One of the most common deformities seen in patients with rheumatoid arthritis is a pronounced ulnar deviation of the MP joints. An effective functional splint minimizes or prevents ulnar drift of the MP joints during work and leisure tasks (Figure 16-13).

Patient with Carpal Tunnel Syndrome

A 43-year-old woman who works long hours as a computer programmer has developed tingling in the hands. She frequently wakes up at night because her hands have "gone numb." Based on her symptoms and the results of electromyographic studies, her physician has diagnosed carpal tunnel syndrome. She is referred to therapy for a splint to position her wrist correctly while she is working at the computer.

Carpal tunnel syndrome is the result of compression of the median nerve as it passes beneath the transverse

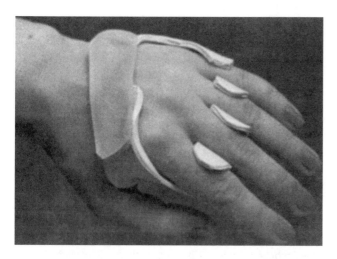

FIGURE 16-13

A static splint, designed to correct the ulnar deviation that is so commonly encountered in patients with rheumatoid arthritis, holds the metacarpophalangeal joints in optimal alignment during functional use of the hand. (Reprinted with permission from BM Coppard, H Lohman. Introduction to Splinting: A Critical Thinking and Problem-Solving Approach. St. Louis: Mosby-Year Book, 1996;15.)

carpal ligament at the wrist. Intervention is determined by the severity of symptoms and chronicity of the condition. In mild cases, when surgery is not required, a volar wrist support that positions the wrist in a neutral position at approximately 10–20 degrees of extension is often an effective conservative interventional strategy. This neutral position allows functional use of the fingers during daily activities (such as typing on a computer keyboard) while minimizing compression and further irritation of the median nerve. A wide variety of splint designs, including many prefabricated versions, can be effective in the management of mild carpal tunnel syndrome. If a prefabricated splint is chosen, the therapist must evaluate and modify fit to the individual patient.

The incidence and prevalence of carpal tunnel syndrome have increased substantially in this age of sustained computer use. It is very important that patients realize how to minimize pressure on the median nerve. Placing a wrist pad at the base of the keyboard, to support the wrist in a relaxed position, is an effective preventive strategy in the workplace and in the home office. In addition, ergonomic assessment of a patient's workstation can prevent worsening of this work-related injury, minimizing risk of functional impairment in the future.

Patient with Surgical Tendon Repair

A 14-year-old boy who was attempting to perform stunts on his skateboard sustained a deep laceration at the base of the ring finger after falling onto a sharp piece of gravel in the road. The injury significantly damaged the tendon of the flexor digitorum protundus (FDP) and required surgical repair. The boy is referred to therapy for fabrication of a splint on postoperative day 3. Because of the "one muscle belly–four tendon" anatomy of the FDP, all three joints of the injured finger as well as the two adjacent fingers must be immobilized after surgical repair. This strategy minimizes the risk of tendon rupture at the site of repair by limiting the patient's ability to use the FDP to move the adjacent fingers.[10]

To manage the postoperative course of patients with tendon repair effectively, the therapist must understand the process of tendon and soft tissue healing and the operative procedure used in the repair. The therapist must also consider the individual patient and the nature of the injury. Important questions to ask when treating patients with tendon injuries and repairs include the following[16]: What was the nature and the extent of the injury to the tendon? What type of tendon repair was performed? Where is the site of the tendon repair? How much can the repair be stressed during motion? How much motion is allowed? Where in the range can motion safely occur? What position will best protect the repair during the early stages of tissue healing?

The four primary goals of splinting for patients in the initial stages of healing after tendon repair surgery are preservation of function, prevention of edema, prevention of contracture, and maintenance of gliding surfaces through motion.[16] It is important to preserve joint mobility so that the tendon can glide freely in its sheath within surrounding tissue.[19] This is possible only if the risk of development of an adherent surgical scar is minimized. A careful balance between protection of healing tissues (by positioning and limiting motion) and the application of a gentle controlled stress (to enhance motion and minimize the loss of muscle strength) must be achieved.

During the protective stage the goal of therapy is to promote a strong tendon repair and to prevent restrictive adhesions. Healing of a repaired FDP tendon can be enhanced with controlled early mobilization via gentle active finger flexion (tendon gliding exercise) along with gentle prolonged tension to increase tendon excursion gently. Early motion helps the tendon to glide over surrounding tissue, gently shearing the tendon away from developing attachments (adhesions). Gentle prolonged tension may also have a positive impact on collagen synthesis, enhancing fiber alignment and minimizing

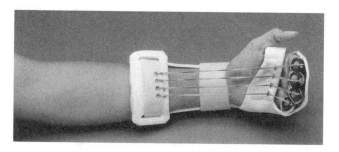

FIGURE 16-14

The Rolyan flexor tendon repair splint is often used in the early postoperative management of patients with flexor digitorum profundus tendon repair. This protective position of the hand reduces the risk of rupture at the site of tendon repair, allowing early gentle mobilization for effective tendon glide and adhesion prevention. (Photo courtesy of Smith & Nephew Rolyan, Inc., Germantown, WI.)

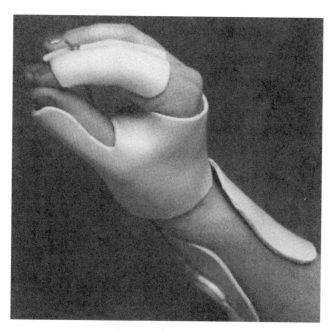

FIGURE 16-15

A tenodesis splint can help a patient with spinal cord injury that is affecting the area of C6 to C7 to use the tenodesis grip functionally. (Reprinted with permission from BM Coppard, H Lohman. Introduction to Splinting: A Critical Thinking and Problem-Solving Approach. St. Louis: Mosby–Year Book, 1996;16.)

cross linkage and associated limitation in tissue mobility.[16] Although limited motion is desirable, the tendon must be protected from excessive active flexion and excessive passive extension.[19] A dorsal protective splint that holds the wrist in 45 degrees of flexion with the MP joints blocked at 40 degrees of flexion and the interphalangeal joints in neutral extension can be used at the base for a dynamic splint[19] (Figure 16-14). Elastic bands are applied to the fingernails to provide protective flexion and to resist active extension to the limits of the dorsal protective splint. The traction from the elastic bands pulls the finger into passive flexion and provides a means of low-stress passive tendon glide to minimize the formation of adhesions.

Patient with Cervical Spinal Cord Injury

A 34-year-old man was involved in a motor vehicle accident on the way home from his job. As a result of the accident, he sustained a complete spinal cord injury at the C6 neurologic level secondary to compression fractures of the C5 and C6 vertebral bodies. In the acute care hospital, he underwent open reduction with internal fixation and bone graft to stabilize the fracture site and was placed in a halo spinal orthosis. Now, 3 weeks after injury, he has been transferred to a rehabilitation center. In physical therapy, he has begun to work on sitting and bed mobility skills. The occupational therapist is focusing on retraining the patient in the use of his upper extremity for functional activities.

With a C6 level of function, this patient is able to extend his wrist actively but does not have active control of his fingers. Tenodesis action will be very important in his ability to use his hand for functional activities. When the wrist is actively extended, passive tension of finger flexors helps to close the fingers, creating a three-jaw chuck grip.[20] A tenodesis splint is designed to take advantage of the patient's available wrist extension to allow for prehension of his thumb, index, and middle fingers to hold objects using the three-jaw chuck grip (Figure 16-15).

Adaptive splinting designs assist patients with quadriplegic spinal cord injury who are unable to extend the wrist to hold and manipulate utensils used in eating and grooming activities (Figure 16-16). The splint supports the wrist in extension. The handle of the utensil is positioned in the splint's universal cuff, which substitutes for a cylindrical grip. With active elbow flexion and shoulder motion, patients are then able to bring a spoon or fork toward the mouth to feed themselves or to bring a comb or brush toward the head for grooming.

Patient with Spastic Hemiplegia

A 68-year-old man has a left hemiplegia with spasticity as a result of an ischemic, thromboembolic cerebrovascular

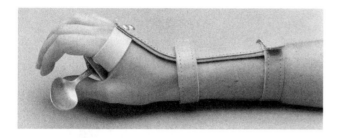

FIGURE 16-16

Dorsal wrist support with a universal palmar cuff attachment to hold utensils for feeding or grooming activities. (Photo courtesy of North Coast Medical, Inc., San Jose, CA.)

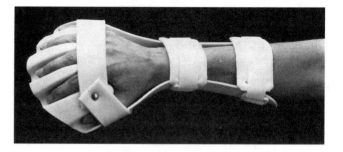

FIGURE 16-17

A volar antispasticity ball splint positions the hand in a reflex-inhibiting posture with abduction of the fingers to decrease hypertonicity. (Rolyan Preformed Antispasticity Ball Splint. Pattern design courtesy of Bronwyn Keller, O.T.R. Photo courtesy of Smith & Nephew Rolyan, Inc., Germantown, WI.)

accident (CVA) of the right middle cerebral artery several weeks ago. He has been in an active rehabilitation program and is making significant gains in mobility and ambulation. One of the problems that remain is a severe hypertonicity at the wrist and finger flexors of his left hand. His fingers are held in a tightly fisted position, with the wrist in flexion and supination. He is unable to open his fingers or lift his wrist into extension actively. The abnormally high tone makes it difficulty to open his hand passively, and it is challenging to clean the palmar surface of his hand.

The use of splinting in managing spasticity in CVA patients has been a subject of significant investigation and some controversy.[21] Splinting can be a successful component in the management of hypertonicity. An antispasticity splint is used for patients with hypertonicity after CVA to

1. Prevent joint contracture as a result of muscle activity imbalance due to flexion hypertonicity
2. Maintain the arches of the hand that are necessary for functional positioning
3. Assist with hygiene by keeping the fingers extended and the palm open
4. Inhibit abnormal tone by holding the limb in reflex-inhibiting postures

One example of a splint design that is used to reduce hypertonicity in the hand and wrist is the antispasticity ball splint. This design holds the fingers and thumb in abduction, with 45 degrees of MP extension and full interphalangeal extension, while positioning the wrist in 30 degrees of extension (Figure 16-17). The antispasticity ball splint can be fabricated with either a volar or a dorsal forearm trough. For patients with hypertonicity of the upper extremity, an antispasticity hand splint alone is insufficient to manage spasticity. Shoulder position is an important determinant of tone as well: Poor shoulder position may not only increase abnormal tone in the arm but also makes it

difficult to fit a splint effectively on the patient. Although a number of different strategies can be used to fit antispasticity splints in patients with hemiplegia and there is some disagreement about the efficacy of dorsal and volar designs,[22–27] McPherson et al.[28] found that volar and dorsal resting hand splints effectively reduced hypertonus in a comparative study of 10 adult patients and suggest that splinting proved a useful adjunctive therapeutic procedure.

SUMMARY

In this chapter, we have introduced the reader to basic principles of upper extremity splinting with special attention to the hand and wrist. We have discovered that splinting is a beneficial therapy intervention for prevention of deformity because it can help to maintain normal tissue length, balance, and excursion. Static splints are used to immobilize, stabilize, or protect the structures of the upper extremity. Dynamic splints use gentle, specifically applied tension to correct deformity or dysfunction by reestablishing normal tissue length and excursion or exercise of a weakened muscle. Splints can be used to control and modify scar formation. They are also helpful in substituting for dysfunctional tissue. Because the hand and wrist are complex functional structures, a thorough understanding of their normal anatomy, physiology, and kinematics is a necessary foundation for effective splint prescription, fabrication, and application. Splint design and fabrication are special skills that can be developed only with advanced instruction and practice. This chapter has given the reader basic knowledge about splinting of the hand and wrist; continuing education workshops and seminars and careful study of the current splinting literature are necessary if the reader is interested in developing effective skills for splinting.

REFERENCES

1. Fess EE, Phillips CA. Hand Splinting Principles and Methods (2nd ed). St. Louis: Mosby, 1987.
2. Brand PW, Hollister A. Clinical Mechanics of the Hand (2nd ed). St. Louis: Mosby–Year Book, 1993.
3. Wynn Parry CB. Rehabilitation of the Hand (4th ed). London: Butterworth-Heinemann, 1981.
4. Cailliet R. Hand Pain and Impairment (2nd ed). Philadelphia: Davis, 1975.
5. Hunter JM, Schneider LH, Mackin EJ, Callahan AD (eds). Rehabilitation of the Hand: Surgery and Therapy, vols. 1–2 (4th ed). St. Louis: Mosby, 1995.
6. Moran CA. Anatomy of the hand. Phys Ther 1989;69(12): 15–21.
7. Malick MH. Manual on Static Hand Splinting (3rd ed). Pittsburgh: Harmarville Rehabilitation Center, 1976.
8. Gribben MG. Splinting Principles for Hand Injuries. In CA Moran (ed), Hand Rehabilitation. New York: Churchill Livingstone, 1986;159–189.
9. Malick MH. Manual on Dynamic Hand Splinting with Thermoplastic Materials (2nd ed). Pittsburgh: Harmarville Rehabilitation Center, 1978.
10. Schultz-Johnson K. Splinting—A Problem-Solving Approach. In BG Stanley, SM Tribuzi (eds), Concepts in Hand Rehabilitation. Philadelphia: Davis, 1992;239–269.
11. Fess EE. Principles and Methods of Splinting for Mobilization of Joints. In JM Hunter, LM Schneider, EJ Mackin, AD Callahan (eds), Rehabilitation of the Hand: Surgery and Therapy Vol II (4th ed). St. Louis: Mosby, 1995;1589–1598.
12. Jacobs ML. Handouts from Static and Dynamic Splinting Workshops. Springfield, MA: Baystate Medical Center, 1995.
13. Nelson N, Reel C. Gentle pressures using dynamic splints in hand rehabilitation. Adv Dir Rehabil 1994;3(5):93–94.
14. Duncan RM. Basic principles of splinting the hand. Phys Ther 1989;69(12):1104–1116.
15. Brand PW. The Forces of Dynamic Splinting: Ten Questions before Applying a Dynamic Splint to the Hand. In JM Hunter, LH Schneider, EJ Mackin, AD Callahan (eds), Rehabilitation of the Hand: Surgery and Therapy Vol II (4th ed). St. Louis: Mosby, 1995;1581–1587.
16. Smith KL. Wound Healing. In BG Stanley, SM Tribuzi (eds), Concepts in Hand Rehabilitation. Philadelphia: Davis, 1992;35–56.
17. Colditz JC. Splinting the Hand with Peripheral Nerve Injury. In JM Hunter, LH Schneider, EJ Mackin, AD Callahan (eds), Rehabilitation of the Hand: Surgery and Therapy Vol 1 (4th ed). St. Louis: Mosby 1995;679–692.
18. Philips CA. Therapist's Management of Patients with Rheumatoid Arthritis. In JM Hunter, LH Schneider, EJ Mackin, AD Callahan (eds), Rehabilitation of the Hand: Surgery and Therapy Vol II (4th ed). St. Louis: Mosby, 1995; 1345–1350.
19. Stewart KM. Tendon Injuries. In BG Stanley, SM Tribuzi (eds), Concepts in Hand Rehabilitation. Philadelphia: Davis, 1992;353–394.
20. Malick MH, Meyer CMH. Manual on Management of the Quadriplegic Upper Extremity. Pittsburgh: Harmarville Rehabilitation Center, 1978.
21. Neuhaus B, Ascher E, Coullon B, et al. A survey of rationales for and against hand splinting in hemiplegia. Am J Occup Ther 1981;35(2):83–90.
22. Zislis J. Splinting of hand in spastic hemiplegic patient. Arch Phys Med Rehabil 1964;45(1):41–43.
23. Kaplan N. Effects of sensorimotor stimulation in treatment of spasticity. Arch Phys Med Rehabil 1962;43(11):565–569.
24. Chariat S. A comparison of volar and dorsal splinting of the hemiplegic hand. Am J Occup Ther 1968;22(2):319–321.
25. Snook J. Spasticity reduction splint. Am J Occup Ther 1979;33(3):648–651.
26. Katz R. Management of spasticity. Am J Phys Med Rehabil 1988;67(3):108–116.
27. Scherling E, Johnson H. A tone reducing wrist-hand orthosis. Am J Occup Ther 1989;43(9):609–611.
28. McPherson JJ, Kreimeyer D, Aalderks M, Gallagher T. A comparison of dorsal and volar resting hand splints in the reduction of hypertonus. Am J Occup Ther 1982;36(10):664–670.

17

Management of Extremity Fractures: Principles of Casting and Orthotics

MELVIN L. STILLS AND KEVIN CHRISTENSEN

Management of injuries to the musculoskeletal system, especially the care of broken bones, has always been a unique specialty. Orthopedics is the medical specialty specifically devoted to the diagnosis, treatment, rehabilitation, and prevention of injuries and disease of the musculoskeletal system: the bones, joints, ligaments, tendons, muscles, and nerves that provide the framework for functional movement and activity. The discipline of orthopedics was once strictly devoted to the care of children with limb and spine deformities. Health professionals in orthopedics now care for patients of all ages, including newborns born with clubfoot deformity, adults and children with broken bones, athletes who require arthroscopic surgery, and older adults with arthritis or osteoporotic fracture. In this chapter, we explore current fracture management strategies, including casting and orthoses.

Today's practice of fracture management requires an extremely complex multidisciplinary team approach, generally under the direction of a physician with training or interest in musculoskeletal limb deformity or injury (orthopedics). Communication between the physician and the rehabilitation specialist is critical in obtaining the most favorable outcomes after skeletal trauma is sustained.

FRACTURES: DESCRIPTIVE CLASSIFICATIONS

Fractures of the upper and lower extremities are classified as either open or closed injuries. In a *closed fracture*, the soft tissue envelope of muscles and skin around the bone fracture site is completely intact. Although muscle around the fracture site may be significantly damaged, the intact skin provides a barrier that prevents bacterial invasion of the injured muscle or bone. When an open *compound* fracture occurs, the soft tissue envelope has been violated: The wound leaves muscle and fractured bone open to the environment and susceptible to infection. In many cases, bone may actually protrude through the skin. Open injuries are orthopedic emergencies: Patients are quickly taken to the operating room for debridement of the wound and fracture. Severely damaged or contaminated tissue is removed, and the wound is carefully cleaned in an effort to avoid infection and provide optimal circumstances for healing. The fracture is then stabilized with a cast or surgical implant.

Classification of Open Fractures

Gustilo and Anderson[1] have developed a classification system that rates the severity of open or compound fractures. The least severe is a type I injury, in which a small wound (1 cm) communicates with the fracture. The wound in a type II fracture is between 1 cm and 12 cm, and significant soft tissue injury may be present underneath the laceration or wound. In a more severe, type III injury, the wound diameter is greater than 12 cm, and barely enough muscle or skin is present to cover the injured or fractured bone adequately. Type III open fractures are subdivided into another three categories, A, B, and C, based on whether the soft tissue can cover the bone and whether neurologic or vascular involvement is present in association with the open fracture.

Locations and Patterns of Fractures

The radiographic or x-ray description of fractured bones is based on the location and the pattern of the fracture. First, fractures are classified as either *metaphyseal* (at or near the end of the bone) or *diaphyseal* (involving the shaft of the bone). They are further described as *intra-articular* (extending into a joint) or *extra-articular* (with no joint involvement). Four terms are commonly used to describe the pattern of a fracture: transverse, oblique, spiral, or comminuted (with multiple bone fragments within the fracture site). The particular location and pattern of fracture determine whether the fracture is stable, and can be effectively managed with an external cast, or unstable, requiring surgical intervention. A fracture with concurrent joint dislocation creates an extremely unstable condition, most often requiring anesthesia or surgery for reduction and management of the fracture/dislocation and a long period of rehabilitation. The use of this type of terminology ensures accurate communication between the managing physician and rehabilitation specialist who are working together to care for patients recovering from fracture.

Complications of Fractures

Two major postfracture complications are of concern to the managing physician: vascular injury and compartment syndrome. Fractures or dislocations around joints such as the elbow or knee may have a concomitant arterial injury that can bruise or completely disrupt an artery, compromising or completely interrupting blood flow beyond the site of fracture. This creates a grave situation: The physician has a window of less than 6–8 hours in which to restore blood supply and nutrition to the distal muscle and bone before significant tissue death occurs. The longer the period of ischemia, the greater the likelihood of delayed healing, infection, and necrosis.

Compartment syndrome evolves when bleeding or inflammation exceeds the expansive capacity of semirigid muscle or soft tissue anatomic spaces (compartments) of the fractured limb. Once interstitial pressure exceeds a critical level, blood vessels and muscle are compressed, and oxygen supply to the muscles is significantly compromised. Irreversible muscle or nerve damage occurs if compartment syndrome continues for longer than 6–8 hours. Presenting signs and symptoms include extreme pain and significant swelling of the extremity with very taut skin. Passive motion of the fingers or toes causes excruciating pain. Compartment syndrome is considered a medical emergency: The treating physician must be notified immediately so that a fasciotomy can be performed to relieve excessive compartment pressures. In some instances, the wound area can be left open until edema subsides, and a skin graft may be required to close the wound adequately.

Each patient who presents to the emergency department with a fracture must be assessed for potential vascular injury and risk of developing compartment syndrome by careful physical examination. Compartment syndrome and vascular injury can occur anywhere in the upper or lower extremity. All health professionals who are involved in the treatment of extremity trauma should be aware of the signs and symptoms of compartment syndrome. If unrecognized and untreated, compartment syndrome has devastating results.

GOALS AND METHODS OF FRACTURE MANAGEMENT

The primary goal of fracture management is to restore musculoskeletal limb function of the injured extremity with optimal anatomic alignment, functional muscle strength, and pain-free joint range of motion. Orthopedic surgeons use a variety of techniques and methods to achieve the goals of fracture management, including the application of splints, circumferential casts, or surgery. In an open reduction internal fixation (ORIF) surgery, the surgeon may use implants such as plates, screws, intramedullary rods, or external fixators to stabilize the fractured bone. Each of these methods of immobilization is designed to allow the normal fracture healing response to occur in a position of function.

Cast immobilization is the most frequently recognized treatment of fractures. To effectively stabilize a fracture, the joints above and below the fracture site are immobilized. The period of immobilization varies with each particular fracture location; in most cases the cast is not removed for at least 6–8 weeks to ensure that bone healing has progressed sufficiently for safe weight bearing and function. Immobilization within a cast often leads to significant joint stiffness; rehabilitation professionals are called on to help the patient who is recovering from fracture to regain preinjury function and range of motion.

External fixation devices have evolved primarily to care for fractures that are associated with open wounds. Pins are placed into bone on either side of the fracture and then clamped onto lightweight rods in an external frame. This maintains skeletal alignment while providing visual access to healing skin and muscle. The external fixator permits active range of motion of the joint above and below the fracture. It is removed when soft tissues have adequately healed and x-rays demonstrate healing of the fracture. Casts or orthoses can be used to provide immobilization after fixator removal to support and protect the fracture until healing is complete.

Fracture Casts

Historically, casts formed from linen bandages soaked in beaten egg whites and lime were used to attempt fracture immobilization. The beginning of the modern era in fracture care may have started with the discovery of plaster of Paris, first used in the Turkish Empire as reported by Eaton in 1798.[2] Plaster of Paris was reportedly used in Europe in the early nineteenth century, and a Flemish surgeon (Mathijsen) is credited with combining the use of plaster of Paris and cloth bandage to form casts for the treatment of fractures in 1852.[2-4]

Plaster Casts

Plaster of Paris (calcium sulfate) is created when heat is used to dehydrate gypsum. When water is added to plaster of Paris powder, the dehydration process is reversed, and crystals of gypsum are re-formed. The new crystals interlock in a chemical exothermic (heat producing) process.[3,5] The setting process is complete when heat is no longer being produced, although the cast remains wet to the touch until the excess water used in the process evaporates. Maximum cast strength is not reached until the plaster is completely dry. Drying time varies with the thickness of the cast, ambient humidity, and the type of plaster used. In most instances, maximum cast strength is reached in approximately 24 hours.

A variety of types of plaster of Paris with different working characteristics are available. Manufacturers may add accelerators to the material that shorten the setting time: The limb has to be held still for less time while the plaster sets. Although this may be advantageous when a cast is applied to the limb of an anxious child or when an unstable fracture is cast, it also means that less working time is available to manipulate the extremity and optimally shape the cast. Setting time can be prolonged slightly if cold water is used. If warm or hot water is used to reduce setting time, care must be taken to protect the limb from injury from the higher heat that can be generated during the setting process.[3] Cast temperatures as high as 68.5°C have been reached with water temperatures of 40°C.[6] Burns can occur if cast temperature is maintained at 44°C for 6 hours or more.[6,7] To minimize any potential for burns in cast or splint application, room temperature tepid water (24°C) is recommended.[6,7] If higher water temperatures have been used, the newly casted limb must not be placed on a pillow or other type of support that is likely to retain or reflect heat. Cast burns can also occur when insufficient padding has been placed between the plaster of Paris and the surface of the skin. Cast burns are avoidable if simple procedures are followed.

Cast strength is determined by three factors: the type of casting material used, the thickness of the cast, and the effectiveness of lamination among the layers of the cast material. The cloth mesh material that serves as the "carrier" for the plaster of Paris provides little strength for the cast. A plaster cast must be kept absolutely dry to prevent it from becoming soft and ineffective in immobilization.

Polyurethane Casts

The difficulties associated with the use of plaster of Paris have led to the development of newer and improved casting materials. Polyurethane-impregnated casting tapes have gained widespread popularity because of their superior strength, light weight, shorter setting time, cleaner application, and low exothermic reaction. Polyurethane casts are also radiolucent, permitting x-ray evaluation of fracture site healing while the limb remains encased in the cast.

Polyurethane is a plastic material that can be impregnated into a fabric substrate. Although the polyurethane bonds the layers of substrate together, it is actually the substrate that determines the strength of the cast. A variety of substrate materials are available. The weave determines how elastic the material will be during cast application and how strong the cast will be when set. Cotton, polyester, fiberglass, polypropylene, and blends of these materials and others are used in synthetic casting tapes.[5,8,9]

Immersing the synthetic casting tape in room temperature water for 10 seconds begins a heat-producing exothermic reaction and causes the material to harden (polymerize). Setting is complete for most synthetic casting materials in 5–10 minutes. Because of this short setting time, the rolls of bandage material cannot be opened until they are ready to be applied as a cast. The application process requires skill and must move quickly to ensure adequate molding time. Unlike plaster of Paris, the plastic bandage does not need to be massaged to ensure proper lamination between the layers of material. Also unlike plaster of Paris, which can easily be washed from the hands or clothing, polyurethane is not easily removed: It is essential that adequate protective padding is placed around the patient's limb and that protective gloves are worn to safeguard the applicator's hands. Polyurethane resin in its natural state is very tacky. An additive may be incorporated into the casting tape to reduce its tackiness. In some cases the manufacturer provides special gloves with an antitacky additive to minimize the tack further.[5] The exothermic polymerization of polyurethane resin produces much less heat (44.9°C in 40°C water) than that of setting plaster of Paris. In addition, heat is quickly dissipated, so that burns are much less likely to occur when synthetic materials are used. To minimize the risk of burns further, immersion of cast tape in room temperature water (24°C) is recommended.[3,7,10]

Other Materials Used in Cast Application

Stockinet is the first layer of a cast, applied over the skin, before any padding is added. The most common stockinet material is cotton. Synthetic materials, such as polyester or polypropylene, can be chosen in place of cotton because they do not retain water like cotton materials do. Stockinet also helps to position dressings over wounds and provides extra circumferential control of soft tissue within the cast. Stockinet is folded over the proximal and distal edges to finish the cast (and prevent inadvertent removal of cast padding by a nonresponsible individual or a child).

Next, a layer of cast padding is added over the stockinet. A variety of materials are available to pad casts.

Sheet cotton comes in various forms and is used to provide a barrier between the rigid walls of the cast and the surface of the skin. Some cast materials have been elasticized for easier application and conformation, and others require more technique to ensure that they uniformly conform to the body part being casted.

Although synthetic cast tapes are not affected by water, cast padding or stockinet can retain water. The risk of skin maceration and breakdown is present if the inside of a cast remains damp for long periods of time. Some manufacturers market cast padding that reportedly permits exposure to water; however, manufacturer recommendations must be followed carefully.

The thickness of cast padding varies between too much and too little. The goal is to protect bony prominences and soft tissue from the rigid walls of the cast while effectively immobilizing the fracture site. The thickness of cast padding varies; $\frac{1}{8}$–$\frac{1}{4}$ in. is sufficient for most patients. Soft tissue usually does well with a fairly thin, uniform two- or three-layer wrap. Extra padding is added to smooth and protect the irregular surfaces around bony prominences. Excessive padding reduces the ability of the cast to provide adequate immobilization. A well-molded cast that accurately follows the anatomic contours of the extremity requires less padding. Cast padding also provides a barrier so that the cast can be removed more easily when it needs to be changed or is no longer needed.

Cast Removal

A cast cutter with a vibrating disk is used to cut the cast during cast removal. Modern cast cutter blades reciprocate back and forth approximately $\frac{1}{8}$ in. in either direction. The vibrating blade easily cuts rigid materials such as metal, wood, plaster, or synthetic cast materials but does not cut through materials that are elastic or mobile. If used properly, a cast cutter does not cut skin. Incorrect or inappropriate use of a cast cutter can seriously cut or burn a patient. To reduce the risk of injury, the blade should not directly contact the patient's skin. Friction between the blade and cast significantly heats the blade, creating a potential for burns. A sharp new blade has less potential for burning the patient than does a blade that has become dull or worn out. The noise of the cast cutter can be quite frightening to children or other particularly anxious patients. A careful explanation and a demonstration of the cast cutter's action are the first steps in the process of cast removal.

To remove a cast safely, the cutter is used in a repetitive in-out motion, progressively opening the cast. This strategy reduces the risk of a cut or burn on the patient's skin.[11] The operator's thumb is used as a fulcrum as downward pressure is applied through the wrist. The thumb also controls the depth of the blade. Care is taken to avoid positioning the cast cutter in areas where skin is vulnerable: over a bony prominence or where significant edema or fragile healing skin is present. As the blade breaks through the inner wall of the cast, the sensation of reduced resistance to downward pressure as well as a change in sound occurs. Once an area of cast has been cut, the blade is repositioned further along the cast, and the process is repeated until the cast can be pried open completely. Bandage scissors are used to cut through padding and stockinet, and the limb is then extracted from the open cast. For infants and young children with small limbs, an alternative strategy can be used: A plaster of Paris cast can be removed by soaking in water. This method works particularly well when a corrective clubfoot cast is removed from an infant's limb.

FRACTURE MANAGEMENT AND POTENTIAL COMPLICATIONS

Benefits and potential complications are associated with each method of fracture management. Whether a splint, cast, surgical ORIF, or placement of external fixators has been used to stabilize the fracture, the condition of the extremity must be monitored carefully by the physician, rehabilitation professional, patient, and family caregivers.

One of the most important considerations for lower extremity fractures is weight-bearing status. A patient's weight-bearing status (full weight bearing, weight bearing as tolerated, toe-touch weight bearing, or non–weight bearing) is determined by the physician based on the stability of the fracture and the immobilization method used. Once a cast is applied and properly set, rehabilitation professionals work with the patient and family on mobility and gait training. The rehabilitation professional selects the appropriate assistive device for a patient's weight-bearing status, given the patient's physical and cognitive status and the characteristics of his or her usual living environment. It is important to communicate quickly to the referring physician any signs of developing complications or difficulty with compliance that might put the fracture site at risk.

Loss of "reduction" of the fracture is a serious complication and can occur whether a splint, cast, ORIF, or external fixator has been used to realign and stabilize the limb. A progressive angular deformity or abnormal position of the limb suggests loss of reduction and must be quickly reported to the managing physician. Even if reduction appears to be appropriate, inadequate immobilization within a splint or cast can lead to delayed union, nonunion (nonhealing), or malunion (healing in an abnormal position).

Any patient who has sustained an open fracture is at risk of developing infection of skin, deep tissue and muscle, or even bone. Infections are serious complications that require aggressive antibiotic treatment or debridement, or both. If an infection occurs after ORIF, the implanted hardware may have to be removed and an external fixation device applied. For patients with external fixation, the pins provide a tract directly into bone. Appropriate wound and pin care is essential to minimize the risk of infection. Osteomyelitis, or infection of bone, is a very serious situation that can result in deformity, joint destruction, and, in some circumstances, amputation.

Patients who have undergone ORIF are at risk of implant failure if repeated loading exceeds the strength of the implant material and design. Loosening or breakage of implanted screws, plates, or other devices also indicates excessive motion of the fracture site and increases the risk of delayed healing or nonunion. The patient's ability to function within weight-bearing limits established by the physician must be carefully assessed and monitored to reduce the risk of implant failure.

Complications also occur in patients whose fractures are managed by casting.[3] The patient's neurovascular function is documented before cast application and carefully monitored while the cast is in place. In the distal lower extremity, the peroneal nerve is susceptible to prolonged pressure (peroneal palsy) as it wraps around the head of the fibula.[11,12] In the upper extremity, the radial nerve is vulnerable to injury at the time of distal humeral fracture or during immobilization.[13,14]

Complaints of edge pressure or toes being squeezed can be solved with cast modifications; however, excessive pressure and discomfort inside the cast often require removal and reapplication of a new cast. On initial application, a cast is designed to have a snug, but not tight, fit. Signs of distal vascular compromise, such as delayed capillary refill on compression of the nail bed, suggest that the cast may be excessively tight.[11]

It is not uncommon for cast fit to loosen over time, as a result of several factors: Initial edema resolves, compressive forces modify soft tissue composition, disuse atrophy occurs, and cast padding compresses over time. Fit must be carefully monitored over time: A loose cast provides less control of the skeleton, and fracture reduction may be lost. Pistoning of a loose cast on the extremity is likely to lead to skin breakdown and shear over bony prominences.

Casts applied postoperatively while the patient is anesthetized are usually univalved (split down the front) to accommodate postoperative swelling.[15] Excessive swelling is accompanied by significant pain. Limb elevation is the first defense against excessive swelling and pain; however, the cast can be opened further or bivalved to relieve extreme pressure.[3] The risk of compartment syndrome must always be considered: If the patient experiences significant pain

on passive motion of the fingers or toes, the physician must be contacted immediately. Failure to recognize and appropriately treat a compartment syndrome results in muscle necrosis and possible loss of the limb.[16]

Occasionally, a window can be cut into a cast to inspect a wound or relieve a pressure area. If the limb is edematous, it is likely that soft tissue will begin to protrude through the window, resulting in additional skin irritation and breakdown. For this reason, any piece of cast that is removed to make a window must be reapplied and secured to the cast after modifications have been made.[3]

Patients with foot pain try to reposition the foot within the cast to make it more comfortable. Inappropriate plantar flexion of the foot within the cast creates excessive pressure on the posterior heel and dorsum of the foot. Discomfort can be reduced if the patient is able to push the relaxed foot gently downward while pulling the cast upward, as if pulling on a boot. If this fails to relieve pressure, the cast must be removed and reapplied.

Foreign objects introduced into a cast are the most common cause of discomfort and pressure. In an attempt to relieve itching of dry skin, patients are sometimes tempted to insert coat hangers, rulers, sticks, pens, and similar objects into the cast to scratch the itchy areas. This strategy often leads to displacement of cast padding, creating lumps and bumps where smooth surface contact is essential. Objects can break off or become trapped within the cast as well. The best way to relieve itching is by tapping on the cast or blowing cool air into it.

Another common complication is skin maceration, which is the result of prolonged exposure to water or a moist environment within the cast. Although, ideally, a cast is kept completely dry, many become wet at some point after application. Plaster casts that become wet lose significant stability and must be replaced. Synthetic casts can be towel dried as much as possible and then further dried using a cool setting on a blower or hairdryer.

EXTERNAL FRACTURE DEVICES

Four commonly used methods of fracture management use externally applied devices: traditional casts, splints, hybrid cast braces, and various fracture orthoses (prefabricated or custom fabricated). In choosing the appropriate external device for a given patient's fracture, several important issues must be considered. The first is the stability of the fracture site and how well a device will be able to maintain fracture reduction and achieve the desired anatomic result. The condition of the skin and soft tissue is also an important consideration, especially if wounds are present that must be accessed for proper care. Limb volume must be

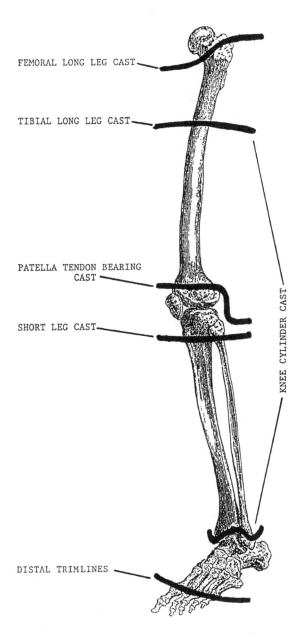

FEMORAL LONG LEG CAST

TIBIAL LONG LEG CAST

PATELLA TENDON BEARING
CAST

SHORT LEG CAST

KNEE CYLINDER CAST

DISTAL TRIMLINES

FIGURE 17-1

Proximal and distal trimlines used in standard lower extremity casts. Typically, the joints above and below the fracture site are immobilized. Trimlines can be extended to provide better control and stabilization.

evaluated, especially if edema is present or anticipated: How will limb size change over time in the device? Length of immobilization time varies as well: Is the device designed for a short-term problem, or will protection of the limb be necessary for an extended period? Will the device need to be removed for hygiene or wound care? Can the patient be unprotected while sleeping or when not ambulating?

How quickly the device will be available may also influence decision making. Casts and cast braces can be applied

quickly. Custom orthoses need additional fabrication and fitting time; an alternative means of protection is often required while the device is being fabricated.

Compliance and Reliability Issues

The patient's ability to comply consistently and reliably with weight-bearing restrictions and other aspects of fracture management must also be considered. Factors such as cognitive ability, emotional status, motivation, and physical ability, as well as the availability of assistance and environmental demands, influence the decision to provide additional external support. An unstable fracture managed by ORIF may not require additional support in patients with sufficient strength and balance who have a clear understanding of the healing process. If a patient is unable to understand the need to protect the involved limb from excessive loading or is physically unable to do so, additional external support is essential. If compliance is questionable, the device of choice is usually a nonremovable cast or cast brace. Pain is not always a deterrent against undesired loading or motion. Deformity can occur slowly over time and may not be detected until it is too late for conservative correction. The use of fracture orthoses requires that the patient be completely reliable and an active participant in his or her own care.

Casts and Splints

As we have already learned, a cast is a rigid, externally applied device that provides circumferential support to an injured body part (Figures 17-1 and 17-2). Casts immobilize a body segment to maintain skeletal alignment optimally. Once a cast has been applied, an x-ray can be used to assess the effectiveness of skeletal alignment. The cast may need to be modified, wedged, or replaced to improve alignment.[3]

A splint is a temporary supportive device, usually fabricated from rigid materials, held in position on the fractured extremity with bandages or straps. Splints can be used for temporary immobilization before casting or surgical stabilization. They can be used to maintain fracture reduction while waiting for swelling to diminish or fracture blisters to clear or to provide comfort. The most commonly used temporary fracture splint is called a *sugar tong splint*, a long, U-shaped, padded plaster splint named for its similarity to the tool used to pick up sugar cubes.[3]

Cast Braces

Cast braces were first developed as a method of fracture management just after World War I but then fell out of use until the mid-1960s.[16-18] They incorporate orthotic components, such as hinge joints and range of motion locks, into a plaster or synthetic cast, in an effort to provide additional stability to the tibia, knee, femur, or

FIGURE 17-2

Proximal and distal trimlines for standard upper extremity casts. Trimlines around the hand are designed to allow normal finger function, unless metacarpal fracture necessitates greater distal stability.

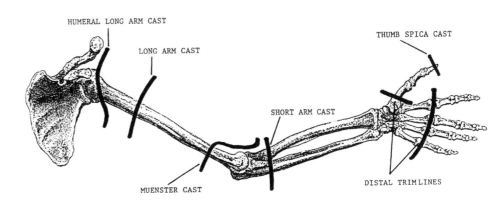

elbow.[17-34] The longer lever arm that is available when the cast is extended above the joint is better able to control varus/valgus and anterior/posterior angulation during motion of the joint. Currently, most cast braces are incorporated into synthetic cast materials because of their superior strength and durability. In most instances, joint motion is supported or guided by a polycentric type joint.[22-25,29,35-39] This joint more closely follows anatomic motion and reduces the torque-related stress that results from a single-axis mechanical joint.[40] Cast braces are often used to aid in controlling nondisplaced fractures about the knee (Figure 17-3) or elbow, to manage flexion contracture, or as an adjunct to internal fracture fixation (Figure 17-4).

Fracture Orthoses

An alternative for fracture management is a custom-fabricated or custom-fit orthotic device designed to maintain a body part in an optimal anatomic position.[29,41-43] Consistent with terminology used for other lower extremity orthotics, fracture orthoses are named by the joints they encompass and the motion that they are designed to control. An ankle-foot orthosis (AFO) with an anterior shell is used to control ankle and distal tibia motion (Figure 17-5); a knee-ankle-foot orthosis with total contact femoral and tibial components is designed to control and support a distal femur or proximal tibia fracture (Figure 17-6). For the most effective fracture orthosis, each prescription must designate the motion to be permitted and controlled, the corrective forces to be applied, and a precise diagnosis and description of the fracture.

The major advantage of a fracture orthosis, as compared to a cast brace, is that the orthosis can be removed for wound or skin care. Fracture orthoses are fabricated from high-temperature thermoplastic materials.[27,29,42,43] They are designed to provide total contact, circumferential control of a fracture while allowing the patient to have functional mobility. Fracture stability is enhanced in two ways: by hydrostatic pressure forces created as the rigid walls of the orthosis compress soft tissue and muscles in the extremity[3,27,29,44] and by the lever arm created by extension of the orthosis above and below the fracture site. Fracture orthoses do not effectively unload the lower extremity during weight bearing. If complete unloading or reduced

FIGURE 17-3

A tibial cast brace with polycentric adjustable range of motion hinges. The patient has undergone an open reduction internal fixation surgery after fracture of the tibial plateau. Note that synthetic cast tape is available in a wide variety of colors and patterns.

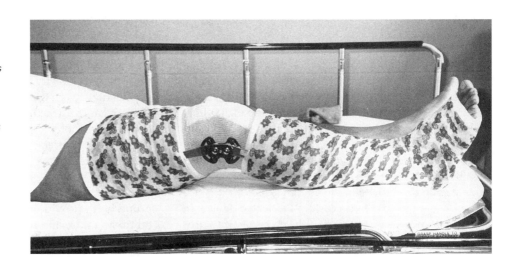

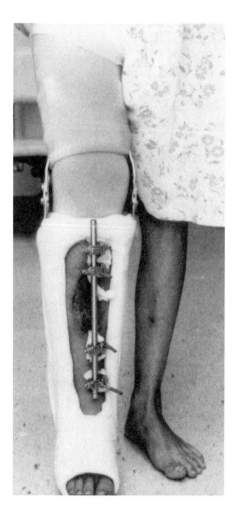

FIGURE 17-4

This cast brace provides medial/lateral stability for a com-minuted grade 3 open tibial fracture. The length of the tibia is being maintained by an external fixation device. The patient also sustained a closed femoral fracture, which has been sup-ported by an intramedullary rod fixation. Because the proxi-mal portion of the cast must not terminate near a fracture line, the femoral portion of the cast has been extended up to the level of the trochanter, to avoid stress on the femoral fixation.

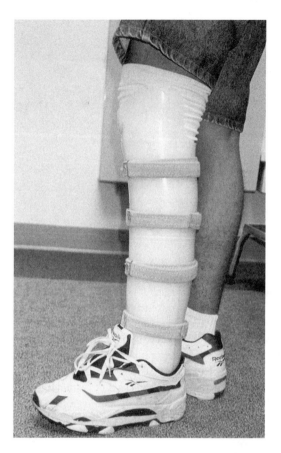

FIGURE 17-5

Ankle-foot fracture orthosis with a patellar tendon-bearing design incorporated to protect the tibia for bending moments during weight bearing. This patient was originally managed with an external fixation device, which had to be removed secondary to pin loosening before union of the fracture was solid. Note that the shoe has been modified with a cushion heel and rocker sole to compensate for a fixed ankle position and to improve forward progression during the stance phase of gait.

loading is required to protect the fracture site, an appro-priate assistive device (crutches or a walker) must be used.[44]

Two types of fracture orthoses are available: (1) those that are custom fabricated from a mold of the patient's limb and (2) prefabricated orthoses that are then custom fit to match the patient's needs. Because of the wide variation in anatomic characteristics among individuals, it is not always possible to use a prefabricated orthosis. Likewise, because of anatomic similarities in the human skeleton, it is not always necessary to create a custom-fabricated device. In certain instances, an orthosis must be precisely fit to pro-

vide the desired stabilization of the fracture; in other cases the orthosis must be heavily padded so that a precise fit is less important. Orthoses that are to be worn under clothes and in shoes require a close fit. The stability provided by the orthosis is directly related to the preciseness of the total contact fit between the orthosis and the skin. Prefabricated components for fracture orthoses usually must be modi-fied by an orthotist to ensure proper fit and function.

A number of prefabricated "short leg walkers" are also on the market today. These devices are designed to sub-stitute for a short leg cast and are intended to be remov-able by the patient. They are heavily padded and, if properly fit, provide excellent immobilization of the dis-tal tibia, ankle, and foot. The various designs are similar, but manufacturers' instructions should be followed to maximize their effectiveness.

SPECIFIC DESIGNS OF EXTERNAL FRACTURE MANAGEMENT DEVICES

In this section, a brief overview of the most commonly encountered casts and fracture orthoses is presented, including function, optimal limb position, and materials and design issues. Readers are referred to Figures 17-1 and 17-2 for examples of the usual trimlines.

Short Leg Casts

The short leg cast is applied when fracture of the distal tibia and fibula, ankle, and foot has occurred. The foot is positioned in a functional neutral ankle position (90 degrees) or in slight dorsiflexion. The foot can be casted in a plantar-flexed position to accommodate repair of an Achilles tendon rupture. Short leg casts are fabricated using either plaster of Paris or synthetic casting materials. The proximal trimline falls at the level of the tibial tubercle; the distal trimline usually encloses the metatarsal heads.[3,11] The area around the fibular head is protected by adding extra cast padding to minimize the risk of entrapment of the peroneal nerve. A cast shoe should be used to protect the bottom of the cast if weight bearing is to be permitted.

Short Leg Walkers

The short leg walker serves the same purpose as the short leg cast, controlling motion at the ankle and foot. Its advantage is that it can be removed for wound and skin care. Its disadvantage may be slightly less effective immobilization. The ankle is positioned at a neutral (90 degrees) angle. Some designs have an adjustable orthotic ankle joint that permits a controlled, limited range of motion, to assist forward progression during walking. The components of a short leg walker include a rigid foot piece that is attached to a pair of metal or thermoplastic uprights and a proximal cuff that helps to suspend a foam liner. Short leg walkers are manufactured in a variety of styles and sizes. To ensure proper fit, the manufacturer's recommendations must be followed carefully.

Ankle-Foot Orthoses with Anterior Shell (Fracture Orthoses)

The AFO with anterior shell is a fracture orthosis that is similar in design to a solid-ankle AFO with an anterior shell. It

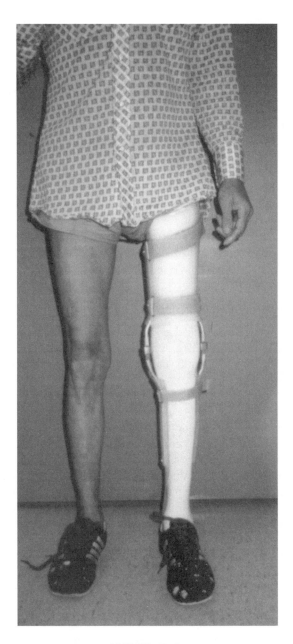

FIGURE 17-6
Knee-ankle-foot fracture orthosis, with a total contact femoral section, drop lock knee, and free ankle joint, prescribed for external support of a chronically infected nonunion of a supracondylar fracture of the femur.

is designed to encase the injured limb completely, absolutely limiting motion of the foot or ankle for patients with distal tibial or fibular fracture (see Figure 17-5). The AFO fracture orthosis has two advantages: It can be removed for wound care and hygiene, and it can be worn with standard lace-up style shoes if weight bearing is permitted. The application of a cushion heel and rocker sole may be necessary on the shoe to compensate for limited heel, ankle, and toe rocker motion during gait. Because total contact is essential, this thermoplastic orthosis is vacuum molded over a positive impression of the patient's limb.[42,43] The anterior shell may be lined with a soft-density foam to accommodate bony deformity or insufficient soft tissue. Perforated thermoplastic material is often used for the anterior section as a means of ventilation for patient comfort. The proximal anterior trimline is at the tibial tubercle. Adequate clearance must be provided for the head of the fibula and the peroneal nerve. The distal posterior section usually extends to just beyond the metatarsal heads on the plantar surface, whereas the anterior section is trimmed just proximally. A stocking or thin sock is worn to protect the skin and for comfort. The anterior section is held in place with a series of Velcro straps. Shoes must be worn if weight bearing is permitted.

Patellar Tendon-Bearing Casts

For patients with midshaft fractures of the tibia, a patellar tendon-bearing (PTB) cast can be chosen. This design incorporates a patellar tendon bar, which directs some of the limb loading force to the external shell of the cast, thus protecting the full length of the tibia against bending moments. This type of cast is not effective, however, in reducing axial loading of the tibia or hind foot. The PTB is most often used when extra stability is desired for patients who will be allowed some degree of weight-bearing activity. The cast is applied with the ankle maintained in neutral or slightly dorsiflexed position, to minimize potential hyperextension moment at the knee in stance. Trimlines are similar to those used for a PTB transtibial socket: at the midpatella (or sometimes suprapatella) anteriorly but trimmed and slightly flared posteriorly to permit knee flexion of at least 90 degrees. Proximally, the cast is well molded to the tibia in the area of the medial flare and around the patella.[3,4,19–21,28] Care must be taken to ensure that no pressure is placed on the peroneal nerve.

Patellar Tendon-Bearing Orthoses

The PTB fracture orthosis is the removable version of the PTB cast (see Figure 17-5), providing significant protection from bending and rotatory torque for the tibia during weight-bearing activities. This thermoplastic orthosis is most often vacuum molded over a positive mold of the patient's limb for optimal total contact fit. Ankle position within the orthosis is often in slight dorsiflexion, once again to minimize hyperextension moment at the knee during the stance phase of gait. Trimlines are similar to those of an AFO with anterior shell, with the proximal trimline extending somewhat more proximally to the proximal pole of the patella anteriorly, medially, and laterally. The pos-

terior trimline should permit free knee flexion beyond 90 degrees. Velcro straps are used to secure the anterior and posterior sections together.[2–4,12,27,42–44] The anterior and the posterior sections can be hinged at the proximal edge for improved anteroposterior control.

Knee Cylinder Cast

A knee cylinder cast is often applied when patients have sustained fractures of the patella or have undergone surgical repair of the knee joint and the knee must be immobilized in full extension. To ensure the necessary stability for the knee joint, the proximal trimline encompasses the lower two-thirds of the thigh and the distal trimline the entire tibial segment to just above the malleoli.[19] The cast can be applied using either plaster of Paris or synthetic casting tape. To limit the risk of pistoning when the patient is standing or walking, the cast is carefully molded to fit the contours of the medial femoral condyle.

Long Leg Cast

Fractures of the upper tibia, knee joint, and/or lower femur require more stability than the knee cylinder can provide. In these circumstances, the long leg cast is often chosen. Depending on the site of fracture and its relative stability, the limb is immobilized in nearly full extension or in a bent knee position.[2,11,12] A straight knee cast is usually applied with a slight (5 degrees) knee flexion angle to enhance patient comfort. Bent knee casts are usually chosen when non–weight bearing must be ensured during ambulation or to aid in controlling rotation of the tibia. With the relatively mobile arrangement of soft tissue that surrounds the femur, it is challenging to provide adequate immobilization, especially for patients who are particularly muscular or overweight. For this reason, control of rotational forces through the femur within a long leg cast is questionable. The cast is applied using either plaster of Paris or synthetic materials. If the cast is being used to stabilize the tibia, the proximal trimline is at the junction of the middle and proximal third of the femur. If the cast is being used to stabilize the distal femur, the proximal trimline is at the level of the greater trochanter. Distally, the cast immobilizes the ankle and extends to a point just beyond the metatarsal heads. The fibular head should be well padded within the cast to minimize the risk of entrapment of the peroneal nerve.

Lower Extremity Cast Braces

An alternative method that is used to control motion while maintaining optimal skeletal alignment of proximal tibial and distal femoral fractures near the knee is the application

of a lower extremity cast brace.[3,5–9,11–14,16,18,19,22,24,25,29–34,36,37,44]
The cast brace is often the method of choice for the management of nondisplaced tibial plateau fractures. It is often used for additional support of fractures near the knee that have been stabilized via ORIF surgery (see Figures 17-3 and 17-4). This method is also used to control motion after knee ligament injury or reconstruction. The cast brace can be applied using either plaster of Paris or synthetic cast materials. Depending on the nature of the fracture and its stability, the orthotic knee joints incorporated into the cast brace may be chosen to provide limited, controlled, or free-knee range of motion. The medial and lateral uprights provide protection against unwanted varus and valgus stress and help to control anterior/posterior displacement of the tibia or femur. Because the anatomic center rotation of the knee moves in an arc centered over the femoral condyles, it is essential that the mechanical joints be carefully aligned with the anatomic knee joint to reduce the abnormal stress that occurs across the joint and fracture site.[26,38,40,45,46] It is often difficult to palpate the condyles on a patient who has recent trauma about the knee; the midpatella is a somewhat less precise alternative landmark for alignment. A properly placed polycentric metal joint will be proximal to the joint line and slightly posterior to the midline.

To control motion for fractures of the tibia and knee, the proximal component encases the lower two-thirds of the femur. If fracture of the femur has occurred, the proximal component extends upward to the level of the greater trochanter. A cast brace is most frequently used to provide additional support for femoral fractures that have been stabilized with internal fixation. To be effective, careful molding of the proximal portion of the cast around the trochanter and medial wall is required. For fractures of the mid to upper femur, an orthotic hip joint and pelvic band must be added to ensure alignment and stability. The trimline of the tibial component is typically at the tibial tubercle; the distal trimline of the femoral component is an equal distance from the midpatella. Posteriorly, both components are trimmed to permit at least 90 degrees of knee flexion. The orthotic knee joints are positioned close to but not quite contacting skin. This is especially important medially, where contact between the knees during functional activity is likely. If warranted, a slight varus or valgus stress can be applied at the time of cast brace application, or a varus/valgus strap can be added to aid in unloading a knee compartment.[43] The distal tibial component holds the ankle in a neutral position and extends distally to encompass the metatarsal heads.

Knee-Ankle-Foot Fracture Orthoses

The purpose of the knee-ankle-foot fracture orthosis is to provide long-term protection for fractures of the dis-

tal to midfemur, or for fractures about the knee (see Figure 17-6). The orthosis is removable for wound care and personal hygiene and when protection is not required. Depending on the location of the fracture, the orthosis can be designed to limit range of motion or to permit full motion of the knee. Drop locks can be used to stabilize the knee in full extension during ambulation. The design of the orthosis also protects the knee from excessive medial/lateral and anterior/posterior sheer stress during ambulation. If maximum stability is necessary, a solid-ankle design can be incorporated; if mobility of the ankle is desired, an articulated ankle joint with an appropriate motion stop mechanism can be used. The orthosis requires total contact within the femoral and tibial components. Proximal trimlines follow the anatomic contours of the proximal femur to the greater trochanter to provide femoral protection. To stabilize the knee or proximal tibia, encasement of the lower two-thirds of the femur is sufficient. The orthosis alone cannot effectively unload the femur, tibia, or foot: If axial unloading is desired, appropriate assistive devices (crutches or walker) must be used.[25]

Hip and Proximal Femur Protection

For patients with proximal femoral fractures, a hip joint and a pelvic band are often incorporated into a femoral long leg cast, cast brace, or total contact knee-ankle-foot orthosis in an effort to control motion and rotational forces. Depending on the patient's specific needs, hip flexion/extension motion can be restricted or free; abduction/adduction is usually restricted. The placement of the orthotic hip joint is approximately 1 cm anterior and 1 cm proximal to the tip of the greater trochanter in most adults.[46] Knee and ankle motion can be free or limited, given the location and stability of the fracture. A variety of single-axis or polycentric orthotic hip joints can be incorporated. A pelvic belt is used to maintain the orthotic hip joint in proper functional position. The belt should fit midway between the crest of the ilium and the greater trochanter.

Hip Spica Casts

A hip spica cast, which encases the hip and pelvis in addition to the lower extremity, is necessary for effective control of fractures of the proximal femur and of the hip joint[3,11,16,47] (Figure 17-7). The hip spica is the primary method of treatment of femoral fractures in children and is used in adults when there is no better alternative. Several variations of the hip spica are available. In a single hip spica, the plaster or synthetic cast material is anchored around the entire pelvis and lower trunk but immobilizes only the hip and proximal femur of the involved side, allow-

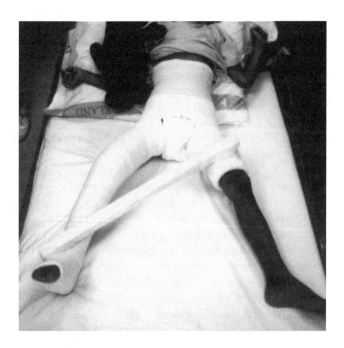

FIGURE 17-7
This child has been placed in a 1 ½ hip spica cast to stabilize a fracture of the proximal femur. Note the opening for personal hygiene and the additional diagonal support bar incorporated between the short and long sections of the cast.

ing fairly unrestricted hip motion of the opposite limb. In a 1 ½ hip spica, the cast encases the entire lower extremity on the affected side, as well as the lower trunk, pelvis, and thigh on the uninvolved side. Usually the knee on the affected side is completely immobilized; however, an articulated knee joint can be incorporated if specific circumstances so dictate. In most instances, the hip joint of the affected limb is immobilized in 30 degrees of flexion and 30 degrees of abduction, and the perineal edges are trimmed back to allow for personal care and hygiene. The knee is usually positioned in 30 degrees of flexion. The proximal cast encases the lower to midtrunk (to the level of the costal margin or nipple line), depending on the amount of spinal immobilization required. The 1 ½ hip spica cast is often reinforced by the incorporation of a lightweight diagonal bar between the short and long extremity segments. Ambulation is possible but often quite challenging, requiring significant upper body strength to manage the adapted crutch-walking gait that the cast position makes necessary.

Hip Abduction Casts

A hip abduction cast can be used for older children and adults who have had reconstructive surgery involving the

hip joint or who have had recurrent hip dislocation and require protective positioning. Well-padded short leg casts, of either plaster or synthetic cast materials, are placed on the individual's lower extremities. The abducted and rotated position of the hip is held by two bars attached to the cast at the proximal and distal trimlines. The amount of abduction and rotation varies. Abduction should not exceed the patient's ability to get through a door. In most cases, patients with hip abduction casts use a wheelchair rather than crutch walking for mobility.

Short Arm Casts

Most fractures of the radius and/or ulna require immobilization of the wrist and forearm but not the hand or fingers. The wrist is usually immobilized in a position of function (slight wrist extension) or in the position that best maintains fracture reduction.[3,48] Radial or ulnar or dorsal or volar molding is often used to facilitate fracture reduction. Careful attention should be given to maintenance of the palmar arch, as well as thumb and finger motion, so that functional use of the hand is preserved: The distal trimlines at the palmar metacarpophalangeal joint should not restrict thumb or finger motion. The proximal trimlines of this cast are tailored to allow supination/pronation and elbow flexion/extension.

Thumb Spica Casts

For patients with fracture or soft tissue injury of the thumb, wrist, or distal radius, a thumb spica short arm cast can be applied.[48,49] In this cast, the wrist is placed in neutral to slight extension, while the thumb is maintained under the second and third finger in an abducted position. With the thumb centered directly under the second and third fingers, the patient is able to use a three-point palmar prehension grasp (three-jaw chuck) for functional activities while in the cast. Finger flexion is unrestricted, but the cast extends to the distal tip of the thumb. In case of a tendon laceration, the thumb can be positioned so that minimal tension is placed on the repair. The proximal trimline can be as long as is necessary to stabilize the fracture without undue restriction of elbow motion.

Muenster Casts

When a forearm or wrist injury requires restriction of supination and pronation, a Muenster cast is applied. This cast effectively immobilizes the wrist and forearm, restricting pronation and supination of the forearm, with preservation of elbow flexion and some limitation of elbow extension (to within 30 degrees of full extension).[50] The forearm is usually positioned in neutral between supination and pronation. The proximal edge of the cast encases the humeral condyles, with careful molding around the medial, lateral, and posterior elbow. The proximal anterior edge is trimmed to permit free elbow flexion.

Forearm Fracture Orthoses

An alternative to a short arm cast, especially for patients with fragile skin or healing wounds, is a forearm fracture orthosis (wrist-hand orthosis; WHO). The major advantage of a WHO fracture orthosis is the ability to take it off for skin care and hygiene.[30] This is also its major disadvantage, as noncompliant patients may choose not to wear the orthosis as much as is indicated. The design of the WHO fracture orthosis is the same as that described previously for a short arm cast. Usually it is custom fabricated or fit, in two pieces, from a low- or high-temperature thermoplastic material (Figure 17-8). The overlapping dorsal and volar pieces are held securely in place with Velcro straps or webbing and buckles. Low-temperature plastics are used when the orthosis will be short term or when modification or changes in position are anticipated. High-temperature materials are used when the orthosis will be worn for extended periods and when no major modifications or changes are necessary.

Long Arm Casts

For patients with fractures of the forearm, elbow, or distal humerus, a long arm cast is chosen. This type of cast cannot adequately control the motion of fractures of the proximal third of the humerus.[1,3,11,14,36,45,48,51] This cast is essentially a short arm cast with an extension above the elbow. The elbow is most often immobilized at 90 degrees of flexion, but this can vary according to fracture patterns and the anticipated long-term result. If control of the elbow is required, the proximal cast extends into the axilla. The proximal trimline may incorporate the acromion if control of the humerus is required. The cast is molded around the shoulder at a comfortable resting position, without limiting internal rotation of the shoulder. Depending on the site and nature of the fracture, the cast can also be used to limit external rotation and abduction of the shoulder.

Upper Extremity Fracture Orthoses

The upper extremity fracture orthosis is an alternative to a long arm cast when control of wrist (flexion/extension), forearm (supination/pronation), and elbow (flexion/extension) motion is desired.[23,30] Its major advantage is the ability to be removed for skin care and personal hygiene. Motion of the elbow can be blocked, limited, or

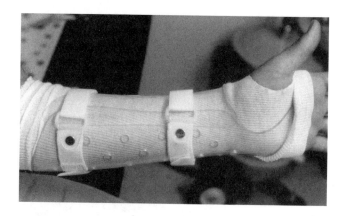

FIGURE 17-8
A wrist-hand fracture orthosis with total contact on the dorsal and ventral surfaces of the forearm is used to control motion of the wrist. Note the stockinet placed between the orthosis and skin for comfort and protection and the position of the palmar trimline that is necessary for thumb opposition during functional activities.

freely allowed, depending on the type of external orthotic elbow joint that is chosen. The orthosis is custom fabricated or custom fit. Either low- or high-temperature thermoplastic materials are used, depending on the degree of modification and the length of use anticipated. Although two orthotic joints (a medial and a lateral) can be used at the elbow, it is challenging to align them with each other and with the anatomic axis of the elbow. In most cases, a single lateral joint, centered over the lateral epicondyle, is sufficient to control motion and provide protection.[39,51] The forearm and humeral sections each have two slightly overlapping pieces, held in place by Velcro straps. Proximal trimlines are similar to those of a long arm cast: For control of elbow motion, the orthosis reaches the axilla, whereas if humeral control is necessary, the orthosis reaches the acromion. Proximal control of the humerus is enhanced by an additional strap around the upper chest.

Arm Cast Braces

For patients who have sustained a fracture near the elbow, an arm cast brace is an alternative to the traditional long arm cast.[39] Depending on the stability of the fracture, orthotic joints can be used to limit motion or to permit free motion. Pronation and supination, however, are usually limited. Fractures distal to the elbow joint are managed in a cast brace that extends to the level of the axilla. If appropriate, anterior trimlines permit flexion, whereas posterior trimlines encompass more of the joint to control extension. For humeral fractures, the cast brace extends to the tip of the acromion. Careful molding of the cast

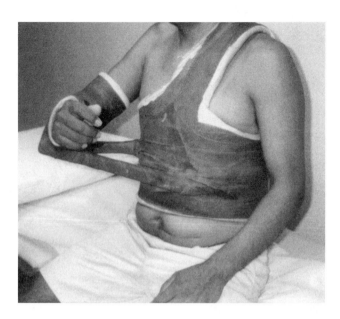

FIGURE 17-9
The shoulder spica cast is used when precise control of all planes of shoulder motion is necessary. This patient has undergone a shoulder fusion. Note the anterior and posterior stabilization bars, which are used to hold the desired upper extremity position with respect to the body cast.

about the shoulder permits a comfortable resting position but does not restrict shoulder motion. The orthotic joint is centered over the lateral epicondyle.[52] The distal trimlines at the hand permit full finger and thumb motion unless the fracture requires distal stabilization. The wrist is held in a straight or slightly extended position, in neutral with respect to radial or ulnar deviation. The forearm is also in neutral with respect to pronation and supination. The thumb is immobilized in a thumb's-up position. In certain fractures, the extremity position can be altered to maintain fracture reduction.

Humeral Cuffs

The humeral cuff is used quite successfully to control humeral motion for patients with isolated humeral fractures.[46,52] Fracture union rates of more than 90% have been reported.[53] In this method of fracture management, shoulder and elbow motion is unrestricted. The cuff is best able to control anterior/posterior and medial/lateral motion of the humerus. It is not effective, however, in controlling a supracondylar fracture of the humerus. For patients with fractures of the proximal third of the humerus, an additional chest strap is used to secure the proximal portion of the orthosis to the humerus. The cuff is fabri-

cated from high- or low-temperature thermoplastic materials, custom fit to the patient. Prefabricated orthoses are effective in the management of humeral fractures because circumference and height can be easily adjusted. Total contact circumferential designs with Velcro closures are recommended. Orthoses must extend proximal and distal to the fracture for effective control of motion.

Shoulder Spica Cast

For patients with complex fractures of the humerus, for which control of all planes of shoulder motion is required, a shoulder spica cast is used.[14,53-55] This method of fracture management immobilizes the shoulder in the position that best maintains fracture reduction or soft tissue repair (Figure 17-9). The most common position is in 30 degrees of forward humeral flexion, 30 degrees of shoulder abduction, and 30 degrees of external rotation. Elbow and wrist motion is often restricted as well. Although complete immobilization of the wrist is not always necessary, the wrist must be well supported. A shoulder spica can be fabricated from either plaster of Paris or synthetic casting materials. In a shoulder spica, a long arm cast is incorporated into a modified body cast, using biomechanical principles to achieve the desired restriction of motion. Humeral adduction is opposed by extending the body portion of the cast distally and laterally on the trunk on the affected side and into the axilla on the contralateral side. Internal rotation of the arm (a result of gravity) is opposed by extending the cast anteriorly and distally as much as possible without restricting hip flexion. The cast is also extended over the shoulder, connecting the anterior and posterior portions of the cast. This extension, which barely contacts the neck on the unaffected side, aids in preventing rotation of the body cast. The arm is held in the desired position by incorporation of a set of stabilizing bars between the body cast and the elbow/forearm sections.

Shoulder-Elbow-Wrist-Hand Orthoses (Airplane Splint)

When fracture reduction requires the upper extremity to be immobilized in a position of shoulder abduction, flexion, and external rotation, an airplane splint, or shoulder-elbow-wrist-hand orthosis, may be necessary.[53] Depending on the stability of the fracture or repair site, external orthotic joints can be used to allow or limit shoulder, elbow, and/or wrist motion. Thermoplastic or lightweight metals are used to fabricate a frame that holds the arm away from the body in the desired position. This orthotic is adjustable to various degrees of shoulder abduction and flexion, and elbow motion may be free or limited. Because of its weight and fit, the shoulder-elbow-wrist-hand orthosis must be well-secured, usually with tightly fit Velcro straps, or it will shift position and become uncomfortable to the patient.

CONCLUSION

Extremity fractures, whether managed by closed reduction or surgical open reduction and internal fixation, usually require a period of immobilization for effective healing (union) of the fracture site to occur. The orthopedic surgeon and orthotist choose from a variety of casts, cast braces, splints, and fracture orthoses to provide the most effective fracture management strategy for each patient, based on fracture type and location, degree of reduction, skin condition, mobility needs, and likelihood of compliance. Geographic and personal preferences regarding design, device selection, and treatment influence the choice of fracture management strategy, as do the training and experience of the health professionals involved. Most fractures can be managed effectively in a variety of ways: Rarely is a single procedure the primary option. The description of the various fracture devices provided in this chapter is meant to serve as a guideline, with the understanding that each must be adjusted to individual needs or preferences.

None of the strategies described can provide 100% rigid fixation: This is only possible with direct skeletal attachment. A variety of factors influence the quality of fit and function of any of the casts, cast braces, splints, or fracture orthoses that we have described. Each of the devices has the potential to contribute to a successful result, but only if used appropriately, with absolute attention to detail by each of the treatment team members.

REFERENCES

1. Gustilo RB, Anderson JT. Prevention of infection in the treatment of one thousand and twenty-five open fractures of long bones. J Bone Joint Surg 1976;58(4):453–458.
2. Bick EM. Source Book of Orthopaedics. New York: Hafner, 1968;286–287.
3. Harkess JW, Ramsey WC, Harkess JW. Principles of Fracture and Dislocations. In CA Rockwood, DP Green, RW Bucholz (eds), Rockwood and Green's Fractures in Adults, vol. 1 (3rd ed). Philadelphia: Lippincott, 1991;1–180.
4. Wytch R, Mitchell C, Ratchie IK, et al. New splinting material. Prosthet Orthot Int 1987;11(1):42–45.
5. Richard RE. Polymers in Fracture Immobilization. In JC Salamore (ed), The Polymeric Materials Encyclopedia CRC Press, 1996.
6. Wytch R, Ashcroft GP, Ledingham WM, et al. Modern splinting bandages. J Bone Joint Surg 1991;73(1):88–91.
7. Lavalette RN, Pope M, Dickstein H. Setting temperatures of plaster casts. J Bone Joint Surg 1982;64(6):907–911.
8. Wytch R, Mitchell CB, Wardlaw D, et al. Mechanical assessment of polyurethane impregnated fiberglass bandage for splinting. Prosthet Orthot Int 1987;11(3):128–134.
9. Wytch R, Ross N, Wardlaw D. Glass fiber versus non-glass fiber splinting bandages. Injury 1992;23(2):101–106.
10. Pope M, Callahan G, Leveled R. Setting temperature of synthetic casts. J Bone Joint Surg 1985;67A(2):262–264.
11. Hilt NE, Cogburn SB. Cast and Splint Therapy. In NE Hilt, SB Cogburn (eds), Manual of Orthopaedics. St. Louis: Mosby, 1980;459–516.
12. Russell TA, Taylor JC, LaVelle DG. Fractures of the Tibia. In CA Rockwood, DP Green, RW Bucholz (eds), Rockwood and Green's Fractures in Adults, 3rd ed, vol 2. Philadelphia: Lippincott, 1991;1915–1982.
13. Curtis RJ, Dameron TB, Rockwood CA. Fractures and Dislocations of the Shoulder in Children. In CA Rockwood, DP Green, RW Bucholz (eds), Rockwood and Green's Fractures in Adults, 3rd ed, vol 3. Philadelphia: Lippincott, 1991;859–920.
14. Epps CH, Grant RE. Fractures of the Shaft of the Humerus. In CA Rockwood, DP Green, RW Bucholz (eds), Rockwood and Green's Fractures in Adults, 3rd ed, vol 1. Philadelphia: Lippincott, 1991;843–870.
15. Chapman MW. Open Fractures. In CA Rockwood, DP Green, RW Bucholz (eds), Rockwood and Green's Fractures in Adults, 3rd ed, vol 1. Philadelphia: Lippincott, 1991;223–264.
16. Pellegrini VD, Evarts CM. Complications. In CA Rockwood, DP Green, RW Bucholz (eds), Rockwood and Green's Fractures in Adults, 3rd ed, vol 1. Philadelphia: Lippincott, 1991;390–393.
17. Connolly JF, Dahne E, Lafollette B. Closed reduction and early cast-brace ambulation in the treatment of femoral fractures. Part 2. J Bone Joint Surg 1973;55A(8):1581–1599.
18. Moll JH. The cast brace walking treatment of open and closed femoral fractures. South Med J 1973;66(3):345–352.
19. Mooney V. Cast bracing. Clin Orthop July Aug 1974;(102):159–166.
20. Brown PW. The early weight-bearing treatment of tibial shaft fractures. Clin Orthop Nov Dec 1974;(105):167–178.
21. Brown PW, Urban J. Early weight-bearing treatment of open fractures of the tibia. J Bone Joint Surg 1969;51A(1):59–75.
22. Connolly JF, King P. Closed reduction and early cast brace ambulation in the treatment of femoral fractures. Part 1. J Bone Joint Surg 1973;55A(8):1559–1580.
23. Kellam JF, Jupiter JB. Diaphyseal Fractures of the Forearm. In BD Browner, JB Jupiter, AM Levine, PG Trafton (eds), Skeletal Trauma, vol 2. Philadelphia: Saunders, 1992;1095–1124.
24. Lenin BE, Mooney V, Ashy ME. Cast-bracing for fractures of the femur. J Bone Joint Surg 1977;59S(7):917–923.
25. Maggot B, Gad DA. Cast bracing for fractures of the femoral shaft. J Bone Joint Surg 1981;63B(1):12–23.
26. Mooney V, Nickel V, Harvey JP, et al. Cast-brace treatment for fractures of the distal part of the femur. J Bone Joint Surg 1970;52A(8):1563–1578.

27. Sarmiento A. A functional below-the-knee brace for tibial fractures. J Bone Joint Surg 1970;52A(2):295–311.

28. Sarmiento A. A functional below-the-knee cast for tibial fractures. J Bone Joint Surg 1967;49A(5):855–975.

29. Sarmiento A. Functional bracing of tibial and femoral shaft fractures. Clin Orthop Jan Feb 1972;(82):2–13.

30. Sarmiento A, Cooper JS, Sinclair WF. Forearm fractures: early functional bracing, preliminary report. J Bone Joint Surg 1975;57(3):297–304.

31. Snelson R, Irons G, Mooney V. Application of cast braces for post acute care of lower extremity fractures. Orthot Prosthet December 1970;21–26.

32. Stills M, Christiansen K, Bucholz RW, et al. Cast bracing bicondylar tibial plateau fractures after combined internal and external fixation. J Prosthet Orthot 1991;3(3):106–113.

33. Thomas T, Megitt B. A comparative study of methods for treating fractures of the distal half of the femur. J Bone Joint Surg 1981;63B(1):3–6.

34. Wardlaw D, McLauchlan J, Pratt D. A biomechanical study of cast-brace treatment of femoral shaft fractures. J Bone Joint Surg 1981;63B(1):7–11.

35. DeCoster TA, Nepola JU, El-khoura GY. Cast brace treatment of proximal tibia fractures. Clin Orthop June 1988;(231):196–204.

36. Hardy AE. The treatment of femoral fractures by cast-brace application and early ambulation. J Bone Joint Surg 1983;65(1):56–65.

37. Hohl M, Johnson EE, Wiss DA. Fractures of the Knee. In CA Rockwood, DP Green, RW Bucholz (eds), Rockwood and Green's Fractures in Adults, vol 2. Philadelphia: Lippincott, 1991;1725–1761.

38. Kapandji IA. The Knee. The Physiology of the Joints, 25th ed. New York: Churchill Livingstone, 1991;64–147.

39. McMaster WC, Tivnon MC, Waugh T. Cast brace for the upper extremity. Clin Orthop 1975;(109):126–129.

40. Norkin CC, Levangie PK. The Knee Complex. Joint Structure and Function—A Comprehensive Analysis (2nd ed). Philadelphia: Davis, 1992;337–378.

41. Pritham CH, Stills ML. Femoral immobilizer. Orthot Prosthet 1979;33(3):39–45.

42. Stills ML. Vacuum-formed orthosis for fractures of the tibia. Orthot Prosthet 1976;30(2):43–55.

43. Wilson AB, Stills ML, Condie D, Pritham C. Lower Limb Orthotics: A Manual. Philadelphia: Rehabilitation Engineering Center Temple-Moss, 1977.

44. Sarmiento A, Sinclair WF. Fracture Orthosis. In American Academy of Orthopaedic Surgeons, Atlas of Orthotics—Biomechanical Principles and Application. St. Louis: Mosby, 1975;245–254.

45. Gschwend NG, Wyss UP. Total Replacement of the Knee in Rheumatoid Arthritis. In J Black, JH Dumbleton (eds), Clinical Biomechanics: A Case History Approach. New York: Churchill Livingstone, 1981;279–306.

46. Weber D (ed). The Knee. In Canadian Association of Prosthetists and Orthotists, Clinical Aspects of Lower Extremity Orthotics. Ontario, Canada: Elgan, 1990.

47. Beatty JH. Congenital Anomalies of the Hip and Pelvis. In AH Crenshaw (ed), Campbell's Operative Orthopaedics. St. Louis: Mosby, 1987;2721–2722.

48. Cooney WP, Linscheid RL, Dobyns JH. Fractures and Dislocations of the Wrist. In CA Rockwood, DP Green, RW Bucholz (eds), Rockwood and Green's Fractures in Adults, 3rd ed, vol 1. Philadelphia: Lippincott, 1991; 563–678.

49. Green DP, Rowland SA. Fractures and Dislocations in the Hand. In CA Rockwood, DP Green, RW Bucholz (eds), Rockwood and Green's Fractures in Adults, 3rd ed, vol 1. Philadelphia: Lippincott, 1991;441–562.

50. Berger N. Upper Limb Prosthetic Systems. In American Academy of Orthopaedic Surgeons, Atlas of Limb Prostheses. St. Louis: Mosby, 1981;99–100.

51. Hotchkiss RN, Green DP. Fractures and Dislocations of the Elbow. In CA Rockwood, DP Green, RW Bucholz (eds), Rockwood and Green's Fractures in Adults, vol 1. Philadelphia: Lippincott, 1991;739–843.

52. Werner FW. Principles of Musculoskeletal Biomechanics—Forearm and Elbow Joint. In CA Peimer (ed), Surgery of the Hand and Upper Extremity. New York: McGraw-Hill, 1996;21.

53. Ward EF, Savoie FH, Hughes JL. Fractures of the Diaphyseal Humerus. In BD Browner, JB Jupiter, AM Levine, PG Trafton (eds), Skeletal Trauma, vol 2. Philadelphia: Saunders, 1992;1177–1200.

54. Curtis RJ, Dameron TB, Rockwood CA. Fractures and Dislocation of the Shoulder in Children. In CA Rockwood, KE Wilkins, RE King (eds), Fractures in Children. Philadelphia: Lippincott, 1991;829–919.

55. Sarmiento A, Kinman PB, Galvin E. Functional bracing of fractures of the shaft of the humerus. J Bone Joint Surg 1977;59(5):596–601.

18

Splinting, Orthotics, and Prosthetics in the Management of Burns

R. Scott Ward

Rehabilitation of a patient with burns involves programs that focus on restoring functions that are compromised by the burn injury.[1] Treatment strategies used by therapists address five important goals: (1) to improve or promote wound healing by reducing wound infection, (2) to prevent or reduce deformity, (3) to increase mobility and strength to achieve maximal function, (4) to reduce the effects of hypertrophic scarring, and (5) to educate patients about their recuperation. The rehabilitation plan for the patient with burns centers on wound care, positioning, range of motion exercises, splinting, strengthening exercises, endurance and functional exercises, gait training, and scar control. Modern burn care emphasizes the need for a comprehensive team approach to achieve maximal clinical results.[1,2]

BURN INJURY

Each year, more than 730,000 people sustain burn injuries that require emergency room visits. Of these, more than 300,000 are seriously injured directly by fire, and nearly 8,000 die as a result of the injury.[3,4] The American Burn Association has developed a process for determining the severity of burn injury; these determinants include etiology of the injury, burn depth, the total body surface area (TBSA) that was burned, the location of the burn, and patient age.[5] A burn injury of any given size is more severe in patients who are very young or very old. The deeper the injury, the more serious the burn is considered. Involvement of the face, eyes, ears, perineum, hands, and feet makes the injury more critical. Associated trauma, smoke inhalation injury, and poor preinjury health status are factors that increase the severity of the injury. An appropriate knowledge of the nature of burn injury and the location and depth of the burn wound is important in understanding and anticipating the possible problems that a patient may face during rehabilitation.

Etiology of Burns

Burn injury can be the result of a variety of causes, including flame, scalds, flash (radiant heat explosions), contact, chemical, electrical, and others (irradiation, radioactivity, etc.).[6] Flame and scald burns are the most common causes of burn injury.[6-8] The elderly and those of preschool age are at the highest risk of suffering scald injuries.[9-11] Chemical and electrical burns present differently than do other burn injuries. Burns resulting from chemical agents require identification of the causative agent so that proper neutralization of the chemical can take place. Assessment of the depth of chemical burns is difficult at first, but these wounds are predictably deep.[12] Areas of significant surface burn may be present with an electrical injury; however, these are often the result of associated flash burns. Small deep wounds where the current enters or exits the body are more typical.[6,13] The major complication with rehabilitative consequence of electrical injury is musculoskeletal necrosis, which frequently results in amputation.[14]

Burn Depth

Thomsen[15] has studied Indian writings that date back to approximately 600 BC, which describe four levels or degrees of burn depth, and declares that deep burns heal slowly and with scarring. Two methods are used to describe burn depth: degree (first, second, or third degree)[16] and thickness (superficial, partial thickness, and full thickness).[17] The thickness terminology is more commonly used in clinical practice. A superficial thickness injury would correspond to a first-degree injury, a partial thickness to a

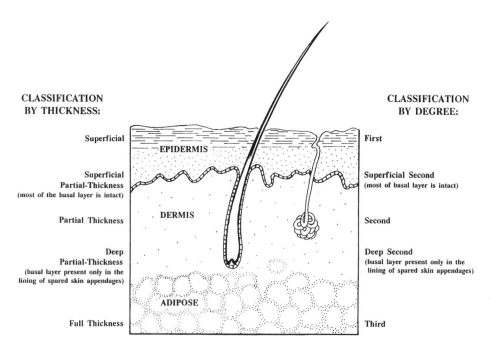

FIGURE 18-1
Representation of the depths of burn injury, referencing the contemporary "thickness" classification with the more traditional "degree" terminology. (Reprinted with permission from RS Ward. The rehabilitation of burn patients. Crit Rev Phys Med Rehabil 1991;2:121–138.)

second-degree injury, and a full thickness to a third-degree injury (Figure 18-1).

A knowledge of clinical characteristics that are associated with the injury thickness is helpful in identification of the depth of the burn. Superficial (first degree) injuries involve only the epidermis. They are often painful, erythematous, and mildly edematous. Superficial burn injuries usually heal in 3–7 days and rarely result in scarring. Superficial partial-thickness (superficial second degree) wounds compromise the epidermis and upper dermis. These burns are very painful, very red, and often have blisters or weeping wounds, or both. Superficial partial-thickness burns usually heal in 14–21 days and rarely develop scar. In deep partial-thickness burns (deep second degree) deeper layers of the dermis are damaged. The wound may or may not be painful, it may be cherry red or pale, and the skin is still pliable. Deep partial-thickness burns require more than 21 days to heal spontaneously and will scar. In full-thickness (third degree) burns destruction of all layers of the skin occurs. The wound generally has a tan or brown appearance and exhibits a leathery texture. Full-thickness wounds are painless and need several weeks to heal without surgical intervention. Deep partial-thickness burns are often managed with skin graft; full-thickness injuries require skin grafting. A deeper burn generally correlates with an increased severity of injury.

Small burn wounds can be excised and closed primarily; however, most burn wounds require excision of the burn followed by coverage of the site with a skin graft.[18] Excision of the burn wound is ordinarily performed tangentially; that is, thin layers of the burn are removed until viable tissue is reached.[19] Autografts (split thickness) are harvested from undamaged areas of the body for coverage of the excised wound.[20] Skin grafts placed on tangentially excised wounds demonstrate good long-term functional results.[21] Full-thickness skin grafts can also be used. Interestingly, split-thickness grafts scar more than do full-thickness grafts.[21]

Progress has been made in the use of skin substitutes and cultured skin for coverage of the excised burn.[22–25] Areas treated in this fashion tend to be fragile and susceptible to breakdown.[26] Further, it appears that wounds treated with cultured epithelium do not scar aggressively; however, little information is yet available about rehabilitative ramifications of this treatment approach.[27]

Burn Size

Burn wound size is reported as a percent of the TBSA that is injured. Lund and Browder[28] describe a method for estimating percent TBSA. Variations in body part ratios during development and diversified proportions of individual anatomic parts are considered in making the estimation (Figure 18-2). A burn injury increases in severity as the percent TBSA burn increases. Large burns usually require longer convalescence, which in turn increases the rehabilitative needs of the patient.

Location of the Burn

Burns of the face, perineum, hands, or feet create special problems. Burns of the face are distressing because of cosmetic disfigurement, the potential for visual impairment,

FIGURE 18-2
The original Lund and Browder chart outlines the accepted method for determining the total body surface area of a burn injury. (Reprinted with permission from CC Lund, NC Browder. The estimation of areas of burns. Surg Gynecol Obstet 1944;79:352–358.)

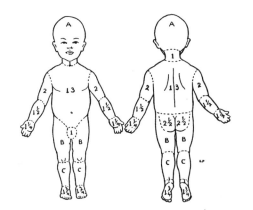
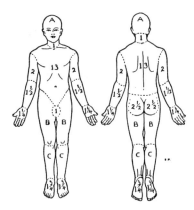

RELATIVE PERCENTAGES OF AREAS AFFECTED BY GROWTH

Area	Age 0	1	5	Area	Age 10	15	Adult
A = 1/2 of Head	9 1/2	8 1/2	6 1/2	A = 1/2 of Head	5 1/2	4 1/2	3 1/2
B = 1/2 of One Thigh	2 3/4	3 1/4	4	B = 1/2 of One Thigh	4 1/4	4 1/2	4 3/4
C = 1/2 of One Leg	2 1/2	2 1/2	2 3/4	C = 1/2 of One Leg	3	3 1/4	3 1/2

and compromised nutrition (intake of food). Injuries of the face are often accompanied by inhalation injuries. The swelling associated with perineal burns can lead to urinary flow obstruction in men. Burns that involve the genitalia produce understandable apprehension and irritation for patients. Hands and feet have broad, sweeping functional importance that can be substantially compromised after burn injury. The severity of injury is magnified significantly as the total surface area of the hand or foot that is encompassed by the burn increases. Any burn that crosses a joint increases the risk of functional compromise and creates challenges in rehabilitation.

WOUND CARE

The time it takes to heal a burn wound is directly related to depth of the injury. The more superficial a wound, the faster it heals. Surgical intervention, such as skin graft, is often used to reduce healing time for deep wounds. Wound infection can significantly delay healing.

Hydrotherapy

Hydrotherapy (whirlpool) is used in acute burn care for three reasons: to cleanse the wound, to remove dressings, and for exercise. The two most common purposes for hydrotherapy are to cleanse the burn wound to control infection and to prepare a wound bed for surgery.[29,30] Water is often used to ease the removal of burn dressings.[30] Immersion in warm water promotes relaxation for patients who are dealing with the stress and discomfort of burns. In addition, the buoyancy of water facilitates the movement of stiff and painful joints, and the "drag" created as limbs move through water provides resisted exercise to minimize loss of strength.[31,32]

Topical Agents and Wound Dressing

In intact skin, the outermost layer of epidermis (stratum corneum) is too dry to support microbial growth and serves as an effective barrier to microbial penetration. As a result, skin infections seldom occur unless the skin is opened.[33] Because this protective barrier is compromised or destroyed in burn injury, the risk of infection is greatly increased. Topical agents can be applied to these open wounds after each cleansing and debridement to prevent or manage infections. Topical agents are particularly important for ischemic wounds, with which systemic delivery of natural substrates to fight infection is compromised.[34]

Antibiotic creams that are commonly used in burn care include silver sulfadiazine and mafenide acetate (Sulfamylon). Although these creams do not completely destroy bacteria in the wound site, they do help to keep bacterial levels down. This decrease in bacterial level allows body defense systems to provide additional control. Silver sulfadiazine is effective against a wide range of wound flora and is the most widely used topical agent for burn care in the United States.[35] This cream is easily applied, comfortable for patients, washes off readily, and exhibits minimal side effects.[33,36] Mafenide acetate is quite effective in bacterial control but necessitates increased wound care time, can cause pain with application, and can result in hyponatremia or metabolic acidosis.[33,37]

Ointments (i.e., Bacitracin, Neosporin, Polysporin) are most often used to cover partial-thickness or open superficial wounds.[33] Because of their lubricating "water-in-oil" preparation, ointments are also used on tendons that are exposed in deep wounds. The most common side effect of ointments is mild hypersensitivity of the normal skin adjacent to the wound. Discontinuance of the ointment typically leads to quick clearance of the reaction.

Mild lotions are important in relieving dryness and itching in maturing healed wounds.[33] The use of moisturizers helps to prevent healed wounds from cracking or splitting. Alcohol is a desiccant to the skin and exacerbates dryness; thus, lotions that contain alcohol should be avoided. Fragrance-free moisturizers are recommended; most hypersensitivity reactions are triggered by perfumes.

After the application of a topical agent, the burn wound is covered with a dressing. The dressing keeps the topical agent in contact with the wound, prevents it from being removed by contact with objects in the environment, and maintains a moist wound environment. Creams are covered with a dry gauze wrap; ointments are overlaid with petroleum-impregnated gauze and then wrapped with dry gauze. Many types of dressings are available, ranging from simple gauze wraps to those that are designed for specific areas of the body or different burn thicknesses. The combination of an appropriate topical agent with a suitable wound covering helps to curtail infection and augment healing.[33] A well-applied dressing minimizes patient discomfort and allows mobility.

Rehabilitative personnel often take an active role in the wound care of a patient with burns. Involvement in wound care provides a better understanding of the reasons for patient complaints of discomfort. Familiarity with wound care procedures is frequently necessary for outpatient therapy sessions.[38] Adjustments in the treatment plan often must be made as the wound heals, and tolerance of certain rehabilitative procedures changes. It is especially important to consider the effects of pressure, shear, and/or friction on a healing wound or newly healed, fragile skin when splints, orthotics, prosthetics, or other types of external devices are being used.

PSYCHOLOGY OF BURN INJURY

An acute burn injury creates emotional distress. The treatment of the burns is often traumatic as well; stress and anxiety continue during the period of recovery. The psychological consequences of burn trauma in the adult include depression, intrusive avoidance and regressive behavior, despair, fear, anxiety, and guilt.[39-44] Children often feel more guilt than do adults and often manifest a loss of interest in play, unpredictable sadness, avoidance, and regres-

sion.[44-47] Malt[44] estimates that 30% of adults will have psychological problems. Even with similar support mechanisms and pre-existing psychological status, psychiatric prognosis is less hopeful for children than for adults.[48]

Psychological adaptation in the early phases after burn injury includes denial (often manifest by a feeling of calmness) and concern about prognosis, pain, personal issues, and dependence on staff (depression).[40,45,49] Patients who become actively involved in the process of rehabilitation and self-care often are more encouraged and optimistic about the future.[45,49]

Rehabilitation professionals can facilitate psychological function and recovery of patients with burns in several ways. Encouraging independence by allowing patients as much control over medical procedures as possible helps to focus them on recovery and empowers them to a certain degree.[49,50] Patients feel more comfortable with caregivers if they have the opportunity to get to know them outside of pain-involving treatment settings.[40,45,50,51] Providing support and understanding demonstrates a caring attitude. Tactful but honest answers to patient questions about prognosis, cosmesis, or functional outcome help to establish trust.[45] Ongoing education about the recovery process is important because it helps the patient to develop realistic expectations about recovery.

REHABILITATION INTERVENTION

Physical therapists and occupational therapists are important members of the burn care team. Early surgical intervention, availability of nutritional support, and pharmaceutical advances have improved survival after burn injury.[52] This, in turn, has increased the emphasis on and need for rehabilitation of patients with burns.

After evaluation, goals are established, and an appropriate plan of care is designed and implemented. Important rehabilitation goals for patients with burns include (1) minimizing the occurrence and adverse consequences of hypertrophic scar formation, (2) minimizing contracture formation and maintenance of full joint range of motion, (3) preserving motor skill function, and (4) improving strength and endurance.[32,53,54] Burn rehabilitation interventions emphasize patient independence through achievement of maximal functional recovery.

Wound Healing and Scar Formation

Unhealed burn wounds can pose challenges during rehabilitation. Most problems in burn rehabilitation are due to the ceaseless contraction and hypertrophy of immature burn scars.[55] Scar contracture leads to visible cosmetic deformity of body parts, especially in the face and hands. Functional limitations are common when the scar crosses over a joint. The contraction of a scar has been classically associated with a type of fibroblast that has contractile properties called *myofibroblasts*.[56]

Burn wound healing has three phases: the inflammatory phase, the proliferative phase, and the maturation or remodeling phase.[57] The *inflammatory phase* includes formation of new blood vessels, an initial defense against infection, and migration of fibroblast and epithelial cells into the injured area. Treatment focuses on proper wound care to encourage vascular regrowth and retard contamination of the site. In the *proliferative phase*, continued revascularization occurs, rebuilding and strengthening the wound site as a result of vigorous synthesis of collagen by fibroblasts and of re-epithelialization. Treatment is directed toward promoting epithelialization and encouraging proper alignment of newly deposited collagen fibers. During *maturation*, the wound site is further strengthened by protracted deposition of collagen fibers by active fibroblasts. Treatment during maturation stresses lengthening the scar, reconditioning of the patient, and a return to preburn functional levels. Activity and rehabilitation interventions aimed at opposing wound and scar tightness and patient education about the process of recovery are critical in all phases of healing.

Although fibroblasts deposit collagen during the proliferative phase, macrophages and endothelial cells release enzymes that degrade collagen. The severity of scar formation is determined by the balance between collagen synthesis and lysis: The more that collagen deposition exceeds its breakdown, the more likely a significant scar will form. A hypertrophic scar is raised above the normal surface of the skin[58,59] (Figure 18-3). A keloid occurs when the scar extends beyond the initial boundaries of the wound.[58,59]

An immature scar is raised, red, leathery, and stiff. As the scar matures, it becomes pale, relatively soft and flattened, and more yielding.[60-62] The process of scar maturation may require from 6 to 18 months after wound closure; scars actively contract during maturation.[60,61] Contraction is most vigorous in the early months of maturation but continues throughout this period of remodeling.

Superficial and partial-thickness burns usually do not scar; full-thickness burns almost always do. Full-thickness wounds closed by skin graft scar significantly less than does a similar wound that is allowed to heal spontaneously. Very dark or very fair-skinned individuals and those with a familial history of susceptibility to scarring are more likely to form hypertrophic scar.[63-65] The larger the burn, the greater the likelihood of scar formation.[64-66] A contracture occurs when a portion or distortion of the shortening scar becomes fixed or semifixed. The face, neck axilla, and hand are the

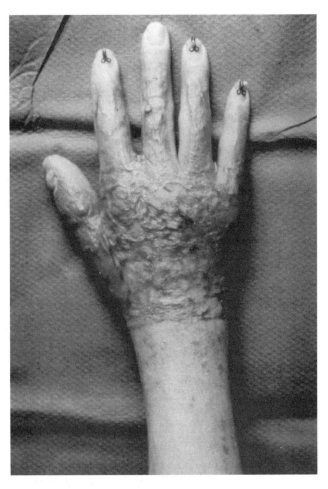

FIGURE 18-3

The dorsum of this patient's hand exhibits hypertrophic scarring. (Reprinted with permission from RS Ward. Pressure therapy for the control of hypertrophic scar formation after burn injury; a history and review. J Burn Care Rehabil 1991;12: 257–262.)

most common and most problematic sites of scar contracture formation.[63,65] One of the most important goals of burn rehabilitation is to counteract and minimize the adverse effects of scar contraction and to prevent scar contracture.

Operative Scar Management

Surgery is used to correct scar contractures that have created specific functional deficits or deformities.[65] Surgical techniques that are used to release scar contracture include split-thickness or full-thickness skin grafts, skin flaps, Z-plasties, and tissue expansion.[65,67] Most surgeries are deferred until at least 6 months after the burn or until the scar is sufficiently matured.[65,68,69] Although surgery alleviates contracture-related problems, it also creates a

TABLE 18-1

Vancouver Burn Scar Scale Ratings for Assessing Burn Scar

Pigmentation
  0 = normal (scar color closely resembles that of the rest of
        the body)
  1 = hypopigmentation
  2 = hyperpigmentation
Pliability
  0 = normal
  1 = supple (flexible with minimum resistance)
  2 = yielding (giving way to pressure)
  3 = firm (inflexible, not easily moved, resistant to manual
        pressure)
  4 = banding (rope-like tissue that blanches with extension
        on the scar)
  5 = contracture (permanent shortening of scar, producing
        deformity or distortion)
Vascularity
  0 = normal (scar color closely resembles that of the rest of
        the body)
  1 = pink
  2 = red
  3 = purple
Height
  0 = normal (flat)
  1 = raised less than 2 mm
  2 = raised less than 5 mm
  3 = raised more than 5 mm

Source: Adapted from Sullivan T, Smith J, Kerrnoda J, et al. Rating
the burn scar. J Burn Care Rehabil 1990;11(3):256–260.

new wound with its own subsequent scar maturation process. Rehabilitation is necessary after a majority of reconstructive surgeries to avert the effects of contraction again.

Nonoperative Scar Management

The nonoperative control of hypertrophic scarring involves pressure therapy or the application of silicone gel sheeting, or both. The use of continuous pressure for the treatment of burn scars was described in 1971 and is still well accepted.[70–72] Pressure has also been shown to relieve other aggravating discomforts of the healing burn wound, such as itching and blistering.[73,74] Range of motion is not significantly impeded with pressure garments despite the restriction felt by patients (particularly initially) when they are fit with these garments.[75] The use of silicone gel sheets has shown some success in controlling hypertrophy.[76–78] This treatment is typically used over small scars or over areas where ample pressure cannot be attained. The mechanism of the effect of pressure or silicone gel is not known.

Pressure therapy is indicated when healing requires more than 14 days or if a skin graft has been performed. Several strategies can be used to assess the burn scar condition. The Vancouver Burn Scar Scale developed by Sul-

livan et al.[79] describes the severity of the scar by rating pigmentation, vascularity, pliability, and height of the scar tissue (Table 18-1).

Early pressure therapy is used to control edema in a wound even if no scar formation ensues. Some of the elastic materials that are most commonly used on newly healing, still fragile wounds include Ace bandages, Coban self-adherent wrap (3M Medical, St. Paul, MN), or elasticized cotton tubular bandages such as Tubigrip (SePro, Montgomeryville, PA). These materials are useful while waiting for the arrival of custom-fit antiburn scar supports.[80]

Patients commonly wear custom-fit pressure garments for the duration of the maturation phase of healing. Custom-fit antiburn scar supports are available from manufacturers such as the Jobst Institute (Toledo, OH), Bio-Concepts (Phoenix, AZ), Barton-Carey Medical Products (Perrysburg, OH), and Gottfried Medical (Toledo, OH). Although the measuring procedures vary by manufacturer, most require measurements at approximately every 1.0–1.5 in. along each extremity, with special guidelines for the torso, face, and hands. Burn scar supports can be fabricated to fit almost any body part, including the face, torso, upper extremity, hand, and lower extremity. Some burn centers fabricate rigid or semirigid face masks in an attempt to gain a better match with facial contours.

Pressure garments and devices are worn through the entire process of scar maturation, to be discontinued only when the scar has completely matured.[1] The fit of pressure garments is reassessed regularly to ensure the desired therapeutic effect. Regular follow-up provides an opportunity for the patient to discuss other ongoing rehabilitative problems associated with the burn.

BURN REHABILITATION TREATMENTS

Many different types of rehabilitation interventions are appropriate in the care of patients with burns. Although many interventions are described briefly in the following section, emphasis is placed on the use of splints, orthoses, and prosthetic devices.

Therapeutic Exercise

Exercise helps to minimize outcomes of burn scar formation by improving the mobility and function of a patient.[81] As important and effective as exercise is in burn rehabilitation, some patients (and some therapists) may be reluctant to exercise because of the anticipation of increased pain or because of anxiety about damaging newly healing tissue. Exercise programs for patients with burns are principally directed at the prevention of burn scar contractures and at the side effects of inactivity and disuse. Additional consequences of immobilization in these patients can include progressive contracture of the joint capsule and pericapsular structures, atrophy and contracture of muscle, deleterious effects on articular cartilage, and possible decrease in bone strength. Exercise is a significant health promotion and disability prevention component in the rehabilitation of patients with burns.

Assessment of location and depth of burn injury identifies those areas that are most at risk of burn scar contracture. This assessment also guides the design of an exercise program to improve mobility, strength, and functional status. Past and present medical conditions influence rehabilitative expectations; a previous orthopedic injury may have already reduced range of motion of a particular joint, and a concomitant inhalation injury may limit a patient's exercise tolerance.

Active Exercise

After a burn, exercise may be difficult because of edema, pain (particularly over areas of partial-thickness burns), the loss of normal skin's elasticity in the burned tissue, and wound contraction.[67] Early on, edema is a major contributor to stiffness of the joints; active exercise is valuable in reducing the edema.[53,82] Positioning and compressive wraps or devices are used in addition to exercise for edema control. Pain tolerance varies widely among patients. The therapist is challenged to help the patient understand the importance of activity despite the pain involved. Many patients experience a relief of pain and stiffness after exercise periods, which may encourage them to participate in the subsequent therapy sessions. Patients who understand the advantages of exercise may be asked to confer with, and encourage, newly injured patients or those patients who have difficulty with their exercises.

General stiffness due to the loss of skin elasticity and wound contraction is not only an acute problem but often persists during the process of scar maturation, especially for those who form a hypertrophic scar. Exercise that targets the areas that are most vulnerable to scar formation as identified in the initial evaluation must begin as early as possible after admission.[54,83] This early presentation of an exercise routine aids edema control, relieves stiffness, and prevents loss of strength and range of motion. The early introduction of active exercise reinforces the importance of exercise to the patient, who will incorporate daily exercise as an important contributor to overall recovery. Because of the wide scope of benefits derived from active exercises, they are the preferred form of range of motion exercises for patients with burns.

Patients are also encouraged to perform independent activities of daily living.[54,82] Self-reliance is important

after burn injury, and independence can increase the level of a patient's self-confidence.[82] It is likely that the more patients can do, particularly in directing their exercise programs, the more compliant they will become.[83] Independence in an exercise program is therefore an important goal for each patient's recovery from burn injury.

The primary goal of active exercise for patients with acute burns is opposition of tissue contraction; the secondary goal is strengthening. For a patient with a burn that crosses the antecubital fossa and weakness of the biceps brachii, exercise is primarily focused on preservation of elbow extension range of motion. If a patient with a burn that encompasses the lower leg and ankle also has weakness and atrophy of the triceps surae, appropriate strengthening exercises can be performed, but not at the sacrifice of active ankle range of motion.

Most of the exercise equipment that is typically found in rehabilitation settings is appropriate for patients with burns. The therapist must decide when certain equipment will be most beneficial and must incorporate the use of this resource into the plan of care. The use of latex rubber tubing for strengthening,[84] overhead reciprocal pulleys for increasing range of motion,[85,86] and hydrotherapy for both of these purposes has been described.[31,32] Bicycle ergometers for either the upper or lower extremities assist with motion, provide resistance, and allow for some cardiovascular workout.

Conditioning exercises are often used to improve the cardiovascular status of the patient. Occupation-specific training programs may be a part of the long-term rehabilitation plan as patients prepare to return to the place of their livelihood. This type of activity can be directed at one or a few specific functions or can incorporate a traditional work-hardening program.

Ambulation

The functional nature of ambulation makes it the most important exercise for burned lower extremities.[87] It assists with edema control, range of motion, and strengthening in all lower extremity joints. Ambulation also helps with the function of other physiologic systems such as the cardiovascular, gastrointestinal, and renal systems. Patients with lower extremity burns exhibit gait deviations related to compromised joint function. They may have incomplete hip and knee flexion in initial swing and incomplete knee extension in terminal swing. Initial contact may be made with the entire foot (foot flat) instead of the heel, and loading response may be compromised by lack of plantar flexion range of motion or an unwillingness to perform the controlled knee flexion that is necessary for shock absorption. Excessive knee flexion is often present in midstance, poor or absent heel-off and weight shift in terminal stance, and inadequate knee flexion in pressing.[38] Differences in individual gait deviations in gait phases are generally based on variations in the location, size, and depth of the burn injury and levels of pain. Any gait deviation secondary to the burn can accentuate the need for vigilant gait training of a patient who also has a lower extremity prosthesis. Exercise is an important adjunct to gait training, addressing specific movement limitations of the lower limbs.

Passive Exercise and Stretching

Passive exercise is included in a therapy regime if a patient is unable to move on his or her own or cannot actively complete normal ranges of motion. Passive range of motion and slow, gentle stretching exercises that elongate healing soft tissues are used to preserve and improve joint range of motion.[88,89] Blanching of the scar indicates an appropriate amount of stretch. Although the scar should be stretched to the point of patient tolerance, joint movement should not be forced because of possible tissue damage and the potential for heterotopic ossification.[90-92]

Positioning or splints can be used after a stretching session to maintain the achieved range of motion. Suitable stretching positions must also consider scars that cross multiple joints and therefore affect a broad kinematic chain. Techniques such as contract-relax or hold-relax have been found to be beneficial stretching approaches.[53]

Physical Agents

Because of the variety of treatment goals that are important for burn rehabilitation, many different types of modalities are used for appropriate intervention. Hydrotherapy, functional electrical stimulation (neuromuscular electrical stimulation), transcutaneous electrical stimulation, ultrasound, continuous passive motion (CPM), and paraffin are physical agents that have been used effectively in burn care. Hydrotherapy is most often used for wound care but can also be used for dressing removal and exercise. If hydrotherapy is chosen as a thermal modality, precautions similar to those used for any open wound care are necessary to reduce the chance of cross contamination.

Functional electrical stimulation has been used successfully to treat recovering hands when those same hands responded poorly to typical treatment.[93] Burn pain has been altered by the use of transcutaneous electrical stimulation in some cases.[94] Ultrasound has been used to treat pain and range of motion impairments in patients with burns.[95-97] However, the efficacy of ultrasound in either decreasing pain or improving motion is still a matter of some debate. More than one-half the major burn treatment centers have used CPM as an adjunct to treatment.[98] Successful use of CPM has been specifically reported on hand burns and lower extremity burns at the knee.[99,100]

The heat provided by paraffin and the potential skin softening secondary to the mineral oil in the paraffin may be reasons for the use of this modality in burn care.[101]

Healing and recently healed skin are often very sensitive. Scar tissue has varying levels of sensory deficit.[102,103] Accordingly, excess heat, cold, coupling agents, and electrode adhesives can lead to skin breakdown. Caution must be exercised when any modality is applied: Thorough pre- and post-treatment inspection of the site is warranted.

Positioning

Positioning is an important component of any burn rehabilitation program. It is used for acute burn and postsurgical edema control as well as to prevent or treat scar contractures. The initial burn therapy evaluation identifies sites that are at risk for contracture formation; appropriate counteractive positions become part of the therapy plan. Contracture prevention is more successful when a program of positioning and activity is instituted as soon after burn as possible.[54,65]

Postexercise positioning extends the effects of activity; positioning is also fundamental for patients who cannot move or exercise. Manufactured positioning devices, such as arm boards that attach to the side of the bed, are available to assist proper positioning of extremities. Positioning need not be expensive or require intricate equipment. Avoiding the use of a pillow behind the head is a simple way of decreasing neck flexion and facilitating a neutral alignment of the head and neck. A pillow or several folded blankets placed under the arms effectively elevate the burned limb, while keeping the elbows extended and supporting the hands. At least some horizontal flexion of the shoulders is indicated to minimize prolonged stretch of the brachial plexus.[104,105] A washcloth, towel, or gauze roll placed in the palm helps to hold the hand in a functional position. Pillows, high-top tennis shoes, towels, blankets, or foot boards help to position the foot with a neutral ankle.[54] Positions of choice for the patient with burns are provided in Table 18-2.

SPLINTING AND ORTHOTICS

Historically, Hippocrates described burn scars as "tetanus," and Wilhelm Fabry illustrated a splint to treat a hand for hyperextension scar contractures.[15] In the early to mid-1900s, patients with burns were placed in splints immediately on admission to the hospital in an effort to prevent contraction; splints were removed for brief periods to permit wound care. Most burns would not have been covered by skin graft until at least 5 weeks after burn injury.

The advent of surgical excision and grafting in the mid-1900s decreased the time required for a burn to heal. As a result, prophylactic splinting became a less common procedure, and in the late 1970s and early 1980s active exercise became the primary treatment method used by burn therapists.[54] The use of splints has, however, become a critical adjunct to active exercise and positioning of the patient with burns. The term *splint* is used in burn care more often than *orthosis* even though the terms and the devices that they represent are basically synonymous.

Splinting is often used to protect fragile wounds or newly grafted burn wounds. Splints are also used to position joints to maintain achieved range of motion or as a dynamic device to apply stretch to increase motion. Splints cannot replace active exercise; contractures form even in desirable positions if a patient is constantly splinted in a particular position. Static splints are designed to maintain a position of choice by immobilizing the joint.[106,107] Dynamic splints are designed to exercise or mobilize a joint.[107] A splint can also enhance the pressure applied to a scar by a pressure support. If unusual pain (other than from gentle tissue elongation or stretch), sensory impairment, or wound maceration occurs at the site of the splint, it must be removed and the fit adjusted.[108]

It is important that a splint be fabricated with a proper secure fit to minimize friction injuries or skin breakdown at pressure points. Pressure points over bony prominences are particularly vulnerable in this regard. Large, broad surface contact areas distribute forces better and reduce the likelihood of pressure-related tissue injury. The splint is worn only when it will not impede the functional activities or requisite exercises of the patient; splints are often donned during rest periods and at night when the patient is sleeping. The corners and edges of the splint are rounded and sometimes padded to avoid shear stresses. The design of the splint may also need to be adapted for orthopedic hardware, such as surgical pins, or for intravenous line sites. The splint design should also, whenever possible, allow for ease of application and removal, to enhance compliance among staff and family members who otherwise might struggle while maneuvering the splint.

Materials used in fabricating splints include thermoplastics, Hexalite (Kirschner Medical Products, Greenwood, SC), plaster, and elastomer compounds. Hexalite and plaster are most often used to make temporary splints. Thermoplastic materials, which can be remolded to adjust fit, make them an ideal splinting material for patients with burns. The amount of material to be used is determined by measuring the area to be splinted and the design of the splint. The splint is then molded to the patient. When the splinting material is set (hardened), the splint should be inspected for correct fit to avoid pressure- and shear-related

TABLE 18-2
Preferred Positions for Patients with Burns

Neck	Extension, no rotation
Shoulder	Abduction (90 degrees)
	External rotation
	Horizontal flexion (10 degrees)
Elbow and forearm	Extension with supination
Wrist	Neutral or slight extension
Hand	Functional position (dorsal burn)
	Finger and thumb extension (palmar burn)
Trunk	Straight postural alignment
Hip	Neutral extension/flexion
	Neutral rotation
	Slight abduction
Knee	Extension
Ankle	Neutral or slight dorsiflexion
	No inversion
	Neutral toe extension/flexion

problems. Splints are often padded with gauze or any of the numerous cushion or foam materials that are available. For areas in which fragile skin is problematic, foam is a soft alternative splinting material; however, it is unable to provide the same resistance to force that more rigid materials do.

Although a number of appropriate splint designs are available for each anatomic site, some are chosen more commonly than others. Our discussion of common splint designs begins with the neck and progresses to the foot and ankle, in the same order as Table 18-2: preferred positioning.

The possible consequences of anterior neck burns include flexion contracture, facial disfigurement, loss of cosmetic contours of the neck, and difficulty with mastication.[108,109] A molded neck conformer splint helps to prevent neck flexion contracture as well as providing compression on the forming scar. A rectangular piece of low-temperature thermoplastic splinting material is cut to span the distance from ear to ear along the jaw line and from below the lower lip to the sternoclavicular notch. After heating, the splint is molded directly on the patient's neck. Padding is added to protect vulnerable areas, and a Velcro strap is attached over the back of the neck to secure the splint.[108] Because this type of splint is occlusive, covering many bony prominences, the splint must be removed frequently to inspect the skin for any areas of irritation or breakdown. For wounds that do not involve much of the chin, soft cervical collars have also been successful in providing positioning, pressure, and contour.[108,109] Although soft collars are more comfortable to wear, they do not extend over the chin for increased moment arm resistance. Commercially available Philadelphia collars may be an alternative.

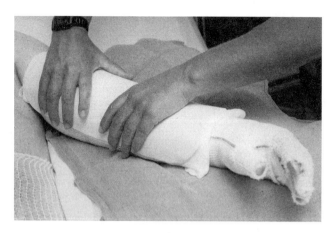

FIGURE 18-4
Thermoplastic anterior elbow gutter splint being custom fit for a patient with burns of the antecubital fossa.

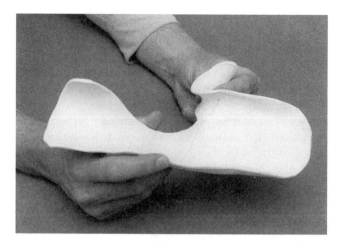

FIGURE 18-5
Thermoplastic pan splint that has been molded to support the wrist in a functional position, with fingers in full extension.

Burns that involve the axilla and shoulder can lead to adduction contracture and webbing of the axillary folds. This type of deformity contributes to difficulty in reaching and overhead use of the arm, components of many functional activities. A custom-fit conforming splint is often used to inhibit development of such contracture and webbing. Conforming splints for axillary burns support the entire arm, from the wrist through the axilla, and extend down the trunk to at least waist level. The splint wraps around the trunk from the umbilicus to the spine, one-third of the circumference of the chest, at the axilla around both folds, and one-half the circumference of the arm at the brachium, elbow, and wrist.[108,110] The splint is molded directly to the patient (flaring at the iliac crest may be necessary), and appropriate padding is applied. Velcro strapping or other wraps around the trunk, shoulder, arm, and wrist secure the splint. A more traditional airplane splint can also be used to counteract the problems at the shoulder. Clavicle straps or soft foam can be used as well, to help conform the axillae.

The most common deformities secondary to burns that involve the elbow and forearm are elbow flexion or pronation contractures. The elbow joint is most often fit with a conformer splint designed as either an anterior or posterior gutter or trough[108-110] (Figure 18-4). The splint is fit to the arm from the proximal third of the brachium to the distal third of the forearm. Partial circumference measurements are taken at the proximal and distal sites and the elbow. The splint is molded directly on the patient with padding added. The splint should be flared or "bubbled" at the bony prominences of the elbow. The splint is held in place by Velcro straps or by circular gauze or elastic wrapping. Commercially available three-point extension or air splints can also be used.

Burns of the wrist can lead to contractures in extension or flexion or in ulnar or radial deviation, depending on the location of the burn. It is extremely important to prevent flexion or extension contractures of the hand and fingers and to maintain the web space of the thumb. Wrist and hand splints are available in many different designs; the best option for a particular patient is based on the anticontracture position of the joint or joint complex that is involved.

The splint that is most commonly used at the wrist and the hand is the antideformity splint.[108-110] This splint is designed to position the wrist and hand in the functional position. A modification of this splint, the pan splint, positions all finger joints in extension (Figure 18-5). Splints that conform to the thumb, thumb web space, and index finger can help to preserve the thumb web space.[108-110] Dorsal or palmar resting extension splints, used when the wrist has been burned but the hand is not damaged, can be custom molded or are commercially available. Finger gutter or trough splints are used to treat individual fingers, based on the same principles used in elbow conformer splints.

Another easily fabricated splint that is useful in minimizing the formation of either flexion or extension contractures when multiple joints of the fingers have been burned is the sandwich splint.[109,111] Foam padding is attached to two pieces of splinting material that have been cut large enough to cover the hand. The burned hand is sandwiched between these two padded supports, which are held in place with a circumferential wrap (Figure 18-6).

Patients with burns that involve the anterior trunk are at risk of developing kyphosis. Clavicular straps in a figure-of-eight design have been used to position the shoulders in retraction and counteract the flexion forces in healing

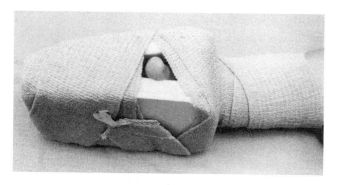

FIGURE 18-6
Sandwich splint for the hand. (Reprinted with permission from RS Ward, WA Schnebly, M Kravitz, et al. Have you tried the sandwich splint? A method for preventing hand deformities in children. J Burn Care Rehabil 1989;10:83–85.)

upper trunk burns.[108,109] Commercially available corsets or thoracolumbar spinal orthotics can be prescribed to help maintain posture for patients with burns of the mid and lower trunk if it is being compromised by scar contracture.

For burns of the pelvis, groin, and hip, the problem is the likelihood of hip flexion and adduction contractures. Hip abduction splints reinforced with a spreader bar or an anterior hip spica splint may be necessary for some patients.[109]

At the knee, flexion contracture is an important concern. Splinting of the knee is similar to that of the elbow, adjusted to fit the longer segments of the lower extremity.[108–110] Although knee conformer splints are most often chosen for patients with burns that involve the knee, three-point extension splints or air splints have also been used to reduce the risk of flexion contracture as the burn scar matures.

Because of the complexity of structure and arthrokinematics, burns of the ankles and feet often present challenges for splinting that are similar to those of the wrists and hands. The location of the burn dictates whether the patient is at risk for contracture in either a plantar flexion or dorsiflexion direction (or both). Posterior foot drop splints or anterior or posterior ankle conformers are the most commonly fabricated ankle splints.[108–110] The distance from toes to calf is measured, and limb half-circumferences determine the width of the splint. After the desired splint pattern is cut from thermoplastic material, the splint is molded directly on the patient. Necessary padding is applied, and the splint is flared at the malleoli and often on the posterior heel. "Bunny boots" and other commercial foot drop splints can also be used for positioning ankles that have been burned.[108] Molded leather shoes can be useful in positioning the ankle and the toes of involved feet.[109] High-top gym shoes provide a less expensive but similar option for foot splinting.[38,109] Toe

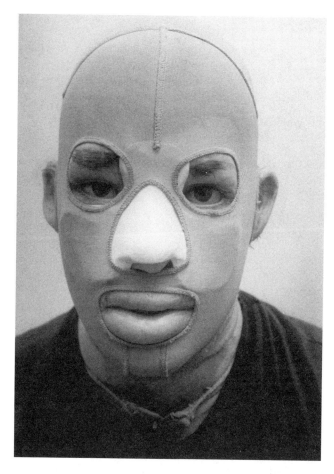

FIGURE 18-7
A splint insert is worn under a face mask pressure garment. In addition to applying pressure more effectively over the irregular surface area of the face, splint inserts can help to minimize ectropion (eversion) of the lower eyelids. (Reprinted with permission from RS Ward. The rehabilitation of burn patients. Crit Rev Phys Med Rehabil 1991;2:121–138.)

conformer splints can be fabricated for the dorsal surface of the foot to prevent toe extension contracture.

Burns of the face can affect the eyes and eyelids, the contours of the face, and the soft tissue around the mouth. Contracture of the mouth (microstomia) is particularly troublesome, as it interferes with feeding (and subsequently nutrition), speaking, and dental care.[112] Splints that are designed to support the functional contours of specific areas of the face are often fabricated. This type of splint helps not only to decrease scar hypertrophy but also to minimize or prevent ectropion (eversion) deformity of the lower eyelids and the lips (Figure 18-7). Microstomia prevention splints, designed to apply pressure or stretch to

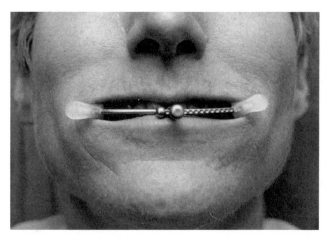

FIGURE 18-8
A microstomia prevention appliance is used to preserve the oral opening.

commissures and fibrotic oral muscles, are commercially available or can be custom made[113-115] (Figure 18-8). This type of splint or appliance is worn at all times when the patient is not eating, receiving oral care, or in conversation.[114] In cases in which contracture affects the actual opening of the mouth, splints of thermoplastic material in the shape of a cone can be used to progressively increase the opening of the mouth. The patient is asked to open the mouth, and the cone is placed between the teeth. As the mouth is able to open wider, the narrower portions of the cone are cut off, and the patient is progressed to a wider part of the splint to widen the opening of the mouth.

Very simple materials such as tongue depressors secured with gauze wrapping have been described as "splints" at various joints for small children.[116] Elastic wraps have also been used to increase range of motion much like dynamic splints.[117,118] These methods may be useful as temporary devices but are not effective substitutes for more stable splinting materials.[117]

For patients with existing contractures, a serial splinting protocol is often used to assist with the stretching of the deformity. Plaster casts, thermoplastic materials, and Dynasplint (Dynasplint Systems, Inc, Baltimore, MD) have been used successfully in this manner.[119,120] Individually fabricated dynamic splints are also very helpful for patients with contracture after burns.

Any splint that is worn over an open wound can be a transfer agent for microorganisms from the burn. In fact, organisms are cultured from splint surfaces 50% of the time.[121] Effective strategies for cleaning burn splints are imperative. Simple washing and drying of the splint is not always effective in clearing all organisms. The use of qua-

ternary ammonia (1 fl oz/gal water) has been found to be 100% effective as a cleaning agent and is the recommended splint-cleaning strategy.[121]

Occasionally, special rehabilitative complications arise after burn injury, especially in patients who have sustained deep thermal wounds or an electrical injury. The most commonly encountered complications are exposed tendons and peripheral neuropathy with motor or sensory deficit. Splints can be useful in protecting or supporting these areas. Exposed tendons must be kept moist with an ointment gauze or biological dressing. The limb is splinted in a position in which the tendon is on slack, and exercise is avoided.[85] Idiopathic neuropathy occurs most often in patients with 20% or more TBSA.[122] Secondary neuropathies may be caused by overelongation or compression of a peripheral nerve; such problems can be prevented by careful systematic monitoring of a patient's position, tightness of dressings, and fit of the splints.[85] Splints can be fit to overcome a temporary or chronic neurologic deficit such as a drop foot.

AMPUTATION AND PROSTHETICS IN BURN REHABILITATION

Electrical burn injuries are more likely than any other types of burns to lead to amputation. Significant damage occurs as electrical current passes through nerve tissue, vascular tissue, and other deep structures. The current can cause destruction of cells, coagulation of tissues, thrombosis of blood vessels, neuropathies, and tissue necrosis. Other types of burn injuries may necessitate amputation if the wound is very deep or because of associated tissue trauma. Some amputations are a result of an unrelenting infection.

Patients with burns who require limb amputation may experience complications that delay prosthetic fitting and training, as a result of multiple wound or scar sites, skin grafting on the residual limb, repeated surgical procedures (not necessarily associated with the residual limb), or burn-induced catabolic atrophy. Patients with burns are also susceptible to the same postoperative complications that are faced by any patient with new amputation: edema, phantom pain, and formation of neuroma or bone spur. Any of these factors can intensify patient discomfort or the amount of work and time that are required for prosthetic training, which can be reasons for limited use or rejection of the prosthesis. Despite these concerns, patients with burn-related amputations are successfully rehabilitated after standard protocols.[123-125]

For patients with skin graft sites on the residual limb, fragility of the skin (its tolerance of pressure and shear forces)

FIGURE 18-9
This patient with burn-related transfemoral amputation has increased risk of hip flexion and adduction contracture secondary to scarring of the graft sites over the anterior surface of the hip and groin. (Reprinted from RS Ward, C Hayes-Lundy, WS Schnebly, et al. Rehabilitation of burn patients with concomitant limb amputation: case reports. Burns 1990;16:390–392.)

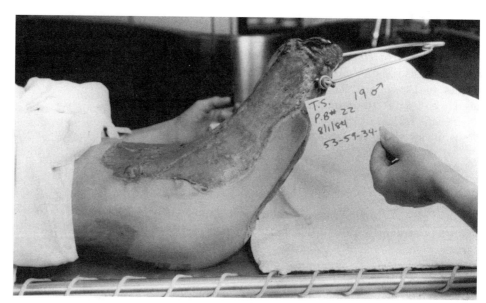

is an important concern. Blisters or small open wounds may appear where a skin graft or a fragile scar breaks down as a result of forces on the residual limb during prosthetic gait. Wearing of the prosthesis is often discontinued until the new wound is adequately healed. Wounds or skin grafts on areas associated with prosthesis use, such as the shoulder or scapula under an upper extremity prosthesis harness, may demonstrate these same initial problems with wound breakdown. Even though the presence of a skin graft or fragile scar can delay or prolong prosthetic training, most patients with burn-related amputation are eventually successful at using their prosthesis on skin-grafted limbs.[123–127] New antishear prosthetic socket suspension and lining materials may be especially helpful for patients with burn-related amputation.

The typical postamputation contracture in patients with burns is a result of muscle and soft tissue shortening related to a decreased moment arm of the affected extremity. When a maturing burn scar or graft site is present over the joint of the residual limb, the risk of contracture increases significantly (Figure 18-9). Such contractures may form more rapidly with the additional shortening force of the contracting scar tissue. The prevention of joint contracture after amputation requires vigilant positioning and stretching, which can be augmented by knee extension splints for patients with transtibial amputation.

For patients with large surface area burns, repeated surgical skin grafting procedures are often necessary to cover the burn wound adequately. Repeated surgical procedures often delay prosthetic fitting and training. Patients can be placed on postoperative bed rest for as many as 7 days to ensure initial healing of the grafted area. To protect the new graft site and promote healing, the limb can be tem-

porarily positioned in a less than optimal position for prosthetic use. Continued monitoring of patients by the therapist, along with conscientious wrapping of the residual limb, can help to overcome some of the problems that are caused by successive surgeries.

It is common for patients with burns to lose weight secondary to hypermetabolism. A large burn can nearly double metabolism above its normal rate. Although patients with significant burns receive nutritional supplementation, this often slows but does not prevent catabolic weight loss. Most patients regain the weight that is lost in the catabolic process; this may require a series of revisions or refabrications of temporary sockets until the weight stabilizes enough to fit a permanent prosthesis.

Patients with amputation as a result of electrical injury may be susceptible to the formation of bone spurs.[128] Otherwise, heterotopic bone formation does not appear to be more prevalent in a burn population. Edema after burn injury is generally an acute problem and seldom creates long-term delays in prosthetic training. No reports have suggested that phantom limb pain is more likely to develop in patients with burns who have had amputations than in other patients with amputation.

PATIENT EDUCATION

The patient is the most important member of the rehabilitative burn care team. Family members and any others who will be caregivers outside the hospital must be included as early as possible to learn about the process of burn recovery and rehabilitation. The effectiveness of patient education is reflected by the patient's and caregiver's ability to demonstrate knowledge and understanding of the rehabilitation program.[53] Skin care, exercise programs, use of pressure supports, positioning techniques, and splint protocols are the obvious items that need to be taught to the patient.[129,130] *Reinforcement, reasoning,* and *reassurance* are key words to remember when designing an educational process.

SUMMARY

Optimal care of patients who are recovering from burn injury taps the knowledge and skills of many different health care providers. Rehabilitation professionals are actively involved in many facets of postburn care, such as wound care after acute burns and surgical grafting procedures, patient and family education about the burn rehabilitation process, and preventative care to minimize the risk of hypertrophic scarring, contractures, and deformity and subsequent disability. Postburn rehabilitation care requires knowledge of and expertise in splint design and fabrication, exercise prescription (stretching and flexibility, strengthening, endurance), adaptive and assistive devices for gait and activities of daily living, and often prosthetic prescription and training. This chapter provides an overview of the many facets of effective burn care and rehabilitation.

REFERENCES

1. Petro JA, Salisbury RE. Rehabilitation of the burn patient. Clin Plast Surg 1986;13(1):145–150.
2. Helm PA, Head MD, Pullium G, et al. Burn rehabilitation: a team approach. Surg Clin North Am 1978;58(6):1263–1278.
3. Frank HA, Berry C, Wachtel TL, Johnson RW. The impact of thermal injury. J Burn Care Rehabil 1987;8(4):260–262.
4. Silverstein P, Lack B. Epidemiology and Prevention. In JA Boswick (ed), The Art and Science of Burn Care. Rockville: Aspen, 1987;11–12.
5. American Burn Association guidelines for service standards and severity classification in the treatment of burn injury. Am Coll Surg Bull 1984;69(10):24–28.
6. Van Rijin OJL, Bouter LM, Meertens RM. The aetiology of burns in developed countries: review of the literature. Burns 1989;15(4):217–221.
7. Lyngdorf P, Sorenson B, Thomsen M. The total number of burn injuries in a Scandinavian population—a prospective analysis. Burns 1986;12(8):567–571.
8. Brodzka W, Thornhill HL, Howard S. Burns: causes and risk factors. Arch Phys Med Rehabil 1985;66(11):746–751.
9. Jay KM, Bartlett RH, Danet R, Allyn PA. Burn epidemiology: a basis for burn prevention. J Trauma 1977;17(12):943–947.
10. Murray JP. A study of the prevention of hot tap water burns. Burns 1988;14(3):185–193.
11. Baptiste MS, Feck G. Preventing tap water burns. Am J Public Health 1980;70(7):727–729.
12. Herbert K, Lawrence JC. Chemical burns. Burns 1989;15(6):381–384.
13. Monafo WW, Freedman BM. Electrical and Lightning Injury. In JA Boswick (ed), The Art and Science of Burn Care. Rockville: Aspen, 1987;241–253.
14. Haberal M. Electrical burns: a five year experience. J Trauma 1986;26(2):103–109.
15. Thomsen M. It all began with Aristotle—the history of the treatment of burns. Burns 1988;(suppl):S1–S4.
16. Solem LD. Classification. In SV Fisher, PA Helm (eds), Comprehensive Rehabilitation of Burns. Baltimore: Williams & Wilkins, 1984;9–15.
17. Choctaw WT, Eisner ME, Wachtel TL. Causes, Prevention, Prehospital Care, Evaluation, Emergency Treatment, and Prognosis. In BM Achauer (ed), Management of the Burned Patient. Norwalk, CT: Appleton & Lange, 1987;3–19.
18. Klasen HJ. Early Excision and Grafting. In JAD Settle (ed), Principles and Practice of Burns Management. New York: Churchill Livingstone, 1996;275–288.
19. Janzekovic Z. A new concept in the early excision and immediate grafting of burns. J Trauma 1970;10(12):1103–1108.
20. Achauer BM. Treating the Burn Wound. In BM Achauer (ed), Management of the Burned Patient. Norwalk, CT: Appleton & Lange, 1987;93–108.
21. Jones T, McDonald S, Deitch EA. Effect of graft bed on long-term functional results of extremity skin grafts. J Burn Care Rehabil 1988;9(1):72–74.
22. Burke JF, Yannas IV, Quinby WC, et al. Successful use of physiological acceptable skin in the treatment of extensive burn injury. Ann Surg 1981;194(4):413–428.
23. Jasik T, Burke JF. The use of artificial skin for burns. Ann Rev Med 1987;38:107–117.
24. Wainwright D, Madden M, Luterman A, et al. Clinical evaluation of an acellular allograft dermal matrix in full-thickness burns. J Burn Care Rehabil 1996;17(2):124–136.
25. Rennekampff HO, Hansbrough JF, Woods V, Kiessig V. Integrin and matrix molecule expression in cultured skin replacements. J Burn Care Rehabil 1996;17(3):213–221.
26. Desai MH, Mlakar JM, McCauley RL, et al. Lack of long-term durability of cultured keratinocyte burn-wound coverage: a case report. J Burn Care Rehabil 1991;12(6):540–545.
27. Stern R, McPherson M, Longaker MT. Histologic study of artificial skin used in the treatment of full-thickness thermal injury. J Burn Care Rehabil 1990;11(1):7–13.
28. Lund CC, Browder NC. The estimation of areas of burns. Surg Gynecol Obstet 1944;79:352–358.
29. Roberts ML, Pruitt, BA. Nursing Care and Psychological Considerations. In C Artz, J Moncrief, B Pruitt (eds), Burns: A Team Approach. Philadelphia: Saunders, 1979;371–389.
30. Marvin JA. Perioperative Care of the Burn Patient. In JA Boswick (ed), The Art and Science of Burn Care. Rockville: Aspen, 1987;93–100.

31. Edlich RF, Towler MA, Goitz RJ, et al. Bioengineering principles of hydrotherapy. J Burn Care Rehabil 1987;8(6):580–584.

32. Nothdurft D, Smith PS, LeMaster JE. Exercise and Treatment Modalities. In SV Fisher, PA Helm (eds), Comprehensive Rehabilitation of Burns. Baltimore: Williams & Wilkins, 1984;96–147.

33. Ward RS, Saffle JR. Topical agents in burn and wound care. Phys Ther 1995;75(6):526–538.

34. Saffle JR, Schnebly WA. Burn Wound Care. In RL Richard RL, MJ Staley (eds), Burn Care and Rehabilitation: Principles and Practice. Philadelphia: Davis, 1994;19–176.

35. Taddonio TE, Thomson PD, Smith DJ Jr, Prasad JK. A survey of wound monitoring and topical antimicrobial therapy practices in the treatment of burn injury. J Burn Care Rehabil 1990;11(5):423–427.

36. Gordon MD. Burn wound care: silver sulfadiazine application. J Burn Care Rehabil 1987;8(5):429–433.

37. Waymack JP, Pruitt BA. Burn wound care. Adv Surg 1990;23:261–280.

38. Ward RS. The rehabilitation of burn patients. Crit Rev Phys Med Rehabil 1991;2:121–138.

39. Steiner H, Clark WR. Psychiatric complications of burned adults: a classification. J Trauma 1977;17(2):134–143.

40. West DA, Shuck JM. Emotional problems of the severely burned patient. Surg Clin North Am 1978;58(6):1189–1204.

41. Wallace LM, Lees J. A psychological follow-up study of adult patients discharged from a British burn unit. Burns 1988;14(1):39–45.

42. Chang FC, Herzog B. Burn morbidity: a follow-up study of physical and psychological disability. Ann Surg 1976;183(1): 34–37.

43. Tempereau CE, Grossman AR, Brones MF. Psychological regression and marital status: determinants in psychiatric management of burn victims. J Burn Care Rehabil 1987;8(4):286–291.

44. Malt U. Long term psychological follow-up studies of burned adults: review of the literature. Burns 1980;6(3):190–197.

45. Goodstein RK. Burns: an overview of clinical consequences affecting patient, staff, and family. Comp Psychiatry 1985;26(1):43–57.

46. Stoddard FJ. Body image development in the burned child. J Am Acad Child Psychiatry 1982;21(5):502–507.

47. Mahaney NB. Restoration of play in a severely burned three-year-old child. J Burn Care Rehabil 1990;11(1):57–63.

48. Andreason NJC. Neuropsychiatric complications in burn patients. Int J Psychiatry Med 1974;5(2):161–171.

49. Watkins PN, Cook EL, May SR, Ehleben CM. Psychological stages of adaptation following burn injury: a method for facilitating psychological recovery of burn victims. J Burn Care Rehabil 1988;9(4):376–384.

50. Tollison CD, Still JM, Tollison JW. The seriously burned adult: psychologic reactions, recovery and management. J Med Assoc Ga 1980;69(2):121–124.

51. Peeling B. One day at a time on a burn unit. Can Nurse 1978;74(10):38–41.

52. Feller I, Tholen D, Cornell RG. Improvements in burn care, 1965 to 1979. JAMA 1980;244(18):2074–2078.

53. Wright PC. Fundamentals of acute burn care and physical therapy management. Phys Ther 1984;64(8):1217–1231.

54. Schnebly WA, Ward RS, Warden GD, Saffle JR. A non-splinting approach to the care of the thermally injured patient. J Burn Care Rehabil 1989;10(3):263–266.

55. Ward RS. Pressure therapy for the control of hypertrophic scar formation after burn injury: a history and review. J Burn Care Rehabil 1991;12(3):257–262.

56. Gabbiani G, Ryan G, Majeno G. Presence of modified fibroblasts in granulation tissue and their possible role in wound contraction. Experientia 1971;27(5):549–550.

57. Hardy MA. The biology of scar formation. Phys Ther 1989;69(12):1014–1024.

58. Ketchum LD. Hypertrophic scars and keloids. Clin Plast Surg 1977;4(2):301–310.

59. Rockwell WB, Cohen IK, Erlich JP. Keloids and hypertrophic scars: a comprehensive report. Plast Reconstr Surg 1989;84(5):827–837.

60. Hunt TK. Disorders of wound healing. World J Surg 1980;4(3):289–295.

61. Clark JA, Cheng JCY, Leung KS, Leung PC. Mechanical characterization of human postburn hypertrophic skin during pressure therapy. J Biomech 1987;20(4):397–406.

62. Rudolph R. Wide spread scars, hypertrophic scars, and keloids. Clin Plast Surg 1987;14(2):253–260.

63. Davies D. Plastic and reconstructive surgery: scars, hypertrophic scars, and keloids. Br Med J 1985;290(6474):1056–1058.

64. Deitch EA, Wheelahan TM, Rose MP. Hypertrophic burn scars: analysis of variables. J Trauma 1983;23(10):895–898.

65. Rudolph R. Construction and the control of contraction. World J Surg 1980;4(3):279–287.

66. Stern PJ, Law EJ, Benedict FE, MacMillan BG. Surgical treatment of elbow contractures in postburn children. Plast Reconstr Surg 1985;76(3):441–446.

67. Parry SW. Reconstruction of the burned hand. Clin Plast Surg 1989;16(3):577–586.

68. Alexander JW, MacMillan BG, Martel L, Krummel R. Surgical correction of postburn flexion contractures of the fingers of children. Plast Reconstr Surg 1981;68(2):218–224.

69. Huang TT, Blackwell SJ, Lewis SR. Ten years experience in managing patients with burn contractures of axilla, elbow, wrist, and knee joints. Plast Reconstr Surg 1978;61(1):70–76.

70. Larson DL, Abston S, Evans EB, et al. Techniques for decreasing scar formation and contractures in the burned patient. J Trauma 1971;11(10):807–823.

71. Kischer CW, Shetlar MR, Shetlar CL. Alteration of hypertrophic scars induced by mechanical pressure. Arch Dermatol 1975;111(1):60–64.

72. Ward RS. Pressure therapy for the control of hypertrophic scar formation after burn injury: a history and review. J Burn Care Rehabil 1991;12(1):257–262.

73. Torring S. Our routine in pressure treatment of hypertrophic scars. Scand J Plast Reconstr Surg. 1984;18(1):135–137.

74. Robertson JC, Druett JE, Hodgson B, Druett J. Pressure therapy for hypertrophic scarring: preliminary communication. J R Soc Med 1980;73(5):348–354.

75. Ward RS, Hayes-Lundy C, Reddy R, et al. Influence of pressure supports on joint range of motion. Burns 1993;18(1):60–62.

76. Gold HM. A controlled clinical trial of topical silicone gel sheeting in the treatment of hypertrophic scars and keloids. J Am Acad Dermatol 1994;30(3):506–507.

77. Perkins K, Davey RB, Wallis KA. Silicone gel: a new treatment for burn scars and contractures. Burns 1982;9(3):201–204.

78. Ahn ST, Monafo WW, Mustoe TA. Topical silicone gel: a new treatment for hypertrophic scars. Surgery 1989;106(4):781–787.

79. Sullivan T, Smith J, Kerrnode J, et al. Rating the burn scar. J Burn Care Rehabil 1990;11(3):256–260.

80. Kealey GP, Jensen KT. Aggressive approach to physical therapy management of the burned hand. Phys Ther 1988;68(5):683–685.

81. Dobbs ER, Curreri PW. Burns: analysis of results of physical therapy in 681 patients. J Trauma 1972;12(3):242–248.

82. Howell JW. Management of the acutely burned hand for the nonspecialized clinician. Phys Ther 1989;69(12):1077–1090.

83. Parrot M, Ryan R, Parks DH, Wainwright DJ. Structured exercise circuit program for burn patients. J Burn Care Rehabil 1988;9(6):666–668.

84. Tafel JA, Thacker JG, Hagemann JM, et al. Mechanical performance of exertubing for isotonic hand exercise. J Burn Care Rehabil 1987;8(4):333–335.

85. Johnson CL. Physical therapists as scar modifiers. Phys Ther 1984;64(9):1381–1387.

86. Richard RL, Miller SF, Finley RK, Jones LM. Home exercise kit for the shoulder. J Burn Care Rehabil 1987;8(2):144–145.

87. Johnson CL, Cain VJ. Burn care—the rehab guide. Am J Nurs 1985;85(1):48–50.

88. Helm PA, Kevorkian CG, Lushbaugh M, et al. Burn injury: rehabilitation management in 1982. Arch Phys Med Rehabil 1982;63(1):6–16.

89. Humphrey C, Richard RL, Staley MJ. Soft Tissue Management and Exercise. In RL Richard, MJ Staley (eds), Burn Care and Rehabilitation Principles and Practice. Philadelphia: Davis, 1994;331–336.

90. Tepperman PS, Hilbert L, Peters WJ, Pritzker KPH. Heterotopic ossification in burns. J Burn Care Rehabil 1984;5(4):283–287.

91. Crawford CM, Vaeghese G, Mani M, Neff JR. Heterotopic ossification: are range of motion exercises contraindicated? J Burn Care Rehabil 1986;7(4):323–327.

92. VanLaeken N, Snelling CFT, Meek RN, et al. Heterotopic bone formation in the patient with burn injuries: a retrospective assessment of contributing factors and methods of investigation. J Burn Care Rehabil 1989;10(4):331–335.

93. Apfel LM, Wachtel TS, Frank DH, et al. Functional electrical stimulation in intrinsic/extrinsic imbalanced burned hands. J Burn Care Rehabil 1987;8(2):97–102.

94. Lewis SM, Clelland JA, Knowles CJ, et al. Effects of auricular acupuncture-like transcutaneous nerve stimulation on pain levels following wound care in patients with burns: a pilot study. J Burn Care Rehabil 1990;11(4):322–329.

95. Bierman W. Ultrasound in the treatment of scars. Arch Phys Med Rehabil 1954;35:209–214.

96. Baryza MJ. Ultrasound in the treatment of postburn skin graft contracture: a single case study. Phys Ther 1996;76:S54.

97. Ward RS, Hayes-Lundy C, Reddy R, et al. Evaluation of topical therapeutic ultrasound to improve response to physical therapy and lessen scar contracture after burn injury. J Burn Care Rehabil 1994;15(1):74–79.

98. Johnson CL. PT/OT forum (editorial). J Burn Care Rehabil 1988;9(4):396.

99. Covey MH, Dutcher K, Marvin JA, Heimbach DM. Efficacy of continuous passive motion (CPM) devices with hand burns. J Burn Care Rehabil 1988;9(4):397–400.

100. McAllister LP, Salazar CA. Case report on the use of CPM on an electrical burn. J Burn Care Rehabil 1988;9(4):401.

101. Head M, Helm P. Paraffin and sustained stretching in treatment of burn contracture. Burns 1977;4(2):136–139.

102. Ward RS, Saffle JR, Schnebly WA, et al. Sensory loss over grafted areas in patients with burns. J Burn Care Rehabil 1989;10(6):536–538.

103. Ward RS, Tuckett RP. Quantitative threshold changes in cutaneous sensation of patients with burns. J Burn Care Rehabil 1991;12(6):569–575.

104. Cooper S, Paul EO. An effective method of positioning the burn patient. J Burn Care Rehabil 1988;9(3):288–289.

105. Heeter PK, Brown R. Arm hammock for elevation of the thermally injured upper extremity. J Burn Care Rehabil 1986;7(2):144–146.

106. Waymack JP, Fidler J, Warden GD. Surgical correction of burn scar contractures of the foot in children. Burns 1988;4(2):156–160.

107. Duncan RM. Basic principles of splinting the hand. Phys Ther 1989;69(12):1104–1116.

108. Malick MH, Carr JA. Manual on Management of the Burn Patient. Pittsburgh: Harmarville Rehabilitation Center, 1982;32.

109. Daugherty MB, Carr-Collins JA. Splinting Techniques for the Burn Patient. In RL Richard, MJ Staley (eds), Burn Care and Rehabilitation Principles and Practice. Philadelphia: Davis, 1994;242–317.

110. Walters C. Splinting the Burn Patient. Laurel, MD: RAMSCO, 1987;9–97.

111. Ward RS, Schnebly WA, Kravitz M, et al. Have you tried the sandwich splint? A method of preventing hand deformities in children. J Burn Care Rehabil 1989;10:83–85.

112. Moore DJ. The role of the maxillofacial prosthetist in support of the burn patient. J Prosthet Dent 1970;24(1):68–76.

113. Heinle JA, Kealey GP, Cram AE, Hartford CE. The microstomia prevention appliance: 14 years of clinical experience. J Burn Care Rehabil 1988;9(1):90–91.

114. Sela M, Tubiana I. A mouth splint for severe burns of the head and neck. J Prosthet Dent 1989;62(6):679–681.

115. Lehman CJ. Splints and accessories following burn reconstruction. Clin Plast Surg 1992;19(3):721–726.

116. Kaufman T, Newman RA, Weinberg A, Wexler MR. The kerlix tongue depressor splint for skin-grafted areas in burned children. J Burn Care Rehabil 1989;10(5):462–463.

117. Wilder RP, Doctor A, Paley RJ, et al. Evaluation of cohesive and elastic bandages for joint immobilization. J Burn Care Rehabil 1989;10(3):258–262.

118. Richard RL, Miller SF, Finley RK Jr, Jones LM. Comparison of the effect of passive exercise vs static wrapping on finger range of motion of the hand. J Burn Care Rehabil 1987;8(6):576–578.

119. Richard RL. Use of the Dynasplint to correct elbow flexion burn contracture: a case report. J Burn Care Rehabil 1986;7(2):151–152.

120. Bennett GB, Helm P, Purdue GF, Hunt JL. Serial casting: a method for treating burn contractures. J Burn Care Rehabil 1989;10(6):543–545.

121. Wright MP, Taddonio TE, Prasad JK, Thomson PD. The microbiology and cleaning of thermoplastic splints in burn care. J Burn Care Rehabil 1989;10(1):79–83.

122. Helm PA. Peripheral neurological problems in acute burn patients. Burns 1977;3(2):123–125.

123. Ward RS, Hayes-Lundy C, Schnebly WS, et al. Rehabilitation of burn patients with concomitant limb amputation: case reports. Burns 1990;16(5):390–392.

124. Ward RS, Hayes-Lundy C, Schnebly WS, Saffle JR. Prosthetic use in patients with burns and associated limb amputation. J Burn Care Rehabil. 1990;11(4):361–364.

125. Meier RH. Amputations and Prosthetic Fitting. In SA Fisher, PA Helm (eds), Comprehensive Rehabilitation of Burns. Baltimore: Williams & Wilkins, 1984;267–310.

126. Rosenfelder R. The below-knee amputee with skin grafts. Phys Ther 1970;50(9):1338–1346.

127. Wood MR, Hunter GA, Millstein SG. The value of stump split skin grafting following amputation for trauma in adult upper and lower limb amputees. Prosthet Orthot Int 1987;11(2):71–74.

128. Helm PA, Walker SC. New bone formation at amputation sites in electrically burn-injured patients. Arch Phys Med Rehabil 1987;68(5, Part 1):284–286.

129. Kaplan SH. Patient education techniques used at burn centers. Am J Occup Ther 1985;39(10):655–658.

130. Neville C, Walker S, Brown B, et al. Discharge planning for burn patients. J Burn Care Rehabil 1988;9(4):414–420.

III

Prosthetics in Rehabilitation

19

Etiology of Amputation

CAROLINE C. NIELSEN

Over the history of medicine, amputation has been a relatively frequently performed medical procedure and has often been the only available alternative for complex fractures or infections of the extremities. The earliest amputations were generally undertaken in an attempt to save lives; however, their outcomes were not often successful: Many resulted in death from shock due to blood loss or onset of infection and septicemia in those who survived the operation. In these early amputations, removal of the compromised limb as quickly as possible was essential. With the advent of antisepsis, asepsis, and anesthesia in the mid-nineteenth century, increased attention could be focused on the surgical procedure and conservation of tissue.[1] With the development of modern medical treatment, alternatives to amputation have become available. When amputation is necessary, the surgery is now undertaken with consideration for the functional aspects of the residual limb. In this chapter, the causes for amputation are defined, the incidence and outcome expectations for particular populations are described, and approaches to rehabilitation are discussed.

INCIDENCE OF AMPUTATION SURGERY

Amputation is a complex problem for a patient, the health care system, and the country. In 1996, there were approximately 1.5 million persons with amputations in the United States. Every year an additional 125,000 people lose a limb as a result of an accident or disease.[2] In addition to immense personal suffering, the costs to the health care system for the care of a patient with an ischemic limb, including wound care, vascular reconstruction, and amputation, are enormous. The more than 50,000 lower extremity amputations performed in the United States in 1985 contributed approximately $500 million per year in direct medical costs.[3] In past years, the incidence of amputation

in the United States reflected the effects of injuries that resulted from war. With a shift in the population to a higher percentage of older adults, an increasing number of amputations are the result of disease.

Current information on the incidence of amputations, particularly lower extremity amputations, is limited by the lack of a standardized approach to gathering data. Differences between studies in case definition, level of ascertainment, and population structure often make meaningful comparisons impossible.[4] Data from two major surveys completed in the 1960s and 1970s using similar definitions are frequently cited. H.W. Glattly surveyed 12,000 persons with amputations, and the Committee on Prosthetics Research and Development and the Committee on Prosthetic-Orthotic Education (CPRD-CPOE) later compared 5,830 cases. Although the numbers have changed, several general indications and trends have continued.

More amputations occur among men than among women. In the Glattly study, using data collected in the early 1960s, the ratio of men to women for amputations related to trauma was 9.2:1, and for amputations related to disease the ratio was 2.6:1. In the Glattly and the CPRD-CPOE surveys, the majority of amputations were a result of a disease process (Figure 19-1). Disease accounted for 58% of all amputations in 1961 and increased to 70% over the next 12 years.[1] The results of more recent studies confirm this trend toward even higher percentages of amputation due to disease. The highest percentage of disease-related amputations occurs in the 61- to 70-year-old age group. Most of these are the lower extremity amputations, which are performed 11 times more frequently than are upper extremity amputations.[5] The disease that is most frequently related to amputation is peripheral vascular disease (PVD) and complications of neuropathy. Although PVD and neuropathy are frequently associated with long-term adult-onset (type II) diabetes, it is impor-

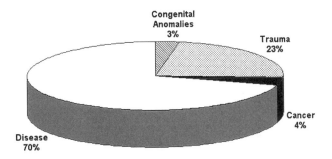

FIGURE 19-1

Causes of amputation by percent. The majority of amputations are a result of a disease process. (Data taken from CP Fylling, DR Knighton. Amputation in the diabetic population: incidence, causes, cost, treatment, and prevention. J Enterostom Ther 1989;1[6]:247–255; and AL Muilenberg, AB Wilson. A Manual for Below-Knee Amputees. Alexandria, VA: American Academy of Orthotists and Prosthetists, 1993.)

TABLE 19-1

Terminology Used to Describe the Site of Lower Extremity Amputation

Site	Terminology
Toe	Phalangeal
Forefoot	Ray resection (one or more complete metatarsal)
	Transmetatarsal (across the metatarsal shaft)
Midfoot	Partial foot (Chopart's, Boyd's, Pirogoff's, etc.)
At the ankle	Syme's
Below the knee	Transtibial (long, standard, short)
At the knee	Knee disarticulation
Above the knee	Transfemoral (long, standard, short)
At the hip	Hip disarticulation
At the pelvis	Hemipelvectomy

tant to note that vascular disease also occurs independent of diabetes. Of disease-related amputations, 50–70% are attributed to complications of diabetes.[6,7]

The increased frequency of amputation for PVD likely reflects the increased growth in the older population. In 1975, the median age of the population in the United States was 29 years; after the year 2000, the median age is expected to rise to more than 36 years. In 1975, 8% of the population in the United States was comprised of people older than 65; by 2020, there will be more than 35 million people age 65 and older, an increase of nearly 59%.[8] The population of the very old, those individuals over the age of 85 years, is projected to increase at the highest rate.[9] Because the prevalence of PVD increases with age, these demographic changes will likely have a large impact on the amount of vascular reconstruction and amputation that will be performed.

The second leading cause of amputation is trauma. According to Glattly, trauma accounted for 33.2% of all amputations between 1961 and 1963. The figure dropped to 22.4% in the CPRD-CPOE 1973–1974 survey.[5] Traumatic amputation was most common in the young adult age group in both studies. The incidence of trauma-related amputation has continued to decrease in the years since the surveys. This reduction in traumatic amputation can be attributed to implementation of new safety regulations, the development of safer farm and industrial machinery, improved safety in work conditions, and medical advancement in techniques for salvaging traumatized limbs.

Amputations related to tumors accounted for 4.5% of amputations in 1974. The tumor most commonly cited was osteosarcoma, which primarily affects children and ado-

lescents in the 11–20 age group. Currently, amputation is no longer the primary intervention for osteosarcoma. With development of new surgical techniques, including bone graft and joint replacement, and advancement in chemotherapy and radiation, the incidence of amputation due to osteosarcoma has decreased significantly.

Congenital limb deficiencies, and the amputations used to adjust or correct them, are relatively rare. Of the total number of amputations reported, congenital limb deficiency accounted for only 4.3% of amputations in Glattly's 1961–1963 survey and 2.8% in the CPRD-CPOE survey of 1973–1974. This percentage has remained relatively stable.

SITE OF AMPUTATIONS

Amputation can be performed as a disarticulation of a joint or as a transection through a long bone. The level of amputation is usually named by the joint or major bone through which the amputation has been made[5] (Table 19-1). An amputation that involves the lower extremity can impact on an individual's ability to stand and to walk, requiring the use of prosthetics, and often an assistive device for mobility. Amputation involving the upper extremity can affect other activities of daily living, such as feeding, grooming, dressing, and a host of activities that require manipulative skills. Because of the complex nature of skilled hand function, prosthetic substitution for upper limb amputation does not typically restore function to the same degree as do lower extremity prosthetics.

The levels of amputation surgery that are most commonly performed at present involve the lower extremity below the knee (including transtibial, foot, and toe amputations), accounting for 65.8% of all amputations (Table 19-2). This high percentage reflects the prevalence of PVD of the lower extremities. Transfemoral amputations account for 27.2% of all amputations. In general, the proportion of lower limb amputations in relation to upper limb amputations is increasing. This most likely reflects an increase in the number of older persons with lower extremity amputations rather than an actual decrease in the number of upper extremity amputations.[1]

Because PVD typically affects both lower extremities, a significant number of individuals will eventually undergo amputation of both lower extremities. Between 25% and 45% of persons with amputations have had amputations of both lower extremities,[1] most often at the transtibial level in both limbs, or a combination of transtibial of one limb and transfemoral of the other.

Today, the majority of transtibial and transfemoral amputations are performed with an understanding of wound healing and the functional needs and constraints of prosthetic fitting, so that rehabilitation outcomes are usually very positive. Other levels of amputation, although less commonly performed procedures, continue to pose challenges for the surgeon, prosthetist, physical therapist, and patient during prosthetic fitting and rehabilitation.

CAUSES OF AMPUTATION

The most likely reasons for amputation at present include (1) complications of peripheral neuropathy and PVD, (2) trauma, or (3) cancer (osteosarcoma). Children with congenital limb deficiencies are a special population group who may require surgical revision during or after periods of significant growth or conversion to a more functional level for prosthetic fitting (see Chapter 30).

Peripheral Vascular Disease

PVD is the most common contributing factor for lower extremity amputations. In epidemiologic studies, two symptoms are classic indicators of vascular insufficiency: intermittent claudication and loss of one or more lower extremity pulses. Intermittent claudication is a significant cramping pain, usually in the calf, that is induced by walking or other prolonged muscle contraction and relieved by a short period of rest. In arteriosclerosis obliterans, at least one major arterial pulse (at the dorsal pedis artery at the ankle, popliteal artery at the knee, or femoral artery in the groin) is often absent or markedly impaired.[3] The major risk factors for development of PVD are the same as those for cardiovascular and cerebrovascular disease,

TABLE 19-2

Incidence of Lower Limb Amputation: Average Annual Number and Percent of Hospital Discharges after Lower Extremity Amputation, 1989–1992

Level of Amputation	Number	Percent
Toe	34,098	32.3
Foot and ankle	10,740	10.2
Transtibial	24,527	23.3
Knee disarticulation	1,482	1.4
Transfemoral	28,640	27.2
Hip and pelvis	473	0.5
Not specified	5,349	5.1
Total	105,309	100

Source: Adapted from GE Reiber, EJ Boyko, DG Smith. Lower Extremity Foot Ulcers and Amputations in Diabetes. In Diabetes in America. Bethesda, MD: National Institutes of Health, National Institute of Diabetes, Digestive and Kidney Diseases, Pub No. 95-1468, 1995;409–427.

most notably poorly managed hypertension, high serum cholesterol and triglyceride levels, and a history of tobacco use and smoking. Peripheral neuropathy and PVD are the major predisposing factors for lower extremity amputation in individuals with diabetes.[3]

The number of hospital discharges, reported in the National Hospital Discharge Survey, which lists diagnoses of amputation and diabetes, increased 29% in the 1980s, from 36,000 in 1980 to 54,000 in 1990.[10] The prevalence of PVD among persons with diabetes, whether men or women, is significantly greater than in those without diabetes. The Framingham Heart Study found a four to five times greater relative risk of intermittent claudication in persons with diabetes, even when controlling for blood pressure, cholesterol, and smoking.[11] The age-adjusted rate of lower extremity amputation among people with diabetes in the United States is approximately 15 times that of the nondiabetic population.[7] More than 50% of the lower limb amputations in the United States are diabetes related, although persons diagnosed with diabetes represent only 3% of the population.[12] In a study of residents of Rochester, Minnesota, persons with non–insulin-dependent diabetes were compared with the general population. The risk of any first lower extremity amputation in individuals with non–insulin-dependent diabetes was nearly 17 times higher than that of the general population.[13] Although major improvements have been made in noninvasive diagnosis, surgical revascularization procedures, and wound-healing techniques, between 2% and 5% of individuals with PVD and without diabetes and between 6% and 25% of those with diabetes eventually undergo an amputation.[6,13,14]

The three most common predisposing factors for lower extremity amputation appear to be (1) concurrent diabetes and hypertension, (2) hypertension without diabetes, and

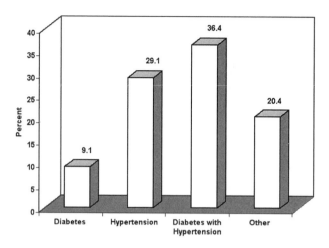

FIGURE 19-2

Lower extremity amputations, classified by predisposing factors. Hypertension, especially in the presence of diabetes, is a very powerful risk factor. "Other" includes a combination of risk factors, including race, gender, cigarette smoking, and previous vascular surgery. (Based on data from CS Lee, J Sariego, T Matsumoto. Changing patterns in the predisposition for amputation of the lower extremities. Am Surg 1992;5[8]:474–477.)

(3) diabetes without hypertension (Figure 19-2). Other predisposing factors include race, gender, history of smoking, and previous vascular surgery.[15] The incidence of lower extremity amputation among persons with diabetes is almost 68% higher for men than for women.[6] The most frequently cited criteria for amputation among persons with diabetes include gangrene, infection, nonhealing neuropathic ulcer, severe ischemic pain, absent or decreased pulses, local necrosis, osteomyelitis, systemic toxicity, acute embolic disease, or severe venous thrombosis.[6,13,16]

In individuals with diabetes, the prevalence and severity of PVD increase significantly with age and with the duration of diabetes, particularly in men.[3,17] Initial amputation may involve toe or foot; subsequent revision to transtibial or transfemoral levels is likely to occur with progression of the underlying disease.[16] In individuals with diabetes, a diagnosis of PVD increases the risk for nonhealing neuropathic ulcer, infection, and/or gangrene, all of which increase the likelihood of amputation. An epidemiologic study in Rochester, Minnesota, examined the relationship between the diagnoses of diabetes and PVD.[13] On initial diagnosis of diabetes, 8% of subjects had clinical evidence of arteriosclerosis obliterans. As the duration of diabetes lengthened, the prevalence of PVD increased to 15% at 10 years and 45% at 20 years. Patients with diabetes who were 65 years old or older accounted for 61% of all diabetes-related lower extremity amputations.[16] In

1990, the estimated amputation rate was 1.4 times higher for persons with diabetes aged 65–74 and 2.4 times higher for those 75 years of age or older, compared with those 0–64 years of age.[10]

Peripheral neuropathy is a common complication of diabetes. Neuropathy is as important and powerful as PVD as a predisposing factor for lower extremity amputation. Peripheral neuropathy is suspected when one or more of the following clinical signs are present: deficits of sensation (loss of Achilles and patellar reflexes, decreased vibratory sensation, and loss of protective sensation),[3] motor impairments (weakness and atrophy of the intrinsic muscles of the foot), and/or autonomic dysfunction (inadequate or abnormal hemodynamic mechanism, tropic changes of the skin, and distal loss of hair). The resulting loss of thermal and pain sensation increases the vulnerability of the foot to acute/high-pressure and repetitive/low-pressure trauma. Patients may also experience significant numbness or painful paresthesia of the foot and lower leg. Individuals with peripheral neuropathy may not be aware of minor trauma, pressure from poorly fitting shoes along the side and tops of their feet, or pressure from thickening plantar callus, all of which contribute to the risk of ulceration, infection, and gangrene. Motor neuropathy and associated weakness and atrophy contribute to development of bony deformity of the foot. The bony prominences and malalignments that are associated with foot deformity change weight-bearing pressure dynamics during walking, further increasing the risk of ulceration.[3] Peripheral neuropathy is one of the most crucial precursors of foot ulceration, especially in the presence of PVD. Nonhealing or infected neuropathic ulcers precede approximately 85% of nontraumatic lower extremity amputations in individuals with diabetes.[12] Conservative management of patients who are vulnerable to neuropathic ulcer due to peripheral neuropathy is discussed in Chapter 20.

Lower extremity amputation continues to be a major health problem for the diabetic population. For this group of patients, amputation is associated with significant morbidity, functional limitation and disability, mortality, and high health care costs. Approximately 54,000 lower extremity amputations were performed on individuals with diabetes in the United States in 1990.[12] The direct medical care costs for all amputations, excluding the cost of rehabilitation, in the diabetic population in the United States was approximately $500 million in 1989.[3] In New Jersey alone, hospital charges for lower extremity amputations averaged almost $30 million annually between 1985 and 1987.[18] According to the U.S. Public Health Service,[9] reducing the incidence of lower extremity amputations in persons with diabetes by more than 40% is a key health care objective in terms of quality of life and containment of health care costs. New amputations in the diabetic population could be reduced by at least 50% through health promotion efforts to minimize the impact of risk factors and by greater access to quality foot care by a multidisciplinary health care team.[3,6]

Incidence among Minority Populations

There is clear evidence that membership in certain racial and ethnic groups holds an increased risk for lower extremity amputation. This increased risk appears to be linked to a higher prevalence of diabetes. Minority groups with the highest incidence of diabetes are (1) Native Americans, (2) Puerto Rican–Americans, (3) African-Americans, (4) Mexican-Americans, and (5) Cuban-Americans. Data collected from 18 hospitals in San Antonio demonstrated the incidence of lower extremity amputations among African-Americans with diabetes to be nearly twice that of Hispanics and almost three times the rate among whites. Similarly, data collected in California in 1991 by hospital discharge records demonstrated that African-Americans were twice as likely as Hispanics and whites to have lower leg amputation due to diabetes (LA Lavery, LB Harkless. Information presented at the American College of Foot and Ankle Surgeons' 53rd annual meeting, San Francisco, March 1, 1995. Personal communication). Other studies report similar discrepancies in the rate of lower extremity amputation among African-Americans.[19,20]

Native Americans have a two to five times higher prevalence of diabetes than the overall population in the United States. This high prevalence is directly reflected in increased amputation rates. Among Pima Indians with diabetes, the rate of amputation is 3.7 times higher than the rate of other persons with diabetes.[21] A survey of lower extremity amputations among patients in the areas served by the Indian Health Service in 1982–1987 found that the age-adjusted incidence rates of all lower extremity amputations among Native Americans with diabetes were substantially higher than the overall rate for the United States.[22] A similar study among Native Americans in Oklahoma found that the incidence of lower extremity amputation, and the associated mortality, was higher than rates reported in the Pima Indian population as well as in other diabetic populations.[23]

It is unclear why these populations have a significantly higher rate of lower extremity amputation. Potential contributors include a genetic or familial predisposition to diabetes and/or a higher prevalence of hypertension and smoking in these populations. Health promotion and education efforts that target this high-risk population (including programs aimed at effective management of diabetes, minimization of other risk factors, and special foot care programs for early detection of neuropathic and traumatic lesions) are effective strategies to reduce the likelihood of amputation.[23]

Outcome of Vascular-Related Amputation

The morbidity and mortality risks associated with systemic diseases, such as diabetes and vascular disease, continue after amputation. As a result, death in the years immediately after amputation is not uncommon. The 3-year survival rate after initial lower extremity amputation for persons with diabetes is only approximately 50%; the 5-year survival rate ranges in various studies from 39% to 68%.[12,24] Because neuropathy and PVD occur in a symmetric distribution, the risk of subsequent amputation of the contralateral lower extremity is high. Data compiled in five studies of persons with disease-related initial amputation (n = 485 patients) indicated that as many as 42% of patients required contralateral amputation within 1–3 years after the first amputation; 56% went on to subsequent amputation within 5 years.[25] The most common causes of death in persons with amputation include complications of diabetes, cardiovascular disease, and renal disease.[23,26]

Evidence is growing that the incidence of lower extremity amputation in persons with diabetes could be significantly reduced through particular kinds of preventive care. Large clinical centers have demonstrated the effect of early intervention for the diabetic population, with a 44–85% reduction in amputation rate reported after the provision of improved foot care.[27,28]

Early interventions to prevent neuropathy and PVD target smoking reduction programs, as well as dietary, exercise, and pharmaceutical interventions, to obtain better control of hypertension, hyperlipidemia, and hyperglycemia. Reduction of these predisposing factors is likely to reduce further the incidence of amputation, heart disease, and stroke among people with diabetes. For those with existing diabetic neuropathy or PVD, intensive foot care programs should focus on prevention of ulceration and early intervention to prevent expansion, infection, or gangrene of a small lesion. Foot care programs are most effective if they are developed in a team setting and are focused on patient education.

The decision to undergo amputation often follows a long struggle to care for an increasingly frail foot by the patient, the family, and health care providers. In this circumstance, elective amputation is often perceived by the patient and family as a positive step toward a more active and less stressful life. The multidisciplinary team approach best addresses the complex needs of the individual with diabetes, including clinical evaluation, determination of risk status, patient education, footwear selection, decision making about amputation, and rehabilitation after surgery.[3]

Traumatic Amputation

Traumatic loss of a limb, the second most common cause of amputation, occurs most frequently in vehicle- or work-related accidents, as a result of violence such as gunshots, or after severe burns and electrocution. Trauma-related amputation occurs most commonly in young adult men but can happen at any age to men or to women.[14] Because the mechanism of injury in traumatic amputation is quite variable, this type of amputation is usually classified or categorized according to the severity of tissue damage. The extent of injury to the musculoskeletal system depends on several factors: (1) movement of the object that causes the injury; (2) direction, magnitude, and speed of the energy vector; and (3) the particular body tissue involved.

In partial traumatic amputations, at least one-half the diameter of the injured extremity is severed or significantly damaged. This kind of injury can incur extensive bleeding, because all of the blood vessels involved may not vasoconstrict. A second type of traumatic amputation occurs when the limb becomes completely detached from the body. As much as 1 liter of blood may be lost before the arteries spasm and vasoconstrict.[29]

For optimal outcome, surgical intervention is usually necessary within the first 12 hours after the accident for revascularization or for treatment of the amputated site. When replantation is considered, the window of opportunity is much narrower. The decision to replant is a difficult one and is influenced by the patient's age and overall health status, the level of extremity injury, and the condition of the amputated part. Replantation has been most successful in the distal upper extremity. The goal of upper extremity replantation is to provide a mechanism for functional grasp rather than cosmetic restoration of the limb. The period of recovery and rehabilitation after replantation is often significantly longer than that after amputation.

Persons with trauma-related amputation undergo extreme physiologic changes as well as psychological trauma. With the sudden loss of a body part, the patient may experience an extended period of grieving. Addressing the patient's psychological needs as well as physical needs are equally important for optimal outcome. An interdisciplinary team approach to rehabilitation is the most effective means to address the comprehensive needs of the patient who has unexpectedly lost a limb to trauma.[29]

Cancer

Amputation due to cancer is generally a result of osteogenic sarcoma (osteosarcoma), which occurs most frequently in the adolescent and young adult years. Since the early 1990s,

the need for amputation in osteosarcoma has been reduced by advances in early detection, improved imaging techniques, more effective chemotherapy regimens, and better limb resectioning and salvage procedures. Tumor resection followed by limb reconstruction frequently provides a functional extremity. Weight bearing is limited, and the limb is protected by an orthosis early in rehabilitation. Once satisfactory healing occurs, full weight bearing and near normal activity can be resumed. With new techniques, 5-year survival rates for individuals with osteosarcoma increased from approximately 20% in the 1970s to 80% in the 1990s.[30-33]

Congenital Limb Deficiencies

The actual incidence of congenital limb deficiencies is difficult to determine because of lack of a common definition and reporting mechanisms. Some estimates suggest an incidence of 1 per 2,000 births; other studies indicate a slightly higher ratio of 1 per 1,692 live births.[34,35] Six categories of limb deficiencies have been recognized[36]:

1. *Failure of formation* of parts, indicating a partial or complete arrest in limb development
2. *Failure of differentiation* or separation of parts, when the basic structures have developed but the final form is not completed
3. Duplication of parts, such as *polydactyly*
4. Overgrowth, also called *gigantism*, and generally caused by skeletal overgrowth
5. Congenital *constriction band syndrome*, characterized by constriction bands, which may compromise circulation to the distal part
6. Generalized skeletal abnormalities

Upper limb deficiencies in children vary from minor abnormalities of the fingers to major limb absences. Embryologic differentiation of the upper limbs occurs most rapidly at 5–8 weeks after gestation, often before pregnancy has been recognized or confirmed. During this period the upper limbs are particularly vulnerable to malformation. The etiology of limb malformation is unclear: Potential contributing factors cited in the research literature include (1) exposure to chemical agents or drugs, (2) fetal position or constriction, (3) endocrine disorders, (4) exposure to radiation, (5) immune reactions, (6) occult infections and other diseases, (7) single gene disorders, (8) chromosomal disorders, and (9) other syndromes with unknown causes.[36] For many children, an upper limb deficiency is their only anomaly. However, as many as 12% of these children have coexisting nonlimb malformations.

Limb deficiencies that are present at birth are classified according to an international standard based on skeletal

TABLE 19-3
Classification of Longitudinal Congenital Limb Deficiencies

Limb Segment	Upper Extremity Bone Segment*	Lower Extremity Bone Segment*
Proximal	Humeral	Femoral
Distal	Radial	Tibial
	Central	Central
	Carpal	Tarsal
	Metacarpal	Metatarsal
	Phalangeal	Phalangeal
Combined	(Indicated by the bone segments that remain)	
	Partial or complete	Partial or complete
	Specific carpal, ray, or phalanx remaining	Specific tarsal, ray, or phalanx remaining

*May be partial or complete.
Source: Adapted from BJ May. Amputations and Prosthetics: A Case Study Approach. Philadelphia: FA Davis, 1996;221.

elements (Table 19-3). These deficiencies are referred to as *transverse* or *longitudinal*. Transverse deficiencies are described by the level at which the limb terminates. In longitudinal deficiencies, a reduction or absence occurs within the long axis of the limb, but normal skeletal components are present distal to the affected bones.[36,37]

The use of prosthetics is a common intervention for children with congenital limb deficiencies. Sometimes surgery is necessary to prepare the existing limb for the most effective use of a prosthesis, especially after periods of rapid growth. The goal of prosthetics training for the child should be to enhance the function of the limb and to provide a cosmetic replacement for a missing limb. Rehabilitation efforts (discussed in Chapter 30) are designed with the child's cognitive, motor, and psychological development in mind.

REHABILITATION ISSUES FOR THE PERSON WITH AN AMPUTATION

Several factors influence the success of rehabilitation after amputation. These include age, health status, cognitive status, sequence of onset of disability, concurrent disease and comorbidity, and the level of amputation.[38]

Progression in rehabilitation has been measured in different ways. Traditionally, physical therapists focus on the person's ability to perform functional activities, such as walking, turning, and managing ramps and other uneven or unpredictable surfaces, safely, independently, and efficiently with and without a prosthesis. Physical therapists assist physicians and prosthetists in determining an individual's readiness for prosthetic fitting and are often involved in the decisions about prosthetic components. After initial fitting, physical therapists coordinate prosthetic training, consulting with prosthetists if problems with prosthetic alignment arise. Once these basic mobility activities are mastered, the therapist can serve as a consultant to assist the person with amputation in returning to pre-

amputation employment and leisure activities. Treatment programs, predictors of outcome, and measures of success or failure are often based on these functional activities.

In one study of progression through rehabilitation (n = 459), between 85% and 89% of persons with lower extremity amputations mastered basic functional activities, such as moving about the bed, moving from supine into sitting position, and sitting balance, within the second postoperative week.[39] Between 65% and 75% of persons with amputation demonstrated independence in transfers and dressing of upper and lower limbs in the third to fifth postoperative week. Although steady gains were made in the ability to doff and don the prosthesis and to walk indoors and outside during the fifth to the twelfth postoperative weeks, just one-third of people in the study achieved independence within this time frame. Optimal rehabilitation outcome, achievement of the highest functional level of which the person with amputation is capable, requires ongoing contact with and support of a multidisciplinary rehabilitation team.

As many as 70% of persons with a lower extremity amputation report using their prosthesis on a full-time basis: putting it on in the early morning, wearing it all day, and taking it off in the evening.[40] Two major reasons for limited use or nonuse are generally cited: physical discomfort when walking with the prosthesis, and psychological discomfort. The wide variation reported (from 29.5% to 100%) in success of functional ambulation with a prosthesis after below-knee amputation appears to be related to age and concurrent disease. Healing time, indicated by time between surgery and fitting for the first prosthesis, correlates with age but not with the cause of amputation. Age is also more important than the etiology of amputation in predicting the total length of time in rehabilitation and achievement of functional ambulation: Older adults with amputation are likely to require a longer rehabilitation period to accomplish an ambulatory status equal to that of the younger group.[41] Although most people who are recovering from amputation achieve some level of

TABLE 19-4

Members and Roles of the Multidisciplinary Team for Rehabilitation After Amputation

Team Member	Role
Physician	Often serves as coordinator of the team
	Assesses need for amputation, performs surgery, monitors healing of suture line
	Monitors and manages patient's overall medical care and health status
	Monitors condition of remaining extremity for patients with peripheral vascular disease (PVD), neuropathy, and/or diabetes
Physical therapist	Provides preoperative education about the rehabilitation process and instruction in single limb mobility
	Designs and manages a preprosthetic rehabilitation program that focuses on mobility and preparation for prosthetic training
	Evaluates patient's readiness for prosthetic fitting; can make recommendations for prosthetic fitting
	Designs and manages a prosthetic training program that focuses on functional ambulation and prosthetic management
	Monitors condition of the remaining extremity for patients with PVD, neuropathy, and/or diabetes
Prosthetist	Designs, fabricates, and fits the prosthesis
	Adapts the prosthesis to individuals, adjusts alignment, repairs/replaces components when necessary
	Monitors fit, function, and comfort of the prosthesis
	Monitors condition of the remaining extremity for patients with PVD, neuropathy, and/or diabetes
Occupational therapist	Assesses and treats patients with upper extremity amputation, monitors readiness for prosthetic fitting, can recommend components
	Assists with problem solving in activities of daily living for patients with upper and/or lower limb amputation
	Makes recommendations for environmental modification and assistive/adaptive equipment to facilitate functional independence
Social worker	Provides financial counseling and coordination of support services
	Liaison with third-party payers and community agencies
	Assists with patient's and family's social, psychological, and financial issues
Dietitian	Evaluates nutritional status and provides nutritional counseling, especially for patients with diabetes or heart disease or those who are on chemotherapy or are recovering from trauma
Nurse/nurse practitioner	Monitors patient's health and functional status during rehabilitation
	Provides ongoing patient education on comorbid and chronic health issues
	Monitors condition of remaining extremity for patients with PVD, neuropathy, and/or diabetes
Vocational counselor	Assesses patient's employment status and potential
	Assists with education, training, and placement

Source: Adapted from B May. Assessment and Treatment of Individuals following Lower Extremity Amputation. In SB O'Sullivan, TJ Schmitz (eds), Physical Rehabilitation: Assessment and Treatment. Philadelphia: FA Davis, 1994;379.

upright mobility, a smaller percentage of older persons with concurrent chronic disease become functional ambulators when compared to younger persons who had amputations because of trauma or osteomyelitis.

The typical age at time of initial lower limb amputation is between 51 and 69 years; therefore, consideration must be given to the special rehabilitation needs of the older patient.[38] The complexity of issues during rehabilitation of the older adult who is undergoing an amputation is often compounded by comorbidity, fragile social supports, and limited resources. In patients with PVD, concomitant cere-brovascular disease can complicate rehabilitation: A pre-amputation history of stroke or occurrence of stroke during the course of rehabilitation is not uncommon.[42] Similarly, cardiovascular disease can limit endurance and exercise tolerance; endurance training becomes a critical component of the postamputation/preprosthetic rehabilitation program. Optimal rehabilitation care begins with consultation and patient/family education efforts before surgery. A specialized multidisciplinary team (Table 19-4) most effectively provides this pre- and perisurgical care. Members of the team often include a surgeon, physical therapist, certified prosthetist, occupational therapist, nurse or nurse practitioner, recreational therapist, psychologist, and social worker.[38] The patient and family members are active and essential members of the team as well. Effective communication provides the team with the necessary information to develop a tentative treatment plan from the time of amputation to discharge home.

With a specialized treatment team and the use of new lightweight and dynamic prosthetic designs, the potential for rehabilitation of the older patient has increased significantly in the last decade. At the time of surgery, special consideration is given to the optimal level of amputation. This is a particularly important concern for the older patient. The selection of the surgical level of amputation is probably one of the most important decisions to be made for the patient who is undergoing an amputation. A lower limb prosthesis ideally becomes a full-body weight-bearing device. However, bony prominences, adhesions of the suture line scar, fragile skin and open areas, shearing forces at the skin/socket interface, and perspiration can complicate this function.[38] The energy cost of ambulation must be considered, especially for older patients with significant deconditioning or comorbid conditions. The higher the level of amputation and loss of joints, long bone length, and muscle insertion, the greater the impairment of normal locomotor mechanisms. This leads to increased energy cost in prosthetic control and functional ambulation and a greater likelihood of functional limitation and disability.

Preservation of the knee joint seems to be a key determinant in determining the potential for functional ambulation and successful rehabilitation outcome. Persons with transtibial amputation, who have an intact anatomic knee joint, demonstrate a more energy-efficient prosthetic gait pattern and postural responses and are more likely to ambulate without additional assistive devices (walkers, crutches, or canes) and to be full-time prosthetic wearers than are those with transfemoral amputation. The benefits of preserving the knee, particularly among older adults, is so crucial that a transtibial amputation may be attempted even with the risk of inadequate healing; this may necessitate later revision to a higher level.[38]

The patient with a bilateral transfemoral amputation faces additional rehabilitation challenges. The significant increase in energy consumption that is required can prevent long-distance ambulation. Many older patients, as well as younger persons with bilateral transfemoral amputation, may choose wheelchair mobility as a more energy-efficient and effective means of locomotion. Ambulation potential is dependent on cardiac function, strength, balance, and endurance.[38]

Options for prosthetic components for the older person with an amputation have increased dramatically since the 1980s. Selecting the most appropriate components for the individual requires the input of the complete rehabil-itation team, in close communication with the patient and the family members.

Rehabilitation Environment

Traditionally, preprosthetic and early prosthetic programs have been housed in rehabilitation departments of acute care hospitals. In this environment, the care may not be specialized for the older person with an amputation. A specialized treatment team is best able to address the complex needs of this group of patients. However, in today's health care environment, it may not be possible for older patients with an amputation to stay in the acute care hospital until they are ready for fitting of the prosthesis. For patients with multiple medical complications, rehabilitation may be continued in a subacute setting or skilled nursing facility. For patients without complications and with a strong social support network, an outpatient rehabilitation program may be preferable. This plan allows them to reintegrate into home and community while maintaining support of the treatment team. The most effective care and rehabilitation for individuals who are undergoing an amputation require the skills and ongoing support of an integrated treatment team.[33,43]

SUMMARY

Although the rehabilitation process after amputation presents many challenges for patients, their families, and the professionals involved in their care, it also allows many opportunities for success and rewards. It is important to understand the risk factors for amputation and the influence of comorbid disease and age on progression of rehabilitation. Optimal outcome after amputation is best achieved through the interaction of a patient-centered, multidisciplinary health care team.[39,44]

REFERENCES

1. Sanders GT, May BJ. Lower Limb Amputations: A Guide to Rehabilitation. Philadelphia: FA Davis, 1988;12–53.
2. American Orthotic and Prosthetic Association. You Can Make a Difference in People's Lives: Become an Orthotist or Prosthetist. Alexandria, VA: Orthotics and Prosthetics National Office, 1995.
3. Bild DE, Selby JV, Sinnock P, et al. Lower extremity amputation in people with diabetes: epidemiology and prevention. Diabetes Care 1989;12(1):24–31.
4. LEA Study Group. Comparing the incidence of lower extremity amputations across the world: the global lower extremity amputation study. Diabetic Med 1995;12:14–18.
5. Shurr DG, Cook TM. Prosthetics and Orthotics. Norwalk, CT: Appleton & Lange, 1990;1–15.

6. Centers for Disease Control. Lower extremity amputations among persons with diabetes mellitus–Washington, 1988. Morbid Mortal 1991;40(43):737–739.

7. National Diabetes Advisory Board. Diabetes, 1989; Annual Report. National Institutes of Health Pub No. 89-1587.1989: Bethesda, MD. U.S. Department of Health and Human Services, April 1989.

8. Campbell PR. Population projections for state by age, sex, race, and Hispanic origin 1993–2020. US Department of Commerce, Bureau of the Census. Washington DC, 1994.

9. U.S. Public Health Service. Healthy People 2000. Washington, DC: U.S. Department of Health and Human Services, 1990;2.

10. Centers for Disease Control and Prevention. Diabetes Surveillance, 1993. Atlanta: U.S. Department of Health and Human Services, 1993;87–93.

11. Kannel WB, McGee DL. Diabetes and glucose tolerance as risk factors for cardiovascular disease: the Framingham study. Diabetes Care 1979;2(2):120–126.

12. Reiber GE, Boyko EJ, Smith DG. Lower Extremity Foot Ulcers and Amputations in Diabetes. In Diabetes in America. Bethesda, MD: National Institutes of Health, National Institute of Diabetes and Digestive and Kidney Diseases, Pub No. 95-1468, 1995;409–427.

13. Humphry LL, Palumbo PJ, Butters MA, et al. The contribution of non–insulin dependent diabetes to lower-extremity amputation in the community. Arch Intern Med 1994;154(8): 885–892.

14. May B. Assessment and Treatment of Individuals following Lower Extremity Amputation. In SB O'Sullivan, TJ Schmitz (eds), Physical Rehabilitation: Assessment and Treatment. Philadelphia: Davis, 1994;375–395.

15. Lee CS, Sariego J, Matsumoto T. Changing patterns in the predisposition for amputation of the lower extremities. Am Surg 1992;58(8):474–477.

16. Fylling CP, Knighton DR. Amputation in the diabetic population: incidence, causes, cost, treatment, and prevention. J Enterostom Ther 1989;16(6):247–255.

17. Moss SE, Klein R, Klein B. The prevalence and incidence of lower extremity amputation in a diabetic population. Arch Intern Med 1992;152(3):610–616.

18. Van Buskirk AH, Barta PJ, Schlossbach NJ. Lower extremity amputations in New Jersey. NJ Med 1994;91(4):260–263.

19. Most RS, Sinnock P. The epidemiology of lower extremity amputations in diabetic individuals. Diabetes Care 1983;6(1):86–91.

20. Miller AD, Van Buskirk AH, Verhoek-Oftedahl W, Miller ER. Diabetes-related lower extremity amputations in New Jersey, 1979–1981. J Med Soc NJ 1985;82(9):723–726.

21. Nelson RG, Ghodes DM, Everhart JE, et al. Lower extremity amputation in NIDDM: 12-year follow-up study in Pima Indians. Diabetes Care 1988;11(1):8–16.

22. Valway SE, Linkins RW, Gohdes, DM. Epidemiology of lower-extremity amputations in the Indian Health Service, 1982–1987. Diabetes Care 1993;16(1):349–353.

23. Lee JS, Lu M, Lee VS, et al. Lower extremity amputation: incidence, risk factors, and mortality in the Oklahoma Indian diabetes study. Diabetes 1993;42(6):876–882.

24. Palumbo PJ, Melton LJ, Harris MI, et al. In MI Harris, RF Hamman (eds), Diabetes in America. National Institutes of Health Pub No. 85-1468. Bethesda, MD: U.S. Department of Health and Human Services, 1985;XVI–XV20.

25. Levin ME, O'Neal LW. The Diabetic Foot: Pathophysiology, Evaluation, and Treatment. In ME Levin, LW O'Neal, JH Bowker (eds). The Diabetic Foot (4th ed). St. Louis: Mosby, 1988;17–60.

26. Stewart CP, Jain AS. Cause of death of lower limb amputees. Prosthet Orthot Int 1992;16(2):129–132.

27. Edmonds ME, Blundell MP, Morris HE, et al. The diabetic foot: impact of a foot clinic. QJM 1986;(60)232:763–771.

28. Assal JP, Mulhauser I, Pernat A, et al. Patient education as the basis for diabetes care in clinical practice. Diabetologia 1985;28(8):602–613.

29. Brown LW. Traumatic amputation. AAOHN J 1990;38(10): 483–486.

30. Lane JM, Kroll MA, Rossbach P. New advancements and concepts in amputee management after treatment for bone and soft-tissue sarcomas. Clin Orthop 1990;July(256):22–28.

31. Yaw KM, Wurtz LD. Resection and reconstruction for bone tumors in the proximal tibia. Orthop Clin North Am 1991;22(1): 133–148.

32. Link MP, Goorin AM, Horowitz M, et al. Adjuvant chemotherapy of high-grade osteosarcoma of the extremity. Clin Orthop 1991;Sept(270):8–14.

33. LaQuaglia MP. Osteosarcoma: specific tumor management and results. Chest Surg Clin N Am 1998;8(1)77–95.

34. Calzolari E, Manservigi D, Garani GP, et al. Limb reduction defects in Emilia Romagna, Italy: epidemiological and genetic study in 173,109 consecutive births. J Med Genet 1990;27(6):353–357.

35. Froster-Iskenius UG, Baird PA. Limb reduction defects in over one million consecutive live births. Teratology 1989;39(2): 127–135.

36. Gover AM, McIvor J. Upper limb deficiencies in infants and young children. Inf Young Children 1992;5(1);58–72.

37. May BJ. Amputations and Prosthetics: A Case Study Approach. Philadelphia: Davis, 1996;219–231.

38. Esquenazi A. Geriatric amputee rehabilitation. Clin Geriatr Med 1993;9(4):731–743.

39. Ham R, de Trafford J, Van de Ven C. Patterns of recovery for lower limb amputations. Clin Rehab 1994;8(4):320–328.

40. Nielsen CC. A survey of amputees: functional level, life satisfaction, information needs, and the prosthetist's role. J Prosthet Orthot 1991;3(3):125–129.

41. Scremin AM, Tapia JI, Vichick DA, et al. Effect of age on progression through temporary prostheses after below-knee amputation. Am J Phys Med Rehabil 1993;72(6):350–354.

42. Phillips NA, Mate-Kole CC, Kirby RL. Neuropsychological function in peripheral vascular disease amputee patients. Arch Phys Med Rehabil 1993;74(12):1309–1314.

43. Ham R, Regan JM, Roberts VC. Evaluation of introducing the team approach to the care of the amputee: the Dulwich study. Prosthet Orthot Int 1987;11(1):25–30.

44. Muilenberg AL, Wilson AB A manual for below-knee amputees. Alexandria, VA: American Academy of Orthotists and Prosthetists, 1993.

20

Conservative Management of Vulnerable Feet

Carolyn B. Kelly

The treatment of foot wounds is not new to rehabilitation professionals. For many years, clients with such problems have been referred for traditional physical therapy treatment, including whirlpool, débridement, and dressing changes. Many of these patients were instructed in crutch walking or asked to minimize their ambulation to limit weight bearing and protect their vulnerable foot. Some of these wounds healed only to recur when the patient returned to function under the same conditions that had caused the problem. Some patients were referred for treatment of wounds so advanced that it was doubtful that conservative intervention would make a difference. We could only ask ourselves, "Couldn't something have been done earlier in the process to prevent this foot from getting so bad?" As we continued with whirlpool treatments and made little progress, we asked, "Isn't there something that can be done that would be more effective?" The answer to both of these questions is "yes," and such interventions are the focus of this chapter.

VULNERABLE FOOT

A patient with a vulnerable foot has an underlying disease process that places the soft tissues of the foot at greater than normal risk for damage. The smallest opening in the skin becomes a potential portal of entry for bacteria, which can lead to deep infection and ultimately amputation.

Diabetes mellitus, although not the only cause, is the diagnosis that is most frequently associated with foot ulceration and lower extremity amputation.[1] One study that followed a large population of patients with diabetes reported that foot problems accounted for 16% of all hospital admissions and 23% of total hospital days.[2] Of the total number of nontraumatic lower extremity amputations performed each year, approximately 50% (54,000 amputations) are performed on patients with diabetes.[3] If the high cost of

medical care is considered, the impact on the health care dollar is tremendous.[4] Just as important, however, is the impact on the quality of life of the patient with diabetes, who may be left with compromised function, permanent disability, and an increased risk of mortality.

The role of physical therapists in treating patients with high-risk feet is to manage their functional rehabilitation programs and to take part, as appropriate, in the evaluation, treatment, and prevention of foot ulcerations that tend to occur in this population. Before one can adequately treat these wounds, however, one must have a basic understanding of the disease processes that cause them. The two disease processes that are most commonly linked to foot wounds are peripheral vascular disease and peripheral neuropathy.[1,5,6]

Many individuals, health care practitioners included, erroneously assume that all patients with diabetes have poor circulation and that most diabetic foot problems are due to vascular compromise. Similarly, many patients with diabetes, when questioned about their circulation, report that it is poor. When asked how they know this, they often answer, "because I am diabetic" or "because my feet feel cold." It is important to recognize that patients with diabetes have a much greater than normal risk for development of vascular disease and that vascular disease alone can cause tissue breakdown or impair wound healing. Vascular screening therefore is an important part of a high-risk foot examination. Poor circulation, although a possible complicating factor, is not the primary cause of most diabetic foot ulcers, however. Most can be attributed to a combination of increased mechanical stress on the foot and sensory loss due to neuropathy.[5,7]

Mechanical Stress

Neuropathy and plantar ulceration have been shown to be related to excessive plantar pressures.[8-11] Pressure on the

337

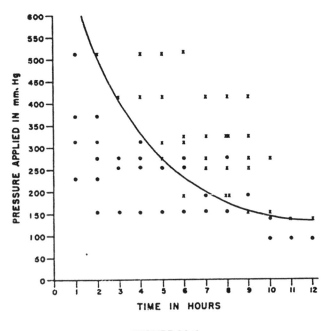

FIGURE 20-1

Results of Kosiak's experiments on dogs show an inverse relationship between amount of pressure applied and the time that it takes to cause ischemic necrosis. x = ulceration; • = no ulceration. (Reprinted with permission from M Kosiak. Etiology and pathology of ischemic ulcers. Arch Phys Med Rehabil 1959;40: 62–69.)

soft tissues of the foot is related to three variables: the magnitude of the force applied to the foot, the amount of surface over which the force is applied, and the length of time over which the force is sustained.[7] Because much of the focus in treating and preventing foot ulcers is on reducing pressure, it is important to understand the relationship of pressure to these three variables. If we consider the formula

$$\text{Pressure} = \frac{\text{force}}{\text{area}}$$

we see that anything that increases the magnitude of the force applied to the foot or decreases the area over which the force is applied increases pressure and makes tissue damage more likely. Immediate injury can occur from extremely high force applied over a very small area: as when a patient steps on a tack or piece of glass. Injury occurs because tremendously high pressure exceeds the tensile strength of the skin. Pressure on the foot can also become excessive when a moderate amount of force is repeatedly applied over a small surface area: when bony deformities cause small localized areas of weight bearing or when partial foot amputation decreases the patient's weight-bearing surface. The force applied to the foot (body weight) remains essentially the same, but the actual pressure on the tissues is greater because of reduction of surface area. In patients with dia-

betes, factors such as limited joint mobility,[12–15] foot deformity,[16] and previous amputation[17,18] can lead to increased force or decreased surface area. All of these have been associated with increased plantar pressures and ulceration.

Further complicating this picture is the time factor. In looking at tissue ischemia and necrosis, Kosiak[19] found an inverse relationship between amount of pressure applied to tissues and length of time that the pressure was sustained (Figure 20-1). Low pressures sustained over long periods of time caused tissue necrosis. This is the mechanism of tissue injury when decubitus ulceration occurs in bedridden, poorly mobile patients. It is also the mechanism of injury in wounds along the medial or lateral borders of the feet when patients wear shoes that are too narrow. Kosiak also found that as the magnitude of pressure increased fewer hours were required to induce injury.

The most common cause of skin breakdown in the neuropathic foot is repeated bouts of moderate pressure during everyday walking.[20] This was demonstrated by Brand[7] in a study of foot pads of anesthetized rats, which demonstrated that repeated bouts of moderate pressure caused inflammatory changes. With continued repetition, this inflammation progressed to ulceration. For health professionals who care for patients with diabetic foot problems, two facts from this research hold particular significance. First, when the inflammatory changes (heat and swelling) began to persist from one day to the next, breakdown of the tissue was prevented by discontinuing the repeated stress. Second, breakdown was prevented by decreasing the amount of pressure per repetition or by reducing the number of repetitions. The findings of Brand and Kosiak suggest that the variables of force, area, and time/repetition contribute to tissue breakdown and that changing one or more of these variables must be considered in the treatment plan for patients with a high-risk foot.

Neuropathy

Peripheral neuropathy has many causes and types[5] (Table 20-1). The most common is the distal symmetric polyneuropathy of diabetes.[1] The etiology of diabetic neuropathy is not fully understood or agreed on. The clinical manifestations often include *sensory, motor,* and *autonomic* components that affect the feet.[5,21]

Sensory Dysfunction in Neuropathy

Sensory changes are often the initial symptoms noted by patients with neuropathy. Common subjective complaints include numbness, cold feet (even though the feet may be warm to the touch and well perfused), and paresthesia (burning, stabbing, pins and needles, or cramping of pain). The pain is often worse at night. It is important to distinguish the pain of neuropathy from the pain associated with vascular problems. Vascular pain often increases with activities such as walking, when the muscles' demand for oxygen increases beyond the available supply. In contrast, walking often improves or diminishes neuropathic pain. The patient with vascular insufficiency is likely to experience increased pain when the lower extremities are elevated and relief when the feet are returned to a dependent position. Elevation or dependent positioning has little impact on neuropathic pain.

The patient with neuropathy often has objective signs of sensory loss in addition to subjective symptoms. These are of particular concern because the patient with such sensory deficit may not perceive dangerous conditions such as a stone in the shoe, hot pavement burning bare feet, the pressure of a hard callus, or friction from rubbing of poorly fitting shoes. Individuals with normal sensation immediately take action to relieve the source of discomfort, sustaining only minor superficial skin damage. The patient with sensory loss, on the other hand, is not aware of the need to take action and unknowingly walks a significant wound into the foot. Patients with a foot ulcer often report, "I didn't know anything was wrong until I saw a blood stain on my sock."

Many objective tests can assist in the diagnosis of diabetic neuropathy.[21] These include electrodiagnostic tests (nerve conduction velocities and electromyography) and quantitative sensory measures (current, thermal, and vibratory perception threshold testing and quantitative esthesiometry). Physical therapists who focus on treating and preventing foot wounds in the high-risk population use sensory testing to identify patients whose sensory deficits correlate with risk for ulceration. Of the sensory modalities, increased vibratory perception thresholds[1,22–24] and loss of protective sensation[6,13,24–26] are strong indicators of risk for ulceration in the neuropathic foot.

An instrument used to measure vibratory perception thresholds is the Biothesiometer (Biomedical Instrument Co, Newbury, OH), an electronic device that delivers varying degrees of vibration to the foot. The point at which the patient begins to feel the vibration is his or her vibratory perception threshold. Although decreased vibratory perception has been correlated with diabetic foot ulcers, a study that compared a variety of quantitative sensory measures found cutaneous pressure perception thresholds, as measured with a Semmes-Weinstein pressure esthesiometer, to have a higher association.[25]

Protective sensation is a term used to describe the amount of sensation that is required for individuals to protect themselves from tissue trauma. In 1986, Birke and Sims[25] used Semmes-Weinstein sensory monofilaments to define quantitatively protective sensation in a group of patients diagnosed with Hansen's disease or with diabetes who had a history of foot ulcers. Semmes-Weinstein filaments are a set of progressively thicker nylon filaments

TABLE 20-1

Diseases and Processes that Result in a Neuropathic Foot

Neuropathy associated with systemic diseases
    Diabetes mellitus
    Uremia
    Amyloidosis
Neuropathy associated with nutritional disturbances
    Alcoholism
    Pernicious anemia
Neuropathy associated with infectious disease
    Leprosy
    Syphilis
    Poliomyelitis
Neuropathy on a vascular basis
    Cerebrovascular accident
    Spinal cord infarction
    Diabetic mononeuropathy
    Arteritis
    Peripheral vascular disease
Hereditary motor and sensory neuropathy
    Roussy-Lévy syndrome
    Charcot-Marie-Tooth disease
Hereditary sensory and autonomic neuropathy
    Hereditary sensory neuropathy
    Congenital sensory neuropathy
    Dysautonomia (Riley-Day syndrome)
Cerebellar degeneration
    Friedreich's ataxia
Motor neuron disease
    Amyotrophic lateral sclerosis
Diseases of the spinal cord
    Spina bifida
    Syringomyelia
Trauma
    Spinal cord injury
    Peripheral nerve injury
    Spinal root trauma
Compressive neuropathy
    Spinal cord tumor
    Peripheral nerve compression
Toxic neuropathy
    Lead poisoning
Other causes
    Cerebral palsy

Source: Reprinted with permission from VJ Heartherington. The Neuropathic Foot. In ED McGlamry, AS Banks, MS Downey (eds), Comprehensive Textbook of Foot Surgery (2nd ed). Baltimore: Williams & Wilkins, 1992;1353.

(much like those of a nylon hairbrush), with one end embedded into a handle. When sufficient pressure is applied against the tip of the filament, the filament bends (Figure 20-2). Each test probe in the set is calibrated so that a different and defined amount of force is needed to bend the filament. The thinner the nylon, the lower the amount of pressure that is required to make it bend.

Using a set of three monofilaments, labeled by the manufacturer as 4.17, 5.07, and 6.10 and equal to a buckling force of 1 g, 10 g, and 75 g, respectively, Birke and Sims[25]

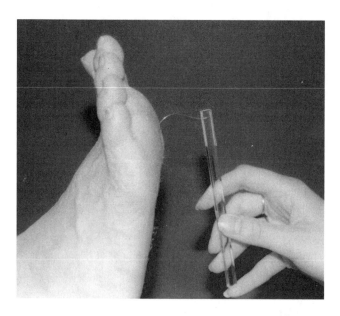

FIGURE 20-2

A monofilament is used to test protective sensation on the sole of the foot. The filament is held perpendicular to the skin surface, and pressure is applied until the monofilament buckles. The number associated with the smallest-diameter filaments perceived at each site is recorded.

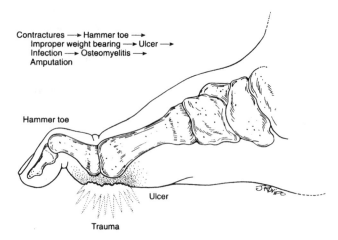

FIGURE 20-3

Progression of motor neuropathy eventually leading to ulceration. (Used with permission from Michigan Diabetes Research and Training Center, University of Michigan Hospital, Ann Arbor, MI, 1983.)

tested 100 patients (72 with Hansen's disease, 28 with diabetes) with the presence or history of plantar ulceration. No patient was able to sense the 5.07 (10 g) monofilament. This finding led these authors to conclude that the ability to perceive the 5.07 monofilament is consistent with the presence of protective sensation. Similar studies in patients with diabetes have confirmed this definition.[6,13,26,27] Overall, research using the Semmes-Weinstein monofilaments has determined that they are a valid and reliable tool for identifying patients who are at risk for foot ulceration.[28] The fact that they are inexpensive, quite portable, and easy to use makes them ideal for use in the clinic.

Motor Dysfunction in Neuropathy

The second component of polyneuropathy is damage to the motor nerves. Motor neuropathy causes weakness of the muscles of the foot and leg, which alters the pattern of force on the foot during walking.[8] At times such weakness is obvious by observing the patient's gait. For instance, in a peroneal neuropathy, weakness of ankle dorsiflexors causes the foot to strike the ground in a plantar-flexed position. The result is increased pressure on the plantar forefoot. The use of an orthosis to assist dorsiflexion and reestablish a more normal force pattern is an appropriate intervention.

More commonly, motor neuropathy in the patient with diabetes leads to foot deformities caused by muscle imbal-

ances. Such deformities are associated with high plantar pressures. The two most common deformities are hammertoes (flexion contractures of the proximal and distal interphalangeal joints) and claw toes (flexion contractures of both interphalangeal joints with extension contracture of the metatarsophalangeal [MTP] joints). Both deformities are the result of weakness of the intrinsic muscles of the foot. The metatarsal heads are very vulnerable because they sustain great pressure from plantar flexion of the metatarsals (Figure 20-3) and distal migration of the plantar fat pad.[29] The dorsal surfaces of the proximal interphalangeal joint (which may rub against the shoe's toe box) and the distal tips of the toes (which do not tolerate the increased weight-bearing forces) are also vulnerable to breakdown.

Autonomic Dysfunction in Neuropathy

Polyneuropathy often also involves autonomic nerves. Damage to sympathetic nerves causes impairment in sweat gland function and results in reduced hydration of the tissues. The skin of the foot becomes dry, less pliable, and much more prone to fissuring. Fissures can prove devastating to the vulnerable foot because they provide a means of entry for bacteria that can lead to serious infection (Figure 20-4).

Autonomic neuropathy also affects vasomotor regulation in the lower extremities. Loss of sympathetic control causes dilation of the arterioles of the foot, with resulting hyperemia of the soft tissues and bone. Increased bone blood flow and arteriovenous shunting due to autonomic neuropathy are factors in the development of Charcot's arthropathy,[30] a condition that can cause severe bony destruction and leave the patient at high risk for ulceration.

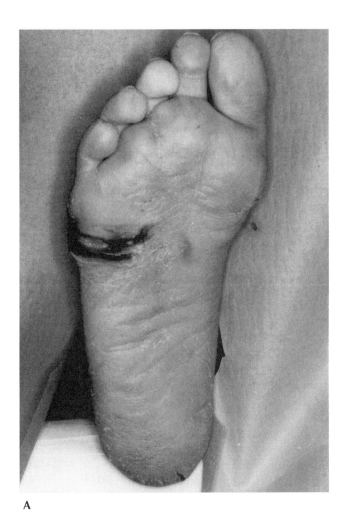

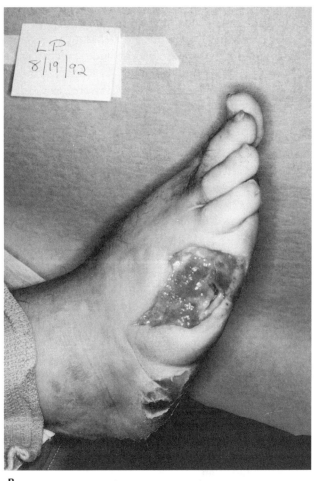

A

B

FIGURE 20-4

What began as a dry fissure (A) turned into significant infection that resulted in loss of soft tissue and bone (B).

EVALUATION OF THE NEUROPATHIC FOOT

A number of factors in addition to those mentioned previously are believed to contribute to the risk for ulceration and amputation in the vulnerable foot.[30-32] In evaluating our patients we need to consider all of these so that we can choose the most appropriate education and treatment interventions. The initial evaluation serves several purposes. It (1) helps to identify factors that have led to or may lead to soft tissue injury, (2) obtains objective data on which to base our recommendations for treatment, and (3) establishes a baseline with which to compare later data.

Patient History

The first component of the evaluation is a review of the patient's overall medical/surgical history. Much can be gathered from the patient interview; however, not all patients are accurate historians or have a thorough understanding of their medical problems. Information should be verified by the referring physician or by the medical record. Questions that are particularly important to consider include the following:

1. Does the patient have diabetes? When was the diabetes diagnosed? How well is blood sugar controlled? How much does it fluctuate? Unexplained, unusually high blood sugars may signal the presence of infection. Patients with diabetes must understand that they are at risk for development of neuropathy and peripheral vascular disease and that these risks increase with the duration of diabetes.[33] A large multicenter study of patients with insulin-dependent diabetes mellitus indicated that patients whose blood glucose levels were intensely and accurately controlled demonstrated

significantly less risk of developing the complications of nephropathy, retinopathy, and neuropathy.[34] Patients with foot wounds should be taught that control of blood glucose levels provides a better environment for wound healing.

2. What other systemic diseases are present? How might these contribute to the patient's lower extremity signs and symptoms?

3. What is the patient's foot health history? Has the patient had previous fractures, foot surgeries, ulcerations, or vascular procedures? If a foot ulcer is present, how long has it been there? How has it been treated? Many patients have been appropriately treated with wound debridement and dressings but have failed to heal because pressure relief was not addressed.

4. What diagnostic testing has been done (x-rays, bone scans, vascular studies, and others)? What have the tests revealed?

5. Does the patient complain of pain? How is the pain described? What makes it better or worse? Answers to these questions may help distinguish between neuropathic, vascular, and musculoskeletal causes.

6. What medications is the patient currently taking? Some may have an effect on healing or contribute to current symptoms.

7. Does the patient have visual deficits? Patients with a history of neuropathic ulceration may have insufficient visual acuity to examine their feet correctly or to recognize early signs of ulceration.[35]

8. Does neuropathy also affect the hands? If so, patients may be unable to perform their own dressing changes or all parts of a foot self-examination. They may require modifications to footwear to allow for independent donning, making compliance with footwear more likely.

9. What has the patient been using for footwear? Could this be contributing to foot problems? Previous studies have recognized poorly fitting footwear as a precipitating factor in diabetic foot ulceration.[35,36,37]

10. What is the patient's occupation? Is this occupation compatible with what the patient's feet will tolerate?

Physical Examination

Vascular disease, polyneuropathy, foot deformity, limited range of motion, previous amputation, and poorly fitting footwear are predisposing factors in the development of foot ulceration. With this understanding, we need to select evaluation procedures that can help us to recognize the presence of any of these risk factors in our patients (Figure 20-5).

Vascular Assessment

Arterial disease must be considered as a potential contributor to foot pathology. It may be the sole cause of soft tissue breakdown, impair the healing of foot wounds caused by other sources, decrease the ability to fight infection, and/or cause ischemic pain. Before clinical vascular screening procedures are performed, a number of observations should be made. If present, they may signal vascular compromise and indicate a need for further workup (Table 20-2).

The vascular examination begins by checking for pulses in the foot. Pulses are palpated at the dorsalis pedis artery on the dorsum of the foot and at the posterior tibial artery located just behind the medial malleolus. If pulses are palpable, the patient likely has adequate blood flow to the foot.

Although lack of palpable pulses is often a sign of peripheral vascular disease, inability to palpate a pulse in the foot does not always mean inadequate blood flow. The extremity may demonstrate reasonably good circulation when further evaluated by Doppler examination or other invasive or noninvasive methods. The Doppler examination uses a Doppler stethoscope to auscultate over the dorsalis pedis and posterior tibial arteries. Assessment of blood flow is based on the number of sounds heard with each pulsation. When audible, sounds are triphasic, biphasic, or monophasic (having three, two, or one sound). Triphasic or biphasic sounds are generally indicative of adequate flow. Monophasic sounds are indicative of compromised circulation and are reason to refer the patient for further noninvasive tests.

Several noninvasive procedures provide general information about the patient's arterial status. The first is the use of segmental systolic pressures[38] (Figure 20-6). Systolic blood pressure is measured at various levels along the lower extremities (proximal and distal thigh, upper calf, ankle, and great toe) and at the brachial artery using a standard pneumatic cuff and Doppler probe. The ankle/arm or ankle/brachial index (ABI) is defined as the ankle systolic pressure divided by the brachial systolic pressure. The ABI has been used as a general measure of arterial insufficiency. In a normal situation the brachial and ankle systolic pressures are approximately equal, so that a normal value for ABI is 1. As the flow of blood in the lower extremity decreases with vascular insufficiency, the ankle pressure decreases. An ABI of less than 0.9 is considered abnormal: the lower the number, the greater the vascular insufficiency. Wound healing is unlikely with ABIs of less than 0.45.[32,39,40]

Patients with diabetes often have stiff lower extremity vessels because of calcification of the medial arterial walls. Because of this stiffness, greater pressure from the blood pressure cuff is required to compress the arteries. Systolic pressure measurements may then be artificially elevated

FIGURE 20-5

A foot evaluation form helps to structure the foot examination and allows for easy recording of data. (Reprinted with permission from WC Coleman, JA Birke. The Initial Foot Examination of the Patient with Diabetes. In SJ Kominsky [ed], Medical and Surgical Management of the Diabetic Foot. St. Louis: Mosby–Year Book, 1994;12.)

OCHSNER FOOT CARE PROGRAM
DIABETIC PATIENT - PHYSICAL EXAM

DATE_____

NAME_____ PATIENT NUMBER _____

PHYSICAL APPEARANCE: Foot type_____ Color_____

Nails_____

Plantarflexed 1st Ray R___ L___   Plantarflexed lesser metatarsal R_____ L _____

LIMITATION OF ANKLE DORSIFLEXION: knee ext. R=____ L=____ knee flex. R=____ L=____
SUBTALAR JOINT ROM: R _____ L _____
REARFOOT: _____   FOREFOOT: _____

Manual Muscle Test:
    Anterior Tibial   R____ L____   Drop Foot R_____ L _____
    Extensor Hallucis Longus R____ L____
    Flexor Hallucis Longus   R____ L____   Intrinsics R_____ L _____
    Posterior Tibial   R____ L____
    Peroneus Longus   R____ L____
    Gastoc/Soleus   R____ L____

D= dryness
S= swelling
R= redness
n = temp. deg. C
callous
P= high pressure point

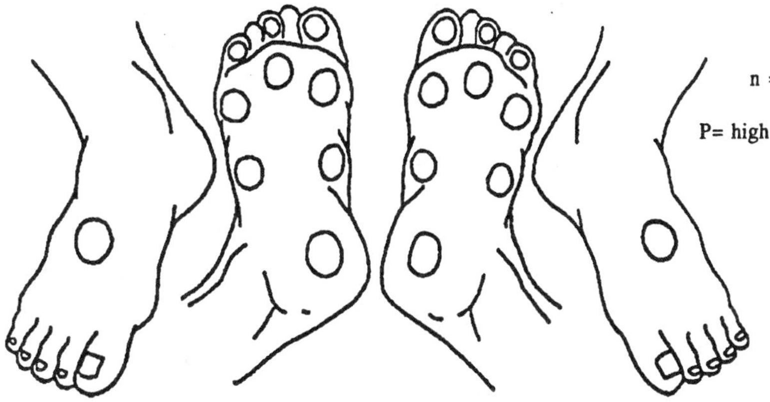

H=Hammered M=Mallet C=Clawed PU =Previous Ulcer site

Sensory Test (Semmes-Weinstein): 1=1 gram 2=10 grams 3=75 grams 4= No perception 75 grams
        Toes L ___ R ___ Forefoot L___ R ___ Heel L ___ R ___ Ankle L ___ R ___
Biothesiometer: R _____ L _____

PEDAL PULSES: Right: DP ____ PT ____   Left: DP ____ PT ____
Ankle/brachial Index: R _____ L _____ After one minute exercise: R _____ L _____
Footwear: Describe _____

and the ABI inaccurate and high.[39,40] For these reasons other measurements are added to the noninvasive examination.

The pulse volume recorder measures variations in the arterial volume at a particular limb segment during each cardiac cycle.[41] These variations are represented by the wave forms that they produce (see Figure 21-2). As blood flow deteriorates the wave forms begin to flatten. For a patient with dia-

betes and arterial insufficiency, the ABI could be read as normal as a result of vessel calcification, but flattening of the pulse volume recorder tracing would identify abnormal flow. Systolic toe pressures[42] and measurements of transcutaneous oxygen pressures[43] have also been reported to be predictive factors in ulcer healing. Generally, no single noninvasive test provides enough information to make decisions about

TABLE 20-2
Clinical Signs of Peripheral Vascular Disease

Absent pulses
Cold feet
Dependent rubor
Shiny skin
Intermittent claudication
Loss of hair on leg and foot
Atrophy of subcutaneous fat
Rest pain relieved with dependency
Delayed capillary filling time
Ischemic lesions

vascular intervention. Judgments are usually based on a combination of two or more tests.

If signs of vascular insufficiency are present and the patient has a foot wound, or if the patient has none of the typical vascular symptoms but has a nonhealing wound in spite of adequate control of infection and external pressure, referral for further vascular evaluation is necessary. Many patients have significant arterial disease but few clinical signs, such as pain or open wounds, that would warrant the risks involved with an invasive vascular procedure. They should still be educated in foot care and proper shoe fit. Because better circulation is required to heal an open wound than to keep unbroken skin intact, the goal for patients with vascular insufficiency is to prevent foot wounds from occurring.

Sensation

Commonly, patients with significant ulcerations on the plantar surfaces of the feet walk into the clinic without any discomfort. Specialized tests are not necessary to determine that significant sensory impairment is present. Many of these individuals are completely unaware of their sensory deficits. Sensory neuropathy does not affect all forms of sensation equally. The ability to feel something touch or brush against the foot may be retained while protective sensation is lost. Because he is able to feel the touch of a hand on his foot or the friction of his sock as he pulls it on, the patient may assume that sensation is normal. Standard tests of light touch and pressure do not reflect the actual risk for ulceration. The sensory examination must include those sensory measures that indicate risk. Increased vibratory perception thresholds and the absence of protective sensation are the neurologic impairments that are most highly correlated with the development of foot ulcers. Quantitative assessment of at least one of these functions is an essential part of the physical examination.

Vibratory perception thresholds are assessed with a Biothesiometer. The patient is positioned prone with the dorsum of the feet supported and the plantar surfaces facing up. The tip of the Biothesiometer handle is placed against the plantar surface of the hallux. The voltage is increased until the patient feels the vibration, and the corresponding number on the unit scale (0–50) is recorded. Three trials are performed, with the speed of voltage increase varied with each trial. The average of the three trials is considered vibratory perception threshold at that site. Risk of ulceration has been associated with a threshold of greater than 25[22,23] and increases as threshold values rise.

Protective sensation is assessed by the use of Semmes-Weinstein sensory monofilaments.[25,26] Before the test is performed, the patient is shown a monofilament, and the test is demonstrated on an area of the body that is known to have intact sensation. This assures the patient that she is being touched with something that will not puncture the skin and allows her to experience the type of stimulus to which she is being asked to respond. The test is performed with the patient supine; the eyes are closed, or she is blindfolded. The monofilament is applied perpendicular to the plantar surface (see Figure 20-2) with enough force to make the filament buckle as follows: 1 second touch, 1 second hold, 1 second lift.[25] Areas that are typically tested include the plantar surfaces of the first, third, and fifth metatarsal heads and tips of the corresponding toes; the medial and lateral midfoot; the heel; and the dorsum of the foot (see Figure 20-5). The patient is instructed to say "yes" each time that she feels the touch of the filament but not to localize the stimulus. If the patient is unable to perceive a particular stimulus in four of five of the trials (80%), she is retested with the next higher filament. The smallest filament to which the patient responds at least 80% of the time is the threshold value.[13,28] Threshold values can vary across areas of the foot that are being tested.

When using the monofilaments care must be taken to avoid areas of thick callus, which could interfere with the pressure perception. The timing between each stimulus should be randomized to minimize patient guessing based on rhythm. The filament should not be allowed to slide, as many patients can sense this sliding but are unable to feel the filament when it is properly applied. Protective sensation has been described as the ability to perceive the 5.07 monofilament.[6,13,25-27] It is appropriate to use this monofilament when screening for the presence of protective sensation. Use of monofilaments on either side of this (4.17 and 6.10) allows us to document improvement or progression of the sensory loss.

Musculoskeletal Examination

Patients with diabetes who have neuropathic feet tend to have abnormally high plantar pressures, and those with a previous history of ulceration show these high pressures at the ulcer sites.[8,9,11] High plantar pressures are thus considered a risk factor in neuropathic foot ulceration. Limited joint mobility,[14,15] foot deformity,[16] and the presence of toe or partial foot amputations[17,18] can contribute to high plantar pressures and need to be evaluated in the physical examination.

FIGURE 20-6

Segmental systolic pressures show a normal condition on the left. A 0.7 ankle/brachial index on the right indicates a reduction in flow. Also of note is the greater than 30 mm Hg drop in pressure between two successive thigh cuffs, which indicates stenosis or occlusion of the segment. (Reprinted with permission from AF Hoffman: Evaluation of Arterial Blood Flow in the Lower Extremity. In J Robbins [ed], Clinics in Podiatric Medicine, Surgery, and Peripheral Vascular Disease. Philadelphia: Saunders, 1999:42.)

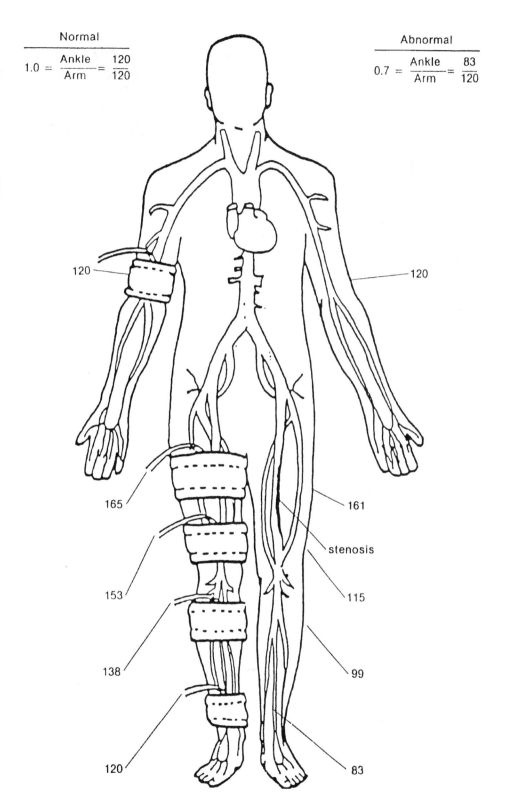

A number of deformities should be considered when one performs the musculoskeletal evaluation. These deformities often alter weight-bearing pressure enough to predispose the insensitive or dysvascular patient to soft tissue damage. They include hammer- and claw toes, hallux valgus, hallux rigidus, hallux limitus, plantar-flexed first ray, prominent bones on the plantar surface, ankle equinus, partial foot resections/amputations, and Charcot's foot.

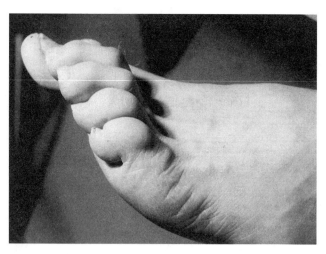

FIGURE 20-7
Claw toe deformity commonly seen in patients with diabetes.

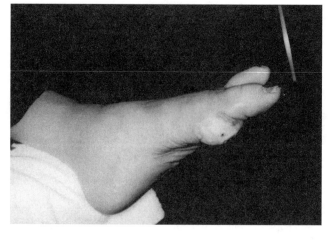

FIGURE 20-8
First ray plantar flexed in relation to the others, causing excessive pressure and leading to ulceration under the first metatarsal head.

Hammertoes and claw toes (Figure 20-7) cause localized pressure at the tips of the distal phalanges, at the dorsum of the toes, or under the metatarsal heads. In patients with diabetes, these deformities are due to intrinsic muscle weakness associated with motor neuropathy. In weight bearing, these deformities decrease loading under the toes while increasing loading under the metatarsal heads.[8,9]

Deformities that involve the first MTP joint include hallux valgus and hallux limitus. Hallux valgus is characterized by marked lateral drifting of the great toe and prominence of the medial surface of the first metatarsal head. As a result, crowding of the forefoot and toes and hammertoeing or overlapping of the lesser toes occur.[44] Excessive medial metatarsal head pressure from a toe box that is too narrow for the foot is a common problem.

Hallux limitus or hallux rigidus is associated with ulceration of the plantar surface of the hallux.[14] In this deformity, limited extension of the first MTP joint is seen. In a normal gait, this joint needs to dorsiflex to at least 45 degrees as body weight moves over the forefoot in late stance.[45] Limitation in range causes increased pressure on the plantar surface of the interphalangeal joint. Excessive pressure occurs when the interphalangeal joint becomes overstretched and hyperextended as it compensates for limited MTP motion.

In a foot with a plantar-flexed first ray, the first metatarsal head lies below the level of the remaining metatarsal heads, making it a likely source of high pressure (Figure 20-8). Any of the bones of the feet may be similarly prominent in relation to the others and a likely target for future ulceration. In the plantar forefoot, prominence of the metatarsal heads is common. The joint destruction of Charcot's arthropathy causes abnormal bony prominences in the midfoot.[30] The plantar prominences that are identified on visual and palpatory examination are often high-pressure areas of the foot, but because of variation in foot function during gait, high-pressure areas may be different than predicted by the non–weight-bearing examination. Soft tissue changes, plantar pressure measurements, and wear patterns of shoes and shoe inserts help to identify areas of high pressure.

High foot pressures and ulceration are associated with limited mobility of the ankle and subtalar joint in patients with diabetes.[12,13,15] Mueller et al.[16] found that the location of ulcers in patients with diabetes is similar to characteristic patterns of plantar callus formation found in healthy patients with the same foot types.[46] Evaluation to identify these biomechanical abnormalities is an important component to include in the examination.

Ankle equinus is frequently seen in the high-risk population. Motor neuropathy or partial foot amputation can reduce dorsiflexor strength of the foot and allow the stronger plantar flexors to dominate, causing the joint to tighten in a plantar-flexed position. Inadequate dorsiflexion is defined as a measurement of less than 10 degrees of dorsiflexion measured with a fully extended knee and subtalar neutral ankle position.[47] In patients with partial foot amputation, this limitation may be hard to evaluate and require a weight-bearing radiograph to detect (Figure 20-9). With insufficient dorsiflexion, pressure on the distal plantar surface of the foot is increased during the propulsive phase of gait. Pressure problems that arise from ankle equinus may improve with stretching or with surgical lengthening of the Achilles tendon.

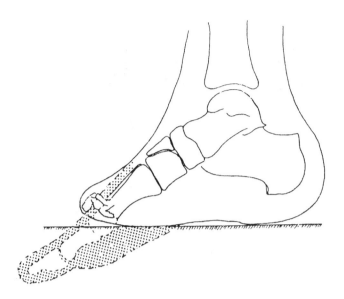

FIGURE 20-9

Tracings of superimposed radiographs showing hidden equinus in a shortened foot as compared with a contralateral normal foot. (Reprinted with permission from JA Birke, DS Sims. The Insensitive Foot. In GC Hunt [ed], Physical Therapy of the Foot and Ankle. New York: Churchill Livingstone, 1988; 133–168.)

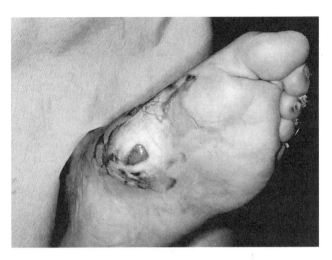

FIGURE 20-10

Charcot's arthropathy causing collapse of the medial midfoot has led to ulceration underlying the bony prominence in the "arch."

Partial foot amputation can have a number of effects that alter plantar pressure distribution. Because the surface area to carry the force of body weight is smaller, pressure on the remaining structures increases. This can lead to ulceration at other sites. Studies that have looked at great toe amputation in patients with diabetes have found an increase in plantar pressure and the development of new deformities and ulcerations after amputation.[17,18] As loss of parts of the foot occurs, the mechanics of the foot change, transferring stresses to new areas.

Diabetic neuropathic osteoarthropathy, also known as *Charcot's foot*, is a highly destructive process that significantly alters the bony architecture of the foot. The severity of the joint changes often leads to significantly high plantar pressures and subsequent ulceration (Figure 20-10). This process was first recognized in the nineteenth century by Jean-Martin Charcot, who described sudden unexpected arthropathies characterized by ligamentous laxity, subluxation of the joints, and enormous wear and tear of the heads of the bones in patients with tabes dorsalis.[30] In 1936, W.R. Jordan first associated neuropathic osteoarthropathy of the foot and ankle with diabetes.[30] Although a large number of neurologic conditions can lead to Charcot's foot, diabetes is currently the most common disease that is related to this process.[48]

Charcot's foot is often misdiagnosed because no one diagnostic test can confirm its presence. Medical history, clinical manifestations, and radiographic findings all must be considered (Figure 20-11). Charcot's foot occurs in the presence of neuropathy and most often in patients with adequate circulation. Autonomic neuropathy can contribute to poorly regulated blood flow, including increased bone blood flow and arteriovenous shunting. This abnormal flow pattern coupled with possible metabolic abnormalities[30] leads to weakening of the bones[49] and ligamentous attachments. Supporting structures of the joints are further weakened by overstretching as insensate joints are subjected to extreme range of motion during gait.[50] With weakening of the bone and ligamentous attachments, minor trauma begins a sequence of events that may include subluxation, dislocation, fragmentation, and fracture.

Clinically, the foot of a patient with an acute Charcot problem shows swelling, erythema, and warmth (Figure 20-12). Because early x-rays are often negative for fracture, patients are frequently misdiagnosed as having a soft tissue injury. Positive findings on bone scan can be misinterpreted as osteomyelitis or arthritis. Charcot's foot should be suspected if a patient with neuropathy presents with sudden onset of localized swelling, warmth, and erythema in the absence of an open wound. Appropriate treatment for Charcot should be initiated until it can be definitely ruled out on further testing. During acute Charcot's arthropathy joint destruction can be minimized by immobilization and non–weight bearing until signs of healing become apparent (decreased temperature, decreased swelling, and improved radiographic findings). If unprotected weight

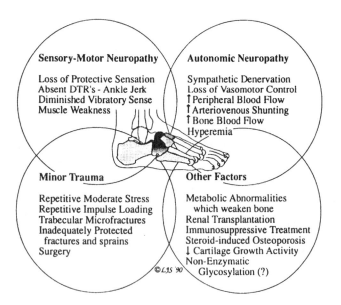

FIGURE 20-11

Multiple possible contributing factors in the development of Charcot's arthropathy. DTR = deep tendon reflex. (Reprinted with permission from LJ Sanders, RG Frykberg. Diabetic Neuropathic Osteoarthropathy: The Charcot Foot. In RG Frykberg [ed], The High Risk Foot in Diabetes Mellitus. New York: Churchill Livingstone, 1991;305.)

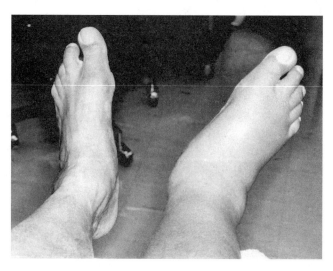

FIGURE 20-12
Acute Charcot's arthropathy affecting the right midfoot.

bearing continues on an acute Charcot's foot, severe deformity often results (Figure 20-13). When cast immobilization is discontinued, the use of an orthotic device for continued protection of the joints during the initial return to weight bearing should be considered.[48,51]

It is common to see patients in the clinic who present with old Charcot's deformities. These patients, as well as those with recently healed Charcot problems, need to be carefully evaluated for all those factors that influence foot pressures and the appropriate healing or preventative measures taken.

Soft Tissue

The abnormal characteristics of soft tissue associated with problems in the vulnerable foot include an increase in soft tissue volume; changes in skin color, temperature, and texture; and the presence of open wounds. Distinct characteristics help to differentiate neuropathic and vascular lesions.

Neuropathic lesions are most often located on the plantar surface of the foot in an area of high pressure[8,16] (Figure 20-14). The body responds to the localized pressure by forming a protective callus. With repeated plantar forces while walking, the callus continues to thicken and becomes a source of additional pressure.[52] Signs of inflammation (heat, swelling, and erythema) begin to appear. If localized pressure is not reduced, the inflammatory symptoms

progress to actual tissue damage marked by maceration, hemorrhage, and ultimately ulceration. The end result is commonly a circular wound with a raised callous border. Because vascular disease often coexists with neuropathy and can compromise the healing of neuropathic ulcers, vascular screening is an important component of evaluation.

Lesions that result from arterial insufficiency are more commonly located on the dorsum of the foot and toes and in the interdigital spaces.[53] They are not associated with callus formation. Early signs may include blue discoloration or mottling of the skin, which may progress to necrosis. Because circulation is compromised, the skin is often cool to the touch. Temperature assessment is performed by using the back of the hand or the first dorsal web space to feel the skin of the foot and ankle. Although some specialized clinics use hand-held infrared thermometers to measure temperatures,[47] the experienced hand is usually capable of detecting temperature differences. Localized temperature increases, particularly if accompanied by redness and warmth, indicate inflammation and possibly infection. Temperature decreases may suggest arterial insufficiency.

While inspecting the skin of the foot for changes in color, it is important to note patterns of the change. Erythema under or over a bony prominence in the absence of a wound often indicates inflammation caused by local stresses. If the erythema persists for 30–60 minutes after the stress is removed, intervention is warranted. Some degree of redness is associated with new open wounds. Redness around the perimeter of a wound may be a normal inflammatory response. If the redness is extensive, or extends some distance away from the wound edges, infection is likely.[54] Lymphangitis is marked by a red streak that runs proximally

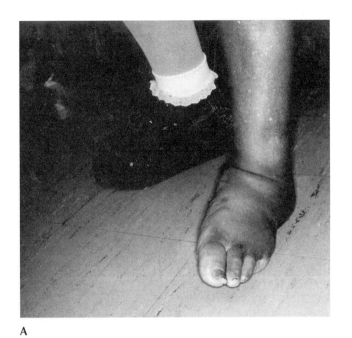

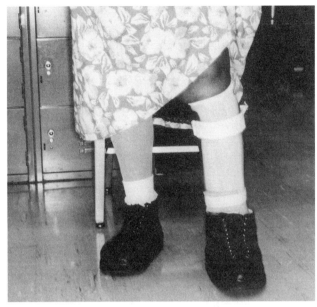

A   B

FIGURE 20-13

(A) Patient with deformity secondary to rear foot Charcot's foot, which was untreated during the acute phase. (B) Appropriate orthotic intervention has kept this patient from ulcerating.

from a wound site.[55] It indicates ascending infection and requires immediate attention by the physician. The redness of dependency (dependent rubor), blue discoloration, and pallor are most often associated with arterial insufficiency.

Evaluation of limb volume or edema includes comparison with the other leg. Bilateral lower extremity edema suggests systemic disease or venous insufficiency rather than a localized foot or ankle problem. Control of the edema is desirable to avoid problems with venous stasis ulceration and shoe fit. Unilateral swelling of the foot and ankle that is unrelated to venous incompetence indicates inflammation caused by injury. If the patient has neuropathy and no open wounds are present, Charcot's arthropathy must be considered.

The skin of the normal foot is well hydrated, soft, and compliant. With aging, vascular disease, or diabetes, the skin is apt to be dry and prone to cracking. Daily moisturizing is an important part of skin care for these patients. Changes in collagen associated with aging[56] and with diabetes[55] reduce tissue compliance and increase the risk of soft tissue injury. Taut, shiny hairless skin is characteristic of patients with significant peripheral vascular disease.[5] Localized callus indicates sites of pressure that must be correlated with other parts of the foot examination. Thin callus is considered to be protective. Excessively thick calluses can cause excessive pressure.[52] Thick callus is often

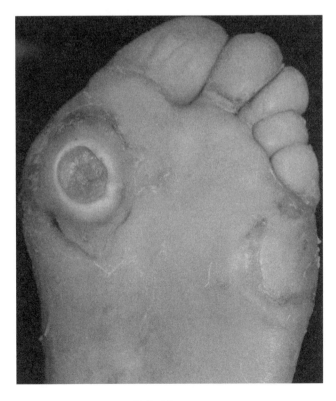

FIGURE 20-14

Typical neuropathic foot ulcer.

trimmed during the examination, because unrecognized preulcerative signs or ulcers may be present underneath.

Preulcerative signs include blisters, maceration, and hematoma. Blisters are the result of shearing forces and are commonly found in areas where a shoe has been rubbing. A poorly fitting shoe most often causes blisters and wounds that appear along the sides of the foot and dorsum of the toes. Preulcerative areas on the plantar surfaces of the feet of patients with sensory neuropathy are usually sites of high pressure during gait. Pressure relief techniques prevent advancement into full ulceration. Often plantar wounds caused by a skin tear or other trauma fail to heal because of continued pressure during walking. Any open wound that is found on examination requires thorough evaluation before the most appropriate intervention strategies are selected.

Footwear

In a study that involved 239 patients with diabetes and foot ulcers, poorly fitting shoes were listed as a precipitating factor in 181.[40] Evaluation of the patient's footwear provides important information. A well-fit shoe accommodates the shape and size of the patient's foot, as well as any protective insole materials. Many patients arrive at the clinic wearing shoes that are too narrow in the toe box. Although rounded or squared toe boxes better match the contours of the foot, many patients find them unfashionable. A patient's shoe style preference may have an impact on compliance if special footwear is necessary for his or her particular foot problem.

Gait

Gait impairment and associated compensation strategies influence foot pressures and joint stability. Patients with peripheral neuropathy secondary to diabetes have problems with gait and stability.[57-60] It is important that evaluation include the patient's foot problems and overall functional status. Recommendations that address safety and function should be included in the treatment plan.

TREATMENT

Patients who present with neuropathic ulcers have two primary goals of intervention: (1) healing of existing foot wounds and (2) prevention of recurrent and new lesions. Effective wound care and application of appropriate relief techniques are key components of the treatment plan.

Wound Care

A thorough wound assessment includes documentation of surface area, depth, appearance of the wound bed, and the quality of the wound exudate. The surface area can be evaluated in several ways.[61] If a wound is circular, measurements of diameter may be adequate in tracking progress toward healing. If the wound has a more irregular shape, tracing the wound perimeter onto transparent film and placing the tracing over metric graph paper provide a more accurate record. Commercially available instant cameras produce a gridded photograph of the wound. Successive color photographs allow for qualitative comparisons as the wound heals. Undermining of the wound is carefully measured using a blunt sterile probe. An undermined wound is larger than is evident by outward appearance.

Wound depth is also assessed by gentle use of a probe. Some wounds may have tracking to the tendon, bone, or joint. Clear bubbly fluid released during probing is most often joint fluid. Bone has a hard scratchy feel when probed. If probing contacts to bone, the presence of underlying osteomyelitis is a strong probability.[62] Infections, particularly those that involve tendon or bone, tend to prevent wound healing and require physician management. The presence of pus or foul odor from a wound is a clinical sign of infection. Absence of granulation tissue or pale or gray color to the wound bed is abnormal and could be related to ischemia or infection.

A comprehensive assessment based on wound evaluation, patient history, and physical examination should be made before an ulcer management plan is established. Generally, three factors prevent a wound from healing: the presence of infection, insufficient circulation, and inadequate relief of pressure. If the findings point to arterial insufficiency, referral is made to a vascular specialist. In such cases, identifying and removing sources of excessive pressure that compound tissue ischemia are also important. If the wound is infected, referral to the physician for local cultures, biopsies, or radiographic studies is necessary. Medical management of wound infection can range from oral antibiotics to surgical removal of infected bone. Once issues involving circulation and infection have been addressed, the focus turns to local wound care and management of pressures.

Wounds should be debrided of necrotic tissue before dressings and pressure relief devices are applied. Thick callus around the perimeter of neuropathic foot ulcers is debrided back to healthy epithelium. Local sharp debridement can be performed efficiently with the use of forceps and scalpel, or with a tissue nipper (Figure 20-15). Very narrow wounds may need to be opened to prevent superficial closing with trapping of underlying fluid. Special caution should be exercised when dealing with patients who have a secondary diagnosis of peripheral vascular disease or who are taking anticoagulants. Because whirlpool causes dependent edema and tissue maceration,[5] it has not been advocated for the treatment of neuropathic foot ulcers. The use of more efficient local wound debridement care techniques is preferred.

After debridement, the wound is cleaned and an appropriate dressing is applied. Although a discussion of topical wound cleansers, antibiotics, and wound dressings is beyond the scope of this chapter, several points should be made. A moist wound environment favors wound healing.[63] This means that a wound needs to be monitored carefully. Alternative dressings must be used if the wound becomes excessively wet or dry. Most wound cleansers and topical agents have ingredients that are cytotoxic to healing tissues.[63,64] This means that the risks and benefits for the individual patient should be weighed before wound cleansers and topical agents are applied. The wound dressing must be compatible with the appropriate pressure relief device. If the dressing must be changed daily, it should not be used with a total contact cast that remains in place for up to 2 weeks. Finally, because neuropathic foot wounds are highly correlated with excessive plantar pressure, pressure relief is often the most important component of the treatment plan. The best wound dressing is unlikely to heal a wound if plantar pressures remain excessive.

Pressure Reduction

Numerous strategies can effectively reduce pressures on the neuropathic foot. No one plan works for all patients. The most appropriate strategy is determined by the patient's coexisting medical and functional problems, the severity of the wound, and the significance of the deformity, as well as the patient's home environment, economic situation, and likely compliance with the instructions associated with the intervention. Choosing the most appropriate strategy is a process of weighing the advantages and disadvantages as they relate to the individual patient.

Bed Rest

Placing a patient on bed rest eliminates all force from the plantar surface of the foot. Historically, patients with foot wounds were admitted to the hospital for the purpose of providing local wound care and keeping them off their feet. In today's health care environment, this occurs only in the case of uncontrolled infection or acute ischemia when other medical or surgical intervention is needed. At home, the patient must be concerned with remaining non–weight bearing while moving short distances from the bed to the bathroom or to the kitchen. For some patients, this is physically impossible. For others, the absence of pain may tempt them to get out of bed and to walk (with the foot unprotected) for short distances, thinking that just a few steps will do no harm. Depending on the condition of the tissues and the degree of deformity,

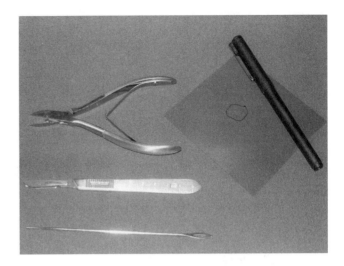

FIGURE 20-15
Instruments used in wound care include tissue nipper, scalpel, probe, transparent film, and marking pen.

a few steps can undo the progress that many hours of protective weight bearing provided.

Total Contact Casting

Total contact casts (Figure 20-16) have been shown to reduce vertical and shear forces that act on the foot.[65,66] Dr. Paul Brand is credited with bringing the total contact cast to the United States after he experienced success with its use on the ulcerated feet of patients with Hansen's disease in India.[67] The total contact cast differs from a conventional fracture cast because little padding is present except over the bony prominences and around the toes. It is designed to reduce pressure at the ulcer site by distributing weight bearing over all areas of the foot. Immobilization of the ankle in the cast eliminates the propulsive phase of gait, which is often associated with high peak pressure. Total contact with the foot and leg prevents movement of the foot, thus reducing the potential for shear. As the cast loosens with the reduction of edema, it must be changed to ensure that total contact is maintained.

Numerous studies report favorable results in healing diabetic foot ulcers with the use of the total contact cast.[65-70] Particularly interesting are the results of a prospective, controlled clinical trial done by Mueller et al.[70] that compared the effectiveness of total contact casting and reduced weight bearing to traditional treatment (debridement, daily dressing changes, the use of accommodative footwear, and instruction to avoid weight bearing through the use of assistive devices). Of 21 ulcers in the total contact cast group, 19 healed, compared to 6 of 19 in the traditional

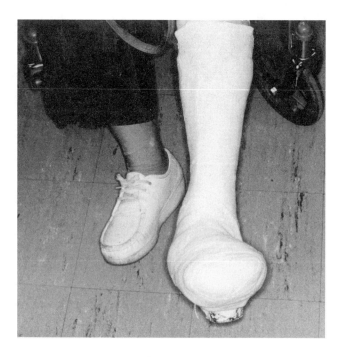

FIGURE 20-16

Total contact cast.

TABLE 20-3

Advantages and Disadvantages of Total Contact Casting

Advantages
 Faster healing times than with traditional treatment
 Reduction in edema
 Decreased opportunity for infection
 No need for daily dressing changes
 Protective weight bearing maintained
 Ambulation maintained
Disadvantages
 Skill required to apply cast
 Time consuming to remove and reapply cast
 Cannot monitor condition of wound
 Possible abrasions of other areas secondary to rubbing
  from cast
 Cast must be kept dry when bathing/showering
 Too cumbersome for some patients to manage
 Patient must maintain non–weight bearing until
  cast is dry
 Difficult to drive if casted foot needed
Contraindications
 Uncontrolled infection
 Fluctuating edema
 Highly fragile skin
 Significant peripheral vascular disease

treatment group. Ulcers treated by total contact casting healed in 42 ± 29 days, whereas the traditionally treated ulcers healed in 65 ± 29 days. Five of 19 patients in the traditional treatment group required hospitalization for infection, versus no one in the total contact cast group.

Because the condition of the foot cannot be monitored while it is enclosed in a cast, it is important that the patient recognizes the warning signs that indicate the need to have the cast removed for examination of the foot. These signs include excessive swelling of the leg that causes the cast to become too tight, loosening of the cast that allows the foot and leg to move within the cast, a sudden increase in body temperature or of blood glucose level, staining and drainage through the cast, excessive odor from the cast, new complaints of pain, or damage to the cast. Advantages and disadvantages of the use of the total contact cast are summarized in Table 20-3.

Walking Splints

An alternative to the total contact cast is the walking splint. Fabrication of the two is similar; however, the walking splint is more heavily reinforced posteriorly. This is necessary to maintain its integrity after the cast is bivalved and the anterior portion is removed. Elastic bandages are used to secure it to the foot and leg. Advantages and disadvantages of the walking cast are summarized in Table 20-4.

Clinical expertise, access to materials, and administrative support are necessary for effective clinical pro-

grams that use splinting and casting techniques. Some patients may not accept splinting or casting or may not be candidates for the use of these devices. Other methods of pressure reduction may better suit the needs and resources of the patient and clinic.

Felted Foam Padding

Felted foam pads are alternative methods of pressure reduction[71] (Figure 20-17). A custom-fit piece of ¼-in. felt-backed foam is adhered to the plantar surface of the foot. A U-shaped aperture is cut in the foam to reduce pressure around the ulcer. The margins of the aperture are positioned close to but not overlapping the wound edge, extending distally beyond the wound. The entire plantar surface of the foot should be examined to identify all vulnerable spots that need accommodation before the pad is applied. The pad is adhered to the foot with rubber cement and reinforced with paper tape or elasticized gauze. For forefoot ulcers, the pad extends proximally along the midfoot to increase the weight carriage in this area. All edges of the foam pad must be beveled to avoid skin breakdown from edge pressure. When a bony deformity is particularly prominent, an additional layer of foam can be used to relieve pressure adequately from the ulcer site. A thin dressing is placed, flat, over the ulcer. If the patient has a draining ulcer, a healing sandal is used for ambulation. If the ulcer is small and shows little drainage, an extra depth shoe can be worn.

TABLE 20-4
Advantages and Disadvantages of the Walking Cast

Advantages
Can be removed for dressing changes, skin inspection, showering
Can be removed for sleeping (increased comfort)
Can be used in most cases in which the total contact cast is contraindicated
Does not require the frequent refabrication of total contact casting
Disadvantages
Skill required to fabricate
Time consuming to fabricate
Can be removed, making unprotected weight bearing more likely
Difficult to drive if splinted foot needed
Too cumbersome for some patients to manage

TABLE 20-5
Advantages and Disadvantages of Felted Foam

Advantages
Easy to apply
Can be used when the total contact cast is contraindicated
Well accepted by patient
Minimal risk
Easier mobility than with cast or splint
Adhered to foot, so some pressure protection afforded when not in shoe
Disadvantages
Must be kept dry—foam shifts when wet
Mobility easier, making excessive activity more likely
Contraindicated with adhesive allergy or if adjacent tissue too fragile
Athlete's foot occasionally develops under the pad

In the author's experience, felted foam has been generally well accepted by the patient. Because this method allows for easier mobility than a total contact cast or walking splint provides, patients tend to walk more. This may not be desirable if decreasing pressure on an ulcerated foot

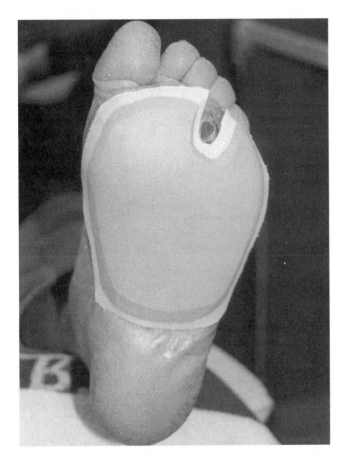

FIGURE 20-17
Felted foam pressure relief pad.

is necessary. The advantages and disadvantages of felted foam are summarized in Table 20-5.

Cutout Sandals
A cutout sandal is another alternative to casting.[71,72] With this technique, the foot bed of a custom-molded Plastazote sandal (Alimed, Dedham, MA) is completely cut out in the area of the ulcer, leaving the outer sole intact. The foot bed must be thick enough so that adequate depth is present to keep the ulcer from contacting the upper surface of the sole after modification. If the fabrication of a custom-molded sandal is not feasible, a more practical solution may be to supply the patient with a thick, custom-molded Plastazote insert to be worn inside a manufactured healing sandal. The insert is then cut out for the ulcer (Figure 20-18). As when using felted foam, care must be taken to bevel the edges of the foot bed or insole to minimize problems with edge pressure. Because Plastazote tends to "bottom out" with repeated loading, the sandal or insert may need to be modified or replaced to be sure that pressure reduction is being maintained. Advantages and disadvantages of cutout sandals are summarized in Table 20-6.

Orthopedic Walkers
The short leg walker is an orthotic device with a rocker-soled walking platform and double uprights fixed at 90 degrees (Figure 20-19). The use of this walking device has been shown to reduce plantar pressures significantly at the forefoot and heel.[73] As with the total contact cast and walking splint, the fixed position of the ankle prevents propulsion at the forefoot, where the greatest pressures tend to occur. Short leg walkers are available from a variety of manufacturers. Because they are not custom made

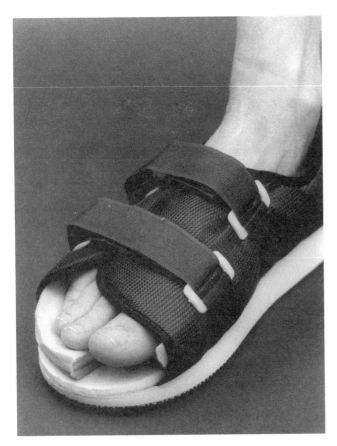

FIGURE 20-18
Custom-molded insert cutout to relieve pressure on plantar surface of hallux.

for each patient, care must be taken when fitting the device to assure that it accommodates the contours of the patient's foot, particularly in the area of the uprights. A custom-molded insert can be added to most manufactured walkers. Advantages and disadvantages are summarized in Table 20-7.

Wedged Sandals

The wedged sandal (Figure 20-20) is used for problems that involve the forefoot. Modification of the sole with a wedge causes the body weight to shift back toward the heel, decreasing forces at the forefoot. In one variation of this sandal, the wedge ends proximal to the metatarsal heads, leaving the forefoot hanging free. Although this removes all pressure from the forefoot, considerable pressure is present where the foot contacts the distal end of the sandal. For the vulnerable foot, the full-length wedge sandal offers support and protection for the forefoot while shifting weight bearing toward the heel. When choosing the correct sandal size, one must be sure that the distal

TABLE 20-6
Advantages and Disadvantages of the Cutout Sandal

Advantages
    Well accepted by patients
    Minimal risk of injury or mobility impairment
    Can be removed for dressing changes, showering, sleeping
    Easier mobility than with cast or splint
    Can be used when total contact cast is contraindicated
Disadvantages
    Can be removed, making unprotected weight bearing more likely
    Mobility easier, making excessive activity more likely
    Can bottom out, reducing effectiveness

end of the wedge remains proximal to the metatarsal heads. Patients must be instructed to take very short steps with the contralateral leg, so that they do not propel over the wedge. Contact between the distal end of the sandal and the ground increases forefoot pressure. Advantages and disadvantages of the wedge sandal are summarized in Table 20-8.

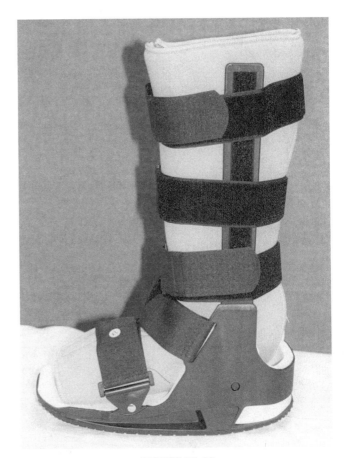

FIGURE 20-19
Example of a short leg walker.

TABLE 20-7
Advantages and Disadvantages of the Orthopedic Walker

Advantages
    Easy to apply
    Can be removed for dressing changes, showering, sleeping
    Minimal risk if properly fit
    Can be used when total contact cast is contraindicated
Disadvantages
    Too cumbersome for some patients to manage
    Can be removed, making unprotected weight bearing
      more likely
    Difficulty in accommodating some midfoot deformities
    Difficult to drive with

TABLE 20-8
Advantages and Disadvantages of the Wedged Sandal

Advantages
    Easy to apply
    Accommodates a bulky dressing, swelling
    Can be used when a cast, splint, foam is contraindicated
    Can be removed for showering, dressing changes, sleeping
Disadvantages
    Unstable for some patients to walk with
    Can be removed, making unprotected weight bearing
      more likely
    Difficult to drive with
    Difficult for some patients to maintain the proper
      gait pattern

Gait Patterns

Although not a primary strategy for healing plantar ulcerations, a change in the gait pattern can help to promote healing by reducing pressures on the foot. A 27% decrease in peak plantar pressures at the forefoot has been demonstrated with a protective gait pattern: The patient is able to minimize push-off by advancing the leg using hip flexors just before push-off.[74] Studies have found higher plantar pressures with increased cadence or stride length.[75,76] Healing can also be facilitated if patients purposefully shorten or slow their steps. Such strategies can augment the pressure reduction that is already offered by other pressure relief techniques.

Follow-Up

All patients with open wounds require frequent follow-up for reevaluation of the wound status and appropriate debridement. Response to treatment may indicate a need to change the type of dressing or the pressure relief technique. Lack of progress may warrant reexploration of the issues of circulation or infection.

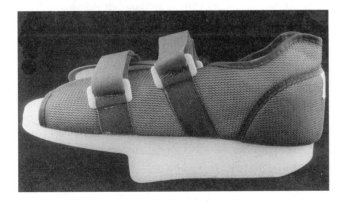

FIGURE 20-20
Wedged sandal.

Once a patient's ulcer has healed, the emphasis of treatment shifts to prevention of recurrent ulceration. Immediately after wound healing, connective tissues are weak and highly vulnerable to stresses on the foot.[7,77] Recurrent ulceration occurs rapidly if the patient returns to unprotected weight bearing. For this reason a program of continued protection (for example, using felted foam or a sandal with a custom-molded foot bed) in combination with an assistive device is recommended for several weeks after initial healing. Patients slowly and progressively increase time and distance of walking, checking their feet often for signs of inflammation. Activity should be limited if signs of inflammation appear.

PREVENTIVE CARE

For all patients with vulnerable feet, with or without a history of ulceration, the primary goal of treatment is prevention. The major components of a preventive program include the prescription of appropriate footwear, timely care of calluses and nails, and patient education.

Definitive Footwear

Birke and Sims[71] categorized patients by level of risk for foot injury based on the following risk factors: loss of protective sensation, presence of deformity, history of ulceration, and history of Charcot's arthropathy. Sims et al.[31] later modified these categories to include high plantar pressure. The primary criterion for risk of foot injury is the absence of protective sensation. As the number of additional risk factors increases, the patient is placed in a higher risk category (Table 20-9). The presence of peripheral vascular disease further increases level or risk. Prospective studies support the use of these risk categories in identifying patients who are at

TABLE 20-9
*Modified Foot Risk Categories**

Risk Category	Definition
0	Protective sensation intact
1	Loss of protective sensation
2	Loss of protective sensation, high plantar pressure, or deformity
3	Loss of protective sensation and history of ulcer
4	Loss of protective sensation, history of ulcer, and high plantar pressure or deformity
5	Neuropathic fracture

*Modification of risk categories originally suggested by Birke and Sims.[71]
Source: Reprinted from DS Sims, PR Cavanagh, JS Ulbrecht. Risk factors in the diabetic foot. Phys Ther 1988;68:1998.

higher risk for ulceration.[78,79] The level of risk serves as a guide when selecting the most appropriate definitive footwear.

A patient who currently has no risk (risk category 0) but has a diagnosis of diabetes needs to understand the relationship of the disease process to possible foot damage. Although special footwear is not indicated for this population, it is important that the patient be instructed in proper shoe fit.[80] The contours of the shoe must closely match the contours of the foot. Necessary shoe width varies across individuals and should be measured at the widest part of the forefoot while weight bearing. The widest part of the forefoot should be positioned at the widest part of the shoe. The length of the shoe should include approximately ½ in. between the end of the longest toe and the end of the shoe. Room within the toe box is also important. Some leather over the dorsum of the forefoot should be able to be pinched between the thumb and index finger if width and depth are adequate.

Patients who lack protective sensation but have no other risk factors (risk category 1) usually do not require specialty footwear. They are instructed in proper shoe fit and also advised to add a thin, nonmolded shoe insert to cushion high-pressure areas. In some cases an extra depth shoe may be needed to accommodate toe and forefoot deformity. Because these patients do not have normal sensation, they need to understand that although a shoe may feel comfortable to them, it may not fit properly and could place their foot at risk for injury. Objective, rather than subjective, measures need to be used when judging fit. Any sense of discomfort is a warning sign to take a closer look at the foot and the shoe fit. Patients sometimes purchase shoes in a larger size to be sure they have plenty of room. A shoe that is too long or too wide, however, allows the foot to slide within the shoe and increases the risk of damage from shear forces. Running shoes appear to decrease plantar pressures as compared to standard leather shoes.[81] Several shoe styles should be avoided due to their potential to cause increased localized pressure. These include shoes with narrow toes which can squeeze the sides of the foot, shoes with thongs which can damage the interdigital space, and high-heeled shoes which increase the pressures on the plantar forefoot where ulceration is the most common.

Patients in the higher risk categories (risk categories 2–5) usually require specialty footwear: either extra depth shoes or custom-molded shoes as well as molded accommodative inserts. Additional modifications to the footwear may also be necessary to reduce pressures further.

Molded accommodative inserts lower plantar pressures in two ways. First, the soft materials used in molding compress as the foot contacts the ground. This compression decelerates the foot, decreasing force on the foot (force = mass × acceleration) in early stance.[82] Second, molding spreads the forces of weight bearing over a greater surface area, decreasing pressure under prominent sites on the plantar surface (Figure 20-21). The ideal insert material to use when fabricating accommodative inserts is a material that molds and cushions and is not so soft that it bottoms out or loses its shape. Because no single material meets all these criteria, inserts are usually made with a combination of materials.[83] The thickness of a multilayer insert requires the use of an extra depth shoe. The combination of molded inserts and manufactured extra depth shoes has been shown to be effective in preventing recurrent ulceration in patients with diabetes.[84]

Custom-molded shoes are required when the shape of the foot is so abnormal that it cannot be accommodated with a standard extra depth shoe. Severe hammertoe, hallux valgus deformities, and changes in shape that result from Charcot's arthropathy are common reasons for such a prescription.

For some patients, extra depth or custom-molded shoes and inserts do not adequately protect the foot from damage. Modifications to the shoe insert or shoe may be necessary to reduce forces further in the high-pressure areas. Inserts can be modified in two ways: Depressions can be incorporated into the insert to protect skin under plantarly prominent sites, or extra material can be "built up" in neighboring pressure-tolerant areas to reduce forces at the higher-risk sites. If such a pressure relief modification is added to the top surface of the insert, special care must be taken to ensure proper positioning and adequately beveled edges to minimize problems with edge pressure. For some patients, biomechanical control of the foot may also be desired. Functional foot orthotics require the use of more rigid materials. All insert modifications and functional orthotics that are aimed at reducing pressure at high-pressure sites do so by increasing pressure in neighboring areas. Careful monitoring is needed to be sure that

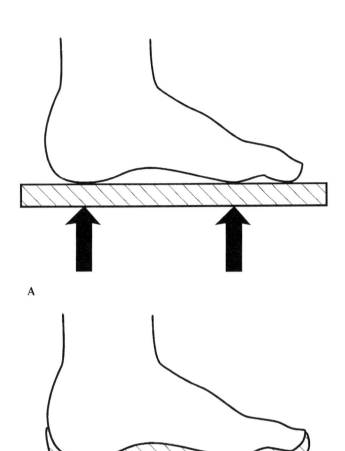

A

B

FIGURE 20-21

(A) Nonmolded insert cushions foot under high-pressure areas.
(B) Molded inserts further decrease pressure at these sites by increasing the weight-bearing area.

these areas are able to withstand this additional pressure. Particular caution is advised when rigid materials are used for patients with an insensitive foot. If movement occurs between the foot and the orthotic in the foot bed of a shoe, damage is likely as bony prominences contact areas of the insert that were not appropriately relieved for them. Lining the functional orthotic with a softer, more accommodative material reduces this risk.

One of the most common strategies used to decrease forefoot pressure during the late stage of gait is the rigid rocker sole (Figure 20-22). Although the sole of this shoe is rigid to prevent bending at the MTP joints, the rocker design allows the center of pressure to roll over the forefoot, minimizing the need for active push-off. One study that measured shear forces showed that the rigid rocker

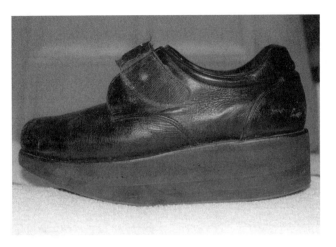

FIGURE 20-22

Rigid rocker soles added to extra depth shoe with molded insert. Used for treatment of a prominent first metatarsal head with history of ulceration.

sole reduces longitudinal shear under all metatarsal heads, except the first, as compared to a standard leather shoe.[65] Studies of vertical pressures in subjects wearing rigid rocker bottom shoes identified significant reductions in plantar pressures at the medial and mid forefoot as compared to conventional footwear.[85,86] Findings at the fifth metatarsal head have varied; evidence to support use of the rigid rocker for pressure reduction here is less convincing.

After transmetatarsal amputation, the shorter foot is at risk for ulceration at its distal end. Two factors that contribute to this risk are the increased plantar pressure caused by the equinus deformity, which is common in this population, and the increased torque that is produced when a full-length shoe is used on a shortened foot.[71] For these reasons, the use of a custom-molded short shoe with a rigid rocker sole is advocated for patients with a higher-risk transmetatarsal amputation foot.

One important point must be remembered: A protective shoe only works when the patient is wearing it. If a shoe's appearance is unacceptable to the patient, it is likely to remain in the closet while the patient wears less protective footwear. In situations such as this, a footwear compromise may be needed. Consideration should also be given to protection of the feet when shoes would otherwise not be worn, for instance, when swimming at the pool or beach or during the night when taking short trips to the bathroom.

Patient Education

The goals of a foot care education program are to eliminate poor foot care habits that otherwise would increase the risk of foot injury and to replace them with habits

TABLE 20-10
Guidelines for Preventive Foot Care

SKIN CARE

Do:

Wash feet daily. Dry them well, especially between the toes.

Apply a thin coat of lubricant to the feet daily, avoiding between the toes.

Trim toenails after washing and drying feet. Cut toenails straight across; any sharp edges should be smoothed with an emery board.

Have a podiatrist handle thickened or ingrown toenails.

Reduce thick corns or calluses with gentle use of a pumice stone or by professional care.

Check water temperature with a thermometer or your elbow before bathing.

Wear socks at night if your feet are cold.

Use sunscreen on the tops of your feet during the summer.

Ask your health care provider to check your feet at each visit.

Do not:

Soak your feet. This can dry them out and cause cracking.

Use moisturizer between your toes. Moisture between the toes creates an environment for germs to grow.

Cut corns and calluses.

Use chemical agents, corn plasters, strong antiseptics, or adhesive tape on your feet—they can damage your skin.

Use hot water bottles or heating pads—they can burn your feet.

FOOT SELF-INSPECTION

Do:

Inspect all surfaces of the feet daily (including between the toes) for signs of irritation, which include reddened areas, blisters, cuts, cracks, or sores. Report these to your health care provider.

Feel for areas of increased temperature.

Palpate the bottom of your feet for tenderness.

Use a mirror if you do not have the flexibility to see the bottom of your feet.

Have a family member, friend, or health care professional check your feet if you don't see well.

Do not:

Wait to report problems to your health care provider. Early attention can often prevent minor problems from becoming major.

FOOTWEAR

Do:

Wear shoes that fit the size and shape of your foot and leave room for any necessary insoles. Ask your health care provider what type of shoes is best for you.

Break in new shoes slowly, checking feet frequently for signs of irritation. Report signs of irritation to your health care provider.

Keep shoes and insoles in good repair.

Always wear socks or stockings with your shoes, wearing a clean pair daily.

Before putting on your shoes, check for rough areas, torn linings, or loose objects that can injure your foot.

Do not:

Walk barefoot (use slippers at night, special shoes or sandals for the beach).

Wear socks that are too baggy or have holes or prominent seams.

Wear socks or stockings that are constricting at the top.

Use sandals with thongs between the toes.

that either prevent injuries or allow them to be detected before they become major problems. Such programs have been shown to reduce the amputation rate effectively in patients with diabetes.[36,87,88] Instructions to the patient must include issues involving footwear, foot self-inspection, and skin care. Although it is important to stress desirable behaviors, it is also important to address behaviors to avoid (Table 20-10).

Professional Foot Care

Patients with high-risk feet frequently do not have the joint mobility or visual acuity to care for their feet ade-

quately.[35] Additionally, impairment in sensation makes it more likely for them to injure themselves while trying to care for their feet. Inadvertent injuries, although most often minor, can be devastating for patients with peripheral vascular disease. Professional follow-up for reevaluation and routine foot care is often advised. Patients who are at low risk for ulceration require a yearly reevaluation to identify any changes in risk factors that require a change in footwear management. Those in the higher risk categories require more frequent care. It is important to include reevaluation of footwear on each visit to be sure that it is retaining its protective qualities.

Use of Technology

Technical devices to measure vertical forces under the foot have been used for a number of years, largely for research purposes.[10] Computerized systems to measure in-shoe pressures have now become available.[82,89,90] Such systems allow visualization of weight-bearing patterns throughout the gait cycle and quantify pressures at specific areas of the foot. They may be of particular use in the clinic to assess change in plantar pressures after surgical intervention, changes in footwear, or adapted gait patterns. Information gathered from these systems may be a useful guide for treatment decisions.

Specialized Foot Clinic

Specialized foot clinics are effective in reducing the rate of amputation in the high-risk foot population.[33,36,87,91] These multidisciplinary foot clinics involve services that cover a variety of specialties, including vascular, podiatric, orthopedic, and plastic surgeries; infectious disease and endocrinology; physical therapy; nursing; orthotics; prosthetics; and pedorthics. The volume of patients seen in such programs often justifies the purchase of technological devices to measure foot pressures quantitatively and influence treatment decisions.

Specialized clinics with advanced technology are valuable resources but are not the only settings in which effective care for high-risk foot problems occurs. Many physical therapists outside of these settings make important contributions to the care of patients with high-risk feet. If health care providers are interested in this population, have knowledge of the principles that surround the evaluation and treatment of vulnerable feet, and use other specialists as appropriate, they can make a significant contribution to preserving the quality of life of the patients they serve.

Acknowledgments

The author acknowledges the contribution of those patients served by the Hartford Hospital Neuropathic Foot Clinic and expresses grateful appreciation to Dr. Larry Suecof, from whom and with whom it has been a pleasure to learn.

REFERENCES

1. Kozak GP, Rowbotham JL. Diabetic Foot Disease: A Major Problem. In GP Kozak, CS Hoar, JL Rowbotham, et al (eds), Management of Diabetic Foot Problems. Philadelphia: Saunders, 1984;1–8.
2. Smith D, Weinberger M, Katz B. A controlled trial to increase office visits and reduce hospitalizations of diabetic patients. J Gen Intern Med 1987;2(4):232–238.
3. Reiber GE. Epidemiology of the Diabetic Foot. In ME Levin, LW O'Neal, JH Bowker (eds), The Diabetic Foot (5th ed). St. Louis: Mosby–Year Book, 1995;1–15.
4. Reiber GE. Diabetic foot care: financial implications and practical guidelines. Diabetes Care 1992;15(suppl 1):29–31.
5. Levin ME. Pathogenesis and Management of Diabetic Foot Lesions. In ME Levin, LW O'Neal, JH Bowker (eds), The Diabetic Foot (5th ed). St. Louis: Mosby–Year Book, 1995;17–60.
6. Mc Neely MJ, Boyko EJ, Ahroni JH, et al. The independent contributions of diabetic neuropathy and vasculopathy in foot ulceration. Diabetes Care 1995;18(2):216–219.
7. Brand PW. The Diabetic Foot. In M Ellenberg, H Rifkin (eds), Diabetes Mellitus: Theory and Practice (3rd ed). New Hyde Park: Medical Examination, 1983;829–849.
8. Ctercteko GC, Dhanendran M, Hutton WC, et al. Vertical forces acting on the feet of diabetic patients with neuropathic ulceration. Br J Surg 1981;68(9):608–614.
9. Boulton AJ, Betts RP, Franks CI, et al. Abnormalities of foot pressure in early diabetic neuropathy. Diabetic Med 1987;4(3):225–228.
10. Alexander IJ, Chao EYS, Johnson KA. The assessment of dynamic foot-to-ground contact forces and plantar pressure distribution: a review of the evolution of current techniques and clinical applications. Foot Ankle 1990;11(3):152–167.
11. Boulton AJ, Hardisty CA, Betts RP, et al. Dynamic foot pressure and other studies as diagnostic and management aids in diabetic neuropathy. Diabetes Care 1983;6(1):26–33.
12. Delbridge L, Perry P, Marrs, et al. Limited joint mobility in the diabetic foot: relationship to neuropathic ulceration. Diabetic Med 1988;5(4):333–337.
13. Mueller MJ, Diamond JE, Delitto A, et al. Insensitivity, limited joint mobility, and plantar ulcers in patients with diabetes mellitus. Phys Ther 1989;69(6):453–459.
14. Birke JA, Cornwall MW, Jackson M. Relationship between hallux limitus and ulceration of the great toe. J Orthop Sports Phys Ther 1988;10(5):172–176.
15. Fernando DJS, Masson EA, Veves A, et al. Relationship of limited joint mobility to abnormal foot pressures and diabetic foot ulceration. Diabetes Care 1991;14(1):8–11.
16. Mueller MJ, Minor SD, Diamond JE, et al. Relationship of foot deformity to ulcer location in patients with diabetes mellitus. Phys Ther 1990;70(6):356–362.
17. Quebedeau TL, Lavery LA, Lavery DC. The development of foot deformities and ulcers after great toe amputation in diabetes. Diabetes Care 1996;19(2):165–167.
18. Lavery LA, Lavery DC, Quebedeau-Farham TL. Increased foot pressures after great toe amputation in diabetes. Diabetes Care 1995;18(11):1460–1462.
19. Kosiak M. Etiology and pathology of ischemic ulcers. Arch Phys Med Rehabil 1959;40:62–69.
20. Brand PW. Repetitive Stress in the Development of Diabetic Foot Ulcers. In ME Levin, LW O'Neal (eds), The Diabetic Foot (4th ed). St. Louis: Mosby, 1988;83–90.
21. Vinik AI, Holland MT, LeBeau JM, et al. Diabetic Neuropathies. Diabetes Care 1992;15(12):1926–1975.
22. Boulton AJM, Kubrusly DB, Bowker JH, et al. Impaired vibratory perception and diabetic foot ulceration. Diabetic Med 1986;3(4):335–337.

23. Young MJ, Breddy JL, Veves A, et al. The prediction of diabetic foot ulceration using vibration perception thresholds. Diabetes Care 1994;17(6):557–560.

24. Sosenko JM, Kato MK, Soto R, et al. Comparison of quantitative sensory-threshold measures for their association with foot ulceration in diabetic patients. Diabetes Care 1990;13(10):1057–1061.

25. Birke JA, Sims DS. Plantar sensory threshold in the ulcerative foot. Lepr Rev 1986;57(3):261–267.

26. Holewski JJ, Stess RM, Graf PM, et al. Aesthesiometry: quantification of cutaneous pressure sensation in diabetic peripheral neuropathy. J Rehabil Res Dev 1988;25(2):1–10.

27. Kumar S, Fernando DJS, Veves A, et al. Semmes-Weinstein monofilaments: a simple, effective and inexpensive screening device for identifying diabetic patients at risk for foot ulceration. Diabetes Res Clin Pract 1995;13:63–68.

28. Mueller MJ. Identifying patients with diabetes mellitus who are at risk for lower extremity complications: use of Semmes-Weinstein monofilaments. Phys Ther 1996;76(1):68–71.

29. Course Materials, Michigan Diabetes Research and Training Center, University of Michigan Hospital, Ann Arbor, 1983.

30. Sanders LJ, Frykberg RG. Charcot Foot. In ME Levin, LW O'Neal, JH Bowker (eds), The Diabetic Foot (5th ed). St. Louis: Mosby–Year Book, 1995;149–180.

31. Sims DS, Cavanagh PR, Ulbrecht JS. Risk factors in the diabetic foot. Phys Ther 1988;68(12):1887–1903.

32. Reiber GE, Pecoraro RE, Koepsell TD. Risk factors for amputation in patients with diabetes mellitus: a case control study. Ann Intern Med 1992;117(2):97–105.

33. Bild DE, Selby JV, Sinnock P, et al. Lower extremity amputation in people with diabetes: epidemiology and prevention. Diabetes Care 1989;12(1):24–31.

34. The Diabetes Control and Complications Triad Research Group. The effect of intensive treatment of diabetes on the development and progression of long term complications in insulin-dependent diabetes. N Engl J Med 1993;329(14):977–986.

35. Crausaz FM, Clavel S, Liniger C, et al. Additional factors associated with plantar ulcers in diabetic neuropathy. Diabetic Med 1988;5(8):771–775.

36. Edmonds ME, Blundell MP, Morris ME, et al. Improved survival of the diabetic foot: the role of the specialized foot clinic. QJM 1986;60(232):763–771.

37. Apelqvist J, Larsson J, Agardh CD. The influence of external precipitiating factors and peripheral neuropathy on the development and outcome of diabetic foot ulcers. J Diabetes Complications 1990;4(1):21–25.

38. Arizona Heart Institute. Cerebrovascular and Peripheral Vascular Disease: Advanced Noninvasive Diagnostic Techniques. Phoenix: Arizona Heart Institute.

39. Raines JK, Darling BC, Buth J, et al. Vascular laboratory criteria for the management of peripheral vascular disease of lower extremities. Surgery 1976;79(1):21–29.

40. Kalker AJ, Kolodny HD, Cavuoto JW. The evaluation and treatment of diabetic foot ulcers. J Am Podiatry Med Assoc 1992;72(10):491–496.

41. Gibbons GW, Campbell DR. Non-invasive Diagnostic Studies. In GP Kozak, CS Hoar, JL Rowbotham (eds), Management of Diabetic Foot Problems. Philadelphia: Saunders, 1984;91–96.

42. Apelqvist J, Castenfors J, Larsson J, et al. Prognostic value of ankle and toe blood pressure levels in outcome of diabetic foot ulcers. Diabetes Care 1989;12(6):373–378.

43. McMahon JHA, Grigg MJ. Predicting healing of lower limb ulcers. Aust NZ J Surg 1995;65(3):173–176.

44. Frykberg RG. Podiatric Problems in Diabetes. In GP Kozak, CS Hoar, JL Rowbotham, et al (eds), Management of Diabetic Foot Problems. Philadelphia: Saunders, 1984;45–67.

45. Fromherz WA. Examination. In GG Hunt (ed), Physical Therapy of the Foot and Ankle. New York: Churchill Livingstone, 1988;55–90.

46. Root ML, Orien WP, Weed JH. Clinical Biomechanics: Normal and Abnormal Function of the Foot. Los Angeles: Clinical Biomechanics Corp, 1977.

47. Coleman WC, Birke JA. The Initial Foot Examination of the Patient with Diabetes. In SJ Kominsky (ed), Medical and Surgical Management of the Diabetic Foot. St. Louis: Mosby–Year Book, 1994;7–28.

48. Banks AS. A Clinical Guide to the Charcot Foot. In SJ Kominsky (ed), Medical and Surgical Management of the Diabetic Foot. St. Louis: Mosby–Year Book, 1994;115–143.

49. Young MJ, Marshall A, Adams JE, et al. Osteopenia, neurological dysfunction, and the development of Charcot neuroarthropathy. Diabetes Care 1995;18(1):34–38.

50. Frykberg RG, Kozak GP. The Diabetic Charcot Foot. In GP Kozak, CS Hoar, JL Rowbotham, et al (eds), Management of Diabetic Foot Problems. Philadelphia: Saunders, 1984;103–112.

51. Morgan JM, Biehl WC, Wagner FW. Management of neuropathic arthropathy with the Charcot restraint orthotic walker. Clin Orthop Nov 1993;(296):58–63.

52. Young MJ, Cavanagh PR, Thomas G, et al. The effect of callus removal on dynamic plantar foot pressures in diabetic patients. Diabetic Med 1992;9(1):55–57.

53. McCulloch JM. Treatment of Wounds Caused by Vascular Insufficiency. In JM McCulloch, LC Kloth, JA Feedar (eds), Wound Healing: Alternatives in Management (2nd ed). Philadelphia: Davis, 1995;213–228.

54. McCulloch JM. Evaluation of Patients with Open Wounds. In JM McCulloch, LC Kloth, JA Feedar (eds), Wound Healing: Alternatives in Management (2nd ed). Philadelphia: Davis, 1995;111–134.

55. McCarthy DJ. Cutaneous Manifestations of the Lower Extremities in Diabetes Mellitus. In SJ Kominsky (ed), Medical and Surgical Management of the Diabetic Foot. St. Louis: Mosby–Year Book, 1994;191–222.

56. Mulder GD, Brazinsky BA, Seeley JE. Factors Complicating Wound Repair. In JM McCulloch, LC Kloth, JA Feedar (eds), Wound Healing: Alternatives in Management (2nd ed). Philadelphia: Davis, 1995;47–59.

57. Cavanagh PR, Derr JA, Ulbrecht JS, et al. Problems with gait and posture in neuropathic patients with insulin-dependent diabetes mellitus. Diabetic Med 1992;9(5):469–474.

58. Cavanagh PR, Simoneau GG, Ulbrecht JS. Ulceration, unsteadiness, and uncertainty: the biomechanical consequences of diabetes mellitus. J Biomech 1993;26(suppl 1):23–40.

59. Simoneau GG, Ulbrecht JS, Derr JA, et al. Postural instability in patients with diabetic sensory neuropathy. Diabetes Care 1994;17(12):1411–1421.

60. Uccioli L, Giacomini PG, Monticone G, et al. Body sway in diabetic neuropathy. Diabetes Care 1995;18(3):339–344.

61. Bohannon RW, Pfaller BA. Documentation of wound surface area from tracings of wound perimeters. Phys Ther 1983;63(10):1622–1624.

62. Grayson ML, Gibbons GW, Balogh K, et al. Probing to bone in infected pedal ulcer. JAMA 1995;273(9):721–723.

63. Feedar JA. Clinical Management of Chronic Wounds. In JM McCulloch, LC Kloth, JA Feedar (eds), Wound Healing: Alternatives in Management (2nd ed). Philadelphia: Davis, 1995;137–176.

64. Alvarez OM, Gilson G, Auletta MJ. Local Aspects of Diabetic Foot and Ulcer Care: Assessment, Dressings, and Topical Agents. In ME Levin, LW O'Neal, JH Bowker (eds), The Diabetic Foot (5th ed). St. Louis: Mosby–Year Book, 1995; 259–281.

65. Pollard JP, LeQuesne LP, Tappin JW. Forces under the foot. J Biomed Eng 1983;5(1):37–40.

66. Birke JA, Sims DS, Buford WL. Walking casts: effect on plantar foot pressures. J Rehabil Res Dev 1985;22(3):18–22.

67. Coleman WC, Brand PW, Birke JA. The total contact cast: a therapy for plantar ulceration on insensitive feet. J Am Podiatry Assoc 1984;74(11):548–552.

68. Helm PA, Walker SC, Pullium G. Total contact casting in diabetic patients with neuropathic ulcerations. Arch Phys Med Rehabil 1984;65(11):691–693.

69. Sinacore DR, Mueller MJ, Diamond JE, et al. Diabetic neuropathic plantar ulcers treated by total contact casting. Phys Ther 1987;67(10):1543–1549.

70. Mueller MJ, Diamond JE, Sinacore DR et al. Total contact casting in treatment of diabetic plantar ulcers: controlled clinical trial. Diabetes Care 1989;12(6):384–388.

71. Birke JA, Sims DS. The Insensitive Foot. In GC Hunt (ed), Physical Therapy of the Foot and Ankle. New York: Churchill Livingstone, 1988;133–168.

72. Birke JA, Novick A, Graham SL, et al. Methods of treating plantar ulcers. Phys Ther 1991;71(2):116–122.

73. Birke JA, Nawoczenski DA. Orthopedic walkers: effect on plantar pressures. Clin Prosthet Orthot 1988;12:74–80.

74. Mueller MJ, Sinacore DR, Hoogstrate S, at al. Hip and ankle walking strategies: effect on peak plantar pressures and implications for neuropathic ulceration. Arch Phys Med Rehabil 1994;75(11):1196–1200.

75. Hongsheng Z, Wertsch JJ, Harris GF, et al. Walking cadence effect on plantar pressures. Arch Phys Med Rehabil 1995;76(11): 1000–1005.

76. Soames RW, Richardson RPS. Stride Length and Cadences: Their Influence on Ground Reaction Forces during Gait. In DA Winter, RW Norman, RP Wells, et al (eds), Biomechanics IX-A. Champaign, IL: Human Kinetics, 1978;406–410.

77. Weiss EL. Connective Tissue in Wound Healing. In JM McCulloch, LC Kloth, JA Feedar (eds), Wound Healing: Alternatives in Management (2nd ed). Philadelphia: Davis, 1995;16–31.

78. Veves A, Murray HJ, Young MJ, et al. The risk of foot ulceration in diabetic patients with high foot pressure: a prospective study. Diabetologia 1992;35(7):660–663.

79. Rith-Najarian SJ, Stolusky T, Gohdes DM. Identifying diabetic patients at high risk for lower extremity amputation in a primary health care setting. Diabetes Care 1992;15(10): 1386–1388.

80. Janisse DJ. Pedorthic Care of the Diabetic Foot. In ME Levin, LW O'Neal, JH Bowker (eds), The Diabetic Foot (5th ed). St. Louis: Mosby–Year Book, 1995;549–576.

81. Ulbrecht JS, Perry J, Hewitt FG, et al. Controversies in footwear for the Diabetic Foot at Risk. In SJ Kominsky (ed), Medical and Surgical Management of the Diabetic Foot. St. Louis: Mosby–Year Book, 1994;441–453.

82. Cavanaugh PR, Ulbrecht JS. Biomechanics of the Foot in Diabetes Mellitus. In ME Levin, LW O'Neal, JH Bowker (eds), The Diabetic Foot (5th ed). St. Louis: Mosby–Year Book, 1995;199–232.

83. Steb HS. Pedorthics and the Diabetic Foot. In SJ Kominsky (ed), Medical and Surgical Management of the Diabetic Foot. St. Louis: Mosby–Year Book, 1994;455–476.

84. Uccioli L, Faglia E, Monticone G, et al. Manufactured shoes in the prevention of diabetic foot ulcers. Diabetes Care 1995;18(10):1376–1378.

85. Nawoczenski DA, Birke JA, Coleman WC. Effect of rocker sole design on plantar foot pressures. J Am Podiatry Assoc 1988;78(9):455–460.

86. Schaff PS, Cavanagh PR. Shoes for the insensitive foot: the effect of a "rocker bottom" shoe modification on plantar pressure distribution. Foot Ankle 1990;11(3):129–140.

87. Davidson JK, Alonga M, Goldsmith M, et al. Assessment of Program Effectiveness at Grady Memorial Hospital-Atlanta. In G Steiner, PA Lawrence (eds), Educating Patients. New York: Springer-Verlag, 1981;329–348.

88. Litzelman DK, Slemenda CW, Langefeld CD, et al. Reduction of lower extremity clinical abnormalities in patients with non–insulin-dependent diabetes mellitus; a randomized controlled trial. Ann Intern Med 1993;119(1):36–41.

89. Cavanagh PR, Hewitt FG, Perr JE. In-shoe plantar pressure measurement: a review. Foot 1992;2:185–194.

90. Mueller MJ, Strube MJ. Generalizability of in-shoe peak pressure measures using the F-scan system. Clin Biomech 1996;11:159–164.

91. Griffiths GD, Weiman TJ. Meticulous attention to foot care improves the prognosis in diabetic ulceration of the foot. Surg Gynecol Obstet 1992;174(1):49–51.

21

When Amputation Is Necessary: Preoperative Assessment and Surgery

FRANCES J. LAGANA AND RICHARD I. WEINER

The etiologies that are associated with the potential for lower extremity amputation include vascular insufficiency, complications from diabetes mellitus, infection, trauma, and malignancy. This chapter begins with a review of the process that determines the need for and extent of lower extremity amputation related to complications of peripheral vascular disease and diabetes mellitus. It outlines the process of clinical evaluation, discusses the role of technical imaging, defines the commonly used surgical levels and approaches, and opens a discussion on the long-term physiologic impact of amputation. Amputation that results from trauma and malignancy, which is usually a local phenomenon in otherwise healthy individuals, may involve a slightly different emphasis in assessment and postoperative healing.

For patients with dysvascular or neuropathic disease, amputation is likely to be the end result of a series of events that began with an attempt to salvage a compromised foot or lower extremity. Inadequate circulation combined with repetitive neuropathic trauma often leads to secondary infection of soft tissue and underlying bone. Systemic physiologic dysfunction associated with acute and chronic illness can further compromise tissue healing after amputation. This may result in an inability to control soft tissue necrosis adequately, leading to revision of amputation to a higher level to prevent septicemia or loss of life.

Seventy-five percent of lower extremity amputations occur in individuals who are in the later years of life, with the largest group falling in the 55–65 age bracket. Ischemic disease is implicated in 80% of these patients, and more than one-half have diabetes mellitus.[1] The 3-year survival rate for patients with diabetes who have undergone a lower extremity amputation is approximately 50%. Of patients who have had any part of the foot or leg amputated, 20% are likely to die within 2 years.[2] Careful clinical evaluation, optimum technical imaging, and skilled surgical intervention are important determinants of sur-

gical outcome and the long-term quality of life of an individual with amputation.

In older patients, foot and lower extremity symptoms and compromise are most often a result of a more proximal cause. Individuals with peripheral vascular disease who are at risk of lower extremity amputation usually have evidence of concurrent cardiac and cerebral atherosclerotic disease. In a study of patients who were undergoing cardiac catheterization at the Cleveland Clinic, a 31% coexistence of abdominal aneurysm, 26% coexistence of cerebrovascular disease, and 21% coexistence of lower extremity ischemia were seen.[3] Patients with diabetes mellitus present an even higher risk of complications related to extensive atherosclerotic disease. Cerebral and coronary artery disease manifest their effects earlier in the diabetic versus the nondiabetic population. Coronary artery disease has the greatest mortality for persons with type II diabetes.[4] Because life expectancy in the United States has increased dramatically in the past several decades, health care providers can anticipate that risk factors for vascular disease (long-term hypertension, tobacco use, and unhealthy diets) will lead to clinical manifestation in increasingly older populations.

ASSESSMENT OF PATIENTS WITH DYSVASCULAR AND NEUROPATHIC DISEASE

Careful clinical evaluation and history taking for patients with lower extremity symptoms are essential tools in establishing a cause and ultimate treatment plan for these individuals. Initial evaluation of a patient who presents with symptoms or pain of the foot or lower extremity must include a comprehensive historical review of systems, exploration of lifestyle, discussion of present complaints, skilled clinical assessment, and vascular status evaluation. Omission of one or more of these avenues can result in a misdiagnosis that could seriously affect the morbidity of the patient.

History Taking and Interview

A systematic focused interview is the first component of a comprehensive assessment to determine the etiology and extent of lower extremity symptoms or pain.[5] An example of an interview progression is presented in Figure 21-1.[3] It is very important that the patient and the clinician understand and use similar definitions of the different types of lower extremity pain. Clear communication assists in differentiating whether signs and symptoms are arterial, venous, or lymphatic in origin. If signs and symptoms present concomitantly, the physical examination determines which system is of primary concern and whether or not the problem is acute or chronic. Commonly encountered arterial, venous, and lymphatic vascular diseases are listed in Table 21-1.

Vascular Pain
The pain that is most commonly described by patients with chronic arterial insufficiency is *intermittent claudication*, a term derived from the Latin word *claudicatio*, meaning "I limp."[5] The patient may report symptoms including but not limited to aching, cramping, tiredness, or tightness that are noted only during exercise and activity. Symptoms typically cease when exercise stops or after a short rest. The pain most often affects calf muscles but can present in the thigh or buttock muscles as well. Patients with acute arterial occlusion may report claudication if spontaneous but limited collateral circulation develops. Boyd describes three categories or classifications of intermittent claudication.[5] In type 2 claudication, the most common type, once pain begins, it remains at a steady level, although the patient can continue walking if necessary.[5] Severity of claudication can be measured by the number of city blocks that an individual can walk before the pain presents.[6] Alternately, time to onset of symptoms can be determined during treadmill testing at a rate of 120 steps per minute.[3]

If an acute arterial occlusion occurs without collateral supply, pain is immediate and unrelenting. The acutely ischemic limb is characterized by sensations of cold, tingling, and numbness. This array of sensory symptoms is a result of an ischemic condition of the peripheral nerves. The skin of the limb distal to the site of occlusion may also appear to be blanched.

Ischemic rest pain associated with chronic arterial insufficiency typically presents at the metatarsal head level on the plantar aspect of the foot. This type of pain may be temporarily relieved by limb dependency and is often exacerbated by limb elevation. Patients with these symptoms may benefit from arterial reconstruction or bypass.

Venous disease, in comparison, is related to the valvular incompetence of varicose veins or to obstruction or vascular incompetence of deep veins. The pain is described as throbbing, sore, or heavy. Increased venous pressure often leads to edema of the lower extremity. This type of edema does not easily "pit" on deep palpation, does not usually involve the feet, and is often seen concomitantly with stasis dermatitis. It is important to note that lower extremity edema may also indicate underlying heart disease, hypoproteinemia, or a malignant process and must be distinguished accordingly to arrive at a correct diagnosis.

Lymphedema, in contrast to venous-related edema, usually begins with swelling of the feet and eventually involves the entire limb. Because lymphedema is the result of an accumulation of lymph in the interstitial space, "pitting" on tissue compression is likely to occur. Lymphedema does not quickly subside with elevation as does venous edema and is usually not painful.[6] Lymphedema occurs when obstruction, inflammation, or removal of the lymph vessels or glands has occurred.

Pain in the lower extremities and feet must be evaluated carefully. Individuals with peripheral neuropathy, especially those with diabetes mellitus, may not experience pain, even in the presence of severe venous or arterial insufficiency. Furthermore, the pain may mimic an orthopedic or neurologic component with similarly found clinical features such as changes in color, temperature, or sensation.

Physical Examination

Physical examination of the patient is the next component of the assessment process. The examination includes observational techniques, palpation of pulses, and positional tests for arterial and venous insufficiency. As in the interview, the physical examination must be consistent, thorough, and easily reproducible. The clinician who is methodical in observing a patient and consistent in recording findings will be efficient and effective in intervention planning. Three key areas should be carefully observed: skin condition, hair distribution, and condition of the nails. Palpation of pulses and noninvasive testing strategies then further evaluate the availability of vascular supply.

Examination of the Skin, Hair, and Nails
The color, texture, and temperature of skin in the foot, ankle, and lower and upper limb should be carefully inspected. The presence of any lesions, open or otherwise, should be noted on a body chart. The color of a patient's skin on the lower extremities and feet should be consistent

Vascular Patient History

Diagnosed Conditions

Diabetes	( )	years:
Hypertension	( )	years:
Hyperlipidemia	( )	Family Health ( )
CVA / TIA	( )	
Heart Disease	( )	
Angina	( )	
Syncope	( )	
Varicose Veins	( )	
Impotence	( )	

Risk Factors

Cigarette / tobacco	( )	PPD:	years:
Alcohol	( )		
Lifestyle: active	( )	sedentary	( )
Oral Contraceptives	( )		

Current Signs and Symptoms

A. **General:**

headache / vertigo / memory loss	( )
SOB / DOE	( )
orthopnea / chest pains	( )
palpitations	( )

B. **Localized:**

extremity muscle weakness	( )
limb / hair loss	( )
skin color changes	( )
stasis dermatitis	( )
trophic nails	( )
ulcerations	( )
gangrene	( )
edema	( )
cellulitis	( )
rubor	( )

C. **Extremity Pain**

	Left Leg	**Right Leg**	
rest pain	( )	( )	
claudication	( )	( )	blocks:
pain location			
thigh / buttock	( )	( )	
calf	( )	( )	
digits	( )	( )	
pain relieved by:			
rest	( )	( )	
exercise	( )	( )	
legs elevated	( )	( )	
legs dependent	( )	( )	

FIGURE 21-1

The vascular history checklist provides a guideline for the patient interview in the initial assessment of patients with dysvascular and neuropathic disease. CVA = cerebrovascular accident; DOE = dyspnea on exertion; PPD = pack per day; SOB = shortness of breath; TIA = transient ischemic attack. (Reprinted with permission from Imex Medical Systems, Golden, CO.)

TABLE 21-1
Common Peripheral Vascular Diseases

Vessel	Acute Conditions	Chronic Conditions
Arterial	Arterial thrombosis	Atherosclerosis obliterans
	Embolic occlusion	Thromboangiitis obliterans/Buerger's
	Vasospastic disease (Raynaud's)	Diabetic angiopathy
Venous	Venous thromboembolism	Varicose veins
		Chronic venous insufficiency
Lymphatic	Lymphangiitis	Primary lymphedema (congenital)
		Secondary lymphedema (acquired)

with his or her age and race. An increase in color, termed *erythema*, may indicate an inflammatory or infective process. The clinician looks for the extent of erythema, whether or not it is present bilaterally, and other accompanying information. Skin pallor, a decrease in color that is most obvious if the limb is elevated, often indicates significantly diminished arterial perfusion. Rubor of dependency, a prolonged intense blush of the sole when the limb is lowered after elevation, also suggests arterial insufficiency. Inconsistencies in color, termed *mottling*, may reflect underlying vascular disease, adaptations in local temperature changes, or both. The presence of any color other than a normal pink (such as purple, blue, or black) may signify vascular disease of an episodic nature (e.g., Raynaud's disease, embolic showers, etc.) or subcutaneous bleeding from any number of clotting disorders, nutritional deficits, or other nonvascular related entities. Uniformity of color, differences related to positional changes, and overall distribution are key in this analysis.

The texture of a patient's skin can be compromised by age, metabolic or vascular disease, or dermatologic conditions. The skin of the lower extremities should move freely, be reasonably supple, and be consistent in thickness throughout. In arterial insufficiency, the skin is often tight, shiny, and/or paper thin. Dry, cracked, or scaling skin may be a result of autonomic neuropathy in patients with diabetes mellitus.

The temperature of the skin, its uniformity as well as its relative measurement, is also important. The backs of the examiner's hands and fingers deliver the best interpretation of skin temperature in manual palpation. Consistent proximal to distal palpation of the skin surfaces, adhering to bilaterally symmetric areas (i.e., lateral, dorsal, medial, plantar), can exhibit differences from one body segment to the other or asymmetric distribution of temperature in a particular area. A "hot" foot in patients with diabetes may suggest underlying infection or may be an indicator of early Charcot's disease. A patient with vascular compromise may exhibit a sharp decrease in temperature over the popliteal or tibial area in one leg only. This may be a clinical sign of the site and severity of occlusion.

If any skin lesion is present, whether a callus, a dermatologic condition, or an open ulceration, its shape, diameter, depth, exact location, and the presence of any drainage must be documented carefully. Description of the wound should include any other significant characteristics that might be helpful in evaluating change in status of the area at a later date or by another individual. Historical review of any lesion (i.e., date of presentation, changes, etc.) should also be documented.

Careful evaluation of a patient's hair growth and nail tissue is important in determining the nutritional status of these features overall. Absence or changes in hair or nail growth reflect a generalized decline in the arterial and venous circulation to the area.

Palpation of Pulses and Positional Tests for Vascular Insufficiency

The next step in clinical evaluation is the palpation of lower extremity pulses. Reliability and reproducibility in evaluating pulses is a skill that develops over time. An appreciation of variable anatomic anomalies that influence distal pulses within the general population is helpful. The lower extremity pulses, including the femoral, popliteal, posterior tibial, and dorsalis pedis, can be graded by the method described by Kidawa[7] as absent (scored as 0/4), weak (1/4), normal (2/4), full (3/4), or bounding (4/4). A bounding pulse at any level can signify an underlying aneurysm or stenosis and should be considered pathologic until proven otherwise.

For optimal palpation of pulses, the patient is positioned in supine with the knees minimally flexed. The femoral pulse is palpable below the inguinal ligament, the posterior tibial pulse is located posterior to the medial malleolus, and the dorsalis pedis pulse is found on the dorsum of the foot just distal to the ankle joint flexure. The popliteal pulse is often difficult to locate; it can be found by using the fingers of both hands to compress the artery within the popliteal space between the heads of the gastrocnemius muscle. A pedal pulse can disappear on examination if the patient exercises to a level of claudication before assessment. Pedal pulses are noted to be absent in approximately 7% of the general population.[6]

Palpation of pulses is often followed by additional clinical tests for assessment of arterial and venous disease. These tests are easy to perform and give immediate information on arterial or venous insufficiencies.

Arterial supply can be evaluated by one of three methods (capillary filling time, venous filling time, and filling time after a temporary proximal occlusion) based on the response of a limb to changes in position. Capillary filling time is assessed by first elevating the limb of a patient for 10–20 seconds, lowering it to a dependent position, and applying and releasing pressure to the plantar aspect of the first toe with finger compression. If capillary refill is normal, the toe blanches but returns to normal color in 1–2 seconds. A shorter filling time suggests venous congestion, whereas a longer filling time may indicate arterial compromise. Venous filling time reflects the time required for filling of veins on the dorsum of the foot after 2 minutes of elevation. In a normal subject, refill occurs within 10 seconds of return of the limb to a dependent position. A delay in filling suggests inadequate arterial perfusion. If the vein has valvular incompetency, filling occurs quickly even in the presence of arterial insufficiency. The third test requires placement of a sphygmomanometer cuff on the patient's thigh, occluding arterial circulation for 5 minutes. When the cuff is released, the time it takes for the skin to flush back to a normal color directly measures the arterial pressure behind the arterioles. It should take no more than 10 seconds for this flush to return down to the level of the digits.

Testing for venous insufficiency is accomplished by positioning the patient in supine, elevating the lower extremity to 90 degrees, and applying a sphygmomanometer cuff around the upper thigh to occlude superficial venous vessels. If, when the patient stands, the veins above the tourniquet fill while those below do not, the superficial system above the tourniquet is likely to be incompetent. If the veins below the tourniquet fill, an incompetent communicating vein is present below the tourniquet. Repeating the test by moving the cuff to different levels helps to locate the site of venous incompetency between the superficial and deep systems. To determine the patency of the deep venous system, a patient with a tourniquet applied above the knee walks in place. If the varices empty, the deep venous system is patent and the valves in the communicating system are competent. If the varices persist after the patient lies down, an abnormality in arteriovenous communication should be suspected.[8]

Noninvasive Vascular Testing

Once a careful history and clinical evaluation have been performed, lower extremity blood flow evaluation by non-invasive methods can be assessed. This most typically is performed by Doppler analysis; however, photoplethysmography, pulse volume recording, magnetic resonance angiography (MRA), and transcutaneous oximetry are also available. These assessments determine the general location and extent of occlusive arterial disease. This is the main guide in assessing severity of the arterial compromise and in selecting the proper treatment intervention.

As blood vessels become compromised with the advancement of atherosclerosis, an accumulation of plaques within the vessels, a loss in elasticity of the arterial wall and an overall narrowing of the vessel leading to a decreased flow to one or more particular areas of the leg or the foot occur. The body can accommodate these changes by increasing its pulse pressure. Before significant blood flow is reduced, 50% of the arterial diameter may be lost. Blood flow varies directly with pressure and indirectly with resistance based on Poiseuille's law: More energy is required to propel blood through a narrowed inelastic vessel. Changes that result include a loss of backward flow initially, followed by a slower blood flow velocity and finally with a decrease in blood flow volume.[8]

Doppler waveform analysis can be performed easily and can be accurately reproduced. This method specifically assesses an analogue signal proportional to the velocity of the blood flow in the vessel being examined. It produces a qualitative and quantitative analysis of the wave form (Figure 21-2). Normally, in the lower extremity, a vessel waveform is triphasic, with a reverse flow in early diastole. It is pulsatile as well and should produce three distinct sounds: the first for forward flow during systole, the second for backward flow during early diastole, and the third for forward flow later in diastole. With decreased flow in a narrowed vessel, because of high resistance, the vessel pitch sound becomes much lower and monophasic (only one sound is heard). Proportionally, the waveforms reflect abnormality in being monophasic, more broadly peaked, and producing a flatter curve formation. The following represents a comparison of normal versus abnormal waveforms in the lower extremity.[9]

Segmental limb pressures can be assessed to provide the location and severity of occlusion in the lower extremity. This is determined by an ankle/brachial pressure index (ABI). The ABI is calculated by dividing the systolic pressure of the pedal artery by the systolic pressure of the brachial artery. See Figure 20-6 for placement of pneumatic tourniquets on the upper and lower extremities in performing a segmental pressure study.

An ABI of 1 or greater, calculated by the pressure of the leg tourniquet reading in mm Hg over the arm tourniquet reading in mm Hg, is "normal," indicating an absence

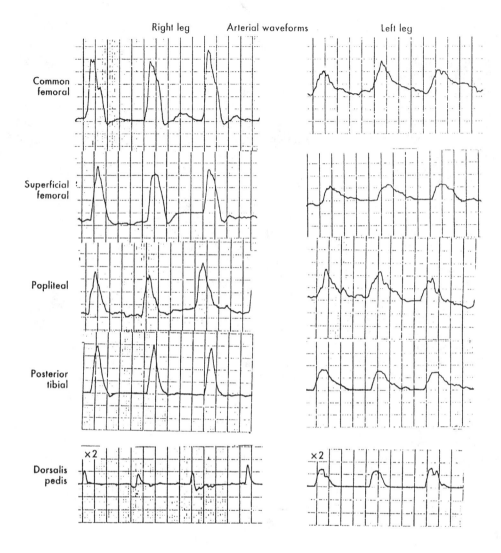

FIGURE 21-2
Doppler waveform analysis. The right leg waveforms show normal triphasic Doppler flow signals. The left leg, with pronounced occlusive disease, shows monophasic waves that are diminished in amplitude. (Reprinted with permission from F Jarrett. Vascular Surgery of the Lower Extremity. St. Louis: Mosby, 1985;14.)

of organic disease. An index of 0.5–0.8 usually suggests one primary arterial occlusion, whereas an index of less than 0.5 points to multilevel occlusive disease.

A pressure gradient difference of greater than 20 mm Hg between cuff levels or at the same level on the contralateral side suggests a significant occlusive lesion. In occluded vessel segments with good collateral flow or in severely calcified vessels that are not easily compressed during the study, false interpretation may exist. If there is a question as to the validity of the results of the segmental tests, the application of exercise can be introduced to challenge it. This is done by choosing the two best pedal arteries, raising the patient's leg 30 degrees, and asking him or her to dorsiflex and plantar flex the foot actively for 1 minute. After this, the foot is returned to the level of the heart, and pressures at 30-, 60-, 90-, and 120-second intervals are analyzed. If a proximal occlusion exists, the ankle pressures will fall more than 20%.

MRA has emerged in the past 57 years as an optional, sole, or combined imaging tool in preoperative vascular surgery in many patients. The gold standard of vessel imaging, arteriography, which is an invasive procedure, carries with it a number of limitations. Because a contrast medium is necessary for arteriography, patients with renal dysfunction or with cholesterol emboli syndrome are placed at considerable risk during the testing procedure.[10] Arterial puncture and the possibility of iodinated contrast allergy approach an overall complication rate of 10%, with life-threatening developments occurring in 0.05% of patients.[11] Although noniodinated compounds are used, the invasive nature of arteriography remains a concern, as many of these patients already possess a high-risk profile with multiple concomitant problems.

MRA is performed by using a body, extremity, or phase array multicoil, dependent on the arterial segment to be analyzed. A 1.5 Tesla, Signa magnet (General Electric Medical Systems, Milwaukee, WI), and two-dimensional time-of-flight technique are used. Imaging in 2-mm slices at 60% flip angles is the usual imaging parameter.[12] This technique is contraindicated for patients with implanted metal (pacemakers, cerebral aneurysm clips) and claustrophobia.[13] Comparison of MRA and arteriography results and applicability are discussed in the following section.

Risks and Benefits of Invasive Vascular Testing

Once noninvasive vascular testing is able to provide information to a multidisciplinary team involved in the management of an individual who is being considered for some portion of lower extremity amputation or bypass, careful selection of invasive vascular imaging can be considered. Most invasive procedures are performed as a staging rather than as a diagnostic process. Information such as the extent of an obstruction, its exact location, and the collateral circulation, distal and proximal to the vessel, can be obtained.[14]

As previously discussed, MRA evaluation may be sufficient to obtain an accurate road map of a patient's arterial tree. However, in those instances in which there is a question as to the accuracy of MRA or contraindications to its use, arteriography remains the definitive technical imaging tool.

Percutaneous catheter insertion was first described by Seldinger in 1953.[15] It uses an 18-gauge, 2.75-in. needle with a hollow, thin outer-walled cannula and a sharply beveled, hollow inner stylet for arterial puncture. A retrograde femoral artery puncture is the most commonly used approach, performed on the contralateral side of the patient's symptoms if possible. A transaxillary approach can also be used. The inner stylet is removed once the artery has been punctured, and a guide wire is inserted through the needle and advanced into the artery. A catheter is then placed over the wire into the artery. Contrast compound is delivered through a power injector with volumes ranging from 40 to 120 ml. Heparinized saline is flushed through the catheter to prevent clotting. Radiographs of the lower extremities can be obtained by a step-table or long-leg changer filming technique.[15] Biplane filming can enhance the value of the arteriogram when viewing paired or distal vessels by angling the x-ray tube in a lateral fashion.[12] Digital subtraction arteriography using electronic recording has been known to amplify the iodinated signal and provide better overall contrast. Its spatial resolution, however, is more limited than that of conventional angiography.[14]

Debate is ongoing about the efficacy of MRA imaging as the only preoperative vascular assessment in place of conventional arteriography. Because of the relative newness of the technique, a limited number of research studies have been performed. Hertz et al.[13] argue for MRA as a sole imaging technique not only because it eliminates the potential complications of contrast arteriography but also because of its ability to observe multiplanar defects, three-dimensional plaque morphology, and vessel wall characteristics that traditional arteriography is unable to appreciate fully. Cambria et al.[10] found 100% agreement between the two imaging systems at the level of the superficial femoral, popliteal, and infrapopliteal runoff vessels. They did indicate, however, that MRA tended to overestimate iliac segment stenosis. Carpenter et al.[11] believe that MRA is more sensitive for patent distal runoff vessels than contrast arteriography and provides reliable images of inflow vessels. All of their initial MRA findings were confirmed by intraoperative intra-arterial pressure measurements performed during bypass surgery.[9] According to Ricco et al.,[16] other noninvasive techniques (e.g., Doppler recordings) helped to establish or substantiate distal runoff vessels in planning bypass procedures for 65% of patients in their study sample. Doppler recordings were able to demonstrate signal flow at the ankle level, where preoperative arteriography could not visualize such flow.[16]

The key to successful imaging by MRA is to standardize the equipment and technique to ensure an accurate preoperative assessment. MRA may, at some point, replace conventional arteriography and reduce the risk of complication to the patient as well as the overall cost, while supplying information to direct a surgeon to the level of impairment and successful levels of reconstruction.

WHEN AMPUTATION IS NECESSARY

Timely intervention by a multidisciplinary team involved with the pre- and postoperative care of patients who are undergoing angioplasty or bypass procedure can restore circulation to a compromised limb. Many times, however, necrosis as a result of trauma in a neuropathic foot, with or without ensuing infection, mandates an amputation. Moreover, necrosis as a result of vascular impairment, with or without concomitant infection, may necessitate a partial foot amputation with the combined intervention of lower extremity bypass.

The level of amputation is determined by three factors: (1) the ability to heal successfully at the incision, based on adequacy of circulation; (2) the removal of all nonviable tissues and structures, especially in the presence of infection; and (3) the ability to achieve a long-term functional residual limb that can restore the individual to some level of activity without pain. The most commonly performed levels of amputation are listed in Table 21-2.

TABLE 21-2
Most Commonly Performed Levels of Amputations

Hip disarticulation
Transfemoral (above knee)
    Short
    Standard
    Long
Knee disarticulation
Transtibial (below knee)
    Short
    Standard
    Long
Ankle disarticulation (Syme's)
Partial foot (pedal)
    Transtarsal (e.g., Chopart's, Pirogoff's, Boyd's)
    Tarsometatarsal (e.g., Lisfranc's)
    Transmetarsal
    Metatarsal ray resection
    Hallux or digit (phalangeal)

Partial Foot/Pedal Amputations

Most pedal amputations occur as a result of overt trauma, trauma complicated by an underlying entity (i.e., peripheral neuropathy), infection, malignancy, or ischemia. The three most commonly performed pedal amputations are those involving the hallux or a digit (phalangeal), a metatarsal ray resection, or a transmetatarsal amputation (Figure 21-3). In many instances, amputation of a necrotic digit or foot is accompanied by concomitant vascular reconstruction. If clear demarcation of necrosis or infection in the foot is present, performing these two surgeries at one time alleviates the need for the patient to return to the operating room and to be subjected to additional anesthesia. The greatest failure in a primarily closed amputation site at any level is a delay in wound healing due to marginal necrosis of skin edges.[17] Therefore, careful planning at determining amputation level, recognition and containment of infection, control of underlying medical problems, and appreciation for tissue handling and technique are paramount in producing a successful amputation.

In amputations of the hallux and of the first ray, a medial to lateral racquet-type incision is made, extending plantarly. In a hallux amputation, this plantar cut extends distally approximately 1.5 cm from the metatarsophalangeal joint and meets on the dorsal aspect of the foot approximately 1 cm proximal to the metatarsal head. This allows for adequate plantar to dorsal soft tissue coverage over the metatarsal head and enough residual tissue to remodel skin edges, if necessary, before closure. In both surgeries, the extensor hallucis longus tendon is compromised. If the tendon is healthy, it can be detached and sutured into the remaining metatarsal proximally. This allows continued

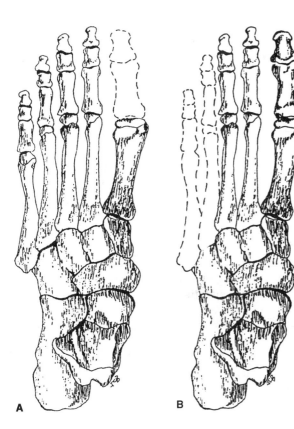
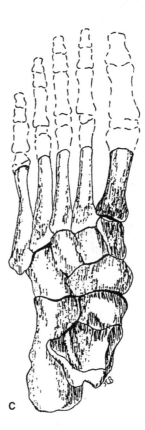

A   B   C

FIGURE 21-3
(A) Amputation of the hallux or a digit can either preserve the base of the proximal phalanx to retain muscle attachments or be disarticulation through the metatarsophalangeal joint (phalangeal, complete). (B) In a metatarsal ray resection, the entire ray (metatarsal and toes) is removed near or through the tarsometatarsal joint. (C) In a transmetarasal surgery, the amputation occurs just proximal to the metatarsal heads. With preservation of a portion of the forefoot, functional gait without a prosthesis is possible.

function of dorsiflexion and weak supination after amputation. If a midshaft metatarsal or first ray amputation is necessary, care in beveling the remaining shaft in a dorsal distal to plantar proximal fashion is recommended. Rounding of prominent bony edges is necessary. When the first metatarsophalangeal joint is compromised and the metatarsal head is removed, the underlying sesamoid apparatus can also be removed to minimize the subsequent risk of ulceration in a neuropathic or dysvascular foot.

The transmetatarsal amputation requires similar planning with a racquet-type incision, fashioning the plantar cut in the sulcus area and the dorsal one just proximal to the metatarsal heads. The digits are disarticulated at the metatarsophalangeal joints, and a similar angled cut with rounding of plantar bony edges is performed. At this level, it is important to identify, pull distally, sever, and allow to retract proximally all nervous supply; this will avoid the complication of a stump neuroma. In all three cases, closure with healthy skin edges and minimal to no tension over the remaining architecture is paramount for a successful outcome. Flaps should always extend in a plantar to dorsal fashion with strict avoidance of placing a dorsal flap on the plantar aspect of the foot. Postoperative care should be directed at limited or protected weight bearing to prevent compromise to the surgical site. Inspection for wound dehiscence (separation of the edges of the incision), hematoma formation, peripheral vascular changes, and infection should continue up to and including the time of suture removal, 10–14 days after operation. As soon as full skin closure and integrity of the wound site are complete, based on clinical evaluation, fabrication of prosthetic devices can be facilitated and implemented. Although additional amputation sites and combinations in the foot can be used, prosthetic intervention with close to normal postoperative ambulation and gait can be achieved using the above procedures.

Amputations at the level of the midfoot or rear foot that involve disarticulation of some or all of the tarsals (e.g., Chopart's, Lisfranc's, Pirogoff's, or Boyd's procedures) have also been described.[18] Theoretically, distal weight bearing and ambulation without prosthesis are possible in a well-healed residual limb; however, altered tendinous attachments frequently result in equinus deformity and a challenging prosthetic fit. Functional outcome and ease of prosthetic fit improve when disarticulation of the ankle (Syme's amputation) has been performed. Rehabilitation of patients with partial foot and Syme's amputation is the focus of Chapter 22.

Transtibial Amputation

Transtibial (below-knee) amputations are most frequently performed when extensive tissue destruction from non-healing ischemic or infected ulceration has occurred, when vascular reconstruction is not possible or not preferred due to other serious medical problems, or when vascular reconstruction has not been successful. Historically, before the use of an antibiotic regimen to control infection was widely available, most lower extremity amputations were performed at the transfemoral (above knee) level, because successful and timely healing was more likely. Three factors have increased the use of transtibial amputation in patients with dysvascular and neuropathic lower limbs. First, antibiotics have greatly reduced the risk of postoperative infection and the likelihood of revision to higher amputation levels. Second, the energy cost of prosthetic gait is significantly lower when the knee joint is preserved. Third, appreciation is growing for the psychological benefits of early postoperative ambulation in supporting physiologic well-being. In a study at New England Deaconess Hospital over a 13-month period, the ratio of transtibial to transfemoral amputations was 4:1.[17] Moreover, the physical requirements (i.e., balance, additional cardiac output, etc.) make ambulation after transfemoral amputation significantly more difficult. Barber et al. note that only 10% of patients with transfemoral amputation used a prosthesis and attempted ambulation.[19]

A transtibial amputation presents as a good surgical choice, because the below-knee prosthesis is an excellent one and cardiac load is only moderately increased with attempts to ambulate. Socioeconomic and emotional problems are less because individuals can be more independent and cosmetic satisfaction with this type of system is higher.[20] Adequate collateral circulation may be present even if femoral or popliteal pulses are diminished or absent. Unless the patient has appreciable proximal skin or tissue compromise, or a fixed knee contracture of greater than 20 degrees, a transtibial amputation should be the treatment of choice.

The four most commonly performed surgical techniques for closure of incision after transtibial amputation are illustrated in Figure 21-4. Many surgeons advocate the use of the long posterior flap, with its preservation of blood supply to the proximal gastrocnemius and soleus muscles (see Figure 21-4D).[21] The length of a standard transtibial residual limb is between 12.5 and 17.5 cm, depending on the patient's height.[22] If the residual limb is longer or shorter, difficulty with comfort, fit, and/or suspension of the prosthesis often occurs. Ultimately, however, the flap selection is based on vascular sufficiency, absence of skin or tissue compromise, and individual anatomic characteristics.

As the surgery begins, regardless of the skin incisions, the anterior and posterior tibial and peroneal vessels are isolated and ligated. The muscles are permitted to retract, and the tibia and fibula are exposed. The anterior skin flap, with its

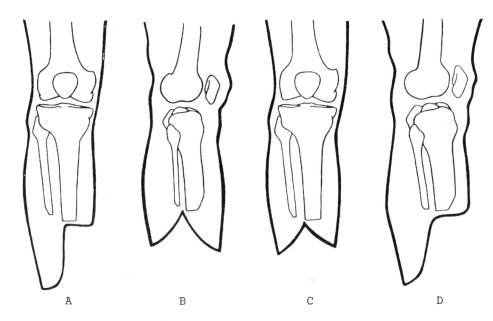

FIGURE 21-4
Examples of transtibial amputation techniques. (A) When a long lateral flap is used, the suture line is on the distal medial aspect of the residual limb. (B) When equal anterior and posterior flaps are used, the suture line lies in the frontal plane, side to side across the distal residual limb. (C) In the case of equal sagittal flaps, the suture line lies in the sagittal plane, front to back across the distal residual limb. (D) When a long posterior flap is used, the suture line crosses the anterior surface of the residual limb, distal to the end of the tibia. (Reprinted with permission from JM Singer. Hershey Board Certification Review Outline Study Guide. Camphill, PA: Philadelphia College of Podiatric Medicine, 1993;640.)

underlying soft tissue and fascia, is elevated from the tibia, and dissection is extended at least 5 cm proximally to allow closure without tension and with maintenance of ample blood supply.[20,21] The fibula is transected first and must ultimately be at least 1.5 cm shorter than the tibia.[22] The tibia is then beveled anteriorly with a 45-degree angle and transected through and through. All bony edges are smoothed with a bone rongeur or rasp. This beveling and smoothing of bony edges are done to reduce the risk of high-pressure areas that are vulnerable to skin irritation and breakdown, to enhance postoperative prosthetic fit and function.

In posterior flap surgery, the remaining gastrocnemius and soleus are contoured to wrap anteriorly without excessive bulkiness and are sutured to the deep fascia of the anterior muscle compartment and periosteum of the anterior tibia.[23] Nerves are usually gently elongated and then transected with a sharp scalpel; the nerve end can be ligated to reduce the risk of neuroma formation. The nerve is then allowed to retract into the residual limb, to reduce the risk of a painful postoperative entrapment that would interfere with prosthetic function. The surgical site is next irrigated using sterile saline and antibiotic lavage. A Penrose or suction drain can be temporarily placed to enhance the drainage of excess fluid away from the incision site in the first few postoperative days. The anatomic layers are gently closed without subcutaneous sutures. Skin edges are closed without tension using interrupted monofilament sutures or surgical staples.

Several types of dressing can be applied in the operating room. A bulky pressure dressing can be used to decrease postoperative edema and pain. A posterior plaster splint can then be applied to hold the knee in full extension. Some surgeons prefer to use a plaster cast that encompasses the knee joint to protect the distal residual limb and control postoperative edema. The cast may incorporate an attachment for an immediate postoperative prosthesis (IPOP).[24] Postoperative care is the focus of Chapter 23.

TRANSFEMORAL AMPUTATION

Transfemoral amputation is performed at or above the knee joint. This higher-level amputation is usually reserved for recalcitrant pathology that involves extensive tissue necrosis, vascular insufficiency, failure of a more distal amputation, or a combination of these factors. Knee disarticulation surgery (Figure 21-5A) results in a residual limb that is quite tolerant of distal end weight bearing; however, incorporation of a knee unit into the prosthesis often compromises cosmesis. Traditional transfemoral (above knee) amputation is performed at the junction of the middle and lower thirds of the femur[17] (Figure 21-5B). As the length of the transfemoral residual limb increases, so does the patient's ability to control and stabilize a prosthetic knee unit during the stance phase of gait using hip extension force within the prosthetic socket. If the resid-

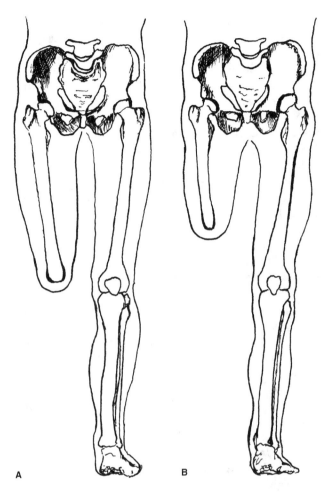

FIGURE 21-5

Amputation at the level of the femur. (A) Knee disarticulation may transect the knee joint or femoral condyles. (B) Traditional transfemoral amputation preserves 50–66% of femoral length. A long transfemoral residual limb (more than 66% of femoral length) provides mechanical advantage for prosthetic use but problems with prosthetic cosmesis due to incorporation of a knee unit. A short transfemoral limb (less than 50% of femoral length) may challenge prosthetic fit and suspension.

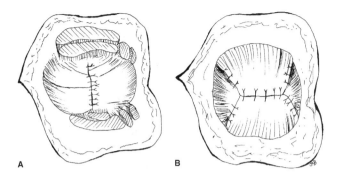

FIGURE 21-6

Myodesis of the thigh musculature is used to stabilize muscle tissue in transfemoral amputation. In this example, the initial layer (A) attaches the medial adductor group to the vastus lateralis and iliotibial band. The second layer (B) connects the anterior quadriceps to the posterior hamstrings. Finally, the two layers are sutured together to stabilize the muscular sling across the bottom of the residual limb.

is located, cut, and permitted to retract proximally to prevent formation of a neuroma. Tissue and muscle are separated from the femur at least 5 cm proximal from the incision line. The femur is transected, and bony edges are beveled and smoothed. A variety of techniques can be used to close the many layers and compartments of thigh musculature.[17,20] Myodesis can be used to protect the distal lateral femoral residuum using the vastus lateralis and iliotibial band. Myoplasty is then used to connect the adductors to the vastus lateralis and iliotibial band and the remaining quadriceps to the hamstrings and across the end of the femur (Figure 21-6). An alternative approach sutures a long flap of quadriceps to a shorter posterior hamstring group. A drain can be temporarily placed deep to the surface suture line before final skin closure. Further closure continues, and again the skin is closed in an interrupted fashion with fine suture or wire staples.[22]

POSTOPERATIVE COMPLICATIONS

Complications after any amputation with a nonhealing presentation most commonly result from improper patient selection or technical error. Obvious control of external factors, including the overall health and nutritional profile of a patient, infection, meticulous postoperative care, and proper fashioning and implementation of a prosthesis, minimizes these problems. The most frequently reported postoperative complications after amputation include phantom limb sensation or pain (5–80%), death (0–35%), pulmonary problems including pneumonia (8%),

ual limb is longer than two-thirds of the normal femur, however, problems with cosmesis occur that are similar to those of knee disarticulation. As the length of the transfemoral limb decreases, stability in stance may be challenged, and suspension of the prosthesis compromised, especially in the sitting position.

If anterior and posterior skin flaps are of relatively equal lengths, the transfemoral suture line is in the frontal plane along the distal residual limb. To minimize postoperative complications, meticulous attention is paid to tissue handling and systematic dissection of tissue layers is performed. Major vessels are identified and ligated. The sciatic nerve infection of the residual limb (12–28%), nonhealing residual limb (3–28%), and pulmonary embolus (4–38%).[20] Haimovici[17] classifies complications into two phases: In the early phase, infection, delayed wound healing, painful stump, phantom sensations, and pressure sores can occur; phantom pain, flexion contracture, and gangrene of the residual limb occur as later complications.

Four factors influence the optimal rehabilitation outcome after lower extremity amputation.[25] First, the level of amputation must be based on clinical and technical information about the likelihood of wound healing, as well as control of external medical and infective factors. Second, the skill of the surgical team in shaping an optimal residual limb for optimal healing and prosthetic fit is critical. Third, in addition to careful and complete preoperative assessment, appropriate postoperative care and follow-up of the healing surgical site after discharge are essential. Finally, the design and fitting of the most appropriate prosthesis for a given patient and access to a comprehensive prosthetic training program complete the rehabilitation process.

SPECIAL CONSIDERATIONS IN TRAUMATIC AMPUTATION

Patients who come to amputation because of trauma differ from those with dysvascular or neuropathic amputation in several important ways. Most are relatively healthy young men who were injured in motor vehicle or industrial accidents. Many have concurrent acute, possibly life-threatening, injuries of multiple systems, including the neuromuscular (e.g., head injury), cardiopulmonary (e.g., pneumothorax or crush injury involving the thorax), or gastrointestinal (ruptured spleen or bowel) systems.[26] The decision as to whether to pursue limb reconstruction or amputation is determined by several key factors. First is the mechanism of the injury itself: Crush injury usually requires amputation, whereas some avulsion or degloving injuries may fit salvage criteria. The condition of the remaining skin, bone, muscle, vascular structures, and nerve must be carefully evaluated. Amputation is usually performed when damage has occurred to three or more of these tissues. The second factor is the status of the wound itself: the greater the degree of contamination, the greater the likelihood of infection and the need for amputation to a "clean" level. Finally, the anticipated functional outcome must be considered: A fragile or insensate salvaged limb often produces greater disability than do amputation and effective prosthetic management. At this time, the functional outcome of amputation and prosthetic training is significantly better than that of lower extremity replantation.[26]

In many traumatic lower extremity injuries, extensive damage occurs to the skin and soft tissue. The availability of skin for wound coverage and closure at the site of amputation may be limited. Excessive skin tension across suture lines, when combined with postoperative edema, increases the risk of dehiscence, necrosis, and compartment syndromes in the days after amputation. Split- or full-thickness skin graft may be necessary to achieve protective skin coverage. Grafted and scarred skin and soft tissue often present particular challenges to subsequent prosthetic fit and function during rehabilitation.

Typically, muscle that has sustained severe damage or prolonged ischemia is debrided until viable tissue remains to reduce the risk of necrosis, infection, and delayed healing. Large amounts of myoglobin released with extensive muscle damage can increase the risk of renal dysfunction and further compromise wound healing.[27] If damaged tendons require repair, the subsequent immobilization can delay prosthetic fit and training. Fractures proximal to the level of amputation must be stabilized adequately and healed before weight bearing in prosthetic training. If nerve damage has been extensive, the ability to perceive areas of excessive pressure within the prosthetic socket must be carefully evaluated. Care must be taken not to compromise arterial vascular repair or grafting in the early phases of rehabilitation. Depending on the degree of wound contamination, surgical wound closure can be delayed until the risk of infection can be minimized by topical and systemic antibiotics.[26]

The goal of amputation after traumatic lower extremity injury is to achieve a well-healed, functional residual limb. In addition to the likelihood of tissue healing, important determinants in choosing the level of amputation include the ability of musculoskeletal structures to support weight bearing and to control prosthetic components during gait and the anticipated shape of the residual limb itself with regard to potential problems in prosthetic fit and suspension. Although wound healing may be possible with a very short, transtibial residual limb, functional outcome is often better in a long transfemoral amputation. The prosthetic fit of a traditional transtibial or transfemoral level amputation may ultimately be more successful than that of an irregularly shaped or significantly scarred forefoot or transtibial residual limb.[26,27]

IMMEDIATE POSTOPERATIVE CARE

All wounds, those compromised by infection or ischemia and those created with intent (i.e., surgical intervention) or trauma, heal by similar wound phase properties. The three general phases to wound healing are the inflammatory, fibroblastic, and maturation phases.[25] The *inflammatory phase* lasts for approximately 3–4 days after operation. During this stage, the two primary treatment goals are to avoid compromise of the vascular framework within the operative site and to keep the area bacteria free by stimulating multiple biochemical factors. This creates a surface for epidermal cells to migrate in an effort to begin wound closure and strength.

The *proliferative phase* lasts from 5 to 20 days. The wound begins to gain strength through epidermal regeneration and ultimately through the synthesizing of collagen. At approximately postoperative day 14, the wound that is healing well has reached 35% of its original strength.[25]

The final phase, *maturation*, may continue for most of the first postoperative year. This is the phase in which remodeling and an equilibrium between the enzymatic processes of lysing and resorbing old collagen and forming new collagen occurs. It takes at least 6 months to determine how a scar will ultimately look.

Infection, uncontrolled or poorly managed edema, poor nutrition, compromised circulation, and a host of other external factors can delay progression through the stages of wound healing. In the first postoperative week, skin edges within the suture line should be carefully assessed for increasing redness, excessive bloody or purulent drainage, discoloration, and separation of suture margins (dehiscence). The area overall should be monitored for edema, and consistent edema management strategies, such as a compressive dressing, should be put into place. The location, amount, and source of any wound drainage must be carefully documented and addressed. When drainage is superficial and localized, sutures may need to be released, allowing the area to drain with a semidependent or intermittently dependent position of the limb or foot. If the infection appears deeper within the fascia, antibiotic coverage, if not already established, should be considered. If infection persists, surgical exploration of the wound and revision to a higher level of amputation may be necessary.

Significant discoloration or a report of intense pressure by the patient often indicates development of an area of hematoma. Location and evacuation of the hematoma may be necessary to prevent serious postoperative complications, including delayed healing and subsequent infection. Depending on the condition of the suture line, sutures or staples can be removed as early as the second postoperative week. Once suture removal is complete, the area can be supported with Steri-Strips to protect the healing wound from the forces of resistive exercise and weight bearing during early prosthetic training. It is important to remember that, early in rehabilitation, the wound has achieved less than 40% of its ultimate strength; time in the prosthesis and full activity must be approached in a systematic and cautious fashion.[28]

The two primary goals in the immediate postoperative period are ensuring optimal wound healing and early preparation of the limb for prosthetic fitting. A variety of strategies are available, depending on the needs of the particular patient and the preference of the surgeon. Petroleum gauze can be layered over the suture line and covered with a soft bulky dressing and an Ace wrap for compression. A posterior splint can be held in place under the Ace wrap to minimize the risk of knee flexion contracture.[17] Although this strategy allows the easiest access to the wound for inspection, it may not effectively control postoperative edema.

Application of a rigid dressing (cast) in the operating room immediately after surgery minimizes edema, protects the healing limb from inadvertent trauma, and minimizes the risk of knee flexion contracture but precludes inspection of the suture line. The initial cast can be left in place for 3–7 days after operation unless the patient has signs of infection (low-grade fever or elevated white blood cell count).[26] If the suture line is healing well when the initial cast is removed, the interdisciplinary team may decide to take a negative mold of the residual limb to use in the fabrication of a training (temporary) prosthesis or to fabricate a removable rigid dressing to continue protection and edema control until the wound is adequately healed.[29]

One of the variations of this cast application strategy is the IPOP, also known as the *immediate postoperative prosthetic fitting*.[1,26,28,29] The IPOP cast is designed not only to protect the healing residual limb but also to enhance prosthetic training and reduce the time required for rehabilitation. A trained surgeon or a prosthetist apply the device in the operating room in three successive steps: application of padding and preparation of the site for the unit, application of the rigid dressing itself, and finally incorporation of the prosthetic system (attachment for the pylon, the pylon, and a prosthetic foot) to the cast.

On the first or second postoperative day, the patient is allowed minimal toe-touch weight bearing with the IPOP during ambulation with a walker. Over successive days, the amount of weight bearing allowed can increase to approximately 20 lb pressure. This small amount of contact with the floor greatly enhances balance, especially among frail, fearful, or older patients.[30] Postoperative pain is also greatly minimized.[1] High rates of successful early rehabilitation have been reported after dysvascular and traumatic amputation.[1,26] The primary complication of IPOP is unrecognized necrosis of the suture line; occurrence of complications appears to be inversely related to the skill of the surgeon or prosthetist who applies the IPOP cast.[24] Results of the Boston Interhospital Amputation Study, although supporting the use of IPOP in settings in which an interdisciplinary team is active, suggest that its practical application in community settings in which such teams are not available is not cost effective or practical.[28]

Not all patients with amputation are candidates for the IPOP early rehabilitation strategy, especially in the presence of a high risk of ischemia or extensive peripheral neuropathy. Because the surgical site cannot be monitored closely in an IPOP cast, insufficient blood supply or trauma from insensitivity can increase the likelihood of complications. Additionally, patients whose cognitive or physical status makes questionable their ability to limit weight bearing to less than 20 lb are not good IPOP candidates.

SUMMARY AND CONCLUSIONS

In this chapter, we have reviewed the typical clinical examination and common signs and symptoms of vascular and neuropathic compromise in the lower extremity. We have also described the most common noninvasive and invasive methods of assessment that are used to determine the necessity of amputation in patients with dysvascular and neuropathic disease. The critical determinants of successful rehabilitation outcome after amputation, regardless of level of surgery, are adequate blood supply for wound healing, minimization of risk of infection, and functional status of the residual limb. The most commonly used surgical procedures for partial foot, transtibial, and transfemoral amputations have been described, and potential postoperative complications have been discussed. The operative care and early rehabilitation of traumatic amputation may be quite different from, and more prosthetically challenging than, those of amputations due to vascular or neuropathic disease. Several concepts of early postoperative wound and postoperative management, including the immediate postoperative prosthesis, have been compared. On completion of this chapter, the reader has developed an appreciation of the complexity and challenges presented by patients who are undergoing lower limb amputation.

REFERENCES

1. Russek AS. Immediate Postoperative Prosthetic Fitting and Rehabilitation. In H Haimovici (ed), Vascular Surgery Principles and Techniques (3rd ed). Norwalk, CT: Appleton & Lange, 1989;1049–1059.
2. Scarlet JJ, Blais MR. Statistics on the diabetic foot (special communication). JAPMA 1989;79(6):306.
3. Nelson JP. The Vascular History and Physical Examination. In J Robbins (ed), Clinics in Podiatric Medicine and Surgery; Peripheral Vascular Disease in the Lower Extremity. Philadelphia: Saunders, 1992;1–17.
4. Peragallo-Dittko V, Godley K, Meyer G. A Core Curriculum for Diabetes Education (2nd ed). Chicago: American Association of Diabetes Educators, 1993;668–670.
5. Boyd CE, Bird PJ. Teates CD, et al. Pain free physical training in intermittant claudication. J Sports Med Phys Fitness 1984;24(2):112–122.
6. Rob CG. Clinical Evaluation of Patients with Peripheral Vascular Disease of the Lower Extremity. In F Jarrett (ed), Vascular Surgery of the Lower Extremity. St. Louis: Mosby, 1985;3–11.
7. Kidawa AS. Vascular Evaluation. Clin Podiatri Med Surg 1993;10(2):187–203.
8. Hoffman AF. Evaluation of Arterial Blood Flow in the Lower Extremity. In J Robbins (ed), Clinics In Podiatric Medicine and Surgery; Peripheral Vascular Disease in the Lower Extremity. Philadelphia: Saunders, 1992;19–55.
9. Jarrett F, Wolfson SK Jr. Use of the Noninvasive Vascular Laboratory. In F Jarrett (ed), Vascular Surgery of the Lower Extremity. St. Louis: Mosby, 1985;12–26.
10. Cambria RP, Yucel EK, Brewster DC, et al. The potential for lower extremity revascularization without contrast arteriography: experience with magnetic resonance angiography. J Vasc Surg 1993;17(6):1050–1057.
11. Carpenter JP, Baum RA, Holland GA, Barker CF. Peripheral vascular surgery with magnetic resonance angiography as the sole preoperative imaging modality. J Vasc Surg 1994;20(6):861–871.
12. McDermott VG, Meakem TJ, Carpenter JP, et al. Magnetic resonance angiography of the distal lower extremity. Clin Radiol 1995;50(11):741–746.
13. Hertz SM, Baum RA, Owend RS, et al. Comparison of magnetic resonance angiography and contrast arteriography in peripheral arterial stenosis. Am J Surg 1993;166(2):112–116.
14. Crummy AB. Arteriography in Peripheral Vascular Disease; Some Technical Considerations. In F Jarrett (ed), Vascular Surgery of the Lower Extremity. St. Louis: Mosby, 1985;28–36.
15. Plecha DM, Plecha FM, King TA. Invasive Diagnostic Imaging of the Lower Extremities. In J Robbins (ed), Clinics in Podiatric Medicine and Surgery; Peripheral Vascular Disease of the Lower Extremity. Philadelphia: Saunders, 1992;57–68.
16. Ricco JB, Pearce WH, Yao JS, et al. The use of operative prebypass arteriography and Doppler ultrasound recordings to select patients for extended femorodistal bypass. Ann Surg 1983;198(5):646–653.
17. Haimovici H. Amputation of Lower Extremity. In H Haimovici (ed), Vascular Surgery Principles and Techniques (3rd ed). Norwalk, CT: Appleton & Lange, 1989;1021–1048.
18. Sanders GT. Lower Limb Amputations: A Guide to Rehabilitation. Philadelphia: Davis, 1986.
19. Barber GC, McPhail NV, Scobie TK, et al. A prospective study of lower limb amputations. Can J Surg 1983;26(4):339–341.
20. Wheelock FC, Gibbons GW. Lower Extremity Amputations. In F Jarrett (ed), Vascular Surgery of the Lower Extremity. St. Louis: Mosby, 1985;273–283.
21. Stephens MM. Amputations Below the Knee. In GJ Sammarco (ed), Foot and Ankle Manual. Philadelphia: Lea & Febiger, 1991;315–325.

22. Litton RR. Atlas of Vascular Surgery. Philadelphia: Saunders, 1973;492–497.

23. Gerhardt JJ, King PS, Zettl JH. Immediate and Early Prosthetic Management: Rehabilitation Aspects. Toronto, Canada: Hans Huber, 1986.

24. Cohen SI, Goldman LD, Salzman EW, Glotzer DJ. The deleterious effect of immediate postoperative prosthesis in below-knee amputation for ischemic disease. Surgery 1974;76(6):992.

25. Singer JM. Hershey Board Certification Review Outline Study Guide. Camp Hill, PA: Pennsylvania Podiatric Medical Association, 1993;108–111.

26. Malone JM, McIntyre KE, Rubin J, Ballard J. Amputation for Trauma. In WS Moore, JM Malone (eds), Lower Extremity Amputation. Philadelphia: Saunders, 1989;320–329.

27. Malone JM, Goldstone J. Lower Extremity Amputation. In WS Moore (ed.), A Comprehensive Review of Vascular Surgery (2nd ed). Philadelphia: Saunders, 1986;1139–1208.

28. Warren R, James RC, Banks HH, et al. The Boston Interhospital Amputation Study. Experience with a community service in immediate postoperative amputation prosthetic fitting. Arch Surg 1973;107(6):861–865.

29. Leonard JA, Andrews KL. Removable Rigid Dressings, Immediate Postoperative Prosthesis, and Rehabilitation of the Amputee. In CB Ernst, JC Stanley (eds), Current Therapy in Vascular Surgery (2nd ed). Philadelphia, PA: Decker, 1991;708–712.

30. Esquenazi A. Geriatric amputee rehabilitation. Clin Geriatr Med 1993;9(4):731–743.

22

Postsurgical Management of Partial Foot and Syme's Amputation

EDMOND AYYAPPA

Partial foot and Syme's level amputations present advantages and challenges to the patient and the prosthetic/rehabilitation team. Preservation of the ankle and heel in partial foot amputation, and most of the length of the lower limb in Syme's amputation, has an important advantage of distal weight-bearing capability: The patient with partial foot or Syme's level amputation is often able to ambulate with or without a prosthesis. The prosthesis also provides protection of a vulnerable distal residual limb for patients with vascular compromise and neuropathy. Suspension of the prosthesis on the residual limb, distribution of weight-bearing forces within the prosthesis, and attachment and alignment of the prosthetic foot are three challenges that must be addressed in the fitting and prosthetic training of patients with partial foot and Syme's amputation. This chapter defines the most common partial foot and Syme's amputations and reviews the prosthetic management options that are currently available. It also identifies specific indications or contraindications for the various prosthetic designs.

DEFINITIONS OF PARTIAL FOOT AMPUTATIONS

Until the advent of antibiotics, disarticulation through the joints of the foot reduced the risk of sepsis and shock and improved the prognosis for healing when compared to amputations that transected bone. The earliest partial foot amputation was recorded in 434 BC by the Greek historian Herodotus,[1] who told of a Persian warrior who escaped death while in the stocks by disarticulating his own foot. He hobbled 30 miles to a nearby town, where he was nursed to health until he could construct a prosthesis for himself. Later he became a soothsayer for the Persian army but ultimately was recaptured by the Spartans and put to death.

At present, partial foot amputations include a wide variety of ray resections, digit amputations, metatarsal transections, and surgical ablation at Chopart's[2] and Lisfranc's levels (Figure 22-1). Chopart's disarticulation involves the talocalcaneonavicular joint and separates the talus and navicular as well as the calcaneus and cuboid.[3] Lisfranc's disarticulation separates the three cuneiform bones and the cuboid bone from the five metatarsal bones of the forefoot.

Pirogoff's amputation is a wedging transection of the calcaneus, followed by bony fusion of the calcaneus and distal tibia with all other distal structures removed. In Boyd's amputation the calcaneus remains largely intact rather than being wedged before arthrodesis with the tibia. Today these amputations are performed infrequently on adult patients. Neither is easily fit with a prosthesis. Boyd's amputation has received positive clinical reviews when used in management of congenital limb deficiencies in children, in which the amputated limb is shorter than the sound limb.[4,5] Few postoperative complications with regard to scarring and heel pad migration occur, and little susceptibility to the bony overgrowth, which is common in children with congenital limb deficiencies, is seen. For most adults, Syme's amputation (Figure 22-2) is performed more frequently because of the ease of prosthetic management at this level. Because of the length of the residual limb in Pirogoff's and Boyd's amputations, the attachment of a prosthetic foot relatively lengthens the limb when a prosthesis is worn. Usually, a heel lift on the contralateral sound limb is necessary to counteract this artificially long limb.

Proximal partial foot amputations often result in equinus deformities because of muscular imbalance created by severed dorsiflexors and intact triceps surae.[6-8] Nevertheless, many individuals with a partial foot amputa-

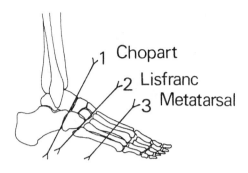

FIGURE 22-1

Chopart's (1) and Lisfranc's (2) amputations are both joint disarticulations, whereas the transmetatarsal amputation (3) is a transection.

tion function extremely well. In one survey, physicians and prosthetists reported that patients with partial foot amputation function better than those with Syme's amputation.[9] Although surgeons and prosthetists have long supported Syme's amputation in preference to Lisfranc's or Chopart's, many patients with midfoot amputation

achieve high levels of function. For example, Jack Dempsey, a professional football player with a midfoot amputation, set several all-time field goal records wearing a custom-designed kicking boot.[10]

GAIT CHARACTERISTICS AFTER PARTIAL FOOT AMPUTATION

A person with a partial foot amputation typically has vascular insufficiency, is usually between the ages of 60 and 70, has compromised proprioception and sensation, and has weak lower limb musculature. After Syme's or partial foot amputation, a patient may be able to ambulate without a prosthesis but experiences a loss of the anterior lever arm in ambulation and has an inefficient, somewhat dysfunctional gait. The primary need immediately after amputation is protection of the remaining tissue. The neuropathic walker developed at Rancho Los Amigos Medical Center locks the ankle in a custom-molded, foam-lined, thermoplastic ankle-foot orthosis (AFO; Figure 22-3). A rocker bottom is contoured to promote a smooth rollover,

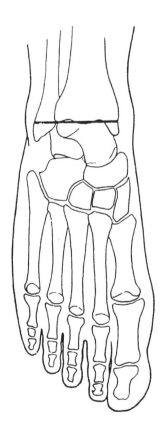

FIGURE 22-2

Syme's amputation involves removal of the inferior projections of the tibia and fibula and all bone structures distally while preserving the natural weight-bearing fat pad of the heel.

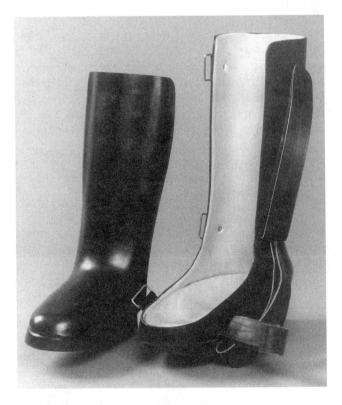

FIGURE 22-3

The neuropathic walker provides maximum protection for the denervated foot at risk for amputation. The combination of custom-molded multidurometer liner, locked neutral ankle, and rocker bottom permits a rollover with minimal plantar pressure.

and the orthosis provides optimum protection for the insensate residual foot. For patients with adequate protective sensation, the risk of tissue breakdown is less, and a custom shoe insert with in-depth or postoperative shoes often provides adequate protection.

A study of gait in four partial foot case histories showed variations in temporal values directly related to the reduction of the forefoot lever arm of a partial foot and consequent increase in the force concentration on the distal end during terminal stance.[11] In the normal person, a fully intact anterior lever arm preserves elevation of the center of mass at terminal stance. With normal quadriceps strength, knee flexion is preserved throughout loading response. The flexed knee acts as a shock absorber from the impact of limb loading (Figure 22-4A). The majority of people with dysvascular partial foot and Syme's amputation demonstrate significant weakness of the quadriceps. This functional weakness threatens eccentric control of the usual knee flexion angle of 20 degrees that occurs during loading response. To compensate, the patient often extends the knee, shifting the ground reaction force anterior to the joint axis to lessen the workload of the quadriceps. This compensatory strategy sacrifices the shock absorption mechanism at the knee and hip joints, increasing the likelihood of cumulative joint trauma at both joints

(Figure 22-4B). Neuropathic impairment of proprioception and sensation further complicates control of the knee in early stance. In addition, compromised forefoot support increases center of gravity displacement. A penalty of higher energy cost results.

Normally, the forefoot lever arm of the trailing limb provides anterior support and results in adequate terminal stance support time (Figure 22-5A). This results in appropriate step length of the advancing limb. By contrast, inadequate anterior support of the trailing limb reduces the lever arm, resulting in premature toe break and forefoot collapse. The step length of the advancing limb is correspondingly reduced (Figure 22-5B).

The relationship between surface area and peak pressure is inverse when body weight is loaded on the foot during stance. This is especially important for individuals with partial foot amputation during terminal stance. As the plantar surface area of the supporting forefoot is reduced, the magnitude of the pressure is increased. The reduced forefoot lever arm also creates abrupt weight transfer to the contralateral side and can reduce step length, stride length, and velocity. Without prosthetic support, the advancing sound side step length diminishes. Fear, insecurity, and pain aggravated by increased pressure near the amputation site can combine to create an abrupt trans-

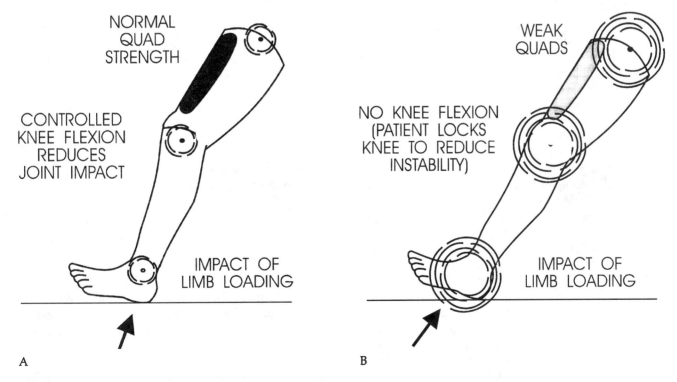

FIGURE 22-4

(A) During loading in normal gait, knee flexion provides a significant shock absorption mechanism to protect the proximal joints. (B) The patient with weakness associated with dysvascular disease avoids knee flexion to increase stability, with a penalty of increased trauma to the proximal joints.

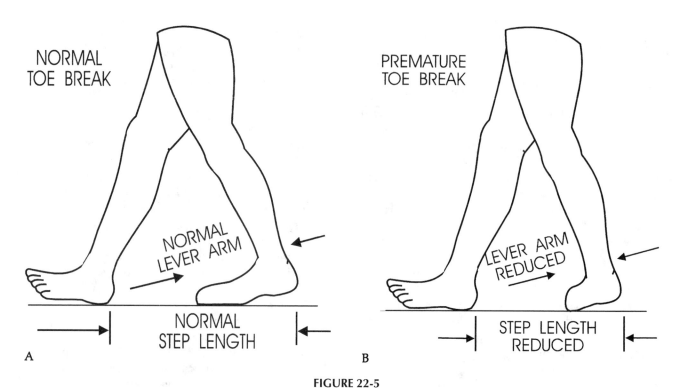

FIGURE 22-5
(A) The forefoot lever arm contributes to a normal step length. (B) Reduction of the forefoot support produces a consequent reduction in contralateral step length.

fer of weight to the sound side, thus increasing the magnitude of the initial vertical force peak.[11]

In normal gait, the weight line falls increasingly anterior to the knee joint during late stance. This results in an energy-efficient passive knee support and increased stability. The length of the forefoot lever arm is a contributing factor to this support (Figure 22-6A). After partial foot amputation the lever arm is reduced, leading to premature loss of support. This shorter level places the ground reaction force closer to or behind the knee. Some passive stability is lost, increasing the energy demands of walking (Figure 22-6B).

Pinzur et al.[12] describe a functional relationship between gait velocity and the level of amputation at the foot. As the amputation level becomes more proximal, changes in temporal and kinetic gait characteristics include reduced sound side step length, decreased velocity, increased energy cost, and increased vertical load on the sound side. The relationship between the length of the remaining portion of the forefoot and the single limb support time is inverse on the amputated side.[11] In partial foot amputation proximal to the metatarsal heads, a loss of medial support at loading response occurs. This may require orthotic "posting" to limit resultant valgus deformity. In patients with partial foot amputations, plantar flexion contracture is also likely to develop, which in turn increases pressure at the distal residual limb during

terminal stance, causing discomfort, pain, and ulceration.[13] This is even more problematic for patients with Hansen's disease or diabetic neuropathy whose sensation is already compromised.[14,15] Without prosthetic care, the shoe quickly becomes disfigured, collapsing at a displaced toe break, further endangering the vulnerable areas of the residual limb.[16] The areas of greatest concern include the distal end, first and fifth metatarsal heads, navicular, malleoli, and tibial crest. The longitudinal and transverse arches, the heel pad, and the area along the pretibial muscle belly are pressure-tolerant areas for loading in a custom shoe or prosthesis.

PROSTHETIC MANAGEMENT IN PARTIAL FOOT AND SYME'S AMPUTATION

During the 1800s, digit amputations were fitted by a wood or cork sandal with leather ankle lacer.[17,18] Partial foot amputations were sometimes fitted with a socket and keel fashioned from one piece of carefully chosen root wood, the grain of which followed the curve of the ankle. This was referred to as the *natural crook technique*. Another commonly used historic design incorporated steel-reinforced leather sockets.[19]

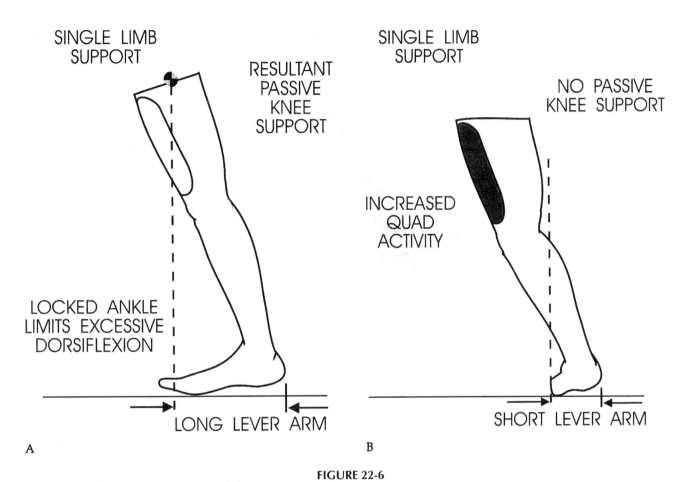

FIGURE 22-6

(A) Normal energy-efficient passive knee support relies on limitations of dorsiflexion at the ankle and a normal forefoot lever arm to maintain the ground reaction force anterior to the knee. (B) After Chopart's or Lisfranc's amputation, the reduced forefoot lever arm may require increased quadriceps activity to compensate for reduced passive knee support.

In recent decades a wide variety of prosthetic options for individuals with partial foot amputation have emerged. The prescribing physician and patient care team must familiarize themselves with the broad array of options that are available in prosthetic components and design so that prescription considerations can best accommodate the special needs of each patient. Because of variability in level of amputation, sensitivity, and/or insensitivity of the residual limb; concurrent foot deformity; and patient activity, no single prosthetic prescription can be used for all patients with foot amputation.[20] As the amputation level becomes more proximal, prostheses are more likely to incorporate supramalleolar containment or more superior support. This is especially true as a patient's activity level increases. Commonly used prosthetic approaches include toe fillers placed inside the shoe, a foot orthosis or an arch support, a University of California Biomechanics Laboratory (UCBL) orthosis to control heel position, a silicone or rubber epoxy resin slipper or boot (e.g.,

Lynadure Medical Prosthetics, Stafford, TX), cosmetic restoration, or several variations of AFOs.

The length and degree of flexibility of the prosthetic forefoot affect the anterior lever arm and consequently foot and ankle motion. The biomechanical goal is to allow anterior support in the area of the lost metatarsals and a controlled fulcrum of forward motion as the foot-ankle complex pivots over the area of the lost metatarsal heads in the third rocker of late stance. An additional goal is to minimize pressure at the amputated distal end within the socket or shoe.

Toe Fillers and Modified Shoes

If a simple filler is prescribed, an extended steel shank or band of rigid spring steel should also be placed within the sole of the shoe, extending from the calcaneus to the metatarsal heads. The challenge that faces the prosthetist is to match the appropriate degree of forefoot flexibility to the needs of each patient. For an energy-efficient and pain or in conjunction with a custom-molded accommodative interface for patients with a neuropathy-related risk of reamputation. Extra depth shoes have 6 to 8 mm or more of space inside the shoe on the plantar surface for accommodation of an orthotic insert or prosthesis and may be useful for patients with digit or ray amputations.[23]

Custom-molded shoes, when used in conjunction with a filler and shank, improve the comfort level and reduce the risk of ulceration in many dysvascular patients with amputation. They are not as subject to forefoot collapse, provide major protection to the endangered foot, and may last longer than stock shoes.

Custom Shoe Inserts and Toe Fillers

A custom-molded, flexible, plantar shoe insert is one of the options for individuals with hallux amputation. This orthotic approach is typically used in combination with extra depth shoes. The goal is to provide a flexible anterior extension to compensate for a missing or shortened first ray to improve the third rocker and yet support and protect the amputation site during the simulated metatarsophalangeal hyperextension.[24] This provides some relief for metatarsal head pressure, supports the arch, and probably assists in normalizing the ground reaction force pattern during terminal stance and preswing. It may incorporate a toe filler to prevent premature forefoot shoe collapse.[25-27] Toe fillers consist of soft foam material such as room-temperature vulcanized elastomer, which fills up the voids in the toe box of the shoe. They provide limited extension of the shoe life and a moderate degree of cosmesis. Toe fillers also act as spacers, keeping adjoining toes properly positioned and reducing abnormal motion that can otherwise lead to ulceration. The toe filler alone provides limited mechanical advantage. A spring steel shank within the sole of the shoe and extending from midcalcaneus to the metatarsal heads is a shoe modification that can further improve gait. An alternative to the spring steel shank is a longitudinal support built into a flexible custom insole. Either support device must terminate at the metatarsal heads to allow hyperextension of the metatarsophalangeal joints. The foot orthotic/arch support with filler is preferable to the simple filler because it can be used in different shoes and because it provides plantar support to an already compromised weight-bearing surface.[28] Custom insoles can also be made in a Birkenstock style of sawdust and epoxy resin instead of foams and thermoplastics.

The UCBL, a foot orthosis that encapsulates the calcaneus, was developed at the University of California Biomechanics Laboratory during the 1960s and was described comprehensively in 1969.[29,30] It is designed to provide better control of subtalar and forefoot position than custom-made shoe inserts, reducing motion and thus

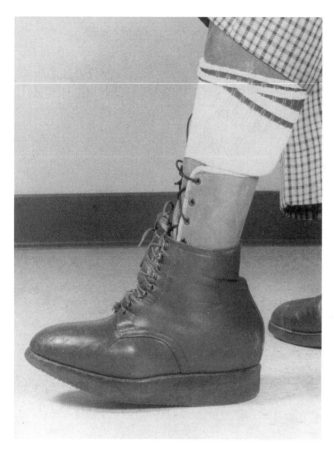

FIGURE 22-7

A supramalleolar leather lacer worn inside a high-top extra depth shoe with toe filler and rocker bottom is an effective prosthetic choice for this patient with Chopart's amputation.

cosmetic gait, relative plantar rigidity should give way to at least 15 degrees of forefoot flexibility distal to the metatarsal heads. The extended steel shank is helpful in providing a limited degree of buoyancy that substitutes for the lost anterior support of the foot.[21] Stiffening the sole using a spring steel shank increases the lever arm support, but often at the expense of additional pressure on the distal end of the residual limb.[22]

For a patient with a more complex partial foot amputation, a rocker bottom shoe modification distributes force over a greater area and advances stance more quickly and efficiently. A curved roll or buildup on the plantar surface of the shoe encourages tibial advancement while minimizing weight-bearing pressures on the distal amputated end (Figure 22-7). For optimum function the plantar contour of a rocker bottom should follow a radius originating from the knee joint center but break or roll more abruptly just distal to the metatarsal heads. Although a rocker bottom assists rollover, it also compromises symmetry of gait. It is often prescribed for patients with chronic friction with a closer fit or purchase over the calcaneus and forefoot[31] (Figure 22-8).

Cosmetic Slipper Designs

The slipper, one variation of which has been referred to as the *slipper-type elastomer prosthesis*, is fabricated from semiflexible urethane elastomer.[32] A similar design in silicone may not provide adequate forefoot support without the addition of an extended steel shank in the patient's shoe. Another similar variation is made from a combination of silicone Silastic, polyester resin, and prosthetic (polyurethane) foam. Both designs probably provide most of the support and control of the UCBL approach but with added cosmesis. These designs may be appropriate for individuals with transmetatarsal amputations or disarticulations. They are ideal for swimming or water sports, because most are water impervious, cosmetic, and capable of providing a flexible whip action, which is useful with swim fins.

Some slipper-type prostheses are cosmetic restorations, made of silicone or vinyl, based on a "life cast," or an alginate impression of a human model (Figure 22-9). This prosthesis is indicated for the patient for whom cosmesis is the paramount consideration. This custom prosthesis is most often produced in special manufacturing centers and frequently requires a considerable amount of time for delivery. It can be ordered with hair, freckles, and a large variety of skin tones; however, it is most often a less than perfect match when compared to the intact contralateral foot. The patient should always share responsibility in the color swatch selection. The material itself is easily stained and changes color with time when exposed to sunlight. The cosmetic restoration provides little ambulation advantage but does increase shoe life. It may be appropriate for patients with transmetatarsal amputations who place a premium on cosmesis.

Prosthetic Boots

The prosthetic boot, with laced or Velcro ankle cuff closures, has greater proximal encompassment to reduce distal motion and increase control (Figure 22-10). This design is appropriate for individuals with Lisfranc's or transmetatarsal disarticulation or amputation. One variation, the Chicago boot, or Imler partial foot prosthesis,[33,34] combines a thermoplastic UCBL-type heel cup using Lynadure. Other designs incorporate Lynadure with a modified solid-ankle cushioned-heel (SACH) foot[35]; some are fabricated from leather, laminated plastic,[36] or Silastic elastomer/Plastazote combinations, as an insert for a boot[37,38] or as an outer boot with inner filler to accommodate bony prominences. These boots often have anterior or medial tongue and laces or some other means of obtaining a firm pur-

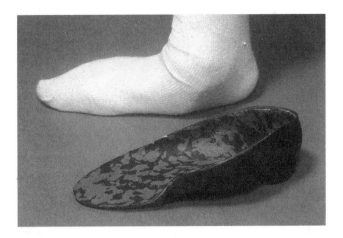

FIGURE 22-8
The custom-molded University of California Biomechanics Laboratory orthosis attempts to obtain a purchase over the os calcis and is thought to influence alignment of the subtalar joint. This patient has Ray resection of the hallux and first metatarsal.

chase above the ankle.[39–42] Some variation of the prosthetic boot may be the general prosthesis of choice for most patients with midfoot amputations.

Ankle-Foot Orthoses

The AFO is another option for patients with partial foot amputation. The polypropylene or copolymer shell supports the plantar aspect of the foot, incorporates the heel, and extends up the posterior leg to the belly of the gas-

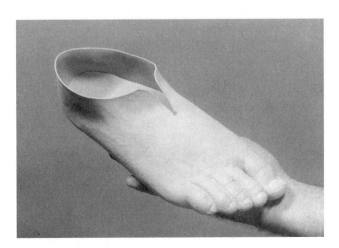

FIGURE 22-9
The life cast prosthesis provides excellent cosmesis with little or no biomechanical assistance. Without additional reinforcement a silicone slipper-style prosthesis does not provide adequate forefoot support.

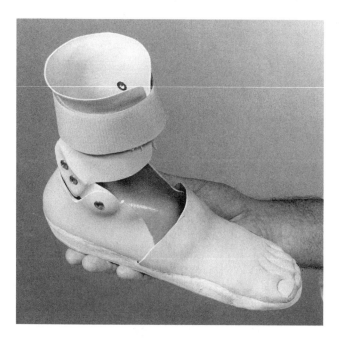

FIGURE 22-10
Epoxy-modified acrylic resin combined with supramalleolar containment and free motion, single axis ankle joints may be helpful at the transmetatarsal level. Without the circumferential containment above the ankle, patients often complain of joint pain toward the end of the day.

trocnemius (Figure 22-11). A circumferential anterior strap stabilizes the limb in the AFO. As an alternative, metal uprights may be attached to a shoe, but this has obvious cosmetic drawbacks. The AFO, whether metal or plastic, provides advantages of the arch support/UCBL and boot with maximum containment and a lever arm for support and substitution of the rocker mechanism. It offers enhanced stability and control because of its high proximal trimline. It has been an excellent solution for many patients with partial foot amputation and may be the prosthesis of choice for the active patient with Chopart's or Lisfranc's amputation. Supramalleolar thermoplastic or laminated versions are fit with Tamarack or Gillette joints to provide free plantar and dorsiflexion motion. This is a popular biomechanical solution for the higher activity level of midfoot amputations. In the presence of acute ankle pain, a patient with Chopart's amputation was successful with a rear entry ground reaction force AFO with rigid ankle.

SYME'S AMPUTATION

In 1867, the Surgeon General of the United States, E. D. Hudson,[43] described Syme's amputation with a litany of

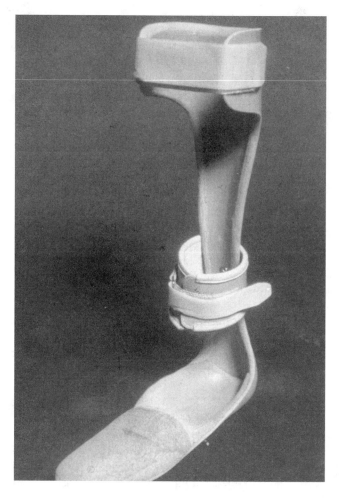

FIGURE 22-11
A posterior leaf spring ankle-foot orthosis with toe filler and anterior strap is successful for many patients with partial foot amputation.

superlatives: "No amputation of the inferior extremity can ever compare in value with that of the ankle joint originated by Mr. Syme. Twelve years of experience with that variety of operation have afforded me assurance that it is a fact complete not capable of being improved in its general character."

The Syme's, or tibiotarsal, amputation is a disarticulation of the talocrural joint. The forefoot is completely removed, but the fat pad of the heel is preserved and anchored to the distal tibia. This allows distal end bearing and some degree of ambulation without a prosthesis[44] (Figure 22-12; see Figure 22-2). It gained popularity during the late 1800s primarily because the patient was more likely to survive with this technique than with other surgical choices, given the reduced degree of sepsis and shock that occurred when the requirement of severing bone

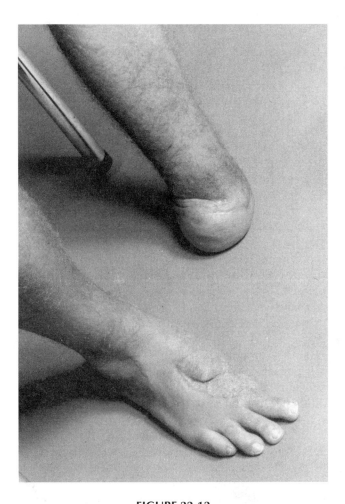

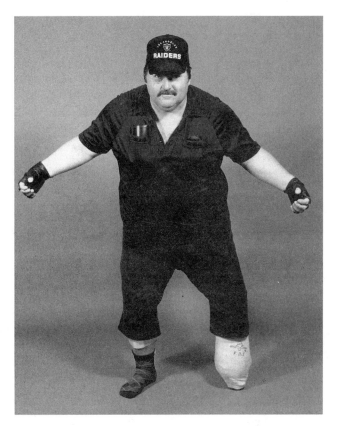

FIGURE 22-13
The patten bottom in a walking cast is used when the clinic team anticipates gross volume changes in patients with Syme's amputation.

FIGURE 22-12
Syme's level amputation on the left lower extremity with first ray resection in the right lower extremity. Early weight bearing before prosthetic fitting can aggravate migration of the heel pad even though migration is primarily a function of surgical technique.

flair, fibula head, and the bony prominence around the distal expansion.[49,50] Pressure-tolerant areas include the midpatella tendon, medial tibial flair, and anterior tibialis.

Walking Casts

To avoid medial migration of the heel pad in the postoperative period, gait training and other therapy that involve weight bearing should be encouraged only after delivery of the prosthesis. The prosthesis is designed to hold the ankle and bulbous distal residual in an appropriate relationship. A fully mature residual limb is less likely to displace. Early prosthetic fitting may involve a definitive prosthesis or a temporary walking cast with a patten bottom (Figure 22-13). This is especially indicated if edema is a problem, in the presence of obesity, or in other medical conditions in which significant volume loss is anticipated. The initial walking cast should be applied as soon as the sutures have been removed, usually within 2 weeks of surgery. The successful application of Syme's walk-

was not involved.[45] Migration of the distal heel pad (which may be surgically avoidable) and poor cosmetic result (which can sometimes be partially addressed by removal of the malleoli) are the primary problems in amputation at the Syme's level. For positive outcome, vascular supply must be adequate to ensure healing. The resurgence of popularity of Syme's amputation today is due to an increased awareness of its energy efficiency in gait compared to transtibial levels, as well as improved vascular evaluation techniques and medical procedures that increase the likelihood of more distal primary wound healing.[46,47] In addition, the dramatic weight-bearing potential of well-performed Syme's surgery (with or without a prosthesis) has always been considered.[48] Pressure-sensitive areas of Syme's residual limb include the tibial crest, lateral tibial

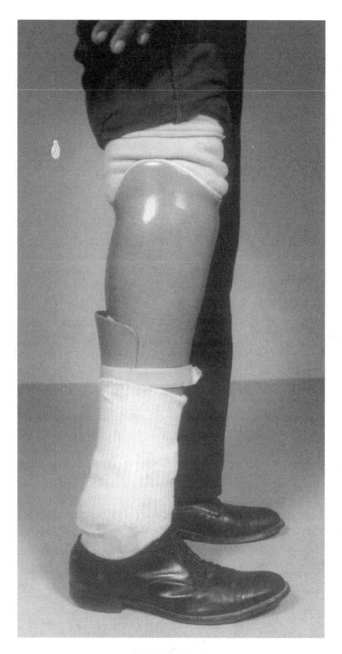

FIGURE 22-14
The Canadian Syme's prosthesis has a posterior opening access panel that diminishes its strength at the ankle. It may be inappropriate for heavy-duty wearers.

ing cast requires a more thorough knowledge base in prosthetics than might be readily appreciated. Application of a walking cast should be done by an individual with a solid prosthetic background.

Prosthetic Considerations

The prosthesis for Syme's amputation must be strong enough at the ankle section to withstand the forces of tension and compression that are produced by the long tibial lever arm throughout the gait cycle, while also providing an acceptable degree of cosmesis over the bulbous expansion at the ankle. All prosthetic designs strive to encompass the tibial section above the distal expansion firmly and still permit donning and doffing. Prostheses designed for Syme's amputations may also be appropriate for Pirogoff's and Boyd's amputations but require that a lift be placed on the contralateral shoe to achieve bilateral limb length symmetry. Before World War II, most patients with Syme's amputations were fit with anterior lacing wooden sockets or leather sockets supported by a superstructure of heavy medial and lateral steel sidebars.[50,51] The prostheses that are most frequently fabricated today include the Canadian, medial opening, sleeve suspension, and flexible wall (bladder) designs.

Canadian Prostheses

The *Canadian Syme's prosthesis* design was introduced during the 1950s as the first major improvement over the traditional steel-reinforced leather[52-55] (Figure 22-14). The Canadian is a relatively cosmetic approach: When viewing the ankle in the coronal plane, no obvious buildups, no windows, and no hardware to increase the ankle diameter can be seen. The Canadian Syme's prosthesis has a removable posterior panel to facilitate donning and doffing. This donning window extends from the apex of the distal expansion, moving proximal as far as necessary to provide clearance for the bulbous end.[56] Breakage may be higher than with other Syme's prostheses because the ankle area, which undergoes the most compression and tension during ambulation, is weakened by the window cutout around the ankle in the posterior region. Modern carbon fiber and acrylic lamination materials and techniques have aided in meeting this challenge.[57,58] However, use of the Canadian design is still limited to patients who are particularly concerned with cosmesis.

Medial Opening Syme's Prostheses

The *medial opening Syme's prosthesis*, also known as the *Veterans Administration Prosthetic Center (VAPC) Syme's*, followed the introduction of the Canadian Syme's and was developed at the New York City Veterans Administration Medical Center in 1959.[59] It has a removable donning door that extends proximally from the distal expansion to a level approximately two-thirds the height of the tibial section on the medial side[60] (Figure 22-15). Like the Canadian, the medial opening is relatively cosmetic at the ankle and compares favorably with it. The

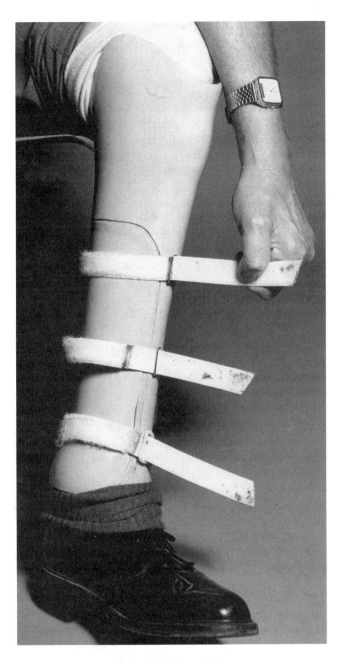

FIGURE 22-15
The Veterans Administration Prosthetic Center (VAPC) Syme's prosthesis has a medial opening window, and has long been a popular approach to fitting the Syme's amputation.

medial placement of the donning panel provides much more opportunity for anteroposterior strengthening of the prosthesis. All other factors being equal, this design is stronger than the Canadian and is the approach of choice for many patients with Syme's amputation.

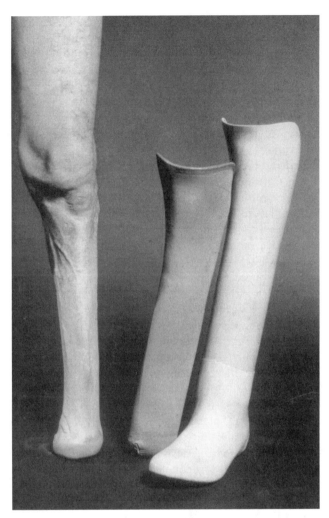

FIGURE 22-16
The sleeve suspension Syme's prosthesis has a full-length liner that accommodates adjustments well. It offers excellent strength at the cost of cosmesis. It is an excellent option for the obese or heavy-duty wearer.

Sleeve Suspension Syme's Prostheses

The *sleeve suspension Syme's prosthesis* is sometimes referred to as the *stovepipe Syme's* because of the cylindrical appearance of its removable liner (Figure 22-16). It is constructed with an inner flexible insert or sleeve that has filler material in the areas just proximal to the distal expansion.[61,62] Before slipping into the outer shell or socket, the patient first pulls on the flexible liner.[63] The outside sleeve then telescopes within the outer prosthetic shell. In another version the leather and foam inner sleeve does not cover the entire residual limb but wraps around the leg and fills up the void areas above the expansion.[64] The sleeve suspension prosthesis is bulky and not very cosmetic, but its strength is significantly better because no window is present to create a structural weakness. It is often chosen for the obese or very heavy-duty wearer or for the patient with recurring prosthetic breakage in other designs. It is more adjustable and forgiving than the other Syme's designs and is often chosen when major fitting problems are anticipated.

Expandable Wall Prostheses

The *flexible, expandable wall*, and *bladder Syme's prostheses*, of which several varieties are available, vary more by materials used than by mechanism of action. All are based on the concept of an inner socket wall just proximal to the distal expansion that is elastic or expandable enough to allow entry of the limb into the prosthesis and still provide a level of total contact around the ankle once donned.[65,66] This design normally requires a double prosthetic wall. The original bladder Syme's prosthesis described by Marx in 1969[67] obtained expansion by using flexible polyester resin in the neck area. The more recent Rancho Syme's prosthesis uses a flexible inner socket, supported by a frame or superstructure of laminated thermosetting plastic. The use of flexible thermosetting plastics and silicone elastomer for expandable wall sockets has gradually eclipsed the use of Surlyn and other thermoplastics as a material of choice for the inner liner. Expandable wall Syme's prostheses are slightly bulkier and less cosmetic at the ankle than their Canadian or medial opening counterparts because they require a flexible inner socket and a rigid exterior superstructure. The fabrication process is more involved, and fitting adjustments to the flexible inner socket can be difficult. Creating either a silicone elastomer or a Surlyn inner socket that is flexible enough for comfortable donning and doffing may significantly limit its durability. Syme's residual limb presents greater pressure distribution challenges to a prosthetist than do other types of lower limb prosthetics. A test socket is especially recommended for all Syme's prostheses. Because the act of donning and doffing with this system is relatively simple, it may be the prosthesis of choice for patients with upper limb dysfunction or cognitive impairment.

The Tucker-Winnipeg Syme's prosthesis, rarely seen in the United States, ignores the traditional requirement of comprehensive total contact by introducing lateral and medial donning slots.[68] The design is well suited for children. It is contraindicated for patients with severe vascular disease and for others who are prone to window edema. A loss of total contact can also affect proprioception and control of the prosthesis. In general, the method permits a prosthesis that is relatively cosmetic, easy to don, and not prone to the noises that are some-times created by rubbing at the window covers of the medial opening and Canadian Syme's prostheses.

Prosthetic Feet for the Syme's Prosthesis

One of the challenges in designing prostheses for patients with Syme's amputation is fitting a prosthetic foot without creating a relatively longer limb. Many prosthetic feet that are used for transtibial amputation have been adapted for Syme's as well. The Canadian Syme's prosthesis was the first to incorporate the use of a SACH foot design, which simulates plantar flexion as the patient rolls over a compressible heel. The SACH foot was the historical foot of choice for patients with Syme's amputation in previous decades but has been eclipsed in function by a variety of more dynamic foot designs. The stationary-ankle–flexible endoskeletal (SAFE) foot provides an inversion and eversion component of motion and is generally thought to be most appropriate for individuals who negotiate uneven terrain. For active walkers, the Carbon Copy II (Ohio Willowwood Co., Mt. Sterling, OH) or Seattle Light (Seattle Orthopedic Group Inc., Seattle, WA) is an excellent choice of similar quality. Other options include the Springlite (Springlite Inc., Salt Lake City, UT) and Flex-Foot (Flex-Foot Inc, Aliso Viejo, CA) Syme's feet. The Steplight (United States Manufacturing Co., Pasadena, CA) is particularly useful when space is limited under the amputation site for the attachment of the prosthetic foot. It can accommodate residual limb lengths as little as 4 cm shorter on the prosthetic side than on the sound side. The Steplight provides a buoyant elastic forefoot but is limited in its heel compression. Nearly all prosthetic feet for Syme's prostheses have ankles that are essentially locked. This results in increased work for the quadriceps for controlled knee flexion during loading response. Incorporation of several degrees of adjustable articulated plantar flexion (at the risk of increasing the weight of the prosthesis) might improve function for certain patients.

Alignment Issues

With most prosthetic feet, the small area between the distal residual limb and floor limits the prosthetist's ability to make dynamic refinements in alignment. Adjustable alignment devices, similar to those that are available for transtibial prostheses, are not compact enough to fit in the available space between the prosthetic foot and the end of the socket. Ohio Willowwood (Mt. Sterling, OH) developed a functional alignment device that permits some degree of dynamic alignment. It allows the prosthetist to adjust the angular positions of the foot during the fitting process. Other manufacturers have since developed similar designs. Slight dorsiflexion of Syme's prosthesis mimics normal gait patterns, encourages a smooth cosmetic and energy-efficient rollover during stance phase, and optimizes the weight-bearing potential of the socket contours. For patients with quadriceps weakness, the dorsiflexion angle can be reduced to minimize excessive demands on the quadriceps. The telltale clinical sign of excessive demand is trembling of the knee during midstance. Early alignment recommendations placed optimal initial dorsiflexion at 12–15 degrees, but most prosthetists today set the foot at a smaller angle, of approximately 5 degrees.[69] The long Syme's residual limb does not easily accommodate itself cosmetically or functionally to more than 5 degrees of dorsiflexion. Alignment is often significantly compromised when knee flexion contracture is present. To prevent breakage and premature wear from the anterior lever arm, the degree of anterior (linear) displacement of the socket over the foot is generally reduced from that of a transtibial prosthesis.

Syme's socket is positioned in an angle of adduction that matches the anatomic adduction angle of the tibia. The adduction of the socket should be positioned to create as smooth a transition as possible at the ankle and knee, so that the prosthetic foot rolls over with the sole flat on the floor. Socket adduction angle, foot eversion angle, and linear displacement affect the external varus moment at the knee during midstance. The optimal spatial relationship in the coronal plane is one that creates a slight varus moment. For an efficient and cosmetic gait, the knee must displace approximately 12 mm laterally at midstance. Insufficient displacement implicates malalignment, most often an inadequate eversion angle. Excessive displacement may be the result of malalignment or lateral collateral ligament laxity at the knee. The most successful strategy to address chronic weight-bearing ulceration that has not responded to a silicone liner, or to address major laxity of the collateral ligaments, is the addition of orthotic components (external knee joints and a thigh lacer) to provide extra support and protection.

CONCLUSION

In this chapter, the options for prosthetic management for patients with partial foot and Syme's amputations have been discussed. Because of the variability in surgical procedures, condition of the residual limb, and altered biomechanics of the residual limb in gait, there is no single best option for prosthetic design. Instead, the characteristics of each patient (weight, skin condition, desired activity level, and length of residual limb) must be considered carefully in prosthetic prescription. The goal is to find the best match of the patient's status and needs with the growing array of prosthetic design options for the partial foot and Syme's amputations. This places an increasing demand on the knowledge base of medical professionals. More than ever the physician, therapist, and prosthetist are challenged to function as a cohesive team, drawing on each others' strengths to achieve the best possible outcome for each patient.

REFERENCES

1. Herodotus. Library IX, 37, Loeb Classical Edition, Vol 4. Translated by Godley. London: Heinemann, 1924;202–205.
2. Bowker JH. Partial foot and Syme amputations—an overview. Clin Prosthet Orthot 1987–1988;12(1):10–13.
3. Bahler A. The biomechanics of the foot. Clin Prosthet Orthot 1986;10(1):8–14.
4. Frankovitch KF, Farrell WJ. Syme and Boyd amputations in children. Int Clin Info Bull 1984;19(3):61.
5. Oglesby DG, Tablada C. The Child Amputee: Lower Limb Deficiencies: Prosthetic and Orthotic Management. In American Academy of Orthopaedic Surgeons, Atlas of Limb Prosthetics (2nd ed). St. Louis: Mosby, 1992;837.
6. Burgess EM. Prevention and correction of fixed equinus deformity in mid-foot amputations. Bull Prosthet Res 1966;10(5):45–47.
7. Pritham CH. Partial foot amputation—a case study. Newsletter Prosthet Orthot Clin 1977;1(3):5–7.
8. Wagner FW. Partial Foot Amputations. In American Academy of Orthopaedic Surgeons, Atlas of Limb Prosthetics. St. Louis: Mosby, 1981;315–325.
9. Wilson AB. Partial foot amputation results of the questionnaire survey. Newsletter Prosthet Orthot Clin 1977;1(4):1–3.
10. Kay HW. Limb deficits no bar to record performance. Int Clin Info Bull 1970;10(3):17.
11. Ayyappa E, Moinzadeh H, Friedman J. Gait Characteristics of the Partial Foot Amputee. Proceedings of the 21st annual meeting and scientific symposium of the American Academy of Orthotists and Prosthetists, New Orleans, March 21–25, 1995.
12. Pinzur MS, Gold J, Schwartz D, Gross N. Energy demands for walking in dysvascular amputees as related to the level of amputation. Orthopedics 1992;15(9):1033–1037.
13. New York University Post Graduate Medical School. Lower Limb Prosthetics. New York: New York University, 1979;233–234.
14. Enna CD, Brand PW, Reed JK, Welch D. The orthotic care of the denervated foot in Hansen's disease. Orthot Prosthet 1976;30(1):33–39.
15. Menon PBM. A new type of protective footwear for anesthetic feet. ISPO Bull 1976;18:4.
16. Veterans Administration Prosthetics Center. Semiannual report of the VA Prosthetics Center. Bull Prosthet Res 1965;10(3):142–146.

17. Marks AA. Manual of Artificial Limbs. New York: AA Marks, 1931;27–36
18. Marks GE. A treatise on artificial limbs with rubber hands and feet. New York: AA Marks, 1888;40–47.
19. American Academy of Orthopaedic Surgeons. Orthopedic Appliance Atlas. Vol 2: Artificial Limbs. Ann Arbor, MI: J.W. Edwards, 1960;212–281.
20. Cestaro JM. Comments on partial foot amputations. Newsletter Prosthet Orthot Clin 1977;1(3):7.
21. Levy SE. Total contact restoration prosthesis for partial foot amputations. Orthot Prosthet 1961;15(1):34–44.
22. Lunsford T. Partial Foot Amputations: Prosthetic and Orthotic Management. In American Academy of Orthopaedic Surgeons, Atlas of Limb Prosthetics. St. Louis: Mosby, 1981; 320–325.
23. Staros A, Peizer E. Veterans Administration Prosthetic Center research report. Bull Prosthet Res 1969;10(12): 340–342.
24. Zamosky I. Shoes and Their Modifications. In Light S, Kampuetz H. (eds), Orthotics Etcetera (2nd ed). Baltimore: Williams & Wilkins, 1980;368–431.
25. Potter JW, Stockwell JE. Custom foamed toe filler for amputation of the forefoot. Orthot Prosthet 1974;28(3):57–60.
26. Young RD. Functional positioning toe restoration. Orthot Prosthet 1985;39(3):57–59.
27. Young RD. Special Chopart prosthesis with custom molded foot. Orthot Prosthet 1984;38(1):79–85.
28. Platts RGS, Knight S, Jakins I. Shoe inserts for small deformed feet. Prosthet Orthot Int 1982;6(2):108–110.
29. Henderson WH, Campbell JW. UC-BL shoe insert, casting and fabrication (first printed as a technical report in August 1967). Bull Prosthet Res 1969;10(11):215–235.
30. Inman VT. UC-BL dual axis ankle control system and UC-BL shoe insert; biomechanical considerations. Bull Prosthet Res 1969;10(11):130–145.
31. Quigley MJ. The present use of the UCBL foot orthosis. Orthot Prosthet 1974;28(4):59–63.
32. Stills M. Partial foot prosthesis/orthosis. Clin Prosthet Orthot 1987–1988;12(1):14–18.
33. Imler CD. Imler partial foot prosthesis IPFP—the Chicago boot. Orthot Prosthet 1985;39(3):53–56.
34. Imler CD. Imler partial foot prosthesis IPFP "Chicago boot." Clin Prosthet Orthot 1987–1988;12(1):24–28.
35. Wilson MT. Clinical application of TRV elastomer. Orthot Prosthet 1979;33(4):23–29.
36. Fillauer K. A prosthesis for foot amputation near the tarsal-metatarsal junction. Orthot Prosthet 1976;30(3):9–12.
37. Pullen JJ. A low profile pediatric partial foot. Prosthet Orthot Int 1987;11(3):137–138.
38. Rubin G, Danisi M. A functional partial-foot prosthesis. ISPO Bull 1972;3:6.
39. Collins JN. A partial foot prosthesis for the transmetatarsal level. Clin Prosthet Orthot 1987–1988;12(1):19–23.
40. Rubin G, Danisi M. Functional partial-foot prosthesis. Bull Prosthet Res 1971;10(16):149–152.
41. Staros A, Goralnik B. Lower Limb Prosthetic Systems. In American Academy of Orthopaedic Surgeons, Atlas of Limb Prosthetics. St. Louis, Mosby, 1981;293–295.

42. LaTorre R. The total contact partial foot prosthesis. Clin Prosthet Orthot 1987–1988;12(1):29–32.
43. Hudson ED. Mechanical Surgery; Artificial Limbs, Apparatus for Resections, by U.S. Soldiers. New York: Commission of the Surgeon-General, 1867 (Library of Congress Call No. RD 756.H86).
44. Jansen K. Amputation—principles and methods. Bull. Prosthet Res 1965;10(4):19–20.
45. Harris RI. The History and Development of the Syme's Amputation; Selected Articles from Artificial Limbs. Huntington, NY: Krieger, 1970;233–272.
46. Burgess EM, Romano RL, Zettl JH. The Management of Lower-Extremity Amputations. Washington, DC: US Government Printing Office, 1969;74–84.
47. Wagner FW. The Syme Amputation: Surgical Procedures. In American Academy of Orthopaedic Surgeons, Atlas of Limb Prosthetics. St. Louis: Mosby, 1981;326–334.
48. Quigley M. The Rancho Syme prosthesis with the Regnell foot. Clin Prosthet Orthot 1987–1988;12(1):33–40.
49. Hanger HB. The Syme and Chopart Prostheses. Chicago: Northwestern University Prosthetic-Orthotic Center, 1965.
50. Wilson AB. Prosetheses for Syme amputation. Artif Limbs 1961;61(1):52–75.
51. Leimkuehler J. Syme's prosthesis—a brief review and a new fabrication technique. Orthot Prosthet 1980;34(4):3–12.
52. Foort J. The Canadian type Syme prosthesis. Abstracts Artif Limbs 1954;4(2):75–76.
53. Murphy EF. Lower Extremity Components. In American Academy of Orthopaedic Surgeons, Orthopedic Appliance Atlas. Vol 2. Ann Arbor, MI: J.W. Edwards, 1960;212–217.
54. Voner R. The Syme Amputation: Prosthetic Management. In American Academy of Orthopaedic Surgeons, Atlas of Limb Prosthetics. St. Louis: Mosby, 1981;334–340.
55. Boccius CS. The plastic Syme prosthesis in Canada. Artif Limbs 1961;6(1):86–89.
56. Department of Veterans Affairs, Prosthetic Services Centre. Syme Amputation and Prosthesis. Toronto: Department of Veterans Affairs, Prosthetic Services Centre, January 1, 1954.
57. Dankmeyer CH, Doshi R, Alban CR. Adding strength to the Syme prosthesis. Orthot Prosthet 1974;28(3):3–7.
58. Radcliffe CW. The Biomechanics of the Syme Prosthesis; Selected Articles from Artificial Limbs. Huntington, NY: Krieger, 1970;273–282.
59. Schwartz RE, Bohne WO, Kramer HE. Prosthetic management of below knee amputation with flexion contracture in the child. J Assoc Child Prosthet Orthot Clin 1986;21(1):8–10.
60. Iuliucci L, Degaetano R. V.A.P.C. Technique for Fabricating a Plastic Syme Prosthesis with Medial Opening (revised and reprinted from 1959 ed). New York: New York University Medical School, 1969.
61. Byers JL. Fabrication of Cordo, Plastizote, or Pelite removable liner for closed Syme sockets. Bull Prosthet Res 1972; 10(18):182–188.
62. Warner R, Daniel R, Lesswing A. Another new prosthetic approach for the Syme's amputation. Int Clin Info Bull 1972;12(1):7–10.
63. Byers JL. The closed Syme socket with removable liner. ISPO Bull 1973;7:4–5.

64. McFarlen JM. The Syme prosthesis, Orthot Prosthet 1966;20:23–27.
65. Eckhardt AL, Enneberg H. The use of a Silastic liner in the Syme's prosthesis. Int Clin Info Bull 1970;9(6):1–4.
66. Meyer LC, Bailey HL, Friddle D. An improved prosthesis for fitting the ankle-disarticulation amputee. Int Clin Info Bull 1970;9(6):11–15.
67. Marx HW. An innovation in Syme prosthetics. Orthot Prosthet 1969;23(3):131–141.
68. Lyttle D. Tucker-Syme prosthetic fitting in young people. Int Clin Info Bull 1984;19(3):62.
69. Hanger of England. Prosthesis for Below-Knee Amputation—Roelite Instruction Manual. Bath: Trowbridges, 1982;20

23

Postoperative and Preprosthetic Care

MICHELLE M. LUSARDI AND LAURA L. F. OWENS

In the days immediately after amputation, the goals of the members of the interdisciplinary team vary, but all ultimately lead toward the patient's independence and return to his or her preferred lifestyle. Surgical and medical members of the team are most concerned about the healing suture line and overall health status, especially for patients with vascular insufficiency or for those at risk of infection after traumatic amputation. The rehabilitation staff focuses on enhancing the patient's early single limb mobility, assessment of the potential for prosthetic use, control of edema, and optimal shaping of the residual limb for prosthetic wear. The prosthetist begins to consider which prosthetic components and suspension systems would be most appropriate, given the patient's individual characteristics and functional needs. The patient and family are often concerned about pain management and what life will be like without the lost limb. Communication among team members, especially the opportunity for patients and family members to ask questions and voice concerns, is as important in this early postoperative/preprosthetic period as it is during the process of prosthetic prescription and training later in the rehabilitation process. This early period sets the stage for the patient's expectations, and ultimately success, as a person with an amputation.

Although the multidisciplinary team can vary in size, depending on patient needs and practice settings, the members at the center are the patient and his or her caregivers. The referring or consulting physician who is familiar with the patient's health history and medical status and the vascular or orthopedic surgeon who performed the amputation are typically members as well. The nurses who will be providing general medical and wound care as the suture line heals and a dietitian who can assess the patient's nutritional needs related to wound healing and exercise demands are important members. Physical and occupational ther-

apists who work with the patient in this early rehabilitation period play an important role in preventing secondary complications, determining rehabilitation potential and discharge needs. The prosthetist serves as a resource for determination of the patient's readiness for prosthetic fitting, especially for patients with potentially hard-to-fit limbs. A psychologist, social worker, vocational counselor, or school counselor is involved as necessary to help the patient adjust psychologically and to organize long-term rehabilitation care or community resources in preparation for discharge. A patient's clergyman can also be a valuable resource for the patient, family, and team. The unique training, clinical expertise, and individual roles of each team member contribute, in a collaborative process, to the development of a plan for rehabilitation that best meets the needs and optimizes the potential of the patient. The team must come to agreement on the timing and prioritization of specific rehabilitative interventions to meet the goals defined for each patient.

In this chapter, we focus on the roles of rehabilitation professionals who work with patients with new amputation in the days and weeks immediately after surgery. We explore how surgical pain and phantom sensation are managed, strategies for controlling postoperative edema, and methods to assess a patient's readiness for prosthetic fitting. We also identify interventions that help a patient gain competence with single limb mobility tasks and exercises that provide the foundation for successful prosthetic use.

PATIENTS WITH A NEW AMPUTATION

In the immediate postoperative period, the patient with a new amputation is likely to experience acute surgical pain and may be grieving the physical loss of the limb. Older patients with dysvascular or neuropathic limb loss often have had time to prepare for an elective amputation after a prolonged period of managing a poorly vascularized foot or nonhealing neuropathic ulcer. Although they may be somewhat less distressed about the loss of their limb than younger patients who have suddenly lost a limb in a traumatic accident or other medical emergency, loss of one's limb requires significant psychological adjustment. The immediacy of pain and feelings of loss may make it difficult for the patient to recognize the potential for a very positive rehabilitation outcome. Early education and discussion about the process of rehabilitation and the patient's ultimate goals are extremely important. Patients need to understand quickly the most effective strategies to manage acute pain (such as edema control and judicious use of pain medications) and to prevent secondary complications (such as joint contracture) that will make rehabilitation more difficult.

POSTOPERATIVE PAIN MANAGEMENT

In addition to reducing the patient's acute discomfort, effective postoperative pain management is important for several other reasons. Pain is a significant physiologic stressor that has an impact on homeostasis, as well as on the patient's ability to concentrate and to learn.[1] In the early postoperative period, patients are faced with learning how to care for their new residual limb, including monitoring for signs of infection, using strategies to control edema, and appropriate positioning to minimize the risk of contracture formation. They must also learn a variety of new motor skills, including exercises to preserve strength and range of motion, and how to protect their healing suture while moving around with crutches or walker on their remaining limb. If postoperative discomfort and pain are kept to a minimum, patients are able to learn and retain these new cognitive and motor skills more effectively. Pain can also be very fatiguing and demoralizing. Patients with significant pain may be reluctant to participate fully in active rehabilitation programs because they fear that movement will only increase their pain. Patients with significant pain may be erroneously labeled as unmotivated or uncooperative, when their primary goal is to find a way to escape their discomfort. It is important to note that although certain types of pain medications (narcotics and other psychogesics) are very effective in providing relief, they may themselves compromise cognitive function or increase the risk of postural hypotension.[2] Therapists must be aware of the actions and side effects of the pain medication prescribed for the patient.

Pain is a subjective sensation; each patient defines his or her own level of tolerance. A number of clinical tools have been developed to assess levels of discomfort and pain; these are often useful in assessing the effectiveness of strategies used for postoperative pain management. Descriptive pain scales based on numeric representation of pain severity or a visual analogue are effective methods of tracking how pain changes over time and after intervention.[3]

In the days immediately after amputation, the goal is to minimize the severity of acute postoperative pain. Prevention is more effective than reduction of significant pain: For this reason, patients are encouraged to request pain medication before pain becomes severe.[3] Preoperative and intraoperative pain management also have an impact on postoperative pain: In patients undergoing amputation due to vascular insufficiency who receive epidural analgesia before surgery, problematic phantom limb pain after amputation may be less likely to develop.[4] Effective management of postoperative edema is an important element in the control of postoperative pain as well.

Phantom Limb Sensation and Phantom Pain

It is common for patients with recent amputation to experience a sense that the amputated limb remains in place in the days and weeks after surgery.[5] Melzak[6] estimates that as many as 70% of patients with new amputation have noticeable phantom limb sensation. Most experience a sense of numbness, tingling, or pressure in the missing limb, and some complain of itching toes or mild muscle cramps in the foot or calf.[7] A small number of patients experience significant phantom pain, reporting shooting pains, severe cramping, or a distressing burning sensation that may be localized in the amputated foot or present throughout the missing limb. Phantom pain is often intermittent, although some patients report constant discomfort.[8] Onset of phantom pain may or may not be linked to activities such as exercise or dressing change. There is evidence that patients who experienced significant dysvascular limb pain in the weeks and months before surgery are more likely to experience phantom pain in the immediate postoperative period and for up to 2 years after surgery.[9] Severity or duration of preoperative pain does not appear to be predictive of long-term phantom pain. Phantom limb sensation and pain tend to decrease over time whether the amputation was the result of a dysvascular/neuropathic extremity or a traumatic injury.[5] Although a number of models or theories for phantom limb sensation and phantom pain have been proposed, the neurophysiologic mechanism that underlies this phenomenon is not well understood.[6,10,11]

It is very important that the likelihood of postoperative phantom limb sensation is discussed with patients before their amputation surgery as well as in the days immediately after operation. Phantom limb sensation is quite vivid; its realistic qualities can be disturbing and frightening to patients with recent amputation. Candid discussion about phantom limb sensation as a normally anticipated occurrence helps to reduce the patient's anxiety and distress should phantom sensation occur. It also alerts the patient to issues of safety in the immediate postoperative period. Patients with recent amputation are at significant risk of falling when they awaken from sleep and attempt to stand and walk to the bathroom in the middle of the night, thinking, in their semialert state, that both limbs are intact. Ecchymosis or wound dehiscence sustained during a fall often causes major delays in rehabilitation and prosthetic fitting; some fall-related injuries require surgical revision or closure.

If a patient reports significant phantom sensation or pain, careful inspection of the residual limb helps to rule out other potential sources of pain, such as a neuroma or an inflamed or infected surgical wound. A variety of interventions are available for patients whose phantom limb sensation or pain is significant, although management of phantom pain is often challenging and frustrating for the patient and the rehabilitation team. Non-narcotic and narcotic pain medications alone are typically ineffective in the presence of phantom pain.[7] Medications that are used to prevent seizure as well as certain antidepressants, prescribed alone or in conjunction with low-dose narcotic agents, may be helpful for some patients. When a clear locus or trigger point is present, some patients receive temporary relief after local injection of a steroid or analgesic. Continuous analgesic infusion to create a nerve sheath or interneural block has been used to control the severity of phantom limb pain in the immediate postoperative period: The success of this intervention varies with pharmacologic agents and the rate of their administration.[12–14] Noninvasive alternatives, such as relaxation techniques or hypnosis, may be effective for certain patients as well.

Physical Therapy Management of Postoperative Pain

The success of early rehabilitation is influenced by the effectiveness of postoperative pain management; for this reason, physical therapists must be aware of medications being used and be involved in assessing the effectiveness of the pain management strategy and its impact on patient learning and function. When epidural anesthesia has been used during surgery or in the immediate postoperative period, it is imperative that the patient's sensory and motor function is carefully evaluated before transfer training and single limb mobility activities are begun. In the acute care hospital, it is important that administration of medications be timed so that pain control is optimal during physical therapy activities. If the patient is experiencing phantom sensation or pain, the physical therapist plays

an important role in educating the patient and family about these sensations and often incorporates imagery and relaxation methods into the treatment program. Transcutaneous electrical nerve stimulation can be an effective adjunct modality for patients with acute surgical pain and may also play a role in the management of troubling phantom sensation or pain in the immediate postoperative period.[15] There is some evidence that transcutaneous electrical nerve stimulation may contribute to wound healing after amputation, reducing the need for revision or reamputation, in addition to reducing the severity of postoperative phantom pain.[15] Physical therapists have also used accupressure, ultrasound, application of cold or ice, and a variety of massage techniques to assist pain management, with varying degrees of success.[7,16,17] Careful attention to the healing status of the wound is imperative: Wound closure must not be compromised by any intervention that is aimed at reducing discomfort or pain.

CONTROL OF EDEMA

The management of postoperative edema is important for four reasons: Edema control strategies are important components of pain control, enhance wound healing, protect the incision during functional activity, and facilitate preparation for prosthetic replacement by shaping and desensitizing the residual limb. A variety of postsurgical dressing and edema control strategies are available. These include soft dressings with or without Ace wrap compression, semirigid dressings, removable rigid dressings (RRDs) applied over soft dressings, or the application of a rigid cast dressing in the operating room. An immediate postoperative prosthesis (IPOP) is a rigid dressing with an attachment for a pylon and prosthetic foot. Each option contributes to pain control, wound healing and protection, and preparation for prosthetic use in a significantly different way. The choice of strategy is determined by the etiology and level of amputation, the condition of the skin, the medical and functional status of the patient, access to prosthetic consultation and care, the preference and experience of the surgeon, and established institutional protocol.

Rigid Dressings and Immediate Postoperative Prostheses

Many patients with elective transtibial amputation are placed in a cylindrical plaster cast immediately after amputation while in the operating room (Figure 23-1). A simple postoperative cast, used as a rigid dressing, is applied in much the same way as a cast that is used to immobilize a fracture of the proximal tibia or distal femur. If the cast is to be used as an IPOP, a prosthetist often joins the surgi-

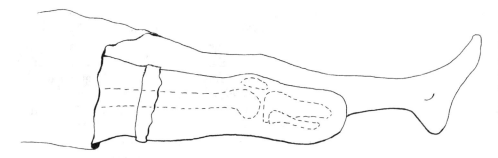

FIGURE 23-1
A plaster cast, applied immediately after amputation in the operating room, is an effective method of edema control, protection of the residual limb, and prevention of knee flexion contracture.

cal team in the operating room during cast application to incorporate the features of a patellar tendon-bearing socket and an attachment for a pylon into the cast (Figure 23-2).

Several steps are necessary in the application of a rigid postoperative dressing.[18,19] First, a surgical dressing is applied over the suture line, and a cotton stockinet or lightly compressive lycra spandex sock is pulled over the limb to the upper thigh. Next, a layer of protective padding is applied, with particular attention to protection of skin over the bony prominences. If the cast will be the socket for an IPOP, several felt pads are positioned on the limb to direct and distribute weight-bearing forces more effectively onto pressure-tolerant areas, including the medial tibial flare, the anterior muscle compartment, and the patellar tendon. The residual limb is then supported with the knee extended, and several layers of elastic or nonelastic plaster of Paris are applied. The proximal edges of the cast are finished at midthigh level. Modifications of the cast (as it is setting) are used to aid suspension or, for an IPOP, to ensure that weight-bearing forces are directed to pressure-tolerant areas. Pressure applied to the outside of the cast just above the femoral condyles captures normal femoral anatomy to create supracondylar suspension. For an IPOP, the prosthetist incorporates a patellar tendon bar, a broad "shelf" for the medial tibial flare, and a stabilizing popliteal bulge by applying manual pressure to these areas as the cast begins to set. He or she also incor-

porates a point of attachment and alignment into the distal cast for subsequent attachment of a pylon and prosthetic foot. Finally, for rigid dressings and for IPOPs, the surgeon or prosthetist can incorporate a suspension attachment, which will connect to a waist belt, into the proximal anterior surface of the cast.

A rigid dressing or IPOP is left in place for 3 or more days postoperatively, depending on the patient's condition and the surgeon's preference. When the cast is removed, the status of the wound is carefully inspected. If the wound is healing well, the physician may opt for reapplication of the cast or IPOP for an additional period. If the status of the wound is questionable, an alternative method of edema control that allows more frequent wound inspection and care must be used. Some physicians opt to replace a rigid dressing with an RRD after the first cast is taken off, regardless of wound status.

Rigid dressings are one of the most effective strategies for controlling postoperative edema and, as a result, reducing postoperative pain.[20] The rigid cast protects the vulnerable suture line from unintentional trauma as the patient moves around in bed, transfers to and from bed (or toilet or mat table), is transported by wheelchair, and begins single limb mobility training. Enclosure of the limb in an extended knee position is also very effective in preventing problematic knee flexion contracture formation. As a result, patients who wear rigid dressings or IPOPs are

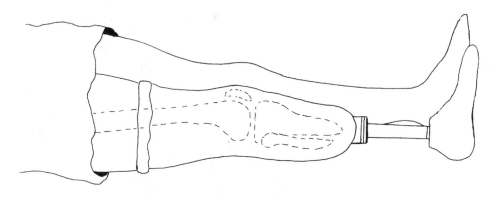

FIGURE 23-2
Incorporation of a pylon and features of a patellar tendon-bearing socket in an immediate postoperative prosthesis can facilitate early mobility in selected patients.

often ready for prosthetic fitting sooner than those managed by other edema control strategies.

Several important disadvantages or drawbacks are associated with rigid dressings and IPOPs, however. Application of a cast precludes visual inspection of the healing incision, and wound care can only occur when the cast is removed or changed. For this reason, a rigid dressing may not be appropriate for patients with significant risk of infection, especially those whose wounds were potentially contaminated during traumatic injury. Wound status can only be monitored indirectly, using body temperature, white blood cell count, size and color of drainage stains on the cast, and patient reports of increasing discomfort and pain as indicators of a developing infection. Application of a rigid cast, especially if it is the base of an IPOP, also requires careful attention to anatomy and alignment, well-developed manual skills, and a clear understanding of prosthetic principles. A poorly applied or inadequately suspended rigid dressing can lead to skin abrasions or pressure-related ulcerations over bony prominences, delaying prosthetic fitting until wound healing occurs. Pistoning or rotation of the rigid dressing on the residual limb can apply distracting forces over the suture line, compromising healing and increasing the risk of ecchymosis or dehiscence.

The early mobility afforded by application of an IPOP may be important for patients who are unable to achieve single limb ambulation with a walker or crutches, especially those who are at significant risk of functional decline, physiologic deconditioning, or atalectasis and pneumonia secondary to inactivity and immobilization. It is important to note that, although an IPOP replaces the amputated limb with a pylon and prosthetic foot, it is most appropriately used with limited, protected, toe-touch partial weight bearing. Shearing forces that result from excessive weight shift and repeated loading of the residual limb in an IPOP can compromise or delay wound healing.[21] Because of this risk, an IPOP is inappropriate for patients who are likely to be unreliable about limiting weight bearing. Many proponents of IPOP suggest that gradual controlled application of mechanical stress to healing connective tissues actually facilitates tissue modeling for better tolerance of the mechanical stresses of prosthetic wear and ambulation.[18,19,21] Although the early application of mechanical stresses is apparently well tolerated by wounds with adequate blood supply, ischemic wounds tolerate only minimum stress in their healing phase.[21]

Removable Rigid Dressings

For some patients with transtibial amputation who were initially managed with a rigid dressing applied in the oper-

ating room, the next step in postoperative edema control may be fabrication of an RRD. In other settings, the RRD can be applied instead of a cylindrical cast in the operating room, or patients who were initially managed with a soft dressing and compressive Ace wrap can be referred for fabrication of an RRD several days after surgery. The physical therapist may be responsible for fabrication of the RRD, working in collaboration with the surgeon, surgical nurse, and/or prosthetist.

The RRD is a cap cast worn over a soft or compressive dressing (Figure 23-3). This edema control strategy effectively protects the healing residual limb and limits the development of edema. One of its major advantages, when compared to a cylindrical cast, is the ability to doff (remove) and don (apply) the RRD quickly and easily to monitor wound healing and provide daily wound care.[22] The RRD is an effective adjunct for pain management. Use of an RRD also facilitates residual limb shaping and shrinkage; patients who wear RRDs are often ready for prosthetic fitting more quickly than those managed with soft dressings or Ace wraps alone.[23] Because the RRD limits the development of edema, it is an important adjunct in the management of postsurgical pain. The protective cap limits shearing across the incision site as the patient moves around in bed or during therapy; this soft tissue immobilization can facilitate wound healing. The RRD is not likely to become displaced or dislodged during activity, a problem that often renders Ace wrap compression ineffective. The ease of donning and doffing means that patients can quickly become responsible for this task component of caring for their residual limb. Because the RRD is removed and reapplied several times a day for wound care, the residual limb quickly becomes desensitized and tolerant of pressure, which facilitates transition to prosthetic wear. Fabrication and use of an RRD provide the opportunity to educate patients about the fabrication of a preparatory prosthesis and the use of prosthetic socks to obtain and maintain socket fit.

The RRD is most appropriate for patients whose transtibial incision appears to be in the initial stages of healing. Although the wound may be inflamed secondary to the trauma of surgery, no signs of infection, significant ecchymosis, or large areas of wound dehiscence should be present.[24] Patients with substantial drainage from their surgical wound that requires bulky soft dressings and frequent dressing changes are often not good candidates for RRD; it is difficult to accommodate distally placed bulky dressings within the RRD shell. Patients with fluctuating edema secondary to congestive heart failure or dialysis can be managed with an RRD if it is fabricated when limb volume is high: Layering prosthetic sock ply over the limb before putting on the RRD accommodates for volume loss.[24] Ideally, distal residual limb circum-

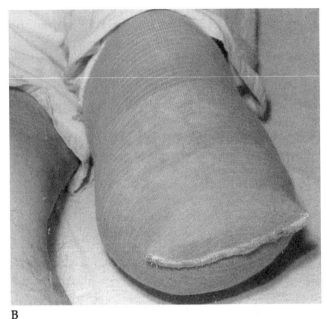

B

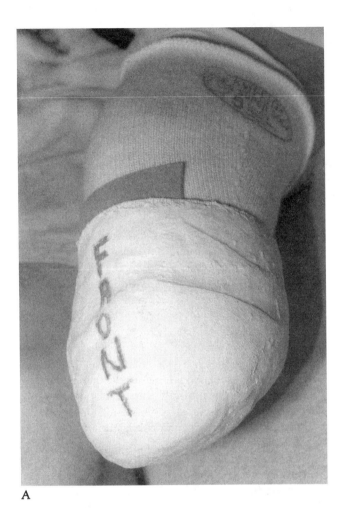

A

FIGURE 23-3

(A) This removable rigid dressing has been donned over a nylon sheath and five-ply wool prosthetic sock, with an additional foam pad at the proximal anterior edge for comfort and protection of the skin. Marking the anterior midline of the cast ensures that it will be applied in optimal alignment. *(B)* The removable rigid dressing is held onto the limb by application of elasticized Tubigrip, sewn closed at one end and pulled up to midthigh level for a sleeve suspension. A Velcro-closing thermoplastic or woven supracondylar strap is applied over the sleeve to ensure suspension.

ference is no more than 0.5 in. larger than its proximal circumference. Compressive dressings may be more appropriate for patients with very bulbous residual limbs

Fabrication of Removable Rigid Dressings

The patient's residual limb is prepared for casting by first placing a protective layer of gauze fluff over the suture line. The limb can be loosely wrapped in plastic wrap to facilitate removal of the completed RRD after casting. Next, a "sock" made from elasticized cotton stockinet or Tubigrip (Seton Health Care Group TLC, Oldham, England) is applied over the limb, with particular care to avoid shearing across the suture line. Pieces of webril or a similar filler material are layered around the limb to create reliefs within the RRD for bony prominences (tibial crest, fibular head, distal tibia) and the hamstring tendons. When the distal residual limb has a larger circumference, additional padding is added proximally to ensure that the RRD will be cylindrical or conical and easily donned. A long sock made from regular cotton stockinet is carefully donned over the padding; this will be the inner layer of the fin-

ished RRD. The outline of the patella marked on the stockinet guides trimlines as plaster is applied. Typically, two rolls of fast-setting plaster cast material are sufficient for an RRD. The patient's residual limb is supported in full knee extension, and successive layers of plaster are smoothed into place, building a cast with an anterior trimline at midpatella and a slightly lower posterior trimline to allow knee flexion without tissue impingement. The cotton stockinet sock is then folded down over the cast at the knee, and several additional circumferential layers of plaster are used to finish and reinforce the proximal brim (to ensure that the RRD can subsequently withstand repeated donning/doffing). An Ace wrap can be applied to provide additional compression while the plaster sets. Once the RRD has hardened sufficiently, the patient is asked to flex the knee slightly, and the cast is carefully and slowly pulled off the residual limb. The extra webril or padding is pulled out of the RRD, and the inner surface is inspected for potentially problematic rough areas or ridges. Because the RRD is almost cylindrical, it is helpful to mark the front of the cast to ensure that it is correctly donned.

Wearing the Removable Rigid Dressing

Before the RRD is applied, one or two gauze pads are placed over the suture line for protection. A prosthetic sock, Tubigrip, elasticized stockinet sock, or commercially manufactured "shrinker" is carefully donned, with minimal shear stress across the suture line. Additional ply of prosthetic socks are used as necessary to ensure a snug fit within the RRD. A small amount of webril or other fluffy padding is placed in the distal anterior RRD to protect the distal tibia and suture line; then the RRD is carefully slipped onto the residual limb, aligning the markings on the front of the RRD with the patella for optimal fit (see Figure 23-3A). A small foam filler or cushion can be placed between the anterior brim and residual limb to minimize the risk of friction during activity. The outer Tubigrip or stockinet suspension sleeve is then rolled over the RRD and onto the thigh, the supracondylar strap is secured in place, and the sock is folded back down over the strap to minimize the risk of loss of suspension.

It is important that the skin be inspected within the first 60–90 minutes of initial fitting with an RRD, to assess skin integrity and identify potential pressure-related problems. If no skin problems develop, routine wound inspection once per nursing shift is usually adequate. The RRD is designed to be worn continuously, even when sleeping, except during routine wound care or bathing.[25] If the patient is expecting to be out of the RRD for more than several minutes, another form of compression (such as a shrinker or several layers of Tubigrip) must be available to minimize the risk of edema. Patients and caregivers must be encouraged to report any localized pain or discomfort as signs of potential problems with RRD fit or function. Patients usually need to layer an additional stockinet, tube socks, or prosthetic socks to assure a snug RRD fit to accommodate progressive shrinkage of the residual limb. Sometimes short distal socks are necessary to provide for distal compression without excessive proximal bulkiness that can prohibit donning. The consistent use of 12- to 15-ply socks to achieve appropriate fit usually indicates the need for fabrication of a smaller RRD. Significant change in the shape or configuration of the residual limb also requires fabrication of a new RRD.

Wu et al. suggest a variety of weight-bearing exercises for patients who are wearing an RRD between the seventh and fourteenth postoperative day, depending on the state of wound healing.[22,25] These exercises are designed to prepare patients for standing and walking in their first prosthesis. In some settings, patients are referred to the prosthetist for fabrication and delivery of the initial (preparatory or training) prosthesis within 12–17 days of surgery if the incision has healed sufficiently. In these

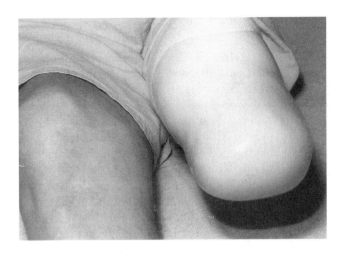

FIGURE 23-4

A flexible, polyethylene semirigid dressing is fabricated by a prosthetist over a positive model of the patient's residual limb. This ensures an intimate fit for effective control of edema, protection of the healing incision, and optimal "shaping" of a new residual limb.

instances, early gait training in the prosthesis can negate the need for preparatory weight-bearing exercises in the RRD. Many patients continue to use their RRD in conjunction with a shrinker for control of edema and limb protection whenever they are not wearing their prosthesis for as long as 6 months after surgery.

Semirigid Dressings

An alternative to a plaster RRD is a polyethylene semirigid dressing (SRD; Figure 23-4). Like the RRD, the SRD is an effective strategy for control of edema, protection of the healing incision, and shaping of the residual limb. Unlike the RRD, however, the SRD requires the skill of a prosthetist for fabrication. The prosthetist may take a negative mold of the patient's residual limb while in the operating room or when the rigid dressing is removed on the third or fourth postoperative day. A positive model is created using the negative mold and is modified to incorporate reliefs for pressure-intolerant areas of the residual limb. The polyethylene is heated and vacuum molded over the positive model, in the same way that a thermoplastic socket would be. The SRD is often ready for delivery in 2 or 3 days after casting. Patients who are initially casted in the operating room may receive their SRD on the day that their rigid plaster dressing is removed.

The polyethylene SRD has several advantages when compared to the plaster of Paris RRD. First, polyethylene is easier to clean; as a result hygiene of the residual limb may be improved. The SRD is lighter in weight and somewhat more durable than a plaster RRD; it does not melt if exposed to liquids. The flexibility of the material makes it easier to don and doff than the stiff plaster RRD. Because the SRD closely resembles a transtibial socket, greater carryover about proper use of prosthetic socks for optimal fit in the socket of the initial (preparatory, temporary, or training) prosthesis is likely.[26] The major disadvantage of a polyethylene SRD is the cost associated with casting and fabrication. Because most residual limbs become progressively smaller with maturation in the weeks and months after amputation, several successfully smaller SRDs may need to be fabricated as the limb shrinks. In some settings, plaster RRDs are used until the initial prosthetic fitting. At that point, the prosthetist makes a polyethylene SRD in addition to the socket for the training prosthesis.

An alternative method for semirigid dressing after amputation is the application of an UNNA paste dressing to the residual limb immediately after wound closure in the operating room.[27,28] The UNNA paste dressing was initially developed for the management of venous stasis ulcers. Zinc oxide, glycerin, calamine, and gelatin are impregnated into a roll of gauze to create a pasty dressing that easily adheres to the skin. The UNNA dressing typically dries to a semirigid leathery consistency within 24 hours.[17] Although not as rigid and protective as a rigid dressing or RRD, UNNA paste dressings are more effective in limiting postoperative edema than are soft dressings and Ace wrapping.[27] The UNNA semirigid dressing can be left on for as long as 5–7 days; if more frequent wound inspection is desired, it can be easily removed with bandage scissors. Because the UNNA dressing remains in place for an extended period of time, fewer opportunities are available for limb desensitization and patient education about socket fit compared to those of the RRD and polyethylene SRD.

Soft Dressings and Compression

The traditional postoperative edema control and wound management strategy is a soft gauze dressing with compressive Ace bandage wrap. This method continues to be the most frequently used immediate postsurgical option for patients with transfemoral amputation. Although Ace wrapping may be the most viable option when significant wound drainage and a high risk of infection are present, this method of compression is not nearly as effective in limiting postoperative edema as those described previously.[7] Soft dressings are not able to protect a healing incision from bumps, bruising, or shearing during activity or from fall-related injury. The other practical disadvantage of elastic Ace bandage compression of the residual limb is the need for frequent reapplication: Movement during daily activities quickly loosens the bandages,

compromising the effectiveness of the compression. Most rehabilitation professionals suggest that Ace bandages should be removed and reapplied every 4–6 hours and should never be kept in place for more than 12 hours without rebandaging.[29]

Effective application of an Ace wrap requires practice, manual dexterity, and attention to details if the desired distal-to-proximal pressure gradient is to be achieved[7,17,19] (Figures 23-5 and 23-6). It may be difficult for patients with limited vision, arthritis of the hands and wrist, limited trunk mobility, or compromised postural control to master this technique for independence in control of edema. It is very important that nurses, residents, surgeons, therapists, prosthetists, and family members (and anyone else who may be taking down the soft dressing to care for the wound) be consistent and effective in reapplication of the Ace bandage if maximal control of edema is to be achieved. Ineffectively applied elastic wraps can lead to a bulbous, poorly shaped residual limb, which is likely to delay prosthetic fitting.[23] Tight circumferential wrapping can significantly compromise blood flow, compromising healing of the incision and even leading to skin breakdown.[23]

Several alternatives are available for elastic compression when Ace wrap proves to be cumbersome or problematic. One method that is effective for patients with a bulbous or pressure-sensitive residual limb is application of a elasticized stockinet or Tubigrip sock. Both materials are available with various levels of elasticity; minimal to significant compression can be achieved, depending on the patient's tolerance of pressure. Wu[25] describes a double-layer method in which a long piece of elastic stockinet or Tubigrip is carefully applied over the transtibial residual limb to midthigh level (Figure 23-7).[5] The extra length of elastic stockinet or Tubigrip is then turned or twisted 180 degrees (to minimize pressure over the new incision) and rolled over the residual limb as a second layer of compression. As the patient's residual limb volume decreases and the limb becomes more pressure tolerant, stockinet or Tubigrip with progressively narrower diameters can be used to increase compressive forces and facilitate limb shrinkage and maturation. These materials are relatively inexpensive, but they are not as durable as commerically available elastic shrinker socks.

Commercially Available Shrinker Garments

Once the suture line has healed sufficiently, many prosthetists and therapists recommend that patients begin to use commercially manufactured elastic shrinker garments whenever the prosthesis is not being worn (Figure 23-8). Most shrinkers are designed to apply significant compressive force to the residual limb, and it may be difficult

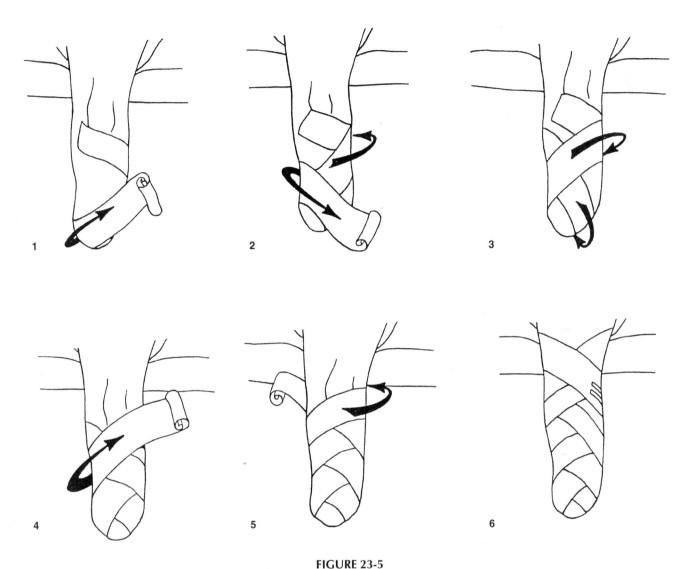

FIGURE 23-5

The application of an effective Ace wrap to a transtibial residual limb uses successive diagonal figure-of-eight loops between the distal residual limb and thigh to create a distal-to-proximal pressure gradient. This creates a distal-to-proximal, tapering, cylindrical residual limb with minimal excess distal soft tissue. (Adapted from LA Karacollof, CS Hammersley, FJ Schneider. Lower Extremity Amputation. Gaithersburg, MD: Aspen, 1992;16–17.)

for patients with limited manual dexterity or upper extremity strength to apply them. Patients with recent amputation must be careful to minimize or avoid excessive shear forces over the incision as the shrinker is being applied. Although shrinkers are very effective for control of edema and limb volume, it is not possible to create "relief" for bony prominences or pressure-vulnerable areas on the residual limb. As with other soft dressings, commercial shrinkers cannot protect the residual limb from trauma during daily activities or in the event of a fall. It is not unusual for patients to continue to use a shrinker for limb volume control, whenever they are not wearing their prosthesis, for 6 months to a year after amputation.

Although a number of edema control options are available for patients with transtibial amputation, those with tranfemoral residual limbs have fewer strategies from which to choose. Commercially manufactured shrinkers are more convenient to don and are more likely to remain in place than the more cumbersome Ace wraps, but patients who choose this option must be just as careful to capture all the soft tissue high in the groin within the shrinker to avoid the development of an adductor roll. Another alternative for patients with transfemoral amputation is a custom-fit Jobst pressure garment. Jobst garments can be fabricated either as a half-panty or full pant garment; the full pant garment achieves a more consis-

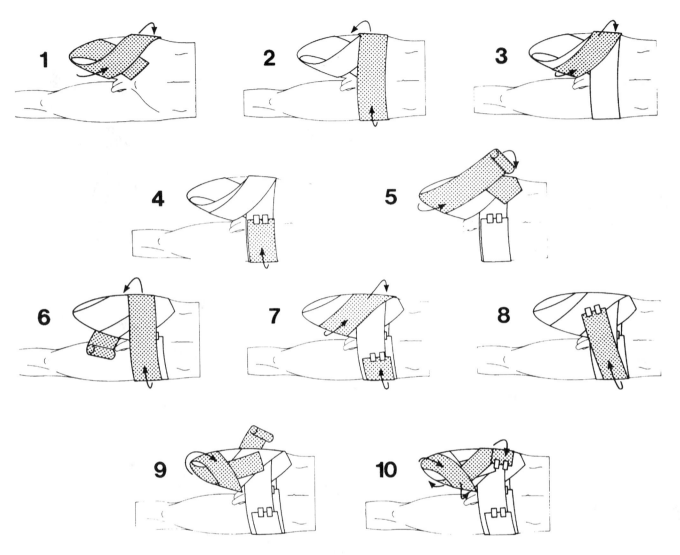

FIGURE 23-6

The application of an effective Ace wrap to a transfemoral limb also strives to create a distal-to-proximal pressure gradient using a modified figure-of-eight pattern. For patients with transfemoral amputation, the wrap is anchored around the pelvis and applied to pull the hip toward hip extension and adduction. Note the importance of capturing soft tissue high in the groin within the Ace wrap, to reduce the risk of developing an adductor roll of noncompressed soft tissue. (Reprinted with permission from BJ May. Amputation and Prosthetics: A Case Study Approach. Philadelphia: FA Davis, 1996;84.)

tent suspension and compression, especially for patients who are obese. A Jobst garment may be the only effective alternative for patients with very short transfemoral amputation.

Selecting the Appropriate Compression Device

In deciding which edema control and limb-shaping strategy is most appropriate for a given patient, the rehabilitation team considers the following questions[23]:

1. Is the patient able to don/doff the device independently? If not, is a family member available who can assist with this task?
2. Given the patient's physical characteristics and likely level of activity, will the device remain securely in place on the residual limb?
3. Will the device apply enough compression for effective progressive limb shrinkage?
4. Will the device apply enough compression for symmetric shaping of the residual limb?

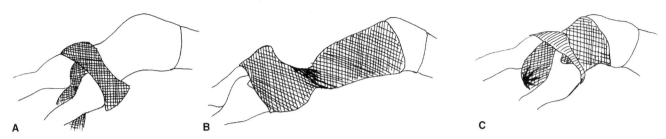

FIGURE 23-7

One strategy to control edema and manage limb volume is to use a double layer of an elastic stockinet or Tubigrip to apply compressive forces to the limb. After the initial layer (A) has been smoothly applied, the stockinet is twisted closed (B) at the end of the limb, and the excess is applied (C) as a second layer of compression.

5. Will the device protect the skin and healing suture line during daily activities, and does use of the device carry any risk of skin irritation or breakdown?

6. Is the device comfortable for the patient to use or wear over the long periods of time that are required for effective control or edema and limb shaping?

7. Is the device relatively cost effective in terms of fabrication, modification, and replacement?

It is important to monitor tissue tolerance and potential areas of pressure closely in whatever edema control method is chosen, especially in the first few days and weeks after amputation. Although rigid dressings, IPOPs, and UNNA dressings remain on the limb for extended periods, each of the other methods of edema control and shaping should be removed and reapplied a minimum of three times each day, to assure appropriate fit and tissue tolerance in the acute phase of healing. When a rigid cast or IPOP is removed, it must be quickly replaced with an alternative compression device so that limb volume does not increase substantially. The patient with recent amputation will wear the compression device at all times, unless walking in a training prosthesis (even time out of compression during bathing should be as short as possible). Most patients find that a compression device is necessary to maintain the desired limb volume for 6 months to a year after surgery. Some patients with mature residual limbs who have fluctuation in volume due to concurrent medical conditions continue to require compression well beyond the first postoperative year. Because some patients experience a transient increase in residual limb volume after a shower or bathing, many choose to bathe in the evening so that volume change does not interfere with prosthetic use. Those who prefer to bathe in the morning may need to use a compression device immediately after bathing to achieve optimal prosthetic fit and suspension, especially

if suction suspension (which requires consistent limb volume) is used. Those who use prosthetic socks may require a few less ply of sock immediately after bathing but need to add a few more ply after a few hours as limb volume decreases.

PHYSICAL THERAPY ASSESSMENT

Ideally, patients who are about to undergo "elective" amputation of a dysvascular or neuropathic limb are referred to physical therapy for a comprehensive preoperative assessment. In some instances, input from rehabilitation professionals may be sought by trauma surgeons to assist patients and families in making informed decisions when faced with amputation after severe crush

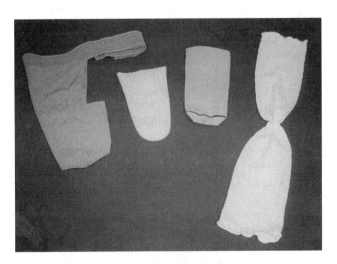

FIGURE 23-8

Examples of commercially available transfemoral (left) and transtibial shrinkers used for edema control and shaping of the residual limb.

injury of the limb. This early contact provides an opportunity to educate patients and their families about the early days of rehabilitation and the process of prosthetic prescription. It also is an opportunity for the physical therapist to collect information about the patient's health, functional status, and home environment important for clinical decision making about the rehabilitation program, prosthetic candidacy, and discharge planning. In some settings, the physical therapist and prosthetist, as members of the interdisciplinary rehabilitation team, may be involved in discussion with surgeons, patients, and family members about surgical levels, in terms of potential for prosthetic use and optimization of rehabilitation.[30] The earlier that the initial assessment can occur, the greater the opportunity to develop a true transdisciplinary assessment and plan of care. Effective communication and strong relationships between the surgeons, orthopedists, or trauma teams who perform the majority of amputations and the rehabilitation team substantially improve the quality of patient care and facilitate the rehabilitation process. If preoperative assessment is not possible, referral to rehabilitation should be made as soon after surgery as possible; delaying referrals often leads to contracture formation, further cardiovascular and musculoskeletal deconditioning, delayed prosthetic fitting and training, and a greater risk of dependency for the patient.[30] The components of a comprehensive assessment for patients with lower extremity amputation are summarized in Table 23-1.

Preoperative Assessment and Education

One of the most important aspects of preoperative assessment is determination of the patient's usual ambulatory status. The therapist is interested in learning about the patient's use of assistive devices and need for assistance, the usual distances walked, the frequency of walking, any factors that limit walking, and the type of walking environment (level inside, uneven outside, stairs and ramps, etc.). Patient and family self-report as well as direct observation of the patient walking provide this information. Preamputation ambulatory status is a strong predictor of functional postoperative prosthetic use.[31] Additionally, the therapist is interested in assessing the patient's postural control during transitional activities, such as rising to standing from a seated position on the bed or chair. Providing an opportunity for the patient to practice moving from sitting to standing and ambulation with an appropriate assistive device allow the therapist to identify potential problems with balance and postural control. This also helps the patient to anticipate what mobility will be like in the early postoperative period.

Assessment of skin condition and the vascular, sensory, and motor status of the patient's limbs (especially the remaining limb) is also important. The opportunity is present during this assessment to introduce the patient and family to the strategies that are likely to be used for pain management and compression/edema control after surgery. It is also very important to instruct the patient and family about proper positioning and the need to maintain knee extension and neutral hip alignment to minimize soft tissue tightness and joint contracture.

Information about the patient's medical and surgical history can be obtained from review of the medical record and an interview with the patient and family members. Information about the circumstances that have led to amputation is important, as are comorbid conditions and associated impairments and functional limitations, pharmacologic regimes, or other medical interventions that are likely to have an impact on rehabilitation and prosthetic use. Potentially important medical conditions include diabetes, cardiovascular disease, cerebrovascular disease, neuropathy, renal disease, congestive heart failure, uncontrolled hypertension, and preexisting neuromuscular or musculoskeletal pathologies or impairments. These conditions potentially have an impact on wound healing, functional mobility, and exercise tolerance during rehabilitation. Healing and risk of infection are also concerns for patients with compromised immune system function, whether from diseases such as human immunodeficiency virus (HIV)/acquired immunodeficiency syndrome (AIDS) or from chemotherapy or steroid use. Wound healing, skin condition, and endurance may be issues for patients who are currently undergoing radiation treatments for cancer. The presence of visual impairment has implications for the patient's ability to self-monitor his or her wound and skin condition and for selection of prosthetic components and suspension methods.

Forecasting the potential for prosthetic replacement and rehabilitation can be challenging; decisions must be informed by several factors:

1. The overall health, cognitive, and preamputation functional status of the patient
2. The level of amputation as it impacts on prosthetic control and the energy cost of walking
3. The likely contribution of prosthetic use to performance of basic and instrumental activities of daily living, for the patient and for the caregivers
4. The resources (financial and instrumental) that are available to the patient

TABLE 23-1

Comprehensive Assessment for Patients with Lower Extremity Amputation

History

Demographics	Age, primary language, race/ethnicity, gender
Social history	Family and caregiver resources, other social support systems
Occupation/social	Employment or retirement status, typical work and leisure activities
Living environment	Characteristics and accessibility of "home" environment, projected discharge destination
Current condition	Reason for referral, current concerns/needs, previous medical/surgical interventions for current condition
Past medical history	Review of systems: cardiopulmonary, endocrine/metabolic, musculoskeletal, neuro-muscular, gastrointestinal, genitourinary
	Prior hospitalizations and surgeries
	Smoking, alcohol, or drug use (past and present)
Family history	Health risk factors for vascular disease, cardiac disease, etc.
Medications	Prescription medication for current and other medical conditions
	Over-the-counter medications typically used
Functional status	Current and prior abilities and functional limitations [activities of daily living/instrumental activities of daily living (IADL)]

Assessments

Vital signs	Blood pressure, heart rate, respiratory rate (resting and in activity), limb vascularity
	Vascular supply (palpation/auscultation of lower extremity pulses)
	Skin temperature and presence of trophic changes
	Skin color and response to elevation or dependent position
	Autonomic responses and risk of postural (orthostatic) hypotension
Aerobic capacity	Perceived exertion, dyspnea, angina, during functional activity
	Claudication and its impact on function
	Overall level of physical fitness and functional capacity
Anthropomorphic assessment	Residual limb length (bone length, soft tissue length)
	Residual limb girth, redundant tissue ("dog ears," adductor roll)
	Residual limb shape (bulbous, cylindrical, conical)
	Assessment of type and severity of edema
	Effectiveness of edema control strategy being used
	Overall height, weight, body composition
Cognition/emotion	Level of consciousness, sleep patterns
	Ability to learn and preferred learning style
	Cognitive dysfunction screening (delirium, depression, dementia)
	Other factors that have an impact on motivation, attention, learning
Mobility	Changing position in bed (rolling, scooting, coming to sitting)
	Dynamic (anticipatory and reactive) postural control in sitting
	Ability to transfer to/from bed, toilet, wheelchair, mat, tub/shower
Assistive devices and adaptive equipment	Assistive devices/adaptive equipment currently being used
	Ability to use ambulatory aid safely for single limb gait
	Ability to use wheelchair safely
	Adaptations/equipment needed for patient's living environment
Gait and balance	Assessment of postural control in quiet standing, reaching, ability to stop/start, change direction, alter velocity while walking
	Reaction to unexpected perturbation, at rest and during activity
	Observational gait assessment, identification of gait deviations
	Kinematic gait assessment (e.g., speed, stride length, cadence)
	Energy cost or efficiency of locomotion/gait
	Ability/safety to manage uneven terrain, stairs, ramps
Skin/integument	Assessment of surgical wound healing
	Assessment/management of adhesions and existing scar tissue
	Other skin problems (other incisions, grafts, psoriasis, cysts, etc.)
	Integrity of remaining foot/limb, especially if neuropathic or dysvascular
Joint integrity/mobility	Range of motion, soft tissue length, and joint contracture
	Ligamentous integrity or joint instability
	Structural alignment or joint deformity
	Integrity or inflammation of synovium, bursae, cartilage
Motor function	Motor control, including dexterity, coordination, agility, tone
	Motor learning, including previous use of ambulatory aids, prostheses

continued

TABLE 23-1 *(continued)*

Muscle function	Current muscle strength of upper extremity, trunk, lower extremity
	Muscular power for functional activity
	Muscular endurance for functional activity
	Potential for improvement
Pain	Presence of phantom limb sensation or pain
	Postoperative pain and pain management strategies
	Muscle soreness related to altered movement patterns
	Joint pain related to motion or comorbid arthritis, etc.
Sensory integrity	Protective sensation of residual and remaining limb
	Superficial sensation: light touch, sharp/dull, pressure, temperature
	Proprioception: kinesthesia, position sense
Posture	Resting posture in sitting, standing, other positions
	Alteration in posture due to loss of limb segment
Prosthetic requirements	Potential for functional prosthetic use
	Readiness for prosthetic fitting/prescription
	Appropriate prosthetic design, components, suspension
Self-care	Ability to perform basic activities of daily living
	Ability to perform IADL
	Availability of assistance and preparation of caregivers
Community/work reintegration	Analysis of roles/activities/tasks
	Functional capacity analysis, determination of essential functions
	Analysis of environment, safety assessment
	Assessment of need for adaptation

Source: Adapted from The Guide to Physical Therapy Practice; Pattern K: Impaired gait, locomotion, and balance, and impaired motor function secondary to lower extremity amputation. Phys Ther 1997;77(11):1354–1367.

Premorbid level of mobility, activities of daily living status, and level of amputation contribute more to an accurate projection of rehabilitation potential and prosthetic use after amputation than does any single or combination of comorbid health factors.[32] A long list of past or chronic illnesses does not predict poor rehabilitation potential: Patients often manage multiple chronic conditions effectively and become highly functional prosthetic users. Long-term outcome is harder to forecast: The relatively high morbidity and mortality for patients with amputation secondary to vascular disease have been well documented.[33–35] Unless clear evidence is found that ambulation will not be possible and that provision of prosthesis will not improve the patient's mobility (for example, reducing the amount of assistance that is necessary to transfer), prosthetic replacement should be considered.

POSTOPERATIVE ASSESSMENT AND INTERVENTION

After amputation surgery, the focus shifts to preparation for prosthetic use. Strategies for control of edema, pain management, and facilitation of wound healing are implemented. The patient receives instruction and the opportunity to practice single limb mobility with an appropriate assistive device. Handling of the residual limb during dressing changes and skin inspection, as well as the consistent use of compression devices, helps to desensitize the residual limb, enhancing readiness for prosthetic use. Exercises to strengthen key muscle groups in the residual and remaining limb and to facilitate effective postural responses are implemented to facilitate function and prepare for prosthetic gait.

Healing of the Residual Limb

In most settings, the surgeon who performed the amputation assesses the condition of the surgical site at the initial dressing change. This can occur as early as the first postoperative day when soft dressings and elastic wraps have been used or on the third postoperative day if the residual limb has been casted in a rigid dressing. After this initial assessment, the status of the surgical wound is assessed by the nurse or physician at each dressing change. The physical therapist also inspects the residual limb to monitor the stage of healing of the incision and the limb's shape, length, sensory integrity, and volume; he or she works closely with the surgeon in postoperative wound management and timing of prosthetic replacement.

With each dressing change, the wound is carefully inspected and the quantity and quality of drainage from the wound are documented. During the first several postoperative days, it is not unusual to note that fair amounts of serosanguineous drainage have been absorbed by the dressing as the surgical wound begins to heal. The amount of drainage is expected to decrease over time as healing occurs. Significant amounts of bright red arterial blood or darker venous blood should be reported to the surgeon for further assessment. Thickening discolored drainage may be a signal of infection of the wound, especially if accompanied by a foul odor.

Wound closure and tissue integrity are also monitored closely. In the first several postoperative days, signs of mild inflammation may be present along the incision line secondary to tissue trauma. The edges of the wound should be closely approximate for effective primary healing; any areas of wound separation, scab or eschar formation, ecchymosis, or other signs of tissue fragility or decreased viability are carefully documented and monitored. Many patients with traumatic or other nondysvascular amputation have achieved sufficient healing by postoperative day 10 to be casted for their training prosthesis. Patients who required amputation secondary to vascular disease may have healed sufficiently for prosthetic casting as soon as 14 days after operation (Figure 23-9). When primary healing has been achieved, the surgeon can begin to remove sutures or staples from the incision. Initially, every other or every third suture/staple can be left in place to guard against wound dehiscence, to be removed several days later. One or two sutures can be left in place for longer periods if healing has been delayed in one or more areas of the incision. The wound is typically reinforced with Steri-Strips when sutures or staples are removed to protect the incision from shearing forces during preprosthetic activity and early prosthetic training. The Steri-Strips can remain on the limb for 2 or more additional weeks after the sutures/staples have been removed. Gait training with a prosthesis can begin, with the approval of the surgeon, when clear evidence of primary healing is found, even if several sutures have been left in place to protect an area along the incision line that has been slow in closing.

Delayed healing of the surgical wound necessarily delays prosthetic use. Patients with diabetes and vascular insufficiency are particularly at risk for delayed healing. The healing process can also be delayed as a consequence of infection, immunosuppression, or traumatic damage sustained during activity or in a fall. Nutritional status is another important determinant of wound healing in the early postoperative and preprosthetic period. Patients with compromised nutritional status are more likely to experience delayed wound healing and are at greater risk of postoperative infection as well as cardiopulmonary and septic complications.[36]

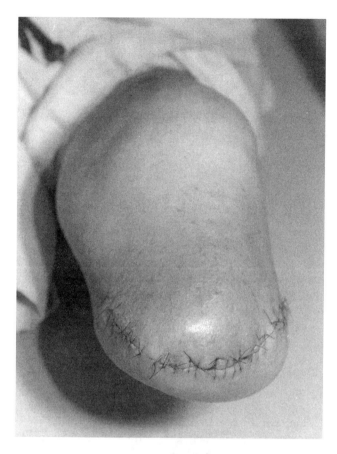

FIGURE 23-9

A well-healed, transtibial residual limb with a "fish mouth" incision 14 days after amputation. The edges of the wound are approximate, and although several small scabs have formed between sutures, primary healing is well established. Strategies for control of edema and initial limb shaping have been successful as well; this residual limb could be described as cylindrical, with very little redundant tissue present.

Skin Care and Scar Management

It is very important that the incision does not adhere to underlying deep tissue or bone as healing progresses. Ideally, enough gliding movement will be present between the skin and the underlying layer of soft tissue that shear forces will be minimal while the prosthesis is donned and used for function. An adherent scar at the distal tibia can be quite problematic: If a point of adherence is present along an incisional scar, the mobility of tissues will be compromised. The resulting traction and shear forces are likely to lead to discomfort, skin irritation, and often to recurrent breakdown of soft tissues with prosthetic use. Once primary healing has been established, the patient can learn to use gentle manual massage to enhance tissue mobility in preparation for prosthetic use. Initially, this is performed above and below, but not across, the incision to minimize the risk of dehiscence. When the wound is well closed and Steri-Strips are no longer necessary to support and protect the incision, the patient can begin to gently mobilize the scar itself. Handling of the limb during soft tissue mobilization and massage not only minimizes adhesion formation but also helps the patient to adapt his or her body image to include the postamputation residual limb and to prepare for the sensory experience of prosthetic use.

Patients with new amputation may have surgical scars from previous vascular bypass or from harvesting veins for coronary artery bypass surgery. These may require carefully applied soft tissue mobilization or friction massage to free adhesions and restore the mobility of the skin. Patients with traumatic amputation may have healing skin grafts or abrasions from road burn, thermal injury, or electrical burns. In such cases, wound care and debridement are important components of preprosthetic rehabilitation. For patients with healing burns or skin graft, the use of an appropriate compression garment or shrinker facilitates healing and maturation of skin, controls postoperative edema, and shapes the residual limb.

Once the sutures have been removed, patients can resume normal bathing and establish a routine for daily skin care. Most physicians, prosthetists, and therapists recommend daily cleansing of the residual limb with a mild nondrying soap. Patting or gently rubbing the limb with a terry cloth towel until it is fully dry also helps to desensitize it in preparation for prosthetic use. A small amount of moisturizer or skin cream can be applied if the skin of the residual limb is dry or flaky. A limb with soft, healthy pliable skin is much more tolerant of prosthetic wear than a limb with tough, dry, easily irritated skin. Patients are taught to inspect the skin of the entire residual limb carefully, using a mirror if necessary to visualize hard-to-see areas. Areas over bony prominences that may be vulnerable to high pressure within the socket are especially important to assess. Patients with amputation are as likely to have other dermatologic conditions (such as eczema or psoriasis) as the general population. Those with hairy limbs or easily irritated skin may be more at risk of folliculitis and similar inflammatory skin conditions once the prosthesis is worn consistently. Effective early management of skin irritation or other skin problems is important: Serious skin irritation or infection precludes prosthetic use until adequate healing as occurred.

Some patients mistakenly assume that something must be used to toughen the skin in preparation for prosthetic use. They may opt to rub the skin with alcohol, vinegar, salt water, or even gasoline, erroneously thinking that this will make the skin more pressure tolerant. In fact, these "treatments" can damage the skin, making it more susceptible to pressure-related problems. Patient and family education about effective cleansing and skin care strategies is essential in the early postoperative/preprosthetic period.[7]

Limb Length and Volume

The length and volume of the residual limb are important determinants of readiness for prosthetic use as well as socket design and components chosen for the training prosthesis. Initial measurements can be made at the first dressing change. Changes in limb volume are tracked by frequent remeasurement during the preprosthetic period of rehabilitation.

The two components of residual limb length are the actual length of the residual tibia or femur and the total length of the limb, including soft tissue. Measurements are taken from an easily identified bony landmark to the palpated end of the long bone, to the incision line, or to the end of soft tissue. In the transtibial limb, the starting place for measurement is most often the medial joint line; an alternative is to begin measurement at the tibial tubercle. In the transfemoral limb, the starting place for measurement can be the ischial tuberosity or the greater trochanter. Clear notation must be made about the proximal and distal landmarks that are used for the initial measurement to ensure consistency in the subsequent measurement process. A standard-length transtibial amputation, which preserves 5–6 in. of tibia (measured from the tibial plateau) ensures sufficient lever arm for effective prosthetic control. Transtibial limbs of less than 3 in. may be insufficient in length for prosthetic control and in surface area for skin tolerance of weight-bearing pressures applied by the socket.[37] Patients with long transtibial residual limbs may be unable to flex the knee beyond 90 degrees in sitting when wearing their prosthesis because of distal anterior discomfort or skin irritation where the limb contacts the socket. For patients with transfemoral amputation, preservation of as much of the length of the femur as possible enhances control of the prosthetic knee unit; however, the choice of knee units may be limited when the transfemoral limb is very long.[38]

Residual limb volume is assessed by serial circumferential girth measurements. For patients with transtibial amputation, circumferential measurement begins at either the medial tibial plateau or the tibial tubercle and is repeated at equally spaced points to the end of the limb (Figure 23-10). For patients with transfemoral amputation, measurement begins at either the ischial tuberosity or the greater trochanter and is also repeated at equally spaced points to the end of the residual limb. The interval between measurements should be clearly documented (i.e., every 5 cm or every inch) for consistency and reliability in the measurement process. One of the determinants of readiness for prosthetic fitting is comparison of the proximal and distal circumference of the limb. Often, referral for prosthetic fit is made when the distal limb circumference measurement is the same (i.e., equal to or no more than ¼ in. greater) than proximal limb circumference. Ideally, with effective control of edema and compression, the transtibial residual limb will mature into a tapered cylindrical shape with distal circumference slightly less than proximal circumference. The transfemoral limb typically matures into a more conical shape, with distal circumference significantly less than proximal ones. A smaller distal circumference is desirable so that shear forces on soft tissue will be minimal when the prosthesis is donned and used.

Range of Motion

Having near normal range of motion in the remaining joints of the residual limb is essential for effective prosthetic use. Patients with recent amputation are very much at risk for development of soft tissue contracture during the preprosthetic period. The risk of hip and knee flexion contracture formation is associated with spending long periods of time sitting in a wheelchair or resting in bed, before and after amputation surgery. Other factors that can contribute to the risk of flexion contracture formation include the protective flexion withdrawal pattern associated with lower extremity pain, muscle imbalances that result from loss of muscle distal attachments, and the loss of tonic sensory input generated by weight bearing on the sole of the foot. Because limitation in lower extremity range of motion can have a significant impact on the quality and energy efficiency of prosthetic gait, it is essential to assess and monitor range of motion. It is equally important to implement strategies to prevent or minimize contracture development as early in the postoperative/preprosthetic period as possible.

For patients with transtibial amputation, definitive measurement of hip range of motion is possible with standard goniometric techniques. With the loss of the malleolus as a distal reference point, accurate measurement of knee extension range of motion can be challenging, especially

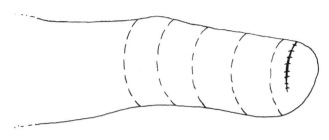

FIGURE 23-10

Limb volume and shape of a transtibial residual limb is assessed by taking successive circumferential measures (dotted lines) from a bony landmark, such as the medial joint line, to the suture line.

when a short residual limb is present (Figure 23-11). Familiarity with the normal anatomy of the tibia improves the therapist's positioning of the mobile arm of the goniometer and the accuracy of measurement. For patients with transtibial and transfemoral amputation, the Thomas test may be an effective tool for determining the severity of hip flexion contracture (Figure 23-12). Full hip extension is critical for prosthetic knee stability when walking with a transfemoral prosthesis. The accuracy of standard goniometric measurement of hip adduction and abduction decreases as residual limb length decreases. There is no effective way to assess rotation of the transfemoral residual limb.

Hip flexor tightness is likely to result in increased lumbar lordosis when the patient is standing and walking with a prosthesis later in the rehabilitation process. Attempts to achieve an upright posture over the prosthesis in the presence of hip flexion contracture can lead, over time, to excessive mobility of the lumbosacral spine. Patients who use a transfemoral prosthesis are very much at risk for this problem: Secondary spinal dysfunction and back pain can be more disabling than the original amputation. Attention to the importance of achieving near normal joint range of motion and soft tissue excursion early in the preprosthetic period has a powerful impact on effective prosthetic use over the long run.

While the patient is sitting or lying in bed, the natural tendency is for the lower limb to roll outward into a slightly

FIGURE 23-11

Measurement of knee extension for patients with transtibial amputation requires an understanding of the normal anatomy of the tibia, to compensate for loss of the distal malleollus as a point of reference for the mobile arm of the goniometer.

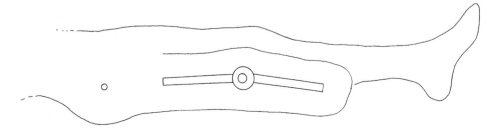

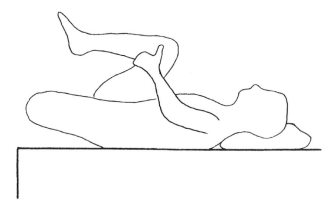

FIGURE 23-12
The Thomas test can be used to assess the tightness or contracture of hip flexors for patients with transtibial and transfemoral residual limbs. The patient is positioned in supine with both limbs flexed toward the chest and the pelvis in slight posterior tilt. While the opposite limb is supported in place, the residual limb is gently lowered toward the support surface. Tightness or contracture of hip flexors causes the pelvis to move into an anterior tilt before the limb is fully lowered.

flexed, abducted, and externally rotated position. Excursion of the hip is important to assess; tightness of external rotators may be masked by apparent tightness of hip flexors or abductors. The functional length of two-joint muscles is also important to consider. Adequate hamstring length is essential if the patient with recent transtibial amputation is to maintain a fully extended knee when seated. If the knee is held in extension by a rigid dressing or thermoplastic splint, hamstring tightness pulls the pelvis into a marked posterior tilt. Instead of sitting squarely on the ischial tuberosities, the patient sits in a kyphotic position with weight shifted onto the sacrum. This compromised postural alignment increases the risk of spinal dysfunction and of skin irritation and decubitus ulcer formation. Tightness in the rectus femoris, satorius, and tensor fascia latae can interfere with advanced mobility skills, such as the ability to kneel while transferring to and from the floor.

Positioning and Stretching

Because of the high risk of knee flexion contracture for patients with transtibial amputation and the negative impact of such contracture on future prosthetic use, proper positioning is a key component of preprosthetic rehabilitation. Prolonged dependence of the residual limb held in knee flexion when sitting also leads to development of distal edema, which can delay readiness for prosthetic fitting. Patients with transtibial amputation must maintain the knee in as much extension as possible, whether

in bed, sitting in a wheelchair or lounge chair, or during exercise and activity. Although it may be comfortable to place a pillow under the knee when sitting or lying in bed, a more effective strategy is to position a small towel roll under the distal posterior residual limb to encourage knee extension. Use of a wheelchair with elevating leg rests helps the patient to keep the residual limb in an extended position, although a "bridge" between the seat and calf support may be necessary for patients with short residual limbs. In some settings, the therapist fabricates a posterior trough splint from low-temperature thermoplastic materials; this splint supports the limb in knee extension when the patient is resting in bed or sitting in a wheelchair. If a patient is able to assume a prone position, the weight of the limb can be used to facilitate elongation of the hamstring muscles and soft tissue of the posterior knee (Figure 23-13). A small towel roll positioned just above the patella effectively positions the limb for elongation. Modalities such as moist heat or ultrasound, followed by manual physical therapy techniques such as manual passive stretching, Proprioceptive Neuromuscular Facilitation (PNF) hold-relax, or deep effleurage massage may be effective in reducing existing knee flexion contracture.[39] Patients also learn to perform home exercises (done at the bedside while an inpatient or at home while an outpatient) that are designed to elongate muscles and soft tissue to counteract the tendency to development of tightness. Performed independently or with the assistance of a family member or caregiver several times a day, these stretching exercises are important adjuncts to physical therapy sessions during preprosthetic and prosthetic rehabilitation.

Significant hip flexion contracture can render a patient with transfemoral amputation ineffective in controlling a prosthetic knee unit and walking with a prosthesis.[37] Because patients with transfemoral amputation spend significant amounts of time in a seated position, development of hip flexor and abductor tightness is almost inevitable. Physical therapy interventions that elongate these soft tissues, including manual stretching, active exercise, and functional postural training, are used to counteract the tendency for tightness to develop.[38-40] Resting in a prone position with a towel roll under the distal anterior residual limb provides prolonged elongation for tight hip flexors. Care must be taken, however, to maintain a neutral pelvis or slight posterior tilt when lying prone. Excessive hip flexor tightness leads to lordosis of the lumbosacral spine.

Muscle Strength and Function

Although assessment of strength and maximization of muscle function are key components of preprosthetic and prosthetic rehabilitation, definitive strength assessment

FIGURE 23-13

Prone positioning for stretching of the posterior soft tissue and prevention of knee flexion contracture. A small towel roll placed just above the patella elevates the residual limb from the surface of the mat or bed. The therapist can use hold-relax or contract-relax techniques, or the patient can actively contract the quadriceps to facilitate elongation of the hamstrings and posterior soft tissues.

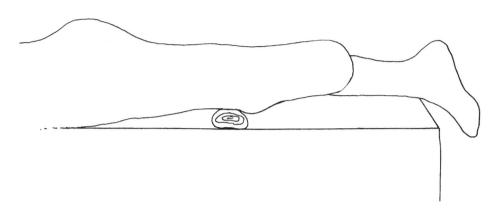

beyond active, nonresisted antigravity motion and progressive resistive exercise must be postponed at the joint just proximal to the amputation until evidence of adequate healing of the surgical site is seen. For patients with transtibial amputation, standard manual muscle testing or hand-held dynamometry techniques are used to assess hip muscle strength and power.[41] Until the surgeon gives clearance, however, observation of active knee flexion and extension strength is used to determine if at least fair (full antigravity) strength is present. For patients with transfemoral amputation, assessment of hip muscle strength beyond active antigravity fair muscle grade must also be postponed pending incisional healing.

Once the surgeon and rehabilitation team are confident that enough healing has occurred so that the incision cannot be compromised by externally applied resistance, definitive strength testing can be implemented. It is important to note that, because of the length of the residual limb, the tester has to apply the resistive force at a more proximal position on the extremity than is defined by standard manual muscle test (MMT) technique. Because of this altered manual contact, the mechanical advantage of the tester is reduced, and the patient's apparent strength grade may be somewhat inflated. This altered point of force application has an impact on the validity of test results. Many therapists attempt to maximize validity by first testing the intact or remaining limb (assuming similarity of strength between the patient's limbs), using the standard technique to assign a muscle grade. The intact limb is then retested with a more proximal hand placement, simulating the position for testing of the residual limb. This grade serves as a point of reference when the residual limb is then tested.

Because a healing suture line may be vulnerable to resistive forces applied during strength testing or strengthening exercise, resistance to knee extension should only be applied if and when the suture line can be observed. According to

this guideline, resistance must not be applied through a soft dressing or compressive garment during the first several weeks of the preprosthetic program. Unless healing has been delayed, most surgeons consider initiation of conservative resistive exercise a few days after sutures have been removed, perhaps as early as the seventh postoperative day for patients with traumatic amputation or 12 or more days for the patient with dysvascular/neuropathic amputation. Surgeon preference, tissue integrity, and the patient's cardiovascular condition must be factored into strength assessment and strengthening exercise programs.

Strengthening programs have two goals: (1) remediation of specific weakness detected in the evaluation and (2) maximization of overall strength and muscular endurance for safe, energy-efficient prosthetic gait. Because functional activities require that patients use their muscles at varying lengths and types of contraction, effective preprosthetic exercise programs include activities that require concentric, holding (isometric), eccentric, and co-contraction in a variety of positions and muscle lengths.[42] In the immediate postoperative period, the specific strengthening program is often a combination of isometric and active isotonic exercise within a limited range of motion of the joint just proximal to the amputation.[7,39,43,44] This strategy minimizes stress or tension across the incision while preserving and improving the strength of key muscle groups. Incorporation of controlled exhalation during isometric contraction minimizes the risks to cardiac function and fluctuations of blood pressure that are associated with the Valsalva maneuver. For patients with transtibial amputation, exercises to strengthen knee extension that are initiated within the first week of amputation might include "quad sets" in the supine position or "short arc quads" performed in supine or sitting. For patients with transfemoral amputation, "glut sets" in the prone or supine position or "short arc" hip extension and abduction in a gravity-eliminated position would be initiated. Gailey recommends an exercise strategy of slow, steadily controlled, 10-second muscular contraction, followed by 5–10 seconds of rest, for 10 repetitions as one that is easily learned and physiologically sound.[39,45] As wound healing is accomplished, exercises can be progressed to include active exercises through larger arcs of motion, active resistive exercise (using weights or manual resistance), or isokinetic training. Application of manual resistance during functional activities, as in PNF, allows the therapist to provide appropriate resistance as muscle strength varies throughout the active range of motion while providing facilitation and augmented sensory feedback to the patient.[46] Isokinetic exercise allows the patient to develop muscular strength and control at a variety of movement velocities.[45]

For patients with transtibial amputation, attachments of the quadriceps and hamstrings are typically intact, and preprosthetic strengthening exercises emphasize control of the knee as well as hip strength for stability in stance. Patients with transfemoral amputation must develop strong hip extension capabilities to control the prosthetic knee unit. They must also have effective hip abduction power if the pelvis is to remain level during stance. It is important to recognize that the distal attachments of the hamstrings, rectus femoris, sartorius, tensor fascia latae/iliotibial band, adductor longus, and adductor magnus are relocated by myodesis or myoplasty or are lost entirely (for patients with short residual limbs) during transfemoral surgery. The combination of an altered line of pull and loss of muscle mass often creates an imbalance of muscle action around the hip.[40,47] The gluteus maximus, gluteus medius, and iliopsoas, with their intact distal attachments, are more powerful in determining resting hip position than the altered adductor group. If the tensor fascia latae/iliotibial band and gluteus maximus become secondarily shortened, function of the adductor group is further compromised. Because of this imbalance, it is important to include activities that strengthen the remaining hip adductors, as well as hip extensors and hip abductors, to prepare the patient for effective postural control in sitting and standing and stance phase stability in prosthetic gait.

General strengthening exercises for the trunk and upper extremities are also essential components of an effective preprosthetic exercise program. Back extensors and abdominal muscles play an important role in postural alignment and postural control. Activities that involve trunk rotation or diagonal movements activate trunk and limb girdle muscles in functional patterns, addressing strength and flexibility for functional activities and enhancing reciprocal arm swing and pelvic control in gait. Upper extremity strengthening, targeting shoulder depressor and elbow extensors, enhances the patient's ability to use an assistive device for single limb ambulation before pros-

thetic fitting. Many patients begin rehabilitation with low endurance: Aerobic exercise programs to improve exercise tolerance and endurance prepare them for the energy demands of single limb and prosthetic ambulation.

Postural Control

Loss of a limb shifts the position of the body's center of mass (COM), moving it slightly upward, backward, and toward the remaining or intact extremity. The magnitude of this shift is determined by the extent of limb loss. The shift may have relatively little impact on postural control and functional ability in patients with Syme's or long transtibial amputation. It may, however, have significant impact on the sitting balance and functional ability of patients with short transfemoral or hip disarticulation amputation. An effective preprosthetic program incorporates activities that challenge patients to improve postural control and equilibrium responses, learning how to control the repositioned COM effectively over an altered base of support. In sitting, this can be accomplished using a variety of reaching tasks, including forward reaching, diagonal reaching across and away from the midline, reaching down to a lower surface or objects, reaching up and away from their center, and turning to reach behind them. Anticipatory and reactive postural responses can also be practiced by throwing and catching games that require an automatic weight shift as part of the activity. The difficulty of the task can be advanced by progressively shifting the location of the catch or toss away from the midline of the patient's trunk; alternating locations from side to side or upward or downward; increasing the speed of the activity; or increasing the weight of the object or ball that is being used.

The effectiveness of postural responses is influenced by the flexibility and strength of the trunk and limb girdles as well as the length and power of the residual limb. The prosthetic replacement of a missing limb increases the functional base of support in sitting; for some patients the weight of the prosthesis serves as a stabilizing anchor during functional activity. For patients with limited flexibility or strength, such a replacement might be essential for effective postural responses and the ability to reach, even if the potential for functional ambulation is small.[47]

Wheelchairs and Seating

Many patients with amputation rely on a wheelchair for mobility during the postoperative and preprosthetic period. Some patients with very short transfemoral amputation or bilateral amputation prefer the relative energy efficiency of wheelchair mobility to ambulation with prostheses. For others, comorbid cardiovascular or cardiopulmonary dysfunction precludes ambulation, and the wheelchair becomes their primary mode of locomotion. The shift in COM after amputation has important implications in choice of wheelchairs.

The design of many standard or traditional wheelchairs is based on the anthropomorphic characteristics of a male adult with intact lower extremities. With the loss of a limb, the COM shifts in a posterior direction; when the patient is seated in a wheelchair, this moves the COM closer to the axis of rotation of the chair's wheels. If the patient with lower extremity amputation turns or reaches backward during a functional activity, the COM shifts even further toward, or even beyond, the wheel axis, and the chair may tip backward. The provision of simple anti-tip devices reduces the risk of posterior tipping during functional activities. For patients with transfemoral or bilateral amputation, a wheelchair with wheels that can be posteriorly offset is recommended. Patients must also be aware of altered dynamics when they are reaching forward while sitting in a wheelchair: High downward pressure on the wheelchair foot plate on the intact side is likely to lead to anterior tipping.

Specific wheelchair assessments and prescription are warranted for all patients who will be using a wheelchair as their primary means of locomotion and mobility. This individual evaluation and prescription process ensures that the wheelchair will provide adequate support of the thighs to increase seating stability and reach, effective seating with an appropriate cushion for pressure distribution, and configuration of components that provides ease of wheelchair locomotion.[47]

Bed Mobility and Transfers

In the acute care setting, physical therapy intervention at the patient's bedside includes instruction about optimal positioning of the residual limb and activities to facilitate the patient's ability to change position in bed and move to or from a seated position. Early mobility and activity significantly reduce the risk of atalectasis, pneumonia, and further physiologic deconditioning.[7] The therapist must, however, be aware of the risk of postural hypotension and of postoperative complications, including deep venous thrombosis and pulmonary embolism. Assessment and monitoring of the patient's vital signs (pulse, respiratory rate, blood pressure, pulse oximetry) is recommend as bed mobility and out-of-bed activity begin. Care must also be taken to minimize the risk of trauma to the newly amputated limb during activity, exercise, or transfers.

Many patients are able to roll from supine to or from the prone position without great difficulty, although those

with transfemoral amputation of the dominant limb may need to develop an adapted movement pattern or sequence. The strategies for transition into sitting are not substantially different from preferred preoperative strategies for most other patients; however, efficiency of postural responses may be challenged by the alteration in body mass after amputation. Patients who have become deconditioned by inactivity in the days and weeks before amputation may find bed rails, a trapeze, bed ladders, or other devices helpful early in rehabilitation. Strategic placement of a bed table or walker near the bedside at night may serve as a reminder of the amputation for patients who are likely to get up during the night to go to the bathroom (without otherwise fully awakening), reducing the risk of falling.

Patient education about the risk of decubitus ulceration and strategies to reduce this risk are also important components of early postoperative care. Patients with vascular disease and neuropathy are particularly at risk, with the heel and lateral border of the remaining foot most vulnerable.[48] Patients with dysvascular limbs may have barely enough circulation to support tissue health in an intact or noninjured foot; once a wound has occurred, circulation may be inadequate for tissue healing. An open wound on the remaining limb would preclude single limb ambulation, increasing the risk of inactivity-related postoperative complications and making prosthetic rehabilitation even more challenging. Pressure-related wounds significantly delay rehabilitation, increase disability, and multiply health care costs for patients with amputation. Vulnerability to pressure increases with sensory impairment; altered mechanical characteristics of injured, calcified, or scarred tissues; poor circulatory status; microclimate of the skin; and (in combination with these factors) advanced age.[49] For patients who have a limited ability to change position, a pressure-distributing mattress and well-designed, carefully applied heel protectors can reduce the risk of decubitus ulcer formation. Helping patients to develop a routine of frequent position change, weight shifting, and exercise reduces weight-bearing pressures and enhances circulation to vulnerable tissues.

An important goal of postoperative preprosthetic rehabilitation is development of the patient's ability to move between seating surfaces or from sitting to standing as safely and independently as possible. Depending on the patient's preamputation level of activity, this may require some degree of assistance or use of adaptive devices or may be accomplished relatively smoothly and easily. Patients who are very deconditioned or who have previous neuromuscular-related postural impairment may require a mechanical lifting aid or multiperson lifting or assistance in the early postoperative period. Other patients may benefit from a strategically placed transfer board as they develop their ability to perform a pivot transfer on their remaining limb. Others may require a walker or crutches for extra stability in single limb stance in the midst of their pivot transfers. Still others quickly master scooting in sitting and pivoting on their remaining limb, to become independent in transfers. Patients with single limb amputation initially prefer transferring toward their remaining limb but should be encouraged to master moving in either direction. Patients with bilateral limb loss or injury that precludes weight bearing on the remaining limb can scoot across a sliding board to a wheelchair or commode that is positioned diagonally from the bed. Patients with bilateral transfemoral amputation (and those with bilateral transtibial amputation who have sufficient hamstring excursion) may prefer the surface-to-surface stability that is provided when the entire anterior edge of the wheelchair seat abuts the side of the bed. Some patients who require significant assistance to transfer without a prosthesis become nearly independent in pivot transfers when a prosthesis is worn: The sensory feedback that is provided to the residual limb within the socket when there is contact between the prosthetic foot and the floor enhances sitting balance during sliding board or pivot transfers.[49] Patients with transfemoral amputation must learn that, although they can wear a prosthesis when seated, the prosthesis cannot be counted on for stability during transfers.

Mastery of single limb or non–weight-bearing transfers in the postoperative period is the foundation for functional transfers whenever the person with amputation is not wearing his or her prosthesis. At times in the future, mechanical problems with the prosthesis, skin problems on the residual limb, or a medical problem (e.g., congestive heart failure or renal failure) may have an impact on socket fit, temporarily precluding prosthetic use. It may be appropriate to provide opportunities for patients to practice transferring between surfaces at different levels (e.g., wheelchair to stool to floor) in the postoperative preprosthetic period, especially if delayed prosthetic fitting is anticipated. Many patients are discharged from the acute care setting to home before their limb is ready for prosthetic fitting and training. It is very important that appropriate adaptive equipment (e.g., tub bench, hand-held shower adapter, raised toilet seat, and grab bars) is identified and correctly installed so that safety in the bathroom is maximized.

Ambulation

Single limb ambulation with an appropriate assistive device provides an opportunity to enhance postural control and to build strength and cardiovascular endurance, in addition to allowing patients with recent amputation to move about in their environment. Some patients quickly master a two- or three-point swing-through pattern with crutches on level surfaces and are ready to build advanced gait skills on uneven surfaces, inclines, and stairs. Others are fearful of using crutches, preferring the stability provided by a walker to the mobility of crutches. A walker may be quite appropriate for patients with limited endurance and balance impairment who would otherwise be limited to wheelchair use. Therapists must be aware, however, of the potential long-term limitation in gait patterns imposed by walkers: The halting hop-to-gait pattern interrupts forward progression of the COM. Patients who have adapted to this pattern of motion may have difficulty developing a smooth step-through pattern or becoming comfortable with a less supportive ambulation aid once they are using their prosthesis. Walkers are also more difficult to use on inclines and are dangerous to use on stairs. Whenever possible, patients are encouraged to use crutches.[7]

Some patients with limited endurance or poor balance spend much time practicing a hop-to or a swing-through gait in the parallel bars before they acquire the confidence and motor skill that are needed to move out of the parallel bars with walker or crutches. It is important to note that single limb ambulation with an assistive device is often more energy intensive than walking with a prosthesis.[50] Achievement of single limb ambulation is not a prerequisite for prosthetic fitting. Patients should be encouraged to ambulate as much as possible, even if they are walking for aerobic exercise rather than for functional activities. For patients with single limb amputation, wheelchair use should be reserved for long distance transportation unless ambulation is not medically advisable. Wheelchairs are appropriate for patients with bilateral amputation; self-propulsion provides some aerobic conditioning as well as an energy-efficient means of locomotion.[51]

An alternative strategy for preprosthetic ambulation for physically or medically frail patients is the use of an air splint and prosthetic frame and foot[52,53] (Figure 23-14). The air splint used is much like those used by emergency medical technicians to stabilize a limb that is suspected of having a fracture. Felt pads are strategically placed over the residual limb's soft dressing, or a shrinker loads pressure-tolerant areas (medial tibial flare and patellar tendon) while protecting pressure-sensitive areas (crest of the tibia and fibular head) after inflation of the air splint. The sleeve is zipped into place around the limb, and the limb is positioned in the frame before inflation. The sleeve is inflated with a hand or foot pump to an air pressure of 35–40 mm Hg. This low pressure sustains toe touch to partial weight without compromising capillary blood flow to the healing suture line. The air splint provides limited mobility for patients who would not otherwise be ambulatory and may be a useful means of assessing the potential for prosthetic rehabilitation.

SUMMARY

Early rehabilitation in the postoperative preprosthetic period lays the foundation for prosthetic rehabilitation. Initial emphasis is placed on wound healing and control of edema, essential prerequisites for prosthetic use. Very early in the process, the patient and family become actively involved in the rehabilitation process and decision making, assuming responsibility for limb compression, skin care, and desensitization. The therapist is alert for postoperative medical complications, such as postural hypotension or deep venous thrombosis, as early mobility begins and implements strategies to prevent secondary impairments and functional limitations, such as further deconditioning and contracture formation. Strengthening exercises, targeting the residual limb and overall fitness, begin in the acute or subacute setting and continue as an aggressive home program to prepare the patient for prosthetic training. Patients are encouraged to become as independent as possible in transfers, single limb gait, and/or wheelchair mobility, depending on their medical status and functional capability. As the wound heals and edema subsides, the patient, therapist, prosthetist, and physician begin discussion about future prosthetic rehabilitation. The postoperative preprosthetic period is a time of transition in which patients may mourn the loss of their limb and question their future yet are challenged and encouraged by the possibilities offered by prosthetic replacement of their limb. If the consensus is that prosthetic fitting is not viable, emphasis shifts to development of wheelchair mobility skills and adaptation of the patient's environment as rehabilitation continues.

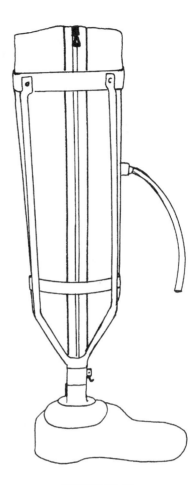

FIGURE 23-14

An air splint and prosthetic frame may provide limited ambulation for patients who are unable to accomplish single limb gait with an assistive device. The splint is inflated within the frame to 35–40 mm Hg, allowing toe touch to partial weight bearing, with minimal risk to the healing incision.

REFERENCES

1. Jackson-Wyatt O. Brain Function, Aging, and Dementia. In DA Umphred (ed), Neurological Rehabilitation (3rd ed). St. Louis: Mosby, 1995;722–746.
2. Ciccone CD. Geriatric Pharmacology. In AA Guccione (ed), Geriatric Rehabilitation. St. Louis: Mosby, 1993;171–200.
3. Acute Pain Management: Operative or Medical Procedures and Trauma. Clinical Practice Guideline. AHCPR Pub. No. 92-0032. Rockville, MD: Agency for Health Care Policy and Research, Public Health Service, US Department of Health and Human Services, February 1992.
4. Bach S, Noreng MF, Tjellden NU. Phantom limb pain in amputees during the first 12 months following limb amputation, after preoperative lumbar epidural blockage. Pain 1988;33(3):297–301.
5. Houghton AD, Nicholls G, Houghton AL, et al. Phantom pain: natural history and association with rehabilitation. Ann R Coll Surg Engl 1994;76(1):22.
6. Melzack R. Phantom limbs. Sci Am 1992;266(4):120–126.
7. May BJ. Postsurgical Management. In BJ May, Amputations and Prosthetics: A Case Study Approach. Philadelphia: Davis, 1996;67–98.
8. Sherman RA. Limb pain and stump blood circulation. Orthopaedics 1984;7(8):1319–1320.
9. Jensen TS, Krebs B, Nielsen J, Rasmussen P. Immediate and long term phantom limb pain in amputees: incidence, clinical characteristics, and relationship to preamputation limb pain. Pain 1985;21(3):267–278.
10. Mouratoglou VM. Amputees and phantom limb pain; a literature review. Physiother Pract 1986;2:177–180.

11. Sherman RA, Ernst JL, Barja RH, Bruno GM. Phantom limb pain: a lesson in the necessity for careful clinical research on chronic pain problems. J Rehabil Res Dev 1988;25(2):vii–x.

12. Elizaga AM, Smith DG, Sharar SR, et al. Continuous regional analgesia by intraneural block; effect on post-operative opioid requirements and phantom pain following amputation. J Rehabil Res Dev 1994;31(3):179–187.

13. Iacono RB, Linford J, Sandyk R. Pain management after lower extremity amputation. Neurosurgery 1987;20(3):496–500.

14. Malawer MM, Buch R, Khurana JS, et al. Post-operative infusional continuous regional analgesia; a technique for postoperative pain following major extremity surgery. Clin Orthop May 1991;(266):227–237.

15. Long D. Fifteen years of transcutaneous electrical stimulation for pain control. Stereotact Funct Neurosurg 1991;56(1):2–19.

16. Mirabella-Susans L. Pain Management. In DA Umphred (ed), Neurological Rehabilitation (3rd ed). St. Louis: Mosby, 1995;872–892.

17. Edelstein JE. Preprosthetic management of patients with lower- or upper-limb amputation. Prosthet Phys Med Rehabil Clin North Am 1991;2(2):285–297.

18. Burgess EM, Romano RL. The management of lower extremity amputees using immediate post-surgical prostheses. Clin Orthop 1968;March April (57):137–156.

19. Harrington IJ, Lexier R, Woods J, et al. A plaster-pylon technique for below knee amputation. J Bone Joint Surg 1991;73(1):76–78.

20. May BJ. Assessment and Treatment for Individuals following Lower Extremity Amputation. In SB O'Sullivan, TJ Schmitz (eds), Physical Rehabilitation: Assessment and Treatment (3rd ed). Philadelphia: Davis, 1994;375–396.

21. Mooney V, Harvey IP, McBride E, Snelson R. Comparison of postoperative stump management: plaster vs. soft dressings. J Bone Joint Surg 1971;53A(2):241–249.

22. Wu Y, Krick H. Removable rigid dressing for below-knee amputees. Clin Prosthet Orthot 1987;11(1):33–44.

23. Mueller M. Comparison of removable rigid dressings and elastic bandages in preprosthetic management of patients with below-knee amputations. Phys Ther 1982;62(10):1438–1441.

24. Palma T, Owens L, Jennings S. Removable Rigid Dressing Protocol. Hartford, CT: Department of Rehabilitation, Hartford Hospital, 1990.

25. Wu Y. Removable Rigid Dressings for Residual Limb Management. Appendix D. In LA Karacoloff, CS Hammersley, FJ Schneider (eds), Lower Extremity Amputation: A Guide to Functional Outcomes in Physical Therapy Management. Rehabilitation Institute of Chicago Procedure Manual. Gaithersburg, MD: Aspen, 1992;241–248.

26. Post-Amputation Care Options. In Prosthetic and Orthotic Currents, Newsletter of Newington Prosthetics and Orthotic Systems, Inc. Newington, CT, Spring 1995.

27. Maclean N, Fick GH. The effect of semirigid dressings on below knee amputations. Phys Ther 1994;74(7):668–673.

28. Sterescu LE. Semi-rigid (UNNA) dressing for amputation. Arch Phys Med Rehabil 1974;55(9):433–434.

29. Muilenburg AL, Wilson AB. A Manual for Below-Knee Amputees (4th ed). American Academy of Orthotists and Prosthetists. Alexandria, VA,1993.

30. May BJ. Amputation and Prosthetics, Then and Now. In BJ May, Amputation and Prosthetics: A Case Study Approach. Philadelphia: FA Davis, 1996;1–14

31. Moore TJ, Barron J, Hutchinson F, et al. Prosthetic usage following major lower extremity amputation. Clin Orthop Jan 1989;(248):227–230.

32. Muecke L, Shekar S, Dwyer D, et al. Functional screening of lower-limb amputees: a role in predicting rehabilitation outcome? Arch Phys Med Rehabil 1992;73(9):851–858.

33. Hubbard WA. Rehabilitation outcomes for elderly lower limb amputees. Aust J Physiother 1989;35(4):219–224.

34. Stewart CP, Jain AS. Cause of death in lower limb amputees. Prosthet Orthot Int 1992;16(2):129–132.

35. Ham R, de Trafford J, Van de Ven C. Patterns of recovery for lower limb amputations. Clin Rehabil 1994;8(4):320–328.

36. Pedersen NW, Pederson D. Nutrition as a prognostic indicator in amputations. Acta Orthop Scand 1992;63(6):675–678.

37. Berger N, Edelstein JE, Fishman S, Springer WP. Lower-Limb Prosthetics. New York: Prosthetics and Orthotics, New York University, Post Graduate Medical School, 1987.

38. Shurr DG, Cook TM. Above Knee Amputation and Prosthetics. In DG Schurr, TM Cook (eds), Prosthetics and Orthotics. Norwalk CT: Appleton & Lange, 1990;83–116.

39. Gaily RS, Gaily AM. Stretching and Strengthening for Lower Extremity Amputees. Miami: Advanced Rehabilitation Therapy, Inc, 1994.

40. Jaegers S, Hans Arendzen J, deJongh HJ. Changes in hip muscles after above-knee amputation. Clin Orthop Oct 1995;(319):276–284.

41. Kendall FP, McCreary EK, Provance PG. Muscle Testing and Function (4th ed). Baltimore: Williams & Wilkins, 1993.

42. Gossman M, Sahrmann S, Rose S. Review of length-associated change in muscle. Phys Ther 1982;62(12):1799–1808.

43. Kegel B, Burgess EM, Starr TW, Daly WK. Effects of isometric muscle training on residual limb volume, strength, and gait of below knee amputees. Phys Ther 1981;61(10):1419–1426.

44. Kisner C, Colby LA. Therapeutic Exercise: Foundations and Techniques (2nd ed). Philadelphia: Harper & Row, 1993.

45. Davies GJ. A Compendium of Isokinetics in Clinical Usage and Rehabilitation Techniques (2nd ed). LaCrosse, WI: S&S, 1985.

46. Knott M, Voss DE. Proprioceptive Neuromuscular Facilitation (2nd ed). New York: Harper & Row, 1968.

47. Burger H, et al. Properties of musculus gluteus maximus in above-knee amputees. Clin Biomech 1996;11(1):35.

48. Czerniecki JM, Harrington RM, Wyss CR. The effects of age and peripheral vascular disease on the circulatory and mechanical response of skin to loading. Am J Phys Med Rehabil 1990;69(6):302–306.

49. Kirby RL, Chari VR. Prostheses and the forward reach of sitting lower-limb amputees. Arch Phys Med Rehabil 1990;71(2):125–127.

50. Waters RL, Perry J, Antonelli D, Hislop H. Energy cost of walking of amputees: influence of level of amputation. J Bone Joint Surg 1976;58(1):42–46.

51. DuBow LL, Witt PL, Kadaba MP, et al. Oxygen consumption of elderly persons with bilateral below knee amputa- tions: ambulation versus wheelchair propulsion. Arch Phys Med Rehabil 1983;64(6):255–259.

52. Little JM. The use of air splints as immediate prostheses after below knee amputation for vascular insufficiency. Med J Aust 1970;2(19):870–872.

53. May BJ. Postoperative Management. In GT Sanders (ed), Lower Limb Amputations: A Guide to Rehabilitation. Philadelphia: FA Davis, 1986;357–384.

24

Prosthetic Feet

JOHN FERGASON

The prosthetic foot is designed to replace many of the functions of the anatomic human foot. As the connection between the prosthesis and the ground, it must mimic the biomechanical characteristics of the human foot as much as possible. Understanding the functions of the anatomic foot enables the clinic team to recommend the type of prosthetic foot that best meets the functional needs of each patient. Prosthetic feet can be classified according to the motions they allow or simulate. Only a few basic foot designs were commonly used until the 1990s, when dozens of options became available. For most members of the prosthetic team, knowledge of the characteristics of groups of prosthetic feet is more efficient for decision making than attempting to remember exact characteristics of each commercially available prosthetic foot. The certified prosthetist understands the complexities of the many prosthetic feet and remains current with the rapid advances in prosthetic foot technology.

New materials for the keel of the foot have been developed to increase the foot's flexibility. The use of carbon composites, with their superior strength-weight ratio, has been successfully applied to the design of high-performance, dynamic-response prosthetic feet. Traditional prosthetic feet were separate components that were bolted to the shank of the prosthesis, but some current designs incorporate the shank, ankle, and foot as one continuous unit. Other articulating ankle components substitute for movement in or about all three planes of anatomic ankle motion. Additionally, cosmetic appearance and durability of the various feet should be considered in formulating the appropriate prosthetic prescription. The primary goal of this chapter is to provide a basic understanding of the classification and function of prosthetic feet.

HISTORICAL PERSPECTIVE

Before commercially produced prosthetic feet became available, prosthetists had to assemble prosthetic feet of their own design. Commonly, these early prosthetic feet included some form of an ankle axis to allow plantar flexion and dorsiflexion, as well as a toe break in the area of the metatarsal heads. The body of the foot was often carved from a block of hardwood such as maple. A compressible bumper was positioned in a recessed area of the heel to simulate ankle plantar flexion motion, which is required for the first rocker of gait (heel rocker). As weight was transferred onto the heel during loading response, compression of the bumper resulted in a controlled lowering of the prosthetic foot toward the floor, substituting for the ankle plantar flexion motion that is required to attain the foot-flat position. Similarly, a compressible rubber bumper placed in a recessed area anterior to the ankle axis was used to simulate dorsiflexion, which is required to complete the second rocker of gait (ankle rocker) from loading response into midstance and terminal stance. As the shank of the prosthesis progressed forward, compression of the bumper allowed controlled dorsiflexion of the foot. A third bumper in the anterior of the prosthetic foot was used to simulate dorsiflexion of the metatarsophalangeal (MP) joints, which is required for the third rocker of gait (toe rocker). As the gait cycle progressed from terminal stance into preswing, compression of the toe bumper facilitated the transition from stance into swing. Often the plantar surface of the prosthetic foot was reinforced with flexible belting or felt to provide additional stability and durability. The unidirectional location of the toe break, which limited motion to a single plane, was the major disadvantage of this early design. Any deviation from this one plane caused an inefficient gait from midstance to heel rise.

The weight, lack of flexibility, and maintenance needs associated with a custom-fabricated foot have prompted the development of commercially manufactured prosthetic feet which are more accommodating to the functional concerns, energy costs, and cosmetic preferences of prosthetic users. The basic characteristics of early prosthetic feet provide the biomechanical foundation for many of the feet that are currently in use. The articulating ankle/single-axis foot uses a similar principle for its axial motion. The early prototypes of the solid-ankle cushioned-heel (SACH) foot developed by Foort and Radcliff in the early 1950s used a slightly different approach to achieve the functional goals of earlier prosthetic feet.[1] This simple and lightweight design was a significant improvement and provided acceptable function for the majority of people with amputation. A wedge of compressible material in the heel replaced the plantar flexion bumper, and a rigid internal keel with a rocker shape at the metatarsal heads replaced the toe-break bumper. Early SACH feet were available in three shoe sizes: The foot was purchased with oversized dimensions that were then reduced by machining to fit in the patient's shoe. Specific adjustment and shaping guidelines were followed to provide the best possible fit and function of the foot within the shoe. The prosthetist could choose one of three levels of heel cushion durometer. This heel compressibility, in conjunction with the patient's weight, determined how quickly the foot-flat position was achieved. Early SACH feet were generally maintenance free and considerably lighter than the conventional wood feet.[2,3]

The SACH foot and the single-axis wooden foot remained the only options for prosthetic users for many years. In the late 1970s, Campbell introduced the stationary-ankle–flexible endoskeletal foot (SAFE). This foot maintained the basic characteristics of the SACH foot, adding a component of flexibility that was missing in previous designs. Although heavier than the SACH foot, it allowed for some multiaxial motion that substituted for the accommodation to uneven surfaces, which is possible in the anatomic foot-ankle complex.

Development of articulated multiaxial foot-ankle assemblies followed the institution of the United States Artificial Limb Program in 1945. Early versions were relatively unsuccessful, but a number of later designs found commercial success.[4] These basic designs were the primary options until the early 1980s.

The "technology boom" for prosthetic foot design began in the early 1980s, sparked by the development of the Seattle Foot by the Prosthetic Research Study at the University of Washington.[5] This foot was the first in the class of dynamic-response energy-storing feet that provided an elastic keel for use in higher-level activities, such as running and jumping. Currently, scores of feet use the original Seattle Foot principle of elasticity to offer a higher level of performance to prosthetic wearers who are involved in athletics and other active functional and leisure activities.

FUNCTIONAL DESIGN CRITERIA FOR THE PROSTHETIC FOOT

The design of a prosthetic foot offers the same functional characteristics that are seen in the human foot-ankle complex. Ideally, the prosthetic foot duplicates each biomechanical motion with a mechanical substitute. Given the complexity of the human foot-ankle complex, however, this goal may be unrealistic. During the gait cycle, the human foot offers adaptation to uneven surfaces, shock absorption at heel strike, torque conversion, knee stabilization, transfer of weight-bearing forces, limb lengthening and shortening to even the arc of the center of gravity in forward progression, and a stable weight-bearing base.[6–8] In the early stance phase, the human foot is flexible to allow accommodation to uneven terrain and to maintain balance. Toward the end of the stance phase, the human foot converts to a rigid lever arm for push-off at preswing. This unique biomechanical progression from a flexible to a rigid position is dependent on the position of the components of the foot as well as on their motion and structure.[9] An individual with an amputation has no physical connection between the musculature of the residual limb and the prosthetic foot: In response, the prosthetic foot must substitute for the function of the bony anatomy as well as the loss of muscle action. Few of the currently available prosthetic feet are designed to dorsiflex during swing phase; most focus on performance in stance. Design variations affect how well the prosthetic foot addresses the functional tasks of stance. These tasks include

1. Shock absorption and controlled plantar flexion in loading response
2. Accommodation to uneven terrain and controlled advancement of the prosthetic shank (shin) during midstance
3. Heel rise and weight transfer during terminal stance
4. Transition through double support and preparation for the swing phase

Initial Contact into Loading Response

The two functional tasks in early stance are shock absorption and transition to foot-flat position. The prosthetic foot is designed to absorb much of the impact of the heel contacting the ground to minimize the forces that are transferred to the residual limb. For those with transtibial amputation, shock absorption must also provide for a normal knee flexion moment and position as the gait cycle progresses to loading response.

In early stance, the ground reaction force vector is posterior to the ankle, creating a plantar flexion moment that drives the foot toward the floor. In the human foot-ankle, eccentric contraction of the foot dorsiflexion or pretibial muscle group allows smooth, controlled plantar flexion of the foot toward the floor during the heel rocker of gait. As the foot progresses to the floor, the tibia begins to advance forward during the ankle rocker of gait, and limb progression is continued. Proper control of plantar flexion prevents the tibia from advancing either too slowly or too rapidly.

Midstance

In early stance, the anatomic foot and ankle are flexible and capable of accommodating variations in terrain. The ability of the prosthetic foot to simulate the inversion and eversion of the subtalar joint mechanically determines how effectively it substitutes for this function.

The momentum of the swing limb and forward fall of the body weight create a dorsiflexion torque that moves the tibia over the weight-bearing foot from 8 degrees of plantar flexion at loading response to 5 degrees of dorsiflexion at end stance. This motion is necessary for the forward progression of the stance leg as the opposite limb moves forward in swing. Eccentric contraction of the gastrocnemius and soleus muscles controls the speed of this progression and helps to maintain stance stability.[6] The prosthetic foot simulates this muscle activity by providing stance phase stability through a rigid, semirigid, or flexible keel within the foot.

Terminal Stance

In terminal stance, the anatomic foot-ankle complex locks into position to provide for heel rise as the tibia continues to advance. The body weight is transferred forward onto the forefoot and rolls over the MP joints during the toe rocker of stance. This allows the foot to roll over at the metatarsal heads instead of at the tips of the toes.[6] The design of the prosthetic foot must provide terminal stance phase support as well as simulate MP dorsiflexion, which is necessary for the toe rocker. Although a true articulation is not necessary, the design of the foot should allow for an amount of forefoot flexibility to provide for a smooth rollover motion.

Preswing

During dual limb support, the weight of the body is transferred from the preswing limb to the opposite side. The

muscle force of the gastrocnemius-soleus complex is reduced as the ankle begins to plantar flex. The well-designed prosthetic foot provides sufficient support of the amputated side to assist in balance and facilitate smooth transfer of weight to the sound side. This is a primary factor in reducing the force placed on the sound side foot[10] and may be particularly important for the individual with compromised vascular and neurologic systems.

Rapid knee flexion during preswing results in relative shortening of the limb to allow adequate clearance as the swing phase begins. A slight spring action of the prosthetic foot at the end of terminal stance simulates this muscle activity.

CATEGORIES OF PROSTHETIC FEET

Prosthetic feet are most often categorized by the combinations of functional tasks that they are designed to simulate. The prosthetic feet that are available in the current market can be grouped into four overall designs:

1. Nonarticulating feet (for example, SACH feet)
2. Articulating designs (for example, single-axis and multiaxial feet)
3. Prosthetic feet with elastic keels (for example, SAFE feet)
4. Dynamic-response or energy-storing designs (for example, the Seattle Foot and the Flex-Foot [Flex-Foot, Inc., Aliso Viejo, CA])

Nonarticulating Designs: SACH Feet

The SACH foot has been available in its most basic form since the late 1950s.[2] Today's SACH foot differs very little in principle from those early designs. It continues to be one of the most widely prescribed feet in the United States because of its simplicity, low cost, and durability. It has no true moving parts or articulations and relies on the flexibility of its structure for joint motion simulation. The internal keel SACH foot is available with soft, medium, and firm heel densities and can be obtained in heel heights ranging from 0 to 3 ½ in.[7] The SACH foot is composed of a firm keel that is surrounded by dense yet flexible foam to give shape to the foot (Figure 24-1). The keel ends distally at the toe-break area of the foot. Molded toes are available if desired. A heel cushion wedge is placed under the keel in the posterior of the foot. Rubberized belting is attached to the distal area of the keel and extends to the end of the toes. This belting simulates the toe flexors and assists in giving a slight resistance to MP extension during preswing, thus preventing a feeling of dropping off of the toe during this phase of gait.

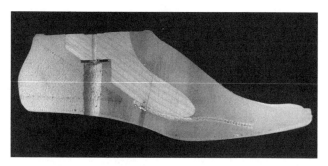

FIGURE 24-1
Solid-ankle cushioned-heel foot in cross section. Note the heel cushion, wooden keel, and belting extending toward the toe.

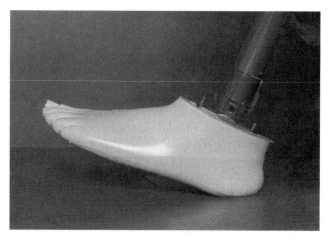

FIGURE 24-2
Compression of the heel cushion in the solid-ankle cushioned-heel foot during loading response simulates controlled plantar flexion of the ankle toward the foot-flat position. The firmness (durometer) of the heel cushion and weight of the prosthetic user determine how quickly the foot-flat position is attained.

Functional Analysis of the SACH Foot during Stance

At initial contact and into loading response, the cushioned heel of the SACH foot adequately provides for shock absorption as body weight is transferred onto the stance foot. The compression resistance of the heel cushion can be varied from very soft to very firm, based on body weight. Compression of the heel cushion also simulates the action of the lost pretibial muscle group in controlling plantar flexion into a foot-flat position (Figure 24-2). This compression of the heel cushion allows for a controlled progression into the early stance phase. For individuals with transtibial amputation, it also provides stability in early stance by limiting the potential effect of rapid knee flexion moment during loading. A soft heel cushion can be chosen for individuals who need to reach a stable foot-flat position very quickly, such as those with transfemoral amputation using a prosthesis with a locked knee or those with balance impairment.

When considering the transition to midstance, it is important to note that the SACH foot has no true inversion or eversion motion to assist in accommodating for uneven terrain. The rubber structure of the outer foot may aid in very small deviations in terrain, but this is not significant and should not be depended on for this function. Simulation of ankle rocker (as the shank of the prosthesis rolls forward over the foot) is controlled through the keel of the foot. The rigid keel offers resistance to tibial advancement until the weight line is past the toe break of the foot.

Control of heel rise during toe rocker in terminal stance and progression onto the forefoot in preswing are functions of the length of the keel in the SACH foot. Although some manufacturers make available SACH feet of various keel lengths or densities, most SACH feet have standard keel lengths that correspond to the size of the foot. In late stance, the prosthetic foot is stable and resists rapid heel rise until the weight line passes the toe break, where the keel ends. As the shank of the prosthesis continues

forward, the end of the keel is reached and toe dorsiflexion begins. If the keel is too short, an early heel rise and an unwanted knee flexion moment occur, often perceived by the prosthetic user as a "buckling" of the knee. If the keel is too long, heel rise and knee extension moment are delayed, interrupting forward progression and smooth weight transfer to the opposite limb.

The toe break on the SACH foot is located at the end of the keel. The toe break simulates dorsiflexion of the toes and shortens the effective length of the foot. Excursion of toe dorsiflexion is controlled by the belting, which is attached to the keel and extends to the toes. This belting allows the toes to dorsiflex so that tibial progression continues smoothly. The dorsiflexed toes of the SACH foot offer little weight-bearing support: The alignment of the foot under the socket determines how effectively the keel provides support as weight is transferred to the sound side. As the prosthetic user moves toward the end of preswing and the limb begins to rise, the flexibility of the belting material adds a small elastic motion to help assist in knee flexion. This motion, however, is minimal compared to the elastic keel and dynamic-response categories of prosthetic feet.

Advantages and Indications of the SACH Foot

Because it has no moving parts, the SACH foot is extremely durable and requires very little maintenance throughout the life of the foot. The wide variety of heel heights that are available often make it the foot of choice. The SACH foot has excellent shock absorption charac-

FIGURE 24-3

Components of a single-axis foot. The ankle axis allows plantar flexion and dorsiflexion during the stance phase of gait. Compression of the rubber bumper posterior to the ankle acts as a shock absorber and mimics controlled plantar flexion toward a foot-flat position in early stance.

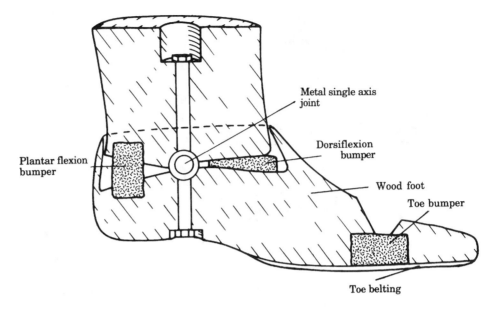

teristics because of its large heel cushion. It is often recommended for use in temporary or preparatory prostheses because of its light weight and low cost. It is most appropriate for prosthetic users at the level of household and limited community ambulation.

Disadvantages and Contraindications of the SACH Foot

The primary disadvantage to the SACH foot is its inherent lack of flexibility, especially its inability to accommodate to uneven surfaces. Proper alignment of a SACH foot is critical because of the very nature of the lack of moveable articulations. Its design and construction target optimal performance during relaxed walking cadence and in a single alignment configuration. Because of these factors it should seldom be recommended for the very active community ambulator. It is also inappropriate for those who are involved in high-level activities and sports or if the user must traverse uneven terrain.

Articulating Designs: Single-Axis Feet

Whereas the SACH foot simulates ankle motion by incorporation of a cushion heel, articulating or axial designs include a simulated ankle joint that actually permits motion about the one or more planes of the joint axis. The single-axis foot design was the first true articulating, or axial, foot. It is a direct descendant of the historic conventional wooden foot. The modern single-axis foot is composed of a keel with a molded rubber foot shell (Figure 24-3). The ankle articulation is most often made of steel, with replaceable plastic bushings surrounding it. The toes are

reinforced with flexible belting that is attached to the keel to give the toes a degree of stiffness while still retaining flexibility. Most single-axis, articulating prosthetic feet allow up to 15 degrees of plantar flexion and 5–7 degrees of dorsiflexion.[1] This is accomplished by foot rotation about the axis located in the ankle area of the foot. Compression of the rubber bumper located posterior to the axis mimics plantar flexion. Its density determines the speed of foot descent in loading response. For dorsiflexion, some single-axis feet have a rubber bumper located anterior to the axis. When compressed, this anterior bumper resists rapid anterior movement of the prosthetic shank. Other designs may instead use a "stop" that limits motion after 5–7 degrees of dorsiflexion is reached.

Functional Analysis of the Single-Axis Foot

A single-axis foot provides excellent shock absorption during initial contact and loading response because of the combined compression of the rubber heel and the plantar flexion bumper. At initial contact, the rubber heel begins to compress and cushion shock. As the heel reaches full compression, the force is transferred to the plantar flexion bumper (Figure 24-4). This rubber plantar flexion bumper begins to compress and continues to absorb the shock of ground contact. It then acts to control the descent of the foot toward the ground. The rate of descent of the foot can be controlled to a certain degree by changing the durometer of the plantar flexion bumper. All manufacturers of single-axis feet supply numerous interchangeable bumpers of varying durometers or firmness. The denser the rubber in the bumper, the more resistance to plantar flexion is experienced by the prosthetic user. If a

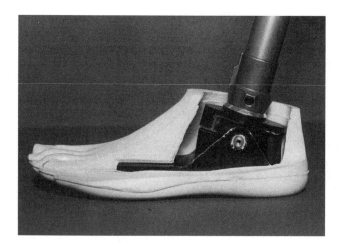

FIGURE 24-4
Compression of the plantar flexion bumper during initial contact and loading response. Note the posterior leaning angle of the pylon as the prosthetic foot approaches the foot-flat position.

firm heel bumper is used, the foot is resistant to plantar flexion, and a knee flexion moment results. If a softer heel bumper is used, the foot reaches foot-flat position quickly. Considerations for determining bumper firmness revolve around patient weight, activity level, and the need for knee stability.

The articulation in the single-axis foot allows movement in the sagittal plane only. This provides more accommodation to uneven surfaces than does a nonarticulated foot but does not allow true articulated movement in the coronal plane when inversion/eversion may be necessary. Any inversion/eversion that is seen is due to the inherent flexibility within the rubber portion of the foot and toe areas. Advancement of the prosthesis' tibial shank during midstance is controlled by the combination of the dorsiflexion bumper (or dorsiflexion stop) and the solid keel in the foot. Once the full range of dorsiflexion is reached, the keel of the foot acts as a rocker to continue the controlled progression of the tibial shank.

Heel rise in terminal stance is determined by the effect of the dorsiflexion bumper or stop. For the prosthetic foot with a dorsiflexion bumper, the firmness of the bumper determines when the tibia stops advancing. Once the bumper is maximally compressed (stopping tibial advancement), the force is applied to the foot and heel rise is initiated. For the foot with a dorsiflexion stop, force is transferred to the foot, and heel rise is initiated once the stop is fully engaged. The length of the keel in the foot also contributes to the control of heel rise. Once the end point of ankle dorsiflexion is reached, the distal portion of the keel acts as a rocker. When the end point of this rocker is reached, toe dorsiflexion begins.

As stance transitions into preswing, the mechanics of the single-axis foot become similar to that of the SACH foot. The toe break of the foot is located where the keel ends. Once the end of the keel is rolled over, the toes begin to dorsiflex. Toe dorsiflexion is controlled by the belting attached at the distal keel that terminates in the toe area. The support necessary to allow smooth transfer of weight to the sound side is determined by the alignment of the foot under the prosthetic socket and the overall length of the keel. As the end of preswing is reached, the elasticity in the plantar belting and the rubber toes offers a slight spring action that encourages knee flexion into the swing phase.

Advantages and Indications of the Single-Axis Foot

The primary advantage of a single-axis foot is its ability to reach a stable foot-flat position quickly in early stance. This may be advantageous for activities that have an impact on knee stability, such as walking down a ramp or other inclines. A single-axis foot reduces the need for strong extension about the knee to control loading response. Although most individuals with amputations at the transtibial level have adequate knee extensor strength for controlled loading response, those who have significant nonremediable strength impairment or a particularly short residual limb may benefit from a single-axis foot. At the transfemoral level of amputation, knee stability during loading response is related to hip extensor strength and length of the residual limb; as a result, knee stability can be more challenging to achieve. A single-axis foot reduces the knee flexion moment placed on the prosthetic knee during loading response and creates an increase in stability during this phase. An additional advantage is the capability of changing the durometer of the bumpers in the foot to suit the needs and activity level of the prosthetic user at transtibial and transfemoral levels of amputation.

Contraindications and Disadvantages of the Single-Axis Foot

The major disadvantages of a single-axis foot include its increased weight (as compared to the SACH and other nonarticulating feet) and its need for occasional maintenance. The benefit of extra stability in early stance may be countered by the increased energy cost of a heavier foot for prosthetic users with significant strength impairment or poor aerobic capacity. Because the foot has moving parts, it needs occasional service for normal wear and tear. Bushings in the joint will show signs of wearing and need to be replaced. With repeated loading, the bumpers can fatigue or harden over time. Any of these situations alters the function of the foot and the efficiency of the gait pattern of the prosthetic user.

Articulating Designs: Multiaxis Feet

The multiple-axis (multiaxis) foot operates in a similar manner to the single-axis foot, using various combinations of rubber bumpers. The multiaxis foot offers coronal and transverse plane motion in addition to motion in the sagittal plane. True inversion/eversion and rotation allow this prosthetic foot to absorb more of the torque forces that would otherwise be transferred to the patient's residual limb. It is important to note that, as a result of the large availability of range, stability is found only at the extremes of each plane of motion.

Feet that offer multiaxial motion are available in a variety of styles. The Greissinger foot (Otto Bock Industries, Minneapolis, MN) has the longest history of commercial availability, with widespread use in Europe and limited but steady success in the United States.[4] It consists of a wooden keel surrounded by a molded rubber foot (Figure 24-5). A wooden ankle interface is connected to the keel of the foot by a U bolt and yoke assembly. Rubber bumpers rest between the ankle block and the U bolt to allow inversion/eversion and rotation. Plantar flexion is controlled by a posterior bumper in the heel, and dorsiflexion is controlled by compression of a rubber block anterior to the ankle axis. The need for maintenance of the rubber and plastic parts and the relative

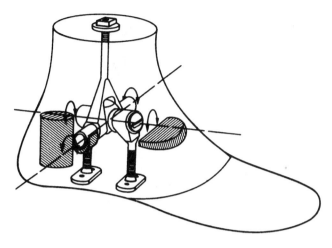

FIGURE 24-5
Internal mechanisms of the Greissinger multiaxial foot. This design allows movement in the sagittal, coronal, and transverse planes.

heaviness of this foot are factors that limit its use in the United States.

A more recent, successful multiple-axis design is the Multiflex ankle-foot (Endolite America, Centerville, OH) (Figure 24-6). This foot has fewer moving parts than the Greissinger foot, with reduced maintenance needs. Motion is obtained by the use of a rubber ball inside of the stem of the ankle tube. As motion in the foot/ankle occurs, the rubber ball compresses against the wall of

FIGURE 24-6
Multiflex ankle-foot assembly. The ball-and-stem assembly and the O-ring mimic inversion and eversion of the foot and ankle, allowing accommodation when the patient is walking on uneven surfaces. (Drawing courtesy of Endolite America, Centerville, OH.)

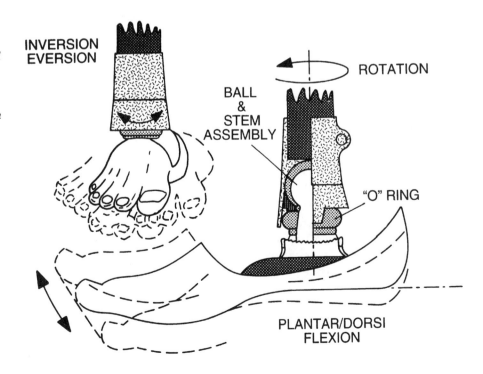

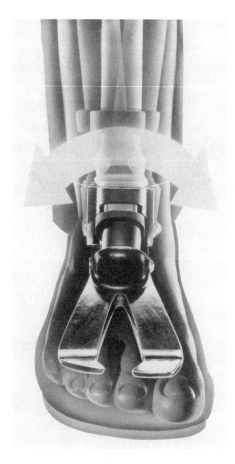

FIGURE 24-7

Multiaxial feet allow movement in the sagittal and coronal planes, giving the person with amputation additional accommodation for uneven terrain. (Photograph courtesy of College Park Industries, Inc., Fraser, MI.)

the ankle tube. A rubber O-ring placed distal to the rubber ball provides secondary resistance to dorsiflexion against a stop on the housing. This O-ring provides limited resistance to all other motions as well. The ring is available in a variety of stiffness levels, so that the prosthetist can tailor overall resistance to motion to the needs of the prosthetic user. The combination of the rubber ball in the ankle stem and the rubber O-ring distal to the ball provides a full range of plantar flexion/dorsiflexion, controlled inversion/eversion, and some rotation. It is important to note that this design does not allow for individual adjustment in a single plane of motion. The rubber ball and the O-ring act continuously for all motions: A change of resistance aimed at one motion affects the other motions as well. As a consequence, this design may have less adjustability for the specific needs of an individual patient. Other multiaxis feet are commercially available, but most function in a manner sim-

ilar to these two designs. The functional analysis of the multiaxial foot takes both designs into consideration.

Functional Analysis of the Multiaxis Foot

As with the single-axis foot, the primary method of shock absorption in early stance occurs from compression of the plantar flexion bumper. Because the ankle components take up the space in the heel that is commonly used for a heel cushion in other foot designs, nearly all shock absorption occurs by this bumper compression. Shock absorption in the multiflex design is provided by compression of the rubber ball and stem against the ankle tube wall and by the O-ring between the ankle tube and foot. As weight is applied to the foot, the plantar flexion bumper or rubber ball and O-ring compress to provide a controlled progression to midstance. Plantar flexion resistance is adjusted to meet specific user needs by changing the plantar flexion bumper or O-ring to one with a different stiffness.

During midstance, the true multiaxial features of the foot become obvious. The multiaxial foot accommodates to uneven ground in the sagittal, coronal, and transverse planes (Figure 24-7). True inversion/eversion is allowed by compression of the rubber rocker insert between the ankle and foot or between the rubber ball and ankle tube and compression of the O-ring (in the Multiflex foot) (see Figure 24-6). Because the multiaxial foot also allows transverse motion, rotational forces are absorbed in the foot-ankle complex rather than being transferred to the residual limb. Tibial advancement is controlled by the stiffness of the rubber components of the ankle. Once full compression of the rubber component is reached, the force is transferred to the foot. The length of the keel determines the continued amount of resistance as terminal stance is reached.

Heel rise in terminal stance is controlled first by the effect of the rubber components in the foot that act to control dorsiflexion and then by the length of the prosthetic keel. For the rocker insert and the ball and O-ring, the component's resistance to dorsiflexion determines when the tibial advancement is slowed and heel rise is initiated. Once the dorsiflexion limit is reached, tibial advancement is slowed, the force is applied to the foot, and heel rise begins. Multiaxial feet have varying keel lengths specific to their design and manufacturer. As in other prosthetic foot designs, the length of the keel also influences heel rise. When the end point of foot-ankle dorsiflexion is reached, the distal portion of the keel serves as a rocker. As the heel rises, the foot pivots over the edge of the keel, and toe dorsiflexion begins. Toe dorsiflexion is controlled by the construction of the foot in the toe area (Figure 24-8). To give the toe area some elasticity, belting can be attached at the distal keel, or the keel can be preformed to include some dorsiflexion. The toe break of the foot is located where the keel ends. Dorsiflexed toes offer little support for the transfer of body weight to the sound side. Prosthetic alignment of the foot under the prosthesis and the overall length of the keel determine how much support is available for smooth transfer of weight from the prosthetic to the opposite limb. As preswing is completed, the elasticity in the rubber toes and their inner supporting structure offer a slight spring action that encourages knee flexion into the swing phase.

Advantages and Indications of Multiaxial Foot Designs

The multiaxial foot has several specific indications for use. The primary advantage is the ability of the foot to accommodate uneven terrain in more than one plane. Although the transverse movement does not mimic normal human motion exactly, it is extremely useful for reducing torque forces on the residual limb during stance. The prosthetic user who anticipates being on uneven terrain would certainly appreciate this feature. Those with mechanical instability of their anatomic knee, poor postural control, or vulnerable skin or fixed adhesions along the incision line of their residual limb would also benefit from reduction of torque forces during stance. The density or resistance of the rubber bumpers can be changed for accommodation to the prosthetic user's weight and activity level.

Disadvantages and Contraindications of Multiaxial Foot Designs

The main advantage of the multiaxial foot can also be considered a disadvantage. Because movement is allowed in all three planes, the multiaxial foot provides less static stability than does the nonaxial foot.[11] An individual with specific muscle weakness may not feel stable or supported when using this foot. These factors can be accommodated by use of a bumper of different durometer, determined by individual needs. Multiaxial feet are often heavier than nonarticulating, elastic keel, or dynamic-response prosthetic feet. It is important to check with the individual manufacturer for weight specifications. The moving parts within the foot make regular maintenance a necessity. Bushings and bumpers wear with use; performance of the foot deteriorates as this occurs. Replacement of worn components in many instances restores performance to acceptable levels. Multiaxial feet should not be used if an individual is unwilling to schedule regular maintenance checks or is inaccessible to the prosthetist.

Elastic Keel Feet

The elastic keel foot is designed to mimic the movement characteristics of the human foot without the use of true articulations and moving parts. Such a task requires the design attention to be placed primarily on the keel of the

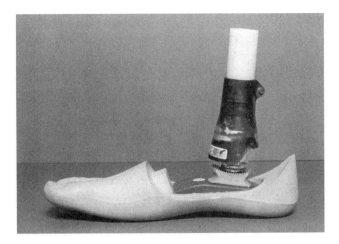

FIGURE 24-8
The preformed keel with dorsiflexed toes of the multiaxial foot's shell facilitates rollover and initiation of heel rise in terminal stance.

foot and the material of the surrounding foot shell. In the anatomic foot, the plantar fascia (plantar aponeurosis) works in combination with the intrinsic muscles of the foot to transmit force across the longitudinal arch of the foot.[12] A "windlass effect" occurs as the MP joints are dorsiflexed and the plantar fascia is tightened. The collagen fibers of the plantar fascia resist the tensile forces and become progressively stiffer. This tension promotes inversion of the calcaneus and supination of the subtalar joint to establish a rigid lever for push-off.[9] The elastic keel foot is designed to mimic this motion by increasing stiffness of the foot as it moves through midstance, terminal stance, and preswing. Several versions of elastic keel feet are commercially available. The SAFE II foot is used to represent this class of prosthetic feet in the functional analysis below, because this design most closely resembles the motion of the anatomic foot. Other feet in the elastic keel category can be analyzed with the same criteria given the variations in design and manufacturing techniques.

Functional Analysis of an Elastic Keel Foot

Most elastic keel feet use a cushioned heel that is similar to the SACH foot for shock absorption in initial contact and loading response. Many of the manufacturers offer the soft-, medium-, and firm-heel durometer to allow for variations in patient weight, activity level, and need for shock absorption. Other feet may not have a separate foam compartment in the heel area, instead using keel flexibility and the foot shell foam to provide shock absorption.

The differences in the design of elastic keel feet become apparent during the transitions from early stance through midstance and into terminal stance. Certain elastic keel feet rely primarily on compression of the heel cushion to con-

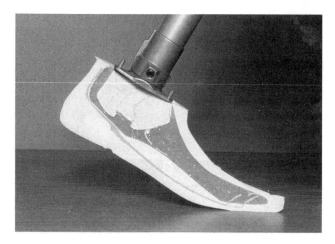

FIGURE 24-9
Elastic keel class, stationary–ankle–flexible endoskeletal (SAFE II) foot. Note the plantar bands originating on the posterior surface of the keel that insert into the distal keel. These bands simulate the action of the plantar fascia in the human foot. As the SAFE II foot is loaded in terminal stance, the tension applied to the plantar bands creates the semirigid level needed for efficient transition from stance into swing.

trol the rate of foot plantar flexion toward foot flat in early stance, using principles similar to those of the SACH foot. Others involve the biomechanical properties of their keel design. The SAFE II has a two-part keel. The most proximal section is a rigid block containing the foot bolt that connects the foot to the prosthesis shank. Inside the foot, this rigid block is connected to the flexible portion of the keel that extends to the distal end of the foot at the toes. Once the cushion heel reaches its limit of compression during loading, the rigid block moves relative to the foot shell and flexible portion of the keel. This movement provides additional cushion to the patient's residual limb.

Inversion and eversion are simulated by the nature of the flexibility in the elastic keel foot. The foot provides moderate accommodation to uneven terrain because of the movement allowed between the keel and its surrounding rubber foot shell. Tibial advancement is controlled by the plantar bands embedded under the keel of the SAFE II foot. These two bands originate at the heel area of the keel. The first band crosses the arch and attaches proximal to the toe break. This band serves to stabilize the arch of the keel and prevent excessive flexibility while standing during midstance. The second band crosses the toe break and attaches in the distal end of the keel. As the tibia advances, the keel begins to bend and the foot starts to dorsiflex. The plantar bands begin to tighten, controlling the rate that the keel bends. This resistance to rapid bending of the keel acts to control

the tibial advancement. Other elastic keel feet achieve the same effect through the use of only a flexible keel within the foot. Most elastic keel feet tend to offer limited rotational ability. Rotation occurs by minimal movement of the flexible keel within the rubber housing of the foot.

Heel rise during terminal stance is controlled by the stiffness of the keel. As the prosthetic tibial shaft advances, the keel continues to flex as the foot dorsiflexes and weight progresses onto the forefoot. The keel in most elastic keel feet extends all the way into the toe area. No rocker effect is created by a rigid, short keel as in the SACH foot or articulating feet. The flexible keel eliminates the need for a rocker effect and provides a considerably smoother rollover throughout this phase. The SAFE II foot has additional control during dorsiflexion and heel rise as tension is applied to the plantar bands (Figure 24-9). These bands allow for gradual stiffening of the forefoot to create a semirigid lever during this phase, as does the aponeurosis in the anatomic foot. In the SAFE II foot (Campbell-Childs, White City, OR), a section is cut into the keel at the metatarsal area to create a toe break and allow for defined MP dorsiflexion as weight is progressed onto the forefoot. The plantar fascia band crosses the toe break and offers control and support as the toes dorsiflex. Other elastic keel feet rely on the flexibility of the keel alone without incorporating a mechanical toe break.

The elastic keel of these feet is compressed as the prosthetic tibial shank advances from midstance to terminal stance. As the prosthetic limb is unweighted during preswing and weight is transferred to the opposite limb, the patient has a sense of "energy return" as the prosthetic foot returns to its uncompressed or resting state. The spring action of this elastic response serves to encourage knee flexion of the amputated side and aid initiation of the swing phase.

Advantages and Indications of an Elastic Keel Foot
Elastic keel feet provide a very smooth gait pattern because no mechanical rocker motions occur during the subphases of stance. Individuals with a moderate need for accommodation to uneven terrain appreciate the flexibility of the foot. The benefit of flexibility of an elastic keel is also evident during activities such as stair climbing or descent and incline negotiation. An elastic keel foot is an alternative for the prosthetic user who would benefit from the features of a multiaxial foot but does not want the maintenance or weight characteristics associated with those designs. Although the range of motion and torque absorption are not as extensive as those in multiaxial designs, the characteristics of the elastic keel foot functionally approximate them for many prosthetic users.

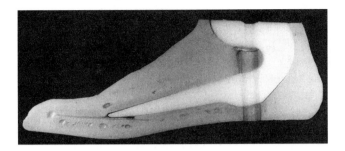

FIGURE 24-10
Seattle Foot (Seattle Orthopedic Group, Seattle, WA) with Delrin (Dupont Inc., Wilmington, DE) dynamic-response keel. The combination of stiffness and flexibility of the keel enhances function in early stance. Compression of the keel in late stance is returned as push-off as the swing phase begins.

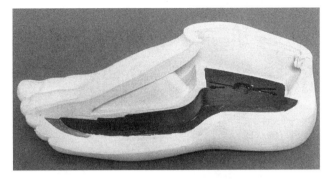

FIGURE 24-11
Carbon Copy II dynamic-response foot (Ohio Willowwood Co., Mt. Sterling, OH). The carbon graphite composite keel acts as a leaf spring, storing energy as it is compressed with forward progression of body weight during stance, and returning that energy as push-off when the foot is unloaded and the swing phase begins.

Disadvantages and Contraindications of an Elastic Keel Foot

The flexibility of the foot, although a major advantage for many prosthetic users, may be a disadvantage for others. The "spongy" feel of an elastic keel foot may be disliked by prosthetic users who are in need of, or accustomed to, a greater sense of stability during stance. Extremely active or athletic individuals often prefer a foot with a more rigid or stiffer keel than those that are available in elastic keel feet, preferring instead those of the dynamic-response class.

Dynamic-Response Feet

The dynamic-response, or energy-storing, class of prosthetic feet is most often chosen for high-performance prosthetic users. An early survey of recreational activities of lower limb prosthetic users by Kegal et al.[13] in 1980 suggested that the major factor that has an impact on performance during and enjoyment of athletic activities is the inability to run effectively. Enoka et al.,[14] in studying performance characteristics and kinetics of running and jumping while wearing a prosthesis, demonstrated that the ground reaction force may be two to three times greater while running than walking. Most prosthetic feet have been designed to substitute for ankle and foot motion during walking; many are unable to meet the increased performance demands of running and jumping. Recognition of these limitations prompted researchers in prosthetics to develop a prosthetic foot with energy-storing capabilities that would absorb and store forces during loading and release this stored energy during push-off or preswing.

One of the first of the dynamic-response designs to become commercially available was the Seattle Foot (Seat-

tle Orthopedic Group, Seattle, WA) (Figure 24-10). This foot has a one-piece keel of synthetic composite material embedded in a foam foot shape.[15] The keel provides a unique combination of stiffness and flexibility to absorb the forces applied early in the gait cycle. As cadence increases from walking speed toward running speeds, the amount of time spent on the forefoot increases. The increasing amplitude of the dorsiflexion moment is accommodated by greater distortion in the keel as it compresses, and absorbs more and more energy, during terminal stance. As the foot is unloaded in preswing, this stored energy is quickly released, simulating push-off and aiding the forward propulsion of the limb into swing.

Since the introduction of this first commercially available dynamic-response foot, many others have followed. Most use similar principles of design but differ in the materials used for the keel. The inherent strength, durability, and light weight of carbon graphite composites have made this the material of choice for recently developed dynamic-response feet. For example, the Carbon Copy II (Ohio Willowwood, Mt. Sterling, OH) foot uses a carbon graphite leaf spring solid keel that is embedded in a foam foot shell (Figure 24-11). Other designs, such as Flex-Foot (Flex-Foot Inc., Aliso Viejo, CA) or Springlite (Springlite, Salt Lake City, UT), use a single carbon graphite component, incorporating the shin, ankle, and foot in a combined design (Figure 24-12). These offer the advantage of increased flexibility because the entire length of the shin and foot deforms under loading conditions. The functional analysis of three dynamic-response foot designs (Seattle Foot, Flex-Foot, and Springlite) illustrates the similarities and differences among dynamic-response designs.

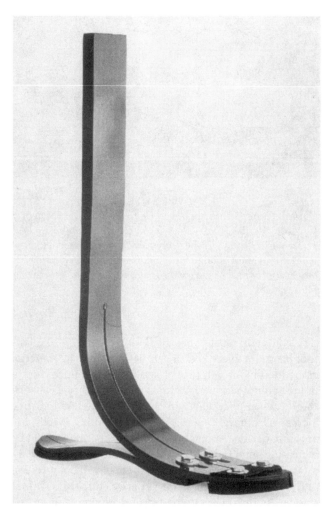

FIGURE 24-12
One-piece dynamic-response carbon graphite design incorporating the shank, ankle, and foot. This type of prosthetic foot can be encased in a foam cosmetic cover. (Photograph courtesy of Flex-Foot, Inc., Aliso Viejo, CA.)

Functional Analysis of Dynamic-Response Feet

Shock absorption during early stance is comparable to that of the other classes. Many dynamic-response feet have a cushioned heel to absorb shock during compression. Control of plantar flexion is also affected by the stiffness of the heel in the foot. Some of the dynamic-response feet, such as the Carbon Copy line, offer feet with various heel foam densities to correspond to the prosthetic user's weight and activity level. The combination systems, such as Flex-Foot and Springlite, provide different degrees of heel stiffness with an interchangeable heel plate and wedge or heel plugs with different densities. These allow the prosthetic user to adjust the stiffness and compress-

ibility of the heel cushion to the various types of activities in which he or she may be involved.

Most dynamic-response feet do not have significant uneven ground accommodation characteristics. Because the keel of dynamic-response feet is designed to be stiffer than that of elastic keel class feet, it is less adaptable to uneven surfaces. The rubber and foam foot shell may absorb a minimal amount of torque forces from stepping on uneven surfaces. Because of the stiff keel, no true inversion/eversion is available in most of these feet. In response to this limitation, several manufacturers have developed alternatives. Flex-Foot offers a split-toe version with a longitudinal separation in forefoot and heel that allows some range of inversion/eversion. The Re-Flex VSP (Flex-Foot, Inc., Aliso Viejo, CA) foot has a vertical compression shaft that is designed to absorb torque forces during high-load activities (Figure 24-13).

The most significant functional differences between dynamic-response feet and other classes of prosthetic feet are found in control of tibia advancement. Dynamic-response feet are chosen for individuals with high activity levels. During these activities, control of the rate of prosthetic tibial shaft advancement is crucial. As cadence increases to running, extra stiffness is necessary during midstance into terminal stance. Tibial shaft advancement is controlled by the stiffness of the keel in the foot. As the shaft advances, the keel deflects, absorbs forces generated during deflection, and resists rapid advancement.

Progression of heel rise is also related to stiffness of the keel in the foot. As the shaft continues to advance, the keel continues to deflect, and the foot dorsiflexes as weight progresses onto the forefoot. The keel in most dynamic-response feet extends into the toe, as in the Carbon Copy product line, or all the way to the distal end of the foot, as in the Flex-Foot and Springlite product lines. The stiffness and deformation qualities of the dynamic-response keel eliminate the need for a rocker effect as seen in the SACH foot. Simultaneously, this extended keel provides stability necessary for support during controlled heel rise during high activity use. In a high loading activity such as running, progression onto the forefoot occurs through a smooth arc of dorsiflexion as the keel continues to deform under the increasing load throughout this phase. Keel deformation and dorsiflexion are now at their maximum point.

The stiffness of the keel now has an effect as body weight is completely transferred to the sound side. Support is provided that allows comfortable transfer of weight to the sound side. Because the stiff yet flexible keel has allowed maximal dorsiflexion without sacrificing support to the amputated side, the runner is allowed a longer sound side stride length. As it is unloaded, the keel begins to decompress as it returns to its original shape, creating a spring action that effectively simulates a true push-off. The spring action of this dynamic response also encourages knee flexion of the amputated side and aids in the initiation of a rapid swing phase.

Advantages and Indications of Dynamic-Response Feet

The primary indication for use of the dynamic-response foot is the potential for and desire to engage in high-demand activities. Many prosthetic users report that they are able to walk with less difficulty and more energy efficiency over a range of grades and speeds.[16] Because the many feet that are available in this class have varying degrees of stiffness, it is critical to match the prosthetic user to the optimal foot for his or her preferred activities. Walking velocity and type of activity directly affect the decision as to which dynamic-response foot to choose. Dynamic-response feet are available in a wide range of stiffness, specific to the weight and activity of the user. Manufacturers are able to custom fabricate a foot to the patient specifications if a standard design is not appropriate.

Dynamic-response feet are indicated when maximum late stance dorsiflexion is desired, for example, during running, when frequent changes in cadence or velocity is necessary, or when walking on inclines.[17,18] The long arc of dorsiflexion and the long flexible keel provided by the Flex-Foot and Re-Flex VSP may also serve to protect the sound limb against excess vertical forces.

Disadvantages and Contraindications of Dynamic-Response Feet

The dynamic-response foot is not appropriate for prosthetic users whose most demanding activity is relaxed gait and household ambulation. The foot is designed to deform under the loading conditions associated with high activity. For users whose activities are unable to generate enough loading force, dynamic-response feet often are perceived as being very stiff and unaccommodating. Because most dynamic-response feet are manufactured from materials such as carbon graphite composite, cost is often significantly higher than for the other classes of prosthetic feet.

Prosthetic Feet that Are Combinations of Classes

Most current prosthetic feet can be placed in one of the four classes. It is important, however, to remember that the prosthetic foot industry is continuously changing. Recent developments have resulted in feet that may combine characteristics from more than one class. For instance, a dynamic-response keel can be combined with a multi-

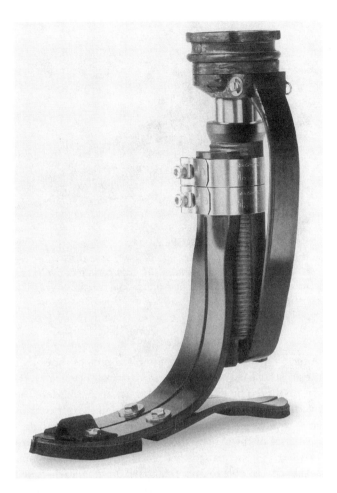

FIGURE 24-13
Carbon fiber side spring and telescoping tubes of the Re-Flex VSP foot absorb shock and return energy for prosthetic users who are involved in high-load activities. Split-foot and heel sections of this dynamic-response foot articulate to allow limited movement in eversion and inversion. (Photograph courtesy of Flex-Foot, Inc., Aliso Viejo, CA.)

axis ankle to give increased accommodation to uneven terrain as well as the spring motion associated with the dynamic-response class (Figure 24-14). In general, the prosthetic foot that combines the characteristics of several classes is likely to be more complicated to use and requires additional maintenance. Each foot must be evaluated on its own merit.

CHOOSING THE APPROPRIATE FOOT

When formulating a prescription recommendation for a prosthetic foot, several additional characteristics should be considered in conjunction with the functional classes

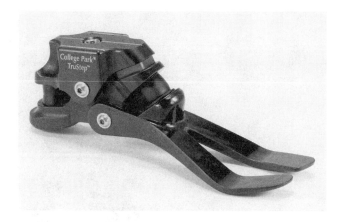

FIGURE 24-14

A dynamic-response keel combined with a multiaxial ankle offers the benefits of two classes of prosthetic feet. Note the plantar flexion and dorsiflexion bumpers and the carbon graphite construction. (Photograph courtesy of College Park Industries, Fraser, MI.)

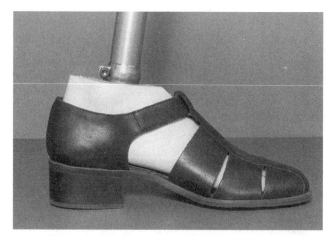

A

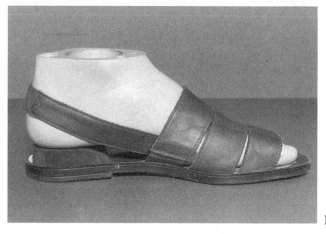

B

FIGURE 24-15

(A) Prosthetic foot in a shoe with excessive heel height. The top of the foot should be level when in a shoe. Gait deviations occur if the heel rise of the prosthetic foot and the heel height of the shoe are mismatched. (B) Firm heel wedge positioned under the prosthetic foot in a flat sandal. This strategy aligns the foot correctly for all phases of the gait cycle.

of feet. The first is heel height and the type of shoes that the prosthetic user desires to wear. For instance, if a Western boot is to be worn, the foot must accommodate the overall height of the heel. If the heel height is not considered, severe gait deviations can occur, and the overall performance of the prosthesis will be compromised (Figure 24-15A). A standard prosthetic foot is designed for a ³/₄-in. heel and is suitable for most standard dress shoes designed for men. If the prosthetic user desires to change to shoes with lower heels, including athletic shoes or sandals, an accommodative wedge can be used to keep the foot level (Figure 24-15B). Changing to shoes with higher heels is not usually possible without changing the prosthetic foot itself.

Another characteristic to consider is the foot's ability to resist moisture. Some feet are essentially waterproof; others should be kept as dry as possible. Many feet can be made water resistant by the prosthetist; however, the manufacturer should always be consulted. The cosmetic appearance of the foot is largely a matter of preference. Some feet appear more life-like, whereas others are very mechanical in appearance by design. Surface features such as toes, veins, and medial and lateral malleoli are available if the patient so desires.

The choice of foot initially centers on the prosthetic user's activity level. The optimal prosthetic foot allows the prosthetic user to walk faster and achieve an equal step length of both amputated and intact limbs.[19] Decisions about the prosthetic foot must consider accommodating not only a user's current activity level but also his or her potential to reach a higher level. Vocational and recreational interests must be considered to ensure that

the foot coincides with the functional needs of the prosthetic user. These needs should be clearly delineated and then balanced with the cost of the desired component. The least expensive prosthetic foot is the simple SACH foot. The most expensive tend to be the sophisticated dynamic-response feet. Many functional and energy-efficient feet that will optimally meet the needs of the prosthetic user fall on a cost continuum between these two extremes. In general, the more sophisticated designs have significantly higher cost and more frequent and complicated maintenance requirements. The prosthetic user who is wearing a foot that requires regular maintenance must be willing to schedule periodic visits to the prosthetist who designed and provided the prosthesis.

CONCLUSION

The choice of foot for any prosthesis should always be a team effort with the prosthetic user as a key participant. The person who is wearing the foot should have a large say in which one is chosen. It is the prosthetist's responsibility to educate the prosthetic user about the options that are available and the characteristics of the feet. The individual with amputation is more vested in the use of the prosthesis if he or she has an active role in decision making regarding components. The proper choice of foot has a drastic effect on the performance of the prosthesis. An improperly prescribed foot leads to poor functional performance and contributes to discouragement on the part of the user. Because many of the feet that are available today are interchangeable, a foot can be changed or upgraded as the needs of the person with amputation change. A SACH foot may be completely appropriate in the early stages of rehabilitation, but as the prosthetic user who becomes more adept in gait desires to resume higher-level activities, a high performance foot may be indicated. This can be accomplished if the prosthesis is based on a modular system that allows for interchangeability of components.

When one is developing a prescription recommendation for a prosthesis, special attention should always be given to the choice of foot. The foot is a critical component because it is the base of the entire prosthesis. A properly prescribed and fitted prosthetic foot can help each prosthetic user reach and maintain his or her desired level of activity and integrate the use of the prosthesis into daily activities.

REFERENCES

1. Sanders GT. Ankle Foot Mechanisms. In GT Sanders, Lower Limb Amputations: A Guide to Rehabilitation. Philadelphia: Davis, 1986;143–162.
2. Radcliff CW, Foort J. The Patellar Tendon Bearing Prosthesis. Berkeley: Regents of the University of California, 1961;104–113.
3. Murphy EM. Lower Extremity Components. In American Academy of Orthopaedic Surgeons, Orthopedic Appliance Atlas. Vol 2. Ann Arbor, MI: Edwards, 1969.
4. Condie DN. Ankle Foot Devices. In G Murdock, RG Donovan (eds), Amputation Surgery and Lower Limb Prosthetics. Oxford: Blackwell Scientific, 1988;52–60.
5. Burgess EM, Wittenberger DA, Forsgren SM, Lindh D. The Seattle Prosthetic Foot: a design for active sports. J Prosthet Orthot 1983;37(1):25–31.
6. Perry J. Gait Analysis; Normal and Pathological Function. New York: McGraw-Hill, 1992;61–69.
7. Cummings D, Kapp SL, MacClellan B. Below Knee Prosthetics. Dallas: University of Texas Prosthetics Orthotics Program, 1987;4/14–4/20.
8. Shurr DG, Cook TM. Prosthetics and Orthotics. Norwalk: Appleton & Lange, 1990;59–62.
9. Donatelli R. The Biomechanics of the Foot and Ankle. Philadelphia: Davis, 1990;9–27.
10. Pitkin MR. Mechanical outcomes of a rolling-joint prosthetic foot and its performance in the dorsiflexion phase of transtibial amputee gait. J Prosthet Orthot 1995;7(3):114–123.
11. Kapp S, Cummings D. Prosthetic Management. In JH Bowker, JW Michael (eds), Atlas of Limb Prosthetics. St. Louis: Mosby–Year Book, 1992;463–466.
12. Perry J. Anatomy and biomechanics of the hindfoot. Clin Orthop 1983;July-Aug(177):9–15.
13. Kegal B, Webster JC, Burgess EM, et al. Recreational activities of lower extremity amputees: a survey. Arch Phys Med Rehabil 1980;61(6):258–264.
14. Enoka RM, Miller DI, Burgess EM, et al. Below amputee running gait. Am J Phys Med 1982;61(2):66–84.
15. Burgess EM. The Seattle Prosthetic Foot. In G Murdock, RG Donovan (eds), Amputation Surgery and Lower Limb Prosthetics. Oxford: Blackwell Scientific, 1988;61–62.
16. Macfarlane PA, Nielsen DH, Shurr DG, et al. Perception of walking difficulty by below-knee amputees using a conventional foot versus the Flex-Foot. J Prosthet Orthot 1991;3(3):114–119.
17. Barth DG, Schumacher L, Thomas SS, et al. Gait analysis and energy cost of below-knee amputees wearing six different prosthetic feet. J Prosthet Orthot 1992;4(2):63–75.
18. Snyder RD, Powers CM, Fontaine C, et al. The effect of five prosthetic feet on the gait and loading of the sound limb in dysvascular below-knee amputees. J Rehabil Res Dev 1995;32(4):309–315.
19. Mizuno N, Aoyama T, Nakajima A, et al. Functional evaluation by gait analysis of various ankle-foot assemblies used by below-knee amputees. Prosthet Orthot Int 1992;16:174–182.

25

Transtibial Prosthetics

GARY M. BERKE

Amputation at the transtibial level occurs at least twice as often as amputation at other levels.[1] Because 90% of all amputations involve the lower extremity, the majority of patients with amputation who are seen by health care professionals has had amputation at the transtibial level. Historically, amputations have been perceived by surgeons as a last resort, perhaps because they view amputation as an admission of failure.[2] Until recently, surgical technique often resulted in residual limbs that were difficult to fit with prostheses, which in turn limited the rehabilitation potential of persons with lower limb amputation. Research and education in the area of amputation surgery have led to more successful surgical and rehabilitation outcomes. Today, many people with transtibial amputations actively participate in professional or amateur sports and leisure activities. These achievements are made possible with a prosthesis that is properly and carefully fit by a qualified prosthetist, in conjunction with gait training and exercise guided by a physical therapist.

A prosthesis is a complex device that must be custom fit to each individual. To achieve optimal fit and alignment, a sequence of several fittings and careful follow-up are necessary to maintain the prosthesis and to make occasional repairs and adjustments as warranted by the individual's activity level and lifestyle. In the last 10 years, the concepts and materials used in fabricating transtibial prostheses have changed dramatically, allowing patients to become much more active and to use their prostheses for longer periods of time. For effective rehabilitation outcomes for patients with new amputation, physical and occupational therapists must be well versed in the mechanical and biomechanical principles of transtibial prostheses.

In this chapter, we (1) distinguish among the various types of transtibial prostheses, (2) discuss the performance characteristics and constraints of the materials and methods that are currently available for rehabilitation inter-

ventions, and (3) identify the biomechanical principles and alignment issues for energy-efficient prosthetic gait.

DETERMINING POTENTIAL FOR PROSTHETIC REHABILITATION

One of the roles of the interdisciplinary rehabilitation team is to determine an individual's potential for limited or functional ambulation with a prosthesis. One of the best indicators of the potential to walk is whether the individual was able to stand and walk before amputation surgery, even if assistance or an ambulatory aid was necessary.[3] Although this suggests that an individual's chance of ambulating with a transtibial prosthesis is highest when ambulation was possible before amputation, it does not imply that a previously nonambulatory patient should be denied a prosthesis. It is important to evaluate all persons with transtibial amputations as candidates for prostheses; many factors (including aerobic conditioning, comorbid medical problems, cognitive status, and motivation and drive) interact to determine the success or failure of prosthetic rehabilitation. Consider the case of an 85-year-old with degenerative joint disease of the hip and bilateral transtibial amputations whose ability to ambulate has been restricted in the 6 months before amputation because of nonhealing neuropathic ulcers. Although this patient may not reach independent ambulation, wearing a prosthesis may enable him or her to transfer independently from a wheelchair to or from a commode or toilet. This functional ability may allow the patient to remain at home with occasional assistance with shopping and cleaning, rather than residing in a long-term care facility.

Medicare has taken the first step in acknowledging various levels of prosthetic use by creating functional level

TABLE 25-1

Medicare Guidelines: Functional Classification for Patients with a Prosthesis

Code	Description
K0	The patient does not have the ability or potential to ambulate or transfer safely with or without assistance, and a prosthesis does not enhance quality of life or mobility.
K1	The patient has the ability or potential to use a prosthesis for transfers or for ambulation on level surfaces at a fixed cadence. With a prosthesis, the patient achieves limited or unlimited household ambulation status.
K2	The patient has the ability or potential for ambulation, including the ability to traverse low-level environmental barriers, such as curbs, stairs, or uneven surfaces. With a prosthesis, the patient is considered a limited community ambulator.
K3	The patient has the ability or potential for ambulation with variable cadence. He or she is likely to achieve community ambulation, with the ability to traverse most environmental barriers, and may have vocational, therapeutic, or exercise activity that demands prosthetic use beyond simple locomotion.
K4	The patient has the ability or potential for prosthetic ambulation that exceeds basic ambulatory skills, exhibiting high impact, stress, or energy levels during activity. This category includes most children, active adults, or athletes with amputation.

Source: DMERC Medicare Advisory Bulletin, Columbia SC, 1994;12:95–145.

codes[4] (Table 25-1). These codes guide the prosthetist in choosing components based on the activity level of the patient. This evaluation process ensures that all patients, regardless of age or functional status, are candidates for a prosthesis that is appropriate to their needs.

COMPONENTS OF A TRANSTIBIAL PROSTHESIS

A transtibial prosthesis has four key components: the socket and its interface, the suspension mechanism, the shank or pylon, and the prosthetic foot. The various types of prosthetic feet and their functional characteristics are discussed in Chapter 24. In this chapter, we focus on the other three components.

Transtibial Socket Design: An Historical Perspective

The socket is the portion of the prosthesis that contacts and disperses pressure around the patient's residual limb. It is designed to contain and support the residual limb during weight bearing and to transmit forces from the limb to control the placement of the foot.[5] The patellar tendon-bearing (PTB) prosthesis, first developed in the 1950s, has been the most commonly prescribed and fabricated transtibial socket. In early versions of the PTB design, the socket was open ended and typically fabricated from carved wood or aluminum. The weight-bearing surfaces of the limb were limited to the patellar tendon and the popliteal space. Pressure in these areas would suspend the residual limb inside

the socket and enable the prosthetic wearer to ambulate with a relatively normal gait. Early PTB designs had problems, however. In some cases, the end of the residual limb was unable to tolerate pressures caused by the movement of the bone within the soft tissue envelope. A lack of distal contact often led to an edematous distal residual limb, making the prosthesis difficult to don and uncomfortable, sometimes impossible, to use.

The concept of total surface bearing has emerged to address the limitations of early PTB socket designs. The total surface-bearing design distributes loading pressures over the entire surface of the residual limb, including the distal end. Distribution of pressure over a larger surface area reduces loading at any one location, making the prosthesis more comfortable to use. Total surface contact also reduces the likelihood of development of distal edema during prosthetic use. It is important to note that, although many areas of the residual limb tolerate considerable pressure, some are quite pressure intolerant. Most modern socket designs incorporate characteristics of total surface bearing and of the original PTB socket design.

Pressure-Tolerant Areas of the Transtibial Residual Limb

The PTB design distributes the loading pressures of weight bearing over six surfaces of the transtibial residual limb (Figure 25-1). These areas include the patellar tendon, the posterior popliteal tissues, along the distal lateral fibular shaft, along the medial tibial shaft and soft tissue of the neighboring anterior compartment, at the medial tibial (metaphyseal) flare, and around the medial and lateral femoral condyles. Pressure-intolerant areas, most notably

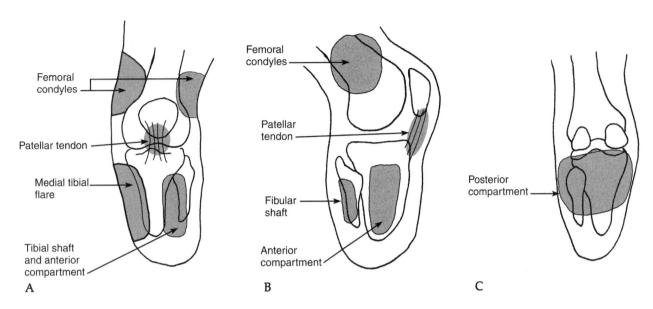

FIGURE 25-1

Pressure-tolerant areas of the transtibial residual limb. **(A)** *On the anterior surface, pressure-tolerant surfaces include the patellar tendon, the medial tibial flare, along both sides of the tibial shaft, and the medial and lateral femoral condyles.* **(B)** *On the lateral view, pressure-tolerant areas include the patellar tendon, anterolateral compartment, and the shaft of the fibula.* **(C)** *On the posterior surface, most structures within the popliteal fossa are pressure tolerant.*

the fibular head and the distal anterior tibia, are protected by relief areas incorporated into the socket.

The PTB design positions the residual limb appropriately within the socket using an anterior bar that loads the patellar tendon above its insertion on the tibial tubercle and a posterior popliteal bulge that is designed to stabilize the limb on the patellar bar (Figure 25-2). Force applied to the pressure-tolerant soft tissue of the posterior compartment pushes the limb forward onto the PTB surface (the patellar bar). This helps to suspend the limb within the prosthesis, minimizing excessive distal weight bearing as the limb is loaded during each stance phase of gait.

Pressure along the lateral fibular shaft (distal to the peroneal nerve) helps to control the distal segment of the residual limb during the stance phase of gait, stabilizing the prosthesis against the varus thrust that normally occurs at the knee at midstance. This distribution of weight-bearing pressures along the shaft of the fibula reduces forces on the pressure-intolerant distal fibula and fibular head.

Pressures applied on either side of midline, along the medial tibial shaft and the anterolateral muscular compartment, are also used to control the tibia during the stance phase of gait; this enhances vertical support of the limb in the prosthesis as well. The PTB design also incorporates a slight relief area for the crest of the tibia and vulnerable anterior distal end of the tibia.

The medial tibial (metaphyseal) flare is one of the most weight-tolerant areas of the residual limb. The PTB socket is carefully contoured so that the medial tibial flare rests against a supporting surface within the socket, to aid vertical support of the limb in the prosthesis during stance.

Pressures along the medial and lateral femoral condyles are used to provide mediolateral stability during the stance phase of gait. The prosthesis is contoured carefully to accept the forces in this area because excessive pressure over either condyle causes discomfort.

Pressure-Intolerant Areas of the Residual Limb

In the evaluation of prosthetic fit, it is probably more important to understand where weight-bearing pressures must be minimized along the residual limb than it is to understand where they are applied most effectively. Excessive pressure over intolerant areas increases the risk of compensatory gait deviation as the prosthetic user attempts to minimize discomfort. Excessive pressure over vulnerable areas also increases the risk of skin irritation or breakdown; waiting for irritated skin or wear-induced open wounds to heal can significantly delay rehabilitation and gait training. The areas that are most vulnerable to excessive pressure include the fibular head and peroneal nerve, used variations are the hard socket, worn with prosthetic socks, various types of soft liners, and a flexible socket supported by a rigid frame.

Hard Socket

For some patients, the prosthetist might recommend a hard socket alone, a rigid plastic interface worn with prosthetic socks but with no additional liner. Often, a soft, closed cell foam pad is placed in the distal end to make the socket more comfortable during weight bearing. This design has several important advantages: First, if an intimate fit is achieved, shearing and friction between the socket and residual limb are minimized, enhancing function. Second, overall cosmesis is enhanced because no liners add bulk around the residual limb, making the prosthesis less obvious when worn under clothing. Third, a hard socket is very easy to clean; the high-temperature thermoplastic materials that are used most often are resistant to bacterial or fungal growth. Finally, the socket is very durable, with no compressible components to pack down or change shape over time.

Several constraints or disadvantages should also be considered: The intimate fit that is necessary for an effective hard socket requires careful skill and exactness on the part of the prosthetist in manufacture, modification, and fitting of the prosthesis. A hard socket is difficult to adjust or modify as the residual limb changes shape or matures. The hard socket alone, without an additional liner, may not be appropriate for patients with fragile skin or significant bony prominences.

Prosthetic Socks

The most common interface that is used between a socket and the residual limb is a prosthetic sock. These prosthetic socks accomplish two goals: (1) they help to cushion the forces that are applied to the residual limb during ambulation, and (2) they help to accommodate for changes in the volume of the residual limb. For most prosthetic users, residual limb volume varies during any given day as a result of normal activity. Minor though these changes may be, they have the potential to compromise the fit of the prosthesis and increase the risk of skin irritation and discomfort. The addition or subtraction of sock layers (ply) accommodates the changes in the limb and helps to maintain the fit. This often presents a challenge to new prosthetic wearers, who may need to add several additional ply of sock in the middle of the day after a morning of moving about in their prosthesis to maintain optimal fit and function. Discerning when and how many ply of sock to add or remove is a skill that is developed during prosthetic training and rehabilitation.

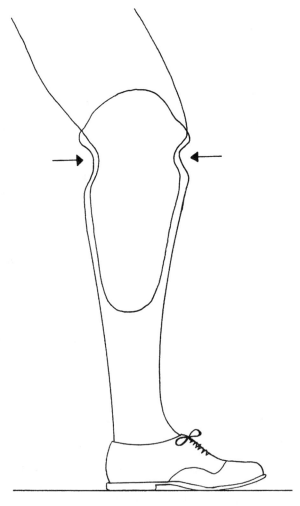

FIGURE 25-2
The patellar tendon bar and posterior popliteal bulge of a patellar tendon-bearing socket apply anteroposterior forces to suspend and stabilize the residual limb within the socket.

the anterior distal tibia (the cut end of the bone), the hamstring tendons, the tibial crest, the anterior tibial tubercle, the distal fibula, the patella, and the adductor tubercle (Figure 25-3). Inspection of the interior surface of a PTB socket reveals relief areas or channels that are designed to protect skin and soft tissue in these vulnerable areas.

TRANSTIBIAL SOCKET

A variety of options are available as an interface between the transtibial socket and the skin of the residual limb. Each material and design has specific advantages and disadvantages that must be carefully considered in the process of prosthetic prescription and fitting. The most commonly

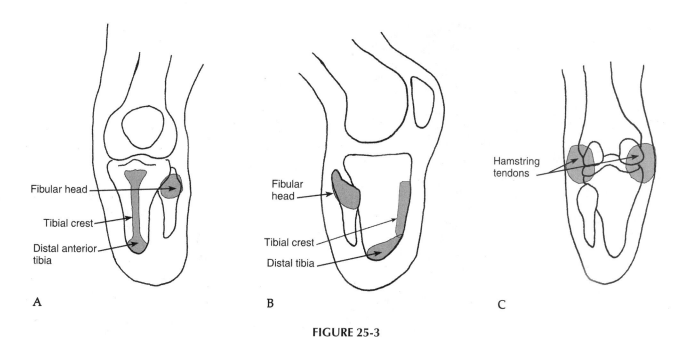

FIGURE 25-3

Pressure-intolerant areas of the residual limb. (A) From an anterior view areas that are pressure intolerant include the head of the fibula, crest of the tibia, and distal anterior tibia. (B) Laterally, the fibular head must be relieved of pressure. (C) On the posterior surface tendons of the hamstring muscles need to be protected.

Prosthetic socks are manufactured from several materials and in multiple thicknesses. They are sized to best fit the circumference and length of the patient's residual limb. The prosthetist usually provides several sets of wool and cotton socks, in one-ply (thin), three-ply, and five-ply (thick) weights. Although prosthetic socks are also available in polyester or cotton-polyester blend, many patients prefer the comfort of wool. During prosthetic training, the new prosthetic user learns to layer socks of various ply to achieve the most comfortable and functional fit in the socket. The thickest sock is worn next to the skin and the thinnest ply as the outer layer, so that ply adjustments can be accomplished easily. Once the layers of sock reach 10–15 ply, however, the fit of the socket is so compromised that a new smaller socket may be necessary.

Socks must be donned and smoothed carefully so that no wrinkles occur in any of the sock layers. A wrinkle increases pressure inside the prosthesis and can lead to skin irritation and ulceration. Many prosthetists design a new prosthesis to fit with one three-ply wool sock. This baseline provides adequate cushioning while preserving intimacy of fit. As the limb shrinks or swells, socks are added or taken off, one ply at a time, until a comfortable fit is possible. For new prosthetic wearers, the distal residual limb may shrink more rapidly than the proximal limb around the knee. In this case, a sock is trimmed to fit only halfway up the residual limb (current sock manufacturing prevents unraveling of cut edges); this improves prosthetic fit distally without compromising proximal fit.

Many people with amputation wear a nylon sheath (similar to a stocking) between the residual limb and the socks. The sheath wicks perspiration away from the skin toward the socks, resulting in a dryer, more comfortable feeling inside the socket.[6] The sheath also helps to decrease the sheer forces between the socket and the residual limb. Daily cleaning and changing of socks are essential, as the bacteria levels in a closed prosthetic environment are often quite high. Wool socks are best hand washed in mild detergent, blotted dry, and then dried flat (the clothes dryer shrinks wool socks to an unusable size and shape).

Soft Liner

For patients with fragile skin or significant bony prominences, and for prosthetic users with high levels of activity, a soft liner may provide additional protection and comfort during gait and other activities. A soft liner is fabricated in conjunction with the rigid outer shell for an exact fit. Some of the materials that are commonly used in the fabrication of soft liners include Pelite, Nickleplast, PPT, silicone gel, Plastazote, and leather. Most commonly, the patient first puts on a sheath and the appropriate ply of sock and then dons the liner. Once all are in place, the residual limb and liner are fit into the socket. This external liner often eases the application of a snugly

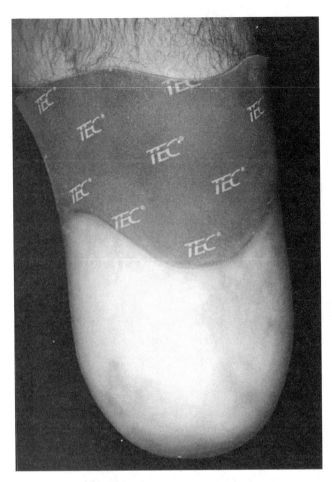

FIGURE 25-4
Total environmental control (TEC) liner. Made of a urethane material, the TEC liner effectively cushions pressure-sensitive areas while dissipating shear forces between the limb and prosthesis during gait. (Courtesy of TEC Manufacturing, St. Cloud, MN.)

fit prosthesis. Sock ply is added or removed between limb and liner as needed to assure comfortable prosthetic fit.

A soft liner provides additional protection and padding for the residual limb and can be easily adjusted or modified. Some liner materials, however, absorb perspiration and may be difficult to clean. Liner materials also compress with repeated loading and use; eventually the quality of prosthetic fit may be compromised. Liners also add an additional layer, increasing the bulk of the prosthesis; this might be problematic for prosthetic users who are concerned about cosmesis. In some cases, especially for very active prosthetic users, the liner presents an opportunity for shearing and friction between the socket and residual limb, and may not be tolerated by some users.

Other Interfaces

Advances in prosthetics have made a third option available as an interface for transtibial sockets. These new liners are designed to absorb some of the shearing forces that normally occur between the limb and prosthesis during gait. Examples of these liners include the urethane Total Environmental Control (TEC; TEC Manufacturing, St. Cloud, MN) liner (Figure 25-4) and silicone liners such as the ALPS liner (ALPS South Corp, St. Petersburg, FL), the ALPHA liner (Ohio Willowwood Corp., Mt. Sterling, OH), and the ICEROSS liner (Ossur USA Inc., Columbia, MD). These liners differ from traditional soft liners because they must be worn directly against the skin, to minimize shearing. Prosthetic socks are still used to accommodate for limb volume changes; however, they are donned over the liner rather than between the liner and the skin. Some liners require that a non–water-soluble lubricant be used for the skin. According to the manufacturer, the TEC liner also has the ability to flow.[7] Pressure on the material causes it to move or cold flow to an area of lesser pressure. The advantage of flow is that with excessive pressure the material actually thins slightly and allows the pressure to decrease. The material returns to the original thickness once the pressure has been removed. Use of a liner provides a true total contact prosthesis.

Silicone liners, also called *silicone suspension sleeves*, are made of a silicone material that is very effective in dampening shearing forces. To don the sleeve, it must first be rolled inside out. The patient then places the distal cup of the sleeve on the end of the residual limb and slowly rolls the sleeve up over the rest of the limb. If a special pin is incorporated distally, these liners also serve as a highly effective suspension mechanism for the prosthesis.

Liners such as the TEC and silicone sleeves have several important advantages when compared to prosthetic socks or other soft liners. First, these liners are extremely effective in dispersion of forces during gait, including shear forces that can irritate or ulcerate the skin, making the prosthesis more comfortable to use. Often these liners also provide a mechanism for suspension of the prosthesis. There is some suggestion that these liners facilitate venous return from the residual limb.[7] These types of liners are especially helpful for patients with fragile skin or recurrent discomfort or breakdown over bony prominences. Some of these liners can accommodate minor changes in residual limb volume without the need for prosthetic socks; moderate to major changes can be addressed by the addition of prosthetic socks over the liner.

As with any of the other interfaces, these antishear liners have disadvantages that must be considered during prosthetic prescription. They require dexterity and upper extremity strength to don; they may be difficult to put on if a patient has arthritis, sensory loss, or other impairments of the upper extremity. Some patients complain about the increased time and attention that are required to don the liner properly. The liner sometimes requires that a special lubricant (such as alcohol) be used on the outside of the liner as it is applied to the skin. Most require greater care in cleaning to reduce odor and bacteria. For some patients, use of this type of liner can cause skin problems, such as contact dermatitis, bacterial infections, or follicular irritation.

Flexible Socket in a Rigid Frame

In a variation of a transtibial prosthesis, a prosthetist can use thin thermoplastic material to create a flexible PTB socket, which is supported within a rigid external frame fabricated from a thicker thermoplastic material or from a fabric or composite material hardened with polymer resin in a thermosetting process (Figure 25-5). The flexible socket is, essentially, the same PTB design described previously, worn with a sheath or prosthetic sock and providing total contact with the residual limb. Its flexibility, however, allows it to change shape slightly as underlying muscle contracts or as the knee joint moves further into flexion range of motion. This flexibility is thought to increase comfort during function, and the thinness of the socket is thought to permit some dissemination of body heat. The external rigid frame is designed to direct forces to the pressure-tolerant areas, particularly the medial tibial flare, the anterolateral muscular compartment and shaft of the fibula, and the patellar tendon. There may be cutaways over pressure-intolerant areas such as the tibial crest and distal tibia and the head of the fibula.

SUSPENSION MECHANISMS

Safe and effective prosthetic use requires that the prosthesis be suspended comfortably and consistently on the limb during the activities in which the user chooses to be involved. All suspension mechanisms must accomplish two things: (1) hold the prosthesis firmly to the limb during gait and (2) allow the patient to sit comfortably. A good suspension reduces the risk of skin irritation or breakdown by minimizing movement (pistoning and torque) between the socket and the limb. In the prosthetic prescription process, the choice of suspension is influenced by the patient's present and predicted activities, his or her goals and physical abilities, and the climate in which the patient lives.

Sleeve Suspension

One of the most commonly prescribed suspension systems is a sleeve made of neoprene, urethane, or latex (Figure 25-6), which is positioned around the shank of the pros-

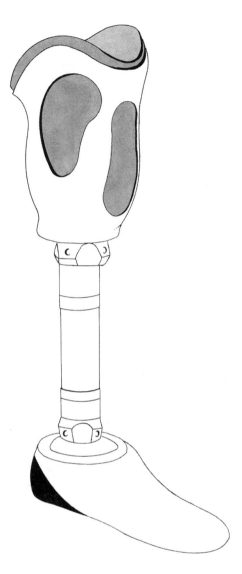

FIGURE 25-5
Example of a flexible socket in a rigid frame (anterolateral view). A thin thermoplastic socket is supported by a rigid external frame that transmits weight-bearing forces from pressure-tolerant areas of the residual limb to the pylon and prosthetic foot while open space around the fibular head and anterior tibia minimizes forces on these pressure-intolerant areas.

thesis and is rolled upward over the thigh once the prosthesis has been donned. Although the outer surface of the sleeve has a smooth covering, the inner surface tends to "grab" the surface of the skin. Sleeves are manufactured in various lengths and diameters to ensure a snug fit against the patient's thigh. To be effective, the sleeve must contact several inches of skin above the top of the prosthetic socks (occasionally, the top of the socks needs to be trimmed). Suspension sleeves use friction, negative pres-

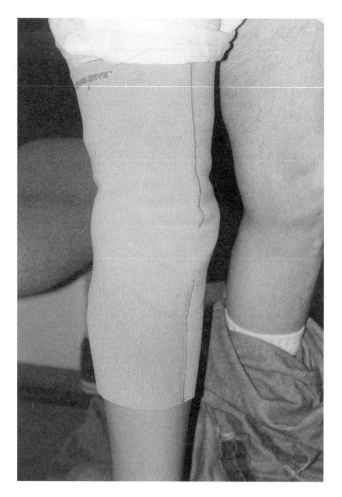

FIGURE 25-6

Neoprene suspension sleeve placed around the shank of the prosthesis and rolled upward against the skin of the thigh to hold the prosthesis in place. Note the seam at the anterior midline and the slight bump where the underlying prosthetic socks have been trimmed to ensure contact with the skin several inches from the top of the sleeve.

sure (a result of the airtight fit), and resistance to stretch to hold the prosthesis on the residual limb. Circumferential constriction is minimal, however, so that suspension sleeves are appropriate even for patients with vascular insufficiency.

Suspension sleeves have a number of advantages over other suspension strategies. Many prosthetic users find these relatively thin sleeves to be more cosmetic than other suspension mechanisms. Because suspension sleeves are fit to be airtight, they are often the suspension of choice for individuals who prefer to wear the prosthesis while

showering or swimming as water does not enter the socket. Although some upper extremity strength and dexterity are required to pull the tight sleeve up into place, many prosthetic wearers find them very easy to use. Suspension sleeves allow unrestricted knee motion during most activities. Some very active wearers dislike the posterior bunching of the material during kneeling or other activities that require maximal knee flexion.

One of the major disadvantages of suspension sleeves is their limited durability: They are susceptible to tearing or stretching from repeated donning and doffing and should be replaced fairly frequently. Even a small hole greatly reduces the sleeve's ability to suspend the prosthesis. Suspension sleeves create a closed environment, which makes them hot to wear for extended periods of time; this is especially problematic if the patient lives where air temperature and/or humidity is typically high. Constant friction against skin can cause skin irritation or hygiene or sweating problems, especially in wearers with significant body hair. Although the sleeve is similar in appearance to an elastic knee orthosis, it does not stabilize the knee directly. For prosthetic users with upper extremity arthritis, weakness, or sensory loss, suspension sleeves may be very difficult to don or doff.

Supracondylar Suspension

Supracondylar suspension captures the femoral condyles as they taper into the shaft of the femur to hold the prosthesis on the residual limb (Figure 25-7). To do this, the medial and lateral walls of a PTB prosthesis rise proximally around the femoral condyles. Because the walls are designed to taper to a narrow mediolateral dimension above the condyles, the prosthesis literally hangs from the condyles. This type of suspension is often abbreviated as *PTB-SC* (patellar tendon-bearing–supracondylar) or *PTS* (patellar tendon–supracondylar) suspension. The high walls of a PTB-SC prosthesis also provide mediolateral stability to the knee joint itself, a major advantage for patients with collateral ligament damage or insufficiency. This suspension is ineffective, however, for obese or muscular patients in whom definition of the condyles is not available.

Most prosthetic users, even those with visual impairment or upper extremity dysfunction, find supracondylar suspension fairly easy to don and doff. The extra medial and lateral support provided by PTB-SD prostheses is important for those with biomechanical instability of the knee. As long as the condyles are accessible, PTB-SC suspension is so effective that no additional means of suspension are necessary. Some wearers, however, are

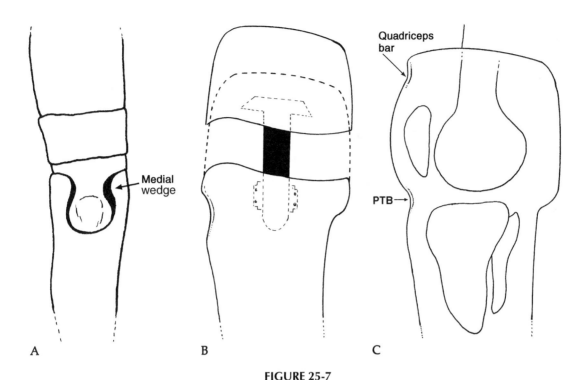

FIGURE 25-7

*Variations of supracondylar suspension. (**A**) The medial and lateral walls of this hard socket extend upward to encompass the femoral condyles. Note the medial wedge incorporated in the soft liner to enhance suspension. (**B**) Some patellar tendon-bearing (PTB)–supracondylar prostheses have a removable medial brim, which opens to facilitate donning and closes once the limb is in the socket to achieve suspension. (**C**) A lateral view of a supracondylar-suprapatellar socket also encompasses the patella within a raised anterior wall. Note the patellar tendon bar and relief for the patella.*

concerned about the cosmesis of this suspension: The proximal walls are quite obvious through clothing when the knee is flexed during sitting. Although this suspension incorporates mediolateral support for the knee, it does not provide stability in the anteroposterior direction and should not be used to address anterior or posterior cruciate ligament problems. Fabrication of the PTB-SC prosthesis is also more time consuming and somewhat more difficult than other forms of suspension.

In a supracondylar-suprapatellar prosthesis (PTB-SCSP) an anterior wall is added to the proximal prosthesis, encapsulating the patella (see Figure 25-7C). This high anterior wall increases the stiffness and stability of the mediolateral walls and facilitates suspension with the addition of a quadriceps bar over the proximal patella. Because this bar maintains the patient's knee in slight flexion during the stance phase, PTB-SCSP suspension may be appropriate for wearers who have a very short residual limb or who tend to abnormally hyperextend the knee in the stance phase of gait. A soft liner is often used with PTB-SCSP sockets to facilitate donning and doffing. This suspension

is, however, even less cosmetic than the PTB-SC in sitting, because of the high anterior wall and patellar relief. Patients may be uncomfortable in the PTB-SCSP prosthesis if they attempt to kneel. Placement of the patellar relief and quadriceps bar requires skill and extra time in fabrication. Finally, the PTB-SCSC may not be appropriate for those who are obese or highly muscular if the condyles cannot be sufficiently "captured" to ensure consistent suspension.

Cuff Suspension

Another method of suspension that captures the femoral condyles is cuff strap suspension (Figure 25-8). In this method, a leather or webbing strap in the shape of a broad "X" is attached to the medial and lateral walls of the prosthesis, slightly posterior to midline. The X of the strap is positioned directly above the patella, and it then wraps around the limb posteriorly above the femoral condyles and is secured with a Velcro, D-ring, or buckle closure. The cuff suspends the prosthesis by being snug over the

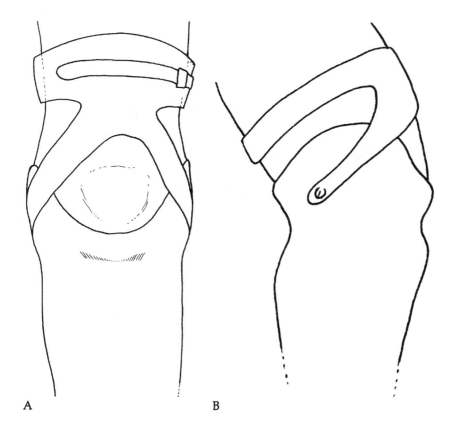

A   B

FIGURE 25-8
*Anterior (**A**) and medial (**B**) views of cuff strap suspension. Note the center of the cuff positioned above the patella (**A**) and the points of attachment slightly posterior to midline (**B**), which are necessary for efficient suspension.*

top of the patella, *not* by circumferential tightness. The quality of suspension is controlled by the cuff's point of attachment on the prosthesis. The attachment points should be posterior to the center of the socket so that the line of pull falls posteriorly at the proximal portion of the patella. This attachment point is also critical if the patient is to sit comfortably. If the cuff is not suspending well, practitioners and patients have an unfortunate tendency to tighten the posterior strap. A tight circumferential pressure compromises circulation and does nothing to enhance the efficiency of prosthetic suspension.

A prosthetist or prosthetic wearer would choose cuff strap suspension because it is easy to don and doff and is readily adjustable. A cuff strap is an efficient suspension system for most individuals with a midlength residual limb. The points of attachment can be varied slightly to help control unwanted knee hyperextension. Some wearers find the cuff to be restrictive when knee flexion is needed for kneeling or sitting. In some cases, inaccurate placement of the points of attachment can lead to rotation of the socket on the limb during gait. In some individuals, especially those who are heavy, impingement of soft tissue may be present between the strap and posterior brim of the socket. In obese or very muscular wearers, it may be difficult to achieve adequate purchase above the patella and around the femoral condyles. Unlike the

PTB-SC suspension, a cuff strap cannot provide any mediolateral or anteroposterior stability to an unstable knee joint. If the cuff is made of leather, it may become misshapen over time and need to be replaced (fortunately, a cuff strap is fairly inexpensive and simple to replace).

Waist Belt and Anterior Strap

An historic method of prosthetic suspension uses a waist belt and anterior strap to suspend the prosthesis from the pelvis (Figure 25-9). The waist belt, usually made of Dacron or leather, can be worn external to clothing during early prosthetic training when frequent skin inspection is warranted, but it is generally worn under the clothes in regular use. An elastic strap extends from the belt toward the prosthesis. This strap can hook or buckle to a cuff strap or can fork to medial and lateral points of attachment directly on the prosthesis. This anterior strap incorporates an elastic material for two reasons: (1) to accommodate for the extra length that is needed for knee flexion from terminal stance to initial swing and when the wearer is sitting and (2) to provide some assistance with knee extension as the elastic recoils from initial swing to initial contact during gait. Although the waist belt has been very effective for suspension, it is bulky and at times difficult to manage under clothing and is now used much less frequently as a primary means of suspension. It may still be used as the first strategy for suspension in patients who are fit with a prosthesis immediately after surgery or for individuals who are frail or deconditioned who would benefit from the assist provided by elastic recoil for limb advancement in swing. Waist straps are also used when other forms of suspension are contraindicated or have proved unsuccessful. Athletes with amputation often opt to use a waist belt as auxiliary suspension, as backup in case their preferred suspension fails during demanding activity or competition.

Although the waist belt and elastic strap provide excellent suspension and are easy to don and doff, the elastic anterior strap can become overstretched over time, and must be occasionally replaced. The various straps and buckles may be difficult to manage for patients with visual impairment, sensory loss, or limited upper extremity dexterity. The waist belt may be difficult to keep clean. Some individuals find it impractical or uncomfortable when worn under clothing but distracting or noncosmetic when worn over their clothes. Although the waist belt and strap is very effective in suspension, it cannot provide any external stability for those with ligamentous instability or weakness of the muscles around the knee.

Suction Suspension

Prosthetists have experimented with various types of suction suspension for transtibial prostheses for a number of years, but until recently most attempts at suction suspension had limited success. Unlike the transfemoral residual limb with its abundant and compliant soft tissue, the irregular topography of the transtibial residual limb presented a challenge for achieving the consistent air lock that was needed for suction. Widespread use of suction suspension became possible only with the development of silicone materials. In 1986, Ossurr Kristinsson presented the first roll-on silicone sleeve that would suspend a prosthesis.[8] Today, several manufacturers market prefabricated silicone suction suspension mechanisms (Figure 25-10). A silicone suspension mechanism has two components. The first is a pliable sleeve, usually made of a silicone polymer, which is 1–9 mm thick and has a short peg or pin incorporated at the distal end. This pin inserts into a locking mechanism embedded at the base of the prosthetic socket. Once the pin is locked in place, the friction between the silicone material and skin suspends the prosthesis. A sock or sheath (with a hole cut in the bottom for the pin) is worn over the sleeve to ease donning into the socket. Additional layers of sock can be added

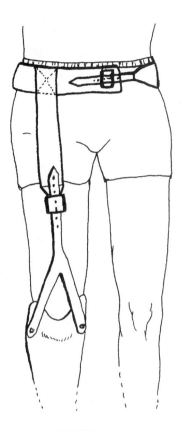

FIGURE 25-9
A waist belt with an anterior elastic strap can be hooked or buckled to a cuff or can attach directly to the prosthesis, as shown here. In either method, the elastic elongates to allow flexion for sitting and for late stance/early swing of gait and then recoils to assist forward progression of the prosthesis during swing.

to adjust for volume change during daily wear or during the period of limb maturation.

Many prosthetic wearers enjoy the increased sense of limb position awareness afforded by silicone suspension. Silicone sleeves attenuate sheer forces and are excellent alternatives for prosthetic wearers with fragile or sensitive skin. Suction suspension sleeves vary in price but tend to be more expensive than some of the other forms of suspension. This is sometimes problematic if sleeves are damaged or torn during frequent donning and doffing. Cleanliness is sometimes a problem as well: Sleeves must be consistently cleaned and maintained to minimize odor and bacterial buildup. Some patients report skin irritation at the liner's proximal edge. Often, this irritation can be reduced by releasing the tension at the skin-liner interface, which occurs when donning or pulling the sleeve up. The problem can be resolved by rolling the sleeve on (rather than pulling), then lifting the edge of the liner, all the way around the limb. The locking

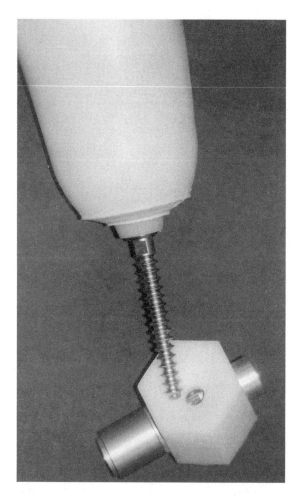

FIGURE 25-10
Silicone suspension sleeve with its distal pin and the locking mechanism to be embedded in the base of the prosthetic socket. Once the sleeve is in place, the wearer steps down into the prosthesis until the pin lock has engaged. When doffing the prosthesis, the wearer pushes a button that is recessed into the wall of the socket to disengage the lock and release the pin.

mechanism can also add weight to the finished prosthesis. Finally, many silicone suspension systems require more frequent maintenance and repair, which will also increase the overall cost of the prosthesis.

"Thigh Lacer" and Side Joints

A prosthesis may be difficult to use for a variety of reasons. If the patient has significant pain, scar tissue, knee instability, a very short residual limb, or an otherwise unsuitable limb for fitting, alternative techniques for fitting and suspension must be investigated. One such alternative is the thigh lacer and side joints prosthesis (Figure 25-11). Although traditional versions use a leather thigh

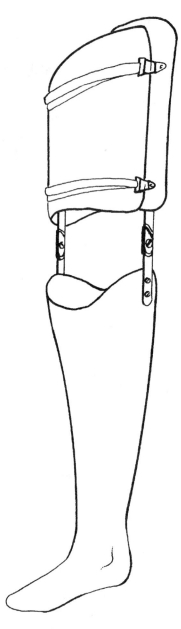

FIGURE 25-11
Example of a transtibial prosthesis with thigh cuff and side joints (also described as a joint and corset prosthesis). Prosthetic knee joints are incorporated at the medial and lateral walls of the prosthesis. Weight-bearing forces are distributed around the thigh through a snugly fit leather or thermoplastic "corset."

corset closed by laces, a long thermoplastic thigh cuff with Velcro closures may be used today. Compression of soft tissue in the thigh by the snugly closed thigh cuff during weight bearing distributes the pressure proximally, relieving forces on the residual limb. The side joints control knee instability in the mediolateral plane. The joints move the varus and valgus forces away from the knee center onto the thigh. If anteroposterior instability of the knee is present, a posterior "check strap" is attached between the posterior distal thigh cuff and the posterior brim of the socket to limit excessive knee extension while the prosthesis is worn. The posterior check strap also reduces noise and limits wear of the prosthetic joint surfaces. The thigh lacer should be worn in conjunction with an auxiliary suspension such as a waist belt and elastic strap.

Although the thigh lacer and side joint suspension provides significant external stability for a biomechanically unstable knee, aids in suspension of the prosthesis, and absorbs vertical loading to deweight the residual limb, many prosthetic wearers find it to be very bulky and heavy. The thigh cuff, if fabricated from leather, may be difficult to keep clean, picking up the smell of perspiration. Although the thigh lacer is designed to be worn under clothing, cosmesis and adjustability may be problematic. For persons with limited flexibility or upper extremity dysfunction, the thigh lacer may be difficult to don. For many users who require the stability and force distribution afforded by a thigh lacer, additional suspension is often necessary, adding to the difficulty of donning and the bulkiness under clothing.

Additional Design and Suspension Variations

Patients who cannot tolerate the thigh lacer or whose residual limb is extremely short (less than 2 in. from knee center to distal tibia) have a limited number of alternatives. The prosthetist may suggest a gluteal-bearing prosthesis, which distributes weight bearing to the gluteus muscles and ischium, or a bent knee prosthesis. Both designs are very difficult to fit and are quite cumbersome to use. Although preservation of the knee joint is associated with reduced energy cost during walking, some patients with very short or extensively scarred residual limbs opt for surgical revision to knee disarticulation or transfemoral amputation so that prosthetic fit can be more effective, comfortable, and cosmetic.

PROSTHETIC PROGRESSION: FROM TEMPORARY TO DEFINITIVE PROSTHESIS

The very first prosthesis received by a patient with a new amputation is a temporary prosthesis (also called a *training* or *preparatory prosthesis*). This type of prosthesis is different from a definitive prosthesis in that it is fabricated fairly quickly in an attempt to get the patient up and moving as soon as healing has occurred. The temporary prosthesis is typically an endoskeletal system, consisting only of a socket, suspension system, pylon, and prosthetic foot, and is usually unfinished cosmetically. This strategy per-

mits interchanging of components and helps to minimize production costs during a time when many adjustments and adaptations to the socket and to prosthetic alignment are anticipated. Typically, the size and shape of the residual limb begin to change once the patient is ambulating on his or her first prosthesis. At some point (which varies from patient to patient), the residual matures or shrinks so much that the patient must wear 10 or more ply of sock to compensate for the loss of limb volume, and prosthetic fit is significantly compromised. For many new prosthetic users, a smaller socket needs to be fabricated within the first 3–6 months of prosthetic use. Because the limb continues to shrink for up to a year after amputation, many patients require several new sockets until limb size and volume stabilize.

The definitive prosthesis is fit when the size of the patient's limb has stabilized, typically indicated when the patient consistently uses the same number of socks with the prosthesis over several weeks or months or when girth measurements remain the same over a similar period of time. Once the residual limb has matured, the definitive prosthesis is fabricated and fit. Most definitive prostheses fit comfortably and maintain their structural integrity for 3–5 years for normal levels of activity.

The definitive prosthesis can be fabricated as either an endoskeletal (having a central pylon with a foam cosmetic cover) or exoskeletal (having a hard outer shell between the socket and prosthetic foot) system. Definitive prostheses are usually cosmetically enhanced to match the contours and skin color of the remaining limb as closely as possible before final delivery to the patient. In deciding whether to use an endo- or exoskeletal system, the prosthetist and person with transtibial amputation must weigh the various advantages and disadvantages of each to determine which system will best meet the patient's individual needs.

Endoskeletal Finishing

In an endoskeletal system, body weight is supported by a central rigid pylon (Figure 25-12), and cosmesis is achieved by a soft contoured foam cover with a nylon stocking, rubberized paint, or latex sheath as a finishing external layer. The pylon (endoskeleton) may be the same steel alloy, titanium, or aluminum tube used in the temporary prosthesis or may be a lighter-weight stiff and durable plastic material. The choice of pylon is influenced by the patient's weight, his or her level of endurance, and the types of activities anticipated; the material must be strong enough to support the patient's body weight and sustain repeated loading during activities. The outer cover, whether nylon, rubberized paint, or latex, is matched as closely as possible to the patient's skin color to maximize prosthetic cosmesis.

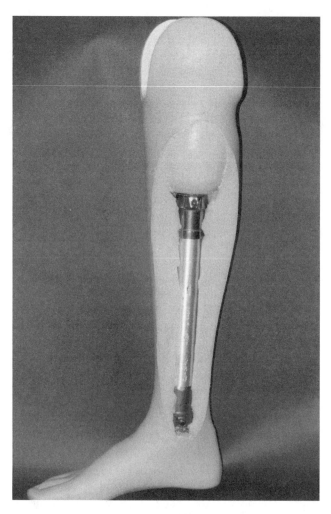

FIGURE 25-12
Cutaway view of an endoskeletal transtibial prosthetic system. Note the hard socket and upright pylon and the foam filler covered by a rubberized "skin." Alignment couplings between the socket and pylon, and between the pylon and prosthetic foot, are used to fine tune alignment for efficient and comfortable gait.

Prosthetic wearers often find that their endoskeletal systems are soft to the touch, much like real skin, and thus are quite cosmetically appealing. The use of a rubber or latex skin over the soft cover increases the durability and water resistance of the prosthesis. The major advantage of an endoskeletal system is its adjustability: Components, such as prosthetic feet, can be interchanged, and realignment of the prosthesis can occur as necessary.

A disadvantage of the endoskeletal system is that the soft foam cover and its protective finish are susceptible to damage during activity and are much less durable than an exoskeletal system. The colored cosmetic hose tends to run or tear and may be somewhat expensive to replace. The soft foam cover itself is not water resistant unless it has a rubberized or latex outer layer. Given the need for a protective finish over the foam cover and the risk of damage or staining, endoskeletal systems may be somewhat more expensive in the long run than the more durable exoskeletal system.

Exoskeletal Finishing

The outer walls of an exoskeletal prosthesis provide support to body weight during stance, in the same way that the pylon does in an endoskeletal prosthesis. The socket is in a fixed position within a skin-colored hard shell, which continues over the entire shank of the prosthesis. The strength of the prosthesis is provided by the hard outer shell. The area below the socket within the shell can be hollow or filled with lightweight foam material. The outer shell (exoskeleton) can be fabricated from multiple layers of materials impregnated with thermosetting plastic resins or from a variety of other plastic materials.

The major advantage of exoskeletal systems is their incredible durability, a feature that is important for prosthetic wearers who are involved in heavy physical activity or athletics. For skilled prosthetists, exoskeletal finishing may be less expensive and require less fabrication time than endoskeletal systems. The hard outer shell assures that the prosthesis is waterproof. Some patients find exoskeletal prostheses to be less cosmetically acceptable and somewhat heavier to wear than endoskeletal systems. The major disadvantage of an exoskeletal system, however, is its fixed alignment and difficulty in adjusting the socket once it has been finished and delivered.

Prosthetic Feet and Footwear

Prosthetic feet are designed to work only when the person with amputation is wearing both shoes. The height of the heel of the prosthetic foot should correspond with the height of the heel of the shoe. A prosthetic foot is well matched with a shoe when the top of the foot is parallel to the surface on which the prosthesis is sitting. If the foot is tilting backward, lifts should be added to the heel on the inside of the shoe to make the top of the foot level. If the foot is tilting forward, the heel height of the shoe is too high, and the patient needs different shoes for the prosthesis to work properly. The foot should fit snugly into the shoe to prevent movement but not so tight that the foot cannot compress properly to achieve normal gait. The prosthetic foot alignment in the shoe affects the entire prosthesis and should be examined carefully before the patient dons the prosthesis.

FIGURE 25-13
Setting the socket in slight flexion rather than in vertical/upright increases comfort and function by distributing weight-bearing forces along the entire anterior surface of the residual limb.

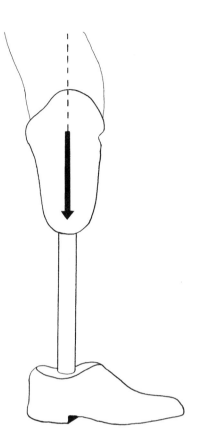
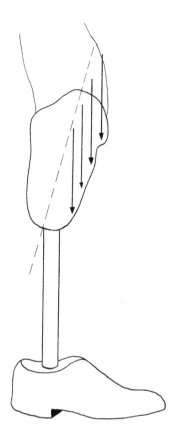

PROSTHETIC ALIGNMENT

Prosthetic alignment is defined as the relationship between the socket and the prosthetic foot. Proper alignment is influenced by the patient's natural gait pattern, the functional characteristics of the prosthetic foot, the condition and force/pressure tolerance of the residual limb, and the functional goals of the patient. Alignment has an impact on comfort and on energy expenditure during gait. Three steps are necessary to achieve optimal prosthetic alignment: bench alignment in the prosthetic laboratory, static alignment while the patient is standing in the prosthesis, and dynamic alignment based on gait analysis. Each step in this process further refines alignment, tailoring the socket-foot relationship to the individual patient. This may take several fittings and trial runs: Proper alignment should be achieved before the prosthesis is finished because changes are difficult or impossible (in exoskeletal systems) once finishing occurs.

Bench Alignment

Bench alignment determines the preliminary relationship between the socket and the foot. Based on knowledge of the patient's musculoskeletal and neuromuscular sta-

tus (such as range of motion, strength, postural stability, and coordination) and well-established initial alignment guidelines, the prosthetist defines the socket-foot relationship in the production laboratory before the patient first dons the prosthesis.

Pressure on the residual limb is greatly affected by the inclination of the supporting surfaces in the socket.[5] When the socket is placed in a slightly flexed position (Figure 25-13), the practitioner can increase the area that provides vertical support for the residual limb, distributing force over the entire length of the tibia, thus minimizing distal end bearing. In contrast, a socket that is mostly vertical relies on the patellar tendon and posterior compartment to support the limb during gait. In bench alignment, the socket is typically placed at 3–5 degrees of flexion. The socket is also placed into a few degrees of adduction to load the medial tibial flare more effectively during stance.

While viewing the prosthesis from the lateral perspective, one places the foot on the prosthesis so that the foot bolt is approximately 1 ¼ in. posterior to the center of the socket; this ensures that weight-bearing forces are balanced between the heel and forefoot of the prosthetic foot. In the mediolateral plane, the foot is placed directly under the center of the socket or up to a ½-in.

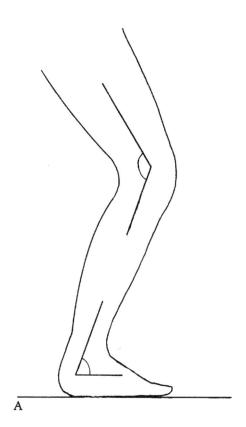
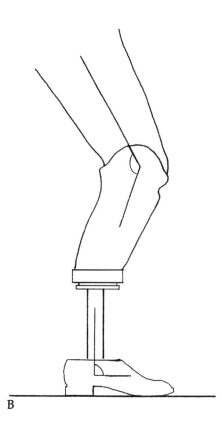

A   B

FIGURE 25-14
(A) In an intact limb, knee flexion is linked to ankle position and dorsiflexion. (B) In a prosthesis, socket position can be changed without altering the balanced position of the prosthetic foot.

inset (medial to the center of the socket) when viewed from behind. This slight medial inset of the prosthetic creates a mild varus thrust at the knee during midstance, similar to that encountered in normal gait.

It is important to note that socket flexion/extension and abduction/adduction occur independently of the position of the foot (Figure 25-14). In an intact limb, when the knee is flexed, the anatomic ankle axis is posterior to the knee, and the ankle has to dorsiflex to maintain contact between the sole and floor. In a prosthesis, however, the knee and socket can be placed in significant flexion, but the prosthetic foot, in its normal 1 1/4-in. position posterior to the socket, is in neutral, flat on the floor. The independence of the socket and ankle position also holds true for socket abduction and adduction. This independence of socket and foot position allows the prosthetist to compensate for fixed deformity or contracture without significant compromise of the quality of prosthetic gait.

Static Alignment

The next step in the alignment process is static alignment. The patient dons the prosthesis and stands while the prosthetist and therapist systematically evaluate fit, comfort, and force distribution in quiet standing (Table 25-2). First, the ability to bear weight equally on both legs without

discomfort is assessed. Patients with recently healed amputations who are receiving their first prosthesis may need encouragement to shift weight toward the prosthetic side until body weight is equally shared by the prosthesis and the intact limb. Next, relative equality of prosthetic and intact leg length is determined. Palpation of the patient's anterior superior iliac spines, posterior superior iliac spines, and iliac crests is used to determine whether the pelvis is level. If the pelvis is not level, it may indicate the need to adjust the length of the prosthetic pylon. Although some patients may not be concerned with slight leg length discrepancy, over time asymmetry in gait may contribute to

TABLE 25-2
Checklist for Evaluation of Static Alignment

Is weight bearing equal between the prosthesis and the intact limb?
Is the patient experiencing any pain or discomfort?
Are the anterior superior iliac spines, posterior superior iliac spines, and iliac crests level?
Is the foot flat on the floor?
Is the top of the foot parallel to the ground in the anteroposterior and mediolateral planes?
Is the knee being forced into flexion or extension?

the development of secondary back pain. Before the length of the prosthesis is adjusted, it is wise to double check the position of the limb within the socket: Inappropriate sock ply can mimic leg length discrepancy.

Attention is then turned to contact between the foot and the floor. Ideally, the foot should be flat on the floor. If obvious differences in weight bearing between the heel and forefoot, or between medial and lateral borders of the foot, are noted, the position of the socket that was established during bench alignment probably needs adjustment or refinement. The prosthetic foot may not be flat on the floor if a knee flexion contracture has developed or if an existing knee flexion contracture has not been well accommodated by initial alignment of the prosthesis. It is not uncommon for knee flexion contracture to reduce with use of the prosthesis as tissues are elongated and remolded over time as frequency and distance of walking increase.

Appropriateness of shoe heel height is also important to evaluate. The top surface of the prosthetic foot is designed to be parallel to the ground when viewed from the side. If this surface is inclined, heel height of the shoe may be incorrect. In an endoskeletal prosthesis, in which a pylon is present between the foot and the socket, the verticality of the pylon is not an appropriate indicator of alignment. A pylon may not be perpendicular to the floor even in a well-aligned prosthesis. The top of the foot, rather than the position of the pylon, is the most important reference in assessing alignment.

Finally, forces that are being applied to the knee while standing are assessed by asking the patient whether the knee is being pushed toward flexion or extension by the prosthesis. A sense that the knee is forced into flexion or extension may indicate incorrect alignment or incorrect heel height of the shoe. If the patient does not exhibit any of the previously mentioned problems, he or she is ready to walk as part of the dynamic alignment process. If the prosthesis does not pass static alignment, however, it is impossible for the patient to ambulate in a normal fashion. Much of the guesswork and time spent in gait analysis can be saved by performing a thorough static alignment evaluation before the patient walks with the prosthesis.

Dynamic Alignment and Gait Analysis

Observational gait analysis is used to evaluate whether the alignment of the prosthesis allows the patient to achieve the most energy-efficient and highest-quality pattern of walking.[9] In the dynamic alignment process, the gait of a person with amputation is compared to the "norms" of able-bodied individuals of the same age and activity level.[10] The goal of the dynamic alignment process is to achieve a gait that is as close to normal as possible. Gait deviations can

be attributed to malalignment of the prosthesis or to the physical limitations (e.g., joint contracture, weakness, skeletal deformities) of the patient.[11] Prosthetic causes of gait problems are numerous and are often easily repaired by adjusting alignment.

For effective gait analysis, the patient must be viewed from the anterior/posterior as well as from the lateral perspectives because certain gait deviations are best observed in each of these planes. Once a prosthetic problem has been identified by the prosthetist or therapist, the prosthetist adjusts the alignment of the prosthesis. In most states, it is the responsibility (and liability) of the prosthetist, rather than the therapist, to make the necessary changes in prosthetic alignment.

TRANSMISSION OF FORCES DURING PROSTHETIC GAIT

When a person with amputation walks in the prosthesis, the forces generated by weight bearing must be absorbed by the residual limb. The amplitude and effect of these forces on the residual limb depend on several interconnected factors: the loading characteristics of the liner and socket materials, the intimacy and quality of prosthetic fit, the health and characteristics of the skin and soft tissue of the residual limb, and the effectiveness of the alignment between the foot and socket. It is often helpful to consider the residual limb and the socket as two separate entities: When force is directed on one, it must be resisted by the other. The residual limb/prosthetic interface can be thought of as a pseudarthrosis with a center of motion at the center of the residual limb.[12] If the residual limb is a stationary object, upward forces from the center of the prosthetic foot are acting on the residual limb during ambulation. If the foot is directly under the residual limb within the socket, the force is applied directly through the center of the residual limb. If the foot is offset from the center of the socket, the socket tends to rotate around the residual limb in the frontal plane or the sagittal plane. Because the residual limb is a stationary object, it resists this rotation with an equal but opposite force. As an example, consider a prosthesis used after transtibial amputation of the right lower extremity. If the prosthetic foot is slightly inset with respect to the socket, the resulting force causes rotation in a counterclockwise direction, which in turn exerts pressures at the bottom left (distal lateral) and top right (proximal medial) surfaces of the residual limb (Figure 25-15). If the foot is instead slightly outset, the direction of the rotational force reverses, with pressures exerted at the top

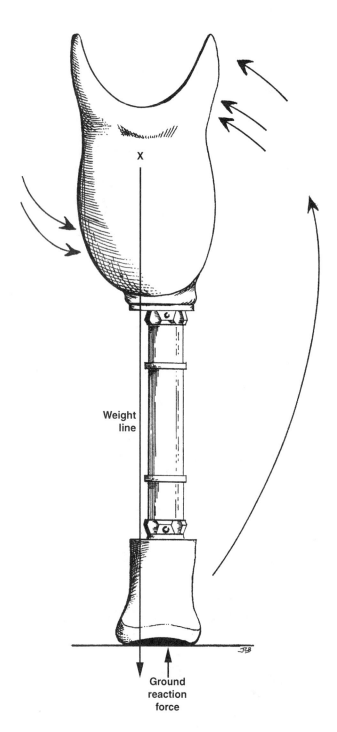

X

Weight
line

Ground
reaction
force

FIGURE 25-15

*Understanding rotation of the socket on the residual limb. If the
residual limb is thought of as a stationary object, the weight-
bearing forces transmitted upward from the center of the foot
during gait and applied at the socket-limb interface can be better understood. For example, when the foot is medially inset,
the resulting force acts to rotate the socket on the residual limb
in the frontal plane. This rotational force creates pressure at the
proximal medial limb (at the medial tibial flare) and distal lateral limb (along the lateral shaft of the tibia).*

left (proximal lateral) and bottom right (distal medial)
surfaces of the residual limb. It is evident that position of the
foot is one of the major determinants of amplitude and location of pressure that the patient feels inside the prosthesis.

Residual Limb/Socket Pressures in the Frontal Plane

The optimum position for the foot in the mediolateral or
frontal plane is directly under or slightly medial to the center of the proximal socket (the reason that the foot is placed
in slight inset during bench alignment). This foot position
imparts a rotation that applies pressure over the medial
condyle of the tibia (medial tibial flare, a very tolerant area)
and the distal lateral shaft of the fibula and tibia (see Figure 25-15). This rotational force also creates a slight varus
thrust to the knee joint, which is necessary for an effective
midstance. Foot position must be adjusted if excessive varus
thrust or a valgus thrust is present, as neither is well tolerated by the patient for any length of time. The contours
of the lateral wall of the socket must protect the distal fibula
and direct pressures to the tolerant fibular shaft.

If the foot is placed too far lateral (outset) to the center
of the socket, the prosthesis rotates on the limb in the opposite direction, such that the patient may experience pressure on the proximal lateral and distal medial portions of
the residual limb. This lateral foot placement loads (exerts
pressure on) the fibular head and peroneal nerve, causing
discomfort in the prosthesis. During gait, the patient also
experiences a valgus thrust of the knee at midstance. The
quality and comfort of gait are significantly compromised
when the prosthetic foot is too far outset or lateral to the
center of the residual limb within the socket.

Residual Limb/Socket Pressures in the Sagittal Plane

The relationship between the socket and foot becomes
more complicated when gait in the sagittal plane is analyzed. The prosthetist must balance heel and toe levers to
provide a smooth and natural gait pattern and to ensure
socket comfort (Figure 25-16). A *heel lever* is the distance
between the back of the heel of the prosthetic foot and the
center of the socket. Functionally, heel lever length is influenced by the density of the prosthetic heel cushion as well
as the position of the socket over the foot. The *toe lever*
is the distance between the center of the socket and the
end of the toe. The toe lever is influenced by the angle of
attachment of the prosthetic foot (relative dorsiflexion or
plantar flexion) and the position of the socket over the
foot. The length of these levers changes as the socket is
moved (in the sagittal plane) relative to the foot, when

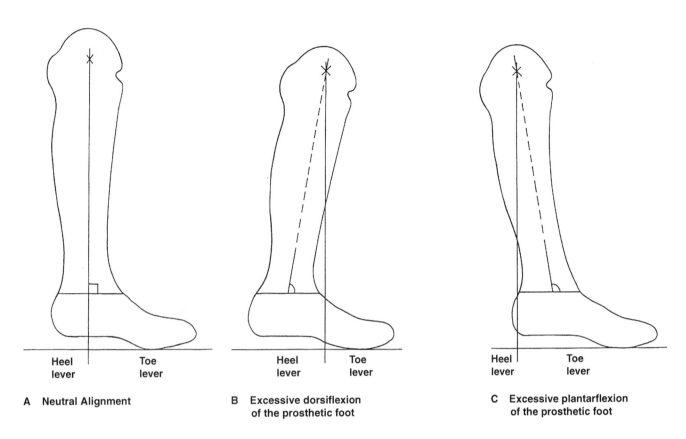

Heel lever	Toe lever		Heel lever	Toe lever		Heel lever	Toe lever

A   Neutral Alignment   **B   Excessive dorsiflexion of the prosthetic foot**   **C   Excessive plantarflexion of the prosthetic foot**

FIGURE 25-16

(A) Toe lever is the distance between the center of the socket and the distal end of the prosthetic foot; heel lever is the distance between the center of the socket and the back of the heel. Both of these levers are influenced by alignment and stiffness of the prosthetic foot as well as relative position of the socket over the foot. (B) The toe lever is relatively shortened and the heel lever is lengthened when the foot is dorsiflexed, the socket is flexed, or the foot is positioned slightly posterior to the socket center. (C) The toe lever is relatively lengthened and the heel lever is shortened when the foot is plantar flexed, the socket is extended, or the foot is positioned slightly anterior to the socket center.

the socket is flexed or extended, or when the foot is dorsiflexed or plantar flexed.

For this discussion, we describe the line that drops from the center of the socket through the foot as the weight line and the point at which the foot contacts the floor as the center of pressure. The relationship between these two landmarks changes as stance phase progresses. In most nonarticulating prosthetic feet, no actual plantar flexion or dorsiflexion is possible. Instead, the heel or posterior portion of the foot must compress with weight bearing to simulate an articulation and provide a natural gait pattern. As weight is transferred onto the prosthesis in loading response, the heel compresses, and the center of pressure and the weight line move together, decreasing rotational forces and facilitating a smooth transition to the next phase of gait.

Forces during Initial Contact and Midstance

At initial contact (heel strike), the center of pressure is behind the weight line, causing a forward moment of the

socket (Figure 25-17A). The larger the difference between the weight line and the center of pressure (i.e., a long heel lever), the more quickly the prosthesis rotates forward. This rotational force increases pressure on the residual limb at the proximal posterior and anterior distal segments as the patient attempts to control the rapid forward movement of the socket (Figure 25-17B). If the heel cushion is too firm or cannot compress because the shoe is too tight, a large difference between the weight line and center of pressure is maintained, forcing the socket rapidly forward. A similar rapid forward progression occurs if the patient does not shift enough weight onto the prosthesis to compress the heel or if the patient is wearing shoes with heels that are too high for the prosthetic foot.

When the heel of the foot is very soft, it lowers the center of the foot to the floor early in the gait cycle. This lowering moves the center of pressure closer to the weight line and decreases the torque around the prosthesis. As the patient moves forward, the reduction in forward rotation

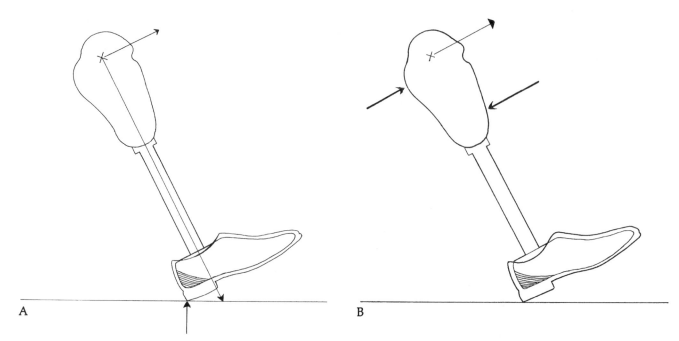

FIGURE 25-17
(A) Because the center of pressure is well behind the weight line at initial contact, the resultant force causes a rapid forward movement of the socket. (B) This creates pressure at the anterior distal and posterior proximal aspects of the residual limb, as the user attempts to slow forward progression of the socket.

of the prosthesis tends to force the knee into extension at heel strike (Figure 25-18). As a result, the patient experiences increased pressure at the proximal anterior and distal posterior aspects of the residual limb within the socket.

During midstance, as the patient moves directly over the prosthesis, little difference is seen between the position of the weight line and center of pressure in the sagittal plane. When patients complain of discomfort during midstance, the most likely problem is improper vertical support within the prosthesis.

Forces from Midstance to Terminal Stance and Preswing

As midstance is completed and the body continues forward over the anterior aspect of the prosthetic foot, the center of pressure moves anterior to the weight line. If the prosthesis has a long toe lever (e.g., a stiff keel, a foot set in plantar flexion, or a foot set too far anterior relative to the socket), the foot begins to resist forward movement of the socket. The center of pressure moves rapidly to the end of the foot, farther from the weight line (Figure 25-19). The resulting rotational force rotates the socket on the residual limb and pushes the proximal tibia posteriorly to extend the knee. The greatest pressures on the limb are found on the anterior proximal and posterior distal portions of the residual limb. The patient most often complains only of excessive pressure at the patellar tendon, because the soft

tissue of the posterior distal residual limb is usually able to tolerate significant pressure. Many patients report a sense of walking uphill, with upward pressure on the patella if the toe lever is excessively long.

A short toe lever (e.g., a soft or short keel or a foot set in dorsiflexion or positioned too far posterior to the socket) does not support the body at the terminal portions of the stance phase. The patient may feel little resistance as the heel rises in terminal stance, reporting a rapid knee flexion (almost a sense of falling into a hole) instead of rolling over the toes as expected in preswing (toe-off). Often, the step length of the contralateral limb is shortened because the lack of anterior support hastens entrance into the period of double support. It is unusual for patients to experience pain or discomfort in terminal stance (heel-off) and preswing (toe-off) of a properly aligned prosthesis because there is too little resistance to forward progression at the end of stance to result in pressures on the residual limb.

OBSERVATIONAL GAIT ANALYSIS FOR TRANSTIBIAL PROSTHETICS

Systematic gait assessment requires evaluation of function in each of the subphases of stance and the swing phase of gait. In performing gait assessment the prosthetist or ther-

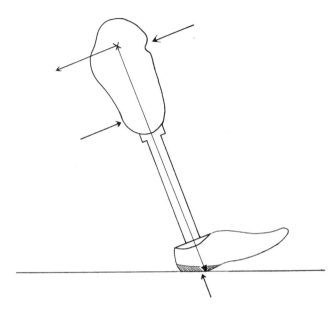

FIGURE 25-18

If the heel of the prosthetic foot is too soft for the patient's weight or activity level, the center of pressure and weight line almost coincide. Without the resultant forward rotation of the socket, the prosthesis fails to move forward, the patient feels high pressures at the proximal anterior and distal posterior socket, and an extension force is imparted to the knee.

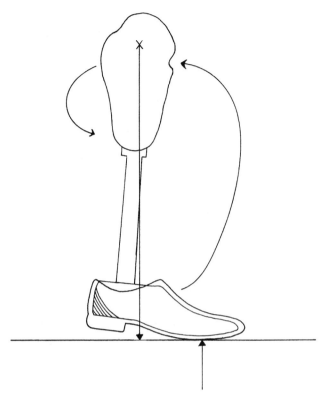

FIGURE 25-19

As the patient moves into terminal stance, the center of pressure moves anterior to the weight line. The resultant rotational forces lead to an extension moment at the knee. If the toe lever is excessive, the patient has to work harder to counteract this backward force and continue with forward progression. The patient often reports a sense of walking uphill if the toe lever is too long.

apist must keep in mind the functional task of the subphase and how that task is accomplished by the components of the patient's prosthesis. If gait deviations are observed, the therapist or prosthetist must first determine the possible prosthetic or nonprosthetic causes of the deviation and then decide on the best strategy to correct the problem.[13]

Initial Contact

Initial contact (*heel strike*) is the moment of transition between the swing and stance phase. Ideally, three conditions are observed for effective early stance phase in prosthetic gait. First, stride length is equal to that of the intact opposite limb. Second, the patient has approximately 5–10 degrees of knee flexion in preparation for limb loading. Third, the prosthetic foot contacts the ground in the line of forward progression, without rotation in the transverse plane. Gait deviations that are common during initial contact are most apparent in the lateral view. Three "classic" deviations are present at initial contact.

Knee Is Fully Extended

If contact is made with the knee fully extended or hyperextended, loading forces on the distal limb can be exaggerated, leading to discomfort or skin irritation, and the

smooth forward progression of the center of mass can be disrupted. When this deviation is observed, two possible prosthetic factors must be considered. First, the suspension system may be inadequate, failing to hold the knee in the desired slightly flexed position. Ensuring appropriate suspension often corrects the problem. This is especially true if cuff suspension is used: In this instance, moving the point of attachment to a slightly more posterior position on the socket better maintains the desired knee flexion. If suspension is not the problem, the focus shifts to a heel lever (the distance between the prosthetic heel and the center of the socket) that may be too short, forcing the knee into extension at initial contact. A short heel lever occurs for several reasons: Initial flexion of the socket may be inadequate, the prosthetic foot may be positioned too far anterior with respect to the socket, or the foot might be positioned in too much plantar flexion. In these cases, the prosthetist would increase socket flexion a few degrees, slide the foot into a slightly more posterior position, or move the foot a few degrees toward dorsiflexion, respectively. Some patients, nervous about knee instability during stance, might purposefully extend the knee more than is desirable to minimize the perceived risk of buckling. Gait training, rather than prosthetic adjustment, is an appropriate strategy for this patient-related problem.

Knee Is Flexed More than 10 Degrees

If initial contact is made with excessive knee flexion, stability in single limb support stance may be threatened. If this gait deviation is observed, two contributing factors must be considered. First, the suspension system may be holding the knee in too much flexion. This is often the case if cuff suspension is adjusted too tightly or if the points of strap attachment are too far posterior on the socket. Adjustment of suspension often solves this problem. Another factor to consider is a possible knee flexion contracture. Although a prosthetist can make prosthetic accommodations for slight contractures, significant limitations in knee range of motion necessarily compromise the quality of gait. Physical therapy interventions to reduce knee flexion contracture may be effective, over time, in improving knee function during early stance. The best strategy, however, is prevention of contracture formation in an aggressive preprosthetic exercise and positioning program. Patients with knee flexion contractures in excess of 40 degrees will find ambulation with a prosthesis impossible.

Unequal Stride Length

Three contributors to unequal stride length are possible. The first, once again, is adequacy of suspension. If suspension limits available knee extension, the prosthetic stride is shorter. If inadequate suspension raises the patient's concern about keeping the prosthesis on, prosthetic stride can be shortened to get the foot on the floor more quickly. Either of these problems is corrected by adjusting the suspension system. The other two factors are patient related. If the patient has pain or dysfunction of the sound limb or pain with pressures on the prosthesis, stance time on that limb may be reduced, thus limiting time in swing on the contralateral side. Careful evaluation of the painful limb identifying the limiting factor, followed by appropriate intervention, often helps to improve the symmetry of stride lengths. Finally, a new prosthetic user who is reluctant to trust the prosthesis can gain confidence and skill from focused gait training.

Loading Response

Three prerequisites must be met for an effective prosthetic loading response. First, the patient's knee must be able to flex an additional 15–20 degrees for shock absorption as weight is transferred onto the prosthesis in preparation for single limb support. Second, approximately ⅜ in. compression of the heel cushion or posterior prosthetic foot should be present to simulate the plantar flexion that is required for an effective first (heel) rocker of gait. Finally, the position of the residual limb in the socket should be consistent as body weight is loaded on the prosthesis, with minimal movement deeper into the prosthesis. Problems that might be observed in loading response include rotation of the foot and socket, poorly controlled or abrupt knee flexion, excessive knee extension, or sinking into the socket.

Rotation of the Foot and Socket

Transverse rotation of the foot at initial contact is best observed from the front or behind the patient as he or she walks. Typically, the foot rotates externally (laterally), pivoting around the point of floor contact at the heel to compensate for difficulty in moving into a foot-flat position. This rotation occurs for a variety of reasons. First, the shoe on the prosthetic foot might be too tight or the heel of the shoe too rigid (e.g., cowboy boots). If the problem persists with different shoes, prosthetic causes must be suspected. A socket that is too loose on the residual limb may rotate as the foot contacts the ground. The addition of more ply of prosthetic sock to improve the fit of the limb in the socket may address this problem. A patient who is very deconditioned or weak may not have adequate strength or endurance of hip and knee musculature to control the prosthesis effectively. A strengthening program that targets improved concentric and eccentric control is necessary in this instance. Early in gait training, a new prosthetic user might be reluctant to load the prosthesis, which limits compression of the heel cushion and can lead to rotation of the prosthetic foot. Similarly, discomfort within the socket can lead to cautious initial contact and inadequate heel cushion compression and result in rotation of the prosthetic foot. If none of these precipitating problems are occurring, the most likely prosthetic problem is a heel cushion that is too stiff. The solution is to replace the prosthetic foot with one that has a heel cushion more appropriate for the patient's weight and activity level.

Poorly Controlled or Jerky Knee Flexion

Patients who are deconditioned or have weak quadriceps may have difficulty controlling the eccentric contraction of the quadriceps that is needed for an effective loading response. Exercises that alternate between concentric and eccentric contraction of the quadriceps muscles within the functional range of motion necessary for loading response, and intensive gait training, are the most appropriate physical therapy interventions to address this gait deviation.

Abrupt or Forceful Knee Flexion

In abrupt or forceful knee flexion, the socket is propelled forward too quickly as the prosthetic foot moves into the foot-flat position. This can happen because of a problem with alignment or a problem with footwear. First, the prosthetist evaluates the relative positions of the foot and of the socket. Quick forward propulsion is the result of an excessively long heel lever. A long heel lever occurs when the foot is positioned too far posteriorly or in too much dorsiflexion, or when the socket is set in too much flexion. The solution is to slide the foot forward (anteriorly), to reposition the foot in a slightly more plantar-flexed direction, or to decrease the amount of socket flexion. A heel cushion that is too stiff and does not compress quickly enough to lower the forefoot to the floor also propels the prosthesis forward and causes abrupt knee flexion. Changing to a prosthetic foot with a less dense heel cushion might be the solution in this case.

Several footwear issues should be considered before changes in alignment are made, however. A shoe with a heel too high for the prosthetic foot, a heel that is excessively stiff, or a shoe that is too narrow or tightly closed on the prosthetic foot also leads to abrupt or forceful knee flexion in loading response. If shoe fit is the source of the problem, changing to a more appropriate heel or better-fitting shoe will improve the quality of gait.

Excessive Knee Extension

If the knee remains in extension when it should be flexing in loading response (sometimes referred to as *riding the heel into midstance*), an abnormal extension moment will act at the patient's knee. Four possible contributing factors should be considered. First, the foot may be positioned too far forward with respect to the socket, creating too short a heel lever for progression to foot flat. This can be addressed by sliding the foot into a more posterior position, moving the foot into a slightly more dorsiflexed position, or increasing the flexion of the socket. Second, if the heel cushion is too soft and is too easily compressed, the prosthesis will resist forward progression and it is difficult for the patient to achieve the desired knee flexion for shock absorption as the knee tends to remain in extension. Changing to a prosthetic foot with a firmer heel cushion addresses this problem. Third, if the heel of the patient's shoe is lower than necessary for his or her prosthetic foot, the knee will also be pushed into excessive extension. This can be solved by putting a heel lift or wedge in the shoe or by changing to a shoe with an optimal heel height for the particular prosthetic foot. Finally, the patient who is new to prosthetic use may activate knee extensor muscles inappropriately because of fear of knee instability in sin-

gle limb support. Gait training activities with an emphasis on controlled knee flexion are often helpful in this case.

Sinking into the Socket

Sinking into the socket is a gait problem most often reported by the patient. If the residual limb feels as if it is sinking into the socket as body weight is transferred onto the prosthesis, the suspension and the number of sock ply should be reevaluated. If adjustment of suspension does not solve the problem, it is likely that the patient is wearing an insufficient number of sock ply and needs to add an additional layer.

Midstance

Stability of the knee and smooth forward progression are the functional goals in midstance. The prosthetist and therapist look for four key components: a level prosthetic foot (top of the foot) as the other limb passes by in its midswing, a varus moment that causes a slight (½ in.) lateral displacement of the knee, an upright trunk with minimal lateral trunk bending, and an equal reciprocal arm swing. Screening for gait deviations in midstance requires a lateral and a posterior viewpoint.

Prosthetic Foot Leans Medially

If at midstance the top surface of the prosthetic foot is not level but leans medially, the prosthetist or therapist considers five possible contributors. This deviation occurs when the socket is set in excessive adduction or the prosthetic foot is set in a pronated position; gait improves if the components are shifted slightly in the opposite direction toward abduction or toward supination. This can also be caused by a foot that is more outset than necessary and corrected by sliding the foot slightly inward or medially. Sometimes this deviation occurs because the sole or heel of the patient's shoes is worn unevenly. It may also be observed in patients new to prosthetic use who are reluctant to shift their weight fully onto the prosthesis because they fear instability, are walking with a wide base of support, or have discomfort or pain in the residual limb within the socket. Gait training activities or the use of an appropriate assistive device helps patients learn to trust their prosthetic limb. When patients report discomfort or pain, however, the fit of the socket must be reevaluated.

Prosthetic Foot Leans Laterally

The possible causes for a laterally leaning foot are the counterparts of those that cause it to lean medially. The foot may be positioned in too much supination or is further inset than is appropriate, or the socket is in less initial adduction than the patient needs. If so, movement of the foot or socket slightly in the opposite direction improves the quality and efficiency of gait. Uneven wear of the sole or heel of the shoes can shift the prosthetic foot laterally, and a new pair of shoes is needed. This deviation also occurs when the patient is walking in a very narrow (less than 2 in.) step width. Gait training activities are often effective in changing step width to a more functional 3- to 4-in. separation.

Inappropriate Varus Moment at the Knee

If, at midstance, the desired varus moment is not occurring, the prosthetic foot is likely positioned too laterally (outset) relative to the socket. To correct this problem, the foot is shifted slightly inward (inset) or the socket moved into a slightly more abducted position. If, instead, the varus moment is excessive (more than $1/2$ in.), the foot is likely too far inset; correction requires the foot to be moved laterally (outset) or set in a slightly more pronated position or the socket to be moved into a more adducted position. Sometimes excessive varus moment can be traced to a socket that is too wide in the mediolateral dimension. In this case, the prosthetist must adjust the width of the socket to improve function at midstance.

Lateral Trunk Bends toward the Prosthetic Side

Excessive trunk bending during stance increases energy expenditure during ambulation and disrupts smooth forward progression. This deviation can occur if the prosthesis is relatively or actually too short or too long as compared to the intact limb. Lateral leaning can be used as a strategy to reduce discomfort by patients who are experiencing pain or skin irritation of the residual limb within the socket. It sometimes occurs if the prosthetic foot is positioned too far laterally (outset) with respect to the socket. Finally, lateral lean may be a compensation for weakness of the abductor muscles of the hip. The fit of the prosthesis should be carefully reevaluated before adjustments to pylon length are made: Too many or too few prosthetic socks can incorrectly position the limb within the socket, resulting in an apparent, artificial leg length problem.

Premature Heel Rise

Most prosthetic feet are designed so that heel rise occurs in terminal stance. If the heel rises during midstance, it is likely that the foot is mispositioned and that the top surface is tipped in an anterior direction. An early rollover at the forefoot and resulting early heel rise occur when the toe lever is too short. The most common prosthetic causes of this deviation are a prosthetic foot positioned too far posterior to the socket or in too much initial dorsiflexion or a socket that is set in too much initial flexion. Sliding the foot forward or into a more plantar-flexed position or moving the socket toward extension a few degrees effec-

tively increases the toe lever and improves the quality of gait. This problem also occurs when the patient is wearing shoes with heels that are higher than appropriate for the prosthetic foot type or when the patient has a knee or hip flexion contracture that has not been adequately addressed by prosthetic alignment. If contracture is a problem, moving the socket into more flexion combined with plantar flexion of the prosthetic foot may enable the prosthetist to establish the desired toe lever.

Prosthetic Foot Leans Posteriorly

When the top surface of the prosthetic foot tilts posteriorly, the forward progression of the body in gait may be compromised. The most common reason for this deviation are shoes with too low a heel for the prosthetic foot. This can be addressed by adding a heel lift inside the shoe or by changing to shoes with a more appropriate heel.

Uneven Arm Swing

Uneven arm swing is most apparent from a lateral viewpoint while the patient is walking. Three factors might contribute to an uneven arm swing during gait. The first, pain or discomfort when wearing the prosthesis, requires careful reevaluation of fit and alignment of the prosthesis. The other two, a sense of insecurity during single limb support and an uneven step length, are often successfully addressed by gait training activities or the use of an assistive device (such as a straight cane) to provide some degree of external support.

Terminal Stance and Preswing

For an efficient and cosmetic gait, heel-off during terminal stance should occur smoothly and effortlessly just before (or simultaneously with) initial contact of the opposite limb. Ideally, a step width of between 2 and 4 in. is present between the medial borders of the feet. The knee should begin to flex as soon as the heel rises, in preparation for toe-off. As the prosthesis is unweighted, the foot should remain within the plane of forward progression with little or no transverse plane rotation of the heel. If these conditions are met, the transfer of body weight from the prosthetic limb to the opposite limb is accomplished smoothly. The socket must remain adequately suspended as the swing phase is initiated. A variety of gait deviations can occur late in the stance phase. Most are best identified from a lateral viewpoint.

Drop-Off and Abrupt, Early Heel Rise

Some patients report a sudden sense of "dropping off" or "falling into a hole" as their weight moves forward over the "toes" of the prosthetic foot. As a result, swing of the opposite limb is shortened for an earlier than normal weight acceptance. Prosthetically, the reasons for this are the same as for an early heel rise in midstance: a short toe lever, most commonly traced to a foot that is too far posterior to the socket or set in too much dorsiflexion, or to a socket that is set in too much initial flexion. These causes can be corrected by moving the socket or foot slightly in the opposite direction. The other potential contributors to this problem are heels that are too high for the prosthetic foot (addressed by changing footwear), a knee flexion contracture that has not been adequately addressed in prosthetic alignment (addressed by combining an increased socket flexion with a more plantar-flexed positioning of the prosthetic foot), or weakness of muscles around the knee that compromises stability in late stance.

Delayed Heel Rise or a Sense of Walking Uphill

Patients sometimes report a sense of walking uphill or a strong knee extension moment, accompanied by a delay in heel rise as they approach the end of the stance phase. This occurs when the toe lever of the prosthetic foot is functionally too long, preventing the normal rollover of the anterior of the prosthetic foot and the initiation of knee flexion in preparation for foot clearance in swing phase. The most common prosthetic causes of this gait deviation are a foot positioned too far forward (anterior) with respect to the socket or in too much initial plantar flexion or the socket that is not adequately flexed. To shorten the toe lever, the prosthetist might move the prosthetic foot slightly backward (into a more posterior position) or a few degrees toward dorsiflexion or might increase the initial flexion of the socket. Rollover and forward progression can also be compromised by a prosthetic foot with a keel that is too firm or stiff given the patient's weight or level of activity or by a shoe that is too stiff. Changing prosthetic feet to a more forgiving keel or changing to more flexible footwear may help to solve the problem.

Very Narrow Step Width

If less than 2 in. is present between the medial borders of the feet, the prosthetic foot may be positioned too far inset (medially) with respect to the socket. Moving the foot laterally (outset) or increasing initial adduction of the socket may help to normalize stride width. If the patient habitually ambulates with a narrow base, gait training activities may be necessary to alter this motor behavior.

Wider than Normal Step Width

Step widths that are wider than 4 in. are associated with increased mediolateral displacement during forward progression of gait. Wide step widths may be related to a problem with alignment (a prosthetic foot that is too far lateral or outset with respect to the socket), or to a fear of instability and reluctance to shift weight completely onto the prosthesis. Abduction of the socket or a medial repositioning of the foot improves efficiency and quality of gait if the deviation is caused by alignment problems. Gait training that reinforces the need for a narrower base of support or the use of an appropriate assistive device may be helpful for patients who are concerned with instability.

Medial or Lateral Rotation of the Heel

Occasionally, the heel appears to rotate as weight progresses forward over the toes of the prosthetic foot. The prosthetic cause of this deviation is a prosthetic foot that has been set in slightly too much pronation or supination. More commonly, the patient-related cause of this deviation is shortening of hip flexor musculature that prevents the femur from rotating with the pelvis in the transition between stance and swing phase. If this is the case, physical therapy interventions that are designed to lengthen hip flexor muscles improve the quality of prosthetic gait. This deviation may also be the consequence of inappropriate cuff strap attachment on the socket; adjusting the point of attachment will improve quality of gait.

Excessive Motion between the Residual Limb and Socket

In preswing, as the prosthesis is unweighted in preparation for initiation of swing, the patient may feel the socket drop away (piston) from the residual limb. Two factors should be considered when this occurs: the adequacy of the suspension and the number of sock ply that the patient is wearing. If adjustment of suspension does not fix this pistoning problem, the patient likely is not wearing enough sock ply over the residual limb and should add another layer or two to improve prosthetic fit.

Swing Phase

Prosthetic gait has two primary goals during swing phase. First, the prosthetic foot should swing forward within the line of progression, without transverse rotations (whips or excessive toe-out/in). Second, toe clearance must be ample as the prosthesis progresses from initial swing into midswing and finally is positioned for the next cycle of gait as terminal swing concludes. Gait deviations during swing phase are evaluated from the lateral and the posterior perspective.

Medial or Lateral Whips

A whip occurs when the prosthetic foot rotates in the transverse plane after toe-off: it may move in a medial arc (toward the stance limb) or a lateral arc (away from the stance limb) during swing. The patient's knee, however, is moving forward within the anteroposterior line of progression. It is important to differentiate whips from abducted or adducted gait, where the entire limb moves in an arc (usually a compensatory deviation when inadequate knee flexion adds relative length to the limb, challenging swing phase clearance). If the patient is using a cuff suspension system, inappropriately placed tabs result in a whip. If the prosthetic foot is aligned (rotated) with slightly too much toe-out or toe-in, it can change the path of forward progression from a straight line into a whip. Adjustment of foot position or suspension usually solves the problem.

"Catching" the Toe during Midswing

Problems with toe clearance during midswing can compromise safe ambulation and challenge the patient's sense of mastery and safety while walking. Catching the toes of the prosthetic foot as the shank of the prosthesis advances forward in midswing is the result of a prosthesis that is either actually or (more commonly) functionally too long. Patients, and sometimes therapists, are quick to assume that the prosthesis is actually too long. No change in length of the prosthesis should be made unless all of the other potential problems have been ruled out and careful reassessment of prosthetic limb length clearly indicates the need to trim length. Prosthetically, the factors that should be investigated include adequacy of the suspension mechanism and of sock ply (pistoning relatively lengthens limb length as the socket drops slightly away from the residual limb) and prosthetic foot position (a foot set in excessive plantar flexion also adds relative length to the prosthesis). An alternate problem might be limitation of the patient's ability to flex the knee in initial swing and midswing, to accomplish the relative shortening of the limb necessary for toe clearance. This may be the result of improper fit of the socket or suspension system, excessive bulkiness of prosthetic socks, the patient's fear of knee instability, muscle weakness, or orthopedic deformity that prevents effective swing phase flexion.

EVALUATION OF PROSTHETIC FIT

The ability to evaluate the fit of a transtibial prosthesis effectively requires attention to detail, training, and cumulative practical experience. Because so many patients with transtibial amputation have sensory impairment of their residual limbs, they are prime candidates for abrasions, skin ulceration, and infection. It is important to assess socket fit objectively and to teach patients to inspect their skin for markings that indicate appropriate force distribution within the socket and for signs of irritation in pressure-sensitive areas.

Initial Evaluation

The first component of assessment of socket fit is visual inspection of the residual limb as the prosthesis is donned and after the patient has stood and walked in the prosthesis for a period of time. Ideally, the residual limb slides smoothly into and out of a snugly fit prosthesis or liner, and the patellar bar contacts the skin at the midpatellar tendon. Although a total contact fit is desired for most patients, for some a small amount of space may be present at the liner's distal end. If the newly delivered prosthesis is comfortably donned, the patient is asked to shift weight onto the residual limb in standing and to walk a short distance, perhaps in the parallel bars if external support is required. After this brief walk, the prosthesis and socks are removed, and the skin is visually inspected once again. The prosthetist and therapists are looking for areas of reactive hyperemia (areas of redness where pressure has been applied by the prosthesis) and the markings from the socks or sheaths over pressure-tolerant areas (the medial tibial flare, the patellar tendon, and the lateral shaft of tibia and fibula), as well as the absence of such redness and markings over pressure-intolerant areas (especially the distal anterior tibia and the fibular head). Areas of significant redness over a sensitive or nontolerant area indicate a potential problem with prosthetic fit, and the patient should not wear the prosthesis until an adjustment can be made. For most patients, reactive hyperemia should blanch on palpation and should dissipate back to normal skin color within a few minutes after this brief ambulation. If redness persists, or any areas of irritation or abrasion are present, the prosthesis should not be worn until the contours of the socket can be appropriately adjusted and the skin is sufficiently healed.

Finding the source of discomfort within a prosthetic socket is sometimes a challenging task. Discomfort may be the result of excessive pressure, or of inadequate contact and too little pressure. Discoloration may be due to too much pressure in one spot or too much pressure proximal to the discolored area. Several "tricks" are used by a prosthetist or therapist to help determine the causes of discoloration or pain noted on initial evaluation: the look-and-see test, the powder test, the ball of clay test, and the lipstick test.

Look-and-See Test

The look-and-see test requires quick visual inspection of the limb immediately after the removal of the prosthesis. Areas that are blanched but quickly turn deep red often indicate areas of excessive pressure. The shape or contour of the blanched area and the patterns of reactive hyperemia (redness) help the practitioner to identify potential problems, based on a knowledge of total surface bearing (total contact) and the areas of support designated by socket design. In many instances, problems are the result of changes in limb circumference or shape and can be successfully corrected by altering the number of socks within the socket.

If a change in sock ply fails to solve the problem, the prosthetist must use other evaluative strategies to identify the source of pain, skin irritation, or excessive pressure.

Powder Test

The powder test works best in cases in which the discomfort is due to the residual limb not touching the bottom of the prosthesis. A small amount of powder (baby powder, cornstarch, or any nontoxic powder) is sprinkled on the sides and bottom of the socket, especially in areas where firm contact between the socket and residual limb is desired. The prosthesis is then donned with care so that the powder within the socket is not disturbed or rubbed away. The patient then stands, walks a short distance, and returns to sitting. The prosthesis is carefully removed, and the socks and interior of the socket are inspected. In a well-fit prosthesis, a minimal amount of powder remains at the bottom of the socket, as most of the powder transfers to the outer surface of the socks. A ring of powder at the bottom or on the sides of the socket indicates loss of total contact fit. The number of sock ply can be adjusted, and the test is repeated. If the powder pattern does not change and the patient is not more comfortable, it may be time to consult the prosthetist about socket fit.

Ball of Clay Test

The clay test helps to identify if the residual limb is seated appropriately within the socket, is descending too far down into the socket (e.g., bottoming out), or is not going deep enough into the socket. A small, penny-sized ball of soft clay (of Play-Doh consistency) is placed in the bottom of the socket before the patient dons the prosthesis. The patient then stands, shifts weight onto the prosthesis, walks a short distance, and sits back down to remove the prosthesis. In a well-fit prosthesis, the clay is compressed into a flat disk approximately $1/8$–$1/4$ in. thick, indicating that proper pressure is being applied around the distal end. If the ball is smashed against the bottom of the socket and is very thin, too much pressure is being borne on the distal end of the limb. If this is the case, the addition of another ply or two of sock often better positions the residual limb within the socket, and discomfort should be reduced. If the clay ball is hardly deformed, the limb is not descending far enough into the socket for proper support. Fit often improves, and discomfort can be eliminated by removing several ply of sock to reposition the limb correctly within the socket. For patients whose distal residual limb is hypersensitive or very pressure intolerant, the prosthesis may be designed with a moderate amount of space at the distal end to enhance comfort. For these patients, the ball of clay test does not give an appropriate analysis of fit.

Lipstick Test

The lipstick test is used when patients are experiencing localized pain. When a patient points to a sensitive area, which is also tender on palpation, the lipstick test is used to determine if the sensitive area is touching the prosthesis. This test is very effective in determining if the pain is referred from another location on the limb. This test also helps the therapist or prosthetist to determine if the limb is correctly positioned within the socket.

A small amount of lipstick is applied to the outer surface of snugly applied prosthetic socks over the pressure-sensitive area. The patient then dons the prosthesis, stands, weight shifts, and walks a short distance. After the patient sits once again, the prosthesis is carefully removed, and the inside of the socket is inspected. The lipstick transfers from the sock to the socket where contact has occurred. If the mark is below the relief for a bony prominence in the prosthesis, the limb is probably positioned too deeply within the socket, and an additional layer of sock may be necessary. Conversely, if the mark is above a relief area for a bony prominence, the limb is not far enough into the socket to fit properly, and a layer or more of sock may need to be removed. The lipstick test can be repeated until comfort is achieved or other problems occur. If changing sock layers does not solve the problem, the prosthetist who designed the prosthesis should be contacted.

If, after walking, no lipstick remains on the liner or interior socket, the patient's discomfort may be referred from pressure in another location on the residual limb. To determine if this is the case, other areas of the residual limb are palpated with moderate pressure. If pain can be reproduced by pressing on a different area (e.g., the peroneal nerve or posterior compartment), it is referred from this other location away from the actual sensation of pain. The possibility of neuroma must also be considered if local discomfort or pain persists when these tests (especially the lipstick test) indicate proper positioning and fit of the prosthesis. Further surgery may be required if discomfort from a neuroma cannot be relieved by adjustment within the prosthesis.

TROUBLESHOOTING

In many instances, problems with prosthetic fit can be solved in a systematic troubleshooting process that considers the location and pattern of pain, the potential prosthetic fit, and patient-related factors that may explain the symptoms. Common problems encountered in new transtibial prosthetic wearers, their most likely causes, and possible solutions are summarized in Table 25-3. Prosthetic problems can often be resolved by the therapist or the patient. If problems persist, however, it is most appro-

TABLE 25-3
Guidelines for Troubleshooting Transtibial Prosthetic Problems

Description	Possible Cause	Other Indicators	Possible Solutions
Inferior patella pain	Knee pathology (patellar-femoral syndrome)	Discomfort duplicated on examination of knee without prosthesis	Refer to physician
	Limb descends too far into socket	Fibular head pressure or redness	Add additional sock ply
		Pressure or discoloration of anterior distal tibia or distal residual limb	
		Inability to flex knee fully	
		Positive ball of clay test	
Anterior tibial tubercle and/or proximal anterior tibial shaft pain	Limb not fitting far enough into socket	Distal discoloration	Remove sock ply
		Distal end pain	
		Pain at fibular head	
		Significant pistoning	
		Difficulty controlling prosthesis	
	Inadequate relief of tibial tubercle	No other problems noted	Refer to prosthetist for socket adjustment
		Positive lipstick test	
Tibial crest pain	Long heel lever	Rapid descent of foot at IC	Check heel height and tightness of shoe
		Anterior distal tibial pain	Instruct patient to fully load the limb in early stance
			Refer to prosthetist for alignment adjustment
	Inadequate relief of tibial crest	No other problems may be noted	Refer to prosthetist for socket adjustment
		Positive lipstick test	
Fibular head pain	Limb descends too far into socket	Anterior distal tibia pain	Add additional sock ply
		Pain at distal pole of patella	
		Feeling of "looseness" within socket	
		Inability to flex the knee fully	
		Positive lipstick test	
	Limb not far enough into socket	Distal discoloration	Remove sock ply
		Distal end pain	
		Lack of control of prosthesis	
		Anterior tibial tubercle pain	
		Increased mediolateral movement of residual limb within socket	
		Positive lipstick or powder test	
	Prosthesis rotates on residual limb	Foot pointing into toe-out or toe-in	Re-don prosthesis with patella centered above patellar tendon bar
		General discomfort	Add or subtract ply of socks
Anterior distal tibia pain	Limb descends too far into socket	Pain on distal pole of patella	Add additional sock ply
		Feeling of looseness within socket	
		Pistoning during gait cycle	
		Inability to flex knee fully	
		Positive ball of clay test	
	Excessively long heel lever	Rapid forward motion at IC	Refer to prosthetist for adjustment of alignment
	Shoes with higher heels	Anterior tilt of foot at MSt	Change to more appropriate heel
	Shoes too tight for prosthetic foot	Inadequate heel compression at IC/LR	Change to larger shoe or smaller foot
Inadequate relief of anterior distal tibia	No other problems noted	Refer to prosthetist for adjustment of socket	
	Pain referred from elsewhere	Positive lipstick test	Address source of problem
		Pain or redness over another area reproduces discomfort at distal tibia	Refer to prosthetist for socket or alignment adjustment

TABLE 25-3
(continued)

Description	Possible Cause	Other Indicators	Possible Solutions
	Limb not far enough into socket	Distal discoloration Distal end pain Pistoning within socket Increased mediolateral movement within socket Anterior tibial tubercle pain Positive powder, lipstick, or ball of clay tests	Remove sock ply
	Bone or skin adhesion at distal tibia	Discomfort with skin traction Decreased skin mobility over tibia	Intervention to reduce adhesion Refer to physician Refer to prosthetist for socket adjustment
Posterior calf pain	Distal socket tightness	Blanching proximal to distal end, turning deep red with observation	Reduce sock ply
	Excessive proximal posterior pressure	Pistoning of limb in socket Popliteal abscess Distal end pain Cramping in limb	Loosen cuff or clothing on thigh Reduce sock ply Refer to prosthetist for further evaluation
	Circulatory disorders	Cool limb Aching residual or contralateral limb (especially after activity) Lack of color in residual limb Patient reports night pain in leg or limb	Refer to physician for evaluation
Vertical movement of limb inside prosthesis (pistoning)	Poor suspension	Old or worn suspension system	Replace or repair suspension system
	Too few socks	Pain at distal patella Loose feeling in prosthesis Inability to flex knee fully Pain on anterior distal tibia or crest	Add additional sock ply
	Too many socks	Distal discoloration Loose feeling in prosthesis Lack of control of prosthesis Anterior tibial tubercle pain	Remove sock ply
Distal looseness with proximal tightness of limb inside prosthesis ("bell clapping")	Normal limb shrinkage with prosthetic use	Distal anterior discomfort Lack of control of prosthesis Patient reports "looseness" Inability to add sock ply comfortably	Cut half-length sock to add ply to distal residual limb only Refer to prosthetist

IC = initial contact; MSt = midstance; LR = loading response.

priate to contact the prosthetist who designed and fabricated the prosthesis for more extensive evaluation and adjustment of prosthetic fit. It is important to remember that the most common causes of new discomfort in a prosthesis that was previously comfortable are often patient related: changes in the volume of the residual limb (e.g., discontinuing use of a prosthetic shrinker when not wearing the prosthesis), changing to shoes with different heel heights or widths, and changes in activity level.

CONCLUSION AND SUMMARY

Most patients with transtibial amputation are candidates for a prosthesis if their functional status and quality of life will be enhanced, whether or not functional community ambulation will be possible. Medicare guidelines have been established to help the prosthetist and therapist determine the appropriate prosthetic components for the patient's anticipated level of function. The PTB socket design is effective for most transtibial prostheses. The decision as to whether to fabricate a hard socket worn with socks or some type of liner as an interface or a flexible socket in a rigid frame is based on the patient's weight, skin condition, bony topography, and anticipated level of activity. The pros and cons of each type of interface must be carefully considered in the prescription process. The ideal suspension system holds the prosthesis securely on the residual limb, minimizing movement of the prosthesis on the residual limb in the transitions between the stance and swing phase, and also allows the patient to sit comfortably. The patient's ability to use his or her upper extremities effectively in donning the prosthesis and securing suspension is an important determinant in choosing among the various suspension systems that are currently available. Although the ability to adjust alignment of an endoskeletal temporary prosthesis is advantageous early in rehabilitation when frequent alignment adjustments are anticipated, prosthetic wearers who are very active may benefit from a more durable exoskeletal definitive prosthesis.

In the process of bench alignment, the prosthetist establishes an initial spatial relationship between the socket and prosthetic foot, based on biomechanical principles that direct forces toward pressure-tolerant areas and enhance a smooth forward progression during gait. Alignment is first refined statically while the patient is standing. If no problems have been identified, dynamic observational gait analysis is used to fine tune alignment until the most energy-efficient and normal-appearing gait pattern is accomplished. Although some problems identified during this dynamic alignment process require adjustment of socket or prosthetic foot position, most can be traced to inadequate suspension, inappropriate sock ply, shoe condition and heel height, or patient-related factors (such as apprehension about shifting weight fully onto the prosthesis). When assessing the effectiveness of a transtibial prosthesis, therapists who are skilled in prosthetic rehabilitation recognize the interplay of many factors: the characteristics of prosthetic components, adequacy of suspension, fit of the socket, alignment of prosthetic components, importance of footwear, and the patient's musculoskeletal and neuromuscular characteristics. Close collaboration between prosthetist, therapist, and patient ensures optimal prosthetic outcome.

REFERENCES

1. Bowker JH, Goldberg B, Poonekar PD. Transtibial Amputation. In JH Bowker, JW Michael (eds), Atlas of Limb Prosthetics: Surgical, Prosthetic, and Rehabilitation Principles. St. Louis: Mosby, 1992;429–452.
2. Brodsky JW. Amputations of the Foot and Ankle. In RA Mann, MJ Coughlin (eds), Surgery of the Foot and Ankle (6th ed). Vol 2. St. Louis: Mosby, 1993;959–990.
3. Penington G, Warmington S, Hull S, Freijah N. Rehabilitation of lower limb amputations and some implications for surgical management. Aust NZ J Surg 1992;62(10):774–779.
4. DMERC Medicare Advisory Bulletin. Columbia, SC: DMERC, 1994;12:95–145.
5. Kapp S. Below Knee Prosthetics Course Manual. Dallas: University of Texas Southwestern Medical Center, 1988.
6. Thompson D. Therapeutic Exercise Course Manual. Oklahoma City: University of Oklahoma Health Sciences Center, Department of Physical Therapy, 1995.
7. Caspers C. TEC Interface Systems (marketing brochure). St. Cloud, MN: TEC Manufacturing, 1995.
8. Fillauer CE, Pritham CH, Fillauer KD. Evolution and development of the silicone suction socket. JPO 1989;1(2):61–72.
9. Waters RL. Energy Expenditure of Amputee Gait. In JH Bowker, JW Michael (eds), Atlas of Limb Prosthetics: Surgical, Prosthetic, and Rehabilitation Principles. St. Louis: Mosby, 1992;381–387.
10. Berger N. Analysis of Amputee Gait. In JH Bowker, JW Michael (eds), Atlas of Limb Prosthetics: Surgical, Prosthetic, and Rehabilitation Principles. St. Louis: Mosby, 1992;371–379.
11. Saunders GT. Static and Dynamic Analysis. In: Lower Limb Amputations: A Guide to Rehabilitation. Philadelphia: Davis, 1986;415–475.
12. 1996 study guide. Arch Phys Med Rehabil 1996;77(suppl):3–5.
13. Kapp S, Cummings D. Transtibial Amputation: Prosthetic Management. In JH Bowker, JW Michael (eds), Atlas of Limb Prosthetics: Surgical, Prosthetic, and Rehabilitation Principles. St. Louis: Mosby, 1992;453–478.

26

Transtibial Prosthetic Training and Rehabilitation

JULIE D. RIES AND KAREN M. BREWER

Many patients who have undergone transtibial amputation approach rehabilitation with a combination of excitement and apprehension. They are often pleased to have healed and are curious about the prosthesis that they are about to receive, but are somewhat distrustful or unrealistic about what they will or will not be able to achieve. To facilitate an individual's optimal rehabilitation outcome, the physical therapist must consider the patient's goals, physical abilities, and mobility needs. In this chapter, we explore the key components of successful rehabilitation for persons with amputation, beginning with evaluation as the patient enters rehabilitation, the delivery and initial use of the prosthesis, and progression through gait training and advanced mobility skills.

A general knowledge of the timeline of the prosthetic rehabilitation process is helpful in projecting goals and educating patients about expected outcomes. A patient with new amputation is ready to be fit with an initial prosthesis (also called a *temporary* or *training prosthesis*) when the surgical incision is healed and girth measurements at the distal residual limb are equal to or less than proximal girth measurements. This can occur as early as 10–14 days postoperatively to as long as 8 weeks or more after surgery. As a new residual limb matures and shrinks in size, the patient will add additional ply (layers) of prosthetic sock to ensure adequate fit in the prosthesis. Typically, when the intimacy of fit within the socket is compromised by 15 or more ply of sock, a new prosthetic socket is indicated. How quickly the initial socket needs to be replaced varies from patient to patient, depending on the pattern of shrinkage of the residual limb. For some, the first replacement socket may be necessary in 2–3 months, whereas others may use their initial socket for 5 or 6 months. The socket may be replaced several additional times as the residual limb continues to shrink in the first postoperative year. A definitive prosthesis is prescribed

when the residual limb size is stable for an 8- to 12-week period, as indicated by girth measurements and by a consistent number of sock ply for prosthetic fit. Although some patients are ready for their definitive prosthesis within 6 months after surgery, others do not achieve stable residual limb size for 12–18 months or longer.

For patients with a new transtibial amputation, physical therapy intervention initially focuses on building tolerance for prosthetic wear and safety in gait and functional mobility activities. As early prosthetic skills are mastered, intervention progresses to more complex, higher-level bipedal activities. Finally, vocational, leisure, and sporting activities can be addressed to aid the patient in returning to a productive and enjoyable lifestyle. In this chapter, we focus on strategies for initial and intermediate-level rehabilitation.

EVALUATION

Effective physical therapy management for patients with amputation begins with a thorough and comprehensive initial evaluation. The S.O.A.P. note format that is commonly used in physical therapy provides a model for comprehensive evaluation. The "S" or subjective heading highlights the importance of the patient's perspective about what will happen during the rehabilitation process. Under the "O" or objective heading, the physical therapist collects data about impairments and functional limitations that may influence the rehabilitation process. This information is used as a basis for the "A" or assessment heading, in which the physical therapist reflects on the patient's present and potential status and begins to formulate specific, outcome-oriented, short- and long-term goals. These goals must be sensible and neither limiting or unrealistic in scope, because they are the measure against which the success of rehabilitation is judged. The final component,

TABLE 26-1

Important Subjective Components for Comprehensive Evaluation of Patients with Amputation

Component	Questions to Consider
The patient's goals	What does the patient want to be able to do?
	What does the family/caregivers expect the patient to be able to do?
	Are these goals realistic and appropriate?
	How important/desirable is the achievement of these goals to the patient? To the caregivers?
The patient's resources	What are the patient's current emotional status, cognitive ability, preferred coping strategies, and preferred learning styles?
	Does the patient have accurate insight into the rehabilitation process?
	What emotional and instrumental support is available to the patient? What emotional and instrumental support is available for the family/caregivers?
Premorbid function	What types and level of activities have been typical for this patient in recent weeks and months?
	What are the patient's current and anticipated mobility goals, and how do they compare to premorbid level of function?
Past medical history	What comorbid impairments or active disease processes involving the vascular, cardiac, pulmonary, endocrine, renal, neuromuscular, or musculoskeletal systems are likely to have an impact on the rehabilitation process?
	What is the patient's overall health status?
	Are visual, auditory, or other sensory deficits present that might influence rehabilitation, communication, and/or self-care?
History of present illness	What is the etiology of this patient's amputation?
	What medications (prescribed and over the counter) is the patient taking?

"P," is the plan of action for rehabilitation: the activities and interventions to be used to meet the goals of the rehabilitation program.

Subjective Information

The patient's perspective of his or her illness, functional limitation, and possible disability has a powerful influence on the rehabilitation process.[1,2] Information about what the patient is thinking and feeling is initially gathered by interview, as well as in conversation during treatment sessions as rehabilitation progresses. A patient's fears and concerns influence determination and motivation and are powerful determinants of the ability to ambulate and perform other important functional activities.[3] An individual with an amputation who is capable of safe and functional ambulation in the community may choose not to venture into public for fear of being identified as disabled or different. In contrast, a person whose clinical picture is less promising for functional prosthetic use but who is determined to return to a busy and productive life "on two feet" may very well do so.

Several important areas must be explored during the subjective component of the patient interview (Table 26-1). It is important to discover what the patient's goals actually are and how strongly he or she feels about achieving these goals. If the patient's initial goals appear to be over- or underambitious, the therapist can address these issues with

patient education and interaction with peers as possible interventions. The patient's emotional status, cognitive abilities, preferred coping strategies, insight into the rehabilitation process, and usual learning style, as well as the availability of emotional and instrumental support systems (assistance with activities of daily living), are important to consider. Information about the patient's preamputation level of activity and mobility, as well as his or her understanding of past medical history and history of present illness, completes the subjective portion of the evaluation. Specific and probing interview questions are often helpful in obtaining a clear and accurate patient history. Although many patients are accurate historians, others may have an incomplete understanding or imprecise memory of what has happened to them. It is always advisable to confirm information by interview with the patient's family and review of the medical record. The physician should be contacted with any outstanding questions.

The patient interview is a means to gather important information that is used to guide intervention and to begin the process of patient education. Many patients do not have a clear understanding of what to expect during rehabilitation or how their disease process might progress. Amputation is not selective to patients of a specific age group, cultural background, educational experience, or socioeconomic rank. All patients benefit by being well educated about their condition and treatment. For many patients, the events that brought them to rehabilitation may be a blur of disjointed experiences and medical jargon or a laundry list of conditions that seem unrelated or independent. The physical therapist can help patients to place their history and experience in a meaningful context, which, in turn, assists them in forming realistic expectations, and may decrease the likelihood of a second amputation.

Objective Examination

The objective examination and evaluation of patients with amputation are based on commonly used measures and assessment strategies at impairment and functional limitation levels.[4] It is important to note that some assessments, such as strength testing or joint play motions, might require modification of technique because loss of limb length necessarily changes where the therapist is able to hold or resist the limb. The therapist selects appropriate tests and measures to assess the following:

1. Cognitive status and preferred learning style
2. Range of motion (ROM) of the residual and remaining limb
3. Motor control and functional strength
4. Sensation and perception
5. Postural control
6. Cardiovascular status and endurance
7. Physical condition of the residual and remaining limbs
8. Adaptive equipment and prosthetic prescription
9. Functional mobility with and without prosthesis
10. The ability to perform self-care and preferred activities

Table 26-2 provides further details of the suggested areas of evaluation.

Assessment

In the assessment (evaluation) component, the physical therapist interprets and integrates subjective and objective information to identify the patient's primary areas of deficiency and uses professional judgment to predict or make a prognosis as to the likely functional outcome and time required for effective prosthetic rehabilitation. Included is a summary of the patient's major problems and the presumed underlying cause(s). Problems should be prioritized, with those that have the most significant functional implications receiving top priority. This is done on an individualized basis, as the same problem may affect different patients in different ways. A patient with poor sensation of the residual limb who is cognitively intact may be easily educated about compensating for the sensory deficit with visual inspection of the residual limb, effectively reducing the risk of compromise of skin integrity. A patient with the same sensory deficit who also has cognitive impairment may require a more extensive educational intervention that is focused on residual limb care. This patient has a much higher risk of problems with skin integrity, and is likely to require the assistance of a caregiver to monitor skin integrity.

Therapists must also be skilled in determining the functional implications of specific problems. For instance, a slight knee flexion contracture can probably be accommodated for in transtibial socket alignment, whereas a significant knee flexion contracture prohibits prosthetic fitting with a conventional prosthesis. Prosthetic prescription and physical therapy intervention may be quite different for two patients who both present with knee flexion contractures.

The prioritized problem list provides a foundation for determination of functional short- and long-term goals that, in turn, direct rehabilitation activities. The physical therapist uses patient history information and specific subjective and objective findings, as well as a knowledge base of outcome measures for patients with transtibial amputation, to predict each patient's rehabilitation potential and probable functional outcome. A young, active, healthy patient with traumatic transtibial amputation who has few postoperative complications is likely to progress through rehabilitation more quickly, achieving a higher level of function in a shorter period of time than an older, medically frail, and deconditioned patient who has had an amputation as a result of vascular compromise or nonhealing neuropathic ulcer. These differences will be reflected in the specific goals set and the rate at which long-term goals are met.

Plan of Care

The physical therapy treatment plan of care includes information about the frequency, duration, location, and specific physical therapy interventions that are to be used. The plan of care is directly related to the goals delineated by the assessment/prognostic process. If independent donning and doffing of a prosthesis are primary short-term goals, the associated treatment plan must include patient education strategies, opportunities to practice this skill, and remediation or adaptation of any movement components that, if missing, would compromise the patient's ability to perform this necessary task (i.e., the patient may need to improve grip strength or intrinsic hand strength to manipulate prosthetic suspension). The plan includes information about equipment to be ordered, referrals to be made, and the ultimate physical therapy discharge plan.

TABLE 26-2

Components of the Objective Evaluation for Patients with Amputation

Component	Issues to Examine
Cognitive status	Orientation Ability to follow commands (multistep) Coping strategies Motivation/emotional status Potential for new learning Problem-solving abilities Safety awareness and judgment
Range of motion	Screening/gross assessment of upper extremity and trunk range of motion Definitive assessment of joints of the residual and remaining limbs
Motor status	Functional strength of upper extremities and trunk Manual muscle test of major lower limb muscle groups Functional strength during lower limb closed chain movements Quality and endurance of eccentric muscle control Overall quality of movement Muscular endurance and/or fatigue Coordination and timing of movement
Sensation	Formal assessment of residual and intact limb (sharp/dull, warm/cold, light touch/deep pressure, proprioception) Patterns of sensory changes (e.g., stocking-glove neuropathy) Phantom sensation and/or phantom pain
Balance (with and without prosthesis)	Static (sitting, standing) and dynamic balance (transitional) Reactive and anticipatory balance
Cardiovascular	Aerobic capacity/endurance as related to functional activity Insight into level of fatigue and ability to initiate rest breaks Vital signs at rest and during activity; recovery to resting level
Condition of intact limb	Hydration of skin Pattern of hair loss Areas of irritation, ulceration, or other open wounds Patterns of callus Skin temperature at foot, ankle, lower leg Palpable arterial pulses (dorsal pedis, posterior tibial, popliteal) Joint mobility at talocrural, subtalar, and forefoot joints Orthopedic deformity (e.g., hallux valgus, claw toe, Charcot's ankle) Condition/adequacy of footwear (wear pattern, fit) Patient's ability to inspect and care for the limb
Condition of residual limb	Integrity/healing of surgical incision (drainage, ecchymosis, dehiscence, necrosis) Integrity of skin (drain sites, skin graft sites, surgical scars from previous vascular bypass) Mobility of soft tissue (adhesion formation) Length of residual limb (tibial length, soft tissue length) Girth of residual limb (proximal, mid, and distal circumference) Shape of residual limb (bulbous/edematous, presence of redundant tissue/"dog ears," cylindrical) Pressure-intolerant areas (bony prominences, distal anterior tibia) Palpable pulses (popliteal, femoral) Skin temperature (distal, midlength, proximal, above the knee)
Equipment	Prosthetic design and components Compression devices (shrinkers) Self-care devices (bedside commode, tub bench, etc.) Assistive devices and mobility aids Wheelchair needs

Functional mobility	Ability to transfer, with and without prosthesis (level of assistance, type of transfer, ability to
	    adapt transfer to different context/setting)
	Bed mobility (level of assistance, preferred movement strategies)
	Wheelchair mobility (level of assistance, technique of propulsion, functional distances, types of
	    terrain)
	Ability to don/doff prosthesis
	Ambulation, with and without prosthesis (level of assistance, ambulatory aid, or assistive
	    device use; gait pattern; functional distances; type of terrain)
	Primary and compensatory gait deviations
	Ability to manage stairs and ramps (level of assistance, technique/preferred pattern of movement)
	Ability to rise from the floor

TABLE 26-2
(continued)

Component	Issues to Examine
Activities of daily living	Self-care skills (level of assistance, preferred pattern of movement, assistive devices required) Home and work responsibilities (possible requirements for adaptation) Preferred/adapted leisure activities Transportation issues (ability to drive, need for adaptation of vehicle, use of public transportation)

IMPORTANT CONSIDERATIONS IN PROSTHETIC TRAINING

A variety of patient skills and physical/functional characteristics create the foundation for successful prosthetic training. These key areas include functional ROM of the hip and knee, functional strength of muscles at the hip and knee, adequacy of motor control and balance, aerobic capacity and endurance, effective edema control and maturation of the residual limb, integrity of the skin and soft tissue, and sensory status of the residual limb. Inability to achieve a certain status or level of performance in one area does not prohibit a good prosthetic outcome; however, difficulties in multiple areas have an impact on prosthetic candidacy and use. Each of these areas should be carefully evaluated and appropriate interventions undertaken to achieve at least minimal requirements for functional prosthetic use, if not optimal status or level of performance.

Range of Motion

Contracture or tightness of hip flexors, abductors, and external rotators and knee flexors of the residual limb can have a significant impact on functional ambulation and mobility. This posture of the residual limb is consistent with the flexor withdrawal pattern associated with lower extremity pain. The flexion withdrawal posture is reinforced if the residual limb is elevated on pillows when the patient is in bed. These factors place patients with recent amputation at significant risk of contracture formation. Maintaining or increasing available ROM at the hip and knee of the residual limb continues to be a primary treatment goal as the patient moves from preprosthetic into prosthetic rehabilitation. Prone positioning is an excellent strategy to combat contracture formation and should be prescribed (at least 30 minutes b.i.d.) for all patients who are able to tolerate prone lying. Although achieving knee flexion ROM is sometimes overlooked in early rehabilitation, full knee flexion ROM is required for step-over-step stair ambulation and for rising from a seated position. Assessment of ROM of the intact limb is also important, as loss of ROM of either limb has an impact on quality and energy efficiency of gait. The importance of functional ROM is also emphasized in patient

education and in daily home exercise routines. The potential prosthetic problems that are associated with loss of functional ROM are summarized in Table 26-3.

Strength and Motor Control

As prosthetic training begins, it is important to evaluate baseline strength in several ways. Standard manual muscle test protocols provide a starting point against which gains can be measured. Assessing knee strength of the resid-

TABLE 26-3
Prosthetic Consequences of Limitations in Range of Motion

Range of Motion Limitation	Potential Functional Implication
Decreased hip extension	Inability to achieve upright posture in stance Chronic low back pain due to compensatory anterior pelvic tilt Compensatory knee flexion causes instability in gait Decreased stride length of contralateral limb in gait
Decreased hip adduction	Abducted stance in gait Abductor lurch on ipsilateral side in gait
Decreased internal rotation	Toe-out stance and gait Knee joint pain and/or pathology due to lack of anterior/posterior orientation of knee joint
Decreased knee extension	Limb functionally shorter, with associated gait deviations Decreased midstance stability in gait Requires prosthetic alignment adjustments to compensate
Decreased knee flexion	Inability to place foot flat on the floor when sitting Inability to weight bear through prosthesis during sit-to-stand transfers Difficulty managing steps and curbs

ual limb becomes somewhat more subjective, as the standard lever arm for providing resistance has been altered by the amputation. Functional strength during closed chain activities and eccentric control are equally important, as they more closely reflect muscle activity during normal gait. Stability of the hip and pelvis, especially in stance on the prosthetic side, is one of the key ingredients in achieving forward progression over the prosthesis. Although preamputation weakness of proximal muscles may not have produced an observable abnormal gait pattern, deviations are often more pronounced when weak muscles are unable to control the distal prosthesis.

The strength and motor control requirements for ambulation with a transtibial prosthesis are similar but not identical to those of normal gait. Both the involved and intact lower extremities display increased muscle activity during their respective stance phases. Specifically, activity of the ipsilateral hip and knee extensors is increased and prolonged during stance as compared to normals.[5,6] The contralateral or intact limb is subject to increased ground reaction forces, presumably a result of the absence of the normal foot and ankle mechanism of the involved side.[7,8] Hip abductors and extensors and knee extensors of the intact limb must respond to these increased forces. It is clear that the therapist must address the strength of the residual limb, as well as the strength of the uninvolved limb.

Balance and Coordination

Postural control, which involves controlling the body's position in space for purposes of stability (maintaining center of mass over base of support) and orientation (appropriate relationship between body segments and between body and environment), is fundamental to functional tasks.[9] Postural control relies on somatosensation (especially proprioception) to provide accurate information about the position of the foot and ankle and the pressures through the lower extremity joints. Visual and vestibular information adds awareness of position in space with respect to objects in the environment and to gravity. Because sensory and proprioceptive input from the distal segment is absent after amputation, a new prosthetic user must learn to compensate for this lack of important postural information. The patient may learn to deduce the position of the prosthetic foot and contact with the support surface by the angle of the knee and pressures felt within the prosthetic socket. Early in gait training, a patient may make an exaggerated effort to dig the heel into the floor at initial contact and early loading response to use the resulting pressure at the posterior residual limb as an indicator of contact with the floor with the knee in extension. The patient may learn to interpret this sensory experience as the secure position for proceeding with loading response and progressing into midstance.

In addition to the loss of direct sensory knowledge of contact with the floor, the loss of muscles at the ankle often compromises postural responses. Nashner[10] describes three stereotypical motor responses that are used to ensure that the center of mass stays within the base of support in response to unexpected anteroposterior perturbations: ankle, hip, and stepping strategies. These postural strategies are also evident during functional activities, such as ambulation.[9] The ankle strategy movement pattern, evident in normal postural sway, requires intact ROM and strength of muscles at the ankle. After amputation, this strategy is no longer available to the transtibial prosthetic user, so that the patient must instead rely on hip strategy (movement of the trunk over the base of support) or stepping strategies when postural responses are necessary.

Patients must be able to respond to environmental demands during ambulation and other functional tasks in anticipatory (feed forward) and reactive (feedback) modes. Therapists can design tasks to assess and encourage each of these types of postural control. For example, catching and throwing a ball allows the patient to anticipate postural demands (in an effort to throw) and react to postural disruptions (in an effort to catch). Reaching activities when standing help patients develop skill and confidence in their anticipatory postural responses and, should the reach distance be excessive, their reactive postural responses as well.

Cardiovascular Endurance

A thorough assessment of a patient's cardiovascular status and cardiovascular endurance training should be integral parts of preprosthetic management. The energy requirements for an individual who is using a prosthesis for ambulation are higher than those of an individual who ambulates on two intact lower limbs.[11,12] The oxygen uptake for patients with unilateral transtibial amputation is correlated to residual limb length and may be 10–40% higher than that of individuals without amputation.[13] Physical conditioning is an essential component of rehabilitation for patients with lower extremity amputation, especially those with cardiopulmonary or vascular compromise. Improving metabolic efficiency (aerobic capacity) has a direct impact on the potential for functional ambulation even for the frailest and most deconditioned patients.[14] Endurance activities during the preprosthetic rehabilitation phase (such as wheelchair propulsion, single limb ambulation with an appropriate assistive device, and upper extremity ergometry) help improve cardiovascular status before the patient is a functional prosthetic user. Patients often continue these activities as they enter into the prosthetic phase of treatment. As the condition of the patient's residual limb and wearing tolerance permit, ambulation with the prosthesis can be used as an additional cardiovascular endurance activity.

For patients whose endurance may be a limiting factor for prosthetic ambulation, the physical therapy plan of care must include a cardiovascular exercise component. Patients who are taught to monitor their own pulse, respiratory rate, and/or perceived rate of exertion are able to participate more fully in prosthetic rehabilitation and prosthetic training. To develop an effective cardiovascular conditioning program, the therapist uses knowledge of the patient's past medical history and cardiovascular pathophysiology, adapting the program to provide an appropriate challenge without surpassing the patient's physiologic capabilities. The therapist must recognize the influence of cardiopulmonary pathologies, such as unstable angina or advanced chronic obstructive pulmonary disease, on the patient's ability to improve his or her endurance and adjust goals and intervention strategies as appropriate.

Edema Control of Residual Limb

Initiation of weight-bearing activities in the prosthetic socket significantly decreases limb edema and accelerates maturation of the residual limb as a result of total contact within the socket and the pumping of muscle contractions during weight-bearing activities and movement.[15,16] A patient who initially wears several ply of cotton or wool socks often needs to add several more layers of socks during the first few weeks of prosthetic use as a result of rapid shrinking of the residual limb. It is important that the patient continues to use a commercial shrinker pressure garment when not wearing the prosthesis to reduce the likelihood of insidious edema when the prosthesis is not being worn. Patients with fluid volume fluctuations (i.e., those with kidney dysfunction or with ongoing congestive heart failure) will need to use such shrinkers indefinitely. For others whose residual limb reaches a stable size and shape, a shrinker may not be necessary once they are using the prosthesis functionally on a daily basis. The decision to discontinue the use of a shrinker permanently is based on two factors: (1) consistency in the number of sock ply worn during the day and (2) the ability to don the prosthesis without decreasing the usual number of sock ply after a night's sleep without the shrinker.

Soft Tissue Mobility of Residual Limb

Soft tissue and bony adhesions that limit tissue mobility around the incision scar and the surrounding area may have an impact on prosthetic tolerance, comfort, and use. The surgical procedure of a transtibial amputation can include muscle-to-muscle (myoplasty), muscle-to-fascia (myofascial), and/or muscle-to-bone (myodesis) surgical

fixations to stabilize the remaining muscle.[17] Scarring or adhesions can occur among any or all of these tissues. The normal stresses and shearing forces of weight bearing and non–weight bearing during gait require that soft tissue throughout the residual limb be mobile. If the soft tissue is not able to move independently of the scar tissue or skeletal structures, the stress can lead to tissue breakdown and discomfort. Deep friction massage (DFM) can be an effective tool in managing scar tissue. Patients can be instructed in the use of this modality with specific guidelines for proper technique. Improper DFM technique is ineffective in managing scar tissue and potentially harmful for the patient with fragile skin and soft tissue. Appropriate DFM targets movements between skin, subcutaneous soft tissue and fascia, and muscle layers.[18] Inappropriate friction generated between the fingers and skin results in skin irritation, blistering, or breakdown and can delay prosthetic use until adequate healing occurs.

Sensory Status of Residual Limb

Residual limb and sound limb sensitivity should be formally assessed using standard sensation testing guidelines (i.e., dermatomal regions, assessing stocking-glove distribution, and testing all sensory modalities—sharp/dull, light touch, deep pressure, warm/cold, proprioception). Several commonly occurring postamputation sensory phenomena can have serious implications for functional outcome in patients with amputation. These include hyposensitivity, hypersensitivity, phantom sensations, and phantom limb pain.

Hyposensitivity

Hyposensitivity is most often encountered among patients with a history of severe neuropathy, traumatic nerve damage, or vascular disease. Patients with amputation who have impaired sensation are at high risk for skin breakdown because they may not recognize discomfort associated with skin irritation resulting from repetitive stresses and pressures. Inclusion of patient education about the preventative need for visual inspection, and practice time to perform visual inspection of the residual limb for signs and symptoms of soft tissue lesions, significantly reduces the risk of skin breakdown. Adaptive equipment, such as mirrors, or the assistance of caregivers may be necessary for patients with concurrent limitations in flexibility or vision deficits.

Hypersensitivity

Early in rehabilitation, it is not uncommon to encounter a generalized hypersensitivity of the residual limb. This hypersensitivity is thought to be a consequence of nerve damage from amputation surgery itself.[18] Hypersensitivity can be effectively managed by bombarding the patient's limb with tactile stimuli using a variety of textures and pressures. Strategies for reducing hypersensitivity include gently tapping with the fingers, massaging with lotion, touching with a soft fabric (i.e., flannel or towel), rolling a small ball over the residual limb, and implementing a specific wearing schedule for shrinker socks and rigid dressings. Intensity of intervention is based on the patient's tolerance to the sensory stimulation. The techniques can be progressed in intensity, type of modality used, and duration of stimulus (i.e., touching the limb with a rougher fabric and increasing wearing time for the shrinker socks). Patients with amputations are encouraged to use these techniques independently as part of their home program.

Localized hypersensitivity is often an indication that a neuroma has developed at the distal end of a surgically severed peripheral nerve. A neuroma is suspected when localized tapping sends a shock sensation up the patient's leg. If conservative clinical treatment is unsuccessful in reducing the pain caused by neuroma, injection of a local anesthetic directly into the region or surgical removal of the neuroma may be necessary.

Phantom Limb Sensations

Phantom limb sensations are also quite common after amputation.[19-23] Many patients report experiencing feelings of tingling or numbness in the toes or foot of the limb that has been amputated. Although the sensation can include the entire missing extremity, it is most often perceived as toe, foot, or ankle sensation. This predominantly distal presentation of phantom sensation is presumably a result of the large area of somatosensory cortex dedicated to the distal portion of the extremity.[2] Phantom limb sensations are considered to be the brain's erroneous interpretation of sensory nerve impulses traveling along the pathway of the nerves that formerly provided sensory feedback from the amputated limb.[2,19] Phantom limb sensation is a relatively harmless condition that has important functional implications for the patient. This sensation may be functionally useful in providing a semblance of proprioceptive feedback from the prosthesis. It may, however, also present a potential danger: Many patients with phantom limb experience nighttime falls when, half asleep, they attempt to stand and walk to the bathroom, expecting their phantom foot to make contact with the floor.

Phantom Limb Pain

Phantom limb pain is a special type of phantom sensation that can have an impact on the rehabilitation of patients with amputation. Although most patients with amputation report phantom sensation, phantom pain is less common. When phantom pain occurs, it is most often described as a cramping, squeezing, or burning sensation in the part of the limb that has been amputated. The spec-trum of patient complaints may vary from occasional mild pain to continuous severe pain. The absence of observable abnormalities of the residual limb is common. Although the etiology of phantom pain is not well understood, it has been theorized to be a product of the central nervous system (central origin theory), spinal cord–mediated mechanisms, or psychological factors.[18] The association between the etiology of amputation (vascular versus traumatic) and the incidence of phantom pain is unclear.[17,22,23] Whatever the etiology, phantom limb pain can be challenging to manage and disabling if the pain is severe. Strategies to address phantom limb pain include desensitization techniques, heat modalities, firm pressure applied to the residual limb, use of analgesics, and consistent use of a prosthesis.[21]

INITIAL PROSTHETIC TRAINING

Several important components of rehabilitation involving prevention of skin breakdown and safe use of equipment, can be effectively addressed in group classes or through printed materials. These components include care of the sound limb, donning and doffing the prosthesis, establishing a prosthetic wearing schedule, management and prevention of skin breakdown, positioning with the prosthesis, and care of equipment.

Care of Sound Limb

Ongoing assessment of the intact lower extremity is the responsibility of the therapist and of the patient. Patients with diabetes, neuropathy, or peripheral vascular disease who have lost one leg as a result of the disease process have a 20% chance of losing the other leg within a 2-year period.[24] To minimize the risk of loss of the remaining limb, close monitoring of limb condition (especially for subtle or insidious trophic, sensory, or motor changes) and optimal foot care are essential. Ongoing, systematic, and frequent assessment of pulses, edema, temperature, and skin is suggested. Education about the importance of a daily routine of cleansing, drying, and closely inspecting the foot (including the plantar surface and between the toes) is crucial. Podiatric care of nails, corns, and plantar callus; appropriately fitting footwear or accommodative foot orthoses; and avoidance of barefoot walking are three additional imperatives for the longevity of the remaining foot. If patients are unable to perform daily foot inspection independently because of disease- or age-related visual impairment or decreased agility, they must be able to direct a caregiver in inspecting the foot. Even if patients are physically incapable of performing certain tasks for their own health and safety, they are ultimately responsible for their own care. Developing or improving on a patient's skill at directing assistance is a useful and realistic physical therapy treatment goal.

Donning and Doffing the Prosthesis

In early prosthetic rehabilitation, prosthetic socks are used to modify the fit between the socket and the shrinking residual limb. Proper use of prosthetic socks enhances residual limb weight bearing in pressure-tolerant areas, decreases the likelihood of skin breakdown in pressure-intolerant areas, and increases patient comfort during ambulation. Many patients use a thin nylon sheath directly over the skin (under the socks) to minimize friction forces and wick moisture away from the skin. Cotton or wool socks of various ply (thicknesses) are then applied before the limb is placed in the socket. These wool or cotton prosthetic socks are available in three different ply: 1 (thinnest), 3, and 5 (thickest). When the patient is using a rigid or flexible socket, the socks are placed over the nylon sheath or directly on the residual limb. When silicone suction suspension is used, the silicone shell is first applied to the limb, and the socks (modified with a small hole for the pin-locking mechanism) are layered on top. Socks of various thicknesses are combined to create a snug and comfortable fit. Patients are encouraged to don the fewest number of socks to achieve the same amount of thickness (i.e., one 3-ply sock is preferable to three 1-ply socks). Prosthetic socks can also be used creatively to solve problems with socket fit. If, for example, the patient's distal residual limb girth has decreased more quickly than proximal girth, creating a pendulum effect within the socket during ambulation, one of the prosthetic socks can be cut to cover just the lower half of the residual limb. When layered between two full-sized socks, the shorter sock helps to fill the extra space within the socket, ensuring total contact between the limb and socket.

Fluctuations in limb volume associated with edema in the first weeks and months after amputation often mean that the appropriate number of sock ply varies from day to day and perhaps within a given day. Because of this variability in limb size, choosing the correct number of prosthetic socks may be challenging for those new to prosthetic use. Limb size can change rapidly: Even a few minutes in a dependent position without a shrinker or Ace wrap in place can substantially increase residual limb size. For this reason, patients should wear their compression device until the moment that they are ready to don the prosthesis. Therapists and prosthetists work with the patient to assist the development of problem-solving skills and strategies to determine the appropriate number of socks to don.

It is important that new prosthetic users understand the principles of prosthetic fit and weight bearing. The optimal prosthetic fit is quite snug, like that of a custom-fit glove on the hand. Total contact between the residual limb and socket is important as well: Significant skin problems occur when total contact is not achieved. Patients must understand where weight-bearing pressures are best tolerated on the limb and where pressure sensitivity is likely to occur. Although they might initially expect to bear weight through the distal end of the limb, they must understand that most sockets are designed to distribute weight-bearing forces across several areas, including the patellar tendon, anteromedial and anterolateral surfaces of the residual limb, medial tibial flare, and distal posterior aspect of the residual limb.

A number of indicators are used to assess the adequacy of sock ply during prosthetic ambulation. If too few socks are put on, the residual limb descends too far down within the socket. The patient may complain of pistoning during ambulation: The prosthesis slips downward when unweighted during the swing phase and is pushed upward on the residual limb during weight bearing in stance. If pistoning is suspected, a pen or marker is used to mark the prosthetic sock at the anterior or posterior trimline of the socket. If the line becomes more visible when the patient lifts the limb (using a hip-hiking motion), it is likely that slippage is occurring, and additional sock layers are indicated. When the prosthesis and socks are taken off for inspection of the skin, reactive hyperemia (redness) is seen at the proximal patellar tendon and at the inferior border of the patella, as well as at the distal anterior residual limb. Redness may also be present on the fibular head, which contacted the socket below its intended relief area. These are signs that thickness of the sock is inadequate and additional sock layers should be added.

A different set of signs indicates that too many ply of sock have been donned. The patient may feel that the prosthetic limb is difficult to don, fits too tightly, and is just slightly longer during forward progression at midstance and in foot clearance in swing. When the skin is inspected after ambulation, reactive hyperemia is seen at the distal patellar tendon and the tibial tubercle. Redness may also be present at the head of the fibula, which contacted the socket above its intended relief within the socket. These are indications that one or more ply of socks should be removed to enhance socket fit.

Most patients become adept at judging the adequacy of sock ply when given the opportunity to practice and problem solve early in their rehabilitation. For the functional prosthetic user, donning and doffing the prosthesis become as second nature as donning and doffing one's pants or shoes. The initial instruction period in this skill, however, requires attention to detail. Patients should be encouraged to establish a careful routine of donning the appropriate number of prosthetic socks, one layer at a time. The socks should be smoothed free of wrinkles, with any seams facing down and out so as to minimize pressure on the surgical scar. Patients then don the soft insert (if applicable) and palpate to assure that the patellar tendon indentation on the insert aligns appropriately with the patellar tendon. The hard socket of the prosthesis is then applied by gradually increasing weight bearing (from the sitting or standing position) to push the residual limb gently into the socket and checking that the alignment of the socket in the horizontal plane is correct. If great force is required to achieve purchase into the socket, the patient should be instructed to stop and start over. Figure 26-1 illustrates an effective strategy for donning the transtibial prosthesis.

Once the patient is comfortably in the socket, adjustment of the suspension device is necessary. Suspension devices for transtibial prostheses include a neoprene sleeve, supracondylar strap waist belt with auxiliary fork strap, supracondylar socket design, supracondylar/suprapatellar socket design, thigh corset with joint uprights, and suction socket with pin or ring suspension. To complete the donning process, the patient stands and weight bears through the socket to ensure proper positioning of the residual limb while adjusting the suspension system.

Prevention and Management of Skin Breakdown

Because prolonged wound healing and development of new skin irritation can delay prosthetic training, the prevention and management of skin breakdown on the residual limb represent an important part of the physical therapist's role. Open areas frequently preclude weight-bearing and gait-training activities. Pressure, friction, or shearing forces are the primary etiologies of skin breakdown related to prosthetic wear.

If, during weight bearing, external pressure exceeds capillary refill pressure (25–32 mm Hg) for an extended period of time, the delivery of oxygen and nutrients and the removal of waste products from active tissues are interrupted. If relief of pressure is provided, this local ischemia is followed by a reactive vasodilation or hyperemia. This is the mechanism that produces the redness over weight-bearing areas, such as the patellar tendon and medial tibial flare and shaft, that is observed in new prosthetic users. A blanchable area of redness over weight-bearing areas, which returns to normal skin coloration within 10 minutes, is to be expected in early prosthetic training and indicates normal reactive hyperemia.[25] If redness persists or does not blanch on firm palpation, tissue damage has likely occurred, and the risk of skin breakdown increases significantly.

It is important that therapists and patients recognize the different implications of redness over pressure-tolerant versus pressure-sensitive areas of the residual limb. If a pressure-tolerant area shows evidence of excessive pressure, socket fit and alignment may be appropriate, but the amount of weight bearing or duration of wearing time may need to be decreased. If pressure-sensitive areas are showing signs of too much pressure, it is more likely that socket fit or alignment needs to be adjusted. When excessive redness is observed, successful problem solving will change a single variable (e.g., wearing time) and assess the impact of this one change on the prosthetic problem. If multiple changes are made at the same time (e.g., wearing time, alignment, and socket fit), it is not clear which change actually solved the problem. If a therapist adds a nylon sheath, removes two ply socks, and changes socket alignment all at the same time and the patient's problem does not subside, it is impossible to know whether the interventions might have been more successful independent of one another. If the patient's problem is eliminated, there is no way of knowing which intervention was key to solving the problem.

An individual's risk for skin breakdown on the residual limb is determined by physiologic and mechanical factors. The vascular, sensory, and musculoskeletal status of the residual limb are the physiologic determinants, whereas socket fit, socket alignment, amount of weight bearing, and duration of weight bearing are the mechanical determinants. Each of these risk factors may have clinical implications for the physical therapist and patient. A conservative prosthetic-wearing schedule and frequent residual limb inspection may be indicated for patients with skin breakdown caused by any of the physiologic risk factors. If poor scar and soft tissue mobility of the residual limb leads to tissue breakdown, DFM over the involved area (after healing) and/or application of a nylon sheath under prosthetic socks may be appropriate interventions.

Improper socket fit or alignment can result in increased weight bearing to pressure-sensitive areas of the residual limb and may result in skin breakdown. If improper fit or alignment is suspected, the first step in problem solving is a thorough reevaluation of donning technique and the number of socks used. Prosthetic fit is then reassessed to determine if total contact between residual limb and socket has been achieved. If all of these areas are sufficient, potential problems with prosthetic alignment are investigated. It is important to note that increasing duration of prosthetic wearing too quickly in a well-aligned and appropriately fit prosthesis can also result in skin breakdown to pressure-tolerant areas of the residual limb. A patient who has been ambulating with partial weight bearing using axillary crutches without any problems with skin integrity may, when progressed to full-time unilateral crutch use, present with skin breakdown over the

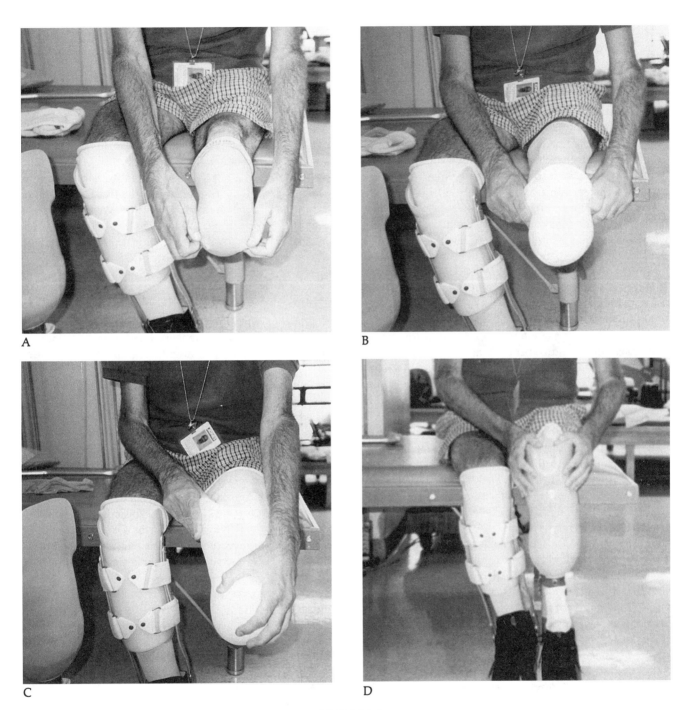

FIGURE 26-1

*This patient with a recent transstibial amputation is practicing the correct sequence for donning his prosthesis. (**A**) First, he applies a nylon sheath, adjusting its fit to prevent formation of wrinkles or folds as additional layers of sock are added. Wrinkles result in uneven distribution of pressure and can increase the likelihood of residual limb discomfort and skin breakdown. (**B**) Once the sheath is positioned, prosthetic socks are added, one at a time, and carefully adjusted for smooth fit until the desired number of ply is reached. The least possible number of socks is used to create a snug, comfortable prosthetic fit. (**C**) This patient's prosthetic design includes a soft Pelite insert. The anterior trimline of the liner is cup shaped to accommodate the patella and is used to guide the position of the liner on the limb during donning. Patients are cautioned against using a twisting motion when applying the insert/liner, to avoid causing wrinkles in the underlying sheath or socks. (**D**) The final step is to insert the residual limb with properly positioned socks and liner into the prosthesis. This patient dons the prosthesis in a sitting position, gradually increasing weight bearing to achieve the desired total contact fit. Note that a patellar tendon-bearing orthosis is used to support and protect his remaining limb, which is vulnerable as a result of Charcot's arthropathy.*

patellar tendon, a pressure-tolerant area, as a result of increased weight bearing.

The presence of skin breakdown is not a direct contraindication to further use of the prosthetic device. The first priority should be to identify the cause of breakdown and eliminate it by making the appropriate changes. Close observation and ongoing assessment and treatment of any lesions using appropriate nonadherent dressings inside the socket should allow prosthetic training to continue. Certainly, if a lesion becomes progressively worse despite clinical management during prosthetic training, a hiatus from prosthetic use may be indicated. In the example presented previously, a return to bilateral crutch use and diminished prosthetic wearing time may be indicated until the lesion is healed. After healing, ambulation time might be divided between bilateral and unilateral crutch use, to build tolerance for increased weight bearing before full-time unilateral crutch use is attempted once more. If the area does not show signs of healing or becomes worse with increasing lesion size or signs of inflammation or infection, prosthetic use may need to be discontinued altogether for healing to occur.

As a patient begins to ambulate over different terrains, the magnitude and direction of weight-bearing pressures within the socket may change as well, presenting additional mechanical risk factors for skin breakdown. Descending stairs using a step-over-step pattern produces a different pattern of pressure distribution on the residual limb than a step-to-step pattern that protects the residual limb by leading with the prosthetic leg. Depth of stairs also has an impact on pressure distribution within the socket: As step height increases, so does the total excursion through ROM necessary to descend the staircase. Ambulation on uneven terrain, such as on the lawn, produces different pressures than walking on a predictable, level floor surface. When evaluating potential causes of skin breakdown, it is important to consider the characteristics of the environment and the task demands of the activity. Changing technique, adapting movement strategies, or adding an assistive device provides just enough protection for the residual limb to prevent skin irritation and breakdown.

If localized increased pressure is determined to be the cause of tissue breakdown, pressure relief is the goal, and socket modification by the prosthetist may be necessary. Certain methods of pressure relief are inappropriate for patients with amputation and should be avoided. The use of "donut" padding around an area of breakdown or potential breakdown is counterproductive for three reasons. A donut pad will (1) increase pressure to the area surrounding the lesion when the limb is placed in the socket, (2) increase the ischemic effect of weight bearing, and (3) may lead to edema or extrusion of the vulnerable tissue through the "hole" of the donut. Any adhesive materials that are in

contact with skin should be used with extreme caution. A nylon sheath often can be used to hold a dressing in place under the prosthetic socks. Finally, the abrasive quality of certain dressings, including standard gauze, must be recognized and avoided for use inside the socket. Nonadherent dressings or non-stick pads tend to be less textured and less abrasive to an area of skin breakdown. Dressings should be used sparingly inside a prosthetic socket, as the socket fit is designed to be snug, and a padded dressing actually increases pressure over the affected area, which is counterproductive to the goal of wound healing. The therapist must reevaluate the prosthetic fit if a dressing is used within the socket, recognizing that the application of even a thin dressing may require the removal of one ply layer of socks.

Wearing Schedule

Once the evaluation of socket fit and alignment has been completed and any adjustments have been made, it is time to begin prosthetic training. Constant reassessment of socket fit and alignment is necessary during the entire training phase because of changes in residual limb shape and size. Each patient needs an individualized wearing schedule to begin prosthetic use. The time for initial prosthetic wearing is usually conservative, especially for patients with a history of skin integrity problems. Often, the first prosthetic weight-bearing activities are closely supervised, lasting no longer than 5–10 minutes. Time in the prosthesis is gradually increased, often in increments of 15–30 minutes, as skin condition permits. Patients with no history of skin integrity problems (i.e., after traumatic amputation or revision of congenital limb anomaly) often progress quickly with wearing activities, whereas those with sensory impairment or peripheral vascular disease need to be progressed much more cautiously. Inspection of the residual limb after the first few minutes of weight bearing should reveal redness of the skin in predictable pressure-bearing regions: at the patellar tendon, medial tibial flare, anterolateral distal tibial shaft, and posterior aspect of the residual limb. Because the socket is intended to have total contact with the residual limb, the entire limb may develop a mild reactive hyperemia when the socket is first removed. Increases in wearing time require continued, frequent skin inspection. It is vital that the patient understand the importance of gradual progression of wearing time. If a patient is allowed to initiate prosthetic wearing unsupervised or does not take the wearing schedule seriously, the potential for skin breakdown is greatly increased.

The optimal plan is for the prosthetist to deliver the prosthesis directly to the physical therapist. The physical

FIGURE 26-2
Example of a wearing schedule used to guide the patient's use of the new prosthesis at home, early in rehabilitation.

PROSTHESIS WEARING SCHEDULE

Patient Name:_____

Your wearing schedule for your prosthesis is _____ on and _____ off

Check your skin every time you take your prosthesis off. You are looking for areas of redness that do not go away within 10 minutes, areas of blistering or abrasions, or pain in your residual limb. If you have any of these problems, or any questions, call your therapist at the number below and do not wear your prosthesis again until the problem is addressed with your therapist.

If you do not have any of the problems above, in two (2) days you can increase the "on time" to _____ and maintain the off time as above.

Next scheduled appointment: _____

Therapist Name & Phone Number: _____

therapist and patient may determine that it is safest to use the prosthesis only in the clinical environment during the first week or more of therapy. Once the patient is cleared to use the prosthesis at home, a written wearing schedule is used to guide the patient and prevent misunderstanding about the time permitted for prosthetic wear (Figure 26-2). The schedule should be individualized to the specific patient's needs.

Positioning

Patients often need instruction about positioning of the lower extremity in the prosthesis when seated. The trimlines of the socket are designed for optimal pressure distribution during weight-bearing activities. The high posterior wall of the socket is necessary to provide counter pressure to the patellar tendon-bearing surface in stance but can provide undue pressure to the hamstring tendons in sitting. The patellar tendon bar in the prosthesis is designed to take weight in standing but can provide pressure to the anterior aspect of the tibial tuberosity if the prosthesis slips down when the patient is seated. When seated, the patient's prosthetic foot should rest flat on the floor or foot plate of the wheelchair so that the residual limb remains in total contact with the socket; thus avoiding the risk of undue pressure and decreasing the chance of gapping between the prosthesis and the residual limb that may allow edema to collect.

Care of Prosthetic Equipment

Patients also require instruction about the proper care and maintenance of their prosthetic equipment. The prosthetic socket and liner should be wiped daily with a damp cloth. Prosthetic socks should be washed daily and laid flat to dry (wool socks shrink in a clothes dryer). When not being worn, the prosthesis should be stored in a flat position to minimize the risk of damage should it fall over (hard sockets are particularly vulnerable to traumatic cracks). Patients also benefit from tips for ease of daily activities, such as dressing the prosthesis with sock, pant leg, and shoe before donning on the residual limb.

PROSTHETIC FIT AND ALIGNMENT

As new prosthetic users become comfortable and confident with their prosthetic limb, changes in socket fit and alignment are necessary to achieve the most energy-efficient and cosmetic gait. Ideally, the prosthetist, patient, and therapist work as an interdisciplinary team to solve problems with socket fit and alignment as they arise. The physical therapist should have a thorough foundational knowledge of appropriate socket fit and alignment to recognize and troubleshoot problems and be ready to refer the patient to the prosthetist should alignment need adjustment.

Socket

An intimate fit between the residual limb and the socket is necessary for successful prosthetic training. The total contact socket is designed to distribute the load of weight bearing over the residual limb to assist in venous blood return from the limb and provide some sensory feedback to the prosthetic user through the residual limb. Although the socket is prepared over a positive model of the patient's limb, either through casting or computerized technology, it is not uncommon for the socket to be modified in the early days of prosthetic training. Frequent and careful inspection of the residual limb and verbal feedback from the patient help to assess socket fit and patient tolerance to prosthetic wear.

Alignment

Prosthetic alignment is evaluated in quiet standing (statically) and during gait activities (dynamically). Static alignment refers to assessment of the relationships between the socket, pylon, prosthetic foot, and floor; the length of the prosthesis; and the overall fit of the socket on the residual limb. Dynamic alignment includes those concepts as well as prosthetic considerations as they relate to suspension, symmetry of gait, and energy requirements of gait.[26] Because static alignment assessment is the first standing activity in which a patient engages, it is prudent to carry this out in the parallel bars or with substantial support if parallel bars are not readily available. Information gleaned from align-

ment assessment can reveal clues about pressure distribution on the tissues of the residual limb inside the socket. Problems with alignment affect not only pressures within the socket but also the biomechanics of gait and the translation of forces from the prosthetic foot up the kinetic chain. Static and dynamic alignment are evaluated from an anterior, posterior, and lateral (prosthetic side) view. For a thorough review of transtibial prosthetic alignment, see Chapter 28; Table 26-4 provides a basic rationale for standard transtibial static prosthetic alignment.

Preparatory Prosthesis

Patients are fitted for a temporary or training prosthesis as soon as the surgical incision is stable, usually from 2 to 6 weeks after surgery. The initial socket is most often fabricated from high-temperature thermoplastic but can be made of plaster of Paris, fiberglass, or laminate. The socket is connected to the prosthetic foot using an alignment system at either end of a metal or plastic pylon (pipe). Endoskeletal modular prostheses are preferred to exoskeletal prostheses because modification of alignment can be expected early in the rehabilitation process. Some patients are fitted with a permanent pylon and prosthetic foot at this early stage and progress through a series of sockets until their residual limb reaches its mature contours. Most often, a foam and stocking prosthetic cover is not provided until the final socket fitting. Because of significant changes in residual limb size and shape, patients may progress through two to three sockets before being fitted for the definitive socket or prosthesis. The three primary benefits of early fitting with a temporary or training prosthesis include (1) early bipedal

TABLE 26-4
Transtibial Static Prosthetic Alignment and Rationale

Alignment	Rationale for Alignment
Posterior view	
Prosthetic height: symmetric leg length	Prevents gait deviations associated with leg length discrepancy
	Prevents orthopedic deformity associated with leg length discrepancy
Plumb line: midsocket to ½ in. lateral to midheel	Creates slight varus moment during stance, as in normal gait
	Directs compressive forces to pressure-tolerant areas at medial proximal (medial tibial flare, medial femoral condyle) and lateral distal (fibular shaft) residual limb
	Minimizes compressive forces on nontolerant areas at lateral proximal (fibular head) and medial distal residual limb
Lateral view	
Socket in 5–10 degrees of flexion (anterior tilt) with top of prosthetic foot parallel to the floor	Distributes compressive forces to anterior aspect residual limb and loads patellar tendon bar
	Limits vertical displacement of center of gravity at midstance to decrease energy cost of gait
	Allows for controlled knee flexion in loading response and late stance, as in normal gait
	Prevents abnormal hyperextension of the knee in midstance
Plumb line: midsocket to anterior edge of heel	Allows for knee flexion from mid- to terminal stance
	Prevents hyperextension of the knee in stance

ambulation with limited weight bearing through the residual limb, (2) improved edema control of the residual limb, and (3) faster shrinking (maturation) of the residual limb.[27]

PROSTHETIC GAIT TRAINING

The ability to move within and over one's base of support with efficient timing and sequencing of muscle activity and appropriate postural control is the key determinant of functional ambulation across the wide variety of environments that are encountered in daily life. Most transtibial prosthetic users have the potential to ambulate with a near normal symmetrical gait pattern that is free of significant gait deviations and walking without the use of an assistive device.[28] To do this, however, the patient must meet a variety of challenges, including (1) building tolerance to prosthetic wear and weight bearing through the residual limb, (2) controlling dynamic weight shifting through the prosthesis in all planes of movement, and (3) reintegrating postural control and balance with respect to the lack of ankle joint sensory and proprioceptive input, muscle control, and ROM.

Initial Training

For the new transtibial prosthetic user, initiation of gait training typically starts with ambulation on level surfaces with few environmental demands. Gait training often begins in the parallel bars, as a protected environment, because they provide a stable and secure setting with minimal challenges, allowing patients the flexibility of progressing from gait activities with significant bilateral upper extremity support to those with minimal or no support. Ambulation in the parallel bars also helps the therapist to identify potential gait deviations early in training before maladaptive habits become problematic. Based on this preliminary gait assessment, individual problem areas can be addressed with preambulation exercise activities. Early gait activities may include dynamic weight shifting (forward/back and medial/lateral), reaching and repeated stepping to challenge postural control and balance, and short-distance ambulation within the parallel bars with frequent skin checks for signs of pressure intolerance and skin irritation.

The prescribed wearing schedule and progressive weight-bearing and weight-shifting activities assist patients in developing tolerance to prosthetic wear. Simple dynamic weight-shifting activities may include loading and unloading body weight through the prosthesis in anterolateral, anteroposterior, and straight lateral directions (as is required in gait and functional activities), and functional reaching

activities that require the patient to reach to a variety of heights and directions within a functional context (Figure 26-3). Early therapeutic activities initially support and later challenge the patient's postural stability, progressing from static standing activities with upper extremity support, to static standing activities without support, to dynamic standing activities with support, to dynamic standing activities without support (Figure 26-4). These activities are most effective if performed within the context of functional tasks. Coordination and sequencing of an appropriate assistive device and activities to promote timing and fluidity of gait (i.e., use of a metronome to facilitate equal stance duration right and left) are other areas that can be included in early prosthetic training.

Patients who are having difficulty accepting weight onto the prosthesis during the gait cycle are reluctant to shift body weight over the prosthetic limb, rely heavily on weight bearing through the upper extremities in the parallel bars, and express great concern about putting all of their weight through the prosthesis. Strategies that might assist them to improve their ability and confidence in weight shifting as preparation for walking include:

1. Verbal cueing to progress the pelvis toward the parallel bars on the prosthetic side over a stable foot
2. Tactile cueing of the therapist's hand placed on the anterolateral aspect of the involved hip to facilitate anterior progression
3. Stepping onto a bathroom scale to give objective feedback regarding weight bearing through the prosthesis
4. Mental imagery of successful mastery of the activity

Repetitive loading of the prosthesis may be an appropriate task, without continuing with the translation of weight over the foot as in the intact gait cycle. Once patients become accustomed to accepting the weight as in the initial components of the stance phase of gait, they may then progress to practicing more full weight-bearing activities in preparation for the single limb support phase of gait. These can be categorized as weight-shifting activities, but they certainly address postural control and balance issues as the therapist strategically progresses activities that provide challenges to the patient's stability and balance control.

Assistive Devices

Assistive devices can provide help with balance only (i.e., single-point cane or quad cane) or with weight bearing and balance (i.e., walker, axillary crutches, or Lofstrand crutches). The goal is to provide only the amount of support that is necessary to protect the healing residual limb

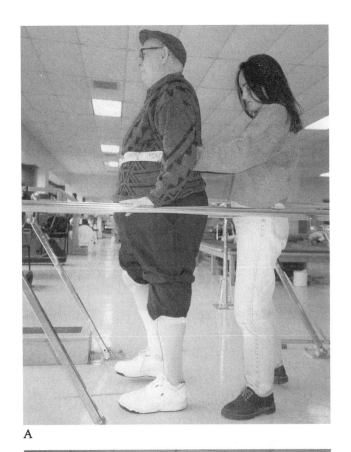

A

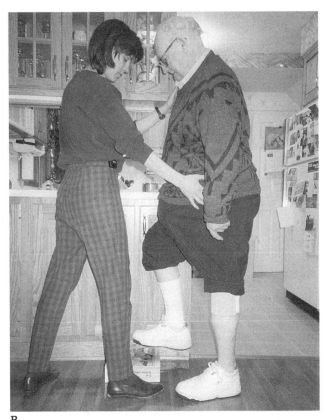

B

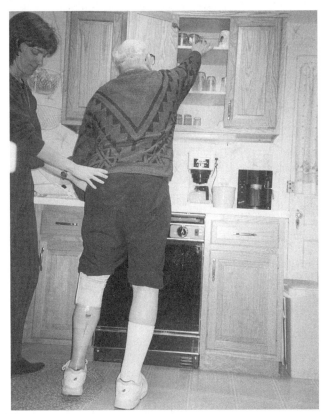

C

D

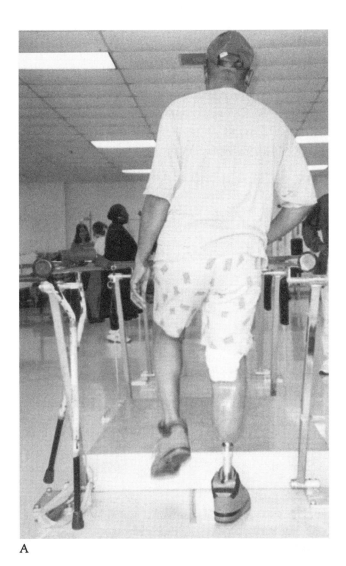

A

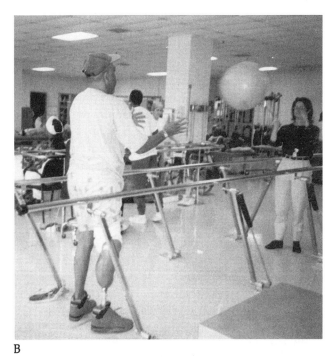

B

FIGURE 26-4

(A) Stepping activities become more challenging without the use of the upper extremities for balance or support. (B) Throwing and catching activities encompass balance (feed forward and feedback), coordination, postural control, and weight bearing through the prosthesis.

◀ **FIGURE 26-3**

(A) New prosthetic users practice loading weight onto the prosthesis by shifting weight and practicing single steps with their other limb. Note full weight bearing through the prosthesis, demonstrating good prosthetic alignment and erect trunk and head posture, with a gentle open-handed grip on the parallel bars. (B) Stepping up onto a phone book or low stool can increase stance time on the prosthesis. (C) Reaching activities, using all planes of movement, encourage weight shifting onto and off of the prosthesis and can challenge balance and postural control. Early on, the opposite hand grip on the parallel bar compensates for decreased balance and postural control. One goal of this activity is to eliminate the need for upper extremity support. (D) Reaching activities in a functional context can be integrated early on in the rehabilitation process.

and reduce the risk of falling without hampering the patient's willingness or ability to load the prosthesis. It may be prudent to spend time on prosthetic weight-bearing and weight-shifting activities in the parallel bars or at a stable surface to allow the patient to progress directly to an assistive device that aids in balance only. Patients are encouraged to use an open hand versus a closed grip on the parallel bars to minimize the stability gained from pulling on the bars. Optimally, the prosthetic limb can tolerate 100% weight bearing, so that upper extremity weight bearing is not necessary. Patients who demonstrate good weight bearing, strength, and coordination may progress directly from the parallel bars to the use of a single-point cane or no assistive device. Use of a quad cane is not recommended, as it is frequently misused as a weight-bearing device and its wide base can create a fall hazard. For patients who are unable to achieve early full weight bearing through the prosthesis and require a weight-bearing assistive device, the devices of choice are axillary or Lofstrand crutches. Crutches allow patients to progress to a two-point gait using a step-through gait pattern, which closely approximates a normal sequence and pattern of gait. Patients who begin with bilateral support progress to unilateral support with crutches as prosthetic weight bearing improves.

Standard walkers limit gait to a step-to pattern, interrupting fluid movement, hampering smooth forward progression of the center of gravity over the prosthesis, and often precluding effective terminal stance and preswing. Walkers are used only when endurance and postural control are significantly compromised. A wheeled walker can minimize this problem if it is advanced between each step or if the patient is weight bearing only slightly through the walker (pushing the walker like a grocery cart). Although some patients, especially those with physical or medical frailty, become functional household ambulators only with the aid of a walker, most individuals with transtibial amputation reach functional independence without any assistive device, or choose to use a cane when walking on unpredictable surfaces or in crowded environmental conditions.

Gait Analysis

An understanding of the biomechanics of normal gait is crucial, as it provides the standard by which prosthetic gait is measured. The main objective of static and dynamic prosthetic alignment and physical therapy intervention is to optimize the energy efficiency and cosmesis of gait. The ultimate goal is a gait that is safe, efficient, and symmetrical. When deviations from the norm are observed, the therapist and prosthetist seek the underlying cause(s) of the problem.

Any one of the commonly observed prosthetic gait deviations has many different potential contributors. Gait deviations may be a product of patient problems (intrinsic), prosthetic problems (extrinsic), and/or environmental factors. The observed deviation may be a primary gait problem or a compensatory strategy. When the gait pattern is less than optimal, the therapist attempts to identify which of these potential contributors is likely to be the root of the problem. Once the primary contributor is identified, the appropriate intervention is undertaken with the goal of minimizing or eliminating the problem's impact on ambulation.

If a new prosthetic user is observed to ambulate with a forward-leaning trunk throughout the stance phase of gait, several possible explanations can be given. This may be a primary gait deviation resulting from a hip flexion contracture that limits the individual's ability to achieve upright posture. It may also be a compensatory strategy of the patient who is fearful of instability during prosthetic stance, using a forward trunk to bring the center of mass anterior to the knee joint quickly, improving stability at the knee by creating an extensor moment around the joint.

Physical therapists who work in prosthetic rehabilitation become skilled at recognizing common prosthetic gait deviations and their possible causes (Table 26-5). When problem solving, the clinician must think about why certain gait deviations might occur and whether they are primary or compensatory. Answering these questions allows the therapist to focus treatment on the most salient issues.

Consider a patient who shows knee instability during loading response and throughout midstance, as evidenced by lack of knee extension or excessive knee flexion. The therapist must use deductive reasoning to identify what the true sources of the problem might be. If the instability is occurring on level surfaces, environmental causes of the problem can be ruled out. If evaluation of the static alignment of the prosthesis reveals appropriate alignment of the foot and pylon but the socket is set in excessive knee flexion, this could contribute to the problem. Thorough evaluation of the problem requires assessment of potential intrinsic or patient causes as well. If evaluation of the patient reveals full, strong, active ROM at the knee and no complaints of pain, the therapist must look to the joints proximal to the problem. Assessment of the hip may reveal a hip flexion contracture that leads the patient to maintain knee flexion as a compensatory strategy to maintain upright posture. If these two distinct potential causes of the problem are found, the therapist can then prioritize and address each cause. Extrinsic causes can be modified immediately: A socket alignment adjustment may improve or eliminate the gait deviation, thus suggesting that this was a primary cause of the problem. If a socket alignment adjustment does not have a significant impact, magnifies the observed gait problem, or leads to a new gait deviation, the focus of treatment should be on the identified intrinsic or patient cause of the problem. In this example, restoration of hip extension ROM through a program of stretching of the hip flexion contracture would be appropriate.

Progression of Level Surface Ambulation and Alternate Surface Ambulation

To adapt to and meet environmental demands, the patient who walks with a prosthesis must be able to adjust his or her step length and cadence while ambulating in response to environmental conditions or circumstances. The physical therapy program might begin with practice opportunities until the patient is able to achieve a normal cadence. It might then progress to activities that demand an increased or decreased cadence, and transitional gait movements, such as sidestepping, turning, and walking backward. These skills can initially be practiced in the clinic with minimal environmental demands and can be progressed to situations in which the environment pre-

TABLE 26-5
Common Gait Deviations in Transtibial Prosthetic Gait

Phase of Gait	Problem	Category[a]	Possible Cause
IC to MSt	Excessive knee flexion	Intrinsic	Knee flexion contracture
			Hip flexion contracture
			Hip extensor muscle strength and/or timing problem
			Knee extensor muscle strength and/or timing problem
			Anterior distal residual limb pain
		Extrinsic	Excessive dorsiflexion of the prosthetic foot
			Excessive socket in flexion/anterior tilt
			Socket positioned anterior to prosthetic foot
			Excessive heel cushion stiffness
			Prosthesis is too long
		Environmental	Walking down inclines
	Absent knee flexion or knee hyperextension	Intrinsic	Cruciate and/or collateral ligament insufficiency
			Quadriceps weakness
			Anterior or posterior distal residual limb pain
			Excessive soft tissue in popliteal area
		Extrinsic	Excessive plantar flexion of prosthetic foot
			Excessive socket extension
			Excessively soft heel cushion
			Inadequate cuff suspension
			Socket positioned posterior to prosthetic foot
			Prosthesis is too short
		Environmental	Ascending inclines/walking uphill
During MSt	Valgus moment at knee	Intrinsic	Collateral ligament insufficiency
			Medial distal residual limb pain
		Extrinsic	Excessive outset of prosthetic foot
			Inadequate socket fit or suspension
		Environmental	Walking on uneven surfaces
	Varus moment at knee	Intrinsic	Collateral ligament insufficiency
			Lateral/distal residual limb pain
			Weakness of hip abductor muscles
		Extrinsic	Excessive inset of prosthetic foot
			Inadequate socket fit or suspension
		Environmental	Walking on uneven surfaces
	Insufficient weight bearing	Intrinsic	Residual limb pain or hypersensitivity
			Excessive upper extremity weight bearing on assistive device
			Instability of the knee joint
			Decreased muscle strength of residual limb
			Fear of falling/lack of confidence in prosthesis
		Extrinsic	Prosthesis is too long
			Poor socket fit
		Environmental	Walking uphill
			Walking on rugged terrain
MSt to PSw	Early knee flexion (quick drop-off)	Intrinsic	Hip and/or knee flexion contracture
			Weakness of hip extensor muscles
			Anterior/distal residual limb pain
		Extrinsic	Excessive dorsiflexion of prosthetic foot
			Socket positioned anterior to prosthetic foot
			Inadequate socket fit and/or suspension
		Environmental	Walking down inclines or hills
	Delayed knee flexion (walking uphill effect)	Intrinsic	Posterior/distal residual limb pain
			Patient locks knee in extension as compensation for instability or weakness
		Extrinsic	Excessive plantar flexion of prosthetic foot
			Socket positioned posterior to prosthetic foot
			Excessively long keel of prosthetic foot
		Environmental	Walking up inclines/uphill

continued

TABLE 26-5
(continued)

Phase of Gait	Problem	Category[a]	Possible Cause
Swing	Inadequate clearance of foot[b]	Intrinsic	Decreased hip and/or knee flexion range of motion
			Decreased hip and/or knee flexion strength or motor control
		Extrinsic	Prosthesis is too long
			Excessive plantar flexion of prosthetic foot
		Environmental	Walking on uneven surfaces

IC = initial contact; MSt = midstance; PSw = preswing.
[a]Intrinsic problems are due to patient-related factors, whereas extrinsic problems are associated with prosthetic alignment or fit issues. Environmental problems are best understood by analyzing the specific conditions or activity in which they are observed.
[b]Compensations for inadequate swing phase clearance include a lateral lean of the trunk toward the remaining limb, circumduction of the prosthesis and residual limb, or a high steppage gait.

sents a challenge, such as crossing a street, getting on and off an elevator or escalator, walking through a crowded corridor in a busy store, or walking to a seat in the middle of an aisle in an auditorium or theater.

Successful community ambulation also requires management of many different ground surfaces, including steps, curbs, ramps, and varied terrain (Figure 26-5). In providing therapeutic practice opportunities for a patient who is new to prosthetic use, the therapist considers the following important extrinsic variables:

1. Level of assistance required for safe performance
2. The specific demands of the environment, such as depth or height of steps and curbs, or degree of slope of a ramp
3. The need for an assistive device or railing
4. The optimal technique for performing the task safely
5. The ability to superimpose an additional activity while walking or moving in the environment

An initial goal might be to decrease the level of assistance on these alternative surfaces, which can be accomplished by simplifying one or more of the other variables of the task, such as decreasing the depth of the step/curb, allowing the use of sturdy rail versus crutch or cane, and/or allowing the sound limb to "lead" or dominate the task. Once skill is consistently demonstrated, the task demands are increased. Early skills in stair climbing are generally developed with the sound limb leading in ascent and the prosthetic limb leading in descent. Advanced gait training activities may instead require the patient to use the prosthetic limb first while ascending and the sound limb first while descending. This allows the patient a repertoire of strategies to respond to environmental demands: For example, when crossing the street, the patient is able to ascend the curb with the prosthetic foot without dis-

rupting gait cadence. The unpredictable surface of uneven terrain, encountered in walking across a lawn, can challenge postural responses significantly if no assistive device is used. Sidestepping is a skill needed in environments such as theaters and can be practiced when the theater is empty or when people are seated. A community outing is an excellent strategy for addressing and achieving high-level ambulation goals.

Superimposing functional activities on gait during therapeutic treatment prepares patients for the daily "real world" challenges that they are sure to encounter. The variety of functional tasks practiced by the patient may be driven by specific patient goals. Safe ambulation while carrying objects of varying weights and sizes is an important functional skill and an appropriate physical therapy goal. The patient's specific goal may be to carry a full laundry basket down the hall or a cup of hot coffee from the kitchen to the living room. As patients become functional prosthetic users, household tasks and leisure or work activities may guide their therapeutic needs. High-level activities, such as running and athletic endeavors, are appropriate and attainable goals for some transtibial prosthetic users.

Functional Activities

Prosthetic training is not just a matter of teaching a patient to ambulate but includes a variety of other functional activities, such as transfer training from a variety of surfaces, kneeling, management of falls, and rising from the floor. Specific functional tasks should also be designed to address the individual patient's goals as they relate to activities of daily living, job-related activities, or recreational activities. The skill of the therapist is in designing activities that are task oriented and work to develop patient problem-solving skills and flexibility.

One movement goal that should be addressed throughout functional tasks is weight bearing through the pros-

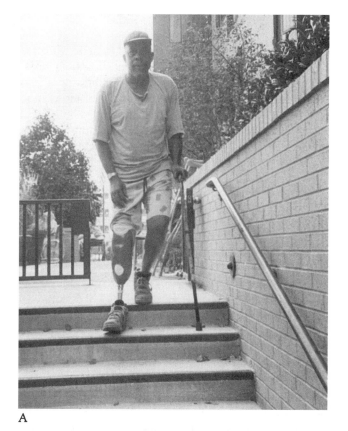

A

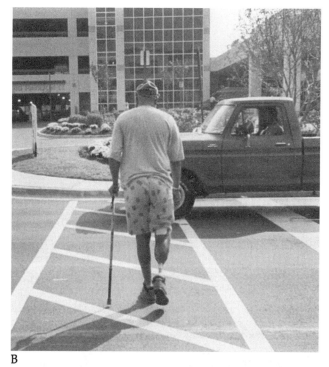

B

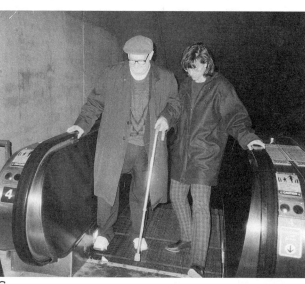

C

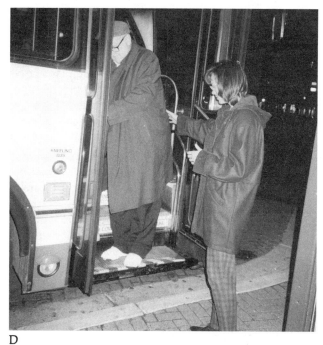

D

FIGURE 26-5

In addition to walking on level surfaces, functional community ambulation requires that the patient be able to adapt movement strategies to meet various environmental demands. (A) When descending stairs, three factors contribute to level of difficulty: the number and depth of steps, the type of upper extremity support (rail, assistive device, or none), and the movement pattern (step-to-step versus step-over-step). (B) Crossing a street requires the patient to adjust cadence in response to a dynamic, somewhat unpredictable environment. (C) Managing an escalator requires a quick adaptation from a stable to a dynamic surface when getting on and from a dynamic to stable surface when getting off. (D) The use of transportation might include developing skill in getting in and out of the front and back seats of a car or ascending and descending steps of buses if using public transportation.

thesis. Although this may be contrary to fundamental motor learning principles of encouraging action-directed performance versus motor performance, improved prosthetic weight bearing allows for decreased mechanical stresses on the sound limb, which is often vascularly compromised.

Prosthetic Prescription

The members of the interdisciplinary team who are involved in the care and rehabilitation of patients with amputation include the orthopedic or vascular surgeon, a physiatrist, a prosthetist, a physical therapist, an occupational therapist, a social worker, a rehabilitation nurse, and a vocational rehabilitation counselor. Many hospitals and rehabilitation centers have established prosthetic clinics that bring together the appropriate professionals to address the needs and problems of prosthetic users. Determining prosthetic candidacy is the first major clinical decision to be made. Although the research literature has identified predictors of outcome of prosthetic use, the team considers the individual patient's needs, motivation, and functional capacity in deciding about prosthetic candidacy.[29-32] The factors that are most often considered in determining whether to fit with a prosthesis include:

1. *The patient's medical history.* Disabling medical conditions may prohibit successful prosthetic use. Advanced cardiac or pulmonary disease that significantly impairs a patient's functional status before amputation has an impact on a patient's prosthetic candidacy. A history of cerebrovascular accident (stroke) with residual hemiplegia of the side opposite to the residual limb may limit functional prosthetic use.

2. *The patient's premorbid and present level of function.* A patient who required substantial assistance for functional mobility before amputation may have limited prosthetic training goals. Patients who are independent with functional activities, activities of daily living, and ambulation with an assistive device after their amputation and before prosthetic fitting usually do well with a prosthesis. If patients are able to dress themselves, transfer independently from bed to chair, and safely stand and walk using an assistive device, their potential for functional prosthetic use is excellent.

3. *The patient's body build and type.* Patients with morbid obesity or fixed deformities (such as extreme kyphotic posture) that interfered with mobility before an amputation present a challenge in prosthetic training activities.

4. *ROM.* Significant hip and knee flexion contractures must be addressed before definitive prosthetic fitting

if the patient is to achieve functional independence with a prosthesis.

5. *Availability of support at home.* Patients who are likely to require assistance when using their prosthesis depend on family members, significant others, or formal caregivers to help with one or more prosthetic tasks. The potential to be a limited household ambulator with a prosthesis may be important in reducing the burden of care for caregivers and may allow a patient to remain at home with a family caregiver as opposed to living in an institutional setting.

Should the patient be deemed a reasonable prosthetic candidate, these same considerations and others are used in determining the specific prosthetic prescription for that individual. Suggestions for prosthetic prescription for patients with special needs are presented in Table 26-6.

The therapist needs to understand the indications and contraindications for the various prosthetic components and design to contribute to the prescription process and be effective in rehabilitation intervention and prosthetic training. Because physical therapists spend a great deal of time working with patients in one-on-one circumstances, they often have a better perspective about the patient's goals or needs than do other members of the team. The therapist may gain insights or information about patients that are important in the decision-making process. If the therapist is familiar with prosthetic components, he or she may be forming an opinion about the best prosthetic prescription for a patient during the early rehabilitation phase. The physical therapist should use the prosthetist and professional literature to stay current with evolving technology in prosthetics. Therapists must be critical consumers of the literature to be able to make decisions that are in the best interest of patients when prescribing prosthetic features. An understanding of the different characteristics of the various prosthetic feet that are available may help to identify the type of foot that is best able to meet the patient's functional needs.[33-37]

Therapists also must be familiar with the special needs of certain clinical populations so that they can assist in the optimal prosthetic prescription to meet the individual patient's needs. Patients with diabetes who are at great risk for additional skin breakdown and poor healing may benefit from a socket with a soft insert or from a silicone sleeve that is designed to reduce friction during prosthetic use. Frail or deconditioned patients may reach higher levels of function if lightweight components are chosen and stability in prosthetic prescription is emphasized. Active children need durable components, but replacement costs must also be considered, as components need to be

TABLE 26-6
Considerations in Transtibial Prosthetic Prescription

Consideration		Potential Prescription Implications
Medical history	Hemodialysis	Socket with removable insert allows for change in residual limb size with fluctuating fluid status
	Ipsilateral hemiplegia	High socket trimlines (supracondylar, suprapatellar suspension) or thigh corset suspension to provide increased knee stability
	Upper extremity involvement	Adaptation of suspension device for ease of donning/doffing
Patient goals	High activity, interest in sports	Energy-storing prosthetic foot
		Use of suction suspension
	Rigorous outdoor work	Exoskeletal prosthesis for durability
Body build and type	Obesity	Supracondylar cuff to achieve purchase on thigh, with auxiliary fork strap
	Cachexia	Soft socket insert to protect bony prominences
	Very short residual limb	High socket trimlines (supracondylar, suprapatellar suspension) or thigh corset suspension
Range of motion	Severe knee flexion contracture	Modification of socket alignment for a bent knee prosthesis

replaced to accommodate growth. Athletes with amputation desire durable, lightweight, high-technology components for a competitive edge.

The time that is required to achieve maturation of the residual limb varies from patient to patient. The decision to fit the patient for a new temporary socket or a definitive prosthesis or socket is guided by several principles. First, an adequate intimate fit is difficult to achieve if the patient is consistently wearing 15 or more ply of sock. Second, the number of sock ply worn must have been consistent for 8–12 weeks. With each new socket, an adjustment period and close monitoring of the residual limb are necessary.

Decisions to change socket design or suspension for long-term prosthetic users must be carefully considered. Some patients who have worn a particular type of prosthesis for a long period of time may have difficulty in acclimating to a new type of device. If a patient has no complaints about a prosthesis other than "it's worn out," it may be prudent to prescribe the same components. If a patient is expressing interest in new goals or activities, however, prosthetic prescription changes may be warranted. A patient who has been using a solid-ankle cushioned-heel foot on the training prosthesis but wants to increase activity (such as trying race walking or jogging) may benefit from the prescription of an energy-storing foot.

CONCLUSION

Prosthetic rehabilitation of patients with transtibial amputation is both challenging and rewarding for the therapist and patient. Early in the rehabilitation process, concerns for the integrity of the suture line and skin are a major determinant of progression of time in the prosthesis and the types of activities that are appropriate. As a patient's limb matures, emphasis is placed on the quality of ambulation and on developing adaptive motor skills that enable the patient to function safely during a variety of activities under many different environmental conditions. The diversity of patients with transtibial amputation requires that the therapist carefully consider individual circumstances to guide prosthetic prescription and progression of the rehabilitation program. Effective patient education strategies and opportunities for practice and appropriate feedback are essential for mastery of mobility skills and optimal outcomes for rehabilitation.

REFERENCES

1. Kemp BJ. Motivation, rehabilitation and aging: a conceptual model. Top Geriatr Rehabil 1988;3(3):41–51.
2. Friedmann LW. The Physiological Rehabilitation of the Amputee. Springfield, IL: Thomas, 1978;109–140.
3. Bandura A. Social Foundations of Thought and Action: A Social Cognitive Theory. Englewood Cliffs, NJ: Prentice-Hall, 1986.
4. Guide to physical therapy practice. Part II: Preferred practice patterns(4K). Phys Ther 1997;77(11):1354–1367.
5. Winter DA, Sienko SE. Biomechanics of below-knee amputee gait. Biomechanics 1988;21(5):361–367.
6. Powers CM, Boyd LA, Fontaine CA, Perry J. The influence of lower-extremity muscle force on gait characteristics in

individuals with below-knee amputations secondary to vascular disease. Phys Ther 1996;76(4):369–377.

7. Powers CM, Torburn L, Perry J, Ayyappa E. Influence of prosthetic foot design on sound limb loading in adults with unilateral below-knee amputations. Arch Phys Med Rehabil 1994;75(7):825–829.

8. Snyder RD, Powers CM, Fontaine C, Perry J. The effect of five prosthetic feet on the gait and loading of the sound limb in dysvascular below-knee amputees. J Rehabil Res Dev 1995;32(4):309–315.

9. Shumway-Cook A, Woollacott M. Control of Posture and Balance in Motor Control: Theory and Practical Applications. Baltimore: Williams & Wilkins, 1995;119–142.

10. Nashner LM. Sensory, Neuromuscular, and Biomechanical Contributions to Human Balance. Balance: Proceedings of the APTA Forum. Alexandria, VA: American Physical Therapy Association, 1990;5–12.

11. Gailey RS, Wenger MA, Raya M, et al. Energy expenditure of trans-tibial amputees during ambulation at self-selected pace. Prosthet Orthot Int 1994;18(2):84–91.

12. Hebert LM, Engsberg JR, Tedford KG, Grimston SK. A comparison of oxygen consumption during walking between children with and without below-knee amputations. Phys Ther 1994;74(10):943–950.

13. Gonzalez EG, Corcoran PJ, Reyes RL. Energy expenditure in below knee amputees: correlation with stump length. Arch Phys Med Rehabil 1974;55(3):111–118.

14. Ward KH, Meyers MC. Exercise performance of lower-extremity amputees. Sports Med 1995;20(4):207–214.

15. Cutson TM, Bongiorni D, Michael JW, Kochersberger G. Early management of elderly dysvascular below-knee amputees. J Prosthet Orthot 1994;6(3):62–66.

16. Redhead RG. The early rehabilitation of lower-limb amputees using pneumatic walking aid. Prosthet Orthot Int 1983;7(2):88–90.

17. Friedmann LW. The Surgical Rehabilitation of the Amputee. Springfield, IL: Charles C Thomas Publisher, 1978.

18. Kempczinski RF. The Ischemic Leg. Chicago: Year Book, 1985;553–568.

19. Melzak R. Phantom limbs. Sci Am 1992;226(4):120–126.

20. Carlen PL, Wall PD, Nadvorna H, Steinbach T. Phantom limbs and related phenomena in recent traumatic amputations. Neurology 1978;28:211–217.

21. Jensen TS, Krebs B, Neilsen J. Immediate and long-term limb pain in amputees: incidence, clinical characteristics and relationship to pre-ambulation limb pain. Pain 1985;21(3):267–278.

22. Houghton AD, Nicholls G, Houghton AL, et al. Phantom pain: natural history and association with rehabilitation. Ann R Coll Surg Engl 1994;76(1):22–25.

23. Weiss SA, Lindell B. Phantom limb pain and etiology of amputation in unilateral lower extremity amputees. J Pain Symptom Manage 1996;11(1):3–17.

24. Defrang R, Taylor LM, Porter JM. Basic data related to amputations. Ann Vasc Surg 1991;5:202–207.

25. Bullock BL, Rosendahl PP. Pathophysiology, Adaptations and Alterations in Function. Boston: Scott, Foresman, and Co., 1988;698–700.

26. Lower Limb Prosthetics. New York: New York University Medical Center, Prosthetics and Orthotics Division, 1983;134–138.

27. Cutson TM, Bongiorni DR. Rehabilitation of the older lower limb amputee: a brief review. J Am Geriatr Soc 1996;44(11):1388–1393.

28. Radcliffe CW. Prosthetics. In J Rose, J Gamble (eds), Human Walking (2nd ed). Baltimore: Williams & Wilkins, 1994;165–199.

29. Campbell WB, St. Johnston JA, Kernick VF, Rutter EA. Lower limb amputation: striking the balance. Ann R Coll Surg Engl 1994;76(3):205–209.

30. Campbell WB, Ridler BM. Predicting the use of prostheses by vascular amputees. Eur J Vasc Endovasc Surg 1996;12(3):342–345.

31. Lundsgaard C. Evaluation of patients with below knee amputation with respect to postoperative prosthesis fitting (abstract). Ugeskr Laeger 1994;156(49):7360–7364.

32. McWhinnie DL, Gordon AC, Collin J, et al. Rehabilitation outcome 5 years after 100 lower-limb amputations. Br J Surg 1994;81(11):1596–1599.

33. Casillas JM, Dulieu V, Cohen M, et al. Bioenergetic comparison of a new energy-storing foot and SACH foot in traumatic below-knee vascular amputations. Arch Phys Med Rehabil 1995;76(1):39–44.

34. Postema K, Hermens HJ, de Vries J, et al. Energy storage and release of prosthetic feet. Part 1: Biomechanical analysis related to user benefits. Prosthet Orthot Int 1997;21(1):17–27.

35. Postema K, Hermens HJ, de Vries J, et al. Energy storage and release of prosthetic feet. Part 2: Subjective ratings of 2 energy storing and 2 conventional feet, user choice of foot and deciding factor. Prosthet Orthot Int 1997;21(1):28–34.

36. Torburn L, Schweiger GP, Perry J, Powers CM. Below-knee amputee gait in stair ambulation: a comparison of stride characteristics using five different prosthetic feet. Clin Orthop 1994 June;(303):185–192.

37. Torburn L, Powers CM, Guiterrez R, Perry J. Energy expenditure during ambulation in dysvascular and traumatic below-knee amputees: a comparison of five prosthetic feet. J Rehabil Res Dev 1995;32(2):111–119.

27

Transfemoral Prosthetics

RICHARD PSONAK

ADVANCES IN TECHNOLOGY

Advances in technology, materials, and prosthetic components have had a greater impact on the quality of life of individuals with transfemoral amputation than on any other level of amputation. As little as 10 years ago, ambulation in transfemoral prostheses was labored and often painful. Only the most physically fit individuals attempted to run with their prosthesis. Now, socket designs better approximate anatomy of the lower limb, materials are more friendly to the residual limb, and dynamic prosthetic feet and knee components offer improved, energy-efficient function. The result has been a significant improvement in quality of gait, allowing more people with transfemoral amputation to walk comfortably and naturally with their prosthesis. In addition, athletes with amputation are now able to run in a natural "step over step" pattern with a higher degree of stability and comfort than previously possible.

To assist the reader in understanding transfemoral prosthetic systems, this chapter presents information about current socket design and materials, the major types of prosthetic knee components, and the suspension systems that are available for individuals with transfemoral amputation. It also provides the reader with a strategy to assess fit and dynamic function, and the major user- and prosthesis-related reasons for commonly observed gait deviations.

PROSTHETIC MANAGEMENT IN TRANSFEMORAL AMPUTATION AND KNEE DISARTICULATION

An amputation proximal to the anatomic knee joint is referred to as a *transfemoral* (above knee) amputation. An amputation through the center of the anatomic knee joint is known as a *knee disarticulation* (Figure 27-1). Individuals with knee disarticulation present with prosthetic challenges and functional advantages when compared with those with transfemoral amputation. The disarticulation residual limb tends to be long and distally bulbous, a result of the preservation of the femur and its condyles. Prosthetically, this creates a challenge in donning the prosthesis and for cosmetically fitting a knee component. The bulbous distal end does, however, facilitate prosthetic suspension. The normal adduction angle of the lower extremity is more likely to be preserved, and the long lever arm of the femur facilitates control of the prosthetic knee. Also, as the proximal component of a weight-bearing joint, the distal femur tolerates end-bearing pressures within the socket. In contrast, the transfemoral residual limb varies in length, depending on how much of the femur has been retained. The shape of the residual limb is likely to be a tapered cylinder, so that donning is less difficult. Suspension can be challenging, however, as a result of the cylindrical shape of the residual limb. The fleshiness of the transfemoral residual limb presents an opportunity for suction suspension. As the length of the residual limb decreases, socket suspension and control of the prosthetic knee (anatomic stability in stance) become more problematic.

The successful prosthetic management of transfemoral amputation and knee disarticulation involves providing a prosthesis which is comfortable in containing the residual limb, stable during the stance phase of gait, smooth in transition to the swing phase of gait, and acceptable in appearance.[1] In choosing components for an individual's transfemoral or knee disarticulation prosthesis, the prosthetic team must consider the inter-relationship between the component's weight, function, cosmesis, comfort, and cost. Often, the most functional or technologically sophisticated components are also the heaviest, most expensive, most likely to need maintenance, and least cosmetic.

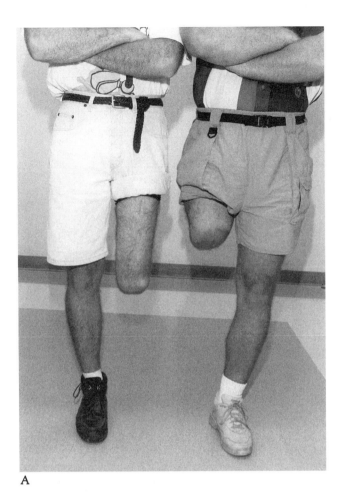

A

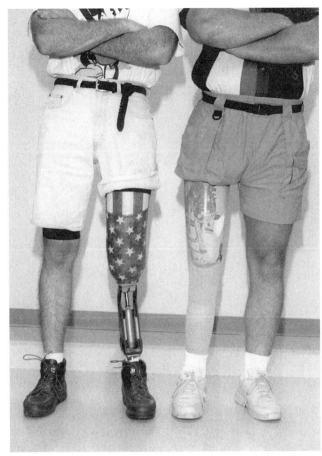

B

FIGURE 27-1

*The similarities and differences in prosthetic fit and function between amputations at transfemoral and knee disarticulation levels are determined, to a large degree, by the length of femur that is preserved. (**A**) The knee disarticulation residual limb is long and bulbous, whereas the transfemoral residual limb is a tapered cylinder. (**B**) In a knee articulation prosthesis, the center of the prosthetic knee is generally lower than that of the intact limb, whereas the knee center of most transfermoral prostheses match that of the intact limb.*

Because of the great variation in physical characteristics and preferred activities of many individuals with high-level amputation, no single material, component, or transfemoral design is appropriate for the majority. The preferences and needs of each individual must be considered carefully, in the context of weight, function, cosmesis, comfort, and cost, for the optimal prosthetic outcome.

ENERGY EXPENDITURE

An individual with a transfemoral amputation faces significant energy expenditure when ambulating with a prosthesis (Table 27-1). The energy cost of gait increases

significantly as the length of the residual limb decreases.[2–5] Fisher and Gullickson[6] report the energy cost of walking for healthy individuals (mean gait speed, 83 m/min) as 0.063 kcal/min/kg (oxygen consumption/physical effort)

TABLE 27-1

Prosthetic Features that Have an Impact on Energy Expenditure

Weight of the prosthesis
Quality of the socket fit
Accuracy of alignment of the prosthesis
Functional characteristics of the prosthetic components

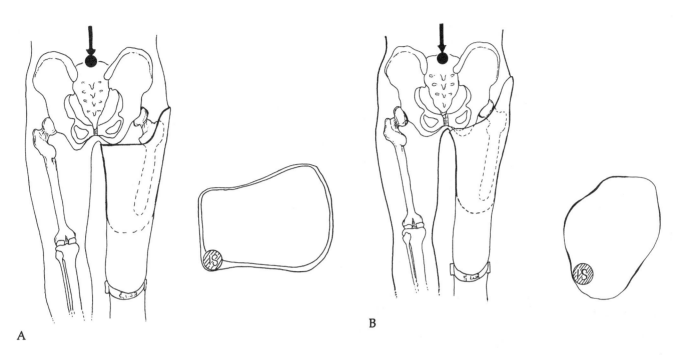

FIGURE 27-2

Comparison of the design of the quadrilateral (quad) socket (A) and the ischial-ramal containment (IRC) socket from a posterior per-spective (B). Note the narrow anteroposterior dimension in the quad socket, and the narrow mediolateral dimension in the IRC socket. Also note that in the IRC socket, the ischium (IS) sits inside the socket; in the quad socket, the ischium sits on the socket brim (seat).

and 0.000764 kcal/m/kg body weight (oxygen cost/energy required to ambulate). Individuals with transtibial amputation walk 36% more slowly, expend-ing 2% more kilocalories per minute and 41% more kilo-calories per meter to cover a similar distance. For individuals with transfemoral amputation, gait speed is 43% slower, whereas energy cost is reflected as 5% less kilocalories per minute and 89% more kilocalories per meter. In other words, the individual ambulating on a transfemoral prosthesis walks more slowly to avoid an increase in energy consumption per minute and is dra-matically less efficient in terms of energy expended over distance (per meter). This increase in energy cost is man-ifested as a higher rate of oxygen consumption, elevated heart rate, and notable reduction in comfortable (self-selected) walking speed.[2,5]

Because of this high energy cost, many older individ-uals with amputation related to vascular disease may be limited in their ability to become functional community ambulators, instead walking slowly with the assistance of a walker or cane.[5] Individuals with bilateral trans-femoral amputation are rarely able to become commu-

nity ambulators with prostheses, instead choosing a wheel-chair for long-distance mobility.

CONTEMPORARY TRANSFEMORAL SOCKET DESIGN

A significant evolution in the design of the transfemoral socket has occurred over the last several decades. Before the 1950s, prosthetists often carved a "plug fit" socket from a block of wood, which, depending on the skill of the crafts-man, was often uncomfortable and cumbersome in walk-ing and in sitting. The traditional quadrilateral (quad) socket, developed at the University of California at Berke-ley in the 1950s, offered a notable improvement in fit and function, and remained the socket design of choice until the mid-1980s. The quad socket, as its name implies, has four distinct walls fashioned to contain the thigh musculature, and to allow the muscles to function at maximum poten-tial[1,7,8] (Figure 27-2A). A flat posterior shelf, the ischial seat, is the primary weight-bearing surface for the ischium and gluteal muscles. The anterior wall contours create a

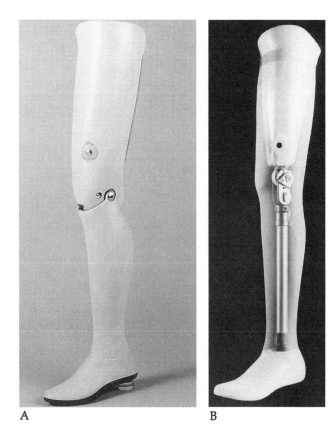

FIGURE 27-3

Comparison of the rugged exoskeletal (A) and the modular endoskeletal (B) transfemoral prosthetic systems. (Reprinted with permission from Otto Bock Orthopedic Industry, Inc, Minneapolis, MN.)

posterior-directed force at the anatomical Scarpa's triangle, which is intended to stabilize the ischium on its prosthetic seat. As a result, the socket is more narrow in its anterior-posterior dimension than its medial-lateral direction.

The most recent design development, which has been evolving since the 1980s, is the Ischial-Ramal Containment (IRC) socket[9] (Figure 27-2B). The IRC socket is designed to stabilize the socket on the residual limb and to control socket rotation by containing the ischial tuberosity and the pubic ramus within the contours of the socket. This socket also attempts to better maintain normal femoral adduction by distributing pressure through the socket along the shaft of the femur.[10,11] When comparing the IRC socket with the quad socket, the most obvious difference is the narrow medial-lateral dimension. According to Long,[10] an additional advantage of the IRC design is that the wider anteroposterior dimension enhances muscle function by providing more room to accommodate

contraction than possible in the crowded anteroposterior dimension of the quad socket. In most cases, the IRC socket is preferred except when the patient is a prior quad socket wearer who has been satisfied with the comfort of the quad socket design. Radcliffe[7] suggests that, regardless of socket design, the primary goals of a transfemoral prosthesis are to achieve comfort in weight bearing, a narrow base of support in standing and walking, and as close to normal swing phase function as possible.

SOCKET OPTIONS: HARD AND FLEXIBLE MATERIALS

Most transfemoral sockets are fabricated from a variety of thermoplastic or thermosetting resin materials. A hard socket consists of a resin-laminated or thermoformed plastic socket that is intended to have an intimate, total contact fit over the entire surface of the residual limb. Prosthetic socks are often worn as a soft interface between the socket and the residual limb. The hard socket is very durable, easy to clean, and often less bulky and less expensive to produce than flexible sockets. In contrast, it is more difficult to adjust the fit of a hard socket, especially for individuals with very "bony" or sensitive residual limbs.

The flexible socket is vacuum formed using any number of flexible thermoplastic materials.[12,13] It is encased in a rigid frame, which provides support during weight bearing and helps to maintain socket shape. The flexible socket accommodates to change in muscle shape during contraction, and can be easily modified after initial fabrication to provide relief for bony prominences. Flexible sockets may also be more comfortable to wear, especially in sitting, because there are no hard edges at the brim to impinge on the groin. Flexible sockets are especially useful if suction suspension is desired. They are, however, somewhat less durable, more bulky to wear (requiring a socket and a frame), and more expensive to produce than hard sockets.

PROSTHETIC SYSTEMS

A transfemoral prosthesis can be fabricated as either an exoskeletal or endoskeletal system. The weight-bearing strength and cosmetic shape of an exoskeletal prosthesis are provided by a laminated shell that incorporates the socket, shin component, and ankle block (Figure 27-3A). This system is very durable and requires little maintenance but cannot be easily realigned or adjusted. In the endoskeletal system, weight-bearing strength comes from an internal pylon that connects the socket to the prosthetic knee unit and then to the prosthetic foot (Figure 27-3B). The cosmetic shape of the prosthesis is provided by a soft foam cover, carved to mirror the remaining limb, which is fit over the socket, knee unit, and pylon. This foam shell is, in turn, covered by several cosmetic stockings or a silicone "skin" to achieve the desired skin color. The endoskeletal system has two distinct advantages: The prosthetist is quickly able to adjust prosthetic alignment, and he or she can easily interchange or replace modular components. This is particularly helpful as new prosthetic users become more competent in controlling their knee unit or when advancing mobility leads to different functional needs (for example, involvement in athletic activities). The durability of the foam and cosmetic coverings may be an issue for some prosthetic users, especially when work or leisure activities are physically demanding.

PROSTHETIC KNEE UNITS

The function of the human knee joint is very difficult to replicate. Henschke Mauch, who developed hydraulic guidance systems for rockets during World War II, turned his considerable knowledge and creativity to designing a hydraulic prosthetic knee for veterans with amputations after the war.[14] He commented that it was far easier to design a large rocket with a guidance system capable of maneuvering hundreds of miles distant than to duplicate the human knee. The knee joint is a modified hinge-type synovial joint. The offset axis of the knee allows rotation in addition to flexion and extension, practically making it three joints rolled into one.[15] Because most prosthetic knees function in a single plane of motion, action of the anatomic knee cannot be fully replicated. As a result, it is more difficult for the individual who is using a transfemoral prosthesis to walk as efficiently and cosmetically as someone using a transtibial prosthesis.

Prosthetic knee mechanisms have two primary functions. First, to simulate normal gait, the prosthetic knee must smoothly flex and extend through the swing phase of gait. The speed or rate of shin advancement during swing is determined by the mechanical properties (friction or resistance) of the prosthetic knee unit. Second, the prosthetic knee must remain stable as body weight rolls forward over the prosthetic foot during stance phase of gait. The major categories of commonly used prosthetic knee units vary with respect to how, and to what degree, they accomplish these two tasks. Most knee units are available in endoskeletal and exoskeletal versions. Advancing microprocessor technology is already changing the functional characteristics of prosthetic knee units as well.

Single Axis Knee

The single axis knee simulates a simple hinge, and allows the prosthetic shin to swing freely in flexion and extension. Stance phase knee stability is achieved by a combination of positioning of the knee unit with respect to the weight line (alignment) and muscular control (activity of hip extensors). This knee is lightweight and durable and requires very little maintenance, but because of its unrestricted movement, it has no inherent mechanical stability. For this reason, it is not appropriate for individuals with relatively short residual limbs who lack the mechanical advantage of a long femoral lever for muscular control of the knee unit or for those whose stability is compromised for other reasons. Although the rate of advancement of the shin during swing phase (determined by the resistance setting of the knee) can be individualized, cadence responsiveness is minimal once the resistance has been set. The shin of the prosthesis will swing forward at the same rate, regardless of gait speed. As a result, an audible terminal impact often occurs as the knee reaches full extension. To run with a single axis knee, the individual must use a skipping pattern on the intact stance limb while waiting for the prosthesis to complete the swing phase and begin the initial heel contact. The single axis knee is primarily for those patients with long residual limbs and who are able to voluntarily stabilize the knee through active hip extension against the posterior wall of the prosthesis.

Polycentric Knee Units

The instantaneous center of rotation of a polycentric knee unit changes through the range of motion because of the linkage provided by its "four bar" design.[16] In addition to simulating the anatomic axis of motion more closely, the mechanical characteristics of this type of knee unit enhance stance phase stability in gait. As the knee unit flexes during swing phase, the polycentric axis of motion leads to relative "shortening" of the distal prosthesis (shin and foot components), which enhances toe clearance throughout swing phase. It is especially helpful for individuals with long residual limbs or knee disarticulation, because the changing center of rotation allows the shin to tuck under the thigh when sitting, resulting in a more natural and cosmetic appearance of thigh and shin lengths. The polycentric knee unit's inherent stance phase stability also makes it an option for individuals who have short residual limbs or significant weakness of hip extensors. The major disadvantage of the polycentric knee, with its multiple mechanical joints, is its durability.

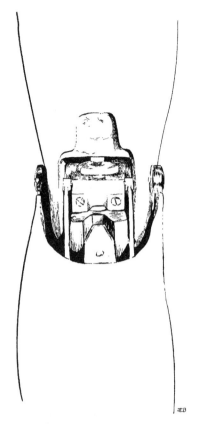

FIGURE 27-4

Example of a stance control knee unit used for an exoskeletal prosthesis. Mechanical knee stability is activated as body weight is loaded through the prosthesis during stance phase of gait. In this exoskeletal design, the wedge segment in the prosthetic shin is pressed into a grooved thigh segment to provide mechanical stability in stance.

Weight-Activated Stance Control Knee Units

The stance control knee has a braking mechanism that is activated when weight is applied through the knee during the stance phase of gait (Figure 27-4). The intent of the braking mechanism is to prevent (or at least retard) unwanted knee flexion during stance. The sensitivity of the braking mechanism can be adjusted to match the individual's level of activity and ability to control the knee voluntarily. If initial contact is made when the knee is not completely extended, as when walking on uneven ground, the braking mechanism provides additional mechanical stability to keep the knee from rapidly buckling. During swing phase, the weight-activated stance control knee unit functions like a single axis knee, and has similar disadvantages. Advancement of the prosthetic shin occurs at the same

rate regardless of changes in gait speed; minimal cadence responsiveness is present. This type of knee unit is most often prescribed for individuals with short residual limbs or nonremediable weakness of hip extensors who would otherwise have difficulty in actively stabilizing their prosthetic knee.

Manual Locking Knee

For patients who must rely on mechanical stability in stance, the knee of choice is often a manual locking knee. This unit is basically a single axis knee with the addition of a locking pin mechanism (Figure 27-5). The pin automatically locks with a distinctive click when the knee is fully extended. Individuals who use a manual locking knee unit walk with their prosthetic knee locked in extension. Although a locked knee provides maximum mechanical stability in stance, it also significantly compromises mobility and toe clearance in swing. The prosthesis is often fit to be slightly shorter than the sound side limb to facilitate toe clearance during swing of the prosthesis. The prosthetic wearer can manually unlock the knee by manipulating a pulley or lever system attached to the outside of the socket. This unit is often used in the initial training prosthesis for patients when balance, endurance, or cooperation may be problematic. For example, a locking knee was used to facilitate early mobilization of a patient with moderate head injury, traumatic amputation of the left lower extremity, and comminuted fracture of the right femur after a motor vehicle accident. The patient was extremely agitated and combative in bed, and could not comprehend the need to limit weight bearing on the fractured side. He was fit (on postoperative day 8) with an IRC socket, locking knee, and solid-ankle cushioned-heel (SACH) foot. When elevated on a tilt table (with a 3-in. lift under the prosthetic side to maintain the non–weight-bearing status of the fractured extremity), his cognitive function and behavior improved rapidly. Within several days, he was able to step off the tilt table, and began to ambulate using a walker for short distances. Eventually he became independent with crutches, and continued to use the locking knee until his fracture site healed enough to safely tolerate full weight bearing safely.

Hydraulic Knee Units

Hydraulic knee units are cadence responsive: The forward progression of the prosthetic shin changes as gait speed changes. This is because the flow of hydraulic fluid through narrow channels within the prosthetic knee unit provides a frictional resistance, which increases with the speed of

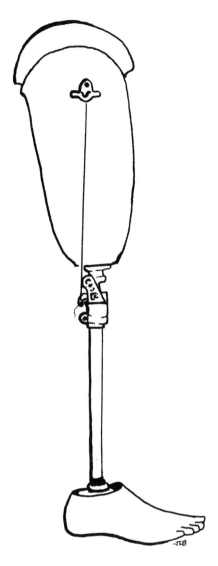

FIGURE 27-5

A manual locking knee provides maximum stability when the knee is in the locked position. The knee can be unlocked manually by manipulating a lever and cable system connected to the knee.

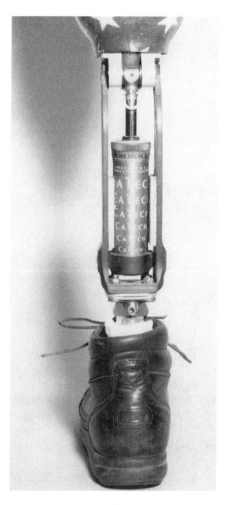

FIGURE 27-6

Example of a swing and stance hydraulic fluid-controlled knee. This type of knee is fit inside the shin (shank) of an exoskeletal prosthesis or within the cosmetic cover of an endoskeletal prosthesis.

compression (Figure 27-6). This variable resistance permits a swing phase that more closely simulates normal gait. As gait speed increases, the shin of the prosthesis also extends more rapidly. Very little swing phase delay is experienced in knee extension as compared with single axis or polycentric knee units. This variable cadence characteristic has been helpful for both young, active individuals, and for older adults with mobility impairment.[17] This enhanced function, however, is associated with increased weight, higher maintenance needs, and higher cost. It should also be noted that with colder tempera-

tures the knee may initially be slow to respond to changes in cadence until the hydraulic fluid warms up from typical daily use.

Some manufacturers offer a variation of hydraulic knee units which offer both variable cadence in swing and mechanical stability in stance (Swing and Stance control/SNS).[14] Stance control occurs as a result of hydraulic resistance to knee flexion during weight bearing or by a braking mechanism that is activated by weight bearing through the prosthesis. This feature allows the individual to ambulate with greater confidence over uneven surfaces and also permits the use of a more natural step over step pattern when negotiating hills and going down stairs.

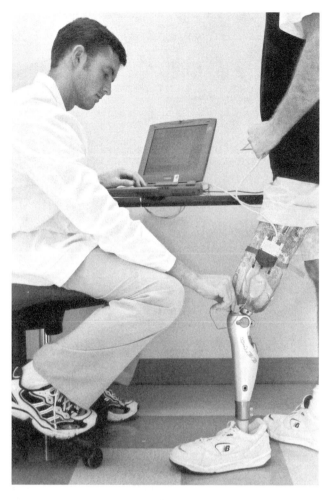

FIGURE 27-7
Customized stance and swing phase adjustments are made to the microprocessor knee using a personal computer.

Pneumatic Knee Units

Pneumatic knee units offer the prosthetic user a varied cadence capability, using air pressure dynamics in much the same way that fluid is used in the hydraulic knee. Because air is compressible, the channels within the knee can be adjusted to have an impact on the rate of swing. Pneumatic knees usually weigh less and are less expensive than their hydraulic counterparts; however, they provide less precise cadence control and require just as much maintenance. This is because hydraulic fluid is denser and has a higher coefficient of viscosity than air.[16]

Microprocessor Technology

The initial theory of microprocessor knee control was developed in Japan in the early 1980s. Charles A. Blatch-

ford & Sons, Ltd, the developer of the Endolite carbon composite prosthetic system, collaborated with a Japanese electronics company to produce the first commercial application of microprocessor control in a transfemoral prosthesis. The microprocessor swing phase control knee is known as the *Intelligent Prosthesis Plus* (IP+).

Another computerized system is the Otto Bock C-LEG (Computer-Leg), the world's first completely computer-controlled artificial limb. This prosthesis is powered by a rechargeable lithium ion battery with 25–30 hours of functional capacity. The C-LEG incorporates an on-board microprocessor, hydraulics, pneumatics, and servomotors. A microprocessor controls the single axis knee with hydraulic stance and swing phase control, as well as the automatic servo-adjustment of the hydraulic resistance valves. The knee position sensor and force sensor in the shin gather data at a frequency rate of approximately 50 times per second.[18] The microprocessor control of the C-LEG is based on scientific gait analysis and biomechanical studies. Electronic sensors in the C-LEG collect real-time data, which is then sent to the hydraulic damper to control stance and swing phase movements. At initial contact with the ground, the user may notice the added hydraulic stance stability, which prevents any unintentional bending of the knee that sometimes occur when walking on uneven terrain. The microprocessor enables the patient with transfemoral amputation to move in a very natural way, which makes it easier to walk downhill or down stairs. Customized adjustments are made to the C-LEG using a personal computer (Figure 27-7). Unique software algorithms determine the phase of gait, then immediately adjust the knee functions to compensate during both the stance and swing phases of gait. The current disadvantage of microprocessor technology in prosthetics is the significant expense of such devices. As the use of such technology becomes more frequent in prosthetics, the cost of microprocessor-based knee units is expected to decrease.

Additional Components

For individuals who require assistance to initiate knee extension in early swing phase, an extension aid can be incorporated into the prosthesis. An extension aid is usually an internal spring or an elastic strap that recoils from an elongated position to accelerate the prosthetic shin into extension during swing. Extension aids may also be useful to control excessive heel rise in early swing phase.

Torque absorbers (axial rotation devices) are designed to simulate the rotation during stance, which would normally occur in an intact anatomic limb. In the absence

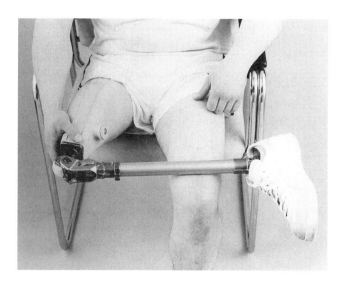

FIGURE 27-8

A transverse rotational unit is generally installed between the socket and the prosthetic knee. When the unit is unlocked, the individual can sit with legs crossed (e.g., to change shoes without having to remove the prosthesis). (Reprinted with permission from Otto Bock Orthopedic Industry, Inc, Minneapolis, MN.)

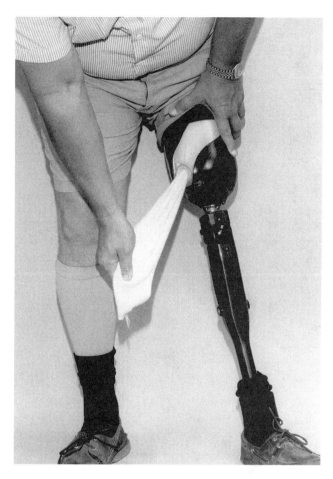

FIGURE 27-9

Patient donning a suction socket using a pull sock. The air expulsion valve has been removed so that the sock can be pulled completely out of the socket.

of the ankle and knee joint, significant shearing forces can occur at the socket–residual limb interface as the prosthetic user pivots on the prosthesis. Torque absorbers are effective in reducing shearing, and may be especially useful for individuals with fragile sensitive skin or with adherent scars. They are also often indicated for those involved with sports or work which requires them to negotiate uneven ground. Although these units reduce shear to the residual limb and increase comfort during functional activities, they also add weight to the prosthesis, and are susceptible to mechanical failure.

Transverse rotational units have been developed to allow prosthetic wearers to passively rotate the shin section of their prosthesis passively (Figure 27-8). An external button is pushed to unlock the limb, allowing a full 360 degrees of rotation. The unit automatically locks once the knee is moved back into its natural position. This type of device allows the prosthetic wearer to sit in a crossed-legged position, change shoes without having to remove the prosthesis, and enter and exit automobiles with greater ease.

TRANSFEMORAL SUSPENSION SYSTEMS

Keeping the prosthesis on in its optimal functional position is more challenging for individuals with transfemoral amputation than with transtibial amputation. The trans-

femoral residual limb is fleshy and cylindrical, lacking the bony prominences which aid in suspending the transtibial prosthesis. The weight of the transfemoral prosthesis with the addition of its knee unit creates an additional challenge for adequate suspension. Five options for suspension are currently being used. Depending on the nature of the prosthetic wearer's normal activities, a single system or a combination of several systems may be chosen.

Traditional Pull In Suction Suspension

Traditional pull in suction suspension uses negative air pressure, skin to socket contact, and muscle tension to hold the socket onto the limb (Figure 27-9). A suction prosthesis can be donned in several ways. One option uses a donning sock or Ace bandage to pull the residual limb down into the socket. Once the limb is well seated in the

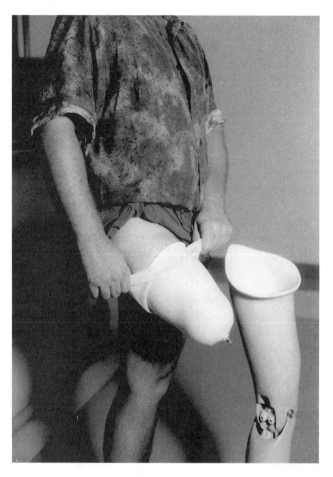

FIGURE 27-10

Roll on liners are an alternative to traditional suspension, especially for wearers who are susceptible to skin breakdown or irritation from shear or friction forces. The pin at the distal sleeve locks into a shuttle lock within the socket, suspending the prosthesis on the residual limb.

socket, the sock or ace wrap is pulled through the valve housing at the distal socket, the air expulsion valve is then screwed back into place. This process requires considerable agility and balance on the part of the wearer. A second option is to add a lubricant to the skin (e.g., liquid powder) to facilitate the residual limb sliding into the socket. The air-expulsion valve is then "burped," by pushing or pulling the valve button, to release any trapped air. The liquid powder dries quickly, and suction is achieved.

The intimate fit required for suction suspension has several additional benefits: The wearer often reports enhanced prosthetic control, and a better proprioceptive sense of the prosthesis during walking. Because an intimate fit is essential, suction suspension is inappropriate for patients with recent amputation who will continue to lose limb volume, or for those with a history of fluctuating edema

or unstable weight. The high shearing forces that are associated with donning a suction socket also may preclude its use for patients with fragile or sensitive skin, painful trigger points, or significant scarring or adhesions.

Roll On Liner Suction Suspension

Recently, suspension liners (Figure 27-10) have become available as an alternative to the standard suction suspension system. Roll on liners are manufactured from a variety of materials, including silicone, urethane, and elastomer. Worn against the skin, roll on liners are donned by first being turned inside-out, and then rolled directly over the residual limb. The roll on liner creates a negative atmospheric pressure and somewhat adhesive bond to the skin. The liner can be fit into the socket like the traditional suction socket method using a release valve or can be attached to the distal socket by a shuttle locking pin. The major advantage of this type of suspension is a significant reduction in the amount of friction and shear on the residual limb. The donning procedure is simple, and can be accomplished while seated. This suspension system has been useful for individuals with short residual limbs and those who have experienced discomfort using the traditional pull in suction method. The disadvantages of this system include its expense and durability. Roll on liners become worn or tear and need to be replaced two to three times a year depending on the wearer's activity level. Some wearers have experienced rashes or other types of skin irritation as a result of these types of liners. Wearers who choose this type of suspension must clean the liners daily to prevent the build up of perspiration and bacteria.[19]

Silesian Belt Suspension

A Silesian belt is usually made from leather or lightweight webbing (Figure 27-11). It is attached to the lateral aspect of the socket, encircles the pelvis, and then runs through a loop or buckle on the anterior of the socket. It is most often used as an auxiliary (backup) for traditional suction suspension systems. The problem with choosing the Silesian belt as the sole means of suspension lies with its inability to control residual limb rotation within the socket. For individuals with long residual limbs who are not expected to be vigorous ambulators, the Silesian belt may provide adequate suspension.

Total Elastic Suspension Belt

The Total Elastic Suspension (TES) belt is made of an elastic neoprene material. The distal sleeve of the TES belt

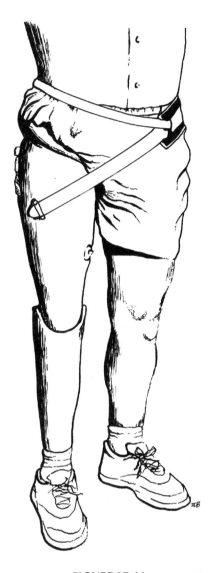

FIGURE 27-11

Example of Silesian belt suspension. Although the belt suspends the prosthesis to the pelvis, it is not able to fully counteract rotary forces between limb and socket during vigorous walking.

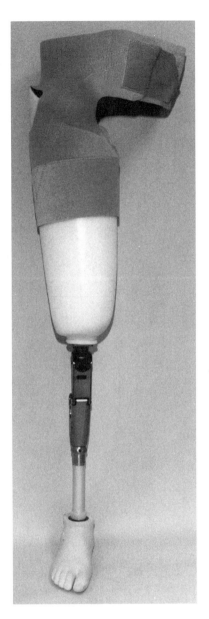

FIGURE 27-12

The total elastic suspension (TES) belt is a simple and comfortable suspension system that is often used for individuals as an auxiliary suspension.

fits snugly around the proximal half of the thigh section of the transfemoral prosthesis. The neoprene belt encircles the waist, and attached in front with Velcro (Figure 27-12). The TES belt is easy to don, comfortable to wear, and maintains good suspension with minimal pistoning between the limb and socket. It is an excellent auxiliary suspension system. This system is generally not recommended for prosthetic users who are very active ambulators, because, like the Silesian belt, the TES belt is unable to control residual limb rotation adequately within the socket. The major disadvantages of the TES system include its limited durability, especially for active ambulators, and its tendency to retain heat. It is often chosen for individuals with recent amputation whose residual limb has not yet matured to a stable size, for older patients who are unable to use the pull in suction or roll on liners due to upper extremity weakness or pain, and for those with easily irritated skin or adhesions who are unable to tolerate suction.

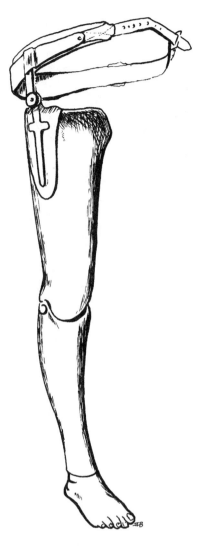

FIGURE 27-13
A pelvic belt with hip joint not only suspends the prosthesis but also helps to control rotation and increases medial lateral stability of the residual limb within the socket.

Pelvic Belt and Hip Joint

For some patients, a pelvic belt and hip joint are used as a means of suspension (Figure 27-13). Generally, the pelvic belt is made of leather and attached to the prosthesis by means of a metal hip joint. Recently, lighter weight plastic materials have been used as an alternative to the metal joint. Whatever the material, the joint center should be positioned just superior and anterior to the anatomic greater trochanter. This system not only suspends the prosthesis but also helps to control rotation and increase

medial-lateral stability of the residual limb within the socket. Traditionally, this has been the suspension of choice for those with very short residual limbs. The major drawbacks of this type of suspension is its bulkiness under the clothes, added weight, and tendency to be uncomfortable when sitting.

CHOOSING A PROSTHETIC FOOT

Individuals with transfemoral amputation and knee disarticulation can use any of the prosthetic feet and ankle options that are available (see Chapter 24). For someone with transfemoral amputation, one of the important considerations in choosing a prosthetic foot is its impact on stability of the prosthetic knee in stance. A foot that is able to reach foot flat quickly (for example, single-axis or multiaxial foot) is preferable because it enhances stance phase stability.[17] Reaching foot flat quickly is especially important for individuals who have a short residual limb or weak hip extensors.

For active individuals, dynamic response feet (e.g., Flex-Foot [Flex-Foot, Inc, Aliso Viejo, CA]; Seattle Foot [Seattle Orthopedic Group, Seattle, WA] etc...) and those with flexible keels (e.g., SAFE II foot [Campbell Childs, White City, OR]) may have advantages. The energy-storing capabilities of these prosthetic feet at push off promote rapid advancement of the shin section during swing phase. This enhances the ability of the individual who is using a transfemoral prosthesis to walk at faster speeds. Most of these feet are much lighter in weight than the articulating feet. Distal weight is one of the most important determinants of energy consumption for individuals using a transfemoral prosthesis.

GAIT CHARACTERISTICS IN TRANSFEMORAL PROSTHETICS

Normal ambulation is a result of dynamic symmetric relationships of the head, spine, and upper and lower extremities. With a transfemoral amputation, an individual's gait pattern wearing a prosthesis becomes significantly asymmetric, regardless of the functional characteristics of the prosthetic components.[20] The more asymmetric the pattern and uneven the cadence, the greater the energy cost of walking. Asymmetry also increases the demand for postural adaptation and balance reactions. For patients with impairment of musculoskeletal and neuromuscular systems, which are common among those with diabetes or advanced age, there is significant increase of instability and falls.

In normal gait, the muscles of the hip, knee, and ankle work in three ways. (1) Muscle contraction provides stability during stance by resisting the effects of gravity. (2) During push off and early swing phase, they act to provide propulsion and accelerate the limb. (3) They also act to decelerate forward progression, especially in late swing in preparation for subsequent initial contact. The loss of ankle and knee musculature as a result of transfemoral amputation compromises energy efficiency and quality of gait.

Knee Stability

The most important goal in transfemoral prosthetics is to obtain optimum knee stability throughout the stance phase. A prosthetic knee that is unstable or difficult to control during stance is a great danger, and could lead to a serious fall. Alternately, a knee that is difficult to flex can cause problems with swing phase clearance, increasing the relative length of the limb and the likelihood of tripping and falling.

Three variables influence knee stability during stance:

1. How well the individual is able to voluntarily control the knee using muscular power
2. The alignment of the knee unit with respect to the weight line (TKA)
3. The inherent mechanical stability of the knee unit

The relationship can be best understood by visualizing the trochanter-knee-ankle (TKA line), representing body weight in stance (drawn from the greater trochanter to the ankle of the prosthetic foot), and considering the position of the knee with respect to the line (Figure 27-14). The most appropriate position of the socket, knee, and ankle components is the one that allows the individual to best use his or her muscle control with the minimum amount of alignment stability, and still consistently stabilize the knee. If the prosthetic knee is positioned slightly behind the TKA line, so that the weight line passes anterior to the knee axis, the resulting extensor moment provides alignment stability during stance so that very little muscular power is required. This alignment also, however, increases the muscular effort and energy required to initiate of knee flexion for swing phase of gait. If the knee is positioned at or slightly in front of the TKA line, so that the weight line passes behind the knee, the resulting flexion moment decreases stance phase stability, making muscular power much more important. It also enhances the ability to flex the knee to initiate swing phase.

An individual's ability to voluntarily control the prosthetic knee is determined by the strength and endurance of muscles around the hip and by the overall length of the residual limb. If stance stability is provided primarily by voluntary control, hip extensors must be forcefully activated at heel strike to create an extensor moment at the knee. For an individual with a knee disarticulation or long residual limb, the long bony lever is a distinct advantage: There is an inverse relationship between length of residual limb and amount of muscular force necessary to control the prosthetic knee. With a long limb, less muscular power is needed to control prosthetic knee extension or to initiate flexion in early swing phase, and the prosthetic knee can be placed at or in front of the TKA line. For individuals with a short residual limb, much more muscular power is needed to achieve the same level of control. For this reason, stance phase stability is provided by using a knee unit with high mechanical stability, or by aligning the knee unit posterior to the TKA line. Voluntary control is also compromised for patients with hip flexion contracture, weakness of hip extensors, or physical frailty.

Prosthetists often attempt to enhance muscular control by placing the socket in a slight amount of flexion. Slight elongation of the extensors enhance their contractile ability just enough to develop an effective force (against the posterior wall of the socket) to keep the prosthetic knee extended[1,17] (see Figure 27-14). This also reduces the individual's tendency to substitute for the weakness of hip extensor muscles with excessive pelvic lordosis. The amount of initial socket flexion is determined by the initial available range of motion at the hip joint. In preparation for initial alignment, the prosthetist sets the socket in 5 degrees of flexion, in addition to the number of degrees of flexion contracture that may be present.

The stability/mobility of the knee is further influenced by the mechanical properties of the prosthetic knee itself. The degree of inherent stability of the knee varies greatly among the different designs of commercially available prosthetic knees. A manually locking knee offers ultimate mechanical stability; therefore, placement with respect to the weight line and muscular power is of lesser importance. At the other end of the continuum, a freely moving single axis knee offers virtually no mechanical stability; stance phase stability must come from voluntary control, alignment, or a combination of the two. The mechanical stability provided by hydraulic swing and stance, pneumatic, and weight-activated stance control knee units fall between these extremes. It is especially important to consider the contribution of mechanical stability for indi-

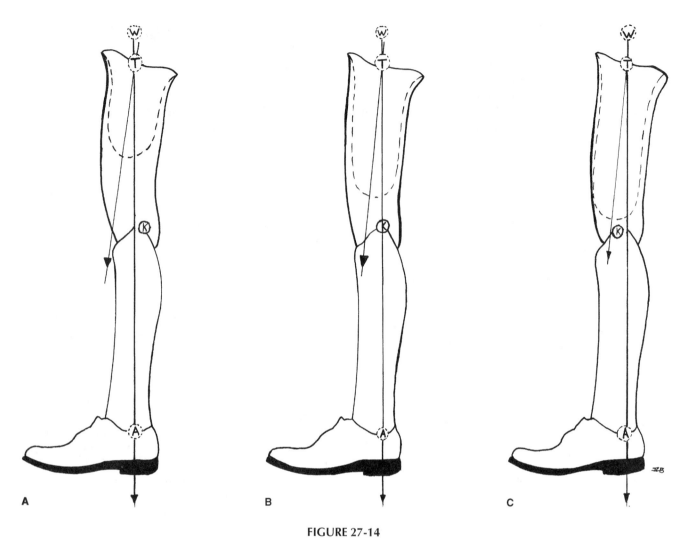

FIGURE 27-14

The imaginary trochanter-knee-ankle (TKA) line is a useful way to understand the components of stance phase stability at the knee. (A) Alignment stability is at its maximum when the weight line (W) passes anterior to the knee axis. This is often important for prosthetic wearers with short residual limbs or weak muscles, or when initial socket flexion is increased more than the typical 5 degrees of preflexion. (B) Alignment stability is minimal when the weight line passes through the center of the knee axis, making additional muscular or mechanical stability necessary. Many prosthetic wearers with midlength residual limbs and good muscular power benefit from the enhanced initiation of swing that this alignment provides. (C) No inherent alignment stability is present when the weight line passes behind the knee axis; all of the stance phase stability must be provided by the mechanical characteristics of the knee unit and/or by muscular activity. Prosthetic wearers with long residual limbs are best able to manage this alignment.

viduals with short residual limbs and weakness of hip muscles, as well as those who routinely negotiate uneven or rough terrain.

Pelvic Stability

Because of transfemoral amputation, the direct anatomic connection between the femur and the ground surface is lost and closed chain medial-lateral stability of the pelvis is significantly compromised. The femur, without its distal attachment at the knee, is susceptible to marked lat-

eral displacement within the socket during weight bearing in stance phase. This lateral shift makes it impossible to maintain a horizontal pelvis, even for individuals with strong hip abductor muscles, and results in an apparent Trendelenburg's sign and compensatory gait deviations. Pelvic stability is especially problematic for those with short residual limbs and those who have developed flexion/abduction/external rotation contracture. The design of a quadrilateral socket primarily applies stabilizing forces in the anteroposterior plane, so that there is little to keep the femur from drifting laterally within the socket. As a

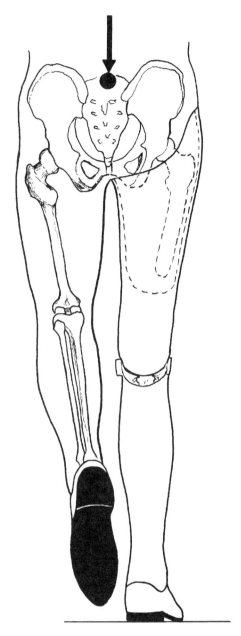

FIGURE 27-15

Lateral stabilization of the pelvis is maintained by positioning the femur as close as possible to its preamputation adduction angle (usually a mirror image of the intact limb). The resultant narrow base of support also significantly reduces the energy cost of transfemoral prosthetic gait.

consequence, the pelvis drops when the intact limb is in swing phase. To compensate, the prosthetic wearer often leans or lurches laterally toward the prosthetic side. This strategy improves swing clearance, but also results in a wide-based, energy-taxing gait. Because the femur is held in an abnormally abducted position, circumduction of

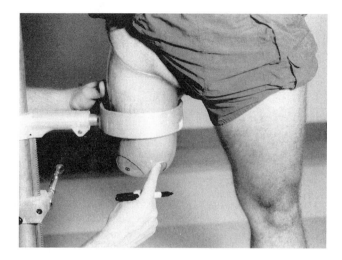

FIGURE 27-16

Clear diagnostic sockets are used to evaluate visually the design of the prosthetic socket. Inspection of the skin at the site of the suction valve provides information about adequacy of residual limb containment within the socket.

the prosthesis during swing is likely to occur. In contrast, the design of the IRC containment socket attempts to hold the femur in its normal adducted position during stance with an upward and medially directed force along the length of the lateral femur. This strategy enhances the prosthetic wearer's ability to maintain a level pelvis and improves the quality of functional gait (Figure 27-15).

EVALUATION OF SOCKET FIT AND STATIC ALIGNMENT

Despite all the technological advances in prosthetic knee units, prosthetic feet, and materials, the single most important influence on functional outcome in prosthetics is the quality of socket fit. The socket is the interface between the wearer and the prosthesis. It must comfortably contain soft tissue when the patient is standing or sitting, furnish adequate relief for bony prominences, distribute stabilizing pressure to the femur and pelvis, and provide an adequate weight-bearing surface for the ischial gluteal region.

Transparent diagnostic sockets (test sockets) are routinely used to assess socket fit.[21] These thermoplastic sockets are molded over the modified positive model of the residual limb as an interim step in socket fabrication. They are donned without a sock, or over a thin nylon sheath so that contact with tissues and bony prominences can be clearly viewed (Figure 27-16). Areas of excessive or inadequate pressure can be detected according to the degree of skin blanching. To make necessary reliefs or to enhance total contact, corrections to the diagnostic socket are made by reheating the socket with a hot air gun or torch. The socket may be tried on and then modified several times before optimal fit and comfort are achieved. Once proper fit has been established, the diagnostic socket is filled with plaster or is digitized to create a new, accurate positive model for fabrication of the definitive socket.

Donning Procedure

The first step in evaluation of socket fit is to ensure that the socket has been donned properly. If the socket is not positioned correctly on the residual limb because of being rotated or partially put on, its fit cannot be accurately assessed. Optimally, the socket fits easily but snugly over the residual limb. If too many ply of prosthetic sock are worn, donning is difficult and the person will feel as if the residual limb is not fully down in the socket. If too few ply of sock are worn, the limb falls more deeply into the socket and the person will feel medial socket pressure at the pubic ramus as well as a high degree of distal end pressure.

When suction suspension is used, the socket is slightly more difficult to don because of the relatively tight total contact fit that is required to maintain suction. Whether Ace wrap, pull sock, or liquid powder is used, the donning procedure must be consistent each time that the prosthesis is donned. Before the air-escape valve is screwed into place, total contact between skin and socket is evaluated. The skin should protrude slightly into the valve housing; however, tissue should not be taut, bulging, painful, or discolored.

The size of the residual limb of individuals with recent amputation vary if adequate pressure management has not been achieved. Inconsistent use of elastic shrinkers or Ace wrapping can lead to increased limb circumference. Even small increases in limb size can compromise the ability to don a prosthetic socket correctly and can significantly alter the quality of functional gait. The importance of the consistent use of a shrinker or Ace wrap whenever the prosthesis is not being worn cannot be overemphasized.

Total Contact Fit

Most prosthetic sockets are designed so that total contact is present between the skin of the residual limb and the socket. Total contact fit distributes socket pressure over the entire surface of the residual limb. Relief areas are used to reduce pressure over bony prominences, bone spurs, a neuroma, or other pressure-intolerant areas, but total contact is maintained. Total contact also promotes venous

return from the tissues of the residual limb and helps to reduce edema. Wherever contact is inadequate, the residual limb is likely to become edematous. Over time, secondary skin problems are likely to develop as well.

Once the socket has been donned, it may be difficult to determine if total contact has been achieved or to locate precise areas of discomfort or excessive pressure. Placing a small amount of clay or powder or a thin film of lipstick inside the socket before donning can assist with assessment of fit. The person dons the socket as usual, and then walks (or, if too uncomfortable, stands) for several minutes. When the prosthesis is removed, relatively even traces of the substance should be found on the socks (or skin) of the residual limb. Alternatively, lipstick can be applied to the sock (or skin for suction suspension users) over the area of discomfort before the prosthesis is put on. After donning as usual and wearing for several minutes, the prosthesis is removed and the inside of the socket is inspected. Traces of lipstick identify the area of the socket that requires modification for pressure relief.

Sitting and Kneeling

To be comfortable in sitting and in kneeling, individuals with transfemoral amputation must be able to reach at least 90 degrees of hip flexion. If the anterior wall of the socket is excessively high, the brim impinges on the abdomen and the anterior-superior iliac spine (ASIS). For those who are using pelvic belt and hip joint suspension, care should be taken to avoid painful pinching of flesh between the socket and belt.

Evaluating Socket Fit and Brim Contours: The Quadrilateral Socket

For the quad socket, the brim shape is rectangular, with a narrow anteroposterior dimension (see Figure 27-2A). The primary weight-bearing surface, the ischial seat, is located on the medial posterior brim. The seat should be widest at the posterior medial corner to adequately support the ischium and gluteal muscles. It should lie parallel to the ground. The overall height of the prosthesis is measured as the distance from this posteromedial corner to the ground with the knee in full extension. A channel for the adductor longus tendon is located at the anteromedial corner of the socket. The anterior brim is higher than the ischial seat as it moves toward the lateral wall. The contours of the anterior wall, at Scarpa's (femoral) triangle, provides a posteriorly directed force to maintain the ischium on its seat.

The medial wall is a flattened surface that represents the line of forward progression. The height of the medial brim is usually the same as that of the ischial seat, fitting well into the groin. It should not, however, create undue pressure on the perineum or pubic ramus. For those persons in whom an adductor roll has developed, the medial brim should be flared to accommodate the extra tissue. The primary function of the lateral wall is to maintain a "normal" femoral adduction angle. This is often difficult to achieve in the quad socket because of the wide mediolateral dimension of the design. Pressure is applied to the limb by flattening the socket along the femoral shaft. A relief area is usually necessary to accommodate pressure sensitivity of the distal lateral femur. The lateral wall completely encases the greater trochanter, and fits snugly around the gluteal muscles as the socket wraps toward the posterior wall.[14]

Evaluating Socket Fit and Brim Contours: The Ischial-Ramal Containment Socket

A proximal cross section of an IRC socket is more oval in shape rather than rectangular, with a narrow mediolateral dimension (see Figure 27-1B). This design more closely resembles the natural shape of the thigh. The brim of this socket captures more of the adductor muscle complex than the quad socket does. The ischial tuberosity and the pubic ramus are contained in a fossa well within the socket. This creates a bony lock that provides mediolateral stability and reduces likelihood of rotation of the socket on the residual limb. The contour of the posterior socket captures gluteal muscles. No ischial seat is present because weight bearing occurs predominantly on the soft tissues of the gluteal region and medial aspect of the ischium.[10,11] Because stability is provided in the mediolateral plane, a buildup into Scarpa's triangle on the anterior wall is not as severe.

The medial wall of the IRC socket incorporates an adductor complex channel designed to contain all medial tissues. This minimizes problems with adductor roll pinching. The lateral socket wall is contoured in adduction, with additional pressure against the posterior shaft of the femur for added stability. A pocket hollow or fossa is incorporated into the lateral wall posterior to the greater trochanter for a snug fit against the lateral gluteal muscles.

Static Evaluation in Standing

When an individual receives a new transfemoral prosthesis, the prosthetist and physical therapist first evaluate fit in a secure standing position. Typically, this evaluation is performed with the patient standing within a set of parallel bars to provide upper extremity support and stability. In addition to evaluating socket fit, the static examination

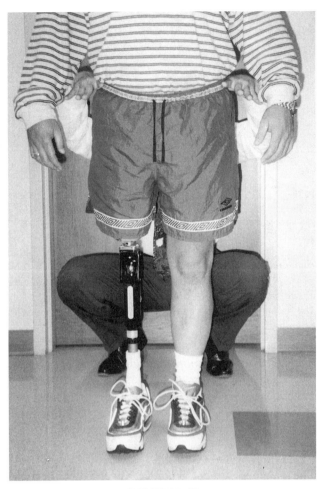

FIGURE 27-17
The overall height of the prosthesis should approximate that of the sound limb. One method of checking for adequate prosthetic height is to assess whether the pelvis is level, by comparing the planes of the examiner's hands as they rest on the patient's iliac crests.

focuses on a level pelvis (to check the height of the prosthesis), knee stability, and the width of the base of support.

Height of the Prosthesis
Patients are encouraged to shift weight mediolaterally until they are comfortable with a symmetric standing position with relatively equal weight bearing on the prosthesis and intact limb. The prosthetist or therapist applies a firm downward force through the iliac crests to assure equal distribution of body weight and then visually evaluates the position of the pelvis. Ideally, the examiner's hands over the iliac crests will be in the same plane, and the pelvis will be level (Figure 27-17). The prosthesis may be up to ¼ in. shorter than the intact side to enhance toe clearance in swing phase. Leg length discrepancy of more than ¼

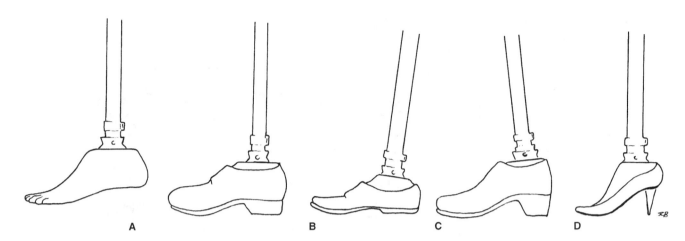

FIGURE 27-18

Shoes with differing heel heights have an impact on knee stability for individuals who are using a transfemoral prosthesis. (A) Most prosthetic feet are designed for a standard ³/4-in. heel. (B) Decreasing heel height creates an extension moment at the knee, leading to an excessively stable knee. (C) Increasing heel height creates a flexion moment, leading to instability of the prosthetic knee. (D) Special prosthetic feet are made especially for shoes with high heels.

in. leads to gait deviation and higher energy cost in gait. The examiner can place one or more shims or boards (cut in various increments of thickness) under the "short" limb to determine the extent of the discrepancy if the prosthesis appears to be too short or too long.

Evaluation of Knee Stability

The examiner must determine if the prosthetic wearer can easily extend the knee and maintain it in a stable position and whether he or she has a sense of security or fears that the knee will buckle in late stance. It is important to note that stability of the knee can be altered significantly if shoes other than those for which the prosthesis has been aligned are worn (Figure 27-18). Shoes with lower heels create an extension moment at the knee; the resulting stability is often excessive and can interfere with the knee flexion that is needed in late stance and early swing phase. If a prosthetic wearer would like to have the option of wearing shoes with lower heel heights, a small, firm heel wedge can be placed inside the shoe to simulate proper heel height and minimize excessive stability. Shoes with higher heels create a flexion moment at the knee, reducing stance stability and increasing the likelihood of buckling or drop-off at midstance. It is difficult to accommodate for higher heels unless the individual uses a prosthetic foot that is specifically designed for high heels.

Base of Support

The ideal distance between heels during comfortable stance is relatively narrow, approximating the normal base of individuals without amputation (2–3 in.). The prosthetic foot and shoe should lie flat on the ground with relatively equal weight bearing on medial and lateral borders. This can be assessed by slipping a piece of paper under both sides of the forefoot and rear foot: The distances should be fairly equal. The individual must also be able to shift weight comfortably between the intact and prosthetic limbs. The adequacy of the suspension system is evaluated by asking the patient to lift the prosthetic foot off of the ground using a hip-hiking motion. Minimal pistoning of the residual limb should occur within the socket.

DYNAMIC EVALUATION

Once appropriate socket fit has been ascertained, a process of dynamic evaluation is used to customize alignment and make adjustments to components to optimize prosthetic function. The goal is to achieve a gait pattern that is safe, comfortable, cosmetic, and energy efficient. The patient's ambulatory history, strength, endurance, usual activity level and preferred activities, concurrent medical conditions or health issues, previous experience in wearing prostheses, and current goals are as important to consider as the prescribed prosthetic components. The dynamic evaluation may occur in the prosthetist's office, physical therapy gym, or "amputee" clinic settings. It begins with a walk down the length of the parallel bars. It is often helpful to have an assistant or aid guard or assist new prosthetic users as they walk so that the examiner can focus on observation of gait characteristics. For a complete understanding of the dynamic interaction of patient and prosthesis, gait must be observed from lateral/sagittal and anterior/posterior perspectives.

Lateral/Sagittal View

The four key areas that are evaluated from the lateral perspective are (1) knee stability throughout stance, (2) transition from initial contact to foot-flat position, (3) symmetry of step length and step duration, and (4) quality of knee flexion during late stance and swing phase.

Stability of the knee is the major determinant of safety in ambulation. The new prosthetic wearer must learn to extend the hip at initial contact (heel strike) to stabilize the prosthetic knee adequately. Optimally, the knee will extend smoothly, with little hesitation.

Initial contact (heel strike) is the most unstable point in prosthetic gait. Stability in stance increases significantly when a foot-flat position is reached. The transition from initial contact to foot flat should occur relatively quickly and smoothly, with the goal of reaching a position that promotes knee stability without obvious "foot slap." Quality of prosthetic gait and commonly occurring gait deviations are discussed further in the section "Quality of Transfemoral Prosthetic Gait."

Optimally, the prosthetic and intact limb's step lengths are equal in distance, symmetric in pattern, and even in cadence. The patient should have little hesitation in initiation of swing on the prosthesis or intact limb. Asymmetry in step characteristics impedes the momentum necessary for energy-efficient forward progression, increasing the work of walking significantly.

Step length and swing phase function are influenced by knee flexion during late stance phase. As the patient moves from midstance into initial swing, a controlled and gradual knee flexion must occur to provide adequate toe clearance during the swing phase of gait. Knee flexion that occurs too early compromises stance stability, whereas excessive knee flexion during swing causes rapid heel rise.

Anterior/Frontal View

When viewing gait from an anterior or posterior perspective, the examiner is most interested in adequacy of suspension, width of the base of support, control of the pelvis during prosthetic stance, and quality and pattern of the prosthetic swing.

Suspension can be only effective if it is donned properly and fit adequately to the individual. The examiner wants to determine if the prosthesis remains in optimal orientation on the limb through all phases of the gait cycle. Pis-toning or rotation of the prosthesis should be minimal on the residual limb at any point in the gait cycle, but especially during unweighted swing. Because pistoning results in a relative lengthening of the prosthetic limb, patients must use a compensatory strategy to achieve toe clearance. One of the most common gait deviations observed when suspension is incorrectly applied or inadequate is circumduction of the prosthetic limb during swing.

Optimally, a normal narrow base of support and swing path will be present with a 2- to 3-in. separation between feet as they alternate between stance and swing. A wide base increases energy expenditure and results in a less cosmetic gait pattern.

The pelvis should remain relatively horizontal during the prosthetic stance phase with a minimal drop of 5 degrees on the intact swing side for optimal cosmetic and energy-efficient gait.[1,7] For those with short residual limbs or weakness of hip abductors, a level pelvis is a challenge to maintain. In these instances, the pelvis drops noticeably on the intact limb during swing. A compensatory pattern, such as lateral trunk bending, can be used to assure adequate toe clearance of the intact swing limb. The frontal plane alignment of socket, knee, and foot plays a significant role in stabilizing the pelvis and trunk. This relationship is established by the prosthetist during diagnostic fitting and alignment sessions before delivery of the finished prosthesis.

The line of progression of the prosthetic foot and knee during swing phase is also assessed. Ideally, the foot and knee move forward in the same plane. If the prosthesis has been donned improperly, evidence of a medial or lateral whip may be seen with the foot circumscribing with an inward or outward arc during swing phase.

Variations in Quality of Gait

The pattern and quality of gait with a transfemoral prosthesis can vary a great deal between treatment sessions, especially for those who are new to their prosthesis or have recently had a change in prosthetic components. Most often, these variations in performance can be traced to intraindividual factors, rather than to malalignment or dysfunction of the prosthesis itself. If unrecognized, some of these quite controllable factors can significantly impede progress in gait training and functional mobility. The most common problems encountered include inadequate volume control/edema management, continued shrinkage of the residual limb as it matures, inappropriate number of sock ply, inappropriate heel heights, skin irritation from overuse of a new prosthesis, improper donning, inadequate suspension, worn or loose components, and "patient innovation." Effective patient education and communication between the prosthetic clinical team and the patient can solve many of these problems.[22]

Edema and Limb Volume

For a new prosthetic user who is having difficulty with prosthetic fit and donning, one of the first questions asked should concern his or her compliance in wearing compression garments. It is not uncommon to have an increase in limb circumference after only 15–30 minutes without wearing a shrinker or compressive Ace wrap. The importance of routine use of a compressive garment whenever the prosthesis is not being worn (including overnight while sleeping) cannot be overstated, especially for those within 6 months of amputation. Even in an experienced prosthetic wearer, limb volume can vary over the course of the day. It is not unusual to have to add or subtract one or more ply of prosthetic socks at some point during the day. For those who need the very snug fit of suction suspension, edema is a serious problem that can prevent donning the prosthesis and achieving suction. In this case, the compression garment or Ace wrap should be applied for 15–20 minutes before donning the prosthesis again.

Maturation and Shrinkage of the Residual Limb

New prosthetic users often experience rapid reduction of limb volume as their time in the prosthesis increases over the first few weeks and months after delivery of the prosthesis. Although this limb maturation may require several socket adjustments until limb size stabilizes, it is a natural and important process that should be supported by the use of compression whenever the prosthesis is not worn. The loss of limb volume is usually accommodated by the need to increase the number of ply of prosthetic socks being worn to a 15-ply maximum. When more than 15 ply of sock are worn, intimacy of fit is compromised and a new socket should be fabricated. Traditionally, the use of suction suspension is not recommended until limb volume has stabilized. For those using suction suspension who experience further reduction in limb size (due to weight loss, increased activity, time in the socket, etc.), the prosthetist can add padding to the socket to restore the intimate skin-socket fit that is needed to restore suction.

Inappropriate Number of Sock Ply

Because of the normal mild fluctuation in limb volume, the number of prosthetic sock ply that are required for appropriate fit also can vary from day to day and within the same day. New and experienced prosthetic users often carry several 1-ply cotton socks with them during the day so that they are prepared should adjustment become necessary. Individuals who are wearing too many ply of sock lose total contact with the distal portion of the socket, complain of tightness at the proximal socket, and feel as if the prosthesis is excessively long (this may be manifested as difficulty with toe clearance in swing). Those who have too few ply of sock applied experience increasing distal end pressure or discomfort in the perineum because they are seated too far down in the socket. It is often helpful to have new prosthetic users keep a record of the number of socks and overall ply (thickness) worn, and the frequency of making adjustments to ply during the day. This helps them to better understand the dynamic nature of limb volume size and enhance proper care of the residual limb.

Changing Footwear: Improper Heel Heights

All prosthetic feet are designed to be worn with shoes of a particular heel height (see Figure 27-18). They are available in a variety of heel heights, ranging from a heel rise of 0 mm for sandals and flats to a 45-mm heel rise for women's high heels. It is essential to match the heel rise of the prosthetic foot to the shoes that are most often worn by the patient. A heel wedge placed inside the shoe can be used to accommodate for the occasional use of shoes with slightly lower heels. Change to a shoe with significantly lower heels results in excessive knee stability in stance. Conversely, a change to shoes with much higher heels compromises alignment stability of the knee, and places much greater demand on the patient for muscular control of knee position during stance.

Impact of Overuse

Whether learning to use a training prosthesis for the first time since amputation or being fit with a new definitive prosthesis, most prosthetic users benefit from a gradual break-in period. This strategy allows the skin, soft tissue, and musculature to grow accustomed to the forces that are acting on the residual limb. Failure to adhere to such a plan can lead to muscle soreness, skin irritation, and, in some cases, skin breakdown. New users should be advised to increase the length of time in their prosthesis gradually, carefully inspecting their skin each time that the prosthesis is removed, and wearing an appropriate compression garment when not in the prosthesis.

Improper Donning

When a prosthesis is not properly oriented on the residual limb as a result of improper donning technique or incomplete donning, it cannot operate efficiently. The wearer may experience discomfort within the socket or may exhibit a variety of gait deviations. Emphasis on developing a careful systematic method of donning is essential when working with new prosthetic wearers. Attention to details when donning the prosthesis can minimize the frustration, inconvenience, and discomfort of having to reapply the prosthesis multiple times until the desired position is achieved.

Inadequate Suspension

Inadequately tightened or badly worn suspension straps, belts, or Velcro closures should be suspected when the wearer experiences pistoning of the residual limb within the socket. The prosthesis drops down slightly when it is unweighted during swing, resulting in a relatively longer swing limb and challenging toe clearance. Additionally, the prosthesis may rotate on the residual limb, leading to a variety of compensatory gait deviations. New prosthetic users should be encouraged to assess the adequacy of suspension carefully and systematically each time that they don the prosthesis. All prosthetic users must periodically inspect belts, straps, or Velcro closures for signs of fraying, stretching, or significant wear and tear.

Worn or Loosened Components

As in any mechanical device that is subjected to daily use, the prosthesis should be periodically inspected for signs of excessive wear or loosening of the components. It is important to schedule periodic maintenance check-ups with the prosthetist, especially if the prosthetic wearer is involved in physically demanding leisure or work activities. In some circumstances, the prosthesis may be misused or abused, increasing the likelihood of damage to prosthetic components. It is much less expensive to fix a small problem in the making than to have to replace major components or to fabricate a new prosthesis because of complete mechanical failure.

Patient Innovation

Prosthetic users, who do not fully understand the intricate alignment and specifics of design of their prosthesis, may attempt to modify it. If a patient who has been progressing well in gait training and has been compliant with compression strategies suddenly has difficulty with socket fit, patient innovation should be suspected. It may be that padding has been added or removed from inside the socket. If knee stability has suddenly changed without any change in footwear, the wearer may have attempted to fine tune alignment or knee unit function. Individuals who have questions about alignment (including most physical therapists) should be cautioned not to make random small alignment adjustments, instead relying on the knowledge, equipment, and skilled experience of the prosthetist if adjustment is necessary.

QUALITY OF TRANSFEMORAL PROSTHETIC GAIT

The goal of a well-designed and accurately fit transfemoral prosthesis is an energy-efficient gait in as natural a pattern as possible. Quality of gait is inconsistent early in the gait-training phase, but improves as the individual becomes more experienced with the prosthesis during therapy. If gait problems persist, especially if the risk of instability and falls or of skin irritation is present, the source of the problem should be identified, and an attempt made to correct it. A number of classic transfemoral prosthetic gait problems may be the result of prosthetic malalignment. Before making changes in alignment or adjusting mechanical settings of the prosthetic knee or foot; it is wise to rule out patient-related factors (such as hip flexion contracture, weakness, or habit) as potential contributors.

Problems in Early Stance Phase

At initial contact, the prosthetic knee should be fully extended to position the prosthetic foot appropriately for smooth loading as body weight is transferred onto the prosthesis. As loading occurs, the prosthetic foot rolls smoothly into a foot-flat position. Problems with either of these functions increase the risk of instability, and shorten the swing time and step length of the opposite limb.

Knee Instability: Initial Contact to Midstance

If the prosthetic knee is unable to maintain the necessary extension as the heel strikes the ground and the prosthesis is loaded, several possible prosthetic and patient-related factors should be considered (Figure 27-19). The most common patient-related problems that lead to knee instability at initial contact include significant hip flexion contracture or weakness of hip extensor muscles, which compromise the patient's ability to stabilize the prosthetic knee using active hip extension. If strength and range of motion are adequate, four different prosthetic factors might lead to knee instability:

1. The knee axis may be aligned too far anterior to the TKA line, promoting a flexion moment.
2. The socket may not have been set in the optimal pre-flexed position, which places the hip extensor muscles at a biomechanical advantage for stabilizing the knee.
3. The prosthetic foot may have been aligned in excessive dorsiflexion.
4. The plantar flexion bumper or SACH heel may be too stiff.

Foot Slap

The speed that the prosthetic foot descends to the floor is determined by the durometer of the heel cushion or stiffness of the plantar flexion bumper, and by how quickly or forcefully the individual loads the heel of the foot. If the prosthetic foot functions with an apparent foot slap,

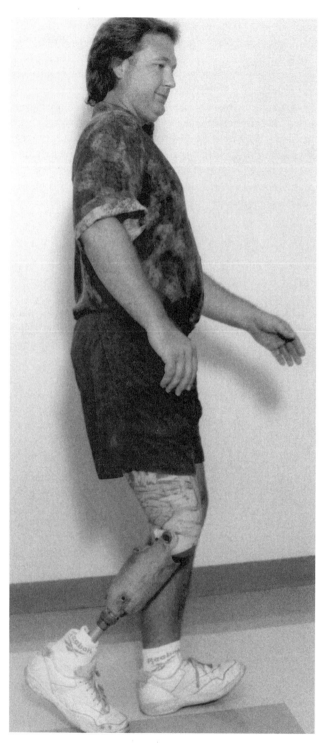

FIGURE 27-19

*An unstable prosthetic knee in the early stance phase may be
due to patient factors (e.g., hip extensor weakness, hip flexion
contracture) or inappropriate alignment of the prosthetic knee,
anterior to the trochanter-knee-ankle (TKA) line. If the knee
is unstable, the opposite swing phase (stride length) is necessarily shortened to regain postural stability.*

two factors should be considered. The heel cushion or
plantar flexion bumper may be too soft for the user's
weight and activity level. Alternatively, those prosthetic
wearers who are fearful of instability in the early stance
phase may be forcefully driving their heel into the ground
to ensure complete knee extension. For those using a locking knee component, the ability to reach a foot-flat position quickly is essential for a smooth transition throughout
the stance phase of gait. For most other knee units, the
goal is to strike a balance between cosmesis and function.

External Rotation of the Prosthetic Foot

One of the gait deviations that is observed in the frontal
plane is an external rotation of the prosthetic foot at initial contact and loading response as weight is transferred
onto the prosthesis. This creates a rotary torque that is
transmitted up the length of the prosthesis to the residual limb/socket interface, and can lead to skin irritation
and discomfort. The most common prosthetic cause of
this deviation is an excessively firm heel cushion or plantar flexion bumper. Inappropriate toe out alignment
of the prosthetic foot must first be ruled out. When girth
of the residual limb is decreasing (for individuals in whom
the whole limb is shrinking as it matures or in anyone who
has recently lost weight), fit within the socket may be too
loose, so that the effect of even a small rotary torque is
manifested. Three user-related factors must also be considered: (1) if there is weakness of hip muscles, the wearer
may be unable to maintain the limb in optimal alignment
as transition to stance phase takes place, (2) if the wearer
is fearful of knee instability in early stance, he or she may
be extending the prosthetic knee too vigorously at heel
strike to ensure full knee extension has been reached, and
(3) the shoe may be too tight for the prosthetic foot.

Problems in Mid- to Late Stance Phase

In early stance phase, the primary goal is to ensure sufficient stability of the knee while body weight is loaded
onto the prosthesis. In mid- to late stance phase, two
additional but equally important goals must be met:
(1) smooth forward progression of the body over the
prosthetic foot and (2) efficient preparation for the
upcoming swing phase.

Pelvic Rise/Hill Climbing

Excessive pelvic elevation during the transition through
mid- and terminal stance is often a compensatory strategy
to achieve a smooth progression from foot flat to heel off.
The prosthetic wearer may make the classic statement: "I
feel as though I am walking up a hill." The individual has
to exert an extra effort, substituting a rise of the pelvis to

roll over the toe-break area of the foot. This is most often a consequence of inappropriate alignment of the prosthetic foot, which may be excessively plantar-flexed. Alternatively, the foot may be positioned too far anteriorly with respect to the knee and socket. Both of these conditions create a relative increase in foot length, moving the fulcrum of the third rocker of gait (toe rocker) farther forward.

Drop-Off at Midstance

When relative shortening of the foot is present, the third rocker is reached prematurely and stability of late stance is compromised, just as relative lengthening of the prosthesis foot leads to delayed forward progression and difficulty in reaching the third rocker of gait. A prosthetic wearer may sense knee instability and report they feel as though they are stepping into a hole. A dropping off or lowering of the pelvis often occurs because roll over takes place too early in the transition between mid- and terminal stance, rather than during terminal stance to preswing. The stride of the swing limb must be shortened to compensate for lack of stability in late stance. Most often, this deviation is a consequence of inappropriate prosthetic alignment. The prosthetic foot may be positioned in too much dorsiflexion. If an articulating/axial foot is used, the dorsiflexion bumper may be worn out or be excessively soft. The durometer of heel cushion on a SACH foot may be inappropriately soft for the patient's weight or activity level. Finally, the transfemoral socket may be positioned too far anteriorly, so that the weight line falls toward the front of the foot at midstance. All of these conditions functionally decrease the length of the prosthetic foot, lead to premature roll over, and instability in later stance.

Lateral Trunk Bending

One of the most common gait deviations observed in the frontal plane is lateral trunk bending toward the prosthetic side during mid- and late stance (Figure 27-20). If the lateral prosthetic wall is not contoured to stabilize the femur in a natural position of adduction, drift of the femur into an abducted position causes a drop of the pelvis on the swinging side. An exaggerated lateral lean toward the stance (prosthetic) side ensures adequate toe clearance. Lateral trunk bending is used to avoid discomfort or excessive pressure in the perineum. This may be a result of a medial wall that is excessively high or rigid when fleshy tissue of an adductor roll is being pinched between the socket and the pubic ramus, or when too few prosthetic socks are worn, and the residual limb is positioned too deeply in the prosthesis. Other possible explanations include a socket that is aligned in excessive initial abduction, or a prosthetic foot excessively outset from the midline position. In both of these instances, the base of support

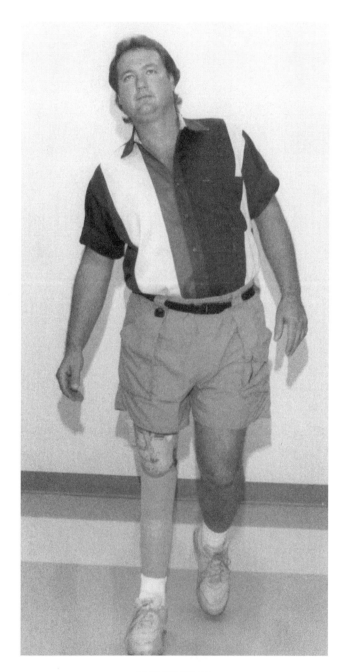

FIGURE 27-20
Lateral trunk bending during prosthetic stance helps to clear the swinging limb. This gait deviation is observed in the frontal plane.

is functionally wider than normal, and the only effective way to shift weight onto the prosthetic side is by leaning laterally. Finally, it is very difficult to provide lateral stabilization within the socket, and to align prosthetic components in the ideal narrow base of support for individuals with very short residual limbs.

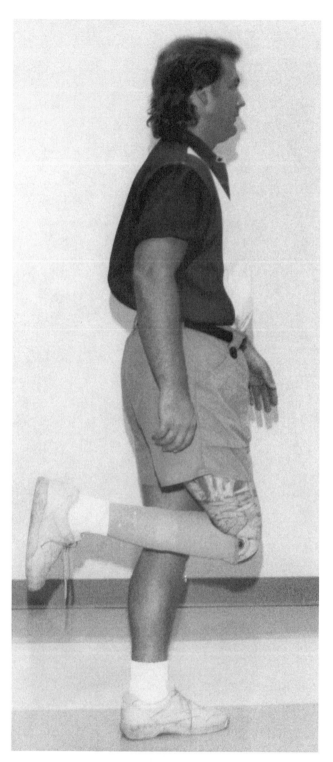

FIGURE 27-21
Uneven heel rise in early swing delays the extension of the knee, which is needed to prepare for the next initial contact.

Problems in Swing Phase

The functional goal of swing phase is advancement of the unweighted limb. The prosthetic wearer has two tasks: (1) to initiate swing with enough hip flexion momentum to achieve the prosthetic knee flexion that is necessary for toe clearance and (2) to position the knee in extension in preparation for initial contact.

Excessive Lumbar Lordosis

Some prosthetic users move into excessive lumbar lordosis in late stance and into the early swing phase. This may be the result of an alignment problem: The transfemoral socket may not have been positioned in an appropriate amount of initial flexion, especially for patients with hip flexion contracture. Patients with weakness of hip flexors or abdominal muscles may compensate by using exaggerated lumbar motion to initiate hip flexion needed for a functional swing. Finally, lumbar lordosis may be a functional compensation for an ineffective femoral lever in those with short residual limbs.

Uneven Heel Rise

Uneven heel rise is a problem that occurs in initial swing phase, and can be observed in the sagittal plane of motion (Figure 27-21). When the knee of the prosthesis flexes as swing phase begins, the prosthetic knee continues in flexion with the foot rising quickly away from the floor. If this heel rise is excessive, it delays extension of the prosthetic knee as the swing phase progresses. Prosthetic causes of this gait deviation include inadequate flexion resistance settings in the knee unit, or inadequate adjustment of the knee extension aid. Adjustment of friction or flexion resistance of the knee unit, or replacement of worn extension aids generally solves the problem.

Vaulting

If the prosthetic wearer must rise up on the toes during stance on the nonamputated limb to provide adequate clearance for the prosthesis through midswing (Figure 27-22), several possible prosthetic factors should be evaluated. First, the adequacy and correct application of suspension should be assessed. Second, if suspension is appropriate, adjustment of swing resistance in the prosthetic knee should be considered. Too much resistance to knee flexion and a foot set in excessive plantar flexion may relatively lengthen the prosthesis and compromise toe clearance in swing. Finally, if suspension and knee unit friction are appropriate, the overall height of the prosthesis should be double-checked to determine if the prosthesis is really too long.

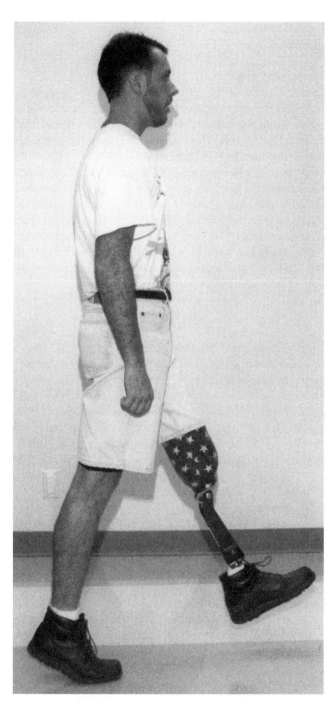

FIGURE 27-22

Vaulting is a compensatory strategy for a prosthesis that is functionally too long. It may be due to inadequate suspension, excessive friction of the knee unit, an excessively plantar flexed foot, or, sometimes, to excessive length of the prosthesis.

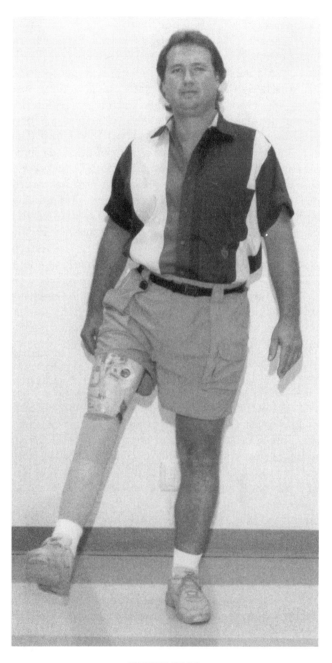

FIGURE 27-23

In a circumduction gait pattern, the prosthesis swings in a wide lateral arc to facilitate toe clearance in swing. Prosthetic causes of circumduction include inadequate suspension, a locked knee unit, or excessive friction in the knee unit.

Circumduction during Swing

Optimally, forward progression of the prosthesis during swing takes place in a straight line with enough knee flexion for adequate toe clearance (Figure 27-23). If the prosthetic knee is maintained in extension instead, one compensatory strategy would be to swing the limb in a wide lateral arc. In this strategy, the peak distance from midline occurs during midswing, but the limb moves back toward midline during terminal swing, in preparation for a normal heel strike at initial contact. This deviation, most easily observed from a position in front or behind the patient (frontal plane), is an attempt to compensate for a prosthesis that is functionally or actually too long. Circumstances that can lead to this compensation are similar to the vaulting deviation and include (1) adequate suspension, in which the prosthesis pistons downward due to the force of gravity when unweighted during swing and (2) a prosthetic knee unit that is locked in extension or set with an excessive friction setting, preventing the knee flexion necessary during swing phase. The pattern is also used by prosthetic wearers who are nervous about catching their toe during swing, or who are reluctant to use knee flexion because of anticipated instability in the subsequent early stance period. Circumduction can also be the result of a foot set in excessive plantar flexion, which makes the prosthesis functionally longer.

Medial and Lateral Whips
Optimally, forward progression of the prosthetic knee and foot occurs in the same line of progression, perpendicular to the floor. A whip occurs when forward progression of the distal parts of the prosthesis follows an oblique path. Whips differ from circumducted gait because the thigh advances in the expected, straight, forward line of progression, whereas the shin and foot travel in an arcing pattern. Whips are most easily observed while evaluating gait in the frontal plane. In a medial whip (Figure 27-24A), the prosthetic knee appears to rotate externally, so that the prosthetic foot moves in an arc of motion that carries the foot toward midline during swing. For some patients, the heels of the swing and stance limbs narrowly miss contact at midstance/midswing. Although this occurs when the prosthetic knee is aligned in too much external rotation, it also can be the result of several user-related factors. Medial whips occur when the prosthesis is donned incorrectly in too much external rotation, or when the Silesian belt is worn too tightly and pulls the socket into external rotation. It also may be the consequence of poor purchase between skin and socket for individuals who are using suction suspension, especially those with "flabby" thigh tissue.

In a lateral whip (Figure 27-24B), the prosthetic knee seems to rotate internally, and the foot traces an arc of motion that moves away from the midline. The possible causes of a lateral whip are the exact opposite of those for a medial whip: The knee unit may be prepositioned in too much internal rotation, or the socket may have

been positioned in a slightly internally rotated position during donning.

Terminal Impact
Excessive terminal impact is a gait deviation that is observed in the sagittal plane during terminal swing. The shin of the prosthesis moves forward so quickly that the fully extended position is reached early, often with an audible or visible impact against the prosthetic knee. Prosthetic factors that contribute to this deviation include insufficient resistance to extension of the knee unit, an excessively strong extension aid, or worn extension bumper. Prosthetic wearers who are fearful of knee instability in early stance may choose to flex the hip forcefully in initial swing to build momentum for knee extension, then forcefully extend the hip in terminal swing to snap the knee into full extension in preparation for initial contact.

Other Issues
Ideally, a reasonably narrow base with minimal sway is present, as well as symmetry and evenness in stride length, cadence, and arm swing, so that the gait pattern appears to be as natural as possible when the transfemoral prosthesis is used. Excessive side-to-side sway and asymmetry in place of fluid reciprocal movements increase the work and energy cost of walking and are obviously different from a normal gait pattern.

Uneven Step Length and Swing Time
Early in prosthetic training, new prosthetic wearers may be cautious and reluctant to use the prosthesis to its full capacity. It is important to emphasize the goal of equal step length and swing time. Patients gain confidence by practicing single limb support on the prosthetic side, and by performing gait training exercises that provide appropriate visual, kinesthetic, and auditory feedback (e.g., equally spaced target marks on the floor, or use of mirrors or videotape). Several possible patient-related issues and/or prosthetic problems should be considered if gait pattern asymmetry persists. First, the fit of the socket and condition of the skin should be examined carefully. Anyone would be reluctant to spend time in weight bearing if tissue is being pinched or irritated within the socket, if relief for bony prominences is inadequate, or if an inflamed or open area or unrecognized neuroma is present. Second, hip flexion contracture on the prosthetic side may limit excursion in hip extension in late stance, compromising forward progression of the opposite swing limb. If fit, skin condition, and ROM are adequate, the mechanical and alignment stability of the knee unit should be reevaluated. If a wearer senses that the knee cannot pro-

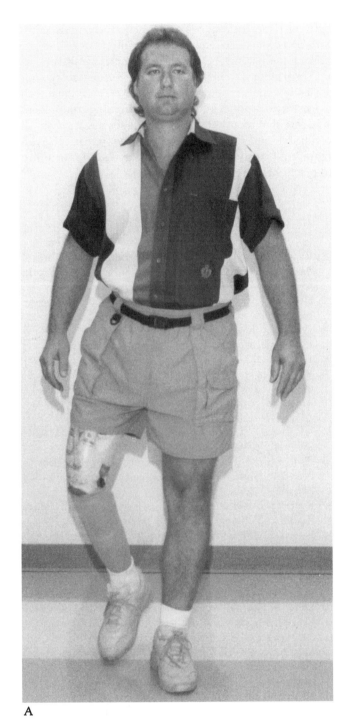

A

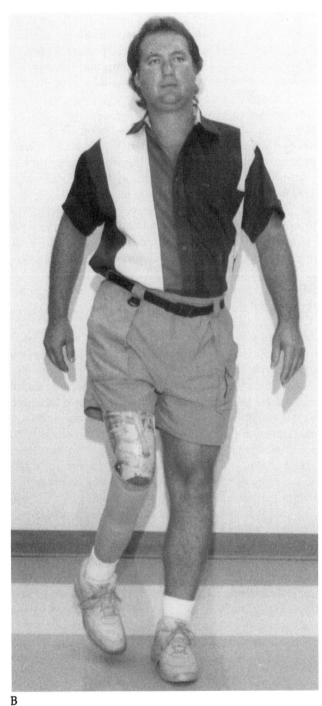

B

FIGURE 27-24

(A) In a medial whip, the thigh moves forward as expected, whereas the shin and foot progress in a medial arc, appearing to be in excessive external rotation. (B) In a lateral whip, the shin and foot describe a lateral arc, appearing to be in excessive internal rotation. Most whips are the consequence of improper donning or suspension.

vide adequate support in stance, he or she will compensate by shortening stance time to minimize sense of security. Finally, individuals with impaired postural responses (poor balance) who are fearful of falling may decrease the time spent in single limb support by reducing step length.

Uneven Arm Swing

Many individuals with amputation demonstrate diminished or absent reciprocal arm swing when walking with their prosthesis. They may hold the arm on the prosthetic side stiffly and relatively still throughout the gait cycle. This is especially common in a new prosthetic user who has not yet developed confidence in the stability of his prosthesis, and for those with a painful residual limb. This behavior is also observed in some proficient prosthetic users. The mechanism that underlies this alteration in motor behavior is not clearly understood, but may be related to loss of sensation from the distal contact between the foot and the ground.

Abducted Gait Pattern

In an abducted gait pattern, the prosthesis is held away from the midline throughout the gait cycle. Functionally, this is most notable in the stance phase of gait. In initial contact, the prosthetic foot lands several inches lateral to the normal or ideal foot position, resulting in a wide base of support, and requiring excessive side-to-side sway to accomplish weight transfer from one limb to the other. This deviation has a number of possible causes. The overall length of the prosthesis may need to be reduced. The socket may be aligned in a position of too much initial abduction. There may be uncomfortable or painful pressure in the groin area (as in lateral leaning). An abducted gait pattern may be a compensatory strategy when pelvic instability is a result of inadequate lateral wall stabilization of the femur or weakness of hip abductors. The prosthetic wearer may be attempting to minimize lateral-distal femoral pain within the socket. Finally, for those who are fearful of falling, an abducted gait pattern may be a habitual movement strategy to minimize feelings of insecurity.

SUMMARY

Advances in technology and improved prosthetic components have greatly benefited individuals with transfemoral amputation. In this chapter, we have learned that the successful functional outcome for individuals needing prosthetic care requires more than advanced technology. A prosthetic team is necessary in which the prosthetist and physical therapist are key contributors. A thorough understanding of the interrelationship

between the prosthesis' weight, function, cosmesis, comfort, and cost is also required. Attention to socket design, knee biomechanics, and prosthetic alignment is also important in providing optimal patient care. The prosthetic clinical team's goal is not merely to present an individual with a prosthetic product but to provide ongoing comprehensive care that focuses on the individual's needs, physical condition, and personal goals. In this way, patients who require a transfemoral prosthesis have an opportunity to reach their full functional potential.

REFERENCES

1. Radcliffe CW. Functional Considerations in the Fitting of Above-Knee Prostheses. In Artificial Limbs. New York: Krieger, 1970;35–60.
2. Huang CT, Jackson JR, Moore, et al. Amputation: energy cost of ambulation. Arch Phys Med Rehabil 1979;60(1):18–24.
3. Waters RL. Energy Expenditure. In J Perry (ed), Gait Analysis: Normal and Pathological Function. Thorofare, NJ: Slack, 1992;443–487.
4. Waters RL. Energy cost of walking amputees: the influence of level of amputation. J Bone Joint Surg 1976;58A:42–46.
5. Waters R, Yakura J. Energy Expenditure of Normal and Abnormal Ambulation. In GL Smidt (ed), Clinics in Physical Therapy: Gait in Rehabilitation. New York: Churchill Livingstone, 1990;65–93.
6. Fischer SV, Gullickson G. Energy cost of ambulation in health and disability: a literature review. Arch Phys Med Rehabil 1978;59(3):124–132.
7. Radcliffe CW. Prosthetics. In J Rose, JG Gamble (eds), Human Walking. Baltimore: Williams & Wilkins, 1981;165–199.
8. Schuch CM. Report from the international workshop on above-knee fitting and alignment techniques. Clin Prosthet Orthot 1988;12:81–98.
9. Pritham CH. Workshop on teaching materials for above-knee socket variants. J Prosthet Orthot 1988;1(1):51–67.
10. Long IA. Normal shape–normal alignment (NSNA) above knee prosthesis. Clin Prosthet Orthot 1985;9:9–14.
11. Sabolich J. Contoured adducted trochanteric-controlled alignment method (CAT-CAM): introduction and basic principles. Clin Prosthet Orthot 1985;9:15–26.
12. Jendrezejczk DJ. Flexible socket systems. Clin Prosthet Orthot 1985;9:27–30.
13. Kristinsson O. Flexible above-knee socket made from low density polyethylene suspended by a weight transmitting frame. Orthot Prosthet 1983;37:25–27.
14. Manual for the Henschke-Mauch Hydraulic Swing-N-Stance Control System. Dayton, OH: Mauch Laboratories, 1976.
15. Moore KL. Clinical Oriented Anatomy. Baltimore: Williams & Wilkins, 1980;553.
16. Mooney V, Quigley MJ. Above Knee Amputations: Prosthetic Management. In JH Bowker (ed), Atlas of Limb Prosthetics. St. Louis: Mosby–Year Book, 1981;381–401.

17. Schuch CM. Prosthetic Management. In JH Bowker, JW Michael (eds), Atlas of Prosthetics: Surgical, Prosthetic, and Rehabilitation Principles (2nd ed). St. Louis: Mosby, 1992;528–529.

18. Otto Bock Orthopedic Industry, INC: Manual for the 3c100 Otto Bock C-LEG. Duderstadt, Germany, 1998.

19. Haberman LJ, Bedotto RA, Colodney EJ. Silicone-only suspension (SOS) for the above knee amputee. J Prosthet Orthot 1992;4(2):76–85.

20. Padula PA, Friedman LW. Amputee Gait. In LW Friedman (ed), Physical Medicine and Rehabilitation Clinics of North America. Philadelphia: Saunders, 1991; 423–432.

21. Quigley M. The role of test socket procedures in today's prosthetic practices. Clin Prosthet Orthot 1985;9(3): 11–12.

22. Nielsen CC, Psonak RP, Kalter TL. Factors affecting the use of prosthetic services. J Prosthet Orthot 1989;1(4):242–249.

28

Rehabilitation for Persons with Transfemoral Amputation

DAVID M. THOMPSON

REHABILITATION OUTCOMES AFTER TRANSFEMORAL AMPUTATION

Rehabilitation specialists sometimes assume that a person's ability to use a prosthesis and be functional after amputation is determined by the level of amputation: Those with transfemoral amputations, for instance, might be more dependent or use their prostheses less frequently than those with transtibial amputations. Although some studies support this assumption, others challenge it. In a retrospective review of 157 records of patients with new lower limb amputation, Moore et al.[1] found that of the 129 patients who were fitted for prostheses, 88 (68.2%) achieved functional ambulation, whereas 41 (31.8%) did not. Functional use of a prosthesis also varied with level of amputation: 66% of those with unilateral transtibial amputation, 46% of those with unilateral transfemoral amputation, and only 19% of those with bilateral amputation used their prosthesis for walking.

A growing number of studies, however, suggest that preamputation functional status is a better predictor of rehabilitation outcome than level of amputation alone. A 3-year study of adults with peripheral vascular insufficiency who were followed in the Veterans Administration health system rated ambulation status before amputation using a seven-level functional grading system based, in part, on the use of assistive devices and distance typically walked.[2] After rehabilitation, 84% of patients walked with their prosthesis within one functional level of their preamputation status. Regardless of level of amputation, patients who walked functional distances before surgery were more likely to use their prosthesis and less likely to require an assistive device than were those with limited ambulation capacity before surgery. Similar studies suggest that any patient who is able to ambulate before

surgery should be considered a candidate for prosthetic fitting and rehabilitation postoperatively.[3]

PREPARING TO DON THE PROSTHESIS

Patients with new transfemoral amputation must understand that their new prosthesis cannot help them to stand or to transfer. It is important that patients gain skill in standing and balancing on the remaining extremity so that they can safely and independently apply the prosthesis to their residual limb. Single limb activities are a very important component of preprosthetic training.

Many training (temporary) transfemoral prostheses are suspended on the patient using a system of straps, bands, or belts. Given the likelihood of frequent adjustments of suspension during early prosthetic training, many patients choose to wear loose-fitting shorts that fit easily over the prosthesis for early gait training sessions. Many elect to don the prosthesis, especially its suspension straps, over these clothes. This strategy is successful only if clothing does not interfere with insertion of the residual limb into the prosthetic socket. With adequate healing of the suture line and increased tolerance of or time in the prosthesis, many patients begin to wear the prosthesis under their clothing. Wearing the prosthesis for extended periods helps patients to incorporate their prosthesis more effectively into daily life. They need not, for example, remove the prosthesis to use the bathroom if it is worn under clothing, as they must if it is worn and suspended over a pair of shorts.

Because transfemoral prostheses are somewhat large and cumbersome, most persons with amputation "dress the prosthesis first" (socks, pants, shoes), donn the prosthesis, then dress their remaining limb. While sitting, holding the prosthesis and clothing in their laps, the patients

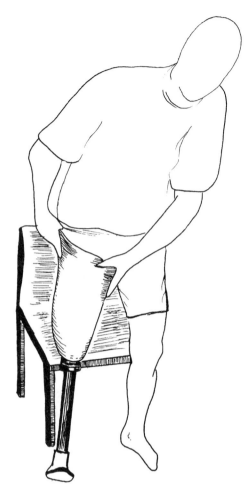

FIGURE 28-1

To don a transfemoral prosthesis with an ischial containment socket, the patient must be stable in single limb support on the intact, nonamputated lower extremity. After application of the appropriate ply of prosthetic socks, the residual limb is inserted into the socket. The patient uses the position of the toes of the prosthetic foot as an indicator of proper placement of the limb within the socket.

insert the prosthesis into the appropriate pant leg. Some persons with amputation prepare their prosthesis before retiring for bed in the evening and joke that they are "already half-dressed" when they arise the next morning. After clothing is applied to the prosthesis, the prosthetic foot is placed on the floor, positioned so that the nonamputated limb can be inserted into its own pant leg. The patient then prepares to don the prosthesis.

Donning Prosthetic Socks

The next step in donning the prosthesis is to apply one or more ply of prosthetic socks. For patients with rela-

tively new amputations, prosthetic socks are worn over the residual limb to accommodate for limb volume changes and to ensure total contact fitting within the prosthetic socket. Prosthetic socks also absorb perspiration and decrease friction between the socket and the residual limb. Unless suction suspension is chosen for the definitive prosthesis once limb volume has stabilized, most patients with amputation wear at least one thin cotton sock or nylon sheath even after they receive their definitive prosthesis.

Prosthetic socks are knit from wool or cotton and are available in one-, three-, or five-ply thicknesses and in a variety of widths and lengths. Some patients apply a nylon sheath as the innermost layer in an effort to wick perspiration away from the skin. Next, each prosthetic sock is rolled smoothly over the residual limb with the thickest sock applied first. Ideally, all layers of sock are applied without dimples or wrinkles on the distal end to minimize areas of high pressure within the prosthesis. For patients whose residual limb is irregularly shaped, however, this "perfect" fit may not be possible. Because distal weight bearing is minimal within the prosthetic socket, small distal wrinkles in the sock do not pose a threat to the integrity of the skin. The way that prosthetic socks are woven during manufacture prevents unraveling if it becomes necessary to trim the sock's proximal (open) end for a better match with the length of the patient's residual limb.

When the residual limb is somewhat conical in shape with a larger proximal than distal circumference, prosthetic socks may migrate distally when the prosthesis is donned, sometimes descending into the socket, where they bunch and wrinkle, interfering with the prosthesis' fit. One strategy used to prevent this problem involves positioning what will be the outermost sock within the socket, lapping its edges over the entire proximal brim. When the residual limb (with the appropriate additional sock ply smoothly in place) is inserted into the socket, this outer sock forms a sling that prevents the additional socks from sliding downward. It may be helpful to anchor this outer sock layer to the socket brim with adhesive-backed Velcro pieces placed on the outer wall of the socket. The woven edges of the prosthetic sock are snagged by the Velcro hooks, preventing the sock from sliding downward into the socket as the prosthesis is donned and during ambulation.

Positioning the Prosthesis

Once socks are in place, most patients rise to a standing position to don the prosthesis effectively (Figure 28-1). Early in prosthetic training, most patients feel secure when using an assistive device, such as a walker, for stability as they don the prosthesis in standing. Some require additional assistance from the therapist or family member. With practice, agile patients can become quite adept at donning the prosthesis without requiring additional stability. Some patients prefer to slip their residual limb into the socket while they are still seated; however, the prosthesis cannot support their weight when they stand, and patients must be careful not to shift weight toward the prosthetic side until suspension has been achieved. They must be taught to balance themselves in standing on the remaining limb. Once in a stable erect position with the residual limb inserted into the socket, the patient positions the prosthesis with a fully extended prosthetic knee, and shifts weight onto the prosthesis to ensure optimal positioning within the socket.

The socket of a transfemoral prosthesis is designed to fit intimately on the residual limb. This fit is most comfortable when the socket is placed on the residual limb in one certain position. Most patients learn to monitor the position of the socket on the limb by noting the angle at which the prosthetic foot rests beneath them. A socket donned in an excessively internally or externally rotated position on the residual limb is likely to become uncomfortable during ambulation. It is important to note that many prosthetists place the foot in slight toe out, an external rotation of the foot with regard to the socket and knee joint axis. With repeated donning and ambulation, the patient learns the optimal neutral position for his or her prosthesis. One of the most common causes of discomfort is a prosthesis that is donned in too much internal rotation: If the socket's relatively high anterior wall is poorly positioned and contacts the sensitive groin area, the patient experiences pressure and discomfort during stance. Early in rehabilitation, it is helpful to cue patients verbally to check for socket rotation during the process of donning.

Another important aspect of proper donning is the position of the ischium. Quadrilateral socket designs nest this important weight-bearing contour on a carefully shaped region on the posteromedial socket border. Patients with recent amputation must learn to discern whether the ischium is optimally seated on this socket surface. Therapists palpate the ischial tuberosity to assist patients to recognize its optimal position on the socket. To palpate the ischial tuberosity, the therapist first instructs the patient to lean forward by flexing the hips. This moves the pelvis into an anterior tilt, lifting the tuberosity from its resting place on the socket. The therapist palpates the tuberosity and then asks the patient to return to an erect standing position. If the socket is optimally positioned, the therapist's fingers will be squeezed between the ischium and the socket wall. If the patient is wearing too many sock ply, the ischium will be above its intended surface. If the patient is wear-

ing too few sock ply, the ischium will fall below its intended surface. In either case, the number of sock ply must be changed until the ischium is optimally positioned.

Another skill that patients with recent amputation must master is the ability to judge the appropriate number and combination of socks to wear inside the temporary prosthesis. On delivery, a temporary or training prosthetic socket is designed to fit with a single three-ply sock. Limb volume often decreases rapidly as ambulation and overall activity level increase and patients use the muscles of their residual limb more effectively. As limb volume decreases, the residual limb slides further down into the prosthesis during use. One of the first signs of this is groin discomfort: Application of additional socks restores optimal positioning of the limb within the socket. Early in prosthetic training, patients use trial and error to determine if groin pressure is a result of inadequate sock ply or of improper rotation of the socket on the limb during donning. With practice, most patients become adept at problem solving and making appropriate adjustments in sock ply and fitting.

Adjusting the Suspension

As patients become more comfortable with their prosthesis and residual limb volume changes, adjustments to suspension often become necessary. Patients with recent amputation must discern whether problems with fit or comfort relate to faulty suspension or the number of socks they are wearing. The goal of all methods of suspension is to hold the prosthesis securely on the residual limb, minimizing pistoning or rotation of the socket on the limb while it is unweighted during swing or bears weight during stance. The cylindrical shape and the mass of soft tissue in a transfemoral residual limb challenge the ability to control rotation of the prosthesis on the limb. Rotation control is complicated by changing limb volume (shrinkage), which is common in early rehabilitation. For patients with recent amputation, prosthetists may use a Silesian belt or total elastic suspension, which encircles the waist to suspend the prosthesis from the pelvis. Although appropriate tightening of these suspension systems minimizes the risk of pistoning, overtightening can cause rotation of the socket on the residual limb. Early in rehabilitation, patients are tempted to tighten suspension systems as much as possible, assuming erroneously that this will prevent pistoning. Patients must develop a sense of what is appropriate tightening versus overtightening of the prosthetic suspension. Once limb volume has stabilized and the patient is ready for a definitive prosthesis, suction suspension may be possible.

The Silesian belt and total elastic suspensions are tightened by pulling the abdominal strap or belt away from the prosthesis toward the body's opposite side. If this adjustment is made without some degree of weight bearing on the prosthesis, the additional tension on the belt causes the prosthesis to rotate inwardly on the residual limb. Overtightening of suspension in this way causes two problems. Donning the prosthesis in an internally rotated position produces socket pressure and discomfort in the groin. Even if the socket does not immediately rotate on the limb, excessive tension in the suspension belt causes internal rotation on the residual limb after a few steps of walking. Signs of an overtightened suspension include a prosthetic toe that moves progressively more medially, and increasing pressure in the groin with repeated stepping. As patients become more comfortable with their prostheses, they learn to tighten the suspension only to the point at which the prosthesis does not piston on the residual limb.

Should pistoning or socket rotation occur, the initial strategy in problem solving should be to examine and appropriately adjust prosthetic suspension. Only if the problem cannot be solved by adjusting suspension should sock ply be altered. If the initial strategy is instead to add prosthetic socks to fill in the gap, the pistoning or rotation may become even more problematic. Even if improved fit is perceived, additional socks increase the circumference of the limb, hampering its descent into the socket and sacrificing the intimate fit between the socket's medial and posterior brims and the ischium and pubis. When the contact between socket and bony contours is compromised, the likelihood of rotation increases, and patients may lose control of the prosthesis as they walk.

EARLY GAIT TRAINING

During final fitting and delivery, the prosthetist ensures that the prosthesis' initial alignment is appropriate for the patient. Therapists must be aware of this initial alignment to verify that the prosthesis has been properly donned and to recognize when adjustments to alignment might be necessary to achieve the most energy-efficient and cosmetic gait. This knowledge also allows therapists to assist new prosthetic users to problem solve when they experience difficulties related to limb volume change or to increased levels of activity as they become more comfortable with weight bearing on their prosthesis.

One of the keys for assessing the fit of a transfemoral prosthesis is orientation or position of the pelvis. The therapist evaluates pelvic orientation while the patient stands comfortably in the parallel bars or with a walker, using the anterior superior iliac spine or iliac crests to judge whether the pelvis is level. To assess fit and alignment accurately, the patient's weight must be equally distrib-

uted between the prosthesis and the intact limb. If the pelvis is not level or is rotated forward or backward on one side, the therapist should first assist the patient to shift weight to achieve equal weight bearing in an erect posture and then reexamine pelvic orientation. If asymmetry persists after these adjustments are made, the length or alignment of the prosthesis may be a problem and the prosthetist should be contacted for further evaluation.

Early in rehabilitation and prosthetic training, many patients with recent amputation are reluctant to trust their prosthesis or find it difficult to bear weight on the prosthesis through the residual limb. Ironically, those who have been most active with walker or crutches during their preprosthetic rehabilitation may have the most difficulty in adapting to prosthetic use. Those who have become adept at single limb mobility, positioning the intact foot directly under the center of gravity while using an assistive device, often alter postural alignment and strategies at the hip. The resultant postural asymmetry, with increased adduction of the intact limb and abduction of the residual limb, becomes comfortable and habitual. Now, to use a prosthesis effectively, they must reposition the center of mass between the heel of their intact and prosthetic limb and resume a more symmetric position of the hip and pelvis.

Traditional approaches to gait training of patients with recent transfemoral amputation include activities and exercises that are designed to equalize weight bearing on either leg while they are standing.[4–6] These exercises are part of a sequential approach that emphasizes the perfection of pre-gait skills, such as weight shifting, alternate knee bending, and repetitive stance and swing drills that simulate components of the total movement pattern of walking.[5,7]

MOTOR LEARNING PRINCIPLES FOR REHABILITATION

Many of the traditional gait-training drills and exercises are valuable in isolated instances in which individuals must remedy specific deficits. Therapists have several reasons to choose a more direct and functional approach. First, researchers who have studied motor learning suggest that practicing specific gait training exercises does not ensure transfer or integration of these isolated skills into the functional task of walking.[8] Winstein et al.,[9] for example, discovered that patients who were recovering from a cerebrovascular accident bore their body weight more symmetrically on either leg by adhering to a standing balance training regime that involved augmented feedback. This skill did not carry over into functional ambulation: Patients also did not increase the single limb stance duration, the amount of time they spent on the paretic limb when they walked.

Other students of the motor learning process question the use of repetitive drills. Schmidt[10] argues that blocked and highly repetitive practice and drills do not effectively facilitate learning, and, in his words, "should almost never be used." Instead, he recommends more random or varied type practice that emphasizes solving of motor problems during functional tasks. Schmidt believes that random practice, even practice in which one makes mistakes, generates motor learning more effectively than does the rote repetition of accurate performance.

Motor learning researchers also caution therapists about assuming that all motor tasks can be effectively divided into a series of learnable subtasks. Walking, in fact, may be a movement pattern in which timing and energy transfers are so critical that persons cannot perform it in discrete parts but must learn it as a whole.[8]

In the current health care practice environment, it is essential to focus on rapid development of functional skills. With the likelihood of early discharge and outpatient-based rehabilitation, it is essential that safety and function be emphasized. The activities that were traditionally used as pre-gait training can be used to address specific difficulties or problems that are encountered during functional gait training. A growing body of research validates the effectiveness of a rehabilitation approach that requires less direct intervention on the therapist's part and more vigilance by the patient.

Research in the field of motor learning suggests that learning and retention of motor tasks are enhanced when feedback is limited, delayed, or intermittent.[11] Subjects in many controlled studies actually learned tasks less well when their feedback was complete, instantaneous, or ongoing.[9]

Patients with recent amputation must learn to improve their function even as they rely less on the therapist for feedback and guidance during their rehabilitation. Therapists must not assume that feedback necessarily promotes motor learning and that the more extensive and rich the feedback, the better the patient will perform. Feedback actually has negative effects if it promotes dependency and if patients rely on it and cannot recall and perform tasks in its absence.[10]

Therapists who are sensitive to tightening constraints on the time that they can devote to patient education and treatment must focus on empowering patients so that they learn quickly to "be the boss" and to "tell the prosthesis what to do." This emphasis also redirects patients' energies appropriately during their prosthetic rehabilitation and training. Persons with amputation must resist the assumption that prosthetic technology alone can make them function independently; instead they must be active and forceful as they learn to walk with a prosthesis.

WALKING WITH AN ASSISTIVE DEVICE

Many older persons with transfemoral amputations have a variety of medical problems that can complicate their functional recovery. Often they must rely initially on an assistive device, such as parallel bars or a walker, for ambulation. Many advance to walking with less assistance, and some eventually walk without any assistive device. Younger patients with traumatic amputation are even more likely to quickly develop the skills that are necessary for ambulation without an assistive device. For young and older patients, rehabilitation must focus not only on the gait patterns practiced in parallel bars in the clinic but must quickly progress to "real" conditions that they are likely to encounter in their homes and community.

Although standard walkers enhance clients' feelings of security as they learn to use their new prosthesis, a walker alters the gait pattern significantly, requiring the patient to develop compensatory movement strategies. To use a walker safely, patients must use a three-point, step-to-gait pattern: First, the walker is advanced a comfortable arm's length, followed by a forward step with the nonamputated limb, and finally with a step with the prosthesis. This sequence necessarily entails that amputees "chop up" the gait cycle, sacrificing some fluidity of motion. A further restriction on the gait pattern involves safety and stability; patients must maintain their center of gravity within their base of support, even when the walker enlarges the dimensions of that base. Patients must learn to position the walker and to place their feet so that the toes of at least one extremity remain within an imaginary rectangle formed by the walker's four legs. This rule of thumb guarantees the patients' safety whether they are walking forward, backward, or sideways, or are turning or changing direction while using the walker. Patients with poor postural control and impaired balance may need to shorten step lengths even more, so that both toes stay within this rectangular area to increase safety and reduce the risk of instability, even though the resulting gait is slower.

Initially, therapists may advise patients to advance the walker so that its rear legs land at (or just slightly beyond) the toes of the intact limb. Once a patient is comfortable and stable during single limb support in stance on the intact and prosthetic limb, the walker can be advanced further. Increasing the height of the walker to a position slightly above the customary level at the greater trochanter may allow patients to take longer steps because they can advance the walker further in front of the foot without a forward lean of the trunk. The elevated hand rests also provide a cue that helps patients stand with an erect trunk as they walk. As patients become secure with their prosthesis, many progress to ambulation with crutches using

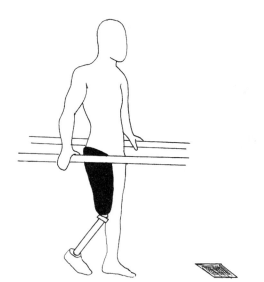

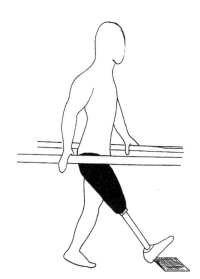

FIGURE 28-2
Repeated and rapid stepping with the prosthesis toward an anterior target provides an opportunity to practice swing limb advancement of the prosthesis. The step is initiated by forceful hip flexion, leading to flexion of the prosthetic knee. A long stride can only be accomplished with forward rotation of the pelvis.

a step-through, reciprocal four-point or two-point pattern, or to a two-point pattern with a single cane. The use of a cane in the hand opposite to the side of amputation increases the functional base of support for safety. May[12] suggests, however, that use of an assistive device on the amputated side during functional training may assist the patient's weight shift onto the prosthesis and improve stability in single limb stance.

GAIT TRAINING

Therapists can analyze a patient's walking patterns most effectively if they concentrate on the aspect of the patterns over which the patient has the greatest control and movement in the lower trunk and pelvis. The critical contribution of pelvic movement patterns to gait efficiency has been long recognized by researchers and rehabilitation professionals. Saunders et al., in 1953,[13] described pelvic movements in the frontal and transverse planes as the "determinants of normal gait," arguing that the quality of the gait pattern depended on the normality of pelvic movement. Proper pelvic movement ensures efficient and proper prosthetic function. Many common transfemoral prosthetic gait deficits are remediable if patients learn to move the pelvis properly.

Swing Phase

To walk comfortably with the new prosthesis and to avoid gait deficits, patients with amputation must regain a normal rhythm of pelvic rotation. Pelvic rotation occurs in the transverse plane, the plane that is parallel to the walking surface. To advance the prosthesis effectively during swing phase, the pelvis on the side of amputation must rotate forward as it would during normal gait. Many patients who are new to prosthetic use instead elevate the pelvis on the prosthetic side, advancing the prosthesis by flexing the hip joint within the socket. Some patients use an even more problematic strategy, rotating the pelvis backward and into a posterior tilt to elongate the hip flexors. In either case, the lack of forward pelvic movement robs the prosthetic socket segment of the velocity that is necessary to produce prosthetic knee flexion. The prosthesis advances slowly with little flexion of the prosthetic knee and with unnatural and inefficient compensatory pelvic and trunk motion.

Patients must learn to use a combination of hip flexion and forward pelvic rotation to advance their prosthesis. Early in gait training, therapists may use manual cues to facilitate the optimal pattern of pelvic rotation. This is one situation in which repeated practice using part-to whole-task training may assist patients in gaining skill and confidence in their ability to rotate the pelvis forward during swing phase. One training strategy for this pre-gait skill is performed in the parallel bars (Figure 28-2). With open palms resting lightly on the parallel bars, patients practice repeated and rapid stepping with their prosthetic limb, emphasizing forward rotation of the pelvis as the prosthetic limb advances. Some patients are better able to perform this task if an anterior and posterior "target" for their prosthetic heel is marked on the floor. The ending position (with the prosthetic heel landing in front of the intact foot) is varied randomly: This simulates situations that require quick stepping in a variety of distances and movement of the prosthesis in a variety of positions medial and lateral to the midline.

FIGURE 28-3
Bridging against a rolled towel or low stool strengthens the muscles of the residual limb in the functional positions that are necessary for stability in the early stance phase.

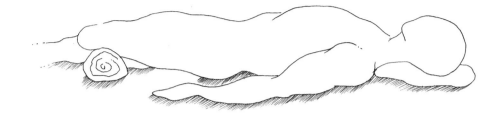

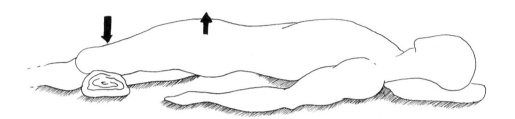

Although this skill is most easily practiced in the parallel bars, patients can also practice at home as their muscle strength and balance improve, using the kitchen counter, a table, or the back of the sofa for support. The drill has two advantages: First, it encourages the patient to use his or her muscles forcefully and aggressively to control prosthetic motion. This is especially important for older patients to master postural control and balance reactions. Second, this exercise provides patients with a simple but important performance cue, signaling sufficient force to produce the pelvic motion that is needed for efficient advancement of the prosthesis in swing. Even while patients who are learning to walk with a prosthesis are focused on conditions of the environment and prosthetic foot movement through space, they must move the pelvis on the amputated side forward so that the pelvis' trajectory is flat and parallel to the floor.

Stance Phase: Loading Response

In persons with intact lower limbs, the flexion moments at the hip and knee that result from ground reaction force as weight is shifted onto the limb at loading response are countered by action of the hip and knee extensors. Patients with transfemoral amputation can activate the hip extensors to counteract the ground reaction force–produced tendency toward hip flexion but cannot directly extend the prosthetic knee. Instead, they rely on a combination of prosthetic alignment, activation of hip extensors within the socket, and the mechanical characteristics of the pros-

thetic knee to achieve stability in early stance. The alignment of the prosthetic knee can be adjusted so that the ground reaction force passes anterior to the prosthetic knee joint during much of the stance phase. Patients also learn that forceful hip extension against the posterior wall of the socket once the prosthetic foot has contacted the ground assists in extension of the prosthetic knee joint.

Hip extensor strength is one of the key components of early stance phase stability. It is usually important that preprosthetic exercises aimed at hip strength and range of motion be continued for several months after delivery of the prosthesis to support and enhance gait training. Therapists who design home exercise programs for patients with transfemoral amputation must keep in mind principles of exercise specificity: Although hip extension performed in side lying resisted by rubber tubing is safe and relatively easy for patients to perform, this activity cannot generate the forceful muscle contractions that are necessary for effective prosthetic use. Similarly, it is difficult to activate hip muscles at the joint angles and muscle lengths that are typical of the phases of the gait cycle. An alternative position is the classic bridging exercise, in which patients lie in the supine position with a firm object (such as a rolled towel or blanket, a firm pad, a short stool, or a phone book) under the distal residual limb[14] (Figure 28-3). With little or no pressure exerted through the intact limb (or while holding it slightly above the mat or bed), the patient activates hip extensors of the residual limb by pushing or pressing the posterior thigh forcefully against the support surface. This action lifts the pelvis off the surface as the hip extends, strengthening hip extensors at the muscle length and range of motion that are typical of the early stance phase. This exercise also helps patients gain control of the pelvis in a closed kinetic chain using the muscles of the residual limb.

Bridging exercises with the intact lower extremity can also be used to assist patients in learning to control pelvic position. Maintaining a bridge on the intact limb, patients slowly lower and raise the pelvis on the amputated side. This exercise strengthens the other muscles around the hip (internal and external rotators, abductors, and adductors), simulating the functional activity of these muscles during gait. It also assists patients with the forward pelvic rotation that is necessary for swing limb advancement of the prosthesis, allowing them to practice control of a motion that is identical in direction and muscle control (although different in terms of postural requirements) to the forward pelvic rotation that is necessary during swing phase.

Ideally, the forward pelvic motion that occurs during an effective swing will continue during loading response as weight is accepted onto the prosthesis. Loading response is an important transition period during which both limbs share the body's weight and muscle activity is widespread throughout the trunk and lower extremities. As weight is accepted onto the prosthesis, the opposite pelvis rotates forward. This rotation is relative: Neither side of the pelvis, whether on the intact or prosthetic side, should move backward in an absolute sense.

Some patients who are concerned about generating enough muscle force to stabilize the knee may use abnormal backward pelvic motion to augment hip extension. In making this motion, they may appear to sit on the posterior brim of the socket. Although this pelvic substitution improves the prosthetic knee joint's stability during this critical weight acceptance phase, it seriously compromises the forward inertia that is necessary for a smooth gait. The energy cost of walking with a prosthesis is high enough without needless sacrifice of energy by interruption of the pelvis' forward progression during every loading response.

Early in prosthetic training, a therapist can facilitate or guide the pelvis in the optimal forward progression using manual contacts to bring deviations from normal pelvic motion to the patient's attention. Manual contacts may also reinforce the desired movement pattern, so that both sides of the pelvis continue to move forward during loading response with the pelvis of the intact limb moving through slightly more excursion as the limb moves through swing. This facilitation is most easily accomplished from a position behind the patient, with the fingers spread wide so that the upward thumb contacts the skin over the paraspinal muscles and the downward-pointing fourth and fifth fingers fall over the gluteus medius. Therapists find that this hand placement works best if the elbows are held close to the sides and the wrists are extended. By maintaining contact with the pelvis in this way, the therapist is able to monitor pelvic movement in the transverse plane, as well as the timing of gluteal activity during loading response and midstance. Therapists have excellent leverage to cue and enforce pelvic movement from this position. Pressure should be directed downward into the gluteus medius on the stance limb with slight anterior and medial components. This downward pressure is best applied when hip abductors are active during stance. This same hand placement can be used to guide the pelvis gently forward when the limb is in swing limb advancement. At the subsequent initial contact and loading response, this gentle forward pressure can cue the patient to maintain forward progression and prevent the "sitting back" that permits the pelvis to drift backward during the loading response. This type of facilitation can be used early in the rehabilitation process, even when a gait belt and guarding are necessary to prevent instability.

The appreciation of pelvic movement and its impact on gait quality helps explain the roots of a gait deviation that is common among patients with transfemoral amputation: external rotation of the prosthetic foot during loading response. This deviation has been attributed to excessive activation of the gluteus maximus as patients attempt to ensure stability of the prosthetic knee. Forceful contraction of this muscle also externally rotates the hip joint, which is translated through the prosthesis to the prosthetic foot. Any interruption of forward progression of the pelvis amplifies this rotational deviation, especially if failure of forward inertia delays the shift of body weight onto the prosthetic foot. If the prosthetic foot is not stable on the floor, it necessarily moves into apparent external rotation when rotational forces are placed on it from above through pelvic or hip joint movement.

Stance Phase: Midstance

Persons with transfemoral amputations frequently exhibit a lateral lean of the trunk toward the prosthesis during the midstance phase of gait. This deviation is a compensatory strategy used to ensure that the pelvis remains level as the intact limb swings forward during prosthetic stance. It occurs when an imbalance of abduction and adduction moments occurs at the residual hip joint and at the interface between the residual limb and the prosthetic socket. Because the distal residual limb is contained within the socket and not connected to the floor by an anatomic knee and foot, some "play" or movement of the femur is present within the socket. Stabilization of the femur in the frontal plane within the prosthetic socket presents prosthetists with one of their greatest challenges.

FIGURE 28-4
A lateral bridge strengthens hip abductors in a functional range that approximates that of the midstance phase of gait.

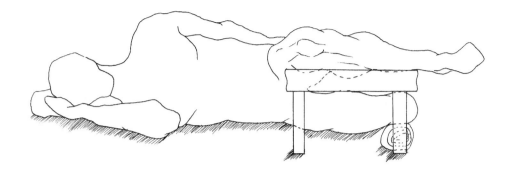

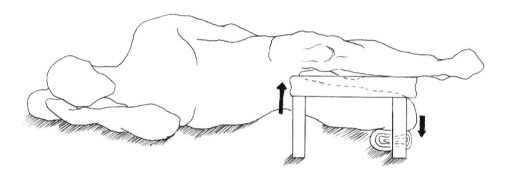

A lateral trunk lean indicates that the patient is having difficulty in controlling adduction at the residual hip joint or where the residual limb meets the prosthetic socket. Although this clinical sign may implicate functional weakness or timing difficulties of the hip abductor muscles (especially of the gluteus medius and the residual tensor fascia lata), it may also indicate inadequate stabilization of the residual femur within the socket. A patient may use a lateral trunk lean to reorient the residual limb within the socket to minimize discomfort due to pressure at the socket's medial proximal brim or its lateral distal wall. If inadequate lateral wall stabilization or excessive pressure is the root of the problem, the socket likely requires modification by the prosthetist. Patients may also use a lateral lean to escape medial brim pressure if residual limb volume has decreased so that the limb descends too far into the socket. In this case, additional sock ply can solve the problem. As the number of sock ply required reaches 15 or more, the prosthetist may consider fabricating a new socket.

If lateral lean persists despite optimal socket fit and lateral stabilization of the femur, attention must focus on the patient's ability to generate hip abductor force. Forceful activation of hip abductors within the socket mini-

mizes or eliminates this gait deviation for patients with a well-fit and well-aligned transfemoral prosthesis.

This is another example of the link between an effective exercise program, muscle strength and endurance, and quality of gait. Hip abductor strengthening is a traditional component of rehabilitation programs for patients with transfemoral amputations. Bridging exercises, described previously for hip extensor strengthening, can be performed while lying on the side of amputation to condition and train hip abductors (Figure 28-4). A small towel roll is placed under the distal lateral residual limb, and the intact limb is flexed at the hip and knee for comfort. Patients then push against the towel roll by forceful activation of hip abductors in an effort to elevate the pelvis off the mat or bed surface. Patients with recently healed limbs may be able to perform three or four repetitions.

This exercise's difficulty is outweighed by the specificity it permits in strengthening the gluteus medius at a point in the range of motion and at a length similar to that encountered during midstance. The therapist and the patient must monitor the optimal position of the trunk and pelvis so that the tendency to substitute with other stronger hip muscles by rolling the pelvis slightly back-

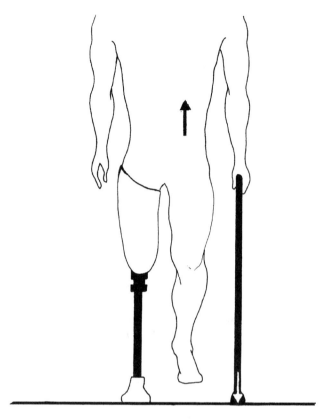

FIGURE 28-5

The use of a straight cane assists patients who have difficulty maintaining a level pelvis during stance on the prosthetic side.

ward or forward can be minimized. As patients become fatigued in performing this difficult exercise, most inadvertently reposition the pelvis in ways that permit them to complete the exercise more easily. If the pelvis shifts posteriorly during a repetition of the exercise, so that the residual hip becomes flexed, the flexion-abduction of the tensor fascia lata substitutes for action of the gluteus medius. Alternately, if the non–weight-bearing pelvis rolls backward so that the weight-bearing pelvis is extended, the hip extensors can substitute for action of the gluteus medius. The goal is to perform sets of effective lateral bridges without substitution and interspersed with other activities or rest periods, increasing the number of repetitions in each set as strength and muscular endurance improve. Patients must learn to recognize early signs of fatigue and to avoid substitution and ineffective exercise.

In addition to practicing effective exercise programs, persons with transfemoral amputation must learn to monitor their pelvic position as they walk throughout the day. Even those who avoid lateral trunk lean to offset inade-

quate hip abductor musculature may demonstrate subtle compensations in their pelvic movement patterns. The pelvis may shift laterally toward the prosthesis during midstance, even if the pelvis remains level (as indicated by the relative positions of the left and right iliac crests). Although this pelvic movement does not involve lateral leaning, it also produces hip adduction during midstance, elongating hip abductors so they can develop additional force. The center of gravity migrates excessively toward the prosthetic limb during midstance as a result of this lateral pelvic shift, cumulatively increasing the energy cost of gait over the course of many walking steps.

Manual cues may again assist the patient who is new to transfemoral prosthetic use to learn how best to achieve appropriate pelvic control throughout the gait cycle. Standing behind the patient with manual contacts on the posterior and lateral pelvis as described previously, the therapist can guide and monitor pelvic motion in the transverse plane (forward rotation) as well as the frontal plane (for lateral shift). If the pelvis begins to drift laterally during midstance, the therapist has sufficient leverage to limit the abnormal motion and to cue the patient to activate muscles to prevent it. To accomplish this most effectively, the therapist applies pressure to the lateral pelvis in a downward, slightly medial and anterior direction. The therapist initially constrains or limits the degrees of freedom within which the pelvis can move and gradually withdraws the facilitation so that the patient assumes control of the pelvis in more dimensions over a larger percentage of the gait cycle.

For patients who have difficulty achieving or maintaining a level pelvis during midstance on the prosthetic side, the use of a straight cane on the side opposite the prosthesis may be helpful. In this case, the biomechanical goal is to produce an upward force on the side of the pelvis opposite the prosthesis (Figure 28-5). To achieve this, patients must create a reaction to the downward "cane on ground force." This reaction force, directed upward, acts through the arm and trunk to elevate the pelvis on the nonprosthetic side. This requires enough strength in the extremities and trunk to transmit force through the cane into the ground.

Instead of leaning their trunk toward the cane, patients should learn to push downward forcefully on the cane handle during prosthetic midstance. Patients should try to push their center of gravity away from the cane, toward the prosthetic stance limb. Although patients may prefer a quad cane, which allows them to take their hands off the handle without having the cane fall to the ground, the use of a straight cane prevents them from developing a habitual lateral lean or bearing weight diagonally through the cane's wide base. With a straight cane, patients must apply force straight downward, in the direction that supports the pelvis most efficiently. Because transfemoral prosthetic gait is energy intensive, patients cannot afford to apply upper extremity muscle force in any but the most efficient direction. A straight cane structures the walking task so that patients must use efficient and proper technique.

Stance Phase: Terminal Stance

In persons with intact lower extremities, activity in the hip flexors and ankle plantar flexors becomes eccentric as the body's mass moves forward over the stance foot. With the loss of the anatomic ankle and knee, stability of the prosthetic knee is influenced by two factors as the patient with transfemoral amputation moves into terminal stance. First, most prostheses are designed and aligned so that the weight line falls anterior to the knee joint axis after midstance. The resultant extensor moment partially counteracts the risk of buckling of the prosthetic knee during mid- to late stance. Second, most prosthetic foot-ankle assemblies have considerable intrinsic stiffness, which prevents the shank of the prosthesis from moving forward as long as direct body weight passes through the foot's solid keel portion. If the ankle mechanism permits some motion (e.g., a single-axis articulating ankle or a multiaxial prosthetic foot), it is usually stiff enough to slow or retard the shank's forward movement, preventing any tendency for the prosthetic knee to bend or buckle during midstance and terminal stance.

To take advantage of these properties, patients must learn to shift and sustain body weight on their prosthesis. The goal of gait training is for prosthetic and intact limb stance to be equal in duration, so that cadence has a regular rhythm and step lengths are approximately equal. Many patients have a tendency to walk with unequal step lengths, especially early in the rehabilitation process. This occurs because they take a relatively short step with the intact limb to shorten the duration of prosthetic stance. Sometimes, shortened prosthetic stance can be traced to weakness of the hip abductors and hip extensors in the residual limb. Because pain also leads the patient to limit prosthetic stance time, it is important to monitor socket fit and skin condition during early gait training. Contracture of muscles and soft tissue around the hip and pelvis that limits functional range of motion also contributes to premature ending of stance on the prosthesis.

Hip flexor tightness is the most common muscle imbalance experienced by those with transfemoral amputations. Hip flexor muscles must have sufficient length so that the prosthetic hip may extend during terminal stance. Shortened hip flexors restrict the prosthetic limb's excursion into hip extension, limiting the step length of the intact limb.

The hip flexor's capacity for elongation is compromised when these muscles remain in their shortened range for significant periods of time. Long periods of sitting or of lying in bed with the affected limb elevated increases the likelihood of problematic shortening as the hip flexors' resting length accommodates to these positions. The therapist can anticipate that many patients with transfemoral amputation will have shortness of hip flexors as they begin prosthetic gait training. Even in those who have diligently performed a program of preprosthetic exercise and stretching, such as daily prone lying and active, antigravity hip extensor strengthening, some hip flexor tightness is likely to develop.

Because transfemoral amputation sacrifices a large portion of hip adductor muscles and their distal attachments, patients are also likely to demonstrate muscle imbalances of the hip adductor and abductors.[15] Whereas in an intact limb hip adductors produce hip adduction and internal rotation, their relative absence in the transfemoral residual limb increases the likelihood of shortening (over time) in the muscles that produces hip abduction and external rotation. The resting length of the gluteus maximus shortens without opposing force (active or passive) of its adductor antagonists. A similar impact on the posterior portion of the gluteus medius occurs because orientation of its posterior fibers near the hip joint is similar to that of the gluteus maximus. For these reasons, many patients with transfemoral amputation demonstrate limitations or contractures in abduction and external rotation, as well as in hip flexion.

The effect of gluteus maximus shortening can be evident when a person sits. Many patients with transfemoral amputations increase their base of support in sitting when not wearing their prosthesis by abducting of their residual limb. If the gluteus maximus has shortened, the hip joint is even more likely to be abducted and externally rotated, and patients have difficulty in bringing their thighs together without changing trunk position by slumping or flexing the lumbar spine. This slumping and the accompanying posterior tilt of the pelvis extend the residual hip joint, affording some length to the gluteus maximus, thus allowing hip adduction to occur.

Gluteus maximus tightness also has an impact on the quality and efficiency of prosthetic gait. During terminal stance, the pelvis normally rotates forward on the side opposite the stance limb. This pelvic rotation is the key to the swinging limb's step length. Pelvic forward rotation in the swing limb produces internal rotation at the hip joint of the stance limb, elongating the gluteus maximus and other hip external rotators and increasing their passive tension. For patients with transfemoral amputation, a shortened gluteus maximus in the residual limb can hamper forward rotation of the pelvis of the swing

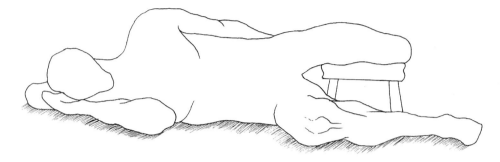

FIGURE 28-6

Active or isometric contraction of the medial residual limb against a low stool can counteract the tendency toward shortening of the gluteus maximus and address muscle strength imbalance between adductor and abductor muscle groups in the residual limb.

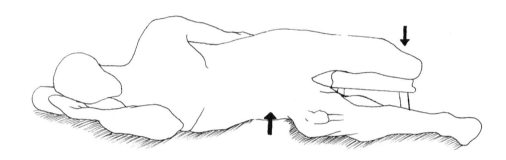

limb because of the passive resistance to internal rotation that develops in the shortened muscles.

Two gait problems are indicators of gluteus maximus shortening. First, the prosthetic foot may rotate externally during terminal stance. This is most obvious if patients have not borne their full body weight on the prosthesis or if they have begun to shift their weight away from the prosthesis very early in the stance phase. Second, the entire prosthesis may rotate inwardly on the residual limb over the course of several steps. This can occur even when patients bear their full weight on the prosthesis. If a shortened gluteus maximus produces enough passive tension to force the residual hip joint to rotate externally during terminal stance, the residual limb may itself rotate externally within the prosthetic socket. Patients and therapists regard this as a relative inward rotation of the socket on the residual limb. Over the course of several steps, the toe of the prosthetic foot points more and more medially as the patient walks. At the very least, this prosthetic alignment is not very cosmetic. If the in toeing is severe enough, it can alter the position of the prosthetic knee joint in space, such that the interaction of the ground reaction and inertial forces may no longer initiate knee flexion in preparation for swing phase. In addition, and perhaps of greater

concern, is the position of the socket on the residual limb. Internal rotation of the prosthetic socket moves its anterior brim medially, and because the medial brim is relatively high, this migration toward the sensitive groin region can cause discomfort during gait, resulting in other gait deviations to minimize discomfort during weight bearing of the stance phase.

Patients can avoid or reverse gluteal shortening by attempting to maintain strength in the residual hip adductor musculature. In one traditional exercise activity, the patient is positioned in side lying on the side opposite the amputation (i.e., residual limb on top) with the intact limb flexed at the hip and knee to create a stable base of support[7,14] (Figure 28-6). The residual limb is supported in an extended position on a low padded stool. The patient pushes the medial surface of the thigh downward into the stool, activating the residual adductor muscle mass against a considerable resistance. As strength improves and soft tissue lengthens, the pelvis may lift slightly from the surface on which the patient is lying. This exercise addresses the strength and length imbalance between the hip adductors and abductors. It can reverse the tendency toward hip abductor tightness by increasing strength in the hip adductors in a range of motion in which they are relatively short.

Transition from Stance to Swing Phase: Preswing

Preswing, which concludes the stance phase and transitions into the swing phase, is a period when many muscle groups are active throughout the trunk and extremities. The effectiveness of movement coordination during preswing determines the quality of movement during the prosthetic swing phase. Patients with transfemoral amputation must initiate flexion in the prosthetic knee joint during preswing so that the prosthesis' overall length shortens sufficiently in early swing to achieve enough toe clearance. If flexion of the prosthetic knee in preswing is inadequate, patients may drag the toe as the swing phase is initiated. The inadequate toe clearance that results from insufficient knee flexion is very dangerous, substantially increasing the likelihood of tripping or falling. Patients use a variety of movement strategies to compensate for inadequate knee flexion to advance the limb safely as the swing phase begins. They may choose to elevate the pelvis excessively on the side of the amputation (hip hiking) to clear the toes without having to flex the knee. Alternatively, they may circumduct the prosthesis away from midline to clear the toe as the limb advances. Finally, they may vault over the contralateral limb during stance, relatively shortening the prosthesis by rising onto the toes of the intact foot by active plantar flexion.

Patients' success in initiating preswing knee flexion depends on four factors: (1) their use of hip flexors, (2) their initiation of forward pelvic rotation, (3) the timing of heel rise, and (4) the way that they control the shifting of weight from the prosthesis to the nonamputated limb. In normal gait at comfortable walking speed, knee flexion is initiated by a combination of forward momentum, hip flexor activity, and limb unweighting, without activation of the hamstrings as knee flexors. The hip flexors are active to lift (pull off) the thigh as swing begins; this muscle activity is an important contributor of propulsive energy to the gait cycle.[16,17] To achieve this propulsive energy, patients who wear a transfemoral prosthesis must learn to activate the hip flexors forcefully inside the prosthetic socket as if they are kicking a ball with the front of the thigh. A rapid but brief concentric activation of these muscles accelerates the prosthesis' socket portion and, through reaction forces at the prosthetic knee, produces knee flexion. Indeed, studies of prosthetic gait patterns suggest that this strategy is an important source of propulsive energy for the walking pattern.[18]

Hip flexion, however strong, may not be enough by itself to flex the prosthetic knee and to initiate swing advancement of the prosthesis. Patients augment the effect of forceful hip flexion with simultaneous forward rotation of the pelvis on the side of the amputation. This forward movement of the pelvis influences the location and orientation of the ground reaction force, which is generated by body weight and inertial forces. Studies of prosthetic gait demonstrate that the ground reaction force vector inclines forward during preswing from its point of origin where the foot contacts the floor.[19] Forward pelvic rotation contributes to the vector's forward inclination, causing it to fall behind the knee joint and produce knee flexion.

Another important event that contributes to knee flexion in normal gait is heel rise, when the heel of the stance limb rises from the floor before preswing at approximately 35% of the gait cycle.[17] Heel rise occurs after the body weight has moved over the forefoot, as gradual dorsiflexion of the ankle, elongation of plantar flexor muscles, and locking of the subtalar joint have occurred.[20] The plantar flexors eventually develop enough passive force that further ankle dorsiflexion is blocked. When this occurs, the lower leg's continued advancement over the foot pulls the heel from the floor. Knee flexion occurs in a closed chain motion as elevation of the heel inclines the tibia forward.

The heel rise of a prosthetic foot is accomplished in a different manner because of the loss of anatomic dorsiflexors and plantar flexors. Most prosthetic ankles (whether in a nonarticulating or articulating prosthetic foot) resist dorsiflexion as body weight advances over the foot because of their mechanical stiffness. For an effective prosthetic heel rise, the ground reaction force must pass anterior to the keel of the prosthetic foot. The timing of this progression beyond the prosthetic keel is influenced by the alignment of the prostheses and the resulting length of the heel and toe levers. If the toe lever is too long, transition beyond the prosthetic keel is delayed, heel rise is late, and patients have difficulty in initiating knee flexion. Patients may report that it feels as if they are constantly walking uphill at the end of each stance phase. If the toe lever is too short and body weight passes anterior to the keel prematurely, an early heel rise and premature knee flexion occur. Patients may report a sense of instability or buckling of the knee, as if they have stepped into an unexpected hole. This can create a precarious situation (drop-off) in which midstance stability is prematurely compromised and a fall may occur.

An effective transfemoral prosthetic gait training program helps the patient to learn to take advantage of proper weight shift and posture during preswing. Initiation of knee flexion during this phase depends on a properly located ground reaction force. Patients must be comfortable and effective in shifting weight completely onto the prosthetic foot early in stance and in maintaining weight on the prosthetic foot through terminal stance into preswing. They must also learn to control the forward movement of their center of mass as it moves over the anterior edge of the prosthetic keel for effective heel rise and initiation of knee flexion in preswing.

Although shifting weight toward the prosthetic limb is a skill that can be accomplished easily, the ability to maintain that weight shift and to remove weight gradually is more challenging. One type of gait exercise that often helps refine these weight-shifting skills is a variety of crossover walking. In crossover walking, patients begin by balancing on the sound limb. They then step with the prosthetic limb, crossing it in front of the sound limb by simultaneously flexing and adducting the hip and rotating the pelvis forward on the prosthetic side. This activity facilitates the patient's ability to use stance limb hip abductor muscles as they control forward pelvic rotation on the prosthetic swing side. Therapists can manually guide the prosthetic-side pelvis through its requisite forward rotation. Patients must be diligent about maintaining an erect standing posture while performing this activity. The tendency to flex the trunk or hips can be minimized by having the patient stand near a wall, and place the hands lightly against it at shoulder height.

USING THE PROSTHESIS FOR ACTIVITIES OF DAILY LIVING

Much more is involved in prosthetic training than donning the prosthesis and developing sound gait habits when walking on level surfaces. In their home, work, and leisure environments, patients will be involved in many activities and will encounter a variety of anticipated and unexpected circumstances. They must manage stairs, curbs, ramps, and slippery or uneven surfaces. They must develop strategies to get up and down from a kneeling position or from lying on the floor. They must get up and down from furniture or car seats of different heights. They also must negotiate spaces that are confined (such as theater seating) or crowded with other people. To return to the lifestyle that they prefer, patients must develop confidence in the stability of their prosthesis and in their ability to use it effectively.

Fear of Falling and Rising from the Floor

Persons with transfemoral amputations often have an understandable fear of falling that can interfere with their becoming confident in walking on inclines, stairs, and uneven terrain. Some therapists advocate teaching patients with amputation how to fall to lessen their fearfulness.

Many patients with transfemoral amputation, however, are older adults who may have a number of interacting medical conditions. For some of these individuals, the actual practice of falling techniques may entail greater risks than rewards. Even a practice fall forward from kneeling, which requires patients to break the fall and absorb the shock of impact on slightly flexed elbows and shoulders and an extended wrist, carries the potential for ligamentous injury, especially at the wrist. An alternative backward fall management technique is to "jackknife" at the waist, landing on the buttocks and then rolling onto rounded back and shoulders.

Because falls are likely, especially in older patients, therapists who choose not to expose patients to the risks of practice falls must at least help them protect themselves should a fall occur. One of the safest responses when the patient has had an irrecoverable loss of balance is to bend at the waist to shift body weight toward the nonamputated side. This strategy lessens the likelihood of being injured by forces that the prosthesis produces if it twists or turns during the fall. This also protects the residual limb because the patient absorbs forces at impact on the intact hip and shoulder.

Many patients are more concerned about being stranded on the floor after a fall than about being injured in the fall itself. An effective strategy to reduce this source of fear of falling is to practice how to rise from the floor. Patients begin to build this skill by first learning how to get down on the floor from a seated or kneeling position while wearing their prosthesis. It is often helpful to demonstrate a possible movement strategy first and then to help patients adapt the strategy based on their individual needs and capabilities. Phrasing verbal cues as questions and using tactile cues to guide movement are helpful in the early stages of motor learning.[10] In the process of mastering this task, patients typically acquire a variety of movement skills that can be applied to other movement problems they may encounter. They learn, for instance, how to kneel on the prosthetic knee, how to arise from kneeling, and how to move between kneeling, side-sitting, and side-lying postures.

Moving into a Kneeling Position

To move from a standing (or seated) position to the floor, patients must first turn toward the piece of furniture that they will use to support their body weight as they descend. Patients shift body weight so that it is balanced between intact limb and their upper extremities leaning on the furniture. The next step is a controlled lowering of their center of mass as they begin to kneel on the prosthetic knee. To accomplish this, a rapid hip extension within the prosthesis moves it as far behind them as possible, and then flexion of the trunk and hip positions the prosthetic knee directly under the pelvis on the floor. Using the arms and hands to balance the upper body, patients then shift their body weight onto the prosthetic knee and move their intact limb into kneeling next to the prosthesis. They may now move into the quadruped or side-sitting position as a transition to sitting on the floor or practicing rising from kneeling.

Rising from Kneeling

For patients with poor endurance and for those whose learning is facilitated by practicing movement patterns in small sequences (part to whole practice), instruction on how to rise from kneeling can begin without descending all the way to a seated position. To prepare to get up, patients must momentarily support body weight between the furniture and the prosthetic knee. This unweights the intact limb so that the patient can reposition the foot flat on the floor by quickly flexing the hip and knee and moving the limb into a half-kneeling position. Next, leaning forward and supporting as much body weight as possible through the upper extremities, the patient extends the intact hip and knee, moving toward upright posture. Once the intact limb is extended enough to provide postural stability, the patient can flex the residual hip to move the prosthesis until the prosthetic foot is beside or slightly behind the intact foot. This ensures that the prosthetic knee is stable as weight is once more shared between the intact and prosthetic limb.

Patients who practice this technique next to a chair, even their own wheelchair, can use it to regain a sitting position if they should be on the floor for any reason, including a fall. Instead of rising all the way to erect stance, they can pivot as they rise to position their ischial tuberosity onto the seat of the chair or wheelchair. As long as patients can maneuver themselves to a piece of furniture and attain a kneeling posture, most can rise in this way without assistance.

To be fully confident that they can get up from the floor should a fall occur, patients must practice more than the transitions between kneeling and standing postures. It is helpful to provide the opportunity for them to practice transitioning between kneeling, quadruped, side-sitting, and supine positions as well.

Lying on the Floor from Standing or Kneeling

Once in a stable kneeling position using a piece of furniture for support and balance, patients are ready to practice getting all the way down to the floor. Most begin by moving the hand on the nonamputated side to a position on the floor that is approximately 12 in. lateral to and slightly in front of the intact knee. A gentle tap by the therapist on the patient's intact limb near the trochanter provides a kinesthetic cue to move into side sitting, resting on the lateral thigh and buttock on the intact limb. From this side-sitting position, controlled elbow flexion lowers the upper trunk until weight bearing occurs along the entire forearm. To complete the transition to the supine position, the patient uses eccentric horizontal adduction at the shoulder to ease into side lying and then rolls into supine.

Rising from the Floor

The easiest way for most patients with a transfemoral prosthesis to initiate rising from a supine or prone position on the floor is to roll into side lying on the body's sound side. Patients then transition into side sitting by flexing both hips and knees and pushing upward with the upper extremity to support their body weight on the forearm and then the hand.

From this side-sitting position with weight borne on the side opposite the prosthesis, patients can maneuver themselves close to the piece of furniture that they will use for support to complete the transition into kneeling and then into erect standing. When positioned next to the furniture, some patients are ready to pivot or swing the pelvis upward to move from side sitting into kneeling. Others may need to move into quadruped as an interim position, sharing some part of their body weight on each of the four extremities. Once the patient is balanced, a hand placed on the seat of the chair, sofa, or wheelchair provides support as the upper body moves into an erect posture and full kneeling (facing the furniture) is achieved. From kneeling, the intact limb is repositioned with the foot flat on the floor, and the transition from half-kneeling to standing is completed, as described previously.

RISING FROM AND SITTING ON FURNITURE

The strategy used to rise from a chair while wearing a transfemoral prosthesis is essentially the same as rising from sitting to standing without the prosthesis in place. The transfemoral prosthesis does not provide stability or assistance during transfers from sitting to standing: Patients must rely only on the intact limb, upper extremities, and, frequently, an assistive device to accomplish this transition.

Early in the rehabilitation process, patients usually prefer to sit in a chair with a seat that is 16–17 in. or more above the floor. They often choose a chair with armrests that they can use for support or balance as they stand and sit. Adequate seat height and firmness, as well as availability of stable armrests, make the task of rising from sitting considerably less taxing. Because most wheelchairs have these characteristics, many patients prefer their wheelchair to other lower and softer seating surfaces in their home (often to the consternation of family members). Simple modifications can make other seating surfaces more "patient-friendly" for transitions between sitting and standing. A wooden two-by-four, cut slightly wider than a kitchen or other household chair, and affixed to the chair's rear legs provides a wider, more stable base of support and raises the chair to make rising less of a challenge. A raised toilet seat may be helpful in the bathroom, and an additional firm foam pad or cushion can be used to elevate the seating surface of a favorite easy chair.

In preparing to stand, patients must first move the pelvis toward the front edge of the seating surface. A visual cue that patients (who wear pants) may find helpful is to move forward until they can no longer see the seat's surface between their thighs; in this position, the ischial tuberosities are resting firmly on the seat. Next, patients must reposition the sound foot by flexing the knee to slide the foot as far under the seat as possible. This positions the foot on the floor close to the vertical projection of the body's center of gravity, so that patients can reach a stable standing posture with a relatively small forward shift in their body weight.

Patients who use a walker for balance during ambulation can place it in front of them as they prepare to rise from a chair. To ensure safety, patients should push with one or both upper extremities from the armrest or seat surface as they stand rather than pull on the walker or other assistive device. Many find the task easiest if one hand is on the armrest (or edge of the bed or mat table) and the other presses directly downward on the walker. If both hands are erroneously placed on the walker, the patient sacrifices stability and control as body weight shifts during the transition to standing; in many instances, the walker tips and the patient falls back into a seated position.

Patients usually do not need advice about which hand to place on the walker and which to leave on the seat surface; trial and error help them to discover a hand placement strategy that is most effective. The relative height of the chair's armrests may influence their decision. Some patients find it helpful to rotate the upper body slightly toward the intact lower extremity to better position that arm to push against the seat surface. If a patient is struggling to discover an effective strategy, the biomechanical aspects of unilateral assistive device use may provide a model for problem solving how best to use the upper extremities when rising from a seated position. Most

patients hold an assistive device, such as a straight cane, in the hand opposite the lower extremity that they wish to assist. Because the prosthesis cannot support body weight during the transition from sitting to standing, the intact limb is the one that requires assistance. For this reason, many find that placing the upper extremity on the side of the residual limb on a stable surface is an effective strategy to help rise successfully from the chair, sofa, or toilet seat.

In addition to discovering which hand placements work best, each patient can experiment with different preparatory postures for seating surfaces that they may encounter, varying their pelvic and trunk postures as well. The common factor in rising from any surface, however, is the forward trunk lean and hip flexion that are necessary to move body weight over the intact foot as the individual prepares to stand. The patient then uses a combination of hip and knee extension in the nonamputated limb, extension of the head and trunk, and upper extremity support to move toward an erect standing posture. Once nearly erect, the patient can use the prosthesis to assist balance if it is positioned directly under the body. Once fully erect with the prosthetic knee in extension, the patient can shift body weight onto the prosthesis.

To sit on a chair, sofa, bed, toilet, or other seating surface, patients with transfemoral amputation learn to reverse the sequence used in standing. The safest way to begin to sit is to make sure that the seating surface is directly behind the patient with the prosthetic foot slightly in front of the intact foot. The patient then shifts body weight onto the intact nonamputated extremity to control the descent effectively into sitting by eccentric contraction of the muscles in the sound limb. Unweighting of the prosthesis also permits unlocking of any stance control mechanism on the prosthetic knee joint. Once weight has been shifted off of the prosthesis, patients who use a locked prosthetic knee joint can manually unlock the knee or move the prosthetic foot forward so that it does not interfere with the ability to lower the body. Before sitting, patients must use one hand to reach for and establish contact with the surface where they will sit, while maintaining the other hand on an assistive device. Many patients feel safer and more comfortable if they turn slightly toward the nonamputated side, reaching for the seat surface with the hand on that side of the body.

Therapists must know the characteristics of the patient's prosthetic knee. Some of the most recently developed knee mechanisms lock the knee during midstance and do not unlock unless some body weight is present on the prosthetic toe. Although these knee mechanisms offer several benefits for safety and quality of gait, they may present a challenge to patients as they unlock the knee to sit. A lateral weight shift away from the prosthesis cannot unlock the knee unit, as it would a standard weight-activated friction knee. Instead, patients must maintain a portion of their body weight on the prosthesis and additionally move that weight to the prosthetic toe. Because the knee quickly flexes once it is unlocked, patients must be ready to respond with the intact lower extremity to control the speed and path of descent into sitting.

While patients experiment to learn the most effective and appropriate way to shift their weight and unlock these newer knee units, therapists can help them to discover a pattern that is natural or cosmetic in appearance. The patient prepares to sit by backing up to the chair and then turns slightly toward the nonamputated side, as if to face the chair. While reaching for the armrest or seat with the hand opposite the prosthesis, the patient uses a forward rotation of the pelvis (which complements the movement of the upper body and shoulder girdle) to shift some weight forward onto the prosthetic toe. With practice, patients can learn to time their pelvic rotation so that their weight reaches the prosthetic toe just as their hand reaches the chair. This unlocks the knee joint when they are prepared to control the sitting motion with the muscles of their nonamputated limb and the support of their upper extremity.

MANAGING CURBS AND STAIRS

The majority of patients who are using a transfemoral prosthesis negotiate stairs in a step up–to–step strategy; few develop the strength and coordination that are necessary to control the prosthetic knee joint for a step-over-step pattern like the one that they used before amputation. The safest and most effective strategy for ascending and descending stairs is the time-honored dictum, "up with the good and down with the bad." To ascend, the patient shifts weight onto the prothesis and then steps up to the next level with the intact limb. Leaning forward and using handrails if necessary, the patient then extends the hip and knee to lift the body up over the intact limb. Finally, the patient lifts and positions the prosthesis on the step to begin the cycle once again. To descend, weight is shifted off the prosthesis, and an eccentric contraction of muscles of the intact limb controls lowering of the center of mass as the prosthesis is placed on the step below. Once the prosthesis is safely positioned to accept body weight, patients may step down to the same step with the intact limb.

Most patients who must routinely manage stairs to enter or move between floors in their home or work environment benefit from the installation of a sturdy handrail. Most often, the handrail is placed so that it is on the side of the amputated limb as the patient ascends the stairs:

Patients who wear a prosthesis on the right benefit most from a handrail to the right of the stairs as they ascend. Many patients are able to ascend using only the handrail (without an additional assistive device) if they ascend the stairs facing the handrail. With the patient placing both hands on the handrail for support, the nonamputated limb is placed "uphill" of the prosthesis; weight is shifted up and over that limb. Elevation of the pelvis lifts the prosthesis onto the same stair, next to the intact limb, and the cycle is repeated. To descend, patients learn to face the handrail once again with their prosthetic limb moving "downhill" first onto the step below. Once the prosthesis is safely positioned and weight is shifted onto it, the intact limb steps down as well and the cycle is repeated. One of the benefits of this sidestepping technique is that the patient's center of pressure falls consistently through the middle of the prosthetic foot. As a result, the ground reaction force passes far enough in front of the prosthetic knee unit to ensure stability in standing. Patients who descend stairs in this manner can shift their weight to this very stable prosthesis and move the sound limb with confidence onto the stair next to the prosthetic foot. During initial training with this method of stair management, a therapist's manual contact is reassuring and effective in providing tactile cues as patients experiment to find their most comfortable foot placements. Depending on the stairs' dimensions, especially their depth, patients must plan to leave space for the nonamputated limb as they step and position the prosthesis.

Not all environments that the patient encounters have a handrail strategically placed on the appropriate side for this sidestepping stair-climbing technique. It is also important for the patient to learn to negotiate stairs using an assistive device. The safest assistive device for stair climbing for patients who are using a transfemoral prosthesis is a simple straight cane. Although there are techniques for use of a walker placed sideways on a set of stairs, the walker's stability depends on whether sufficient downward force is exerted on the uphill handle. Patients must be able to direct this force so that its line of application falls within the walker's base of support. Although patients may perfect this technique in a controlled situation, such as on the practice stairs in the physical therapy clinic, the same technique used on a flight of stairs with different dimensions may be disastrous. When the pitch or dimensions of a staircase are different, the patient's walker-based stair-climbing strategy may produce forces that fall outside the walker's base of support; the walker topples, and a fall is the likely outcome.

With practice, most patients become comfortable and adept at using a straight cane to accompany their prosthesis as they negotiate stairs. When ascending a step or curb, patients learn to stabilize the prosthetic limb by extending the hip joint within the prosthetic socket in preparation for stepping up with the nonamputated limb. The cane, held in the hand opposite the prosthesis, remains on the same step as the prosthesis. Once body weight is lifted up and over the sound limb on the step above, the prosthesis and (finally) the cane are also moved up to that step and the cycle is repeated.

To descend a step or curb safely, the cane is first placed on the downhill step to prepare for movement of the prosthesis. Then, using the nonamputated limb muscles eccentrically, the patient lowers the pelvis to place the prosthesis on the same downhill step. Patients who wear a transfemoral prosthesis must ensure the prosthetic knee joint is stable by extending the residual hip joint within the prosthetic socket before they bring the nonamputated limb down to this step.

Therapists should reinforce the benefits of maintaining an erect posture as patients shift weight onto the prosthesis during stair descent. When standing in erect posture, the patient's ground reaction force moves forward so that it extends the prosthetic knee. If, however, a patient "sits back," letting the residual hip flex and the pelvis move backward in preparation for stepping down with the nonamputated limb, the ground reaction moves posteriorly, creating a flexion moment at the prosthetic knee unit. Ideally, patients should stand in an erect posture and allow the pelvis to rotate forward so that it "follows" their prosthesis to the step below.

Some patients with transfemoral amputation learn to descend stairs in a step-over-step pattern; most of them are very strong, quite skilled with their prosthesis, and rather brave. The step-over-step strategy is a modification of the basic step-to-step technique. When patients begin the sequence by placing their prosthesis on the downhill step, they carefully position the heel of the prosthetic foot close to the edge of the step so that the prosthetic toes overhang slightly. Without anterior support of the prosthetic forefoot, the prosthetic shank does not incline far enough forward to load the forefoot and flex the prosthetic knee. Patients must compensate for this lack of anterior support by extending the residual hip very forcefully inside the prosthetic socket to ensure that the prosthetic knee remains in extension. As weight is shifted onto the prosthesis, the intact limb is advanced beyond the step's edge. At this point, the patient relaxes the extension of the residual limb in the prosthesis (or may even flex the hip slightly), which allows the prosthetic knee to "jackknife" in a quick flexion so that the sound limb can land on the step below. Patients must then flex the residual limb within the socket with sufficient force to swing the prosthesis forward and place the prosthetic heel on the edge of the next lowest stair; they then repeat the process.

Ascent of stairs in a step-over-step pattern is rarely possible for patients with a transfemoral prosthesis. It requires tremendous muscle strength and endurance in the residual limb and upper body to propel the body's center of mass up and over a prosthesis placed on an uphill step in a position of hip and knee flexion. Some athletic and determined individuals may be able to do this if a set of handrails is available. To be successful in lifting the body over the prosthesis, patients must activate the residual gluteal muscles to develop a hip extensor moment that is sufficient to extend the joint, and, in a closed chain, the prosthetic knee unit. Even patients whose long transfemoral residual limbs provide advantageous leverage still find this very difficult. This activity, performed in a controlled environment, might be a reasonable training technique for patients who wish to improve coordination and timing as well as the strength of their residual musculature. The energy requirements of a step-over-step ascent are so substantial that this technique is rarely used in routine daily activities.

MANAGING INCLINES, SLOPES, RAMPS, AND UNEVEN TERRAIN

In the discussion of strategies to manage stairs, we discovered that stability of the prosthetic knee is influenced by the position of the ground reaction force. When this force passes behind the prosthetic knee, a flexor moment results and knee stability is compromised. When this force passes anterior to the prosthetic knee, the resulting extension moment makes knee flexion difficult. The inclination of the prosthetic shank has a similar impact: Forward inclination enhances knee flexion, whereas backward inclination enhances knee extension. Ascending a ramp, hill, or other uneven surfaces with an upward slope causes the prosthetic shank to lean backward or posteriorly, creating an extensor moment at the prosthetic knee and slowing forward progress. Patients find themselves able to take only short steps with the prosthetic limb and may feel unpleasantly at risk of sliding or falling backward down the incline.

Patients can use several strategies to ascend a ramp or incline. One is to extend the residual hip more forcefully, pressing the residual thigh into the socket's posterior wall. Another is to lean forward slightly with the trunk to overcome the angle of the incline. Patients with very short residual limbs or very weak hip musculature, however, may not be able to generate enough force to be successful with these strategies.

Another alternative is to adapt stair-climbing techniques and ascend inclines on a diagonal, leading with the nonamputated side. On extremely steep inclines, patients may need to sidestep, placing the nonamputated limb uphill of the prosthetic limb. More modest slopes can be effectively ascended by a partial turn toward the side of prosthesis. This angled orientation is advantageous because the intact limb is positioned ahead of the prosthetic limb, requiring less hip flexion and allowing the patient to compensate for the inability to dorsiflex the prosthetic ankle. Patients are able to take more symmetric steps with either limb without encountering difficulty in shifting weight up and over the prosthesis.

Descending inclines or ramps present a different problem: As the anterior part of the prosthetic foot contacts the downward sloping surface, the prosthetic shank inclines forward and the prosthetic knee is likely to buckle into flexion. Patients may not be confident that they can effectively use their hip extensors to overcome this knee flexion and may hesitate to commit their weight to the prosthesis. By leading with the prosthesis, placing it ahead of the sound limb in the same way that they descend stairs, patients can grade their weight shift onto the prosthesis, feel more stable, and gain confidence.

With practice on ramps and other inclining surfaces, patients learn to anticipate and appropriately time the strong hip extensor action that is necessary to extend the prosthetic knee in closed chain tasks. Those with weak hip muscles or short residual limbs can compensate for their difficulty in generating sufficient muscle force by turning sideways toward the intact limb as they descend slopes. This orientation permits the prosthesis to lead more easily, eliminating the tendency for the prosthetic toe to drop, the shank to incline, and the knee to flex. On extremely steep inclines, patients can choose to truly sidestep, leading with the prosthesis, or they can descend by taking a series of very short steps.

Patients also must develop skill and confidence in negotiating uneven or unpredictable surfaces and in avoiding obstacles or unsafe walking surfaces by stepping around or over them. Most learn to step over small holes, bumps, or objects in their path as if they were a curb or step that they must ascend. Using this approach, patients can face the obstacle over which they wish to step with the prosthetic foot positioned slightly behind the sound foot. This foot position produces a ground reaction force that falls in front of the prosthetic knee, stabilizing it in extension. As long weight is shifted onto the prosthesis, this stable alignment assists patients in maintaining control and balance as they step over the object with the sound limb. Once the sound limb contacts the ground after stepping over the object, patients learn to flex the residual hip forcefully inside the prosthetic socket to whip the prosthesis forward over the obstacle.

Patients may hesitate to use technique if the ground is sloped or if they do not trust their ability to stabilize their prosthetic knee as they bear full weight on the prosthesis. An alternative is to move over an obstacle in a less direct manner by modifying the sidestepping pattern that is used on ramps or inclines. During advanced gait training, patients practice by approaching the obstacle sideways with the nonamputated limb nearest it. Shifting their body weight onto the prosthesis once again, they flex the sound hip, swinging the sound limb forward and over the obstacle. After shifting weight to the sound limb (now on the other side of the obstacle), quick hip flexion swings the prosthesis up and over the obstacle. With experience, patients can pivot on the sound limb as they bring the prosthesis over the obstacle. They can then swing the prosthesis through, stepping onto it in a continuous motion as they move away from the obstacle.

PICKING UP OBJECTS FROM THE FLOOR

Another activity of daily living that requires practice is the ability to pick an object up from the floor when wearing a prosthesis. Patients with amputation, like other individuals, find it frustrating if they have to ask for assistance to retrieve something from the floor. One strategy that permits them to do so involves first shifting body weight to the sound limb and taking a step backward with the prosthesis. If the prosthetic foot is placed slightly behind the sound foot and weight is then distributed over both extremities, the resulting ground reaction forces stabilize the prosthetic knee in extension. From this stable prosthetic position, patients flex the sound hip and knee and bend forward at the waist to reach for the object that they intend to pick up.

Picking up an object in this manner requires considerable knee and hip strength in the sound limb. For those with less strength, an alternative strategy is to use the skills learned in kneeling to get up and down from the floor. Some individuals can kneel without upper extremity assistance, but most prefer to use a piece of furniture for support and balance. In either case, they balance on the sound limb and then extend the residual hip quickly within the prosthetic socket to place the prosthesis as far behind them as possible. By flexing the trunk and the sound hip and knee, they then lower the prosthetic knee joint gently to the floor. Once it is down, weight can be shifted between both limbs in a half-kneeling position and the object can be retrieved. To return to standing, the patient must shift the center of mass over the sound limb by leaning the trunk toward that side and extending the hip and knee to rise into standing.

MOVING QUICKLY AND RUNNING

Most patients learn to move quickly using a skipping motion rather than by running in the familiar step-over-step pattern. This movement, familiar from childhood games, involves taking two steps (actually hops) on the sound limb for each step with the prosthesis. The extra step is necessary because most non–cadence-responsive prosthetic knee units are designed to swing the shank forward at a comfortable gait speed, not at running speed. The extra step gives the prosthesis time to swing through and be in a position to accept the patient's weight when it touches the ground. To begin this modified running, the first step is taken with the sound limb. Once body weight has been transferred completely to that limb, patients take a forward hop on the sound and, simultaneously, begin to swing the prosthesis forward with quick and forceful residual hip flexion. They "land" on the prosthesis when its knee is fully extended. Body weight is momentarily supported on the prosthesis and then is quickly transferred to the sound limb, and the sequence begins again.

Athletic patients who wear prostheses with knee units that are designed to be cadence responsive can learn to run in a step-over-step pattern. In cadence-responsive knee units, the rate of forward swing of the prosthetic shank is determined by the patient's current gait speed: As gait speed increases, so does the rate of forward swing of the prosthetic shank. Running in a step-over-step pattern is an advanced gait skill.

DEFINITIVE PROSTHESIS

Patients with transfemoral amputation may wear their training prosthesis from 3 to 6 months, until the volume of their residual limb has stabilized. During this time, the limb's volume decreases gradually and may even fluctuate from day to day or between morning and afternoon during a single day. Patients learn to add or subtract prosthetic socks to maintain a proper fit between socket and residual limb. When the patient reports wearing a consistent number of prosthetic socks over a period of several weeks, it may be time to consider transition to the definitive or permanent prosthesis.

One of the major advantages of the definitive prosthesis is its improved appearance; a cosmetic cover conceals the pylon, knee unit, and other prosthetic hardware, which had to be accessible for adjustments in alignment to be accomplished in the temporary prosthesis. Another advantage is a significant improvement in socket fit because the definitive socket is designed specifically for the mature shape of the residual limb. The fit in the tem-

porary socket is likely to have become less and less intimate as the shape of the residual limb changed over time. In many instances, the definitive prosthesis is also lighter in weight (and therefore more energy efficient) than the temporary prosthesis, as adjustable components of a temporary prosthesis are replaced with lighter or more streamlined components. However, if patients choose certain components (such as a hydraulic knee unit) or cosmetic finishes for their definitive prosthesis, the difference in weight may be negligible.

Only if the volume of the residual limb has stabilized is fabrication of the definitive prosthesis advantageous to the patient. The therapist and patient must use the opportunity to improve strength and range of motion and to develop motor skills and gait quality while wearing the training prosthesis so that the transition to a definitive prosthesis proceeds smoothly.

REHABILITATION OF PERSONS WITH BILATERAL AMPUTATION

Patients with vascular insufficiency rarely require bilateral transfemoral amputations unless their disease is very advanced. These patients may have had a previous unilateral amputation, been successful prosthetic users, and subsequently required amputation of the other limb. It is also likely that patients who have lost their limbs because of vascular disease have some degree of compromised cardiac function. Any patients who had been walking in the period just before amputation, including those with bilateral transfemoral amputation, should be considered candidates for prosthetic rehabilitation. Patients with bilateral transfemoral amputation are most successful if their training prostheses are foreshortened or stubby prostheses (Figure 28-7). These special transfemoral prostheses have no knee unit and a modified prosthetic foot with a posterior extension. This gives the patient an opportunity to learn to balance the trunk over the prostheses without having to worry about controlling the prosthetic knee. The limbs are constructed with posterior socket brims that rest approximately ½ to 1 in. higher than the seat of the wheelchair. The patient is then able to step directly into these sockets from the wheelchair (using the upper extremities to support body weight) and "stand" while adjusting the suspension device. Upper extremity strength is necessary to resuming a sitting position, as the patient performs a "wheelchair pushup" to lift the pelvis onto the seat. This can occur with the prostheses still in place or after loosening the suspension to doff the prostheses as the patient returns to sitting. Although traditional prostheses may be more cosmetic, because they permit patients to be near their preamputation height, most patients with bilateral transfemoral amputations cannot stand in them without significant assistance.

SUMMARY

Many patients with transfemoral amputation have the potential to ambulate with a prosthesis, depending on their health and preamputation functional status. For successful prosthetic rehabilitation, patients must learn to don and doff the prosthesis, using the appropriate sock ply to ensure an intimate fit within the socket. They must have ample opportunity to practice and become confident in weight shifting onto the prosthesis and to learn to control the prosthetic knee using a combination of muscle action of the residual hip, and prosthetic and body alignment. Patients with transfemoral amputation often must deal with strength and length imbalances in the muscle groups of the residual limb: Muscle strength and endurance, joint excursion, and soft tissue flexibility are key ingredients for functional prosthetic use. The primary goal of rehabilitation is to help the patient walk with the prosthesis in a gait pattern that is energy efficient and cosmetic, using the least cumbersome assistive device possible. In addition to walking and changing direction on a variety of level surfaces, patients need the opportunity to discover how best to manage uneven terrain, crowded environments, stairs, and ramps and inclines. Because the risk of falling, although real, can lead to a disabling fear of falling, the opportunity to practice getting down to and rising from the floor can be empowering for patients with transfemoral amputation. Successful rehabilitation not only helps the patient develop the skills and abilities necessary to work, self care, and leisure activities, it also enhances the quality of life and is tremendously rewarding.

REFERENCES

1. Moore TJ, Barron J, Hutchinson F, et al. Prosthetic usage following major lower extremity amputation. Clin Orthop 1989;238(Jan):219–224.
2. Pinzur MS, Littooy F, Daniels J, et al. Multidisciplinary preoperative assessment and late function in dysvascular amputees. Clin Orthop 1992;281(Aug):239–243.
3. Penington G, Warmington S, Hull S, Freijah N. Rehabilitation of lower limb amputees and some implications for surgical management. Aust NZ J Surg 1992;62(10):774–779.

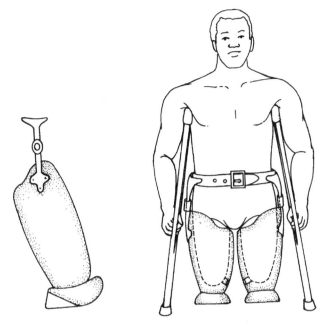

FIGURE 28-7

Diagram of a pair of foreshortened prostheses, sometimes called stubbies, for early gait training for patients with bilateral transfemoral amputation. In these prostheses, patients can develop postural control without having to worry about the stability of prosthetic knee units. (Reprinted with permission from BJ May. Assessment and Treatment of Individuals following Lower Extremity Amputation. In SB O'Sullivan, TJ Schmitz [eds], Physical Rehabilitation: Assessment and Treatment [3rd ed]. Philadelphia: Davis, 1994;392.)

4. Lower Limb Prosthetics for Therapists (course manual). Chicago, IL: Northwestern University Medical School Prosthetics-Orthotics Center, 1989.
5. Schmidt TJ. Pre-ambulation and Gait Training. In SB O'Sullivan, TJ Schmitz (eds), Physical Rehabilitation: Assessment and Treatment (3rd ed). Philadelphia: Davis, 1994;251–276.
6. May BJ. Assessment and Treatment of Individuals following Lower Extremity Amputation. In SB O'Sullivan, TJ Schmitz (eds), Physical Rehabilitation: Assessment and Treatment (3rd ed). Philadelphia: Davis, 1994;375–396.
7. Gailey RS, Garley AM. Prosthetic Gait Training Program for Lower Extremity Amputees. Miami, FL: Ther Ed Resource, 1999.
8. Shumway-Cook A, Woollacott M. Motor Learning and Recovery of Function. In Motor Control: Theory and Practical Application. Baltimore: Williams & Wilkins, 1995;23–43.
9. Winstein CJ, Gardner ER, McNeal DR, et al. Standing balance training: effect on balance and locomotion in hemiparetic adults. Arch Phys Med Rehabil 1989;70(10):755–762.
10. Schmidt RA. Motor Learning Principles for Physical Therapy. In Contemporary Management of Motor Control Problems: Proceedings of the II-STEP Conference. Alexandria, VA: Foundation for Physical Therapy, 1991;49–64.

11. Winstein CJ. Designing Practice for Motor Learning: Clinical Implications. In Contemporary Management of Motor Control Problems: Proceedings of the II-STEP Conference. Alexandria, VA: Foundation for Physical Therapy, 1991;65–76.

12. May BJ. Lower Extremity Prosthetic Management. In Amputations and Prosthetics: A Case Study Approach. Philadelphia: Davis, 1996;139–185.

13. Saunders JB, Inman VT, Eberhart HD. The major determinants in normal and pathological gait. J Bone Joint Surg 1953;35:543–558.

14. Eisert O, Tester OW. Dynamic exercises for lower extremity amputees. Arch Phys Med Rehabil 1954;35(11):695–704.

15. Gottschalk FA, Kourosh S, Stills M. Does socket configuration influence the position of the femur in above knee amputation? J Prosthet Orthot 1990;2(1):94–102.

16. Perry J. Gait Analysis; Normal and Pathological Function. Thorofare, NJ: Slack, 1992.

17. Inman VT, Ralston HJ, Todd F. Human Walking. Baltimore: Williams & Wilkins, 1981.

18. Winter DA, Sienko SE. Biomechanics of below-knee amputee gait. J Biomech 1988;21(5):361–367.

19. Cerny K. Pathomechanics of stance: clinical concepts for analysis. Phys Ther 1984;64(12):1851–1859.

20. McPoil TG. The Foot and Ankle. In TR Malone, TG McPoil, AJ Nitz (eds), Orthopedic and Sports Physical Therapy (3rd ed). St. Louis: Mosby, 1997;259–293.

29

Prosthetic Options for High-Level and Bilateral Amputation

JOHN W. MICHAEL

Although relatively uncommon in the developed world, high-level and bilateral lower limb amputations present unique rehabilitation challenges. It is obvious that such a significant limb loss presents a substantial challenge to the person with amputation, to the prosthetist, and to other rehabilitation professionals. While successful prosthesis fitting is often time-consuming and difficult, there is clear evidence that, for many individuals with high or bilateral amputation, prostheses can serve a useful purpose by increasing functional independence and mobility. This chapter summarizes key concepts from the clinical and research literature, so that we all may learn from the collective experience of our predecessors.

HIGH-LEVEL LOWER LIMB LOSS

The first part of this chapter focuses on options for patients with a unilateral high-level limb absence; an amputation at or above the hip joint. It has been estimated that hip disarticulation, transpelvic, and translumbar losses comprise less than 2% of all amputations in the United States.[1] As a result, only those clinicians associated with specialty centers, such as major trauma hospitals, have the opportunity to see significant numbers of such cases. Most prosthetists, therapists, and physicians see only a handful of people with such high-level loss in a practice lifetime. One result of treating each individual high-level amputee as "one of a kind" is that many differing approaches can be found in the literature.

Etiology

Although vascular impairment and neuropathy, whether or not they are associated with diabetes mellitus, are the most common causes for all lower limb loss in the devel-oped world, these risk factors rarely lead to high-level amputation.[2] Dysvascular and neuropathic symptoms are generally most pronounced in the distal (peripheral) limb, leading to non-healing ulceration, infection, gangrene, and ablation. Usually, the trunk and a portion of the upper thigh is spared even in the presence of severe peripheral vascular disease. The assumptions about healing, cardiovascular limitations, and tolerance of activity derived from our experience with patients with dysvascular amputation do not apply to those with high-level amputation. A very large percentage of the population with high-level amputation is healthy, has reasonable cardiopulmonary reserves, excellent cognition, and a strong desire to attempt prosthetic fitting. Most patients with hip disarticulation or other high-level amputation should be offered the opportunity for prosthetic fitting and rehabilitation.

Many high-level amputations are performed when there is a tumor, such as osteosarcoma, in the femur, although the frequency of tumor-related high-level amputation is decreasing with advances in limb salvage procedures and more effective chemotherapy and radiation therapy. Patients who require amputation secondary to tumor can be divided into two groups: those with benign or fully contained tumors who require no further oncological intervention, and those undergoing chemotherapy and/or radiation after amputation. Those with benign or fully contained tumors are typically in excellent physical condition after the amputation, eager to return to their former lifestyle as much as possible, and are ready for early prosthetic fitting. The benefits of early prosthetic fitting are well established, and include both physical and psychological benefits for the patient with amputation.[3] Early mobilization and single-limb gait training on the contralateral limb with an appropriate assistive device is recommended to reduce the risk of deconditioning, which occurs even after a few days of hospitalization.[4] The rehabilitation and prosthetic

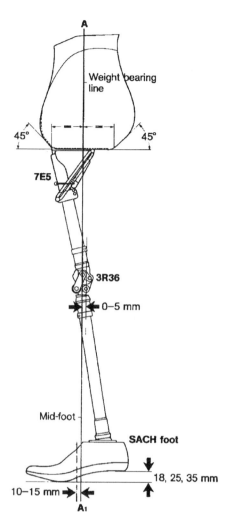

FIGURE 29-1

Static balance with a high-level lower limb prosthesis is achieved when the ground reaction force passes behind the hip joint and in front of the knee and ankle joints. The resulting extensor moments at the hip and knee, and dorsiflexion moment at the ankle make the prosthesis stable. Mechanical stops in the prosthetic joints prevent further movement, and the patient is able to stand without exertion. SACH = solid-ankle cushion-heel. (Courtesy of Otto Bock Orthopedic Industry, Inc, Minneapolis, MN.)

management of patients requiring chemotherapy or radiation therapy may have to be adapted or delayed, depending on the patient's physical condition, energy level, tolerance of activity, and healing of the surgical site.

Biomechanics

Although historically it was assumed that the loss of the entire lower limb would require the use of locked joints

in the prosthesis, there is now ample clinical evidence that locked prosthetic joints are seldom necessary. Since the 1950s, free motion hip, knee, and ankle joints for hip disarticulation and transpelvic prostheses have become the norm. The "Canadian design" hip disarticulation prosthesis was introduced by Colin McLaurin,[5] and the biomechanics of this prosthesis were clarified by Radcliffe in 1957.[6] These same biomechanical principles are also used in the functional design of prostheses for patients with higher level amputation,

In essence, the high-level prosthesis is stabilized by the ground reaction force (GRF), which occurs during walking. For example, when standing quietly in the prosthesis, the person's weight-bearing line falls posterior to the hip joint, anterior to the knee joint, and anterior to the ankle joint. The resultant hip and knee extension moments are resisted by mechanical hyperextension stops of the prosthetic hip and knee joints, while the dorsiflexion moment is resisted by the stiffness of the prosthetic foot (Figure 29-1). This is precisely the same principle that permits the person with paraplegia using bilateral Scott-Craig knee-ankle-foot-orthoses (KAFOs) to stand without external support.[7]

Ambulation with a high-level prosthesis also relies on the GRF (Figure 29-2). When an experienced prosthetic wearer walks with an optimally aligned hip disarticulation or transpelvic prosthesis, the dynamic gait is suprisingly smooth and consistent. Patients with hip disarticulation or transpelvic amputations who have sufficient balance and strength can learn to walk without any external aids, although the use of a single cane is also common.

The basic functions of the GRF during ambulation with one type of high-level prosthesis can be summarized as follows. At initial contact, as the prosthetic heel touches the ground, the GRF passes posterior to the ankle axis, the heel cushion compresses and the foot is lowered to the ground. At the same time, an extension moment is created at the prosthetic knee as the GRF passes anterior to the knee joint axis (Figure 29-2A). By midstance, alignment stability is maximal as the GRF now passes posterior to the prosthetic hip joint axis and anterior to the prosthetic knee joint axis, just as it does during quiet standing (Figure 29-2B). As forward progression continues into preswing, the GRF moves posterior to the knee joint axis, allowing the knee to passively bend to facilitate swing phase foot clearance, while weight is being shifted onto the opposite limb (Figure 29-2C).

There are, however, two major biomechanical deficits inherent with hip disarticulation and transpelvic prostheses that should be noted. First, the prosthetic limb is always fully extended at midswing due to the loss of active hip flexion. As a result, the prosthesis must be slightly short to assist

FIGURE 29-2

*The ground reaction force (GRF) at initial contact. (**A**), from loading response through midstance and terminal stance (**B**), and just prior to preswing (**C**) of the gait cycle for patients using a unilateral high-level prosthesis. Once properly aligned, the prosthesis will move in a consistent, predictable fashion and permit slow but steady ambulation. The patient uses trunk motion to initiate and control prosthetic movements. (Reprinted with permission from T Van der Waarde, JW Michael. Hip Disarticulation and Transpelvic Management: Prosthetic Considerations. In JH Bowker, JW Michael [eds], Atlas of Limb Prosthetics: Surgical, Prosthetic, and Rehabilitation Principles [2nd ed]. St. Louis: Mosby–Year Book, 1992;539–552.)*

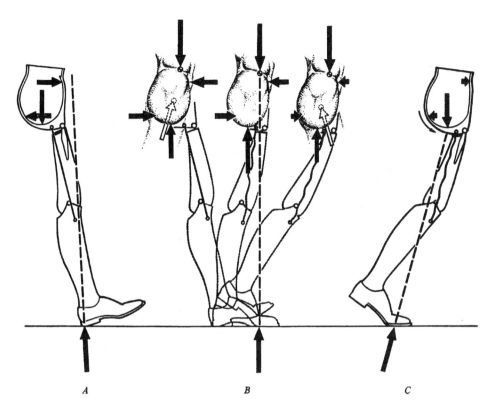

A   B   C

in toe clearance during swing phase of gait, creating the second biomechanical deficit: a limb length discrepancy.[8]

Component Selection

The earliest hip disarticulation prosthesis designers insisted on locking all prosthetic joints. Later, proponents of free axis joints for hip disarticulation prostheses advocated the use of only basic components, such as a single-axis knee and ankle. In recent years, a strong consensus has emerged that components for patients with hip disarticulation and transpelvic amputations should be selected for the same reasons and with the same criteria as for those with transfemoral and transtibial amputation: to fully meet the patient's functional needs and goals.[9] The majority of patients benefit from a free motion hip joint, although locking joints are still sometimes chosen for those with very limited ambulation capabilities.

The prosthetist selects a particular knee unit based on the patient's functional needs. When stability is a primary concern, stance control or polycentric knees may be most appropriate. Single-axis knees, when properly aligned, also work well. The prosthetist might choose a pneumatic or hydraulic knee unit to provide fluid swing phase control for patients who are active and desire to be able to change cadence.[10] Because of the biomechanical stability of these prostheses, locked knee designs are rarely necessary. Locked knee designs have two additional drawbacks: They must be unlocked before sitting, and they may increase the risk of injury in the event of a fall.

The prosthetist selects a prosthetic foot from among the many that are available: All have been used successfully at these high levels. Non-articulating designs, such as the solid-ankle cushion-heel (SACH), are often chosen because of their dependability, durability, and low maintenance; these designs rarely require servicing as a result of wear and tear. Single-axis feet (which allow the patient to quickly attain a stable foot-flat position) are used when enhanced knee stability is a concern. Multiaxial and dynamic response designs are usually reserved for higher activity individuals who will appreciate the added mobility of such components.[11]

A number of efforts have been made to provide some measure of active hip flexion motion in these prostheses, as this would reduce or eliminate the key biomechanical deficits noted previously. The use of a flexible carbon fiber thigh "strut" is now being tried clinically in selected cases. Initial reports suggest that this increases cadence and that the improved swing clearance achieved by better prosthetic hip and knee flexion eliminates the need to shorten

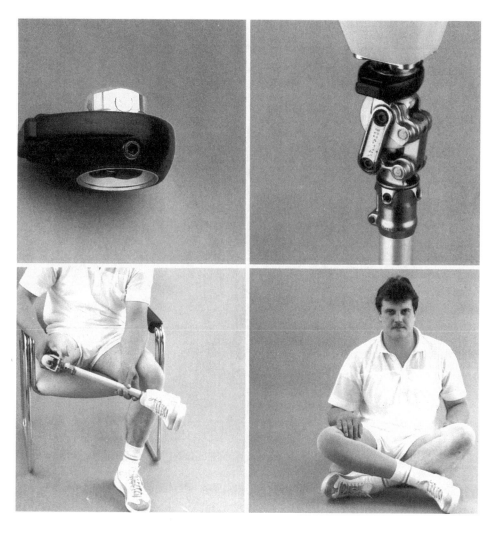

FIGURE 29-3
A lockable turntable (upper left) positioned in the prosthesis above the prosthetic knee (upper right) makes dressing, entering an automobile, and similar daily tasks much easier for individuals with high-level amputation (lower left and right). Torsion adapter absorbs the torque forces generated during gait and decreases the stress on both the wearer's skin and the prosthetic components. Such ancillary components should always be considered for persons with high-level amputation. (Courtesy of Otto Bock Orthopedic Industry, Inc. Minneapolis, MN.)

the prosthesis.[12] Use of vertical shock-absorbing shin elements and knees with stance flexion features are also being explored, with encouraging clinical acceptance.

With the loss of three biological joints of the lower limb, there is a corresponding loss of the ability of the body to compensate for rotary motions inherent in gait. For this reason, many prosthetists strongly recommend that a torque-absorbing device be included in these high-level prostheses. Torque absorbers typically improve both stride length and comfort by absorbing transverse forces that would otherwise be transmitted to the socket as skin shear.[13] Incorporation of a lockable turntable above the prosthetic knee is also suggested to facilitate such common daily activities as dressing and entering an automobile (Figure 29-3).

Energy Consumption

The major unresolved drawback to prosthetic fitting for those with high-level amputation is the tremendous increase in effort required to control a prosthetic limb with passive joints. Walking with a hip disarticulation or transpelvic prosthesis is much like controlling a flail biological leg. The concentration and energy required to ambulate makes short distance ambulation much more practical than distance walking for all but the most vigorous adult wearers.

Gait studies suggest that use of a hip disarticulation prosthesis requires approximately 200% more effort than unimpaired walking.[14] This is approximately the same effort required when using axillary crutches in single limb gait. Because single limb amputation with crutches tends to be faster than walking with a hip disarticulation prosthesis, the relatively high rejection rate of such prostheses is not surprising.

Most rehabilitation professionals believe that any individual with an amputation who is physically and mentally capable of prosthetic use should, if interested, be fitted with an initial prosthesis. This is particularly true

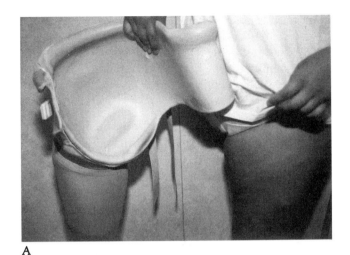

A

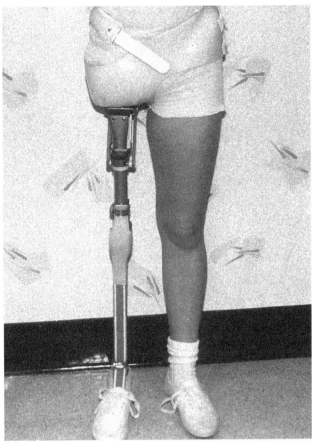

B

FIGURE 29-4
The interior of a hip disarticulation socket (A) fabricated from flexible silicone rubber. Note the contouring of the proximal brim to encase the crest of the ileum. Thermoplastic sockets (B) are also used for hip disarticulation prostheses. (Reprinted with permission from JW Michael. Component selection criteria: lower limb disarticulations. Clin Prosthet Orthot 1988;12[3]: 99–108.)

for those with high-level amputation, who may feel "cheated" and become depressed if the clinic team refuses to allow them to try prosthetic ambulation.

Socket Design

A variety of socket designs have been described in the clinical literature. The most critical factors for successful use are careful fitting and secure suspension, regardless of which socket design is selected. For patients with hip disarticulation, encapsulation of the ascending pubic ramus may add stability, although not every patient is able to tolerate a proximal trimline in the perineum.[15] Use of flexible thermoplastic or silicone materials within a rigid laminated frame is a more comfortable and increasingly popular design than the more common hard plastic sockets (Figure 29-4).[16]

Suspension is achieved by carefully contouring the socket just proximal to the iliac crests whenever possible. In the presence of obesity, or the absence of the ileum, shoulder straps may be necessary to minimize swing phase pistoning of the prosthesis.

The transpelvic socket must fully enclose the gluteal fold and perineal tissues and completely contain the soft tissues on the amputated side. Full enclosure permits a quasi-hydrostatic weight bearing, despite the absence of hemi-pelvis, as the incompressible viscera are fully encased in the socket. Early transpelvic sockets extended upward to contain the lower ribs.[17] Clinical experience has shown that this may not always be necessary for relatively muscular or lean individuals. Failure to adequately contain the transpelvic residuum results in obvious protrusion wherever the trimlines are insufficient. Prosthetists modify the positive plaster model of the transpelvic residuum to incorporate a diagonally directed compressive force in the socket design to support and contain transpelvic tissues and to eliminate the risk of perineal shear and tissue breakdown.[18]

For patients with translumbar amputation, weight bearing is achieved with a combination of soft tissue compression and thoracic rib support. Because of the loss of more than one-half of the body mass in this amputation, weight-bearing tolerance is better than might be expected.

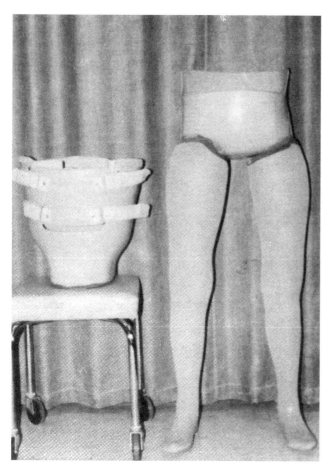

FIGURE 29-5

For patients with translumbar amputation, a laminated adjustable socket provides a stable base for sitting balance and wheeled stability (left). The socket can be positioned within an outer shell with bilateral prosthetic limbs (right) for cosmesis in sitting and for limited prosthetic ambulation. (Reprinted with permission from G Gruman, JW Michael. Translumbar Amputation: Prosthetic Considerations. In JH Bowker, JW Michael [eds], Atlas of Limb Prosthetics: Surgical, Prosthetic, and Rehabilitation Principles [2nd ed]. St. Louis: Mosby–Year Book, 1992;563–568.)

Long-term follow-up demonstrates positive prosthetic outcomes; return to work or school is usually a realistic goal.[20] For most patients, polycentric knees provide sufficient stability for the household ambulation typical of this population, making locking joints unnecessary.

Rehabilitation Outcomes after High-Level Amputation

Despite the obvious challenges that face individuals with high-level amputation, a substantial percentage are able to manage a prosthetic device with appropriate training and long-term follow-up. Although the rate of prosthetic use varies, the trend is toward increasing functional use of a prosthesis.[21] Fitting by an experienced prosthetist with the support of a specialty clinic team is believed to enhance the likelihood of success.

BILATERAL LOWER LIMB LOSS

The loss of both lower limbs complicates the rehabilitation process, especially if the loss occurs simultaneously. In North America, simultaneous bilateral loss is infrequent; such cases are typically the result of traumatic transportation or industrial accidents. In the developing world, simultaneous limb loss is more frequent; in post-war zones landmines are a major factor.[22] Fortunately, most individuals with traumatic amputation are healthy and strong, and generally have a good prognosis for successful use of a prosthesis.

Because vascular disease affects both limbs, patients with a single dysvascular amputation face a significant risk of eventual bilateral limb loss. An incidence as high as 50% contralateral limb loss over 5 years has been reported.[23] Clinical follow-up suggests that successful use of a unilateral prosthesis increases the likelihood of success with bilateral artificial limbs. For this reason, early fitting after initial amputation is strongly advocated, even when amputation of the opposite limb seems imminent.[24]

Energy Cost

The effort required to use a unilateral prosthesis increases in direct proportion to the level of amputation: the longer the residual limb the lower the energy cost of walking with a prosthesis.[25] Saving as much functional limb length as possible is therefore an axiom in amputation surgery. Although preservation of the anatomic knee joint is important for patients with unilateral amputation, it is a critical consideration when there is bilateral limb loss: when

Designs that allow the patient to vary the compression via adjustable straps are often useful.[19]

Patients with translumbar amputation require a socket for effective seating and wheeled mobility (Figure 29-5, *left*). Many individuals with translumbar amputation successfully progress to ambulation for short distances with a prosthesis (Figure 29-5, *right*). Many patients with translumbar amputation choose to wear prosthetic limbs to enhance their cosmetic appearance and self-image.

at least one biological knee joint remains, the chances for practical ambulation increase significantly.[26]

Energy cost of ambulation is also related to etiology of limb loss.[27] In general, patients with dysvascular amputation have lower energy reserves and expend more effort walking than those with traumatic amputation (Figure 29-6). Long-term use of bilateral transfemoral prostheses is uncommon, but not impossible, for elderly patients with dysvascular amputation.[28] In contrast, a significant number of those with traumatic bilateral transfemoral amputation successfully use prostheses long term. Patients with bilateral transtibial ambulation tend to do well with prostheses, regardless of etiology or amputation. It is interesting to note that the use of bilateral transtibial prostheses requires less effort than use of a unilateral transfemoral prosthesis; this finding emphasizes the importance of retaining biological knee function whenever possible.

Components

Selection of components for persons with bilateral lower limb amputation is based on the same guidelines as for unilateral limb absence; there are no "bilateral" components. It is important, however, to consider both prostheses together rather than to simply generate a "right side" and a "left side" prescription recommendation. Prosthetists generally recommend that the same ankle-foot device be used on both sides in order that gait mechanics will be consistent, but this is not an absolute necessity. Some patients will do best with different prosthetic feet, depending on the level of amputations, the length and consideration of the residual limbs, the nature of their preferred activities, or other individual characteristics.

Bilateral Transtibial Amputations

In North America, a solid-ankle prosthetic foot is often chosen for patients with bilateral transtibial amputation because such feet offer predictable standing balance. Most patients with bilateral amputation are concerned about falling backward. The prosthetist often chooses to use a slightly stiffer heel resistance to minimize the risk of backward falls. When there is concern about forward falls as well, the prosthetist may also choose to use a slightly stiffer keel to offer additional resistance to falling forward. Patients classified as limited ambulators, those with poor postural responses, and those who walk with a very slow cadence often find this approach useful.

Active individuals walk well with elastic keel and dynamic response feet, or with multiaxial designs, as long

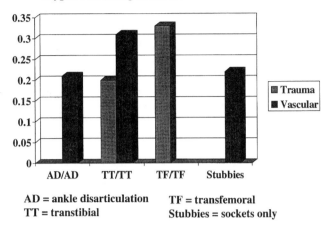

Oxygen Cost (ml/kg-meter) for Bilateral Prostheses

AD = ankle disarticulation
TT = transtibial
TF = transfemoral
Stubbies = sockets only

FIGURE 29-6

The energy cost of ambulation with bilateral prosthesis is compared for patients with ankle disarticulation (AD), transtibial amputation (TT), and transfemoral amputation using traditional transfemoral prostheses (TF) and "stubbies" (simplified prostheses consisting only of the transfemoral sockets attached to a stable base, without any prosthetic knee). Note that energy costs increase as the level of amputation moves proximally. Energy cost is also higher in dysvascular amputation as compared with traumatic amputation. Ambulation requires less effort for patients with at least one anatomic knee joint than for those with bilateral transfemoral amputation. Preservation of an anatomic knee joint increases likelihood of independence in ambulation. (Adapted from RL Waters. The Energy Expenditure of Amputee Gait. In JH Bowker, JW Michael [eds], Atlas of Limb Prosthetics: Surgical, Prosthetic, and Rehabilitation Principles [2nd ed]. St. Louis: Mosby–Year Book, 1992;381–387.)

as they have sufficient strength and postural responses to manage these flexible components. Theoretically, single-axis feet are designed to generate an abrupt hyperextension moment at midstance, which loads the cruciate ligaments of the residual limb. In practice, there is little evidence that this loading is harmful; some patients with bilateral transtibial amputation prefer single-axis feet, choosing them over solid-ankle or dynamic response designs. Patient preference is an important consideration in prosthetic prescription; preference is even more critical for patients with bilateral amputation who, literally, have no "good foot" to stand on other than prosthetic devices. If a patient expresses a definite dissatisfaction with a particular foot during the fitting process, it is best to try an alternative component before proceeding further.

It is important to consider the use of ancillary components, such as torque absorbers or shock absorbing pylons, for all patients with bilateral amputation. Because patients with bilateral amputation must bear all of their body weight on prosthetic devices all of the time, components that increase comfort or protect the skin are particularly appropriate.

It is also important to keep the weight of the prostheses as low as possible, particularly at the ankle-foot area, as this seems to make it easier to control the prosthesis and increases acceptance of the device. Whenever possible, heavier components should be placed as close to the socket as possible.[29]

Bilateral Transfemoral Amputation

Because patients with bilateral transfemoral amputation have lost both anatomic ankles and knees, postural responses are compromised. For this reason, one of the primary goals of prosthetic prescription is stability in the stance phase of gait. One of the most effective prosthetic components for stance phase stability is a polycentric knee unit. For those patients who have the potential to walk at varying speeds, the addition of fluid swing phase control is recommended. Hydraulic stance and swing control units are also quite successful for this population. The risk of injury in a fall is greater if locking or stance control knees are used in both prostheses. For patients with significant stability issues, a locking or stance control knee may be used on one side. Because single-axis knees are stabilized by muscle control and postural responses at the hip, bilateral single-axis knees are often difficult for older adults with dysvascular amputation to use safely. Bilateral single-axis knees may be appropriate for small children because their short stature reduces the balance required to manage such components.

Ankle-foot components that emphasize stability and standing balances are typical for this group with bilateral loss. Solid-ankle designs predominate. Articulating designs are used less often, usually only those with very long transfemoral residual limbs and good muscle strength are able to control the added mobility provided by articulating ankle components. Many patients with bilateral transfemoral amputation use crutches or canes to assist with balance and postural control. Single-axis or multiaxial feet become easier to control if the patient leans forward slightly, shifting the center of gravity forward, so that the weight line falls anterior to the ankle axis at all times and there is no risk of falling backwards.

Ancillary components, such as torque absorbers, will often make walking easier and more comfortable for patients with bilateral transfemoral amputation; use of locking rotation devices will make many activities of daily living easier to accomplish.[30] While the weight of such ancillary

components must be considered, the perception of the artificial limb feeling heavy is minimized if they are positioned as far proximally within the prosthesis as possible.

Transfemoral-Transtibial Amputation

For patients with one transfemoral and one transtibial amputation, the preservation of one biological knee makes prosthetic use much easier, and successful ambulation more likely.[31] For most patients, the transtibial side will be the propulsive and balance limb while the transfemoral side will supplement these functions. Based on these functional differences, the prosthetist may choose to use different prosthetic feet in the prostheses. When the transfemoral amputation is relatively short, for example, a single-axis foot and stance control knee might be recommended for the transfemoral prosthesis, while a dynamic response foot might be used in the transtibial prosthesis.

Socket Designs

The person with bilateral lower limb loss is constantly bearing full weight on artificial limbs while walking or standing. All options to increase skin protection and comfort should be actively considered, and suspension must be as secure as possible. A soft insert and/or flexible sockets may be used to enhance comfort during wear and to reduce the likelihood that shear forces will be problematic for the skin. Suction suspension, using silicone sleeves or inserts as necessary, minimizes pistoning during swing, and should be considered for the majority of patients with bilateral amputation.

Cotton or wool prosthetic socks are often used as an interface between the residual limbs and the sockets when suction suspension is not feasible. In that event, supracondylar wedge or cuff suspensions are typically used in transtibial prostheses; Silesian belts are often used in transfemoral designs. Because most patients with bilateral amputation use a pair of prostheses, suspension belts are usually integrated into a single assembly. Because thigh corsets with metal side joints, hip joints and pelvic bands, and waist belts can be cumbersome for donning and doffing, they are typically avoided unless absolutely necessary.

Ischial containment sockets are as effective for patients with bilateral amputation at the transfemoral level (of one or both limbs) as they are for patients with a single transfemoral amputation. Patients who have previously worn a quadrilateral transfemoral socket, and those who are limited ambulators, may be satisfied with a traditional quadrilateral design. Total contact of the residual limb in the socket is important in both ischial containment and quadrilateral sockets for skin integrity.

The loss of both feet and both knees makes the use of bilateral transfemoral prostheses very challenging. For many adults with acquired limb losses, an initial fitting with sockets attached to special "rocker platforms" may be advocated to facilitate initial gait training (see Figure 28-7). Such "stubbies" require less energy and balance than full-length prosthetic limbs and give the patient new to bilateral prosthetic use the best chance for successful ambulation.[32] Once the patient is able to balance effectively on the stubbies, the prostheses can be converted to use artificial feet with solid pylons, which are gradually lengthened to increase the height of the prostheses. If the patient is able to manage full-length prostheses, prosthetic knees can be incorporated, and definitive prostheses with full componentry provided.

Not all patients with bilateral transfemoral amputation choose to pursue ambulation with prostheses. Some are unable to build the necessary muscular strength or postural control for a safe gait. Others find the energy cost of ambulation with prostheses excessive. In these circumstances, patients choose wheelchair mobility as a much less strenuous means of mobility, and willingly adopt wheelchair use for the independence it provides. Many patients with bilateral transfemoral amputation find a wheelchair most practical for long distance mobility and use their limbs for walking short distances at home and work. Some patients will accept the stubbies for long-term use, particularly if these devices allow them to remain independent in their home setting. Others choose to use their stubbies at home (because they take less effort) but wear full prostheses in public if cosmesis is an important consideration for them.

SUMMARY AND CONCLUSIONS

Individuals with high-level or bilateral lower limb amputations are rare in the developed world. In North America, they are believed to represent less than 5% of all persons with amputation.[33] Given these statistics, most prosthetists and therapists have limited opportunity to work with patients with such significant levels of limb loss. Although successful prosthetic training and rehabilitation for these patients are challenging, a large body of clinical information about managing such cases is available in the literature. This chapter has highlighted the key principles involved in rehabilitation of the person with high-level or bilateral lower limb amputations.

Surgical technique during the amputation largely determines the potential for long-term ambulation. The reader is referred to the consensus document on surgical principles, published by the International Society for Prosthetics &

Orthotics, for specific recommendations.[34] Gentle handling of soft tissues combined with careful preservation of all functional joints and bony length is essential. Anchoring functioning muscles to bone (myodesis) at their normal resting length is strongly encouraged whenever possible.

It is important that the socket design and suspension methods chosen for patients with high-level or bilateral amputation incorporate strategies to protect the skin and to maximize patient comfort, especially for individuals with bilateral amputation. Components reflect each individual's need for stability and responsiveness, at the ankle-foot, knee, or hip joint level.[35] Use of ancillary components to make using the prosthesis more comfortable and easier to manage is advocated. As a rule, these individuals benefit most from the best technology we have to offer.

Although patients with bilateral transfemoral amputation secondary to vascular disease often have difficulty mastering dual prosthetic devices, long-term use of functional prostheses is a realistic goal for patients with traumatic or tumor-related amputation who are otherwise healthy.[36] With appropriate fitting and rehabilitation, many patients with hip disarticulation and transpelvic amputations continue to use their prostheses definitively. Even patients with translumbar amputation are able to return to productive education or work activities with an appropriate prosthesis for sitting, or for limited ambulation.

Despite the obvious physical and psychological challenges faced by patients with high-level or bilateral lower limb amputation, prosthetic rehabilitation must always be considered, and is often successful, especially when offered by an experienced clinic team in a supportive setting.[37] Although the sequelae from amputations of this magnitude present significant challenges, advances in surgical technique, prosthetic design and componentry, and rehabilitation contribute to successful outcomes for patients with high-level and bilateral amputation.

REFERENCES

1. Glattly HW. A preliminary report on the amputee census. Artif Limbs 1963;7(1):5.
2. Stern PH. The epidemiology of amputations. Phys Med Rehabil Clin North Am 1991; March-April (67):145–157.
3. Burgess E, Romano RL. The management of lower extremity amputees using immediate postsurgical prostheses. Clin Orthop 1968; March-April (57):137–146.
4. Cutson T, Bongiorni, Michael JW. Early management of elderly dysvascular below-knee amputees. J Prosthet Orthot 1994;6(3):62–66.
5. McLaurin CA. The evolution of the Canadian-type hip disarticulation prosthesis. Artif Limbs 1957;4:22–28.

6. Radcliffe CW. Biomechanics of the Canadian-type hip disarticulation prosthesis. Artif Limbs 1957;4:29–38.

7. Lehmann JR, Wareen CG, Hertling D. Craig-Scott orthosis: a biomechanical and functional evaluation. Arch Phys Med Rehabil 1976;57(9):438–442.

8. Van der Waarde T, Michael JW. Hip disarticulation and transpelvic management: prosthetic considerations. In JH Bowker, JW Michael (eds), Atlas of limb prosthetics: surgical, prosthetic, and rehabilitation principles (2nd ed). St. Louis: Mosby–Year Book, 1992;539–552.

9. Michael JW. Component selection criteria: lower limb disarticulations. Clin Prosthet Orthot 1988;12(3):99–108.

10. Michael JW. Prosthetic knee mechanisms. Phys Med Rehabil State Art Rev 1994;8(1):147–164.

11. Michael JW. Prosthetic feet: options for the older client. Top Geriatr Rehabil 1992;8(1):30–38.

12. Littig DN. Gait patterns in the unilateral hip disarticulation. AAOP Proc 1995;42.

13. Knoche W. Welche vorteile bringt der einbau eines torsionsadapters in beinprosthesn? Orthop Tech 1979;30:12–14.

14. Huang C-T. Energy cost of ambulation with Canadian hip disarticulation prosthesis. J Med Assoc State Ala 1983;52(11):47–48.

15. Sabolich J, Guth T. The CAT-CAM HD: a new design for hip disarticulation patients. Clin Prosthet Orthot 1988;12:119–122.

16. Madden M. The flexible socket system as applied to the hip disarticulation amputee. Orthot Prosthet 1987;39(4):44–47.

17. Hampton F. A hemipelvectomy prosthesis. Artif Limbs 1964;8(1):3–27.

18. Hampton F. Northwestern University suspension casting technique for hemipelvectomy and hip disarticulation. Artif Limbs 1966;10(1):56–61.

19. Carlson MJ. A double socket prosthesis design for bilateral hip-to-hemi corporectomy amputation levels. AAOP Proc, 1997.

20. Gruman G, Michael JW. Translumbar Amputation: Prosthetic Considerations. In JH Bowker, JW Michael (eds), Atlas of Limb Prosthetics, Second Edition 1992; Mosby–Year Book, St. Louis, 563–568.

21. Shurr DR. Hip disarticulation prostheses: a follow up. Orthot Prosthet 1983;37(3):50–57.

22. Korver AJH. Amputees in a hospital of the International Committee of the Red Cross. Injury 1993;24(9):607–609.

23. Anderson SP. Dysvascular amputee: what can we expect? J Prosthet Orthot 1995;7(2):43–50.

24. Sener S, Uygur F, Yakut Y, et al. Quality of life of rehabilitated lower limb amputees. Physiotherapy 1995;81:455 [abstract].

25. Waters RL. The energy expenditure of amputee gait. In JH Bowker, JW Michael [eds], Atlas of Limb Prosthetics, Second Edition; Mosby–Year Book, St. Louis; 381–387.

26. Schuling S, Greitemann B, Seichter C. Gehfahigkeit Beidseits beinamputierter nach prosthetischer versorgung. Z Orthop 1994;132(3):235–238.

27. Pinzur MS, Gold J, Schwarz D, et al. Energy demands in walking for dysvascular amputees as compared to level of amputation. Orthopaedics 1992;15(9):1033–1037.

28. Moore TJ, Barron J, Hutchinson F, et al. Prosthetic usage following major lower extremity amputation. Clin Orthop 1989; Jan (238):219–224.

29. Bach TM. Optimizing mass and mass distribution in lower limb prostheses. Prosthet Orthot Aust 1995;10(2):29–35.

30. Schmidl H. Torsionadapter im kunstbein aus der sicht des technikers und des amputierten. Orthop Tech 1979;30:35–38.

31. Torres MM, Esquanazi A. Bilateral lower limb rehabilitation: a retrospective review. West J Med 1991;154(4):583–586.

32. Kruger LM. Stubby prostheses in the rehabilitation of infants and children with bilateral lower limb deficiencies. Rehabilitation 1990;29(1):12–15.

33. Torres MM. Incidence and causes of limb amputations. Phys Med Rehabil State Art Rev 1994;8:1–8.

34. Murdoch G, Jacobs NA, Wilson AB. A Report of ISPO Consensus Conference on Amputation Surgery. Denmark: ISPO Copenhagen, 1992.

35. Lehnies HR, et al. Prosthetic management of the cancer patient with high-level amputation. Orthot Prosthet 1981;35(2): 10–28.

36. Collin C, Wade DT, Cochrane GM. Functional outcome of lower limb amputees with peripheral vascular disease. Clin Rehabil 1992;6:13–21.

37. Saadah ESH. Bilateral below-knee amputee 107 years old and still wearing artificial limbs. Prosthet Orthot Int 1988;12: 105–106.

30

Rehabilitation for Children with Limb Deficiencies

JOAN E. EDELSTEIN

Children with limb deficiency, whether congenital anomalies or acquired amputations, confront the clinic team with skeletal, neuromuscular, learning, and psychosocial challenges that are not found in adults. Some rehabilitation issues are similar to those of adults, particularly the basic components of the prosthesis and the essential elements of postoperative care. Other considerations are unique to children. Because youngsters are smaller than adults, the choice of prosthetic components is not as broad as for adults. Children grow and develop through the rehabilitation process. In addition, young people depend legally, financially, and emotionally on adults for their medical, surgical, and rehabilitation care.[1]

This chapter examines the considerations that pertain to comprehensive management of children with limb anomalies, particularly the relation of developmental milestones to prosthetic selection and use and the psychosocial factors that affect children's rehabilitation. Specific issues regarding children with upper-limb, lower-limb, and multiple amputations are intended to enable clinicians to design rational rehabilitation programs. Care of the infant born with a limb anomaly is habilitation, whereas management of an infant or child who acquires amputation because of trauma or disease is rehabilitation. Unless the distinction is relevant, however, *habilitation* and *rehabilitation* are used interchangeably in this chapter. The overall goal of physical therapy is to facilitate the normal developmental sequence and to prevent the onset of secondary impairments and functional limitations, such as contractures, weakness, and dependence in self-care.[1]

COMPREHENSIVE CONSIDERATIONS IN CHILDHOOD

The philosophy of this chapter is that the child with a limb deficiency is first and foremost a child, with the beauty, delight, and promise that are inherent in all young people.

Developmental Milestones

Infants develop motor skills in a predictable sequence, with well-established milestones that mark achievement of important functional abilities. In the absence of cerebral maldevelopment or malformation, the infant born with a limb anomaly or the young child who acquires amputation demonstrates physical control at approximately the same time as an age mate does. Limb deficiency, however, can alter the mode of performance. For example, the 5-month-old baby who has one intact leg will discover a distinctive style of crawling. Therapists who conduct the initial evaluation of the child focus on the child's muscle strength, range of motion, gross motor patterns, coordination, attention span, and interests. They must recognize that much variation is found in the rate of neuromuscular development and that chronologic age does not provide a complete picture of the child's developmental level. In this chapter, milestones pertaining to upper- and lower-limb development are related to habilitation of youngsters with those disorders.

Children with limb deficiency, regardless of etiology, tend to have lower energy output than their age mates. The problem is aggravated by the energy demands of using a prosthesis. Consequently, physical conditioning programs are important to enhance general health and endurance. Play and games increase coordination and improve strength. Youngsters need to engage in active sports. Swimming is particularly beneficial because it does not traumatize the limbs and does not require use of prostheses; nevertheless, some children may be reluctant to display the anomalous limb.

Accommodating Growth

Whether the limb deficiency is congenital or acquired, the child will grow. Prosthetic planning should incorporate measures to maintain comfortable socket fit and symmetric limb length. The preschool-aged child may need a new prosthesis almost yearly. Those in grammar school often require a new larger prosthesis every 12–18 months, and teenagers outgrow prostheses every 18–24 months.[2]

Linear growth is typically more rapid than circumferential growth. This is troublesome for children with lower-limb deficiency: A short lower-limb prosthesis disturbs the quality and increases the energy cost of gait. An upper-limb prosthesis that is slightly short probably will not present a noticeable asymmetry and will have little effect on bimanual activities. Endoskeletal prosthetic components facilitate lengthening and substitution of more sophisticated components.

Vigorous play causes considerable wear of the mechanical parts of the prosthesis. These parts are additionally vulnerable because of their small size. The child is likely to wear out the prosthesis from everyday use before circumferential growth compels a change. Signs of an outgrown socket include a tendency of the amputation limb to slip out of the socket, pain or skin reddening caused by socket tightness, and a flesh roll around the margin of the socket. To accommodate for circumferential growth, socket liners are convenient; as the child grows, a liner is removed. Alternatively, the prosthesis can be fitted with several layers of socks; the child eventually wears fewer socks to accommodate the added residual limb girth.[3] Flexible sockets fitted to extra-thick frames are another means of accommodating growth. To fit the larger residual limb, a new flexible socket is made, and material is ground from the frame.[4,5]

Prosthetic alignment should complement the immature skeleton and joint capsules. For example, infants usually have genu varum, which becomes genu valgum by the third year.[3] Children with amputations through the bony diaphysis or metaphysis may experience terminal bony overgrowth. As the youngster grows, terminal periosteal new bone protrudes beneath the terminal subcutaneous tissue and skin. Without treatment, a bursal sac forms, and the skin becomes ecchymotic and hemorrhagic. The underlying bone then ruptures the bursal sac, and infection can occur.[2] Overgrowth is a particular problem when the adolescent growth spurt commences. Customary treatment is excision of the periosteal sac, transection of the distal 2–3 cm of bone, and primary closure of the incision. Children may require the procedure several times during the growth period. Another approach is continuous skin traction, which can be used to maintain skin and soft tissue coverage over the distal end of the amputation limb until skeletal growth is complete. The emotional difficulties of keeping distal force on the limb day and night usually preclude this method. Disarticulation preserves the distal epiphyseal plate and thus is not associated with overgrowth. In children, as in adults with acquired amputation, availability of near normal range of motion is an important determinant of effective prosthetic use. For children, active therapeutic exercise that is designed to increase joint excursion is preferable to passive stretching, especially in the presence of congenital contractures.[6]

For young children with acquired amputation, postoperative care is simpler than it is for adolescents and adults. Ordinarily the amputation limb presents little or no edema, and the wound heals rapidly. Phantom pain has been reported to be relatively common among those with acquired amputation, and is associated with the extent of preoperative pain.[7] A pain diary may help older children and adolescents to cope with phantom pain.[8]

Psychosocial Factors in Habilitation and Rehabilitation

Habilitation amounts to more than selecting a suitable prosthesis and devising rational training. All children have developing personalities, together with their physical growth and development. Optimal emotional development occurs when parents and professional health caregivers promote wholesome interactions. The essential message is that the child can have a vivacious personality and that independence commensurate with age can be fostered.

Infants

Infants learn trust when their basic needs are met.[9] The baby with limb anomaly has as much need for trusting responsive care as does the infant who has normal limbs. In contrast, if the family cannot accept the infant's appearance, the baby will learn to mistrust others. For successful habilitation, parents must replace the expectation of a picture-perfect infant with the reality of a baby who has a limb deficiency. Infants are very susceptible to the anxiety of parents and others who interact with them. The birth of an infant with a limb deficiency is a period of intense emotion. Because such a birth is a rare event in any hospital, medical staff may react with shock and feelings of helplessness and revulsion. Mothers have described the atmosphere of the delivery room as being "electrified" as staff react with silence or disgust.[10] Parents characterize the first few weeks after birth as nightmarish, a bad dream from which they wish to awaken. They feel that they are alone with a unique and hopeless problem when questions go unanswered or evaded. Mourning for the loss of the ideal child is part of the coping process.[2] Parents are bombarded by the child's grandparents, siblings, and other family members who comment and influence habilitation.

Although the newborn infant is too young for prosthetic fitting, early referral to a specialized clinic is highly desirable. The core team is composed of a pediatrician, physical therapist, occupational therapist, and prosthetist. The team should be able to draw on the expertise of a psychologist, social worker, orthopedist, and engineer, depending on the needs of the child and family.[2] Effective clinic team management involves the family in rehabilitation decisions and weighs management recommendations in light of the immediate impact on the child's welfare and the long-term consequences on the individual's appearance and function as an adult. An important resource for clinicians is the Association of Children's Prosthetic-Orthotic Clinics (6300 North River Road, Suite 727, Rosemont, IL 60018-4226). The association, founded in 1958, has held an annual interdisciplinary conference since 1972.

The clinic team can help parents realize that they and their baby are acceptable. Families need time to talk about their feelings and obtain answers to their questions.[10] The team's approach takes into consideration motives such as hiding the deformity, maximizing function, and the parents' style of dealing with unexpected events. Team members should be empathetic to the parents' shock and grief, which bear little relation to the amount of the infant's disability.[2] Some parents resist holding the baby, avoid direct contact, or withdraw into silence. When professional staff members hold the baby, parents usually realize that the infant is lovable. The team fosters the attitude that, "Yes, I know he is different, but I recognize and accept him for what he is and what he can do," rather than denying any difference.

Families may be interested in seeing pictures or examples of the type of prosthesis that the baby will use. Expectations regarding the extent of prosthetic restoration, however, may be unrealistic. Parents should understand what prosthetic and surgical possibilities exist so that they can make rational decisions for their child. Infants usually receive the first prosthesis at approximately 6–9 months of age.[3,6,11–16] Some parents find it difficult to accept the prosthesis, feeling that it draws attention to the limb deficiency.

The team can also help parents of children who sustain amputation because of trauma or disease to cope with feelings of guilt and shock. Team members assist the family in realizing that they were not negligent in protecting the child against injury or not recognizing symptoms of a disease process early enough to prevent amputation.

In addition to clinic team management, families benefit from membership in a peer support group in which they can share concerns, exchange information, and observe children of various ages playing with and without prostheses. Some groups publish newsletters that disseminate information to those who live too far from the meeting site. For example, *Superkids* (60 Clyde Street, Newton, MA 02160) is a newsletter for families and friends of children with limb differences. *Reach* is a newsletter published by the British Association of Parents Concerned with Children with Upper-Limb Anomalies (Reach Head Office, 25 High Street, Wellingborough, Northamptonshire, NN8 4J2, England).

Parental acceptance of and active cooperation in the training program are the most important factors in its success and largely determine whether the child regards the prosthesis as a tool in daily activities.[2] Families need to learn skin care, prosthetic operation, maintenance, and the capabilities and limitations of the prosthesis. Outpatient training is preferable to avoid homesickness, which can interfere with the child's learning. In addition, the constant presence of one or both parents enables the entire family to learn about prosthetic use and maintenance.[12] Putting a prosthesis on an active child is a skill that takes time for parents to master. Scheduling appointments after nap time or mealtime generally is more productive than attempting to coerce a tired and upset child to participate in therapy. Clinicians need to recognize that infants have short attention spans and, thus, should incorporate many brief activities in the treatment session.

Toddlers

Toddlers must develop self-control to acquire the autonomy that will allow them to cope with their environment. The interval between 1 and 3 years of age is a time of language and functional communication, assertion of independence, and interpersonal control.[10] Children as young as 3 years old should be informed of any impending surgery, whether to revise a congenital anomaly or to treat disease or injury. Doll play can help the child in understanding surgery and rehabilitation.[17,18] Special dolls that depict amputations at various levels, with and without prostheses, are available through Hal's Pals for Challenged Kids (P.O. Box 3490, Winter Park, CO 80482).

The child must resolve feelings of deprivation and resentment that attend the visible alteration of the body.[2] Mobility, control, exploration, initiative, and creativity are prime emotional developmental milestones for older toddlers and kindergartners.[9] Parents and professional staff should encourage the child's independence. Facile use of a prosthesis can help youngsters to maximize their psychological potential. Children compare themselves with others and inquire, "Where is my other hand [or leg]?" Youngsters form two body images, one with and the other without the prosthesis. Parents should be able to give a simple and truthful answer, making it clear that the child will not grow another hand: "You were born this way."[2] Similarly, children who acquire an amputation need a realistic answer to the question, "What happened to you?" The child may engage the parent in a power struggle regarding prosthetic wearing. A firm, yet gentle, approach with a range of acceptable choices usually enables the child to incorporate autonomy needs while gaining prosthetic proficiency.[10]

The clinic team should value the parents' comments about their child and involve the family in all aspects of care. The waiting room should have a variety of safe toys to make visits more pleasant. Parents should be present during the child's examination and prosthetic fitting to reduce anxiety.[10]

School-Aged Children

The developmental task for school-aged children is to become industrious[9]; the upper or lower-limb prosthesis can be instrumental in fostering this important psychological step. Teachers, scout masters, clergy, and other adults now participate in the child's social milieu. The clinic team can help to prepare the child and family for these encounters.

In group experiences, the child has to deal with feelings of social devaluation, which members of minority groups experience. The teacher or other group leader can bolster the child's sense of self-worth. The first encounter at school and camp is the occasion for having the child display the prosthesis and demonstrate its function. The presentation usually dispels the mystery of the appliance and shows that the prosthesis is simply a tool that makes it easier for its wearer to engage in certain activities. The teacher should be aware of the appearance of the amputation limb, the child's function with and without the prosthesis, any environmental or programmatic adaptations that the child may need, and how to cope with prosthetic malfunction. Anticipating awkward situations helps to develop coping strategies. For example, in a circle game, classmates may be reluctant to hold hands with a child who wears an upper-limb prosthesis. If the teacher holds the child's terminal device (hook or mechanical hand), the other pupils are likely to realize that it is not scary or unacceptable to do so. School officials may be concerned about the ability of a child who uses a leg prosthesis to maneuver in the classroom and playground. Classmates' natural curiosity should be dealt with through honest simple answers. Although teasing is inevitable, the youngster who feels secure can understand that taunts are merely crude expressions of interest.

Among school-aged children with limb deficiencies, demographic variables (such as age, sex, socioeconomic status, and degree of limb loss) are not significant predictors of self-esteem. In contrast, social support, family functioning, self-perception, and microstressors explain the child's adaptation to the handicap that is imposed by amputation. Perceived physical appearance is strongly predictive of general self-esteem.[19–21]

Many school-aged and older children respond favorably to scouting, camping, and other group recreational activities. Sports programs, such as skiing, horseback riding, and track events, are fun and give youngsters with disabilities pride in athletic achievement.

Older Children and Adolescents

Adolescents face the critical step of forming a satisfying identity within themselves and with their peer group. The teenager may select times when prosthetic wear is not desirable, for example, eschewing an upper-limb prosthesis during a football game or discarding the leg prosthesis when swimming or playing beach volleyball. Adults should nurture young adults so that they develop sufficient self-esteem to make satisfying decisions. Teenagers who have an amputation must cope with being visibly different. Young adults have to adapt to an environment that is designed for those who do not have handicaps and must evaluate whether people relate to them as persons or as people with handicaps.[22] During adolescence, questions of "Why did this happen to me?" are often intensified. Adolescents constantly reexamine their body image; group showering after physical education class may be especially stressful for the individual with amputation. Other developmental concerns in which amputation plays a role are vocational selection and obtaining a driver's license. The clinic team needs to be sensitive to concerns about privacy, confidentiality, and independence.[10]

Adolescents with bone cancer who undergo an amputation typically pass through a stage of initial impact when they learn that the treatment plan includes amputation. The news may be met with despair, discouragement, passive acceptance, or violent denial. Informing the adolescent of the rehabilitation process and the achievements of others can be helpful. The next stage is retreat, during which the adolescent experiences acute grief. Anger may be part of the process. The goal of grieving is giving up hope of retrieving the lost object. The staff can reinforce the patient's strengths and encourage maximum independence. The third stage is acknowledgment, when the adolescent is willing to participate in rehabilitation and has incorporated the changed appearance into the body image. Reconstruction, the final stage, involves the return to developmentally appropriate activities, such as school, sports, camp, and dating.[22]

REHABILITATION AND PROSTHETIC DECISION MAKING

Not all children with limb deficiency benefit from a prosthesis. With certain upper-limb anomalies, the remaining portion of the limb is more functional than it would be if it were covered by a prosthesis.[2,23] Children who are born with bilateral arm absence generally use their feet to play and do almost everything, without recourse to complicated and heavy prostheses.[12]

Rehabilitation of Children with Upper-Limb Amputation

Because functional use of an upper prosthesis often involves control of a terminal device, it is important that the prosthetic design and the rehabilitation program be appropriate for the child's stage or level of motor, cognitive, and perceptual development.

Infants

Prosthetic fitting and training should complement the infant's development. Although a prosthesis usually is not fitted until the baby is at least 6 months of age, earlier developmental accomplishment paves the way for successful prosthetic use.

The average 2-month-old infant can hold objects with both hands. The baby who lacks one or both hands will attempt to hug a stuffed animal with the forearms or upper arms, capitalizing on the tactile sensitivity of the skin. The 3-month-old can bring grasped objects to the mouth. Three months is also the age when babies attempt two-handed prehension, although this skill is not perfected until the child attains sitting balance at 6–9 months of age.[1]

The 4-month-old baby props on the forearms, shifts weight to reach, and usually enjoys shaking noisy rattles by rapid elbow flexion and extension. An important developmental step is reached at approximately the same age, when the child can manipulate objects with one hand while the other hand stabilizes the toy; simultaneous sitting and manipulating are still challenging at this age.[1] Increased trunk strength enables the baby to reach unilaterally and bilaterally. Bilateral coordination at 4 months allows the infant to reach objects at the midline.[24] Two-handed hold of a bottle typically occurs at approximately 4.5 months.

By the fifth month, the child can transfer toys from one hand to the other and is thus aware of the usefulness of holding objects.[24] The child's dominant interest is in getting food, exploring his surroundings, and social contact with those who feed, hold, and care for her. Holding a large ball encourages clasping between the arms. Manipulating blocks or beads promotes stabilization of proximal body parts to allow fine movements with distal parts. Although a baby with intact limbs can get to the quadruped position and shift weight from side to side,[24] the infant who is missing one or both arms will probably find that creeping is impossible and will have difficulty coming to sitting and pulling to standing.[6]

Six months is generally considered to be the optimum age for upper-limb prosthetic fitting.[2] The baby with unilateral amputation has achieved good sitting balance, can free the sound hand for manual activities while sitting, and is actively engaged in exploring the environment. The prosthesis restores symmetric limb length and enables the infant to hold stuffed animals and similar toys at the midline. The prosthesis also accustoms parents to the concept that a prosthesis will likely be a permanent part of their child's wardrobe. Fitting can assuage parental guilt or shame regarding their infant's abnormal appearance by replacing negative reactions with a constructive device that enhances the baby's development. Many parents seek a prosthetic hand to disguise the limb anomaly. Early fitting provides experience that will be the basis for the child's decision as to whether to continue with prosthetic use.

Some advocate fitting a simple prosthesis between the ages of 3 and 6 months.[11,25] The rapid growth of younger infants, however, makes it difficult to maintain socket fit. In addition, a younger baby would find the prosthesis a hindrance during rolling maneuvers. Infants who are much older than 6 months may resist a prosthesis that deprives them of using the tactile sensation at the end of the amputation limb. Initial fitting after age 2 years tends to result in greater rejection of the prosthesis because of the development of compensatory techniques.[25]

At 8 months, most babies sit while manipulating objects with both hands, using gross palmar grasp and controlled release. A prosthesis aids in clasping large objects and in stabilizing smaller ones while the sound hand explores them.[26] By 15 months, most children can place a pellet in a small container and use crayons for scribbling and a spoon for feeding. These skills can also be performed with a prosthesis.

Babies are usually fitted with a passive prosthesis, that is, one that does not have a cable or other operating mechanism. The terminal device may be a hook or a passive mitt. The hook is covered with pink or brown resilient plastic to disguise its mechanical appearance. The plastic also blunts the impact of the hook as infants explore with it, swiping themselves and others in the vicinity. The hook may be voluntary-opening, without a cable. Parents can place a rattle or other object in the hook to acquaint the baby with prehension on the amputated side. Some infants have a voluntary-closing hook on the first prosthesis; in

TABLE 30-1

Prosthetic Training Goals for Infants

Therapy sessions are designed to increase the infant's:
  Comfort with the prosthesis
  Wearing tolerance
  Ability to clasp large objects
  Use the prosthesis to aid in sitting and crawling
Parents of infants with prostheses should:
  Apply and remove the prosthesis correctly
  Care for the child's skin
  Care for the prosthesis
  Recognize and report any problems with the prosthesis

the absence of a cable, the hook holds the toy by means of tape or a rubber band. A few children start with the CAPP terminal device (developed by the Child Amputee Prosthetic Project, Los Angeles, CA), which functions on the voluntary-opening mode. A fourth terminal device option is the infant passive mitt. The mitt has a less mechanical appearance than other terminal devices but has no prehensile function; consequently, very few objects can be taped or otherwise secured to it for the amusement of the baby. The absence of a hooked configuration hampers use of the mitt when the baby attempts to pull into standing at the side of the crib or playpen. Whatever the design, the terminal device is fitted into a friction or washer-type wrist unit at the distal end of the socket.

The thermoplastic socket is custom molded to a plaster model of the child's limb. It is worn over a cotton sock that protects the skin from pressure concentration. A snug fit is needed about the humeral epicondyles to stabilize the prosthesis on the child's residual limb. Depending on the rate of growth, changes may be needed every 2–4 months. The first prosthesis usually does not have an elbow unit, even if the anomaly is comparable to transhumeral amputation.

Regardless of amputation level, the prosthetic socket is suspended on the infant's torso by a harness, which probably will have more straps than would be needed for an adult. The toddler harness inhibits the infant's attempts to remove the prosthesis, whether deliberately or inadvertently during rolling and crawling.

Clothing problems arise when a prosthesis is worn. The rigid parts of the prosthesis eventually cause holes in clothing. Shirts and blouses worn over the prosthesis should be rather loose fitting; raglan sleeves are preferable to sleeves that are set at the natural shoulder line, which can interfere with cable operation.

Training the infant who is fitted with a passive prosthesis usually begins with two sessions within the same week, and then periodic follow-up appointments. The first session should be deferred until the baby is well rested and content. The therapist or parent puts the prosthesis on the baby and places her on the floor with various toys. The therapist encourages the parents to play with the baby and handle her while she is wearing the prosthesis. The infant may ignore the prosthesis because its socket diminishes the sense of touch and because the length of the prosthesis makes her feel awkward. Parents should present large toys that require the use of both arms. The basic prosthesis allows the infant to cuddle a teddy bear, swat at a mobile and similar hanging toys, and use both upper limbs for rolling and crawling. Training involves instructing the parents and other caregivers to gain familiarity with the prosthesis, to care for the infant's skin by making certain that the socket and harness do not exert undue pressure, and to provide toys that require bimanual prehension (Table 30-1). Placing a rattle in the terminal device is another way of acquainting the infant with grasp on the side of limb deficiency. At the end of the session, therapist and parent remove the prosthesis to inspect the child's skin for signs of irritation from the socket or harness. Parents learn how to apply the prosthesis and how to encourage full-time wear, except during baths, naps, and bedtime. The baby may be rather awkward when sitting and moving while adjusting to the weight of the prosthesis. Toys that are suitable for the infant's developmental level, such as large balls, dolls, stuffed animals, balloons, a toy xylophone, and other noisy and colorful objects, provide incentives for enjoying the prosthesis. Parents can put a mallet or other toy in the hook so that the infant can obtain pleasure from using the prosthesis. Push and pull toys are appropriate when the child is able to stand and cruise.[27-31]

Parents may be concerned when children catch the prosthesis on chair and table legs or use it to strike themselves or others; children recover balance readily, and peers are usually able to defend themselves successfully. Printed instructions, augmented with audiotaped or videotaped recordings, are useful guides for the family.

At the second training session a few days later, the therapist can review with parents their experiences. Donning and doffing the prosthesis should be reviewed. Initially, the infant may tolerate the prosthesis only for a few minutes. It should be applied frequently during the day. Eventually, the child should be able to wear it most of the day, except when sleeping and bathing.

Subsequent follow-up sessions focus on the adequacy of prosthetic fit and the child's readiness for the addition of a cable to the prosthesis or substitution of a myoelectrically controlled prosthesis for a passive one and, in the case of the child with transhumeral amputation, the addition of an elbow unit.

FIGURE 30-1
This group of youngsters is learning that shoulder flexion produces terminal device operation, because flexion tenses the control cable. (Courtesy of T.R.S., Inc, Boulder, CO.)

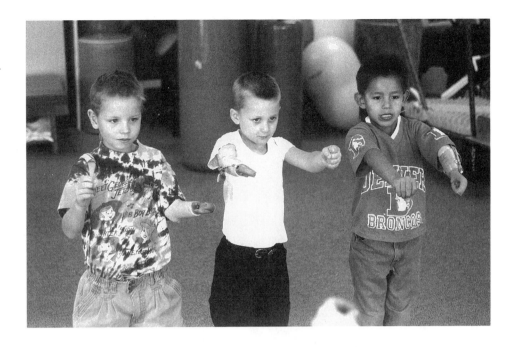

Toddlers

Between the ages of 15 and 18 months, the child has a control cable added to a traditional, body-operated prosthesis. It may not be until the child is 2 ¹/₂ years of age that active control becomes reliable; this is the age when the understanding of cause and effect is established[12] (Figure 30-1). Readiness for the cable is indicated when the child wears the prosthesis full time, can follow simple instructions, has an attention span of at least 5 minutes, and will allow the therapist and prosthetist to handle her. Toddlers who resist instruction from someone other than the parent may be too immature to learn to control the prosthesis.

If the prosthesis has a voluntary-opening hook, it should be fitted with a half- or a quarter-width rubber band to facilitate opening. The tension in the terminal device should be sufficient to let the child hold objects but not so great that it is difficult to open the hook. Young children appear to use the voluntary-closing hook with as much ease as the more traditional voluntary-opening terminal devices. Goals of prosthetic training for toddlers are summarized in Table 30-2.

Training should be conducted in a quiet setting. Therapist and child sit at a low table with toys that require bimanual grasp, such as large beads and a string with a firm tip. For the child with unilateral amputation, the terminal device serves to hold an object, such as a bead, while the child threads the string through the bead. The therapist is on the child's prosthetic side, holding the child's forearm at 90 degrees of elbow flexion, the optimal position of cable operation. This position also keeps the ter-

minal device and the grasped object within view. The adult moves the child's forearm forward, flexing the shoulder, tensing the cable, and causing the hook to operate. When the arm is moved back (shoulder extension), the terminal device changes position. Thus, a voluntary-opening hook opens with shoulder flexion, whereas a voluntary-closing hook closes with shoulder flexion. The child is encouraged to help with the control motion. With either design, the initial training involves placing a toy in the hook and encouraging the child to discover how to keep it in place. With a voluntary-opening hook, the child simply relaxes to allow the rubber bands or springs to keep the hook fingers closed. The voluntary-closing hook requires that the wearer exert tension on the control cable via the harness to keep the hook closed. Children use the same control motions as do adults, namely, shoulder flex-

TABLE 30-2
Prosthetic Training Goals for Toddlers

Therapy sessions are designed to increase the toddler's:
    Control of the terminal device
    Control of the elbow unit
    Use of the prosthesis in bimanual prehension
    Use of the prosthesis in functional activities
Parents of toddlers with prostheses should:
    Provide toys that require bimanual prehension
    Encourage use of the prosthesis as an assistive device
    Inspect the skin to determine whether the prosthesis causes
        undue irritation

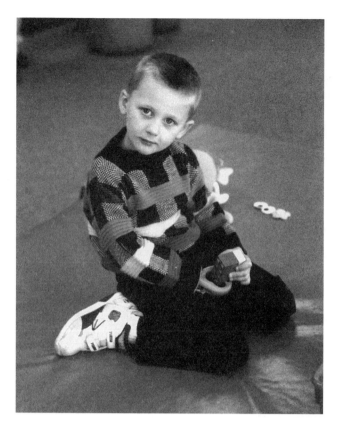

FIGURE 30-2
Large objects or toys such as Duplo (Lego Systems, Inc., Enfield, CT) blocks that require bimanual prehension allow the child the opportunity to incorporate the prosthesis in functional activities. (Courtesy of T.R.S., Inc, Boulder, CO.)

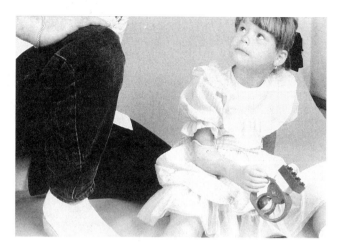

FIGURE 30-3
Young children can learn to contract the forearm muscles to operate the myoelectrically controlled terminal device. (Courtesy of Otto Bock Orthopedic Industry, Inc, Minneapolis, MN.)

ion or shoulder girdle protraction for terminal device operation. The toddler will revert to the earlier practice of opening the terminal device with the sound hand; eventually he or she will find that cable operation is more efficient, allowing more complex play maneuvers.

The natural inclination of the child is to reach for objects with the sound hand. To afford the child the necessary practice with the prosthesis, the therapist or parent should offer the youngster large objects or toys that require bimanual grasp to operate (Figure 30-2). Another technique to encourage prosthetic use is to have the child hold one object in the sound hand and another in the prosthesis. For example, two hand bells make twice as much sound as does one. With some children, prosthetic training merely involves using the terminal device as a stabilizer rather than as a prehensile tool; the youngster may lean the prosthesis onto a replica of a mailbox while placing objects in the slots with the sound hand. The prosthesis also serves to stabilize paper while the child draws and colors pictures.

Although children as young as 18 months have been fitted with myoelectrically controlled transradial prostheses,[32] those who are at least 3 years of age have an easier time learning to contract the appropriate flexors and extensors to effect closing and opening of the hand (Figure 30-3). The prosthesis is relatively heavy, susceptible to breakdown, and needs more maintenance than does a cable-operated device.[12] To prepare the child for a somewhat heavier myoelectric prosthesis, weight should be gradually added to the passive prosthesis. Rudimentary training begins with practice with the prosthesis off the arm. At first, the therapist may place an electrode on the sound forearm and ask the child to flex and extend the wrist to close and open the fingers of the prosthetic hand. The therapist then places an electrode on the forearm on the amputated side and encourages the child to discover that contraction of the forearm musculature on that side achieves the same results. Motorized toys can be used to help the child practice deliberate contraction of flexors and extensors to cause an electric train, for example, to go backward and forward, depending on which electrode was stimulated. When the child gains reasonable proficiency, the prosthetic socket can be made with the electrodes embedded in it. Care must be taken to achieve and maintain snug fit so that the electrodes are in constant contact with the skin.[33]

Practice to gain prosthetic proficiency is the same whether the prosthesis is cable or myoelectrically controlled. The beginner experiences many instances of dropping objects until she learns the amount of muscle contraction or tension on the cable that is needed to maintain suitable terminal device closure. The ability to close the terminal device around an object develops before active release. Grasping an object from the tabletop is difficult. As the young boy attempts to put objects into his mouth, he discovers that the change in shoulder position alters the tension on the control cable. Similarly, a little girl who drops a toy and tries to retrieve it also finds how she must hold her shoulder so that adequate cable tension is maintained. Those who are wearing myoelectrically controlled prostheses also notice that the prosthesis is easier to operate in some positions of the forearm than in others.

Practice in opening and closing the terminal device may involve moving pegs on a board. Tossing a beanbag is useful for teaching terminal device opening, as is playing cards. Cutting paper is another satisfying activity. The child holds the paper in the terminal device and uses the scissors in the sound hand. Prosthetic training should acquaint the child with objects of various textures, sizes, and shapes. Resilient foam toys are easier to grasp than are those made of rigid plastic, wood, or metal. Functional activities with readily available toys such as sewing cards, nested barrels, and snap-apart beads; removing a toy from a drawstring bag; opening a zipper; removing loose clothing; opening small boxes of raisins; opening and closing felt-tipped pens; or playing the xylophone entice the youngster to attempt grasping, holding, and releasing motions with the terminal device.[26] Moving checkers from one location to another on a game board is a good drill. The prosthesis is helpful when swinging and climbing in the playground, rolling a wheelbarrow or doll carriage, jumping rope, and riding a tricycle. Children with unilateral amputation usually regard the intact limb as the dominant one. Many children with unilateral amputation refer to the prosthesis as the helper, which correctly identifies its role as a device that assists the intact hand.

Functional training depends on the child's ability to reach the mouth, waist, hips, feet, and perineum. Feeding, dressing, writing, and personal hygiene are incorporated at the appropriate times. Thirty-month-old youngsters can throw and catch a ball, start uncomplicated dressing, and eat with a spoon with little spillage. Children play in sand, dirt, and water and engage in rough and tumble activities, which can damage the prosthesis. Daily inspection and attention to minor problems help to avoid the loss of wear time that is associated with major prosthetic repairs.

A 2-year-old with transhumeral amputation will have a prosthesis that has an elbow unit, although mastery of the elbow-locking cable is unlikely to occur before the third birthday.

Strategies to self-manage donning and doffing the prosthesis can be introduced to children as young as 3 years of age. Children find removing the prosthesis easier than applying it.

At 3 years of age, the youngster may begin to be curious about the rotational possibilities of the wrist unit. Objects of various shapes within reach oblige the child to turn the terminal device in the wrist unit to the suitable position. Most objects can be manipulated with the terminal device in the pronated position; however, thin disks are more easily managed with the terminal device in midposition, and small balls are best cradled in the terminal device that is rotated to the supinated position. Holding the handlebars of a tricycle or manipulating hand controls in other wheeled toys helps the child to learn how to use terminal device rotation in the wrist unit (Figure 30-4). Prosthetic activities for the toddler should include eating, drinking, dressing, and managing crayons and other school implements. Three-year-olds blow soap bubbles, pull up trousers, pull a belt through loops in trousers, and fill a cup with water from a spigot.[26]

Throughout the toddler phase, work periods should alternate with free play that may or may not involve the prosthesis. Weekly training sessions are effective. Parents should inspect the axilla; persistent redness indicates that the harness is applying undue pressure. The home program should include written suggestions regarding activities to promote bimanual prehension, instructions concerning the care of the prosthesis and the care of the child's skin, terminology pertaining to parts of the prosthesis, and ideas regarding clothing that will not impede prosthetic function.

School-Aged Children

An important consideration for the growing child is a socket that is large enough for comfortable fit yet adequate prosthetic control.

The 4-year-old child is usually coordinated enough to maintain grasp on fragile objects. With a voluntary-opening hook, the child must maintain tension on the control cable to prevent the hook fingers from snapping shut. A voluntary-closing terminal device necessitates application of gentle tension on the cable, rather than forceful shoulder motion. With a myoelectrically controlled hand, the child must contract flexors minimally so that the fingers close on the object without undue pressure. Four-year-olds can pour from containers, peel a banana, sharpen a pencil with a hand-held sharpener, sew, hammer nails, and apply adhesive bandages (Figure 30-5). The average 5-year-old can open a milk container and sweep with a brush and dust pan.[26] Goals of prosthetic training for school-aged children are summarized in Table 30-3.

The pediatric prehension assessment provides a standard clinical assessment of children with transradial amputation by objectively scoring activities of daily living that compel repetitive use of a terminal device. Three test bat-

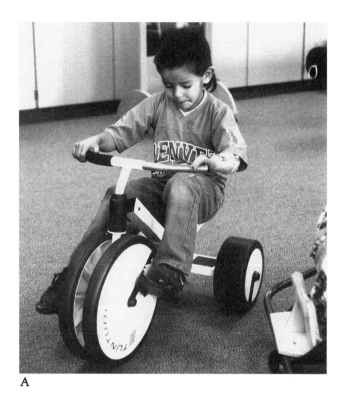

A

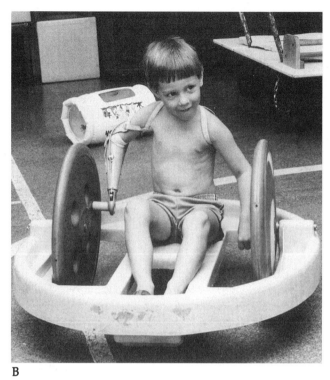

B

FIGURE 30-4
*Steering a tricycle using the handlebars **(A)** or other wheeled riding toy **(B)** provides excellent practice for using the prosthesis to assist the sound hand. (Courtesy of T.R.S., Inc, Boulder, CO.)*

teries correspond to age groups 2–3, 4–5, and 6–7. In test 1, the child is asked to string four large beads, open four 35-mm film cans, separate three nested screw-top barrels, assemble 10 interlocking beads, and separate a five-piece notched plastic block. In test 2, the child uses a sewing card, strings 10 small beads, sticks an adhesive bandage to the table, cuts a paper circle and glues it to another paper, and opens a small package of tissues. In test 3, the child is asked to cut modeling plastic with a knife and fork, cut paper, discard 5 playing cards from a hand of 10 cards, lace a shoe and tie a bow, and wrap a book.[26]

Children in elementary school are often fascinated by playing card games. Maintaining several cards in the terminal device and then releasing the desired card involves a gradation of tension on the control cable for prostheses equipped with a voluntary-opening or -closing terminal device. Card playing is more difficult with a myoelectrically controlled prosthesis because the child must contract the forearm flexors and extensors with the correct amount of force at the appropriate time.[34–36] The 5-year-old should be independent in dressing, except for buttons, shoelaces, and managing pullover shirts and sweaters.[1] As compared with their peers, children who wear a unilateral transradial prosthesis may be slightly delayed in the development of bimanual functional skills, regardless of the age of prosthetic fitting; the delay may be due to the insensate and nondexterous mechanical characteristics of the prosthesis.[37]

The child also needs to learn how to take care of the prosthesis, how to keep it clean, and to ask for help when parts malfunction. Skin inspection is an essential part of training.

Older Children and Adolescents
Many older children are able to incorporate the prosthesis into school activities. Sports prostheses, such as one with a terminal device that is designed to hold a basketball, give the wearer more opportunities to participate in group activities (Figure 30-6). Teenagers may find that playing a musical instrument is pleasurable. Simple adaptations, such as fingering a trumpet with the sound hand and supporting it with the prosthesis, can open a world of enjoyment to the musician.[38] Older adolescents should have prevocational exploration, vocational assessment, and, where indicated, job training.

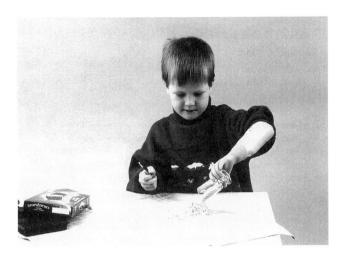

FIGURE 30-5
Preschool- and school-aged children develop manipulation skills as they incorporate their prosthesis into fine motor activities. Emptying a glass requires that the child generate the appropriate myoelectric signal to the forearm flexors to hold the container, while positioning the limb to pour. (Courtesy of Otto Bock Orthopedic Industry, Inc, Minneapolis, MN.)

Some adolescents with unilateral amputation seek to flee from parental control by abandoning their prostheses, preferring to manage with the intact hand. A few young people ultimately resume prosthetic wear either on a full-time or occasional basis. Certain activities are more easily accomplished without the prosthesis or are unsuitable for performing with a prosthesis. For example, one does not wear a prosthesis when showering. Individuals with transradial amputation may prefer to stabilize objects in the antecubital fossa, using elbow flexion, rather than use a prosthetic terminal device. Sometimes simple equipment adaptation facilitates one-handed performance, such as a book holder, guitar pick, or camera grip. Some individuals become very facile with the remaining upper limb, learning to bat a baseball, manage a keyboard, and fold laundry with one hand.[23]

Rehabilitation of Children with Lower-Limb Amputation

Care of children who have lower-limb deficiencies, whether congenital or acquired, is similar to that described for those with upper-limb amputations. Management should suit the patient's developmental stage, so that prosthetic use fosters achievement of key milestones. Parents serve as the primary instructors of their child, with the guidance of the physical therapist and other members

TABLE 30-3
Prosthetic Training Goals for School-Aged Children

Therapy sessions assist the school-aged child to:
  Maintain proper prosthetic fit
  Grasp firm and fragile objects without dropping or crushing them
  Open and close the terminal device reliably
  Don and doff the prosthesis independently
  Dress independently
  Recognize when the prosthesis needs repair or alteration
Parents of school-aged children with prostheses should:
  Encourage the child's independence in daily activities and play

of the clinic team. Early referral to a clinic team is equally important for the family with a child who has a leg amputation. Peer support is also valuable for parents who need to share concerns, suggestions, and camaraderie with others who have to cope with the same situation.

Infants
Achievement of sitting balance is the major guide to lower-limb prosthetic fitting.[2] The average age when healthy babies accomplish independent sitting is 6 months. Sitting depends on postural control and antigravity muscle strength. Sitting balance and trunk stabilization are also important for freeing the hands to explore the environment.[24,26] The goals of rehabilitation of infants with lower-limb malformation or amputation are summarized in Table 30-4.

Nondisabled infants who are 5–7 months of age discover the mobility possibilities of crawling and creeping, moving from supine to four-point and sitting positions and moving to the hands and knees from the sitting position.[39] Creeping on the hands and knees involves alternate action of the opposite arms and legs in a manner similar to that needed for walking. Hip extensors strengthen during creeping and kneeling. Rocking on four points before launching into creeping is another important precursor to walking.

Most babies are able to overcome gravity to pull up to standing and to rise from kneeling to standing at approximately 8 months of age. When pulling to stand, the baby expends great energy bouncing and actively disturbing balance. Bouncing gradually gives way to shifting weight from side to side. The initial standing posture is wide based with the hips abducted, flexed, and externally rotated. The base accommodates the child's new center of gravity position, which is higher than when creeping. Maintaining upright posture depends on sufficient maturity of the visual, proprioceptive, and vestibular systems.

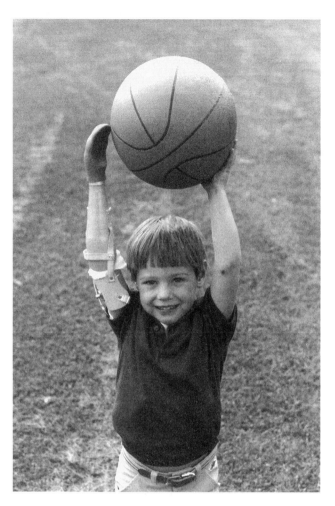

FIGURE 30-6
A variety of terminal devices are available for use in sports and recreational activities. This flexible mitt is shaped to enable participation in activities that require catching, manipulating, or throwing balls. (Courtesy of T.R.S., Inc, Boulder, CO.)

TABLE 30-4
Prosthetic Training Goals for Infants with Lower Extremity Amputation

Therapy sessions are designed to facilitate the infant's:
    Comfort with the prosthesis
    Wearing tolerance
    Ability to stand by leaning against a table
    Ability to cruise around furniture
    Ability to walk with and without support from a doll
       carriage or other supporting toy
Parents of infants with lower extremity prostheses should:
    Apply and remove the prosthesis correctly
    Care for the child's skin
    Care for the prosthesis
    Recognize and report any problems with the prosthesis

Although the 7-month-old displays stepping movements when supported, it is not until the youngster is approximately 10 months old that cruising along furniture becomes a preferred mode of locomotion. Cruising is usually the first form of independent walking and builds strength of the hip abductors. The average nondisabled child stands alone at approximately 11 months and walks alone at 12 months.[40] The urge to walk is the culmination of the endless pulling and standing activity that has occupied the baby for several preceding months.

Prosthetic fitting aims to facilitate the child's attainment of motor milestones. The infant who is missing a lower limb should have prosthetic restoration at approx-imately 6 months of age, when the baby has enough trunk control for sitting and is ready to pull to stand. A simple prosthesis fosters symmetric sitting balance and aids the baby's attempts to pull to standing. In addition, the prosthesis equalizes leg length, adds weight to the anomalous side, and obviates the tendency to compensate with a one-legged standing pattern. Reducing the weight asymmetry that is inherent in amputation facilitates rotational control of the trunk. The prosthesis enables standing and walking. Otherwise, the world is circumscribed by the confines of the stroller or playpen, and the amputation becomes a source of shame to be hidden. Fitting before 6 months is undesirable because the prosthesis would hinder the baby's efforts to turn from prone to supine position and back again.

The first prosthesis includes a solid-ankle cushion-heel (SACH) foot and, for the youngster with transfemoral amputation, a locked-knee unit. The SACH foot is the smallest foot that is manufactured. Unlike leather-soled shoes, rubber-soled shoes give the infant more traction and are therefore preferable. The prosthesis must be comfortable when the baby stands, sits, squats, creeps, and climbs. By age 3, most children can manage an unlocked knee.[3]

Equipment that is useful when working with young children with amputation includes a play table, an elevated sandbox, a floor mat, a rolling stool, a full-length mirror, steps, and a ramp. During the first training session, the therapist and parent confirm that the prosthesis fits comfortably, without redness of the amputation limb. Most of the handling of the child should be done by the parent, rather than the therapist, so that the family gains confidence in managing the child at home. A child-sized table and rolling and stacking toys should be available. The parent should encourage the child's standing on both feet by first supporting the trunk and then gradually reducing the support. The young child gains prosthetic tolerance and standing balance by being near the table. Initially, the child may lean the torso against the table while manipulating the toys. Eventually, the youngster will move along the periphery of the table to place objects in the desired location. The table enables the infant to gain prosthetic tolerance, cruise, get up and down to the floor, and play with the toys on the floor and on the table. Playing with toys on the table requires the use of both hands, thus enabling reliance on standing balance. The SACH foot causes the center of standing pressure to be more posterior than is the case with the anatomic foot.[41] Toys should be moved to places on the table where the child has to reach in different directions, shifting weight.

When first learning to walk with a prosthesis, the child moves like someone maneuvering on a slippery surface, being rather cautious about balance. Initially, the youngster takes small steps and has a wide base, keeping the trunk upright and arms abducted. The new prosthetic wearer resembles normal peers who begin walking with increased hip and knee flexion, full-foot initial contact, short stride, increased cadence, and relative foot drop on the sound side in swing phase.[42–46]

At home, a sturdy table that is chest high to the child encourages standing balance and cruising as he or she plays with toys that are placed on the table. Raised sandboxes, blocks, finger paints, and pans of water with floating toys all promote standing balance. A playpen is a good environment to enable the baby to pull to standing, cruise the perimeter, and sit whenever he or she wishes. Balls are useful in habilitation. Kicking the ball requires balance on one leg and flexion of the other leg. The baby starts by holding onto a stable object with both hands, then with one, and eventually without holding. Throwing a ball requires good balance and usually sustains the infant's interest. Wheeled toys, such as a doll carriage, enable the child to walk with the prosthesis with a modicum of support. Independent ambulation is encouraged by placing toys where the child must take a few steps to reach them.

Young children frequently revert to crawling and sitting on the floor as they grow accustomed to the prosthesis. Falling is seldom a problem, inasmuch as the youngster generally lands on the buttocks, as does a child with intact lower extremities. When the child falls or tries to retrieve a toy on the floor, parents and therapist should let the infant explore the movement, rather than being overly protective. Just as other children learn to walk by supporting themselves on furniture, the child who wears a prosthesis should have the same experience to develop confidence. Parallel bars, walkers, and harnesses are seldom

TABLE 30-5
Prosthetic Training Goals for Toddlers with Lower Extremity Amputation

Goals of rehabilitation for toddlers with lower limb amputation include:

    Full-time wear of the prosthesis, except for bathing and sleeping

    Use of the prosthesis in age-appropriate ambulatory activities

Parents of toddlers with lower limb prostheses should:

    Encourage use of the prosthesis

    Provide toys and equipment that require age-appropriate activities

    Inspect the skin to determine whether the prosthesis causes undue irritation

advisable for children with unilateral amputation or bilateral transtibial amputation,[47] although some fearful children may benefit from their use.[15] These youngsters can also be expected to become very proficient in ambulation.

Because the prosthesis imposes weight-bearing loads on portions of the leg that are not ordinarily used for this purpose, it is important to build tolerance to prosthetic wear gradually so that skin over weight-bearing areas can adjust to the pressure. During the first week most infants tolerate an hour of wear, after which the prosthesis should be removed and the skin examined. After a 10- to 15-minute rest period, the prosthesis can be replaced for another hour. Signs of fatigue, limping, and avoiding standing on the prosthesis indicate that the prosthesis is irritating and should be removed. The infant with a transfemoral prosthesis should be checked to determine whether skin near the proximal part of the prosthesis is irritated by urine or feces, which may leak from the diaper.

Toddlers

By 15 months of age, toddlers are upright and mobile. The heel-toe sequence replaces flat-foot contact during the second year. Neurologic maturation, changes in physique, and improved strength are evident as the child's base of support narrows and stability improves.[44] Muscular activity has matured into the adult pattern.[45] Goals for rehabilitation (Table 30-5) reflect the developmental activities of a preschool-aged child.

Another developmental milestone that is expected of all children, including the child with a prosthesis, is running, which is acquired between 2 and 4 years of age. The flight phase (double float) occurs by strong application of propulsive force during late stance. The prosthetic foot offers much less energy storage and release as compared

TABLE 30-6

Goals for School-Aged Children and Adolescents with Lower Extremity Amputation

In later childhood and adolescence, rehabilitation includes:
> Monitoring and maintaining proper prosthetic fit
> Inspection of the skin
> Donning and doffing the prosthesis independently
> Dressing independently
> Engaging in the full range of ambulatory activities with the prosthesis
> Recognizing when the prosthesis needs repair or alteration

Parents of school-aged children and adolescents with lower limb prostheses should:
> Encourage the young person's independence
> Provide opportunities for sports participation

with the gastrocnemius. Consequently, the child with a prosthesis adopts an asymmetric running gait that emphasizes propulsion on the sound side. Two-year-olds can kick a ball accurately, steer a push toy, and jump.[39] As with running, jumping with a prosthesis is primarily an action of the sound side. Games of throwing and catching a ball or beanbag and tossing darts help the toddler to refine balance with the prosthesis.

The 3-year-old can leap, jump, gallop, climb stairs step over step, and manage a tricycle. The youngster with a prosthesis has an easier time if the tricycle pedal has a dorsal strap to secure the prosthetic foot. Jumping from a step and hopping are other toddler stunts. Playground equipment, such as a jungle gym, slide, swing, seesaw, sandbox, and tunnels, is enticing. Children with unilateral transtibial amputation achieve an almost normal gait and have no difficulty in climbing inclines and stairs.[12] Opportunities for kneeling, managing various types of chairs, and getting to and from the floor are additional elements in rehabilitation. The child will need help in removing and donning the prosthesis.

School-Aged Children and Adolescents

By 4 years of age, most children can descend stairs step over step, bicycle, and roller skate. Skates that clip onto the shoe are preferable to shoe skates; the latter require that the prosthetic foot accommodate the height of the heel in the shoe skate. Five-year-olds skip rope and play dodge ball. Accurate kicking demonstrates balance on one foot while transferring force to the ball.[40] By age 6, children can start, stop, and change direction with ease, as well as skip and hop for long distances.[39] The child moves toward independence in prosthetic management as well, taking more responsibility for donning/doffing, skin inspection, and maintenance of the prosthesis (Table 30-6).

Children who acquire lower-limb amputation after the age of 5 may respond more favorably to balance and gait training similar to that which is appropriate for adults. Physical therapy emphasizes balance, weight shifting, control of the prosthetic foot, and, in the case of the child with transfemoral amputation, the knee unit.

Sports are particularly useful to develop self-esteem, as well as strength and coordination.[48,49] The prosthesis needs carbon acrylic or graphite reinforcement to withstand extremely high stresses.[3] The child should understand that shoes must always be worn: The plantar surface of most prosthetic feet is not durable enough to withstand abrasion by a sidewalk, and the alignment of the foot is intended for a shoe.

Some activities are more easily performed without a lower-limb prosthesis or do not require a prosthesis. Children should learn how to use crutches as an alternate mode of locomotion when the prosthesis must be repaired. Bathing is facilitated either by sitting on the shower floor or by use of a sturdy bath seat. Most people prefer to swim and scuba dive without a prosthesis. They hop or use crutches to get from the dressing room to the water's edge. Sports prostheses, such as a swimming prosthesis with a fin in place of the foot, can be constructed. Bicycling, skiing, and mountain climbing are other sports that can be enjoyed with or without a prosthesis.[23]

Rehabilitation of Children with Multiple Limb Amputation

Babies who have anomalies of one or both upper limbs, together with lower-limb deficiency, generally do best by being fitted first with simple lower-limb prostheses to foster sitting balance. It is undesirable to introduce upper- and lower-limb prostheses simultaneously. Subsequently, upper-limb prostheses should be provided.

When both upper limbs are anomalous, a simple bilateral fitting counteracts the tendency toward development of positional scoliosis. The baby with bilateral upper-limb amputation should receive prostheses after independent walking is established; otherwise, prostheses make it more difficult to creep, move about on the floor, and pull to stand using the chin for support. Those with bilateral upper-limb amputation or anomaly become very skillful with foot prehension. The extent to which foot use should be encouraged is controversial. Foot prehension is so rarely observed in public that the child may experience unwanted stares. Nevertheless, feet have the tactile sensation and considerable dexterity that prostheses lack. Children with bilateral longitudinal deficiencies have partial or complete hands; they would be encumbered by wearing prostheses. Functional activities with and without prostheses should be introduced according to the physical and emotional maturity of the child. Adaptive aids may be required for some functions, such as personal hygiene.[50]

Infants with tri- or quadrimembral limb deficiency move about by rolling along the floor. They need opportunities to look at objects and manipulate toys with their mouth and their residual limbs. Most infants develop good sitting balance and can scoot along on their buttocks. Because of the drastic reduction in body surface, such children can easily become overheated. They should be dressed very lightly to enable heat dissipation.

Children with bilateral transfemoral amputations may require manually locking knees until they are age 6 or older.[3] They progress more rapidly after practice in the parallel bars if they have a pair of forearm or axillary crutches. Depending on the length of the amputation limbs, the child may eventually feel comfortable with a pair of forearm crutches or canes. Young children with bilateral transfemoral amputations may walk indoors without any assistive devices; however, few are willing to venture outdoors and across streets without at least one cane. In adolescence, many find that a wheelchair provides more efficient mobility.

SUMMARY

Rehabilitation of children with amputations can be very gratifying. The physical therapist, together with all members of the clinic team, should design the rehabilitation program to assist the child in achieving the developmental milestones that are associated with maturing upper- and lower-limb function. Psychosocial factors govern the behavior of the child and family; team members need to recognize the basis for parental distress yet foster realistic expectations for the child's function while demonstrating that the child is lovable regardless of the condition of the limbs. Peer support is a most helpful way of facilitating constructive response to the child.

REFERENCES

1. Stanger M. Limb Deficiencies and Amputations. In SK Campbell (ed), Physical Therapy for Children. Philadelphia: Saunders, 1994.
2. Blakeslee B (ed). The Limb-Deficient Child. Berkeley, CA: University of California Press, 1963.
3. Cummings DR, Kapp SL. Lower-limb pediatric prosthetics: general considerations and philosophy. J Prosthet Orthot 1992;4(4):196–206.
4. Fishman S, Edelstein J, Krebs D. ISNY above-knee prosthetic sockets; pediatric experience. J Pediatr Orthop 1987;Oct(5):557–562.
5. Fishman S, Berger N, Edelstein J. ISNY flexible sockets for upper-limb amputees. J Assoc Child Prosthet Orthot Clin 1989; 24:8–11.
6. Setoguchi Y, Rosenfelder R. The Limb-Deficient Child. Springfield, IL: Thomas, 1982.
7. Krane EJ, Heller LB. The prevalence of phantom sensation and pain in pediatric amputees. J Pain Symptom Mgt 1995; 10(1):21–29.
8. McGrath PA, Hillier LM. Phantom limb sensations in adolescents: a case study to illustrate the utility of sensation and pain logs in pediatric clinical practice. J Pain Symptom Mgt 1992;7(1):46–53.
9. Erikson EH. Identity, Youth and Crisis. New York: Norton, 1968.
10. Novotny M, Swagman A. Caring for children with orthotic/ prosthetic needs. J Prosthet Orthot 1992;4(4):191–195.
11. Challenor YB. Limb Deficiencies in Children. In GE Molnar (ed), Pediatric Rehabilitation. Baltimore: Williams & Wilkins, 1985;400–424.
12. Marquardt EG. A holistic approach to rehabilitation for the limb-deficient child. Arch Phys Med Rehabil 1983;64(6): 237–242.
13. Fischer AG. Initial prosthetic fitting of the congenital below-elbow amputee: are we fitting them early enough? Int Clin Information Bull 1976;11–12:7–10.
14. Patton JG. Developmental Approach to Pediatric Prosthetic Evaluation and Training. In DJ Atkins, RH Meier (eds), Comprehensive Management of the Upper-Limb Amputee. New York: Springer-Verlag, 1988;137–164.
15. Radford J, Steensma J. The lower extremity toddler amputee: training procedures. Phys Ther Rev 1957;37:32–41.
16. Robertson E. Rehabilitation of Arm Amputees and Limb-Deficient Children. London: Bailliere Tindall, 1978.
17. Letts M, Stevens L, Coleman J, Kettner R. Puppetry and doll play as an adjunct to pediatric orthopedics. J Pediatr Orthop 1983;3(5):605–609.
18. Svoboda J. Psychosocial considerations in pediatrics: use of amputee dolls. J Prosthet Orthot 1992;4(4):207–212.
19. Varni JW, Rubenfeld LA, Talbot D, Setoguchi Y. Determinants of self-esteem in children with congenital/acquired limb deficiencies. J Dev Behav Pediatr 1989;10(1):13–16.
20. Varni JW, Rubenfeld LA, Talbot D, Setoguchi Y. Stress, social support, and depressive symptomatology in children with congenital/acquired limb deficiencies. J Pediatr Psychol 1989;14(4):515–530.
21. Varni JW, Setoguchi Y. Psychosocial factors in the management of children with limb deficiencies. Phys Med Rehabil Clin North Am 1991;2:395–404.
22. Boren HA. Adolescent adjustment to amputation necessitated by bone cancer. Orthop Nurs 1985;4(5):30–32.
23. Edelstein JE. Special Considerations: Rehabilitation without Prosthetics: Functional Skills Training. In JH Bowker, JW Michael (eds), Atlas of Limb Prosthetics: Surgical, Prosthetic, and Rehabilitation Principles (2nd ed). St. Louis: Mosby–Year Book, 1992;721–728.
24. Cech D, Martin S. Functional Movement Development across the Life Span. Philadelphia: Saunders, 1995.

25. Jain S. Rehabilitation in limb deficiency. 2: The pediatric amputee. Arch Phys Med Rehabil 1996;77(3 Suppl):S9–S13.

26. Krebs D (ed). Prehension Assessment: Prosthetic Therapy for the Upper-Limb Child Amputee. Thorofare, NJ: Slack, 1987.

27. Angliss VE. Habilitation of upper-limb-deficient children. Am J Occup Ther 1974;28(7):407–414.

28. Krebs DE, Edelstein JE, Thornby MA. Prosthetic management children with limb deficiencies. Phys Ther 1991;71(12):920–934.

29. Shaperman J. Early learning of hook operation. Int Clin Information Bull 1975;14:11–18.

30. Sypniewski BL. The child with terminal transverse partial hemimelia: a review of the literature on prosthetic management. Artif Limbs 1972;16(1):20–50.

31. Weiss-Lambrou R. A Manual for the Congenital Unilateral Below-Elbow Child Amputee. Rockville, MD: American Occupational Therapy Association, 1981.

32. Sorbye R. Myoelectric prosthetic fitting in young children. Clin Orthop 1980;May(148):34–40.

33. Glynn MK, Galway HR, Hunter G, Sauter WF. Management of the upper-limb–deficient child with a powered prosthetic device. Clin Orthop 1986;Aug(209):202–207.

34. Trost FJ. A comparison of conventional and myoelectric below-elbow prosthetic use. Int Clin Information Bull 1983;18:9–16.

35. Weaver SA, Lange LR, Vogts VM. Comparison of myoelectric and conventional prostheses for adolescent amputees. Am J Occup Ther 1988;42(2):87–91.

36. Edelstein JE, Berger N. Performance comparison among children fitted with myoelectric and body-powered hands. Arch Phys Med Rehabil 1993;74(4):376–380.

37. Thornby MA, Krebs DE. Bimanual skill development in pediatric below-elbow amputation: a multicenter, cross-sectional study. Arch Phys Med Rehabil 1992;73(8):697–702.

38. Edelstein J. Musical Options for Upper-Limb Amputees. In M Lee (ed), Rehabilitation Music and Human Well-being. St. Louis: MMB Music, 1989.

39. Campbell SK. Understanding Motor Performance in Children. In SK Campbell (ed), Physical Therapy for Children. Philadelphia: Saunders, 1994;1–38.

40. Tecklin JS. Pediatric Physical Therapy. Philadelphia: Lippincott, 1994.

41. Clark LA, Zernicke RF. Balance in lower limb child amputees. Prosthet Orthot Int 1981;5(1):11–18.

42. Higgins S, Higgins JR. The Emergence of Gait. In RL Craik, CA Oatis, Gait Analysis: Theory and Application. St. Louis: Mosby, 1995;15–24.

43. Leonard EL. Early Motor Development and Control: Foundations for Independent Walking. In GL Smidt GL (ed), Gait in Rehabilitation. New York: Churchill Livingstone, 1990;121–140.

44. Stout JL. Gait: Development and Analysis. In SK Campbell (ed), Physical Therapy for Children. Philadelphia: Saunders, 1994;79–104.

45. Sutherland DH. Gait Disorders in Childhood and Adolescence. Baltimore: Williams & Wilkins, 1984.

46. Woollacott M, Shumway-Cook A (eds). Development of Posture and Gait across the Life Span. Columbia, SC: University of South Carolina Press, 1989.

47. Kitabayashi B. The physical therapist's responsibility to the lower extremity child amputee. Phys Ther Rev 1961;41:722–727.

48. Burgess EM, Rappoport A. Physical Fitness: A Guide for Individuals with Lower Limb Loss. Baltimore: Department of Veterans Affairs, 1992.

49. Kegel B. Physical Fitness: Sports and Recreation for Those with Lower Limb Amputation or Impairment. Journal of Rehabilitation Research and Development Clinical. Supplement no. 1. Washington, DC: Department of Veterans Affairs, 1985.

50. Friedmann L. Functional Skills Training in Multiple Limb Anomalies. In DJ Atkins, RH Meier (eds), Comprehensive Management of the Upper-Limb Amputee. New York: Springer-Verlag, 1988;150–164.

31

Upper Extremity Amputations
and Prosthetic Management

ROBERT D. LIPSCHUTZ

Few people, whether lay, medical professional, or rehabilitation professional, have a clear understanding of upper limb prosthetics. Many people are familiar with fictional characters with upper extremity amputation, such as Captain Hook, the Six Million Dollar Man, or Luke Skywalker, or have seen upper limb prostheses presented in the remake of *The Fugitive*. Although the development of upper limb prostheses has far surpassed the single hook used by Captain Hook, current upper extremity components are unable to duplicate the complex functions of the human hand. The human hand is a magnificent instrument with highly sophisticated movements, elegant structure, precise sensory capabilities, and an incredible array of functional capabilities.

Lower extremity prosthetics can effectively restore mobility and locomotion to those with transtibial and transfemoral amputation; using a prosthesis is often more efficient and cosmetically acceptable than using a wheelchair or single limb gait with crutches. Current technology, however, cannot yet fully substitute for the many ways that we use our hands. Many individuals learn to compensate for the loss of a hand by using the forearm, elbow, or mouth. Terminal devices (TDs), such as a hook, may be very functional but are not cosmetically appealing. Mechanical hands often have very lifelike cosmetic covers but have limited functional applications. For these reasons, the rate of dissatisfaction or rejection of upper extremity prostheses is significantly higher than that of lower extremity prostheses.[1] Nevertheless, thousands of individuals with upper extremity amputations successfully use upper limb prostheses to assist them in bimanual tasks, activities of daily living, and psychosocial peer acceptance.

In this chapter we provide an overview of prosthetic options, postoperative and preprosthetic management, and prosthetic training for persons with congenital and acquired upper limb amputations. We introduce commonly chosen components, suspensions, control systems, and prosthetic designs and assist the reader in developing strategies for clinical decision making in choosing among the available design and component options.

HISTORY OF UPPER LIMB PROSTHETICS

The earliest historical record of an attempt to replace an amputated upper extremity dates from the second Punic War (218–201 B.C.), when the Roman general, Marcus Sergius, was fitted with an iron hand to replace his right hand and allow him to return to the battlefield.[2] Little record is available of further advancement or development in upper extremity prosthetics until the early nineteenth century. The iron hands and armor upper limb prostheses that have survived and are now artifacts in museum collections suggest that most of these passive devices were used to conceal the missing limb of a warrior when he went into battle. This cosmetic role of a prosthesis is often as important to persons with upper limb loss today as it was in previous centuries. As with the passive iron hands of previous centuries, function must often be sacrificed to achieve a lifelike cosmetic appearance.

The first major development in upper extremity prosthetics occurred in 1812, when Peter Balif, a dentist from Berlin, developed a mechanism that controlled an artificial hand without the use of the contralateral hand.[2] A strap system harnessed proximal body motions to open and close a prosthetic hand. This early mechanism has evolved and improved into the cable control system that is currently used for body-powered upper extremity prostheses.

The next major development in upper extremity prosthetics was the introduction of the split hook TD, patented by D. W. Dorrance in 1912.[3] This device enhanced the ability to grasp and hold objects and was well received by many persons with upper limb loss. Many variations of the original split hook design have been developed to meet specific functional needs of the prosthetic wearer: One version, designed for plumbers, is shaped to hold pipes. Another version, designed for farmers and ranchers, incorporates a tool to manage baling wire.

Much of the research and development in upper extremity prosthetics that has taken place since the introduction of the split hook has been government funded, in response to the rehabilitation needs of veterans injured in the major wars. In the late 1950s and early 1960s, an alarming increase in congenital limb deficiencies occurred related to the use of thalidomide for morning sickness. Unfortunately, this medication, when taken during the first trimester, disrupted development of the limbs, and many children were born with multiple limb deficiencies or absent limbs. Thalidomide was most widely prescribed in Canada, Denmark, Holland, Scotland, Sweden, England, and Germany. These countries have since become leaders in the research, design, and development of upper limb components for children.

Well-funded government-supported research has led to many technological advances in upper extremity prosthetics. After World War II, pneumatic and electronic switch controls became an alternative to earlier body-powered cable systems. The 1960s saw the development of strategies to harness electromyographic (EMG) signals with electrodes placed on the skin surface over a muscle belly. This amplified signal could be used to control a terminal device and an elbow unit. The myoelectric revolution began with the introduction of the first functional myoelectric prosthesis, the Russian Arm, which allowed on-off switching of a prosthetic hand.[4] In recent decades, the emphasis in upper extremity prosthetic research and development has clearly shifted to externally powered components.

Other significant advances that have improved the outlook for persons with upper extremity limb loss include innovative socket designs, improved surgical techniques, and adaptations of components used in electronics and aerospace for upper extremity prosthetics. Greater emphasis is placed on patient education and training, so that individuals are better able to use their prosthesis to its maximum capabilities. The fact remains that, despite advancements, the upper extremity prosthesis cannot completely replace a lost limb, although it is an effective assistive tool that makes daily tasks less difficult and enhances the quality of the patient's life.

ETIOLOGY OF UPPER EXTREMITY AMPUTATION

Almost 90% of upper limb amputations are the result of traumatic injury.[5] Only a small number of upper extremity amputations are the consequence of peripheral vascular disease, tumor, infection, and congenital limb deficiencies. The distribution of these etiologies is vastly different from that of the lower limb. Traumatic amputation occurs primarily in young men between the ages of 20 and 40; the ratio of men to women with new upper limb loss is approximately 4:1.[5] Although as many as 12,000 new upper limb amputations occur each year, nine times as many lower limb amputation surgeries are performed.[6]

Many traumatic amputations of the upper extremity are a result of carelessness when using machinery or equipment or of tampering with safety features that have been installed on equipment to prevent such injuries. Farming accidents in the Midwestern states account for most new traumatic upper limb amputations in the United States. Many of these accidents occur when an individual attempts to clear a chute without turning the equipment off or tries to force vegetation through the chute manually, such that clothing becomes entangled and draws the limb into the machine. Other accidental amputations may result from being caught in industrial presses, from frostbite, or from electrical burns. The latter frequently require high proximal debridement and bilateral amputation because of the pattern of electrical injury in the human body.

SURGICAL ISSUES IN UPPER EXTREMITY AMPUTATION

Microsurgical limb salvage protocols, external fixation technology, and improved surgical techniques have had two effects on upper limb amputations: reducing the rate of upper limb amputations, and facilitating positive outcome when amputation is deemed necessary. As is the case in lower extremity amputation, the surgical team has two goals: to preserve as much limb length as possible (without the need for revision), and to create a pain-free, functional limb. These goals are often tempered by the emergency presentation of the patient: Little time may be available to prepare for surgery, and preservation of life is usually the primary focus. Debridement and closure may be a secondary or tertiary focus.

Whether the amputation surgery is an emergency or a planned procedure, six factors influence functional outcome[7]:

1.   Optimal skin closure and healing result in a nonadherent suture line and soft tissue coverage that is neither too taut or hypermobile. The residual limb then

has the potential of being pain free and with intact sensation.

2. Attention to the contour of residual muscle bellies increases the likelihood of maintaining bulk and motor power. Early activation and mobilization of muscles and their supportive soft tissues minimize the risk of contracture and disuse atrophy, especially for those with thermal injury.

3. Good surgical technique ensures that nerves are effectively resected, ligated, buried, or anastomosed, to reduce the likelihood of development of a problematic neuroma.

4. Vascular supply must be adequate to support tissue viability, wound closure, and the healing process. In some cases, vessel repair or grafting may be necessary.

5. Distal edges of bone must be beveled or rounded, and fractures, if present, must be adequately stabilized.

6. Joint range of motion (ROM) must be preserved as much as possible for effective prosthetic use once healing has occurred. The use of splints, attention to proper positioning, and exercise (passive and active) are strategies that are used to address ROM issues.

PREPROSTHETIC MANAGEMENT

One of the most important factors in prosthetic management is effective patient education that engages the patient as an active participant in postoperative care. The areas which must be part of preprosthetic care for patients with new upper limb amputation include: wound healing, pain management and edema control, skin care and desensitization, effective shaping of the residual limb, range of motion and strength, single limb skills, psychological adjustment to limb loss, and informed decisions about their prosthetic choices.

Wound Healing, Pain, and Edema Control

The primary goals in the immediate postoperative period are to promote healing, to control edema, and to reduce postoperative pain and phantom sensation. For most patients, a compression garment or an elastic bandage is applied soon after amputation to minimize postoperative edema. Although the prosthetist may measure and deliver the shrinker, nursing and therapy staff are responsible for ensuring proper donning and wear and monitoring the condition of the residual limb and status of the healing suture line.

The use of a compression garment or shrinker to minimize edema is also a key component of postoperative pain control. Patients who consistently wear a shrinker or elastic wrap tend to have less difficulty with phantom sensation or phantom pain. Compression also minimizes the risk of reflex sympathetic dystrophy (RSD) in the postoperative period. For certain patients, an immediate postoperative prosthesis can be fit soon after amputation, although this strategy is far more common after lower extremity amputations. Early prosthetic fitting also helps to reduce the intensity or duration of phantom sensation and RSD.

Nurses and therapists who work with the patient monitor the level of discomfort, evaluate the condition of the skin and wound, and watch for early signs of RSD. Although the nurse or therapist initially assists the patient in donning and doffing the compression garment, patients must learn to manage these routines safely and precisely by themselves. When postoperative pain is significant or problematic, the therapist might use transcutaneous electrical nerve stimulation (TENS) to help the patient better manage the pain. Various pain medications are often prescribed by the surgeon or attending physician for management of acute postoperative pain.

Skin Care and Desensitization

In learning to care for the residual limb, the patient first must understand the process of wound healing and develop good habits for hygienic skin care. These early routines are the foundation for effective skin care long after healing has occurred. The patient must also prepare the residual limb for enclosure in a firmly fitting socket. This desensitization is often best accomplished by the patient, especially if the residual limb is hypersensitive or if RSD has developed. The therapist might provide verbal instruction and demonstrate the desired technique on the patient's intact limb and provide encouragement and feedback as the patient uses gentle or deep massage, tapping, firm pressure, or vibration to desensitize or loosen adhesions on the residual limb. For patients in whom RSD develops in the postoperative period, the desensitization process may be quite challenging.

Shaping of the Residual Limb

Edema control strategies, such as wrapping with an Ace bandage or wearing a commercially available shrinker or other compression garment, also facilitate proper shaping of the residual limb. Aggressive edema control greatly decreases the time between amputation and initial fitting of a prosthesis. Patients who are fit with a prosthesis soon after amputation are much more likely to accept fully and integrate their prosthesis into daily activities than are those whose fitting is delayed by edema and healing problems.[8]

Range of Motion and Strength

Preservation of ROM and of muscle strength are also important components of limb care in the postoperative/preprosthetic period. Patients are likely to hold their healing residual limb in a flexed and protected position. Without stretching and strengthening exercises, flexion contracture at the elbow, and adduction/internal rotation tightness at the shoulder can develop. Until the suture line has closed securely, gentle active and isometric exercise is the most appropriate strategy. Once the incision is adequately healed, resistance exercise can be added to the routine. Loss of full ROM and strength has a significant impact on how facile the patient can become with the prosthesis.

Prosthetic Prescription

An important component of patient education is the introduction of the various components for upper limb prostheses. Although specific recommendations for prosthetic design and components are made by the rehabilitation team, involvement of patients and family members in the decision-making process ultimately facilitates acceptance and functional use of the prosthesis after delivery and training. Discussion of the patient's goals and expectations for the prosthesis must include a truthful representation of the capabilities of prosthetic components and design. It is often helpful to use demonstrations with mock devices, to show videos of individuals using their prosthesis, or to provide the opportunity for interaction with experienced upper limb prosthetic users to assist patients with recent amputation and their families to understand the possibilities and limitations of upper extremity prostheses.

For patients who are candidates for myoelectric control of a TD or elbow component, the final task of preprosthetic management is determination of appropriate EMG electrode placement sites. Patients must also learn to activate their muscles in the sequence and with the force necessary to control the opening or closing of a prosthetic hand or the flexing and extending of a prosthetic elbow unit. It is often beneficial to practice these skills before prosthetic fitting by placing electrodes over muscle bellies to control a remote mock prosthesis to ensure that the patient fully understands the principles of myoelectric prostheses.

Single Limb Skills

It is very important to assist individuals with a unilateral amputation to develop skills and abilities in one-handed activities, especially if the dominant hand has been amputated. Children with a single congenital limb deficiency often become more adept with their intact limb alone

than with their prosthesis. Persons with bilateral upper limb amputations have a more difficult time adapting to independence without prostheses, especially when the amputations are not congenital. A prosthesis that is necessary for or enhances success in performance of prehensile tasks is more readily accepted by patients.

Psychosocial Issues

It is important for the rehabilitation team to be aware of the feelings and emotions that are experienced by patients and family members after the traumatic loss of an upper extremity. The relief and thankfulness of surviving may be quickly replaced by uncertainty and a sense of hopelessness or despair when the future is considered. It is often very helpful to introduce patients with recent amputation to others who have been through similar experiences, either in the context of a support group or a one-on-one encounter. Many individuals who have become successful prosthetic users attest to the importance of supporting each other and obtaining the appropriate device and training.

EARLY PROSTHETIC MANAGEMENT

Patients fit with a prosthesis within 30 days of upper extremity amputation have a much greater rate of acceptance of the prosthesis than do those whose prosthetic fitting is delayed or occurs more than 30 days after amputation.[8] As soon as adequate wound closure and effective edema control have occurred, the patient can be casted for a training or temporary prosthesis. Patient education continues with an orientation to the specific components of the prosthesis: the harness or suspension system, the socket, the elbow unit (for those with transhumeral amputation), the wrist unit, and the TD (hook or prosthetic hand). Patients must also learn about the control system selected for their prosthesis and how to use their passive prosthesis or to activate their cable-driven (body powered) or externally powered prosthesis. It is not uncommon for patients to try a variety of components and tasks during this training or temporary prosthetic period. In this way, the most appropriate prescription for a definitive prosthesis can be determined.

Attention to skin care and hygiene continues to be important: The patient assumes responsibility for skin integrity, keeping the socket and socks free of dirt and debris. The factors that most clearly influence the success or failure of prosthetic intervention are the fit and comfort of the socket, the effectiveness of training, the patient's satisfaction with the cosmesis of the prosthesis, and the patient's psychosocial adaptation after amputation.

Prosthetic options and rehabilitation strategies vary with the level of amputation and the length of the residual limb. The following sections explore the most commonly chosen components, control systems, and training programs for patients with partial hand amputation, wrist disarticulation, transradial amputation, transhumeral amputation, and shoulder disarticulation.

DIGIT AND PARTIAL HAND AMPUTATIONS

For patients who have lost middle or distal phalanges, prosthetic restoration can be accomplished by placing a prosthetic digit over the remaining phalange(s). This covering reduces the patient's ability to feel with the residual limb, however, and may somewhat compromise precision hand function. The transition between even the most cosmetic prosthetic finger and the anatomic hand is often somewhat obvious.

For patients who have lost multiple digits, the most common prosthetic option is a cosmetic glove, which covers the remaining hand and often extends beyond the wrist for adequate suspension. This glove, however, covers the intact skin of the residual limb: The resulting compromise of sensation often has a significant negative impact on functional use of the hand. As cosmetic gloves become more lifelike (some have air-brushed veins and freckles), cost increases significantly. A functional prosthesis for patients with multiple digit loss is the Robin-Aids design (Vallejo, CA). Some Robin-Aids hands enable the prosthetist to design a prosthetic hand with actively positioned digits. Individual digits can be removed from the "hand" to accomodate the remaining fingers. These devices are challenging to fit, and many patients are not well satisfied with the degree of function that is possible.

Partial hand amputations often are the result of a crush or explosion injury. The surgeon is challenged to create a functional hand in the face of missing digits or thumb and a significantly injured palm. This may be as simple as shaping the residuum to best accept a prosthesis or as complex as surgically recreating a thumb from one of the remaining digits so that opposition and grasp can be preserved. The prosthetist is challenged to design a custom prosthesis that enhances function and is acceptably cosmetic. When cosmesis is the patient's primary goal, the prosthetist can fashion a lifelike glove with passive fingers and fillers for the palm. As in the cosmetic gloves used for patients with multiple digit loss, covering the skin of the partial hand residuum reduces the use of sensation during functional activities. Many patients with partial

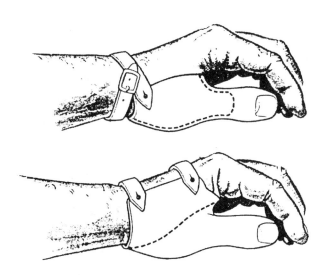

FIGURE 31-1
A thumb post prosthesis set in some degree of opposition can assist the patient with partial or complete thumb amputation to use the hand for grasp and object manipulation. (Reprinted with permission from American Academy of Orthopaedic Surgeons. Orthopaedic Appliances Atlas. Vol 2. Ann Arbor, MI: Edwards, 1960;91.)

hand amputation develop functional strategies to use their residual limb without a prosthesis or cosmetic glove.

It is very important to replace a thumb that has been amputated either prosthetically or surgically. Without a thumb, hand function is seriously compromised, and the hand cannot be effectively used to hold or grasp objects or tools. A passive prosthetic thumb is an effective post for grasp and object manipulation by the remaining digits (Figure 31-1).

Patients with single digit amputation often do not require occupational or physical therapy. Those with multiple digit or partial hand amputation who wear a cosmetic glove may or may not be referred for rehabilitation, depending on their functional goals. Those who have plastic or reconstructive surgery to create a new thumb (pollicization) or to deepen web spaces to improve their grasp often require intensive postoperative therapy to preserve ROM and muscle strength and to learn how best to maximize function of their restored hands.

WRIST DISARTICULATION AND TRANSRADIAL AMPUTATION

The vast majority of upper extremity prostheses are fabricated for patients with wrist disarticulation or transra-

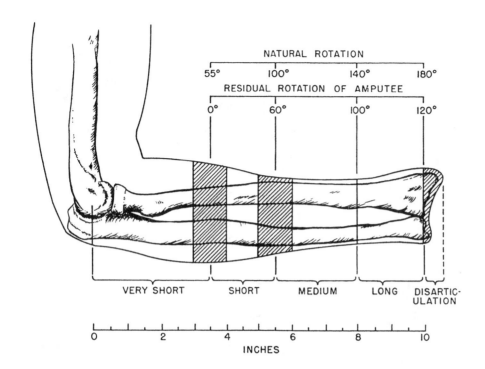

FIGURE 31-2
Potential for pronation/supination of upper extremity residual limbs of differing lengths. (Reprinted with permission from CL Taylor. The biomechanics of control in upper extremity prosthetics. Orthot Prosthet 1981;35:20.)

dial amputation. In designing and fabricating a prosthesis for patients with wrist disarticulation or transradial amputation, the prosthetist must consider the appropriate socket design and the optimal TD and wrist unit for a given patient's functional goals and capabilities. The prosthetist must also decide whether to use endoskeletal or exoskeletal construction and the type of hinges, suspension or harness mechanism, and control system that can best enhance the patient's function. Because of the many options that are available, upper extremity prostheses are uniquely developed for individual patients.

TRANSRADIAL SOCKET DESIGN

One of the most important determinants of socket design for patients with wrist disarticulation and transradial amputation is residual limb length, specifically the preservation of pronation and supination of the forearm. Most people with transradial amputation have full elbow motion in the sagittal plane (elbow flexion and extension); however, the ability to pronate and supinate diminishes as the length of the residual limb decreases (Figure 31-2). Patients with wrist disarticulation, in whom the length of the radius and ulna is preserved, have nearly full pronation and supination ability. Those with long transradial residual limbs may retain much of their pronation/supination

ROM. Those with a midlength transradial residual limb have lost much of their ability to pronate or supinate. Awareness of how much pronation and supination are possible is crucial in the initial casting of the residual limb and trimlines of the prosthesis.

When a transradial residual limb is in the neutral position, it is as if the limb were held in a thumbs-up position. Patients with wrist disarticulation or long transradial residual limbs are positioned in this neutral forearm position for initial casting. The prosthetist pays particular attention to the distal one-third of the limb to create a "screwdriver" purchase of the socket on the limb, so that any residual pronation/supination can be harnessed by the socket design. The narrow dorsal-ventral dimension ensures that the prosthesis will move as the radius and ulna move into pronation or supination (Figure 31-3). If the socket had a rounded contour, the motion of the radius and ulna would not be adequately captured by the socket, and effective pronation or supination would be impossible.

The radial and ulnar styloids create a somewhat bulbous distal end in limbs with wrist disarticulation. Socket design must accommodate for this enlarged distal contour for donning and for suspension. The same ideas used in a Syme's (ankle disarticulation) prosthesis are applied to wrist disarticulation sockets and prostheses. The prosthetist might choose an overlapping socket, a socket with an expandable wall, or a bivalve socket design, among others.

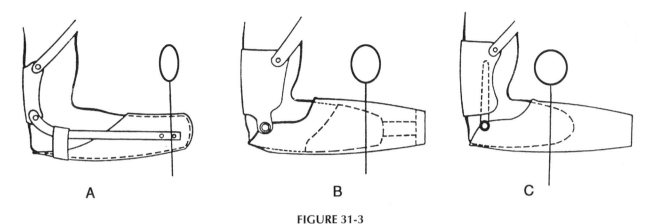

FIGURE 31-3

*Comparison of the shape and cross-sectional area of transradial sockets for a long residual limb (**A**), a midlength residual limb (**B**), and a short residual limb (**C**). (Adapted from American Academy of Orthopaedic Surgeons. Orthopaedic Appliances Atlas. Vol 2. Ann Arbor, MI: Edwards, 1960;71.)*

The conical or cylindrical shape of a long, transradial residual limb requires few special materials or fabrication techniques. As the length of the residual limb decreases, its transverse plane cross-sectional area transitions from a flattened oval to a somewhat round shape, and pronation/supination is greatly diminished if not completely eliminated (see Figure 31-3). As the contour of the distal limb becomes more rounded, the prosthetist is challenged to control rotation of the socket around the residual limb. Two strategies are currently used to control this potential rotation of the prosthesis on the residual limb: The prosthetist can use a self-suspending socket design with proximal trimlines that enclose the distal humerus or can use a triceps pad and rigid hinges to prevent socket rotation. Self-suspending designs can be worn without prosthetic socks, especially if contact between electrodes and skin is necessary in a myoelectric control system.

The Muenster-style self-suspending socket, designed for short transradial limbs, straddles the biceps tendon anteriorly and encloses the proximal olecranon posteriorly (Figure 31-4). Its very narrow anterior-posterior dimension suspends the prosthesis on the residual limb. The high proximal trimlines into the antecubital fold compromise elbow ROM, preventing full elbow flexion and slightly increasing the carrying angle of the arm. Some prosthetists "preflex" the prosthetic forearm with respect to the socket to maximize functional range of elbow flexion; excessive preflexion can compromise cosmesis of the prosthesis.

Another self-suspending socket design that prevents rotation of the socket on the forearm and effectively suspends the prosthesis is the Northwestern University supracondylar design. Similar in design principle to a transtibial supracondylar suspension, the transradial supracondylar socket has narrow proximal medial-lateral dimensions, extending proximally to capture the humeral epicondyles. Unlike the Muenster prosthesis, the supracondylar design does not limit sagittal plane elbow motion and does not always require pre-flexion of the prosthetic forearm.

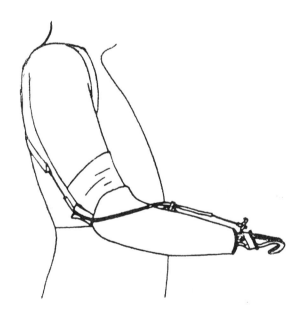

FIGURE 31-4

The high proximal trimlines of this Muenster-style prosthesis stabilize the socket on a short transradial residual limb and provide suspension. If it is used with a myoelectric control system, no further suspension or harnessing is required. (Redrawn from Staff, Prosthetics and Orthotics, New York University Post Graduate Medical School. Upper Limb Prosthetics. New York: New York University Post Graduate Medical School, 1982;50.)

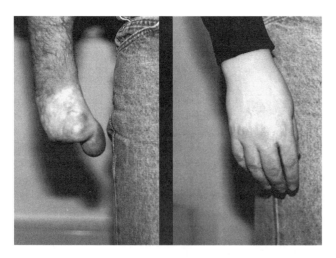

FIGURE 31-5
Example of a custom silicone glove fit over a partial hand residual limb. (Photographs courtesy of Michael Curtain.)

Because suspension is accomplished in the medial-lateral dimension, the anterior trimline is significantly lower than in the Muenster design. As a result, this socket and suspension design can be used for mid to long transradial limbs as well as short transradial limbs.

An alternative method of rotation control is the use of a pair of rigid hinges, attached proximally to a triceps cuff and distally to the proximal forearm of the prosthesis. Hinges are also important when cables are used to control opening and closing of the TD in a body-powered, cable-driven prosthesis and are discussed in greater detail below. There is no specific socket design for prostheses with triceps pads and external hinges; the non–self-suspending socket should, however, approximate the anatomic shape of the residual limb to minimize pistoning of the prosthesis or uneven weight distribution on the residual limb during normal upper extremity activity.

Terminal Devices

The TD is the prosthetic substitute for the hand and fingers. It can be a passive hand or recreational device, a mechanical cable-driven (body powered) hook or hand, or an externally powered (switch controlled or myoelectric) hook or hand. In selecting a TD, the prosthetist and patient must consider the functions that it is designed to perform, the weight of the device, its durability and need for maintenance, and its cost.

Some patients choose to use a passive, often highly cosmetic TD. Many of these passive TDs can also be used as an aid during bimanual activities. Babies who are initially fit with passive TDs quickly learn to stabilize their bottles

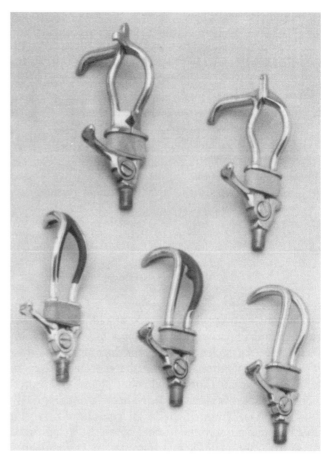

FIGURE 31-6
Examples of terminal devices that are available for patients who choose body-powered, cable-driven systems. (Courtesy of Hosmer Dorrance Corp, Campbell, CA.)

between their intact and prosthetic hands and to support themselves in quadruped position when learning to creep and crawl. Most passive hands are covered with a cosmetic glove; those that are made of polyvinyl chloride achieve a fairly cosmetic result, and the more expensive custom silicone glove provides an even more accurate anatomic appearance (Figure 31-5). Many of the materials used are vulnerable to staining, however. Other special passive devices have been designed to facilitate participation in sports such as basketball, volleyball, gymnastics, skiing, and climbing.

A variety of TDs are available for patients who choose to use a body-powered, cable-driven prosthetic system. Cables and harness systems can be used with hooks and with prosthetic hands. One of the major manufacturers of prosthetic hooks is the Hosmer Dorrance Corporation (Campbell, CA; Figure 31-6). Voluntarily opening (VO) and voluntarily closing (VC) TDs are available. In a VO system, the TD is held in a closed position by elastic bands around its base or by a spring. An operating cable is attached to the device, which opens the device via a cable pull, initiated by shoulder motion. Maximal pinch force of VO TDs, which is analogous to grip strength, is determined by the number of elastic bands used or the amount of spring tension that is present. To open the hand, the user must create enough tension in the cable to overcome the closing force of the rubber bands or spring. Patients are also able to modify pinch force when holding fragile objects (to some degree) by maintaining tension through the cable system. In VC TD, the elastic cords or spring hold the device in an open position unless the prosthetic wearer activates the cable system to close the device. Patients who use a VC TD are capable of a graded prehension force, because pinch force is directly related to the excursion of the cable as it travels from the harness to the TD. Functionally, this means that a patient using a VCTD can carry a sturdy hardcover book and a fragile uncooked egg without having to add or remove rubber bands.

Most body-powered prosthetic hands are designed to allow the prosthetic wearer to use a three-jaw chuck grip between the thumb, index, and middle fingers. Typically, the fourth and fifth fingers are passive, set in a slightly curved or flexed position. If the hand is configured as a VO device, increasing cable excursion would open the fingers; rubber bands or springs within the unit would passively close the device around an object or tool. If it is configured as a VC device, patients would learn to grade prehensile force in the same way that they would control a VC hook.

Hooks and prosthetic hands can also be controlled by an externally powered system, such as switch controls or myoelectric systems, rather than by a cable system. A variety of special externally powered TDs have been designed for use when a strong closing force is required by a patient's employment or recreational activities. Externally powered systems use a battery as a power source to control the TD and/or the elbow unit in a transhumeral prosthesis. Although a high degree of cosmesis and grip strength that is quite close to normal muscle-generated pinch force are positive aspects of externally powered systems, there are several drawbacks to consider when choosing these systems. Because of the weight of externally powered hands, and the fact that the battery pack is often positioned within the prosthetic forearm, many of these systems add significant distal weight to the prosthesis, increasing the energy cost of prosthetic use. Batteries require recharging or replacement. Myoelectric systems must also incorporate an amplifier for the muscle-generated signals that control the opening and closing of the TD. The cost of externally powered systems is often significantly higher than that of traditional body-powered systems, as a result of the supportive technological components and the additional time required for fabrication and prosthetic training.

Wrist Units

The wrist unit is the interface between the TD and the prosthetic forearm. It is used to position the TD for optimal function. A hook that is positioned one way for a work-related task may need to be repositioned to better orient a fork or spoon toward the mouth at mealtime. The patient and prosthetist choose one of three types of wrist units (friction, locking/quick release, or flexion varieties), depending on the patient's typical daily activities and physical capabilities (Figure 31-7). The most frequently prescribed wrist units are either constant friction or variable friction units. These friction-style wrist units allow the user to pre-position the TD in the most appropriate location for the task at hand and ensure that the TD stays in the desired position through full cable excursion or TD function. If the friction is adjusted too tightly, the user will have difficulty when he or she tries to pre-position the TD with the intact hand or against a table or other stable surface in the environment. If friction is insufficient, the TD may rotate during cable operation or when a "heavy" object is being held.

A second alternative is a locking or "quick disconnect" wrist unit. A release button unlocks the TD from one functional position, allows the user to passively rotate the device to a new position, and then lock it back into place in another functional position. By pushing the button in and down, the wearer can completely remove one TD to insert a different device that is better suited to the task at hand. This quick release feature is much appreciated by prosthetic users who use a hook for their job, a mitt for participation in sports, or a cosmetic prosthetic hand for social events. Locking and quick release units are somewhat heavier than friction units; this extra weight may be problematic for those with short transradial or transhumeral levels of amputation.

Flexion wrist units also are available in two styles, one that is incorporated directly into the prosthesis and one that is added to the other types of wrist units. These units orient the TD in slight wrist flexion, toward the midline of the body. This type of wrist unit enhances function for those with bilateral upper limb amputations. Flexion units are activated by pushing a switch or lever with the intact hand or the contralateral TD or by applying pressure against a stable object (such as the edge of a table).

Endoskeletal and Exoskeletal Prosthetic Systems

Upper extremity prostheses can be fabricated either as an endoskeletal system with a socket, pylon, and cosmetic cover or as an exoskeletal system with a socket embedded in a rigid external shell. Although endoskeletal systems permit interchange of components and adjustment of alignment (hence their frequent use in lower extrem-

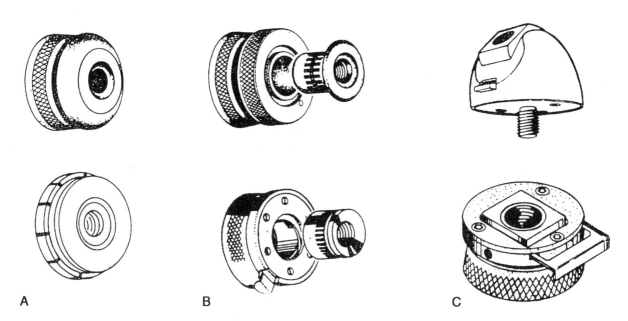

FIGURE 31-7

Examples of the three types of wrist units: (A) friction wrist units, (B) locking/quick release wrist units, and (C) a flexion wrist unit. (Reprinted with permission from Staff, Prosthetics and Orthotics, New York University Post Graduate Medical School. Upper Limb Prosthetics. New York: New York University Post Graduate Medical School, 1982;48.)

ity prostheses), the soft cosmetic covers can be significantly damaged during many common upper extremity activities. One of the reasons that exoskeletal systems are used most frequently for patients with upper extremity amputation is their inherent durability. A lightweight endoskeletal prosthesis may be most appropriate for patients with transhumeral amputation or shoulder disarticulation, especially when the energy cost of prosthetic use and cosmesis are both important concerns.

External Hinges

For patients who are wearing traditional, rather than self-suspending, sockets, a triceps pad and external hinges are used to stabilize the position of the socket on the residual limb. Patients with long transradial amputation or wrist disarticulation are most often fit with a set of flexible hinges, so that the ability to move into pronation/supination is preserved (see Figure 31-3A). When a socket's proximal trimlines do not enclose the humeral epicondyles, the hinge and triceps pad arrangement allows motion in the transverse plane.

For patients with mid to short transradial residual limbs who are not able to wear a self-suspending socket, a set of rigid hinges might prove necessary. Rigid external hinges are available in single-axis or polycentric versions. Rigid

hinges are important components in systems that are designed specifically for those with short, transradial residual limbs. In addition to controlling rotation of the socket on the limb, a step-up system has a split socket, which moves the prosthetic forearm through 2 degrees of motion for every 1 degree of actual elbow motion (Figure 31-8). One potential drawback of step-up/split socket prostheses is that significant force production by the biceps is necessary to accomplish the augmented forearm flexion. Additionally, because movement of the limb and of the prostheses are not directly connected, the quality of proprioceptive feedback during functional activities is somewhat compromised.

Limb-activated locking hinges applied to split socket prostheses are also useful for patients with very short transradial residual limbs. These individuals may have difficulty controlling the position of the prosthesis because of poor leverage. In this instance, it may be necessary to add a cable-driven elbow unit to assist elbow function. When a quick elbow extension motion of the residual limb locks the elbow unit, the cable system activates the TD. When motion of the residual limb unlocks the elbow, the cable system flexes the prosthetic forearm or allows controlled elbow extension.

The drawbacks or tradeoffs of any prosthetic component must also be considered. Most of the commercially available, rigid external hinges are made from metal, which adds to the overall weight of the prosthesis. Many are not particularly cosmetic, are rather bulky, and can damage the sleeves of the patient's shirt, sweater, or jacket.

Harness Systems

Unlike the Muenster and supracondylar self-suspending designs, most traditional transradial prostheses require a harness system to suspend the prostheses and to allow the patient to control the TD. The two harness systems that are used for patients with transradial and wrist disarticulation are the figure-eight harness and the figure-nine harness. The axillary loop of a figure-eight harness loops around the contralateral arm and serves to stabilize the prosthesis on the patient's residual limb (Figure 31-9). A Northwestern ring or the crossing point (where the webbing of the harness overlaps) is positioned just below the spinous process of the seventh cervical vertebrae and offset slightly toward the nonamputated limb. Two additional straps complete the harness. The control attachment strap continues from the axillary loop in an oblique caudal direction over the lower scapula on the amputated side, to a hanger for the cable control for the TD on the posterior surface of the triceps pad. The anterior support strap (also called an *inverted-Y strap*) continues from the axillary loop in an obliquely upward direction, across the ipsilateral deltopectoral groove. After it crosses this groove, the anterior support strap bifurcates to attach to the proximal medial and lateral edges of a triceps pad, which is, in turn, attached to the prosthesis via a pair of flexible or rigid hinges. This harness arrangement ensures efficient suspension, control of rotation, and the ability to tolerate axial load bearing.

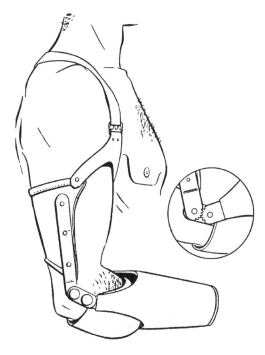

FIGURE 31-8
Rigid hinges and a split socket system are arranged to double the excursion of the prosthetic forearm with respect to active elbow flexion or extension. (Reprinted with permission from American Academy of Orthopaedic Surgeons. Orthopaedic Appliances Atlas. Vol 2. Ann Arbor, MI: Edwards, 1960;45.)

A slightly different harness system, the figure-nine, is appropriate for patients with self-suspending, cable-driven transradial prostheses or with switch-controlled transradial prostheses. The figure-nine system is basically a

FIGURE 31-9
Anterior and posterior view of a figure-eight harness system, illustrating the axillary loop (a), which anchors the harness system; the anterior support strap (b), which provides stability during a downward pull; and the control attachment strap (c), which is the point of attachment for the TD control cable. (Reprinted with permission from Northwestern University Printing and Duplicating Department, Evanston, IL, 1987.)

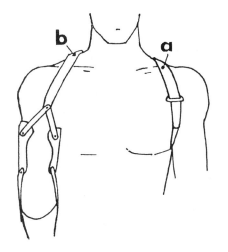
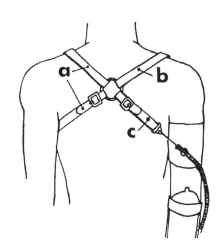

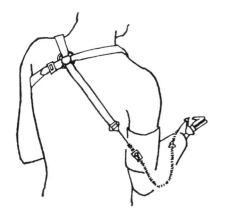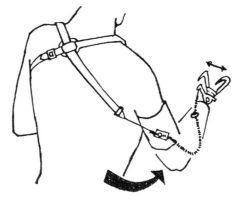

FIGURE 31-10
Glenohumeral flexion and scapular abduction increase tension on the control cable to operate the terminal device during activities that are performed away from the center of the body. Bilateral scapular (biscapular) abduction increases cable tension for fine motor activities performed near the midline or close to the trunk. (Adapted from Northwestern University Printing and Duplicating Department, Evanston, IL, 1987.)

figure-eight system without the anterior support strap. Self-suspending prostheses do not need a traditional triceps cuff for rotational stability. Instead, a modified triceps cuff can be used to provide an interface between the harness and the posterior proximal brim of the prosthesis.

Body-Powered Cable Control Systems

Patients with transradial limbs or with wrist disarticulation who use a body-powered cable-driven system to control the operation of their TD learn to change the tension in the cable, via its control strap and harness system, using volitional motion of the shoulder and arm. With the axillary loop of the harness around the opposite shoulder as a point of stability, three motions effectively increase tension in and excursion of the cable: glenohumeral flexion, unilateral scapular abduction on the prosthetic side, or bilateral scapular abduction (Figure 31-10). These motions create a greater distance between the crossing point or Northwestern ring of the harness and the prosthesis, thus pulling on the cable to activate the TD. If the TD is a VO design (i.e., the device is closed at rest), these motions open the hook or hand in preparation for grasping or holding an object. Relaxation or return to normal shoulder position reduces tension on the cable, and the TD passively closes. If the TD is VC (i.e., the device is open at rest), tension in the cable begins to close the hook or hand; the tension in the cable is translated into closing force, allowing a graded prehension. As the shoulder or arm returns to its normal position, the closing force diminishes, and the hand opens once again. Many individuals with transradial or wrist disarticulation prostheses discover that biscapular abduction is necessary for effective control of their TD when they are involved in activities or tasks that are performed close to their body. This scapulothoracic motion

requires little gross body movement and allows the user to perform finite tasks in this limited arena.

TRANSHUMERAL AMPUTATION

Any amputation that involves loss of the elbow joint has a more significant impact on the person's ability to position the arm and hand in space than does amputation at the transradial level. In an elbow disarticulation, 90–100% of the humerus is maintained. In a standard transhumeral amputation, 50–90% of the humerus remains. Any surgery that removes more than 50% of the length of the humerus is classified as a short transhumeral amputation.

Transhumeral Socket Designs

For patients with an elbow disarticulation, the medial and lateral epicondyles of the humerus are often used to assist suspension of the prosthesis on the residual limb, using designs that are similar to those of wrist and ankle disarticulation prostheses. An elbow disarticulation prosthesis may make use of inserts, an expandable wall socket, a bivalve socket design, or a screw-in socket design to position or capture the epicondyles effectively within the socket and to suspend the prosthesis. The intimate fit and anatomic definition of the elbow disarticulation socket enhance the patient's ability to control the prosthesis during functional activities.

The cross-sectional, almost circular shape of a transhumeral residual limb is similar whether the residual limb is standard or short in length. Because of this shape, control of rotation of the socket on the residual limb can be challenging, especially for those with short residual limbs. Two socket designs are available for persons with stan-

FIGURE 31-11
Utah dynamic transhumeral socket with an elastic V harness system. (Reprinted with permission from JH Bowker, JW Michael [eds]. Atlas of Limb Prosthetics: Surgical, Prosthetic, and Rehabilitation Principles [2nd ed]. St. Louis: Mosby–Year Book, 1992;263.).

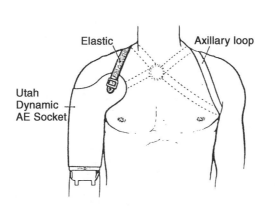
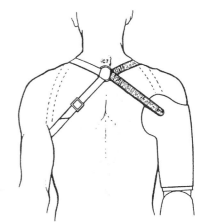

dard and short transhumeral limbs: the standard design, and the narrow mediolateral (Utah dynamic casting) design. In standard socket design, distortion of the soft tissue during casting or wearing is relatively minimal; the socket follows the contour of the residual limb. If the prosthetist uses the Utah dynamic casting technique, the transhumeral socket will have a narrow mediolateral dimension and anterior and posterior wings (Figure 31-11). This socket is designed to provide better rotational control of the socket on the limb and better anteroposterior stabilization.

Transhumeral Terminal Devices and Wrist Units

The same TDs and wrist units that are used in transradial prostheses are used in transhumeral prostheses. The major difference is that the overall weight of the distal prosthesis is much more of a functional concern in transhumeral prostheses. Weight becomes more of a concern as the level of amputation moves proximally. As residual limb length decreases, so does the lever arm and mechanical advantage that are necessary for effective prosthetic control. For patients who are using body-powered control systems, as lightweight a transhumeral prosthesis as possible is preferable. Distal weight has an impact on suspension and on the energy cost and ability to operate the elbow unit and TD. Distal weight may not be as problematic for those who use externally powered and myoelectric control systems.

Prosthetic Elbow Units

A transhumeral prosthesis also must incorporate a prosthetic elbow unit to substitute for the lost anatomic elbow. Two types of elbow units are currently available: those

with external (outside) locking hinges and those with internal locking elbows. In either system, the elbow can be locked at a designated point in the range between full extension and flexion, as appropriate for a particular task or activity. In body-powered prostheses, two cables are necessary to use or control the prosthesis effectively. One cable is used to lock or unlock the elbow. If the elbow is locked, the second cable controls the TD. If the elbow is unlocked, the second cable is used to change elbow position.

External locking hinges are most often chosen for patients with elbow disarticulation or long transhumeral limbs. These units do not add significant length to the prosthesis, so that better congruency between the joint axis of the prosthesis and the intact limb is obtained. External locking hinges are mounted on the outside of the socket in alignment with the humeral epicondyles (Figure 31-12). When external locking hinges are used, however, the wearer is not able to pre-position the prosthetic forearm passively in relative internal or external rotation for functional activity. Instead, the rotational position of the arm must be controlled by the position of the anatomic shoulder.

Internal locking elbow units are most often chosen for patients with a standard or short transhumeral residual limb. At these levels of amputation, enough room is present to incorporate the elbow unit distal to the socket within the humeral portion of the prosthesis and still maintain congruency between the prosthetic and intact elbow axes of rotation (Figure 31-13). Most internal locking elbow units have a built-in turntable, which serves as the point of proximal attachment for the elbow and establishes a "table" for passive positioning of the prosthesis in internal or external rotation.

An elbow flexion assist mechanism can be added to a transhumeral prosthesis to counter the force of gravity so that cable-controlled elbow motion and initiation of elbow

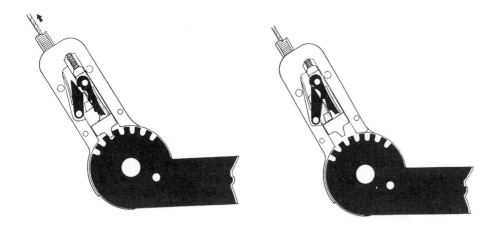

FIGURE 31-12
Example of an external locking hinge. When the elbow is locked (left) a cable pull disengages the lock and allows elbow flexion (right). A second cable pull relocks the elbow unit in a new position. (Reprinted with permission from American Academy of Orthopaedic Surgeons. Orthopaedic Appliances Atlas. Vol 2. Ann Arbor, MI: Edwards, 1960;47.)

flexion are less difficult. Traditionally, these assist mechanisms were simple coil springs mounted on the outside of the prosthetic elbow. However, an automatic forearm balance elbow unit was introduced by Otto Bock Orthopedic Industry (Minneapolis, MN). The automatic forearm balance elbow incorporates an adjustable flexion assist cam mechanism into the forearm. Because of the cam design, the level of assistance provided varies with the elbow ROM, motion more closely resembles the biomechanical action of the human elbow, and wearers do not have to rely entirely on the cable control system to initiate or to maintain elbow flexion.

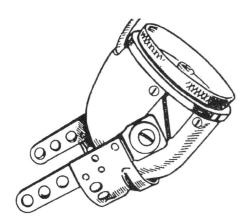

FIGURE 13-13

Example of an internal locking prosthetic elbow unit for transhumeral prostheses. (Reprinted with permission from Upper Limb Prosthetics. New York: New York University Post Graduate Medical School, 1982;57.)

Transhumeral Harness Systems

The transhumeral harness system is very similar to the figure-eight harness used in transradial prostheses. It has an axillary loop, a crossing point or Northwestern ring, and a control attachment strap. The anterior support strap, however, is different in design and purpose. It is used to assist suspension and as part of the locking/unlocking mechanism for the prosthetic elbow. Whereas the transradial anterior strap is an inverted Y, the transhumeral anterior strap has two overlapping components (Figure 31-14). The first is an elastic strap attached to the humeral portion of the prosthesis, which helps to suspend the prosthesis and to return the locking mechanism to its resting position. The second is a nonelastic strap attached to the elbow-locking hanger and cable system, which is used to lock and unlock the elbow. Most elbow lock functions are based on an alternator principle: If an initial cable pull has locked the elbow unit, a period of no tension and return to its resting cable position (usually with the aid of the elastic strap) must occur. A subsequent cable pull unlocks the elbow so that it can be repositioned. To lock the elbow in the new position, a period of no tension must again occur to allow the elbow unit to cycle back and be ready to lock the elbow on the next cable pull.

Another addition to the transhumeral figure-eight harness is a lateral suspensor strap, which originates from the axilla loop or Northwestern ring and attaches on the anterolateral proximal brim of the prosthesis. In addition to suspending the prosthesis, this lateral suspensor strap controls the tendency for the prosthesis to rotate externally as the cable systems are activated. Additional cross-back straps can be used if better distribution of the weight of the prosthesis is needed, for greater efficiency (less fatigue) during prosthetic function, or for prevention of the harness system from riding proximally during use.

FIGURE 31-14

Suspension straps of a transhumeral prosthesis. The elastic posterior component helps to suspend the prosthesis, and the nonelastic anterior component is part of the elbow-locking/-unlocking mechanism. Note the long posterior cable reaching the terminal device, similar to that of a transradial prosthesis. If the elbow unit is locked, this cable operates the terminal device. If the elbow unit is unlocked, this cable is used to change the position of the prosthetic forearm. (Reprinted with permission from Northwestern University Printing and Duplicating Department, Evanston, IL, 1987.)

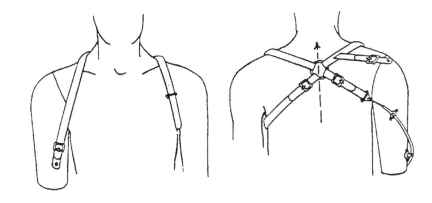

Transhumeral Control Systems

Transhumeral cable-driven control systems require the patient to learn to use two distinct body motions to control each of the cables in a dual-cable control system: one to control the elbow lock and the other to operate the TD (if the elbow is locked) or to flex or extend the elbow (if the elbow is unlocked). The combination of two cables, controlled by antagonistic movements, with functions determined by the status of the elbow lock can be intimidating and frustrating to a new prosthetic user. With practice, however, most persons with transhumeral amputation master the control system and perfect the required movements so well that they are often unnoticed by the casual observer.

To lock or unlock the elbow unit, the distance between the proximal part of the anterior elbow-locking cable, which runs between the nonelastic anterior strap and the elbow unit and its distal attachment, must be elongated (Figure 31-15). To create this tension, the wearer quickly and forcefully extends the shoulder (glenohumeral extension), abducts the arm, and depresses the shoulder (scapular depression) in a downward and backward direction. Some may also add a little shoulder protraction to increase tension in the elbow lock control cable. The key to locking the elbow unit successfully is to perform these motions quickly enough to engage the elbow lock. Inadequate cable tension or slow force production does not lock the elbow unit in the desired position. Instead, the force of gravity may pull the prosthetic forearm into extension during function or the elbow locks in less flexion than was originally desired. Once the elbow is locked and the cable has returned to its resting position, the next downward-backward thrust unlocks the elbow unit.

The second cable system is essentially the same as that of a transradial prosthesis but either controls the TD (if the elbow unit is locked) or flexes the elbow (if the elbow unit is unlocked). The body motions that are used to control this cable are the same ones that are used to control the TD

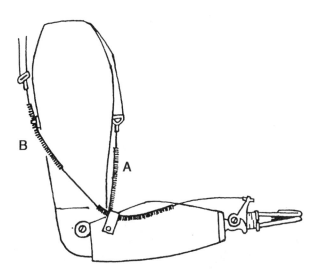

FIGURE 31-15

Dual-control cable system and lift loop of a transhumeral prosthesis. Quick and forceful downward/backward shoulder motion operates the elbow-locking mechanism via the anterior cable (A). The second cable system (B), activated by glenohumeral flexion or scapular abduction, operates the terminal device if the elbow unit is locked or lifts the forearm if the elbow unit is unlocked. (Adapted from Northwestern University Printing and Duplicating Department, Evanston, IL, 1987.)

in transradial prosthetic limbs: glenohumeral flexion, scapular abduction, or biscapular abduction (especially for activities near the trunk). The cable housing assembly for this cable is fed through a forearm lift loop; the location of this lift loop has an impact on the force and cable excursion that are required to control the prosthesis.

When the elbow is unlocked, the amount of force that is required to operate the TD is frequently more than the force needed to move the prosthetic forearm; as a result, any tension exerted through the cable causes the elbow to flex. When the elbow is locked, a cable pull operates the TD. To grasp and lift an object, the patient must first unlock the elbow to allow elbow flexion into the most functional position. He or she then must lock the elbow and then operate the TD to grasp the object. Once the object is in place in the TD, the patient once again unlocks the elbow and attempts to lift the object with the second control cable. Given the added weight and distal position of the object in the TD, it is often more difficult to raise the arm than to operate the TD. If the patient is using a VO TD, the hook or hand opens and the object drops when the force that is required to lift the arm exceeds the force needed to operate the TD. Patients who use a VC device may have difficulty in achieving enough cable excursion to close their TD fully and perform this task of flexing the elbow while holding an object.

SHOULDER DISARTICULATION

Because of the loss of the hand, wrist, elbow, and shoulder joints as a result of shoulder disarticulation, functional prosthetic replacement is difficult to achieve. A true shoulder disarticulation occurs at the glenohumeral joint, with the scapulothoracic joint remaining intact. Patients who have had amputation at the level of the humeral neck are managed as if they had shoulder disarticulation because the residual humerus is very short. Those with forequarter (intrascapulothoracic) amputation are managed in much the same way. Given the extent of limb loss and the resulting difficulty in controlling the prosthesis, many individuals with shoulder disarticulation choose to wear a passive prosthesis for a symmetric and cosmetic appearance. Some choose not to use a prosthesis of any kind. With the recent development of new cable-driven and externally powered components and ongoing research in myoelectric control systems, the possibility of designing a functional shoulder disarticulation prosthesis has become more likely.

Shoulder Disarticulation Socket Designs

Sockets for shoulder disarticulation amputations are commonly referred to as shoulder caps. The more proximal

the level of amputation, the more the socket must encompass the chest and back. Because the contours of the shoulder are preserved after humeral neck and shoulder disarticulation amputation, the prosthesis can be securely positioned and suspended. For patients with forequarter amputation, it is often very difficult to achieve purchase and suspension against the rounded thoracic wall. For all three levels, a total contact design with an intimate fit between the residuum and socket helps to distribute the weight of the prosthesis more evenly. In some externally powered prostheses, inclusion of a switch or pad (activated by remaining shoulder motions) might require a slightly oversized socket where the device has been located.

Components for Shoulder Disarticulation Limbs

In addition to a TD, wrist unit, and elbow unit, the shoulder disarticulation prosthesis must include a mechanism to replace the shoulder joint and a system to control each of these components. Many incorporate mechanical activation switches and excursion amplifiers. A variety of prosthetic shoulder joints are available, ranging from a monolithic shoulder with no shoulder motion to a universal shoulder joint with 6 degrees of freedom. A recently introduced shoulder can be locked in selected flexed or extended positions with a cable pull and spring assist system. A strategically placed switch (for example, the paddle nudge switches that are available from Hosmer Dorrance Corp.) can be activated with a chin tuck to lock or unlock the elbow unit. Pulley- or lever-based excursion amplifiers may assist persons with shoulder disarticulation to operate their TD. By doubling the force put into the system by scapular abduction of the contralateral shoulder, the cable excursion is doubled.

Harness Systems for Disarticulation Limbs

Most harness systems for patients with shoulder disarticulation are custom designed to best match the preference by the wearer and the prosthetic design. Most require a chest, waist, or abdominal strap (or a combination of such straps) to stabilize the prosthesis on the upper trunk. Harness design also depends on the control mechanism that is used to operate the TD or elbow and shoulder units.

Control Systems

For those with shoulder disarticulation, the primary motion used to control operation of the TD and the elbow-locking mechanism is contralateral scapular abduction. A chin-operated nudge switch provides an alternative method for locking/unlocking the elbow if scapular abduction is insufficient. Other elbow-locking alternatives include a chest strap that creates tension in the control cable when the chest is expanded by forceful inspiration or a waist belt linked to ipsilateral shoulder elevation. Both of these require relocation and rerouting of the lock/unlock control cable to maximize possible cable excursion. As in transhumeral cable control systems, activation of a second cable controls the TD when the elbow unit is locked or changes elbow position if the elbow unit is unlocked.

BILATERAL UPPER EXTREMITY AMPUTATION

Many of the traumatic circumstances that lead to upper extremity amputation, such as explosion or electrocution, often damage both upper extremities. Congenital limb deficiencies are as likely to involve both limbs as a single limb. Many individuals with bilateral limb loss are more accepting of a prosthesis, without which grasp would be impossible, than are their peers with single limb loss. The adaptation of the cable control harness system for persons with bilateral amputation may make the devices more comfortable to suspend and to control. Persons with bilateral transradial amputation are quite successful at learning to use prostheses. Feeding, grooming, writing, and other tasks that are performed close to the body are facilitated if wrist flexion units are incorporated into the prostheses. As the level of amputation moves higher, fitting and the use of prostheses become more of a challenge for the prosthetist and the patient. Patients with traumatic limb loss who have at least one long transhumeral limb often opt to use a single prosthesis. Those with high-level, bilateral congenital limb deficiencies may instead develop motor strategies to use their feet as a substitute for their missing upper extremities, becoming quite adept at performing tasks that require grasp and fine manipulation.

KRUKENBERG'S TECHNIQUE

Krukenberg's technique was developed in Germany in 1917 as a means of restoring some capacity for prehension to persons with long transradial limbs. In this reconstructive surgical procedure, the radius and ulna are separated, and muscles and soft tissues are reattached to allow volitional motion (opening and closing) of these long bones. Although the arm can once again be used to hold objects, many patients and families have difficulty with the markedly noncosmetic aspects of the postsurgi-

cal limb. The surgery is not often performed in the United States, as a high level of function and cosmesis can be achieved with traditional transradial prostheses. Under some circumstances, however, this procedure is appropriate. Successful use of conventional and externally powered prostheses requires intact vision to substitute for sensory feedback when a TD replaces the anatomic hand. For patients with visual impairment and upper extremity limb loss, a conventional prosthesis would be difficult, if not impossible, to use and control. Krukenberg's technique might be an alternative for those with severe visual impairment and bilateral traumatic amputation to achieve some degree of independent upper extremity function. The technique can also be used in areas of the world where prosthetic and rehabilitation resources are significantly lacking, as a means of restoring function that would otherwise be unattainable.

CHILDREN WITH UPPER EXTREMITY LIMB LOSS

When working with children who have upper extremity limb loss, the prosthetist and therapist must be aware of the special needs of the growing child and adapt prosthetic design and prosthetic training to the child's motor and cognitive development. Children who have lost a functional upper extremity to trauma or disease, like their adult peers, may be anxious to replace the limb with a prosthesis that is cosmetic and functional. Parents of children with congenital limb deficiencies are often very much concerned with achieving a cosmetically acceptable prosthetic replacement for the child's missing limb. Children with congenital limb deficiency perceive themselves as complete or whole, even without the missing limb, and develop adaptive motor strategies to accomplish the activities that are important to them. The expectations of parents and the desire to be better accepted by peers may convince the child that a prosthesis is necessary. Although a prosthesis may be helpful for bimanual activities, most children are functional with and without a prosthesis.

Infants with transradial or long transhumeral congenital upper limb deficiencies can be fit with a passive prosthesis when they are as young as 6 months old. This early fitting helps the child with sitting balance and with crawling, prepares the child for future fitting with an active prosthesis, reduces the likelihood of stump dependence, and begins to ease parental anxiety about the child's development. When a child reaches 18 months of age, an active prehensile system is first introduced. At this age, children's cognitive development and ability to focus allow them to learn how to operate a simple TD to pick up, hold, and eventually manipulate objects. Children of this age are capable of adapting to either a conventional cable control system or a myoelectric system. Successful training with either device depends, to a large extent, on parental support and involvement. Prosthetic fitting and training may be delayed for children with short transhumeral limbs, shoulder disarticulation, or phocomelic limbs because these prostheses are more complex to fit and to operate.

The components for pediatric upper limb prostheses are very much like those that are used for adults, scaled to be child sized. Most research and development of pediatric components have occurred in countries in which thalidomide has had an impact. In the United States, the Association of Children's Prosthetic Orthotic Clinics sponsors scientific meetings that are focused on clinical research and development of prostheses and orthoses for children, advances in surgical procedures, and the social, psychological, and economic aspects of caring for children with special needs.

Among adults, the volume and length of a mature residual limb are quite stable, so that an upper extremity prosthesis has a long functional life. In children, however, physical growth and development necessitate frequent revision, accommodation, or refabrication—all expensive processes. A number of strategies have been used to stretch the functional life of a child's upper limb prosthesis. The child can be initially fit with several ply of prosthetic sock, so that thin layers of sock can be removed as the child grows. Overlapping "onion skin" sockets, with several layers that can be peeled from the inside to accommodate increasing limb volume and length, have been successfully used to manage the impending growth of the child and residuum.

A child's willingness to use a prosthesis is likely to vary as he or she moves from early childhood into and through adolescence. At times the prosthesis will be perceived as absolutely necessary, and at others it will be rejected entirely. Because prostheses are hot to wear, many are left in the closet, under the bed, or on the living room floor during the summer months. An upcoming important social event, such as the prom, may be the catalyst for a new prosthetic hand or glove. These swings are "normative" and best accepted as such by the child's parents, prosthetists, and therapists.

EXTERNALLY POWERED PROSTHESES

Externally powered systems, as alternatives to the traditional body-powered cable-driven prostheses, were first developed in the 1950s, when pneumatic chambers used in industry and military applications were adapted to drive TDs or elbow-locking mechanisms. Early pneumatic systems added significant weight to the prosthesis and required frequent recharging, making them impractical. Advances in battery technology led to the development of electrically driven components. Early electrically based systems were activated by switches that the patient had to turn on or off mechanically. More recent technological advances have seen the development of myoelectric systems, in which surface electrodes translate electrical activity of muscle into action of a TD or prosthetic elbow unit.

Switch-controlled prostheses are often used for patients with a very short residual limb, when electrical activity of muscles in the residual limb is below the threshold for effective myoelectric control, or when the intimacy of fit that is required for effective electrode placement cannot be easily accomplished. Many types of switch controls are available; the choice of switch is determined by individual abilities or needs. A child with phocomelic digits near the shoulder may be able to use a pull switch to activate an elbow unit or a TD; if the digits are strong enough, the child might instead activate a push or rocker switch. Sophisticated electronic components, such as force-sensing resistors or a Servo-Pro unit (Motion Control, Salt Lake City, UT), can be incorporated so that speed of movement becomes proportional to the level of input to the device. The challenge for the prosthetist is to place the switch for optimal access for activation and minimal interference from other body movements.

Myoelectric control systems are significantly different than the cable control systems described earlier in the chapter. For those with transradial limbs who are using a myoelectric system, harnesses and cable are often unnecessary. For those with elbow disarticulation and transhumeral limbs, a harness can be used for suspension, but no cables are necessary. To be successful with a myoelectric system, the person must volitionally contract a muscle enough that the contraction's electrical potential can be detected by a pair of electrodes placed on the surface of the skin. The change in potential must reach a threshold of more than 10–15 μV (the minimum voltage potential) to activate the system. The potential generated by muscle contraction can be measured and recorded with the use of a myotester or other EMG reading equipment. The surface electrodes (contacts) are aligned along the long axis of the muscle. When the muscle contracts, the difference in electrical potential between the proximal and distal contacts is the signal to activate the system.

The most effective electrode placement is determined by careful mapping of the muscle during the preprosthetic assessment period. Most often, electrodes are placed so that physiologic muscle function and TD activity are congruent (Figure 31-16). In a transradial prosthesis, electrodes that close the TD are placed over wrist and finger flexor muscle groups, whereas those that open the TD are located over wrist and finger extensor muscle groups. If a dual-channel system is desired (allowing volitional control of opening and closing of the TD), the patient must be able to isolate contraction of flexors from that of extensors, as well as generate at least threshold potential at the flexor and extensor contact sites.

Once the optimal contact sites have been identified and marked with indelible ink, the limb is casted to create a negative mold. When the positive model is poured, the precise location of the ink-marked electrode sites is transferred onto the surface of the model. The prosthetist then can incorporate an opening for the electrodes into the socket wall. It is important to note that direct contact must occur between the electrodes and the skin; no prosthetic socks or sheaths are worn in myoelectric prostheses.

When young children are first fit with a myoelectric prosthesis, a single-site, single-control system is usually chosen. Children learn to control a VO TD operated by a single electrode site. Muscle contraction (input) opens the hand, and with muscle relaxation, the hand automatically closes. When the child is developmentally ready, a dual-site, dual-control system is introduced, and the child begins to practice graded prehension in addition to volitional opening of the TD. Dual-site, dual-control systems are available as a digital control (single speed) system or as a proportional control system in which speed of movement is determined by the magnitude and duration of muscle contraction (Figure 31-17).

For those with transhumeral amputation, dual-site, quad control systems have been developed. The electrodes that close the hand or flex the elbow are placed over the

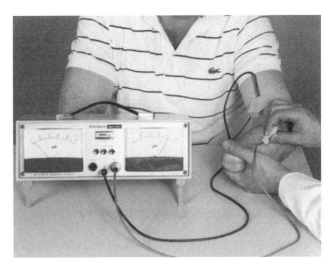

FIGURE 31-16
Locating the optimal site for electrode placement for natural physiologic control of the terminal device for a transradial prosthesis. (Reprinted with permission from M Näder, F Blohmke. Otto Bock Prosthetic Compendium: Upper Extremity Prostheses. Berlin: Schiele & Schön, 1990;30.)

remaining biceps brachii, whereas the electrodes that open the hand or extend the elbow are placed over the triceps brachii. In one design, patients learn to use a forceful co-contraction to deactivate the elbow lock. If the elbow lock is engaged, contraction of the biceps closes the TD, whereas contraction of the triceps opens it. If the elbow lock is disengaged, contraction of the biceps activates

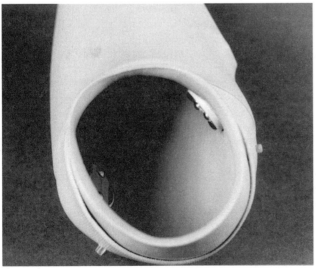

A

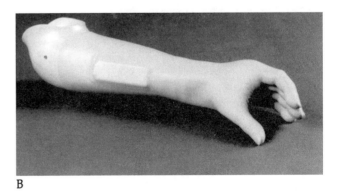

B

FIGURE 31-17
(A) Electrode placement within the socket of a dual-site, dual-control myoelectric prosthesis. (B) The battery pack is positioned in the forearm, under the cosmetic glove. A dual-control system allows voluntary opening and graded prehension of a terminal device. (Photographs courtesy of Robert Lipschutz, C.P.)

elbow flexion, whereas contraction of the triceps activates elbow extension. The optimal configuration of the system varies with the patient's ability to activate muscles of the residual limb volitionally.

A wide variety of TDs and other components are available for myoelectric and switch-controlled externally powered prostheses, and new devices are introduced frequently. Pediatric and adult hooks and hands are available in many sizes, styles, weights, and function-related designs. Wrist rotators and electronic elbows are also available for the child and adult. Sometimes it is helpful to use a hybrid system, which combines components that are for externally powered and cable-driven designs to achieve the desired functional result.

The major difficulties of myoelectric and other externally powered systems are the increased weight of the prosthesis, the need for careful and consistent maintenance, and the high cost of the components. The development of lightweight components and the use of microswitch technology have done much to address the issue of weight. Patients and families who are interested in externally powered systems are usually willing to comply with maintenance schedules and follow-up visits. They must also understand how and when to use the device and the environments or circumstances that can damage the control system. These issues are best addressed during pre- and postprosthetic training and education and reinforced in routine follow-up visits. The expense of the prosthesis is one of the major factors to consider during the prosthetic prescription process. Patients and families may be faced with significant out-of-pocket costs if their health insurance does not routinely cover myoelectric devices and no alternative funding source is available. Dialogue, education, and negotiation between patients and families, rehabilitation professionals, and decision makers in the health insurance industry are often necessary to provide a clearer understanding of the use and necessity of these devices.

SUMMARY

Upper extremity prostheses are helpful tools for individuals who have lost part or all of their limb due to trauma or to disease, as well as those with congenital limb deficiencies. Despite recent advances in technology, no prosthesis can completely substitute for the function of the human arm and hand. Although continued research and development hold the promise that upper limb prostheses will become more hand-like, this requires cooperation and funding from many sources. True sensory feedback, real-time response, and improved battery technology are just a few current research projects that are likely to close the gap between the human limb and prosthetic replacements. Now, as in the future, persons with upper extremity amputation, as well as their prosthetists and therapists, must understand and carefully evaluate the options that are available to arrive at the most appropriate prosthetic prescription. Once the limb has been fabricated and delivered, appropriate training in the use of the device enhances functional ability and satisfaction with the prosthesis. It is also important that patients learn to function without the prosthesis. The optimal outcome can be achieved when careful preprosthetic assessment, appropriate prescription, and effective training have been accomplished. Each of these components is important and necessary if individuals with upper extremity amputation are to be successful with the prosthesis, functioning to the fullest of their capabilities.

REFERENCES

1. Leblanc MA. Patient populations and other estimates of prosthetics and orthotics in the USA. Orthot Prosthet 1973;27(3):38–44.
2. Edwards JW. Historical Development of Artificial Limbs. In American Academy of Orthopaedic Surgeons, Orthopaedic Appliances Atlas. Vol 2. Ann Arbor, MI: American Academy of Orthopaedic Surgeons, 1960;1–22.
3. Hosmer Dorrance Corporation, 561 Division Street, Campbell, CA, 95008.
4. Kobrinski AE, Bolhovitin SV, Voskoboinikora LM. Problems in bioelectric control. In Automatic and Remote Control: Proceedings of the 1st IFAC International Congress, Moscow, USSR. Vol 2. London: Butterworth, 1961;619–623.
5. Ouellette EA. Surgical Principles: Wrist Disarticulation and Transradial Amputation. In JH Bowker, JW Michael (eds), Atlas of Limb Prosthetics: Surgical, Prosthetic, and Rehabilitation Principles (2nd ed). St. Louis: Mosby–Year Book, 1992;237.
6. Kay HW, Newman JD. Relative incidence of new amputations. Orthot Prosthet 1975;29(2):3–16.
7. McAuliffe JA. Surgical Principles: Elbow Disarticulation and Transhumeral Amputation. In JH Bowker, JW Michael (eds), Atlas of Limb Prosthetics: Surgical, Prosthetic, and Rehabilitation Principles (2nd ed). St. Louis: Mosby–Year Book, 1992;252.
8. Brenner CD. Prosthetic Principles: Wrist Disarticulation and Transradial Amputation. In JH Bowker, JW Michael (eds), Atlas of Limb Prosthetics: Surgical, Prosthetic, and Rehabilitation Principles (2nd ed). St. Louis: Mosby–Year Book, 1992;241.

Index

Note: Page numbers followed by *f* indicate figures; page numbers followed by *t* indicate tables.